REVIEWERS OF THE UK EDITION

Keith Booles BSc Hons, RGN, RNT, RCNT, PGCE
Senior Nurse Lecturer, Faculty of Health, Staffordshire University

Donal Deehan RN, BA (Hons), MSc, PGCE
Senior Lecturer/Programme Lead Non-Medical Prescribing, Liverpool John Moores University

Susan Jordan Mb BCh, PhD, PGCE (FE)
Reader, Department of Nursing and Institute of Health Research, School of Health Science, Swansea University

Aidín McKinney MSc, BSc (Hons), PGCE, RGN
Teaching Fellow, School of Nursing and Midwifery, Queens University, Belfast

Ronnie Meechan RNA, RNMH, BSc, MSc, PGCertEd
Programme Leader Pre-Registration Nursing Studies, University of Worcester

Valarie Ness MN, PGCert (TLHE), RNT, BN, ENP, RN
Lecturer/Year 3 leader (Adult branch, DipHE(Nursing)/BN Programme), School of Nursing, Midwifery & Community Health, Glasgow Caledonian University

Tristan Pocock BSc (Hons), PhD, PGCE
Teaching Fellow (Pharmacology), University of Manchester

Eugene Quirk MEd, BSc, DipEd, RGN, RMN, FHEA
Lecturer, School of Nursing, Midwifery & Community Health, Glasgow Caledonian University

Peta Reid MSc, BSc, Dip Teach (Nursing), Dip Applied Science (Nursing)
Lecturer, School of Health Sciences, University of Southampton

Billiejoan Rice BSc (Hons) inclusive of RGN, PGDip in Education, MSc
Teaching Fellow, School of Nursing and Midwifery, Queen's University, Belfast

Paul Warburton MSc, RN, Cert Ed,
Independent & Supplementary Nurse Prescriber Senior Lecturer and Non-Medical Prescribing Programme Co-ordinator, Faculty of Health, Edge Hill University

REVIEWERS OF THE US EDITION

Joanne Bonesteel RN, MSN
Nursing Faculty
Excelsior College
Albany, New York

Gina S. Brown RN, PhD
Chair and Professor
Columbia Union College

Edyth T. James
Department of Nursing
Takoma Park, Maryland

Susan Buchholz RN, BSN, MSN
Associate Professor of Nursing
Georgia Perimeter College
Lawrenceville, Georgia

Barbara M. Carranti RN, MS, CNS
Instructor—Nursing
LeMoyne College
Syracuse, New York

Cynthia L. Dakin RN, PhD
Assistant Professor
Northeastern University School of Nursing
Boston, Massachusetts

Loretta B. Delargy RN, MSN
Assistant Professor
North Georgia College and State University
Dahlonega, Georgia

Carol Fanutti RN, EdD, MSN
Director of Nursing
Trocaire College
Buffalo, New York

Mary-Margaret Finney RN, MSN
Assistant Professor, Department of Nursing
North Georgia College and State University
Dahlonega, Georgia

Charlene Beach Gagliardi BS, RN, MSN
Instructor
Mount Saint Mary's College
Los Angeles, California

Nancy B. Hartel RN, MS
Nursing Faculty St. Joseph's College of Nursing at St. Joseph's Hospital
Syracuse, New York

Annette Hutcherson RN, MN, EdD
Professor of Nursing
Polk Community College
Winter Haven, Florida

Jodie Lane RN, MSN
Nursing Faculty NSC and Critical Care Educator
Summerlin Medical Center
Nevada State College
Henderson, Nevada

Cynthia L. Lapp BS, RN
Practical Nursing Instructor
Jefferson-Lewis BOCES
Lowville, New York

Rhonda Lawes RN, MN
Instructor
University of Oklahoma
College of Nursing Tulsa, Oklahoma

A. Renee Leasure RN, PhD, CCRN, CNS
Associate Professor and Deputy Director, Evidence Based Practice Center Oklahoma
University of Oklahoma
College of Nursing
Oklahoma City, Oklahoma

Barbara Lee-Learned RN, MSN
Nursing Faculty
Technical College of the Lowcountry
Beaufort, South Carolina

Colleen Ley RN, BSN, MSN
AD Instructor
Madison Area Technical College
Watertown, Wisconsin

Linda McIntosh Liptok RN, BMus, MSN, APRN, BC
Assistant Professor
Kent State University, Tuscarawas
New Philadelphia, Ohio

Robin D. Lockhart RN, MSN
Assistant Professor of Nursing
Midwestern State University
Wichita Falls, Texas

Angela Phillips-Lowe RN, EdD
Associate Professor of Nursing
Mount Carmel College of Nursing
Columbus, Ohio

Janet Massoglia BSN, MSN
Instructor
Delta College
University Center, Michigan

Dorothy Mathers RN, MSN
Associate Professor
Pennsylvania College of Technology
Pittsburgh, Pennsylvania

Jeffrey C. McManemy
Associate Professor
University Center, Missouri
St. Louis Community College at Florissant Valley
St. Louis, Missouri

Cathy Michalenko RN, MN, GNC(c)
Instructor
Red Deer College
Red Deer, Alberta, Canada

Patricia J. Neafsey RD, PhD
Professor
University of Connecticut
Storrs, Connecticut

FOCUS ON
Nursing Pharmacology

FIRST UK EDITION

ng
ırsing

Fellow, University of Manchester
ow, University of Manchester

, Bury Primary Care Trust,

tkins

First UK edition
Acquisitions Editor: Rachel Hendrick
Proofreader: Ann Stevens
Cover Design: Julie Martin
Compositor: Thomson Digital
Printer: C&C Offset Printing Co – China

US edition
Acquisitions Editor: Margaret Zuccarini
Senior Managing Editor: Helen Kogut
Managing Editor: Michelle Clarke
Senior Managing Editor, Production: Erika Kors
Senior Production Manager: Helen Ewan
Design Coordinator: Holly Reid McLaughlin
Indexer: Ellen Brennan
Compositor: Thomson Digital
Printer: R.R. Donnelley—Willard

The author and the publisher have endeavoured to ensure that Web sites listed in the text were active prior to publication. However, due to the Internet's evolving nature, Web addresses may have changed or sites may have ceased to exist since publication.

British Library Cataloguing in Publication Data. A catalogue record for this book is available from the British Library.

ISBN-13: 978-1-901831-01-6
ISBN-10: 1-901831-01-9

Care has been taken to confirm the accuracy of the information presented and to describe generally accepted practices. However, the authors, editors, and publisher are not responsible for errors or omissions or for any consequences from application of the information in this book and make no warranty, express or implied, with respect to the contents of the publication.

The authors, editors and publisher have exerted every effort to ensure that drug selection set forth in this text is in accordance with current recommendations and practice at the time of publication. However, in view of ongoing research, changes in government regulations, and the constant flow of information relating to drug therapy and drug reactions, the reader is urged to check the current edition of the British National Formulary (BNF) for each drug for any change in indications and dosage and for added warnings and precautions. This is particularly important when the recommended agent is a new or infrequently employed drug.

To our families and friends for their endless support and encouragement.

CCS0410

Winifred A. Olmstead BSN, MSN
Nursing Faculty
St. Joseph's College of Nursing at St. Joseph's Hospital
Syracuse, New York

Nola Ormrod RN, MSN
Nursing Director
Centralia College
Centralia, Washington

Eva Ann Pihlgren BSN, MN
Professor of Nursing
Antelope Valley College
Lancaster, California

Susan L. Piva RN, MSN, BSN
Associate Professor of Nursing
Brevard Community College
Cocoa, Florida

Loretta G. Quigley RN, MS
Associate Dean
St. Joseph's College of Nursing at St. Joseph's Hospital
Syracuse, New York

Luanne G. Richardson
Assistant Professor
Duquesne University
Pittsburgh, Pennsylvania

Patricia Roper RN, MSN
Professor of Nursing
Columbus State Community College
Columbus, Ohio

Carol A. Sheldon RN, MS, CEN
Nursing Faculty
St Joseph's College of Nursing at St. Joseph's Hospital Health Center
Syracuse, New York

Thomas J. Smith
Faculty-BSN Program
Nicholls State University
Thibodaux, Louisiana

Fran Soukup
Faculty
Madison Area Technical College
Reedsburg, Wisconsin

Martha A. Spies RN, PhD
Professor
Deaconess College of Nursing
St. Louis, Missouri

Carol A. Storm MSN, APRN, BC
Director
B. M. Spurr School of Practical Nursing
Glen Dale, West Virginia

Scott Carter Thigpen, RN, MSN, CCRN, CEN
Assistant Professor of Nursing
South Georgia College, Division of Nursing
Douglas, Georgia

Dina L. Wilson RN, MN
Professor, Nursing
Johnson County Community College
Overland Park, Kansas

Regina L. Wright RN, MSN, CEN
Clinical Assistant Professor
Drexel University
Philadelphia, Pennsylvania

Carolyn Johnson Wyss RN, MSN
Associate Professor of Nursing, Technology Coordinator
Walters State Community College
Morristown, Tennessee

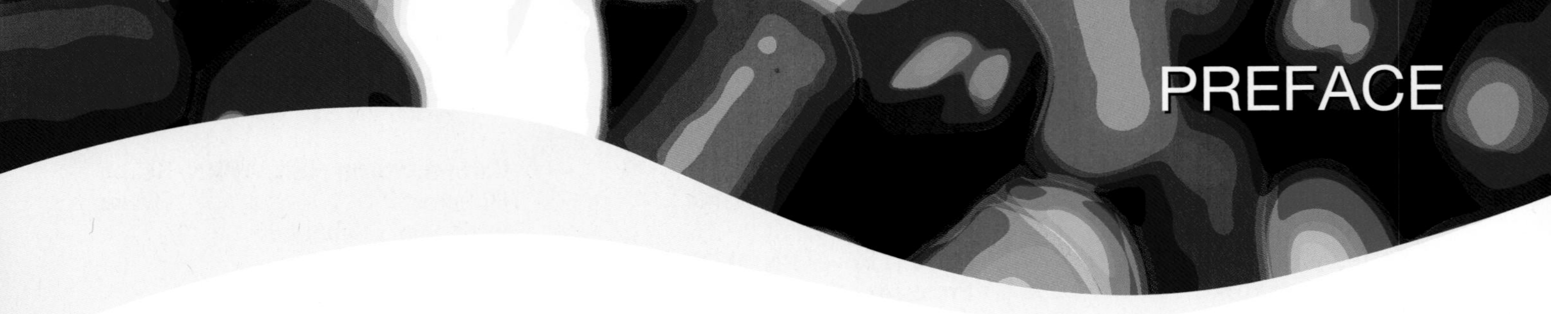

PREFACE

The role of nurses in medical care delivery has changed significantly over recent years – more outpatient and home care, shorter hospital stays and more patient self-care. This has resulted in additional legal and professional responsibilities for nurses, increasing their responsibility for the safe and effective delivery of drug therapy.

Nurses, both in training and those qualified, can find the field of pharmacology a challenging one. Students in the United Kingdom enter undergraduate nursing programmes with diverse educational backgrounds. Many students are introduced to the fields of physiology, pathophysiology, chemistry and microbiology for the very first time when they enter higher education. The study of drug therapy requires a solid understanding of the inter-relationships between these areas and students lacking basic bioscience knowledge can therefore struggle. The objective for teaching staff is to help alleviate their student's fears and to provide an integrated approach to enhance their students learning.

The first edition of *Focus on Nursing Pharmacology* adapted for students on United Kingdom nursing programmes is based on the premise that students first need to have a solid and clearly focused understanding of the principles of drug therapy before they can easily grasp the myriad details associated with individual drugs. The text takes an integrated approach and provides appropriate supporting information on the relevant bioscience fields to enhance a student's understanding of pharmacology. This text will support students who are studying pharmacology either as part of an integrated course in biosciences or as a stand-alone course.

Focus on Nursing Pharmacology provides a concise, user-friendly and uncluttered text. This difficult subject is presented in a streamlined, understandable, deliverable and learnable manner and continues to emphasise 'need-to-know' concepts. This book is designed to be used in conjunction with a current issue of the British National Formulary.

The text reviews and integrates previously learned knowledge of physiology, chemistry and nursing fundamentals into chapters focused on helping students conceptualize what is important to know about each group of drugs. Illustrations and highlighted sections sum up concepts to enhance learning. Special features further focus student learning on clinical application, critical thinking, patient safety, lifespan issues related to drug therapy, evidence-based practice, patient teaching and case study-based critical thinking exercises that incorporate nursing process principles. The text incorporates study materials that conclude each chapter. *Check Your Understanding* provides sample multiple choice (MCQ) and extended matching questions (EMQ).

Organization

Focus on Nursing Pharmacology is organized following a 'simple to complex' approach, much like the syllabus for a basic nursing pharmacology course. The text is divided into distinct parts.

Part I begins with an overview of basic nursing pharmacology. Each of the other parts begins with a review of the physiology of the system affected by the specific drugs being discussed. This review refreshes the information for the student and provides a quick and easy reference when reading about drug actions.

Part II of the text begins with the most basic element of human physiology, the cell; providing students with the background information required to understand the mechanism of action of chemotherapeutic drugs described in the subsequent chapters.

Part III focuses on drugs affecting the immune system. Research knowledge in this area has expanded over recent years allowing pharmaceutical companies to develop new drugs that target the immune system.

Parts IV and **V** of the text address drugs that affect the nervous system, the basic functioning system of the body. Following the nervous system, and closely linked with it in **Part VI**, is the endocrine system. The sequence of these parts introduces students to the concept of control, teaches them about the interrelatedness of these two systems and prepares them for understanding many aspects of shared physiological function and the linking of the two systems into one: the neuroendocrine system.

Parts VII, VIII and **IX** discuss drugs affecting the reproductive, cardiovascular and renal systems, respectively. The sequencing of cardiovascular and renal drugs is logical because most of the augmenting cardiovascular drugs (such as diuretics) affect the renal system.

Part X covers drugs that act on the respiratory system, a logical progression from the cardiovascular system.

Part XI addresses drugs acting on the gastrointestinal system. The gastrointestinal system stands alone; it does not share any actions with any other system.

Text Features

The features in this text are designed to support the text discussion, encouraging the student to look at the whole patient and to focus on the essential information that is important to learn about each drug class. Important features in this new edition focus on incorporating basic nursing skills, patient safety, critical thinking and application of the material learned to the clinical scenario, helping the student to understand the pharmacology material.

Special Elements and Learning Aids

Each chapter commences with a list of learning objectives, helping the student to understand what the key learning points will be. A list of featured drugs and key terms is also found on the opening chapter page.

- In the *Nursing Considerations* section of each chapter, *italics* highlight the *rationale* for each nursing intervention, helping the student to apply the information in a clinical situation. Elsewhere in the text, the rationale is consistently provided for therapeutic drug actions, contraindications and adverse effects. In the *Drug List* at the beginning of each chapter, a special icon appears next to the drug that is considered the prototype drug of each class. In each chapter, *Pharmacokinetic Tables* spotlight the pharmacokinetic information for each prototype drug. A *Glossary* found in the back of the book defines all of the key terms listed in each chapter.
- *Focus on Clinical Skills* points to accurate drug administration practices and the salient and sometimes life-preserving nursing interventions for a specific drug or drug therapy.
- *Focus on the Evidence* boxes compile information based on research to identify the best nursing practices associated with specific drug therapy.
- *Herbal and Alternative Therapies* displays highlight known interactions with specific herbs or alternative therapies that could affect the actions of the drugs being discussed.
- *Focus on Patient Safety* points alert the student to potentially serious drug–drug interactions, common dosing errors associated with specific drugs and reported unsafe drug practices.
- *Focus on Calculations* reviews are designed to help the student hone calculation and measurement skills while learning about the drugs for which dosages might need to be calculated.
- *Drug Therapy Across the Lifespan* tables concisely summarize points to consider when using the drugs of each class with children, adults and older adults. Similarly, where appropriate, discussion of *gender and cultural considerations* encourages the student to think about cultural awareness and to consider the patient as individuals with a special set of characteristics that not only influence variations in drug effectiveness but could influence a patient's perspective on drug therapy.
- *Points to Remember* end each chapter with a bulleted list which summarizes important concepts.
- *Critical Thinking Scenarios* tie each chapter's content together by presenting clinical *scenarios* about a patient using a particular drug from the class being discussed. Included in the case study are hints to guide critical thinking about the case and a discussion of *drug- and nondrug-related nursing considerations* for that particular patient and situation. Most importantly, the case study provides *a plan of nursing care* specifically developed for that patient and specifically based on the nursing process. The care plan is followed by a checklist of *patient teaching points* designed for the patient presented in the case study. This approach helps the student to see how assessment and the collected data are applied in the clinical situation.
- *Check Your Understanding* includes MCQ and EMQ used in many assessment processes.
- *Web Links* alert the student to electronic sources of drug information and sources of drug therapy information for specific diseases.

To the Student Using This Text

As you begin your study of pharmacology, don't be overwhelmed or confused by all of the details. The study of drugs fits perfectly into your study of the human body – anatomy, physiology, chemistry, nutrition, psychology and sociology. Approaching the study of pharmacology from the perspective of putting all of the pieces together is the most effective tactic. Work to understand the concepts and all of the details will fall into place, easier to remember and apply to the clinical situation. This understanding will help you in creating the picture of the whole patient as you are learning to provide comprehensive nursing care. This text is designed to help you accomplish all of this in a simple and concise manner. Good luck!

ACKNOWLEDGMENTS

A big thank you to our friends and families for supporting us throughout this book adaption – we are particularly grateful for the endless supply of tea and biscuits that kept us going! We would also like to thank all our colleagues who have taken the time to make suggestions to improve this first UK edition including Ingrid Gouldsborough, Michelle Keown, Liz Andrew and Michael Hollingsworth at The University of Manchester. Special thanks go to Michael Donnelly and to go Billiejoan Rice and Aidin McKinney of Queens University Belfast for their incredibly useful and timely feedback. We would also like to thank Cathy Peck and Rachel Hendrick from Lippincott Williams & Wilkins for their continuous support and direction.

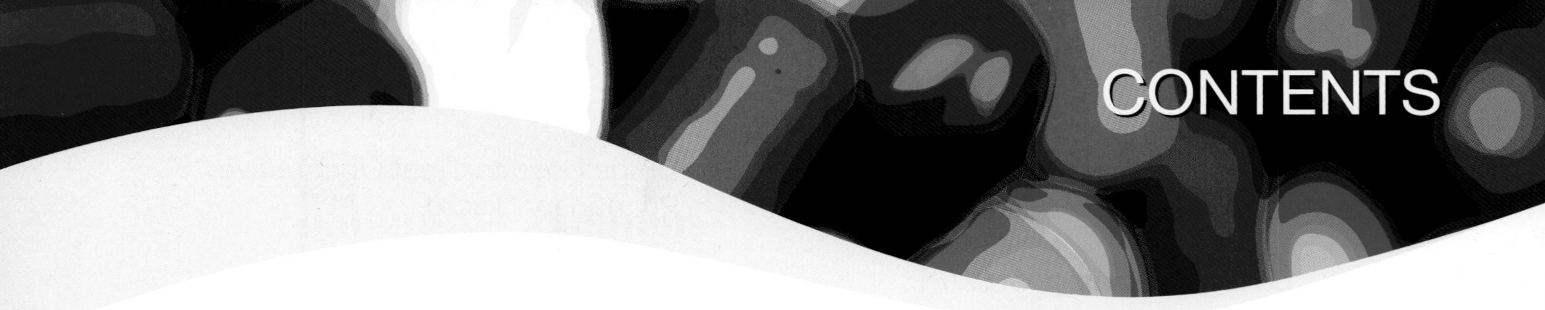

CONTENTS

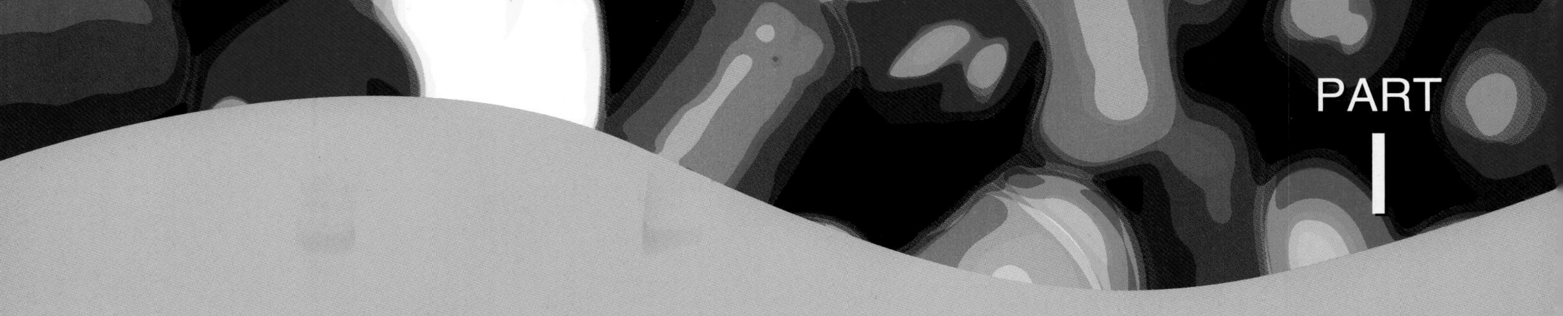

PART I

Introduction to Nursing Pharmacology

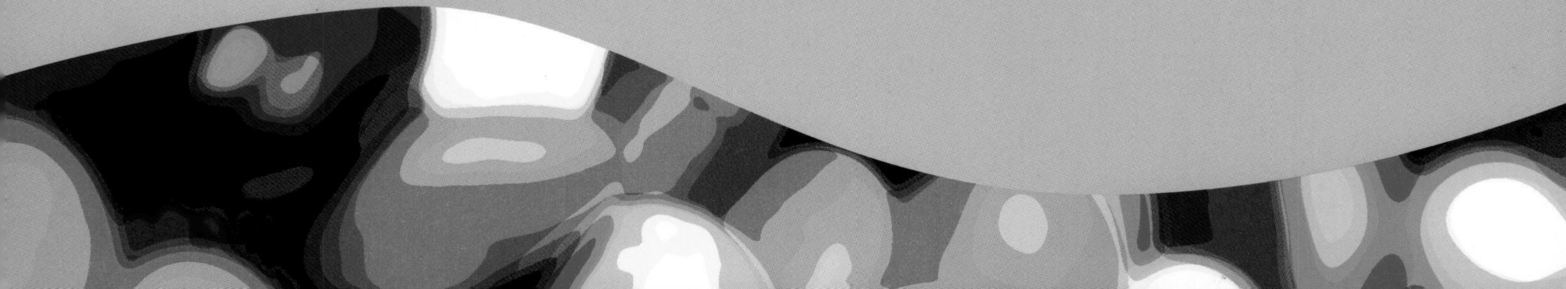

CHAPTER 1

Introduction to Drugs

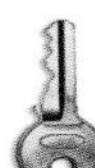

KEY TERMS

adverse effects
biopharmaceutical
British National Formulary
chemical name
concordance
drugs
generic drugs
generic name
genetic engineering
Medicines and Healthcare products Regulatory Agency (MHRA)
mutagenic
National Institute for Health and Clinical Excellence (NICE)
over-the-counter (OTC) drugs
pharmacodynamics
pharmacokinetics
pharmacology
pharmacotherapeutics
phase I studies
phase II studies
phase III studies
phase IV studies
placebo
preclinical tests
teratogen
trade name

LEARNING OBJECTIVES

Upon completion of this chapter, you will be able to:

1. List the standards set by the Nursing and Midwifery Council for the management and administration of drugs.
2. Define the word pharmacology.
3. Outline the steps involved in developing and approving a new drug in the United Kingdom.
4. Describe the controls on drugs that have abuse potential.
5. Differentiate between generic and trade name drugs, over-the-counter drugs and prescription drugs.
6. Explain the benefits and risks associated with the use of over-the-counter drugs.

The human body functions through a complicated series of chemical reactions and processes. **Drugs** are chemicals that are introduced into the body to cause a biological effect. When drugs are administered, there are a sequence of processes that handle the new chemicals including the breakdown and elimination of the drugs from the body.

For many reasons, understanding how drugs act on the body to cause changes and applying that knowledge in the clinical setting are important aspects of nursing practice. For example, patients often follow complicated drug regimens and receive potentially toxic drugs. In addition, some drugs interact with other drugs and some foodstuffs. Many patients also manage their own care at home. Therefore, the nurse is in a unique position regarding drug therapy because nursing responsibilities include the following:

- Administering drugs
- Assessing drug effects
- Intervening to make the drug regimen more tolerable
- Providing patient teaching about drugs and the drug regimen
- Monitoring the overall patient care plan to prevent medication errors.

Understanding the mechanism of action of drugs makes these tasks easier to handle, thus enhancing drug therapy and ultimately patient **concordance**.

This text is designed to provide the pharmacological basis for understanding drug therapy. The physiology of a body system and the related actions of many drugs on that system are presented in a way that allows clear understanding of how drugs work and what to anticipate when giving a particular type of drug. Thousands of drugs are available for use, and it is impossible to memorize all of the individual differences among drugs in a class. However, it is important to know and understand the most common drugs prescribed and administered on a daily basis. When using unfamiliar drugs, the nurse should first seek out the relevant information [e.g. from the British National Formulary (BNF)] prior to drug administration.

The Management and Administration of Drugs by Nurses

For many years, nurses in clinical settings have administered drugs in accordance with instructions given by the hospital pharmacist. The Nursing and Midwifery Council set standards for safe practice in the management and administration of drugs. The council's up-to-date guidelines are included in Standards for Medicines Management (2008).

As a registrant (nurse or midwife), in exercising your professional accountability in the best interests of your patients, you must:

- Be certain of the identity of the patient to whom the medicine is to be administered.
- Check that the patient is not allergic to the medicine before administering it.
- Know the therapeutic uses of the medicine to be administered, its normal dosage, side-effects, precautions and contraindications.
- Be aware of the patient's plan of care (care plan/pathway).
- Check that the prescription or the label on the medicine dispensed is clearly written and unambiguous.
- Check the expiry date (where it exists) of the medicine to be administered.
- Have considered the dosage, weight where appropriate, method of administration, route and timing.
- Administer or withhold in the context of the patient's condition (e.g. digoxin not usually to be given if the pulse is below 60 beats per minute) and coexisting therapies (e.g. physiotherapy).
- Contact the prescriber or another authorized prescriber without delay where contraindications to the prescribed medicine are discovered, where the patient develops a reaction to the medicine, or where assessment of the patient indicates that the medicine is no longer suitable.
- Make a clear, accurate and immediate record of all medicines administered, intentionally withheld or refused by the patient, ensuring the signature is clear and legible; it is also your responsibility to ensure that a record is made when delegating the task of administering medicine.

In addition:

- Where medication is not given the reason for not doing so must be recorded.
- You may administer with a single signature any Prescription Only Medicine (POM), General Sales List (GSL) or Pharmacy (P) medication.

(Taken from Standards for Medicines Management, 2008).

It is important to remember that nurses are legally and professionally responsible for any error that might occur.

In the past, the role of nurses in prescribing has been restricted to community nurses who were allowed to prescribe from a limited range of medicines, and appliances and dressings. However, from May 2006 the government permitted all nurses who had completed the relevant nurse prescribers' course and assessments to become Nurse Independent Prescribers. These qualified nurses are permitted to prescribe any licensed medicine within their competence; this includes some controlled drugs for use in palliative care, for example. The prescribing responsibilities of nurses are dependent on where the nurse is currently working. For example, the responsibilities of a nurse working in England may vary from the responsibilities of a nurse working in Scotland, Wales or Northern Ireland.

Nurses should have a clear understanding of how the responsibilities have been implemented in their country.

Pharmacology

Pharmacology is the study of the biological effects of chemicals administered to a living organism. Nurses deal with **pharmacotherapeutics**, or clinical pharmacology, the branch of pharmacology that uses drugs to treat, prevent and diagnose disease. Clinical pharmacology addresses two key concerns: the effect(s) of the drug on the body (**pharmacodynamics**) and the way in which the body handles the drug (**pharmacokinetics**).

A drug can have many effects; therefore, the nurse must know which ones may occur when a particular drug is administered. Most of these effects are therapeutic, or helpful, whereas others can be undesirable or potentially dangerous and are known as **adverse effects** (see Chapter 3 for a detailed discussion of adverse effects).

Sources of Drugs

Drugs are available from varied sources, both natural (e.g. plants, fungi, animals or inorganic compounds) and synthetic.

Plant Products

Plants and plant extracts have been used as medicines for many centuries. Even today, plants are an important source of chemicals that are developed into drugs. For example, digitalis products from *Digitalis purpurea* (foxglove plant) used to treat cardiac disorders; opiates such as morphine, codeine and papaverine from *Papaver somniferum* (opium poppy); and the taxanes derived from the bark of *Taxus brevifolia* (yew trees) are used in cancer chemotherapy. Plant extracts have also become the main component of the growing alternative therapy movement.

Fungi

The most well-known example of a drug derived from fungi is the antibiotic penicillin used to treat a number of communicable diseases. Penicillin and other β-lactam antibiotics are derived from the mould *Penicillium chrysogenum*. The immunosuppressant drug, ciclosporin, used to reduce the activity of a patient's immune system following organ transplantation, was also originally derived from a fungus.

Animal Products

Animal products are used to replace human chemicals that are not produced because of disease or genetic problems. Until 1982, insulin for treating diabetes was obtained exclusively from the pancreas of cows and pigs. Now **genetic engineering**, the process of altering deoxyribonucleic acid (DNA), permits scientists to produce human insulin by altering *Escherichia coli* bacteria, making insulin without some of the impurities that come with animal products. The insulin produced using genetic engineering procedures is known as a **biopharmaceutical**, a protein or nucleic acid prepared using genetic engineering technology.

Table 1.1 Elements Used for Their Therapeutic Effects

Element	Therapeutic Use
Aluminium	Antacid to decrease gastric acidity
	Management of hyperphosphataemia
	Prevention of the formation of phosphate urinary stones
Fluoride	Prevention of dental cavities
	Prevention of osteoporosis
Gold	Treatment of rheumatoid arthritis
Iron	Treatment of iron deficiency anaemia
Lithium	Treatment of mania

Inorganic Compounds

Salts of various elements can have therapeutic effects in the human body. Aluminium, fluoride, lithium, iron and even gold are used to treat various conditions. The effects of these elements were usually discovered accidentally when a cause–effect relationship was observed. Table 1.1 shows examples of some elements used for their therapeutic benefit.

Synthetic Sources

Even today, many drugs are developed from chemicals in plants, animals or the environment that have been screened for signs of therapeutic activity. Most new drugs are purely synthetic. Technical advances allow scientists to alter a chemical with proven therapeutic effectiveness to make it better. Sometimes, a small change in a chemical's structure can make that chemical more useful as a drug – more potent, more stable, less toxic. These technological advances have led to the development of groups of similar drugs, all of which are derived from an original prototype, but each of which has slightly different properties, making a particular drug more desirable in a specific situation.

Biopharmaceuticals

As mentioned above, biopharmaceuticals are proteins (including antibodies) or nucleic acids produced by genetic engineering for therapeutic purposes. There is a large range of biopharmaceuticals, including thrombolytic agents such as tissue plasminogen activator; hormones (insulin, growth hormone); vaccines; interferons used in the treatment of leukaemia and multiple sclerosis; and also monoclonal antibodies, such as trastuzumab (Herceptin), used to target specific proteins on cancer cells.

Drug Evaluation

To become a drug, a chemical must have demonstrated therapeutic value or efficacy without severe toxicity or damaging properties. Once a chemical that might have therapeutic value is identified, it must undergo a series of tests to evaluate its actual therapeutic and toxic effects. The need for extensive testing was reinforced by the 'thalidomide disaster' in the early 1960s. The hypnotic drug thalidomide was regarded as suitable for use during pregnancy. However, the drug had not been tested on pregnant animals and was subsequently found to be a potent **teratogen** (i.e. causing adverse effects on the foetus). This resulted in more than 10,000 children born with severe malformations.

This process of evaluation significantly reduces the number of potential drugs that actually make it to the end stage: for every 5000 chemicals that are identified as being potential drugs, only one will become an approved drug. Before receiving final approval for marketing to the public, drugs must pass through preclinical tests on animals and phase I, II and III studies on humans. Figure 1.1 highlights the various phases of drug development.

Preclinical Tests

In **preclinical tests**, chemicals that may have therapeutic value are tested on cell cultures and laboratory animals. Whole animal testing is an important part of the drug development process; however, there is significant public opposition to the use of animals in experiments. A comment often quoted is that the physiological processes animals undergo are so different from our own. Although there are recognized differences in the way humans and laboratory animals (e.g. rats, rabbits) metabolize drugs (Berthou *et al.*, 1992) for example, these differences are far outweighed by the similarities between species (Research Defence Society, 2009). It should also be recognized that the number of experiments using live animals has decreased by over 35% in the past 30 years (Home Office, 2009).

Preclinical tests have several purposes:

- To assess if they are likely to have beneficial effects in models of disease.
- To evaluate any toxic effects in the short and long term.
- To assess their teratogenic and **mutagenic** affects, that is their potential to cause adverse effects on the foetus and genetic material, respectively.
- To determine how the animal handles the drug: How is it absorbed? How is it metabolized? How long does it take to eliminate the drug from the body?

At the end of the preclinical testing, some chemicals are discarded for the following reasons:

- The chemical lacks therapeutic activity when used with living animals.
- The chemical is too toxic to living animals to be worth the risk of developing into drugs.
- The chemical is highly teratogenic or mutagenic.
- The safety margins are so small that the chemical would not be useful in the clinical setting.

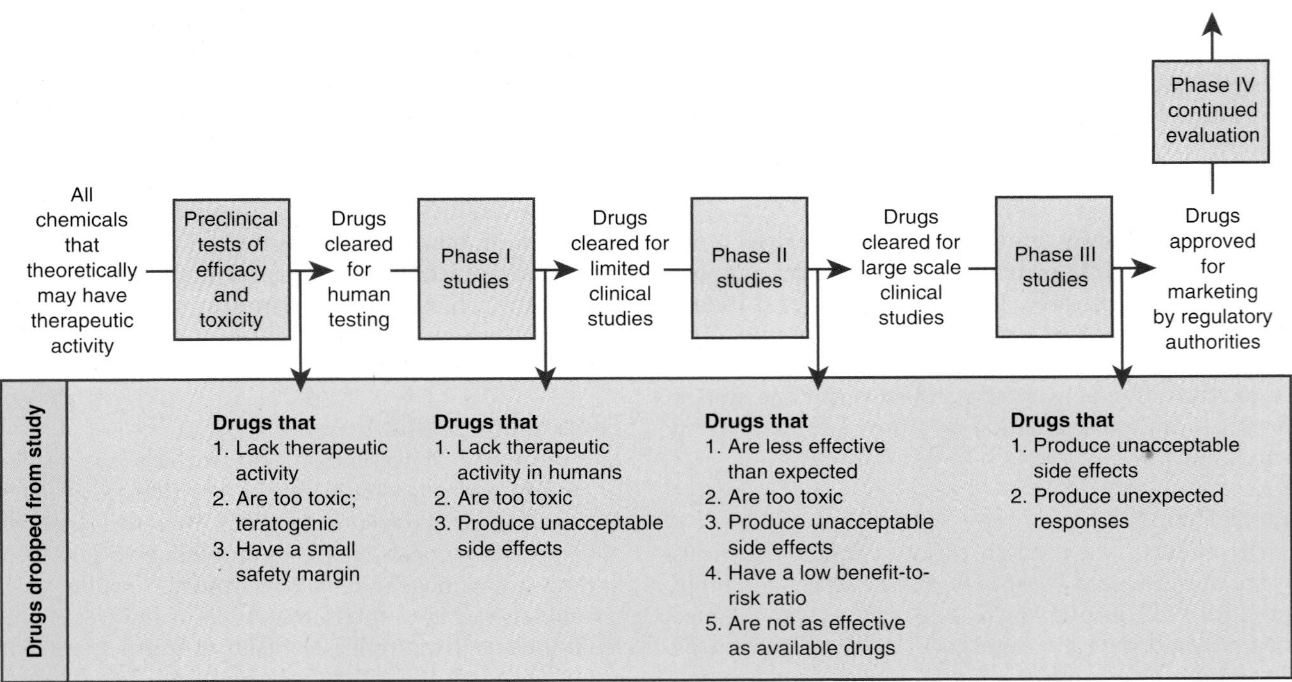

FIGURE 1.1. Phases of drug development.

Some chemicals, however, are found to have therapeutic effects and acceptable safety margins. This means that the chemicals are therapeutic at doses that are reasonably different from doses that cause toxic effects. Such chemicals will pass the preclinical trials and advance to phase I studies.

Phase I Studies

Phase I studies are the first occasion where the drug is tested on humans and the aim is safety evaluation not effectiveness in disease control. Permission to enter phase I studies must be granted by the local ethics committee and also the National Drug Regulatory Authority. The ethics committee will evaluate the risks to the volunteers, the process of recruiting volunteers, the experience of the clinical investigators and the design of the study. The regulatory authorities will determine if there is a scientific need to carry out the study. The overriding authority in control of this regulatory procedure is the **Medicines and Healthcare products Regulatory Agency (MHRA)**.

In phase I studies small groups of between 40 and 60 individuals volunteer to test the drugs. These studies are performed by specially trained clinical investigators. The volunteers are fully informed of possible risks and are paid for expenses and for any inconvenience caused. Generally, the volunteers are healthy, young men. Women are not usually candidates for phase I studies because the chemicals may exert unknown and harmful effects on their ova. In addition, the cyclical changes in female hormones can add further complexity. However, some studies will recruit women provided they are using contraceptives, have produced a negative pregnancy test or are postmenopausal. Men produce sperm daily, so there is less potential for complete destruction or alteration of the sperm.

Single doses of the drug under test are given to the volunteers. Investigators obtain data on how the drug is absorbed, distributed, metabolized and excreted; the biological effects of the drug; adverse effects and toxicity and also the appropriate dosage for subsequent studies. At the end of phase I studies, many drugs are dropped from the process because they may cause unacceptable adverse effects, for example. If phase I studies are successful, then investigations move on to phase II studies.

Phase II Studies

Phase II studies are the first opportunity for clinical investigators to try the drug on patients who have the disease that the drug is designed to treat. Patients are told about the possible benefits of the drug and are invited to participate in the study. Those patients who consent to participate are fully informed about possible risks and are monitored very closely to evaluate the drug's effects. Usually, phase II studies are performed at various sites across the country – in hospitals, clinics and GPs' surgeries – and are monitored by representatives of the pharmaceutical company studying the drug. These studies provide information on the optimal dose and also the therapeutic potential of the drug. The therapeutic potential is often determined in comparison with a **placebo**, a substance or treatment the patient believes will have a therapeutic effect; or to the existing standard treatment.

At the end of phase II studies, a drug may be removed from further investigation for the following reasons:

- It is less effective than anticipated.
- It is too toxic when used with patients.
- It produces unacceptable adverse effects.
- It has a low benefit-to-risk ratio, meaning that the therapeutic benefit it provides does not outweigh the risk of potential adverse effects that it causes.
- It is no more effective than other drugs already on the market, making the cost of continued research and production less attractive to the drug company.

A drug that continues to show promise as a therapeutic agent receives additional scrutiny in phase III studies.

Phase III Studies

Phase III studies involve use of the drug in a larger patient group (250 to >1000 subjects) for a period of 2 to 5 years. As in phase II studies, the drug under test will be compared with either a placebo or an existing treatment.

The larger group size enables evaluation of the efficacy of the drug in patients from different groups, for example age, ethnicity, and others. Patients are observed very closely and monitored for any adverse effects. It is possible that more adverse effects are recorded from a wider sample of the patient population and following long-term drug administration. Prescribers sometimes ask patients to keep journals and record any symptoms they experience. Prescribers then evaluate the reported effects to determine whether they are caused by the disease or by the drug. This information is collected by the drug company that is developing the drug and is shared with the MHRA. A drug that produces unacceptable adverse effects or unforeseen reactions is usually removed from further study by the drug company. In some cases, the MHRA may have to request that a drug be withdrawn from the market.

Final Drug Approval

Drugs that successfully complete phase III studies are evaluated by regulatory authorities in the country where approval is sought. These authorities rely on committees of experts familiar with the specialty area in which the drugs will be used. Only those drugs that receive approval and are granted a product licence may be marketed.

These preclinical tests and clinical trials may take up to 12 years to complete, resulting in a so-called drug lag. However, public safety is paramount in drug approval, so the process remains strict. In certain instances involving the treatment of deadly diseases, the process can be accelerated. For example, efavirenz was thought to offer a benefit to patients with acquired immune deficiency syndrome (AIDS), a potentially fatal immune disorder; and was pushed through because of the progressive nature of AIDS and the lack of a cure. All literature associated with these drugs indicates that

BOX 1.1 Generic, Chemical and Trade Names of Drugs

1-(4-Chlorophenyl)-5-isopropylbiguanide hydrochloride	←	**Chemical name**	→	9α-Chloro-11β,17α,21-trihydroxy-16β-methylpregna-1,4-diene-3,20-dione 17,21-dipropionate
Proguanil hydrochloride	←	**Generic name**	→	Beclometasone dipropionate
Malarone	←	**Trade names**	→	*Beconase*

long-term effects and other information about the drug may not yet be known.

The drugs listed in this book will have undergone rigorous testing and approval for sale to the public, either with or without a prescription from a health care provider.

An approved drug is given a **trade name** by the pharmaceutical company that developed it. The **generic name** of a drug is the original designation that the drug was given when the drug company applied for the approval process. **Chemical names** are names that reflect the chemical structure of a drug. See Box 1.1 for examples of drug names. Some drugs are known by all of the three names. It can be confusing to study drugs when so many different names are used for the same compound. In this text, only the generic name will appear.

The European Union requires manufacturers to use the Recommended International Nonproprietary Name (rINN) for all medicines. In many cases, the rINN was identical to the British Approved Name (BAN). Wherever the two were different, the BAN was changed to the rINN. There are two exceptions to this general rule: adrenaline and noradrenaline are the BANs, whereas epinephrine and norepinephrine are the rINNs. In this text, the BAN names adrenaline and noradrenaline are used as does the **British National Formulary**.

Continual Evaluation

After a drug is approved for marketing, it enters a phase of continual evaluation or **phase IV study**. Prescribers are required to report any untoward or unexpected adverse effects associated with drugs they are using to the MHRA. The MHRA continually evaluates this information. Some drugs cause unexpected effects that are not seen until wide distribution occurs. Sometimes, those effects are therapeutic. For example, patients taking the antiparkinsonism drug amantadine were found to have fewer cases of influenza than other patients, leading to the discovery that amantadine is an effective antiviral agent.

In other instances, the unexpected effects are dangerous. In 1997, the diet drug dexfenfluramine was withdrawn from the market only months after its release because patients taking it developed serious heart problems. In 1998, the antihypertensive drug mibefradil was removed from the market not long after its release because patients taking it were found to have more cardiac morbidity. These problems were not seen in any of the premarket studies.

Licensed and Unlicensed Drugs

There are occasions when an unlicensed drug, that is a drug which has not completed the entire clinical trials programme, is used to treat a patient. For example, an unlicensed drug may be used as drug treatment as part of a clinical trial. Alternatively, the doctor may consider that the patient will benefit from the new treatment because other treatment approaches have failed. The doctor must apply to the pharmaceutical company to use the drug on what is known as a 'named patient' basis. The doctor takes responsibility for the unlicensed drug treatment and the patient must be made aware of the potential risks associated with the drug.

Drugs that have successfully passed through clinical testing are granted a product licence by the MHRA. This licence permits the pharmaceutical company to market this drug for the treatment of specific diseases or medical needs covered by the license. If it becomes apparent that the new drug could be useful in another clinical situation, for example to treat another form of cancer, the pharmaceutical company will need to conduct further clinical trials and obtain another license for the second condition. In the meantime, doctors can use this unlicensed form of the drug to treat a patient for an indication that is not covered by the original license. This is known as 'off-label' use.

The National Institute for Health and Clinical Excellence

The **National Institute for Health and Clinical Excellence (NICE)** was established in 1999 to provide guidance to health care professionals and also members of the public through the sharing of best practise. This organization provides information on three key areas: (1) promotion of good health and prevention of ill health; (2) new and existing medicines, treatments and procedures available within the National Health Service (NHS); and (3) the most suitable treatment for patients with specific diseases and conditions (NICE, 2008) to maximize resources by evaluating the cost to the NHS against the benefits to the patient. NICE uses current published evidence about the intervention to evaluate whether or not it would be cost effective for the NHS to use a particular medical intervention (e.g. the use of inhaled corticosteroids in the treatment of asthma for adults). When NICE recommends a specific medicine or treatment, the NHS is legally obliged to provide the funding.

Legal Regulation of Drugs

The Medicines Act (1968) controls the manufacture and supply of medicine. Newly marketed drugs can be allocated to one of four categories:

1. Prescription-only medicine controlled drugs (POM CD) can be supplied only by authorized individuals.
2. Prescription only medicine can be sold only by a pharmacist in receipt of a prescription from a doctor.
3. Pharmacy-only drugs (P) can be sold without the need of a prescription by pharmacists.
4. General sales list drugs can be sold without a prescription in any shop.

Controlled Substances

Drugs with abuse potential are called controlled substances. The Misuse of Drugs Act (1971) regulates the manufacturing, distribution and possession of drugs that are known to have abuse potential. This act established categories for ranking the abuse potential of various drugs, where Class A drugs are considered to be the most harmful. Examples of drugs in each class include:

- Class A – ecstasy, lysergide (LSD), diamorphine (heroin), morphine, opium, pethidine, cocaine, crack, magic mushrooms, methylamphetamine (crystal meth) and other amphetamines if prepared for injection.
- Class B – oral amphetamines, barbiturates, codeine, pholcodine, ethylmorphine, glutethimide, pentazocine and phenmetrazine.
- Class C – drugs related to amphetamines, cannabis (including resin), most benzodiazepines and androgenic and anabolic steroids.

A second act, the Misuse of Drugs Regulations (2001) specifies those individuals who are authorized to supply drugs from these categories to their patients. The Home Office is responsible for the enforcement of these regulations.

Generic Drugs

When a pharmaceutical company has synthesized and carried out some preclinical testing it applies for a patent. A patent is usually valid for 20 years and only that company can sell the drug during that time. When the patent runs out on a trade name drug, the drug can be produced by other manufacturers. **Generic drugs** are medicines that are produced by companies that just manufacture drugs. These companies do not have the research or the advertising that pharmaceutical companies have and can, therefore, produce the generic drugs more cheaply. In the past, some quality control problems were found with generic products. For example, the binders used in a generic drug might not be the same as those used in the trade name product; as a result, the way the body absorbs and uses the drug may differ. In that case, the bioavailability of the drug is different from that of the trade name product.

Many hospital trusts require that a drug be dispensed in the generic form if one is available. This requirement helps keep down the cost of drugs and health care. Some prescribers, however, specify that a drug prescription be 'dispensed as written'; that is, the trade name product be used. By doing so, the prescriber ensures the quality control and bioavailability expected with that drug. These elements are particularly important in drugs that have narrow safety margins, such as digoxin, a heart drug, and warfarin, an anticoagulant. The initial cost may be higher, but some prescribers believe that, in the long run, the cost to the patient will be less.

Over-the-Counter Drugs

Over-the-counter (OTC) drugs are products that are available without prescription for self-treatment of a variety of complaints. Some of these agents were approved as prescription drugs but were later found to be very safe and useful for patients without the need of a prescription. Although OTC drugs have been found to be safe when taken as directed, nurses should consider several problems related to OTC drug use:

- Taking these drugs could mask the signs and symptoms of underlying disease, making diagnosis difficult.
- Taking these drugs with prescription medications could result in drug interactions and interfere with drug therapy.
- Not taking these drugs as directed could result in serious overdoses.

Many patients do not consider OTC drugs to be medications and, therefore do not report their use. Nurses should always include specific questions about OTC drug use when taking a drug history and should provide information in all drug-teaching protocols about avoiding OTC use while taking prescription drugs.

Sources of Drug Information

The fields of pharmacology and drug therapy change so quickly that it is important to have access to sources of information about drug doses, therapeutic and adverse effects and nursing-related implications. This text addresses *general* drug information and provides valuable background and basic information to help in the understanding of pharmacology, but in clinical practice it is important to have access to up-to-the-minute information. Several sources of drug information are readily available.

The British National Formulary

The nurse must refer to the latest edition of the BNF to obtain the *specific* details required for safe and effective drug administration. Updated on a 6-monthly basis, the BNF provides an up-to-date and comprehensive drug guide for use by prescribers and other health care professionals in the clinical setting. The BNF is also available on the Internet. The prescriber is provided with details of:

- *Indications*, that is the disease(s) the drug is approved to treat.
- *Contraindications*, that is those individuals where taking a specific drug could affect a pre-existing medical condition.
- *Cautions*, where taking the drug could increase the risk of unwanted effects in certain patients, for example those patients who are pregnant or have diabetes.
- *Interactions* lists the possible interactions with any medicines the patients may be taking.
- *Side-effects* include the side-effects observed in patients taking this drug.
- *Costs* of all of the drugs available on the NHS.

The BNF for Children provides equivalent information on medicines approved for children.

Package Inserts

All drugs come with a package insert prepared by the manufacturer according to regulations laid down by the regulatory authorities. The package insert contains information for patients on:

- what the medicine is,
- how the medicine works,
- the infections/diseases the medicine can be used to treat,
- cautions to patients regarding pre-existing conditions or potential interactions with other medicines,
- how to administer the medicine together with any possible cautions to be taken into consideration, for example do not wear contact lenses while you are using an antibacterial treatment for conjunctivitis,
- possible side-effects,
- how to store the medicine.

Nurses should encourage their patients to read these inserts before commencing treatment.

Publications

- The *Journal of Advanced Nursing* is an international, peer-reviewed, scientific journal. The published articles aim to advance knowledge in a number of areas, including practice, education, management and policy.
- The *British Journal of Nursing* is a peer-reviewed scientific journal published fortnightly. The evidence-based articles are written by nurses and provide practical recommendations.
- *Drug Safety Update* is a monthly newsletter from the MHRA and the **Commission on Human Medicines (CHM)**. This newsletter provides updated information on specific medicines and key points on studies of the safety of medicines.
- *Nursing Times* is published on a weekly basis and provides information on research studies and clinical articles to nurses at all levels, including those in training.

Internet Information

There are many Internet sites available for obtaining drug information, patient information or therapeutic information related to specific disease states. Many members of the public now use the Internet as a source of medical information and advice. It is a good idea for the nurse to become familiar with what is available on the Internet and what patients may be referencing. Information presented on Internet sites is less likely to be peer-reviewed and therefore the accuracy of the information must be questioned.

In each chapter the reader is guided towards appropriate and reliable Internet sites related to the chapter content.

WEB LINKS

Health care providers may want to consult the following Internet sources:

http://bnfc.org.uk The BNF for Children provides UK health care professionals with information on suitable drugs for treating children.

http://cks.library.nhs.uk The NHS Clinical Knowledge Summaries provides evidence-based practical information on the common conditions observed in primary care.

http://www.bnf.org.uk The BNF provides UK health care professionals with authoritative and practical information on the selection and clinical use of medicines.

http://www.dh.gov.uk The Department of Health site provides information on many areas to health care professionals.

http://www.direct.gov.uk The information on medical rules for all drivers can be found here (originally found under Driver and Vehicle Licensing Agency site).

http://www.hpa.org.uk The Health Protection Agency provides support and advice on public health issues to the NHS and other authorities.

http://www.mhra.gov.uk The MHRA are an agency of the Department of Health and are responsible for ensuring that medicines and medical devices are safe for the public.

http://www.mhra.gov.uk/mhra/drugsafetyupdate The MHRA and the CHM produce a monthly newsletter giving advice and information on the safe use of medicines.

http://www.nhsdirect.nhs.uk The NHS Direct service provides patients with information and advice about health, illness and health services.

http://www.nice.org.uk The National Institute for Health and Clinical Excellence provides guidance on public health, new and existing treatments within the NHS and also information on the most appropriate care for patients.

http://www.nmc-uk.org The Nursing and Midwifery Council sets standards for training and education and ensures that those standards are maintained.

http://www.travax.nhs.uk This database provides travel health information for health care providers. This site can be accessed only by registered NHS users.

http://www.understandinganimalresearch.org.uk This site for the Research Defence Society provides information on the use of animals in research.

http://www.yellowcard.gov.uk Health care professionals and the public are encouraged to report unwanted or unexpected adverse reactions using the yellow card system.

Points to Remember

- All nurses must abide by the standards set by the Nursing and Midwifery Council for the safe administration of drugs.
- Drugs are chemicals that are introduced into the body to bring about some sort of change.
- Drugs can come from many sources: plants, animals, inorganic elements, synthetic preparations and biopharmaceuticals.
- Preclinical testing of potential drugs involves the use of laboratory animals to determine their therapeutic and adverse effects.
- Phase I studies test potential drugs on healthy human subjects to assess safety.
- Phase II studies test potential drugs on patients who have the disease the drugs are designed to treat.
- Phase III studies test drugs in the clinical setting to determine any unanticipated effects or lack of effectiveness.
- Phase IV studies assess the safety and efficacy of the newly approved drug on a wider population.
- The MHRA regulates the development and marketing of drugs to ensure safety and efficacy.
- Generic drugs are sold under their chemical names, not trade names; they may be cheaper but are not necessarily as safe as trade name drugs. OTC drugs are available without prescription for the self-treatment of various complaints.

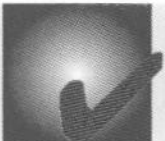

CHECK YOUR UNDERSTANDING

Answers to the questions in this chapter may be found in the answer key in the back of the book.

Multiple Choice

Select the most appropriate answer to the following.

1. Clinical pharmacology is the study of
   a. the biological effects of chemicals.
   b. drugs used to treat, prevent or diagnose disease.
   c. plant components that can be used as medicines.
   d. binders and other vehicles for delivering medication.

2. Phase I drug studies involve
   a. the use of laboratory animals to test chemicals.
   b. patients with the disease the drug is designed to treat.
   c. mass marketing surveys of drug effects in large numbers of people.
   d. healthy human volunteers.

3. The generic name of a drug is
   a. the name assigned to the drug by the pharmaceutical company developing it.
   b. the chemical name of the drug based on its chemical structure.
   c. the original name assigned to the drug at the beginning of the evaluation process.
   d. often used in advertising campaigns.

4. The storing, prescribing and distributing of controlled substances – drugs that are more apt to be addictive – are monitored by the
   a. NICE.
   b. Department of Health.
   c. Committee for the Safety of Medicines.
   d. Home Office.

5. Healthy young women are generally not involved in phase I studies of drugs because
   a. male bodies are more predictable and responsive to chemicals.
   b. females are more apt to suffer problems with ova, which are formed before birth and not formed in later years.
   c. males can tolerate the unknown adverse effects of many drugs better than females.
   d. there are no standards to use to evaluate the female response.

6. A patient has been taking fluoxetine for several years, but when picking up the prescription this month, found that the tablets looked different and became concerned. The nurse, checking with the pharmacist, found that fluoxetine had just become available in the generic form and the prescription had been filled with the generic product. The nurse should tell the patient that
   a. the new tablet may not work and the patient should carefully monitor response.
   b. generic drugs are available without a prescription because they are very safe.
   c. the law requires that prescriptions be filled with the generic form if one is available to cut down the cost of medications.
   d. the pharmacist filled the prescription with the wrong drug and it should be returned to the pharmacy for a refund.

Extended Matching Questions

Select **all** that apply.

1. When teaching a patient about OTC drugs, which points should the nurse include?
   a. These drugs are very safe and can be used freely to relieve your complaints.
   b. These compounds are called drugs, but they aren't really drugs and don't need to be reported to your health care provider.
   c. Some of these drugs were once prescription drugs, but are now thought to be safe when used as directed.
   d. Reading the label of these drugs is very important; the active ingredient is very prominent; you should always check the ingredient name.
   e. It is important to read the label to see what the recommended dose of the drug is; some of these drugs can cause serious problems if too much of the drug is taken.
   f. It is important to report the use of any OTC drug to your physician, because many of them can interact with drugs that might be prescribed for you.
   g. It is important to check an OTC medication with the pharmacist if you are taking other medication.

2. A patient asks what generic drugs are and if he should be using them to treat his infection. Which of the following statements should be included in the nurse's explanation?
   a. A generic drug is a drug that is sold by the name of the ingredient, not by trade name.
   b. Generic drugs are always the best drugs to use because they are never any different from the familiar trade names.
   c. Generic drugs are not available until the patent expires on a specific drug.
   d. Generic drugs are usually cheaper than the well-known trade names.
   e. Generic drugs are forms of a drug that are available over the counter and do not require a prescription.
   f. Your physician may want you to have the trade name of a drug, not the generic form, and DAW, or 'dispense as written', will be on your prescription.
   g. Generic drugs are less likely to cause adverse effects than trade name drugs.

Matching

Match the word with the appropriate definition.

1. ________________ genetic engineering
2. ________________ MHRA
3. ________________ pharmacology
4. ________________ phase I study
5. ________________ OTC drugs
6. ________________ preclinical study
7. ________________ teratogenic
8. ________________ pharmacotherapeutics
9. ________________ generic drugs
10. ________________ drugs

A. The study of the actions of chemicals on living organisms
B. Medicines that can be produced by any pharmaceutical company once the drug's patent has expired
C. Having adverse effects on the foetus
D. Chemicals that are introduced into the body to bring about some sort of change
E. A drug that is available without a prescription
F. Regulatory authority responsible for the evaluation and monitoring of new and existing medicines
G. Process of altering DNA to produce a chemical to be used as a drug
H. Initial study of a potential drug conducted with a small number of selected, healthy human volunteers
I. Initial trial of a chemical believed to have therapeutic potential; uses laboratory animals, not human subjects
J. Clinical pharmacology, the branch of pharmacology that deals with drugs

Bibliography and References

Berthou, F., Guillois, B., Riche, C., Dreano, Y., Jacqz-Aigrain, E., & Beaune, P. H. (1992). Interspecies variations in caffeine metabolism related to cytochrome P450A1 enzymes. *Xenobiotica, 22*(6), 671–680.

British Medical Association and Royal Pharmaceutical Society of Great Britain. (2008). *British National Formulary*. London: BMJ & RPS Publishing. *This publication is updated biannually: it is imperative that the most recent edition is consulted.*

British Medical Association and Royal Pharmaceutical Society of Great Britain. (2008). *British National Formulary for Children*. London: BMJ & RPS Publishing. *This publication is updated annually: it is imperative that the most recent edition is consulted.*

Golan, D. E., Tashjian, A. H., Armstrong, E. J., & Armstrong, A. W. (2005). *Principles of pharmacology: The pathophysiologic basis of drug therapy*. Philadelphia: Lippincott Williams & Wilkins.

Home Office (2009). *Statistics of Scientific Procedures on Living Animals. Great Britain 2008*. Available from http://www.homeoffice.gov.uk/rds/

Howland, R. D., & Mycek, M. J. (2005). *Pharmacology* (3rd ed.). Philadelphia: Lippincott Williams & Wilkins.

National Institute for Health and Clinical Excellence (2008). Available from http://www.nice.org.uk/

Nursing and Midwifery Council. (2008). *Standards for Medicines Management*. Available from http://www.nmc-uk.org/

Rang, H. P. (2006). *Drug discovery and development: Technology in transition*. Edinburgh: Churchill Livingstone.

Rang, H. P., Dale, M. M., Ritter, J. M., & Flower, R. J. (2007). *Rang and Dale's pharmacology* (6th ed.). Philadelphia: Churchill Livingstone.

Research Defence Society (2009). *Understanding Animal Research*. Available from http://www.understandinganimalresearch.org.uk/

Scott, W. N., & McGrath, D. (2009). *Nursing pharmacology made incredibly easy*. Philadelphia: Lippincott Williams & Wilkins.

Simonsen, T., Aarbakke, J., Kay, I., Coleman, I., Sinnott, P., & Lysaa, R. (2006). *Illustrated pharmacology for nurses*. London: Hodder Arnold.

CHAPTER

2

Drugs and the Body

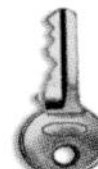

KEY TERMS

absorption
active transport
carrier molecules
chemotherapeutic agents
competitive antagonists
concordance
distribution
effective concentration
excretion
first-pass effect
G-proteins
half-life
ligand
ligand-gated ion channels
loading dose
metabolism
noncompetitive antagonists
nuclear receptors
passive diffusion
pharmacodynamics
pharmacogenomics
pharmacokinetics
placebo effect
protein kinase
receptor sites
selective toxicity
therapeutic index

LEARNING OBJECTIVES

Upon completion of this chapter, you will be able to:

1. Describe how body cells respond to the presence of drugs.
2. Outline the process of dynamic equilibrium that determines the actual concentration of a drug in the body.
3. Explain the meaning of half-life of a drug.
4. List six factors that can influence the actual effectiveness of drugs in the body.
5. Define the terms pharmacodynamics, pharmacokinetics and therapeutic index.
6. Define drug–drug, drug–alternative therapy and drug–food interactions.

To understand what happens when a drug is administered, the nurse must understand **pharmacodynamics** (how the drug affects the body) and **pharmacokinetics** (how the body acts on the drug). These processes form the basis for the guidelines that have been established regarding drug administration; for example, why certain agents are given intramuscularly (IM) and not intravenously (IV), why some drugs are taken with food and others are not and the standard dose that should be used to achieve the desired effect. Understanding the basic principles of pharmacodynamics and pharmacokinetics helps the nurse to anticipate therapeutic and adverse drug effects and to intervene in ways to ensure the most effective drug regimen for the patient.

Pharmacodynamics

Pharmacodynamics examines interactions between the chemical components of living systems and the foreign chemicals, including drugs, which enter those systems. All living organisms function by a series of complicated, continual chemical reactions. When a new chemical enters the system, multiple changes in cell functioning may occur. To avoid such problems, drug development works to provide the most effective and least toxic chemicals for therapeutic use.

Drug Actions

Drugs usually work in one of four ways to:

1. Replace or act as substitutes for missing chemicals.
2. Increase or stimulate certain cellular activities.
3. Depress or slow cellular activities.
4. Interfere with the functioning of foreign cells, such as invading micro-organisms or neoplasms. Drugs that act in this way are called **chemotherapeutic agents**.

As described below, drugs can act in several different ways to achieve these results.

Receptor Sites

All cells in the body possess **receptor sites**, specific proteins expressed either on the plasma membrane or within the cell to which endogenous molecules such as hormones, neurotransmitters and growth factors bind to cause an effect within the cell. Many drugs also bind to these receptor sites. The binding of either endogenous molecule or drug to the receptor is often related to how a key works in a lock. The specific drug (the key) finds a perfect fit (the lock) at a receptor site on the plasma membrane (Figure 2.1). The interaction between the drug and the receptor site can then produce certain effects, such as changes in plasma membrane permeability, increased or decreased cellular activity, or alterations in cellular metabolism. In many situations nearby enzymes break down the reacting drugs and the receptor site is then ready for further binding.

Some receptor sites, **ligand-gated ion channels**, are coupled directly to ion channels and lead to a change in the permeability of the cell to different ions. For example, when the neurotransmitter acetylcholine (a **ligand**) binds to nicotinic acetylcholine receptors present on the neuromuscular junction, sodium channels in the central pore of the receptor open allowing sodium ions to enter the cell. Other membrane receptors are linked to **G-proteins**, for example noradrenaline binding to adrenoceptors. Upon binding of the ligand to the receptor, there is a change in the conformation or shape of the attached G-protein on the inside of the plasma membrane ultimately leading to a change in the activity of either intracellular enzymes or other ion channels. Some receptors, for example those for peptide hormones such as insulin, cytokines and growth factors, incorporate an enzyme known as a **protein kinase**. Activation of these receptors stimulates a cascade of events leading to alterations in gene transcription and thus synthesis of proteins. **Nuclear receptors** can also cause changes in gene transcription; however, in contrast to the other receptors described, these receptors are located within the cytoplasm of the cell. After the drug has bound to the receptor the drug–receptor complex translocates into the nucleus to initiate alterations in gene expression. Examples include receptors for steroid hormones such as oestrogen and glucocorticoids.

Some drugs interact directly with receptor sites to cause the same activity that natural chemicals would cause at that site. These drugs are called **agonists** (see Figure 2.1). For example, salbutamol binds to adrenoceptors in the lungs to cause relaxation of smooth muscle in the bronchioles.

In contrast, other drugs bind to receptor sites to block normal stimulation, producing no effect. For example, curare (a poison used on the tips of hunters' spears in the Amazon to paralyse and kill prey) occupies receptor sites for acetylcholine, which is necessary for muscle contraction and movement. Curare prevents muscle stimulation, causing paralysis and is similar in structure to drugs used to induce paralysis in anaesthesia, for example atracurium. Curare is said to be a **competitive antagonist** of acetylcholine (see Figure 2.1). Some drugs bind to specific receptor sites on a cell and by remaining there, prevent the binding of another chemical to a different receptor site on that cell. Such drugs are called **noncompetitive antagonists** (see Figure 2.1).

Ion Channels

Ion channels are 'pores' spanning the plasma membrane which selectively allow ions including sodium, potassium and calcium to enter and leave the cell. In addition to the ligand-gated ion channels mentioned above, other types of ion channels exist and are regulated by changes in the voltage of the plasma membrane. Regardless of their mechanism of regulation, all types of ion channels are important targets for drugs. For example, local anaesthetics 'plug' voltage-gated

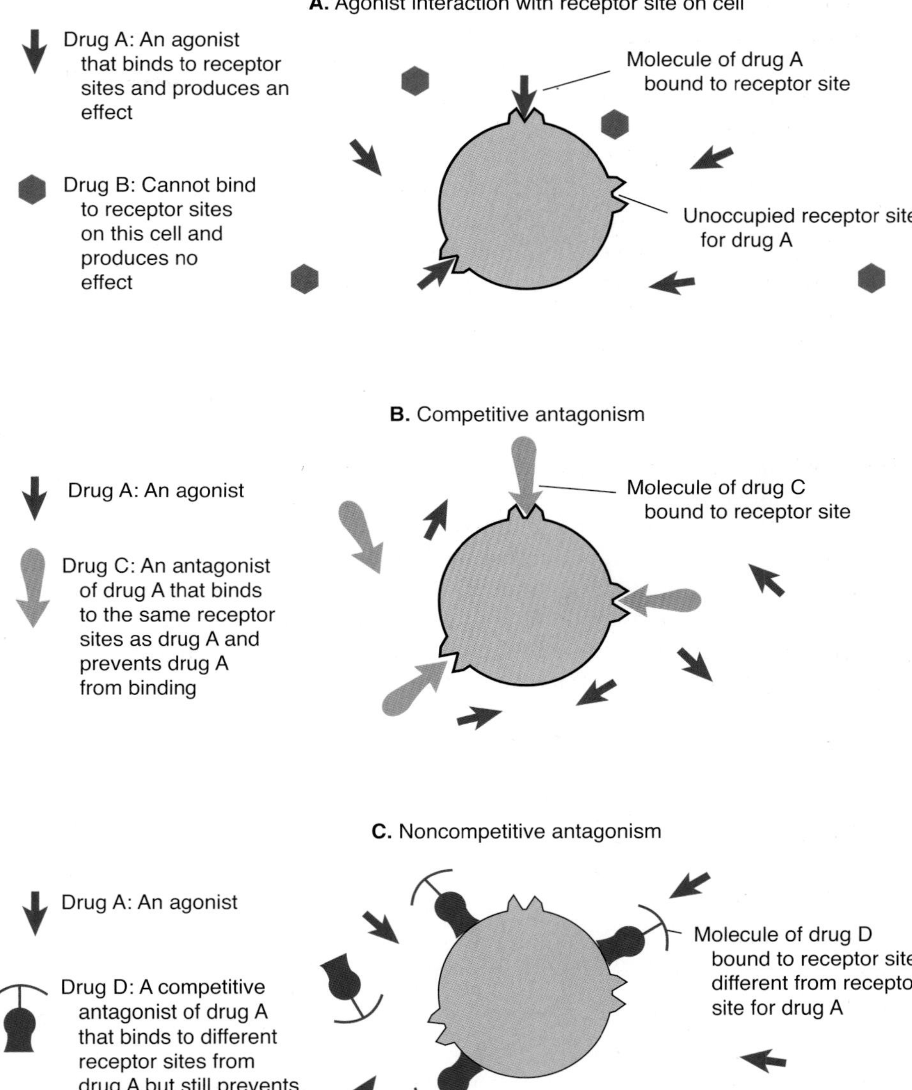

FIGURE 2.1 Receptor theory of drug action. (A) Agonist interaction with receptor site on cell: molecules of drug A react with specific receptor sites on cells of effector organs and change the cells' activity. (B) Competitive antagonism: drug A and drug C have an affinity for the same receptor sites and compete for these sites; drug C has a greater affinity, occupies more of the sites, and antagonizes drug A. (C) Noncompetitive antagonism: drug D reacts with a receptor site that is different from the receptor site for drug A but still prevents drug A from binding with its receptor sites. Drugs that act by inhibiting enzymes can be pictured as acting similarly to the receptor site antagonists illustrated in B and C. Enzyme inhibitors block the binding of molecules of normal substrate to active sites on the enzyme.

sodium channels and prevent the entry of sodium into nerve cells and thus propagation of nerve impulses.

Drug-Enzyme Interactions

Drugs can also cause their effects by interfering with the enzymes that break down the natural chemicals that stimulate the receptor. For example, monoamine oxidase (MAO) inhibitors block the breakdown of noradrenaline by the enzyme MAO. Normally, MAO breaks down noradrenaline, removes it from the receptor site and recycles the components to form new noradrenaline. The blocking action of MAO inhibitors allows noradrenaline to remain bound to the receptor site, stimulating the cell longer and leading to prolonged noradrenaline effects. Those effects can be therapeutic (e.g. relieving depression) or adverse (e.g. increasing heart rate and blood pressure).

Enzymes are also important catalysts for various chemical reactions. Enzyme systems work in a cascade effect, with one enzyme activating another and eventually causing a cellular reaction. If a single step in one of the many enzyme systems is blocked, normal cell function may be disrupted.

Carrier (Transporter) Molecules

Many ions and small polar (i.e. possesses a charge) molecules, for example calcium and glucose, must be transported across the plasma membrane using **carrier molecules** or transporters because they are not sufficiently lipid-soluble. These carrier proteins possess a recognition site to ensure that they only transport specific molecules. Carriers are also responsible for the uptake of the starting materials required to make neurotransmitters or for the reuptake of neurotransmitters themselves. The selective serotonin reuptake inhibitors block the reuptake of serotonin from the synaptic cleft leading to prolonged stimulation of certain brain cells, which is thought to provide relief from depression.

Selective Toxicity

The ability of a drug to attack only targets found in foreign cells is known as selective toxicity. Penicillin, an antibacterial used to treat bacterial infections, has **selective toxicity**. It affects an enzyme system responsible for making cell walls that are unique to bacteria, causing bacterial cell death without disrupting normal human cell functioning.

Ideally, all chemotherapeutic agents would act only on pathogenic or neoplastic cells and would not affect healthy cells. Unfortunately, some chemotherapeutic agents also destroy normal human cells, causing many of the adverse effects associated with chemotherapy. For example, some antibacterial agents can affect the functioning of human cells; e.g. the aminoglycosides can cause irreversible vestibular damage, hearing loss and tinnitus through their toxic effects on cranial nerve VIII. Some antineoplastic agents used to treat cancer also target cells that reproduce, or are replaced, rapidly; for example bone marrow cells, gastrointestinal cells, hair follicles. Consequently, the goal of many chemotherapeutic regimens is to deliver a dose that will be toxic to the invading cells yet cause the least amount of toxicity to the patient.

Pharmacokinetics

Pharmacokinetics involves the study of absorption, distribution, metabolism and excretion of drugs. In clinical practice, pharmacokinetic considerations include the onset of drug action, drug half-life, timing of the peak effect, duration of drug effects, metabolism and excretion of the drug. Figure 2.2 outlines these processes, which are described in the following sections.

Effective Concentration

After a drug is administered, drug molecules must first be absorbed into the body before distribution to the target site. If a drug is going to work effectively at these active sites, and thereby have a therapeutic effect, it must attain a sufficiently high concentration in the body. The amount of a drug needed to cause a therapeutic effect is known as the **effective concentration**. The recommended dose of a drug is based on the amount that must be given to eventually reach the effective concentration: too much of a drug

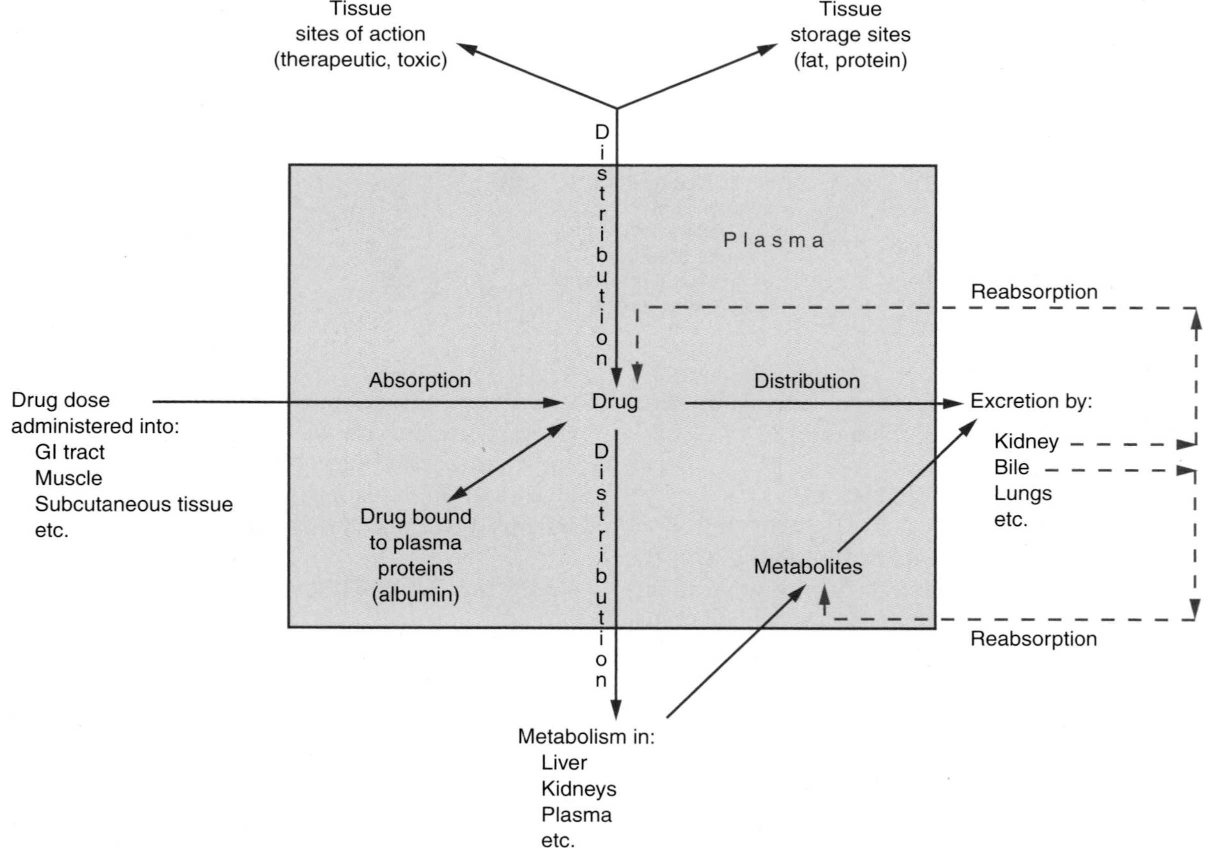

FIGURE 2.2 The processes by which a drug is handled by the body. *Dashed lines* indicate that some portion of a drug and its metabolites may be reabsorbed from the excretory organs. The dynamic equilibrium of pharmacokinetics is shown.

will produce toxic effects and too little will not produce the desired therapeutic effects.

Loading Dose

If a drug takes a long time to reach the effective concentration in the plasma, and its effects are needed quickly, a **loading dose** may be recommended. This is a higher dose than that usually used for treatment. For example, when preparing a patient for emergency angioplasty, the antiplatelet drug clopidogrel can be administered as a loading dose (300 mg) to reach the effective concentration. The effective concentration is then maintained using the recommended dosing schedule (75 mg daily).

Dynamic Equilibrium

The actual concentration that a drug reaches in the body results from a dynamic equilibrium involving several factors:

- Absorption from the site of entry
- Distribution to the target site
- Metabolism in the liver and other tissues
- Excretion from the body.

These factors are key elements in determining the amount of drug needed (dose) and the frequency of dose repetition (regimen) required to achieve the critical concentration for the desired length of time. When administering a drug, the nurse needs to consider the phases of pharmacokinetics so that the drug regimen can be made as effective as possible.

Absorption

To reach the target site, a drug must first make its way into the circulating fluids of the body. **Absorption** refers to what happens to a drug from the time it is introduced to the body until it reaches the circulating fluids and tissues. Drugs can be absorbed from many different regions in the body: through the gastrointestinal (GI) tract – taken either orally or rectally; through mucous membranes, the skin and lung, or through muscle or subcutaneous tissues (see Figure 2.2).

Drugs can be absorbed into cells through various processes, including passive diffusion, active transport and filtration. **Passive diffusion** is the major process through which drugs are absorbed into the body. Passive diffusion occurs down a concentration gradient. When there is a greater concentration of drug on one side of a plasma membrane, the drug will move through the membrane to the area of lower concentration on the other side. This process does not require any cellular energy. It occurs more quickly if the drug molecule is small, soluble in lipids (plasma membranes are made of lipids and proteins – see Chapter 6), and has no electrical charge that could repel it from the plasma membrane.

Unlike passive diffusion, **active transport** is a process that uses energy to actively move a molecule across a plasma membrane. The molecule may be large, or it may be moving against a concentration gradient. Filtration is less important in the absorption of drugs, but is often involved in drug excretion in the kidney.

Administration

The main routes of administration are:

1. Oral
2. Injection (intravenous, intramuscular, subcutaneous, intrathecal); also referred to as the parenteral route
3. Inhalation
4. Rectal
5. Topical
6. Sublingual

The oral route is the most frequently used drug administration route in clinical practice. Figure 2.3 outlines the pharmacokinetic processes that are undergone by a drug administered orally. Oral administration is not invasive and, together with topical application, is one of the safest ways to deliver drugs.

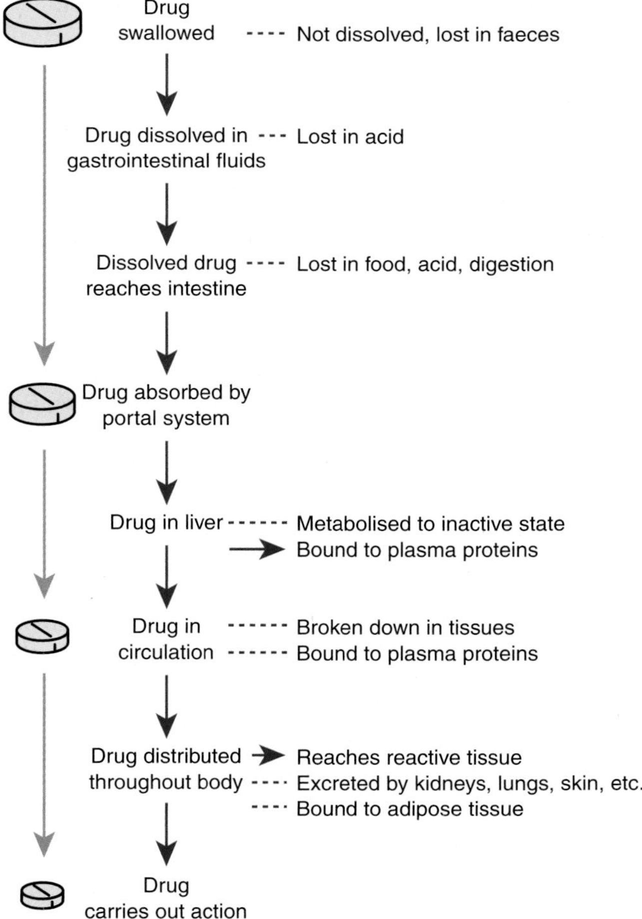

FIGURE 2.3 Pharmacokinetics affect the amount of a drug that reaches reactive tissues. Very little of an oral dose of a drug actually reaches reactive sites.

Patients can relatively easily continue their drug regimen at home when they are taking oral medications (although this can become more challenging if a patient is prescribed a large number of medications). However, oral administration subjects the drug to a number of processes aimed at breaking down ingested foreign chemicals. The acidic environment of the stomach breaks down many compounds and inactivates others. This fact is taken into account by pharmaceutical companies when preparing drug capsules or tablets. The binders used are often designed to break down at a certain acidity value and release the active drug to be absorbed, for example drugs which are enteric-coated (e.g. aspirin) break down in the less acidic environment of the small intestine rather than the stomach.

When food is present, the environment of the stomach is more acidic and the stomach empties more slowly, thus exposing the drug to the acidic environment for a longer period. Certain foods that increase stomach acidity, such as milk products, alcohol, and protein, also speed the breakdown of many drugs. Other foods may chemically bind drugs or block their absorption. To decrease the effects of this acid barrier and the direct effects of certain foods, oral drugs should ideally be given either 1 hour before or 2 hours after a meal.

Some drugs that cannot survive in sufficient quantity when given orally need to be injected directly into the body. Drugs that are injected IV avoid initial breakdown and reach their effective concentration at the time of injection. However, these drugs are more likely to cause toxic effects because the margin for error in dosage is much smaller. Drugs injected IM are absorbed directly into the capillaries in the muscle and sent into circulation. This takes time because the drug must be collected by the capillary and delivered to the veins. Because men have more vascular muscles than women, intramuscular drugs reach a peak level faster in men than in women. Subcutaneous injections deposit the drug beneath the dermis and into the subcutaneous tissues, where it is slowly absorbed into the circulation. Timing of absorption varies with subcutaneous injection, depending on the fat content of the injection site and the state of local circulation. Common injection sites include the patient's upper arm, thigh or abdomen.

Drugs administered by inhalation can have an effect locally on the lungs, for example salbutamol which is used to dilate the airways during an asthma attack, or centrally, for example general anaesthetics used during surgery. Similarly, drugs administered via the rectum can have an effect locally, for example anti-inflammatory drugs used to treat irritable bowel syndrome, or on the rest of the body. Other drugs are applied directly to a surface such as the skin, nasal cavity and eye. A number of drugs are now applied using transdermal patches whereby a stick-on patch containing the active drug is applied directly to the skin, for example nicotine in nicotine-replacement therapy. The drugs in these patches need to be lipid soluble to pass through the skin.

Absorption from the oral cavity is achieved using the sublingual or buccal route. Here the drug is maintained under the tongue (sublingual) or in the pouch between the cheek and the teeth (buccal). The drug is allowed to dissolve and be absorbed across the epithelial cells lining the mouth. This route enables the drug to enter the bloodstream at a faster rate than by the oral route and also prevents the drug from becoming broken down either in the stomach or by the liver.

Table 2.1 outlines the various factors that affect drug absorption via these different administration routes.

First-Pass Effect

Drugs that are taken orally are usually absorbed from the small intestine directly into the portal venous system (the blood vessels that flow through the liver on their way back to the heart). Aspirin and alcohol are two drugs known to be absorbed from the lower end of the stomach. The portal veins deliver these absorbed molecules into the liver, which immediately metabolizes most of the chemicals delivered to it by a series of liver enzymes. These enzymes break the drug into metabolites, some of which are active and cause effects in the body and some of which are deactivated and can be readily excreted from the body. As a result, a large

Table 2.1 Factors That Affect Absorption of Drugs

Route	Factors Affecting Absorption
Intravenous	None: direct entry into the venous system
Intramuscular	Perfusion or blood flow to the muscle
	Fat content of the muscle
	Temperature of the muscle: cold causes vasoconstriction and decreases absorption; heat causes vasodilation and increases absorption
Subcut (subcutaneous)	Perfusion or blood flow to the tissue
	Fat content of the tissue
	Temperature of the tissue: cold causes vasoconstriction and decreases absorption; heat causes vasodilation and increases absorption
PO (oral)	Acidity of stomach
	Length of time in stomach
	Blood flow to gastrointestinal tract
	Presence of interacting foods or drugs
PR (rectal)	Perfusion or blood flow to the rectum
	Lesions in the rectum
	Length of time retained for absorption
Mucous membranes (sublingual, buccal)	Perfusion or blood flow to the area
	Integrity of the mucous membranes
	Presence of food or smoking
	Length of time retained in area
Topical (skin)	Perfusion or blood flow to the area
	Integrity of skin
Inhalation	Perfusion or blood flow to the area
	Integrity of lung lining
	Ability to administer drug properly

FOCUS ON **PATIENT SAFETY**

The liver is very important in metabolizing drugs, and the kidneys are responsible for a large part of the excretion of drugs. In certain circumstances, for example when the therapeutic dose of a drug is close to its toxic dose, it is essential to check a patient's liver and renal functions before a patient starts the drug. If the liver is not functioning properly, the drug may not be metabolized correctly and may reach toxic levels in the body. If the kidneys are not functioning properly, the drug may not be excreted properly and could accumulate in the body. Dosage adjustment must, therefore, be considered if a patient has reduced function of either the liver or the kidneys. Older patients may be particularly susceptible as metabolism and organ function decreases in older age.

percentage of the oral dose is destroyed at this point and never reaches the tissues. This phenomenon is known as the **first-pass effect**. The recommended dose for oral drugs can be considerably higher than the recommended dose for parenteral drugs (i.e. routes avoiding the GI tract), because this higher dose takes the first-pass effect into account. Drugs with a high first-pass rate must be given via another route, for example glyceryl trinitrate which causes relaxation of vascular smooth muscle is administered sublingually or via a patch or spray.

Injected drugs and drugs absorbed from sites other than the GI tract undergo a similar metabolism if they pass through the liver first. However, as some of the active drug has already had a chance to reach the target site before reaching the liver, the injected drug is more effective at a lower dose than the oral equivalent.

Distribution

The portion of the drug that gets through the first-pass effect is delivered to the circulatory system for transport throughout the body. **Distribution** involves the movement of a drug to the body's tissues (see Figure 2.2). As with absorption, factors that can affect distribution include the drug's lipid solubility and ionization (i.e. whether the drug molecule is either positively or negatively charged) and the perfusion of the active site. For example, tissue perfusion is a factor in treating a diabetic patient who has a lower leg bacterial infection and requires an antibacterial drug. In this case, systemic drugs may not be effective because part of the disease process involves changes in the vasculature and decreased blood flow to some areas, particularly the lower limbs. If there is inadequate blood flow to the area, less of the drug can be delivered to the tissues and a reduced antibacterial effect is seen.

In the same way, patients in a cold environment or in shock may have constricted blood vessels (vasoconstriction) in the extremities, which would prevent blood flow to those areas. The circulating blood would be unable to deliver drugs to those areas, and the patient would receive reduced therapeutic effect from drugs intended to act upon those tissues.

Protein Binding

Most circulating drugs are bound to some extent to proteins in the blood (e.g. albumin). This helps to prevent immediate excretion by the kidneys. The protein–drug complex is relatively large and renders the drug inactive because it cannot enter tissues to act. The drug must first be freed from the protein's binding site to become the active form. Some drugs are tightly bound and released very slowly. These drugs have a very long duration of action because they are not freed to be broken down or excreted and are, therefore, released very slowly at the active site. Loosely bound drugs tend to act quickly and are also excreted quickly. Other drugs compete with each other for protein-binding sites, altering effectiveness or causing toxicity when the two drugs are given together, for example aspirin and warfarin.

Blood–Brain Barrier

The blood–brain barrier is a protective layer of endothelial cells, joined by tight junctions, which keep many foreign substances away from the central nervous system (CNS). Drugs that are highly lipid-soluble (e.g. diazepam, alcohol) are more likely to cross the blood–brain barrier and reach the CNS, whereas lipid-insoluble drugs (e.g. anticancer drugs, some antibacterials) are not able to cross the blood–brain barrier. This is clinically significant in treating a brain infection such as bacterial meningitis with antibacterials. Almost all antibacterials are lipid insoluble and, therefore, cannot cross the blood–brain barrier. Chloramphenicol is one antibacterial that can cross the barrier, which although it can be toxic to bone marrow, is still in use. However, the inflammation associated with an infection of this kind can disrupt the blood–brain barrier making it more leaky, allowing other antibacterials to cross.

Placenta and Breast Milk

The physiological changes occurring during pregnancy can affect the way drugs are distributed. For example, the concentration of albumin in the plasma is reduced due to the increase in circulating blood volume in pregnancy, which will increase the amount of free and active drug present in the blood. Many drugs readily pass across the placenta, especially lipid-soluble drugs, and affect the developing foetus. As stated earlier, in some situations it is best not to administer any drugs to pregnant women because of the possible risk to the foetus. Drugs should only be given when the benefit clearly outweighs any risk. Many other drugs are secreted into breast milk and, therefore, have the potential to affect the neonate. The ability of a drug to pass into breast milk must always be considered when giving a drug to a breast-feeding mother.

Metabolism

The body is well prepared to detoxify a wide selection of foreign chemicals. The process by which drugs are converted into less chemically active substances that can be more easily excreted from the body is known as drug **metabolism**. The liver is the most important organ responsible for drug metabolism, but the kidney, gut mucosa, lung, plasma and skin also play a role (see Figure 2.2).

Liver Enzyme Systems

The liver detoxifies many chemicals and uses others to produce enzymes and structures required by the body. Since orally administered drugs enter the liver first, the enzyme systems present in the liver immediately work on the absorbed drug to metabolize it. The smooth endoplasmic reticulum of the liver hepatocytes is packed with drug-metabolizing enzymes, including the large family of enzymes known as the cytochrome P450 (CYP450) enzymes.

There are two phases of drug metabolism: phase I and phase II reactions. Phase I metabolism involves oxidation, reduction or hydrolysis of the drug either via one of the CYP450 enzymes or another enzyme. Phase II metabolism usually involves a conjugation reaction whereby the drug molecule is attached to another large molecule (e.g. an amino acid), making the drug more polar (charged) and, therefore, more water-soluble and more readily excreted by the kidneys.

A number of drugs and some foods are known to increase the activity of specific enzyme systems. This process is referred to as *enzyme induction*. Only a few basic enzyme systems are responsible for metabolizing most of the chemicals that pass through the liver. When the activity of a particular enzyme system is increased, the metabolism of any drugs that are metabolized via that same enzyme system will be increased. This prevents the drugs from reaching their therapeutic levels and explains why some drugs and foods cannot be taken together effectively, for example St. John's wort (for depression) and some antiviral agents used for treating AIDS and antineoplastic agents.

Other drugs and some foods are known to inhibit an enzyme system, making it less effective. This is known as *enzyme inhibition*. As a consequence, any drug that is metabolized by that system will not be broken down for excretion, and the blood levels of that drug will increase, often to toxic levels. For example when the calcium channel blocker felodipine is taken with grapefruit juice, the liver enzymes responsible for metabolizing felodipine are inhibited by the grapefruit juice and blood levels of felodipine can rise to dangerous levels. These observations also explain why liver disease is often a contraindication or a reason to use caution when administering certain drugs. If the liver is not functioning effectively, the drug will not be metabolized as it should be and toxic levels could develop quickly. Table 2.2 gives some examples of drugs that induce or inhibit liver enzyme systems.

Table 2.2 Examples of Drugs That Alter the Effects of Drug Metabolizing Enzymes

Drugs That Induce or Increase Activity	Drugs That Inhibit or Decrease Activity
Carbamazepine	Chloramphenicol
Ethanol (chronic use)	Corticosteroids
Phenobarbital	Erythromycin
Phenytoin	Ketoconazole
Rifampicin	Quinidine

Excretion

Excretion is the removal of a drug from the body. The kidneys play the most important role in drug excretion (see Figure 2.2); however, the skin, saliva, lungs, bile and faeces are also excretion routes. Drugs that have been made water-soluble in the liver are often readily excreted from the kidney by *glomerular filtration*, the passage of water and water-soluble components from the plasma into the renal tubule.

Other drugs are secreted or reabsorbed through the renal tubule by active transport systems. The acidity of the urine can play an important part in drug excretion. The active transport systems that move a drug into the tubule often do so by exchanging it for acid or bicarbonate molecules. This is an important concept to remember when trying to clear a drug rapidly from the system, for example during a drug overdose: by altering the pH of the filtrate in the kidneys, some drugs can be made more water-soluble and are therefore more readily excreted in the urine. Kidney dysfunction can also lead to toxic levels of a drug in the body because the drug cannot be excreted. In contrast, blood flow to the kidneys is enhanced during pregnancy, increasing the rate of drug excretion.

Half-Life

The **half-life** of a drug is the time it takes for the amount of drug in the body to decrease to one-half of the peak level it previously achieved. For instance, if a patient takes 20 mg of a drug with a half-life of 2 hours, 10 mg of the drug will remain 2 hours after administration. Two hours later, 5 mg will be left (half of the previous level); in 2 more hours, only 2.5 mg will remain. This information is important in determining the appropriate timing for a drug dose or determining the duration of a drug's effect on the body, for example in determining dosage intervals, to achieve the most effective drug therapy. Nurses can use their knowledge of drug half-life to explain the importance of following a schedule of drug administration in the hospital or at home. Figure 2.4 shows the effects of drug administration on the effective concentration of a drug. Changes due to ageing can affect the normal half-life of a drug, for example the half-life of diazepam in young adults is 15 to 20 hours and in the older person can be as long as 50 to 150 hours.

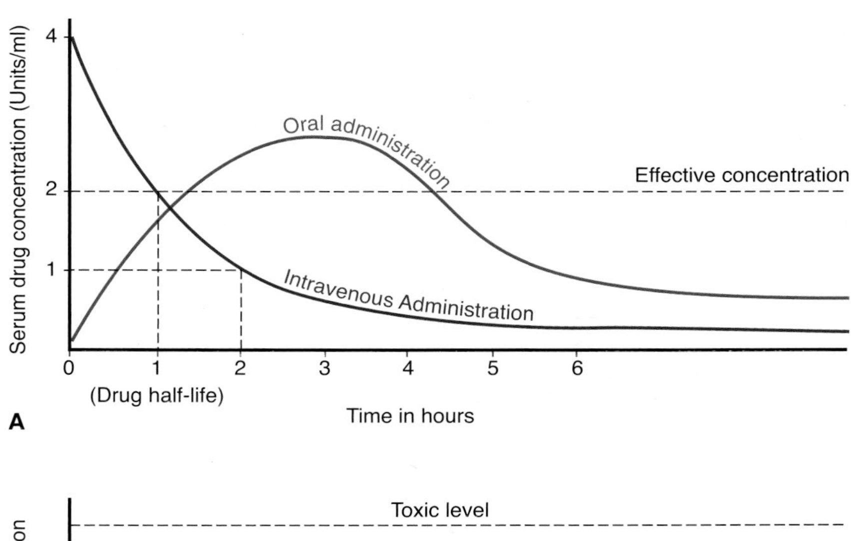

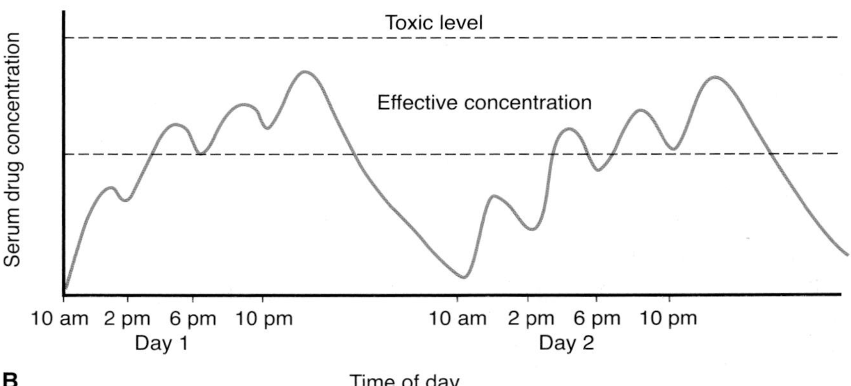

FIGURE 2.4 Influence of half-life, route of administration, and dosage regimen on serum drug levels. (A) Influence of route of administration on time course of drug levels after administration of a single dose of a drug. The *dashed lines* indicate how the half-life of the drug may be determined from the curve of drug concentration after an intravenous dose. At time 0, immediately after the injection, there were four units of the drug in each millilitre of serum. The drug concentration fell to half this amount, 2 units/ml, after 1 hour, the drug's half-life. (B) Influence of dosage regimen on serum drug levels (drug given four times daily, at 10 am and at 2, 6, and 10 pm). The drug accumulates as successive doses are given throughout each day; the drug is given at a rate greater than the patient's body can eliminate it. This dosage regimen has been chosen so that the patient will have a therapeutic level of the drug for a significant portion of the day, yet never reach toxic levels of the drug.

The absorption rate, the distribution to the tissues, the speed of metabolism, and how fast a drug is excreted, can all affect the half-life of the drug (Table 2.3). The half-life that is indicated in any drug monograph is the half-life of the drug in a healthy person. Using this information, the half-life of a drug for a patient with kidney or liver dysfunction (which could prolong the metabolism and the time required for excretion of a drug) can be estimated and changes made in the dosage schedule by the prescriber.

Table 2.3 Factors Affecting the Half-life of Drugs (adapted from Golan *et al.*, 2008)

Factor	Effect on Half-life	Explanation
Obesity	Increased	The increased number of adipocytes in obese individuals permits a greater proportion of a lipid-soluble drug to distribute into the adipose tissue. Transfer of drug from the blood to adipose tissue reduces the amount of drug that can be delivered to the liver or kidneys for metabolism and excretion.
Ageing	Increased	Metabolism and organ function tends to decrease as individuals age. These factors will decrease the rate of drug metabolism and excretion and consequently drugs remain in the blood for a longer period of time.
Increased metabolism, e.g. induction of liver enzymes	Decreased	An increase in the rate of drug metabolism will remove the drug more quickly from the body. As a result the length of time the drug remains in the blood is increased.
Decreased metabolism, e.g. inhibition of liver enzymes	Increased	A decrease in the rate of drug metabolism will reduce the rate at which the drug is removed from the body. Consequently, the length of time the drug remains in the blood is extended.
Hepatic failure	Increased	The ability of the liver to metabolize drugs will be reduced. Consequently, the rate at which the drug is removed from the body will decrease therefore increasing the time the drug remains in the blood.
Renal failure	Increased	The ability of the kidneys to excrete and remove the drug from the body will be reduced leading to an increased length of time the drug remains in the blood.

Factors Influencing Drug Effects

When administering a drug to a patient, the nurse must be aware that individuals have a tremendous influence on what actually happens to a drug when it enters the body. No two people react in exactly the same way to any given drug. Even though textbooks and drug guides explain the pharmacodynamics and pharmacokinetics of a drug, it must be remembered that such information is usually based on studies of healthy, adult males. The clinical setting may be very different and, consequently, the nurse must consider a number of factors before administering any drug. These are discussed in detail in the following sections and summarized in Box 2.1.

Weight

The recommended dosage of a drug is based on drug evaluation studies and is targeted at the average 70-kg person. People who are much heavier than that may require larger doses to achieve a therapeutic effect from a drug because they have increased tissues to perfuse and increased receptor sites in some reactive tissues. People who are much lighter may require smaller doses of a drug to avoid potential toxic effects occurring at the recommended dosage.

Age

Age is a factor primarily in children and older adults. Children metabolize many drugs differently from adults, and they have immature systems for handling drugs. Many drugs come with recommended paediatric dosages, and others can be converted into paediatric dosages (see Chapter 5).

BOX 2.1 Factors Affecting the Body's Response to a Drug

- Weight
- Age
- Gender
- Physiological factors: diurnal rhythm, electrolyte balance, acid–base balance, hydration, diet
- Pathological factors: disease, hepatic dysfunction, renal dysfunction, gastrointestinal dysfunction, vascular disorders, low blood pressure
- Genetic factors
- Immunological factors: allergy
- Psychological factors: placebo effect, health beliefs, concordance
- Environmental factors: temperature, light, noise
- Drug tolerance
- Cumulative effects

Older adults undergo many physical changes that are part of the ageing process. Their bodies may respond very differently in all aspects of pharmacokinetics: less effective absorption, less efficient distribution because of fewer plasma proteins and less efficient perfusion, altered metabolism of drugs in the tissues due to the change in muscle-to-fat ratio or metabolism of drugs because of liver changes with age and less effective excretion owing to less efficient kidneys. Many drugs now come with recommended dosages for older persons. Other drugs may also need decreased dosages in the elderly and serum levels of drugs with low therapeutic index should be monitored regularly.

When administering drugs to a patient at either end of the age spectrum, the nurse should monitor closely for undesired effects. If the effects are not what would normally be expected, a dosage adjustment should be considered.

Gender

Physiological differences between men and women can influence a drug's effect. Women have more adipocytes (fat cells) than men, so drugs that deposit in fat may be slowly released and cause effects for a prolonged period. For example, gaseous general anaesthetics have an affinity for depositing in fat and can cause drowsiness and sedation sometimes weeks after surgery. Women who are given any drug should always be questioned about the possibility of pregnancy because, as stated previously, the use of drugs in pregnant women is not recommended unless the benefit clearly outweighs the potential risk to the foetus.

Physiological Factors

Physiological differences such as diurnal rhythm of the nervous and endocrine systems, acid–base balance, hydration, diet and electrolyte balance can affect the way a drug works on the body and the way the body handles the drug. If a drug does not produce the desired effect, review the patient's acid–base and electrolyte profiles, the timing of the drug administration and other aspects such as diet and lifestyle, for example a high-fat diet will affect the absorption of some drugs, and certain foods and fruit juices and alcohol interact with medications.

Pathological Factors

Drugs are usually used to treat disease or pathology. However, the disease that the drug is intended to treat can change the functioning of the chemical reactions within the body and thus change the response to the drug. Other pathological conditions can change the basic pharmacokinetics of a drug. For example, GI disorders can affect the absorption of many oral drugs. Vascular diseases and low blood pressure alter the distribution of a drug, preventing it from being delivered to the active site and rendering it nontherapeutic. Liver or kidney diseases affect the way that a drug is metabolized and excreted and can lead to toxic reactions when the usual dose is given. An underactive thyroid gland can also affect the metabolism of a drug allowing it to build up to potentially toxic levels in the body.

Genetic Factors

Genetic differences can sometimes explain patients' varied responses to a given drug. Some people lack certain enzyme systems necessary for metabolizing certain drugs, whereas others have overactive enzyme systems and break down drugs very quickly. Still others have differing metabolisms or slightly different enzymatic make-up that alters their chemical reactions and the effects of a given drug. Some predictable differences in the pharmacokinetics and pharmacodynamic effects of drugs can be anticipated with people of particular ethnic backgrounds because of their genetic make-up. **Pharmacogenomics** is a new area of study that explores the unique differences in response to drugs that each individual possesses, based on genetic make-up. The mapping of the human genome has accelerated research in this area. It is thought that in the future, medical care and drug regimens could be personally designed based on the person's own unique genetic make-up. Trastuzumab (see Chapter 13) was developed to treat breast cancer when the tumour expresses human epidermal growth factor receptor 2, a genetic defect seen in some tumours. The drug has no effect on tumours that do not express this growth factor. This drug was developed as a personalized or targeted medicine, based on genetic factors. Such differences are highlighted throughout this book.

Immunological Factors

People can develop an allergy to a drug. After exposure to its components, a person can develop antibodies to a drug; with future exposure to the same drug, that person may experience a full-blown allergic reaction. Sensitivity to a drug can range from dermatological effects to anaphylaxis, shock and death. Drug allergies are discussed in detail in Chapter 3.

Psychological Factors

The patient's attitude about a drug has been shown to have a real effect on how that drug works. A drug is more likely to be effective if the patient thinks it will work than if the patient believes it will not work. This is called the **placebo effect**.

The patient's personality also influences **concordance** with the drug regimen. Some people who believe that they can influence their health actively seek health care and willingly follow a prescribed regimen. These people usually trust the medical system and believe that their efforts will be positive. Other people do not trust the medical system; they may believe that they have no control over their own health and may be unwilling to comply with any prescribed therapy. Knowing a patient's health-seeking history and feelings about health care is important in planning an educational programme that will work for that particular patient. It is also important to know this information when arranging for necessary follow-up procedures and evaluations and to involve the patient in decision-making. The nurse must respect the patient's wishes regarding medication and if the patient refuses administration the nurse should accept that the patient has made an informed decision and continue to provide advice and support.

Environmental Factors

The environment can affect the success of drug therapy. For example, antihypertensives that are working well during cold, winter months may become too effective in warmer environments, when natural vasodilation to release heat tends to lower the blood pressure. If a patient's response to a medication is not as expected, the nurse might look for changes in environmental conditions.

Tolerance

Some drugs become tolerated by the body over time. Tolerance may come about because of increased metabolism of the drug, increased resistance to its effects, or other pharmacokinetic factors. Drugs that are tolerated no longer produce the same effect, and they need to be taken in increasingly larger doses to achieve a therapeutic effect. An example of this type of drug is morphine, an opiate used for pain relief. The longer morphine is taken, the more tolerant the body becomes to the drug, so that increasingly larger doses are needed to relieve pain. Clinically, this situation can be avoided by giving the drug in smaller doses or in combination with other drugs that may also relieve pain. Note that decreasing the dose of morphine is not appropriate for patients with terminal illness. Resistance to drugs within the same class may also occur in some situations.

Accumulation

If a drug is taken in successive doses at intervals that are shorter than recommended, or if the body is not able to eliminate a drug properly, the drug can accumulate in the body, leading to toxic levels and adverse effects. This can be avoided by monitoring blood levels and observing patients carefully for potential side-effects. In reality, with many people managing their own therapy at home, strict concordance with a drug regimen may not occur. Some people take all of their medications first thing in the morning, so that they don't forget to take the pills later in the day. Others realize that they have forgotten a dose and then take two to compensate. Many interruptions of everyday life can interfere with strict adherence to a drug regimen. If a drug is causing adverse effects, take appropriate action, for example reduction in dose or withdrawal of the drug.

Drug–Drug Interactions

When two or more drugs are taken together, there is a possibility that the drugs will interact with each other to cause unanticipated effects in the body. Alternative therapies, such as herbal products, act as drugs in the body and can cause these same interactions. Usually this is an increase or decrease in the desired therapeutic effect of one or all of the drugs or an increase in adverse effects.

Clinically significant drug–drug interactions occur with drugs that have small margins of safety, that is a narrow **therapeutic index**. The therapeutic index is the difference between the therapeutic dose of a drug and its toxic dose. If there is very little difference between a therapeutic dose and a toxic dose of the drug, interference with the drugs pharmacokinetics or pharmacodynamics can produce serious problems.

Drug–drug interactions can occur in the following situations for example:

- *At the site of absorption*: One drug prevents or accelerates absorption of the other drug. For example, the antibacterial tetracycline is not absorbed from the GI tract if calcium or calcium products (milk) are present in the stomach and taking tetracycline with calcium prevents the absorption of the calcium. Tetracycline should, therefore, be avoided by pregnant women (negative effects on foetal bone and teeth development) and also young children (negative effects on secondary teeth development).
- *During distribution*: One drug competes for the protein-binding site of another drug, so the second drug cannot be transported to the reactive tissue. For example, aspirin competes with the oral anticoagulant warfarin for protein-binding sites. Because aspirin is more competitive for the sites, the warfarin is dislodged, resulting in increased release of warfarin and increased toxicity to the tissues.
- *During metabolism*: One drug stimulates or blocks the metabolism of the other drug. For example, warfarin is metabolized more quickly if it is taken at the same time as barbiturates, rifampicin or many other drugs. As the warfarin is metabolized to an inactive state more quickly, higher doses will be needed to achieve the desired effect.
- *During excretion*: One drug competes for excretion with the other drug, leading to accumulation and toxic effects of one of the drugs. For example, digoxin and quinidine are both excreted from the same sites in the kidney. If they are given together, the quinidine is more competitive for these sites and is excreted, resulting in increased serum levels of digoxin, which cannot be excreted.
- *At the site of action*: One drug may be an antagonist of the other drug or may cause effects that oppose those of the other drug, leading to no therapeutic effect. This is seen, for example, when an antihypertensive drug is taken with an allergy drug that also increases blood pressure. The effects on blood pressure are negated, and there is a loss of the antihypertensive effectiveness of the drug.

Whenever two or more drugs are being given together, the nurse should first consult the latest copy of the British National Formulary and the information provided with the drug for a listing of clinically significant drug–drug interactions. Sometimes problems can be avoided by staggering the administration of the drugs or adjusting their dosages. Observed drug–drug and drug–food interactions should be reported.

Drug–Food or Drug–Alternative Therapy Interactions

Certain foods can interact with drugs in much the same way that drugs can interact with each other. This interaction can occur when the drug and the food are in direct contact in the stomach. Some foods increase acid production, speeding the breakdown of the drug molecule and preventing absorption and distribution of the drug. Some foods chemically react with certain drugs and prevent their absorption into the body. The antibacterial tetracycline cannot be taken with iron products for this reason. Tetracycline also binds with calcium to some extent and should not be taken with foods or other drugs containing calcium. Oral drugs can usually be taken with or without food. If the patient cannot tolerate the drug on an empty stomach, the food selected to be taken with the drug should be something that is known not to interact with it.

Certain foods and beverages can also affect the metabolism of drugs by the liver either by inducing or inhibiting hepatic enzymes (Harris *et al.*, 2003). Some vegetables, including cabbages and Brussel sprouts, are known to induce hepatic enzymes and accelerate drug metabolism. Conversely, grapefruit juice inhibits the action of specific CYP450 enzymes, slowing the rate of metabolism of drugs metabolized by the same enzymes, for example the dihydropyridine calcium channel blockers, ciclosporin, saquinavir (Bailey *et al.*, 1998). The reduced drug metabolism can lead to potentially toxic plasma drug concentrations. There is also potential for harmful interaction when drug therapy is combined with alternative therapies such as medical herbs. The most well-known interaction occurs with St. John's wort (*Hypericum perforatum*), one of the most commonly used herbal antidepressants. St. John's wort induces several of the CYP450 enzymes known to metabolize drug groups including antivirals used to treat HIV, benzodiazepines and immunosuppressants (Zhou & Lai, 2008). By increasing the rate of drug metabolism, the duration of the therapeutic effect of the drug is shortened. Patients should be advised not to combine herbal remedies without consulting their prescriber first. Further useful sources of information are the drug monographs accompanying the treatment; these usually list important drug–food interactions and give guidelines to avoid problems and optimize the drug's therapeutic effects.

Achieving the Optimal Therapeutic Effect

Despite the information described above, most patients can follow a drug regimen to achieve optimal therapeutic effects without serious adverse effects. Avoiding problems is the best way to treat adverse or ineffective drug effects. The nurse should incorporate basic history and physical assessment factors into any care plan, so that obvious problems can be spotted and handled promptly. If a drug just does not do what it is expected to do, the nurse should further examine the factors that are known to influence drug effects (see Box 2.1). Frequently, the drug regimen can be modified to deal with that influence. Rarely is it necessary to completely stop a needed drug regimen because of adverse or intolerable effects. In many cases, the nurse is in the best position to assess problems early.

Points to Remember

- Pharmacodynamics is the study of the way drugs affect the body.
- Most drugs work by replacing natural chemicals, by stimulating normal cell activity or by depressing normal cell activity.
- Chemotherapeutic agents work by interfering with normal cell functioning, causing cell death. The most desirable chemotherapeutic agents are those with selective toxicity to foreign cells and foreign cell activities.
- Drugs frequently act at specific receptor sites on or in cells to stimulate or inhibit enzyme systems within the cell and to alter the activity of the cell.
- Pharmacokinetics, the study of the way the body deals with drugs, includes absorption, distribution, metabolism and excretion of drugs.
- The goal of established dosing schedules is to achieve an effective concentration of the drug in the body. This effective concentration is the amount of the drug necessary to achieve the drug's therapeutic effects.
- Arriving at an effective concentration involves a dynamic equilibrium among the processes of drug absorption, distribution, metabolism and excretion.
- Absorption involves moving a drug into the body for circulation. Oral drugs are absorbed from the small intestine, undergo many changes, and are affected by many factors in the process. Intravenous drugs and drugs administered through the skin and oral mucosa are passed directly into the circulation and do not need additional absorption.
- Drugs are distributed to various tissues throughout the body depending on their solubility and charge. Many drugs are bound to plasma proteins for transport to reactive tissues.
- Drugs are metabolized into less toxic chemicals by various enzyme systems in the body. The liver is the primary site of drug metabolism. The liver uses a series of enzymes to alter the drug and start its metabolism.
- The first-pass effect is the breakdown of oral drugs in the liver immediately after absorption. Drugs given by other routes often reach their target site before passing through the liver for metabolism.
- Drug excretion is removal of the drug from the body and occurs mainly through the kidneys.
- The half-life of a drug is the period it takes for an amount of drug in the body to decrease to one-half of the peak level it previously achieved. The half-life is affected by all aspects of pharmacokinetics. Knowing the half-life of a drug helps in predicting dosing schedules and duration of effects.
- The therapeutic index indicates the margin of safety of a drug.
- The actual effects of a drug are determined by the pharmacokinetics, the pharmacodynamics and many human factors that can change the drug's effectiveness.
- To provide the safest and most effective drug therapy, the nurse must consider all of the interacting aspects that influence drug concentration and effectiveness.

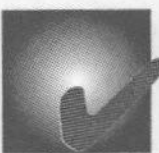

CHECK YOUR UNDERSTANDING

Answers to the questions in this chapter may be found in the answer key in the back of the book.

Multiple Choice

Select the best answer to the following.

1. Chemotherapeutic agents are drugs that
   a. are used only to treat cancers.
   b. replace normal body chemicals that are missing because of disease.
   c. interfere with the functioning of foreign cells, such as invading micro-organisms or neoplasms.
   d. stimulate a cell's normal functioning.

2. Receptor sites
   a. are a normal part of enzyme substrates.
   b. are proteins on plasma membranes or within the cell that specific chemicals bind to resulting in a physiological effect.
   c. can usually be stimulated by many different chemicals.
   d. are responsible for all drug effects in the body.

3. Selective toxicity is the ability of a drug to
   a. seek out a specific bacterial species or micro-organism.
   b. cause only specific adverse effects.
   c. cause foetal damage.
   d. attack only those systems found in foreign or abnormal cells.

4. The absorption of a drug taken orally can be affected by the
   a. blood flow to muscle beds.
   b. acidity of the gastric juices.
   c. weight and age of the patient.
   d. temperature of the peripheral environment.

5. Much of the metabolism that occurs when a drug is taken orally occurs as part of the
   a. protein-binding effect of the drug.
   b. functioning of the renal system.
   c. first-pass effect through the liver.
   d. distribution of the drug to the reactive tissues.

6. The half-life of a drug
   a. is determined by a balance of all of the factors working on that drug: absorption, distribution, metabolism and excretion.
   b. is a constant factor for all drugs taken by a patient.
   c. is influenced by the fat distribution of the patient.
   d. can be calculated with the use of a body surface nomogram.

7. Jack has Parkinson's disease that has been controlled for several years with levodopa. After he begins a health food regimen with lots of vitamin B_6 his tremors return, and he develops a rapid heart rate, hypertension and anxiety. The nurse investigating the problem discovers that vitamin B_6 can speed the conversion of levodopa to dopamine in the peripheral tissues, resulting in less drug reaching the brain and a return of his symptoms. The nurse would consider this problem a:
   a. drug–laboratory test interaction.
   b. drug–drug interaction.
   c. cumulative effect.
   d. sensitivity reaction.

Extended Matching Questions

Select all that apply.

1. When reviewing a drug to be given, the nurse notes that the drug is excreted in the urine. What points should be included in the nurse's assessment of the patient?
   a. The patient's liver function tests
   b. The patient's bladder tone
   c. The patient's renal function tests
   d. The patient's fluid intake
   e. Other drugs the patient might be taking that could affect the kidney
   f. The patient's dietary intake

2. When considering the pharmacokinetics of a drug, what points would the nurse take into consideration?
   a. How the drug will be absorbed
   b. The way the drug affects the body
   c. Receptor site activation and suppression
   d. How the drug will be excreted
   e. How the drug will be metabolized
   f. The half-life of the drug

3. Drug–drug interactions are important considerations in clinical practice. When evaluating a patient for potential drug–drug interactions, what should the nurse consider?
   a. Adverse drug effects on the body
   b. The need to adjust drug dosage or timing of administration to ensure effective drug therapy because of the actions of one drug on the other
   c. The need for more drugs in the drug regimen to balance the effects of the drugs being given
   d. A new therapeutic effect not encountered with either drug alone
   e. Increased adverse effects because of the action of both drugs in the body
   f. The use of herbal or alternative therapies, which could act to affect the pharmacokinetics or pharmacodynamics of the drugs being given

Fill in the Blanks

1. ______________________ describes how drugs affect the body.

2. ______________________ describes how the body acts on drugs.

3. Drugs that interfere with the functioning of foreign cells, such as invading micro-organisms or neoplasms, are called __________________.

4. The amount of a drug that is needed to cause a therapeutic effect is called the __________________.

5. The dynamic equilibrium that must be considered when administering a drug considers four main factors: ______, _______, ______ and _______.

6. Drugs taken orally are absorbed from the GI tract and delivered directly to the liver for metabolism. This phenomenon is called the _______________.

7. The presence of a chemical that is metabolized by a particular enzyme system often increases the activity of that enzyme system. This process is referred to as __________________.

8. The ______________________ of a drug is the time it takes for the amount of drug in the body to decrease to one-half of the peak level it previously achieved.

Bibliography and References

Bailey, D. G., Malcolm, J., Arnold, O., & Spence, J. D. (1998). Grapefruit juice–drug interactions. *British Journal of Clinical Pharmacology, 46*(2), 101–110.

Golan, D. E., Tashjian Jr, A. H., Armstrong, E. J., & Armstrong, A. W. (2008). *Principles of pharmacology: The pathophysiologic basis of drug therapy* (2nd ed.). Philadelphia: Lippincott Williams & Wilkins.

Harris, R. Z., Jang, G. R., & Tsunoda, S. (2003). Dietary effects on drug metabolism and transport. *Clinical Pharmacokinetics, 42*(13), 1071–1088.

Howland, R. D., & Mycek, M. J. (2005). *Pharmacology* (3rd ed.). Philadelphia: Lippincott Williams & Wilkins.

Laroche, M. L., Charmes, J. P., Nouaille, Y., Picard, N., & Merle, L. (2007). Is inappropriate medication use a major cause of adverse drug reactions in the elderly? *British Journal of Clinical Pharmacology, 63*(2), 177–186.

Rang, H. P., Dale, M. M., Ritter, J. M., & Flower, R. J. (2007). *Rang and Dale's pharmacology* (6th ed.). Philadelphia: Churchill Livingstone.

Scott, W. N., & McGrath, D. (2009). *Nursing pharmacology made incredibly easy*. Philadelphia: Lippincott Williams & Wilkins.

Simonsen, T., Aarbakke, J., Kay, I., Coleman, I., Sinnott, P. & Lysaa, R. (2006). *Illustrated pharmacology for nurses*. London: Hodder Arnold.

Zhou, S. F. & Lai, X. (2008). An update on clinical drug interactions with the herbal antidepressant St. John's wort. *Current Drug Metabolism, 9*(5), 394–409.

CHAPTER 3

Toxic Effects of Drugs

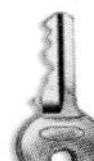

KEY TERMS

adverse drug reaction
anaphylaxis
drug allergy
poisoning
superinfections
therapeutic index

LEARNING OBJECTIVES

Upon completion of this chapter, you will be able to:

1. Define the term adverse drug reaction and explain the clinical significance of this reaction.
2. List four types of allergic responses to drug therapy.
3. Discuss five common examples of drug-induced tissue damage.
4. Define the term poison.
5. Outline the important factors that should be considered in the application of the nursing process to selected situations of drug poisoning.

All drugs are potentially dangerous. Even though chemicals are carefully screened and tested in animals and in people before they are released to the general public, drugs can cause unexpected or unacceptable reactions. Drugs are chemicals, and the human body operates by a vast series of chemical reactions. Consequently, many effects can be seen when just one chemical factor is altered.

Adverse Drug Reactions

Adverse drug reactions (ADR) are undesired effects that occur with the normal use of a particular drug. These effects may be particularly unpleasant or even dangerous. They are a significant cause of morbidity and mortality and account for approximately 5% of all acute hospital admissions in the UK (Pirmohamed *et al.*, 2004). A recent study in the UK noted that approximately one in seven in-patients experience an ADR; over half of these could have been avoidable (Davies *et al.*, 2009).

Adverse drug reactions can occur for many reasons, including the following:

- The drug may have other effects on the body besides the therapeutic effect.
- The patient has a history of allergy and is more likely to be sensitive to other drugs.
- The drug's action on the body causes other responses that are undesirable or unpleasant.
- The patient is taking too much or too little of the drug, leading to adverse effects.
- The way in which the patient's body handles the drug (absorption, distribution, metabolism or excretion) places them at risk.
- A reaction to an inactive component of the drug, for example binding agent.

The nurse must be constantly alert for signs of drug reactions of various types. Patients and their families need to be taught what to look for when patients are taking drugs at home. Some adverse effects can be countered with specific comfort measures or precautions. Knowing that these effects may occur and what actions can be taken to prevent or cope with them may be the most critical factor in helping the patient to comply with drug therapy (Box 3.1).

Adverse drug reactions can be classified according to the interaction between the drug and the patient (Ferner & Butt, 2008). These are (1) the relationship between the reaction and the dose of drug used, (2) the time-course of the effect and (3) the patient susceptibility.

Relationship With Dose Administered

This classification can be further subdivided into *toxic*, *collateral* and *hypersusceptibility* effects. Toxic effects occur where there is an exaggerated quantitative response to a drug. The observed effects can be predicted from the known pharmacological (or toxicological) actions of the drug. In such cases, the patient suffers from effects that are merely an extension of the desired effect. For example, a patient taking an antihypertensive drug may become dizzy, weak or faint when taking the 'recommended dose' but will be able to adjust to the drug therapy with a reduced dose. Toxic effects can be avoided by adjusting the prescribed dose to fit that particular patient's needs.

Collateral effects are where a drug has therapeutic actions in tissues other than the target tissue. These can occur either because the drug has a different pharmacological effect from the therapeutic action; or because the drug exerts its therapeutic pharmacological effect on another tissue, for example the analgesic morphine can cause constipation.

Hypersusceptibility reactions occur in susceptible patients and may result from a pathological or underlying condition. For example, many drugs are excreted through the kidneys; a patient who has kidney problems may not be able to excrete the drug and may accumulate the drug in the body, causing toxic effects. This is particularly relevant for drugs with a narrow **therapeutic index**, for example digoxin, theophylline. The therapeutic index compares the amount of a drug that causes a therapeutic effect to the amount causing a toxic effect. The difference between therapeutic and toxic doses is small in drugs with a narrow therapeutic index and these drugs can reach toxic plasma levels in patients who cannot excrete the drug effectively.

Time-Course

Adverse drug reactions can be either time-independent or -dependent. Time-independent reactions can occur at any time during treatment with the drug, whereas time-dependent reactions occur at specific times during treatment. For example, an adverse reaction that becomes apparent when a drug is administered too rapidly, or occurs with the first dose of a drug but is not observed with subsequent doses. Other time-dependent reactions can occur following continued exposure to a particular drug, for example anaphylaxis following a second dose of penicillin.

BOX 3.1 Safety and the Nursing Process

Before administering any drug to a patient, it is important to review the contraindications and cautions associated with that drug, as well as the anticipated adverse effects of the drug. This information will direct your assessment of the patient, helping you to focus on particular signs and symptoms that would alert you to contraindications or to proceed cautiously and to establish a baseline for that patient so that you will be able to identify adverse effects that occur. When teaching the patient about a drug, you should list the adverse effects that should be anticipated, along with the appropriate actions that the patient can take to alleviate any discomfort associated with these effects. Being alert to adverse effects – what to assess and how to intervene appropriately – can increase the effectiveness of a drug regimen, provide for patient safety and improve patient compliance.

Patient Susceptibility

Some patients are more susceptible to adverse drug reactions than others. For example, genetic variation between patients and the patients' age, gender and disease status. Many drugs are excreted through the kidneys; therefore patients with kidney dysfunction may not be able to excrete the drug. The drug may accumulate in the body causing toxic effects. There is also a reduction in the ability to metabolize and excrete drugs as individuals get older.

If your patient does experience an adverse reaction to either a prescribed drug or one obtained for self-medication, health care professionals, patients and carers are encouraged to inform the Commission on Human Medicines (CHM) and Medicines and Healthcare products Regulatory Authority (MHRA) using the Yellow Card scheme. These cards can be found at the back of the British National Formulary (BNF). Alternatively, the information can be supplied via the web address: www.yellowcard.gov.uk. Nurses have been allowed to report adverse reactions since October 2002, and since then nurses have submitted proportionally more yellow cards than other health care professionals. The role of the nurse in pharmacovigilance is therefore of great importance.

Drug Allergy

A **drug allergy** occurs when the body forms antibodies to a particular drug (or a metabolite of the drug), causing an immune response when the person is re-exposed to the drug. A patient cannot be allergic to a drug that has never been taken, although patients can have cross-allergies to drugs within the same drug class as one formerly taken. Many people state that they have a drug allergy because of the effects of a drug. Patients who state that they have a drug 'allergy' should be further questioned as to the nature of the allergy. Many patients do not receive needed treatment because the response to the drug is not understood by the patient.

Drug allergies fall into four main classifications of hypersensitivity (Table 3.1):

1. Type I reactions – immediate or anaphylactic;
2. Type II reactions – cytotoxic reactions;

Table 3.1 Classification of Drug Hypersensitivities

Allergy Type	Assessment	Interventions
Type I: *Immediate or Anaphylactic Reactions*		
This reaction involves IgE immunoglobulins bound to mast cells and leukocytes. Binding of the drug to the IgE molecules causes the release of chemicals, including histamine, that produce immediate reactions (mucous membrane swelling and constricting bronchi) that can lead to respiratory distress and even respiratory arrest. The reaction can develop within 5–10 min of administering the drug.	Urticaria, rash, difficulty breathing, hypotension, dilated pupils, diaphoresis, 'panic' feeling, increased heart rate and respiratory arrest.	Avoid the drug in the future. Intramuscular (IM) administration of adrenaline (epinephrine; 0.3 ml of a 1:1000 solution). Massage the site to speed absorption rate. Repeat the dose every 15–20 min, as appropriate. If the patients' circulation is inadequate, adrenaline can be given by slow intravenous (IV) injection. Antihistamines, bronchodilators or corticosteroids may also be beneficial. Notify the prescriber and/or primary caregiver and discontinue the drug. Be aware that prevention is the best treatment. Recommend patients with known allergies to wear MedicAlert identification and, if appropriate, to carry an emergency epinephrine kit.
Type II: *Cytotoxic Reactions*		
This allergy involves antibodies that circulate in the blood and attack antigens (the drug or metabolite) bound to the cell surface, causing death of that cell. This reaction is not immediate, but may be seen over a few days.	Full blood count showing damage to blood-forming cells (decreased haematocrit, white blood cell count, and platelets); liver function tests show elevated liver enzymes and renal function test shows decreased renal function.	Blood transfusion or plasmapheresis (removal of antibodies from plasma. The plasma is then returned to the patient). Administer immunosuppressant drugs. Notify the prescriber and/or primary caregiver and discontinue the drug.
Type III: *Immune Complex-Mediated Reactions*		
The antigen forms large complexes with the antibody that circulate in the blood and cause damage to various tissues by blocking blood vessels. An inflammatory reaction occurs at the site of damage. These reactions take between 4 and 12 h to develop and include serum sickness, glomerulonephritis and pulmonary disease.	Itchy rash, high fever, swollen lymph nodes, swollen and painful joints and oedema of the face and limbs.	Administer anti-inflammatory agents (corticosteroids and immunosuppressants). Plasmapheresis. Notify the prescriber and/or primary caregiver and discontinue the drug. Provide comfort measures to help the patient cope with the signs and symptoms (cool environment, skin care, positioning and ice to joints).
Type IV: *Delayed Reactions*		
This reaction occurs between 48 and 72 h after exposure and involves antibodies that are bound to specific white blood cells.	Rash, urticaria and swollen joints.	Administer immunosuppressant drugs or corticosteroids. Notify the prescriber and/or primary caregiver and discontinue drug.

3. Type III reactions – immune complex-mediated reactions;
4. Type IV reactions – delayed reactions.

The nurse, as the primary caregiver involved in administering drugs, must constantly assess for potential drug allergies and must be prepared to intervene appropriately.

Drug-Induced Tissue and Organ Damage

Drugs can act directly or indirectly to cause many types of adverse effects in various tissues, structures and organs (Figure 3.1). These drug effects account for many of the cautions that are noted before drug administration begins. The possible occurrence of these effects also accounts for the fact that the use of some drugs is contraindicated in patients with a particular history or underlying pathology. The specific contraindications and cautions for the administration of a given drug are noted with each class of drugs discussed in this book and in the BNF. For example, the antibacterial chloramphenicol can cause bone marrow suppression and its use is limited to life-threatening infections such as meningitis. These effects occur frequently enough that the nurse should be knowledgeable about the presentation of the drug-induced damage and about appropriate interventions that should be used if they occur.

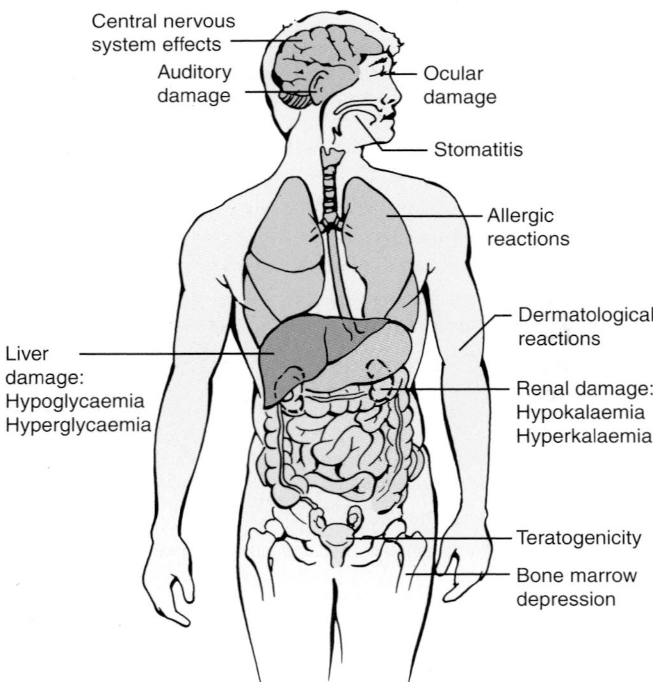

FIGURE 3.1 Variety of adverse effects and toxicities associated with drug use.

Anaphylaxis

Anaphylaxis is the most severe form of Type I hypersensitivity reaction and cannot only be triggered by an adverse drug reaction, but also by insect bites or stings or a food allergy. In these reactions the body recognizes the drug (or other trigger) as an antigen and mounts an immune response and produces antibodies. On the second exposure to the drug, the antibodies trigger the release of chemical mediators (histamine, prostaglandins, leukotrienes) and there is systemic vasodilation leading to a sudden drop in blood pressure. The bronchial smooth muscle also constricts reducing airflow into the lungs. If left untreated, the sustained hypotension and constriction of airways can be fatal. The management of Type I hypersensitivity reactions is detailed in Table 3.1.

Dermatological Reactions

Dermatological reactions are adverse reactions involving the skin. These can range from a simple rash to potentially fatal exfoliative dermatitis. Many adverse reactions involve the skin because many drugs are deposited there or cause direct irritation to the tissue.

Rashes, Urticaria

Urticaria (hives or 'nettle rash') is characterized by itchy swellings in the skin and is a common hypersensitivity reaction to penicillin or aspirin. Procainamide, used to treat cardiac arrhythmias, causes a characteristic skin rash in many patients.

Assessment

Hives, rashes and other dermatological lesions may be seen. Severe reactions may include erythroderma, which is characterized by a red rash over most of the skin, fever and enlarged lymph nodes; and toxic epidermal necrolysis with widespread skin blistering and sloughing of skin layers. This rash often results from a reaction to penicillins, carbamazepine or nonsteroidal anti-inflammatory drugs (NSAIDs) and can extend to internal epithelial surfaces, possibly leading to multiorgan failure. Erythema multiforme, where the skin and mucous membranes are inflamed, can also be caused by an adverse reaction to some antibiotics and barbiturates. Stevens–Johnson syndrome is a severe form of erythema multiforme characterized by inflammation of the oral mucosa, respiratory tract and genitalia.

Interventions

In mild cases, or when the benefit of the drug outweighs the discomfort of the skin lesion, provide frequent skin care; instruct the patient to avoid rubbing, tight or rough clothing, and harsh soaps or perfumed lotions; and administer antihistamines, as appropriate. In severe cases, discontinue the drug and notify the prescriber and/or primary caregiver. In addition to these interventions, topical corticosteroids, antihistamines and emollients can be used. If severe, the use of systemic corticosteroids is advised.

Stomatitis

Stomatitis, or inflammation of the mucous membranes of the mouth and throat, can occur because of a direct toxic reaction to the drug or because the drug deposits in the end capillaries in the mucous membranes, leading to inflammation. Fluorouracil, an antineoplastic agent, causes mouth ulcers or stomatitis in most of the patients who take it. Other examples include antimalarials, tolbutamide and methyldopa.

Assessment

Symptoms can include swollen gums, inflamed gums (gingivitis) and a swollen and red tongue (glossitis). Other symptoms include difficulty swallowing, bad breath and pain in the mouth and throat.

Interventions

Provide frequent mouth care with a mouthwash solution and if necessary, arrange for a dental consultation. Offer nutrition evaluation, for example deficiencies in iron, folic acid or vitamin B_{12}.

Superinfections

One of the body's protective mechanisms is the wide variety of bacteria that live within or on the surface of the body. This bacterial growth is called the *normal flora*. The normal flora protects the body from invasion by other bacteria, viruses and fungi. Several kinds of drugs (especially antibacterials) destroy the normal flora, leading to the development of **superinfections** or infections caused by the usually controlled organisms, for example the development of oral or vaginal thrush when taking antibacterials.

Assessment

Symptoms can include fever, diarrhoea, black or hairy tongue, glossitis, mucous membrane lesions and vaginal discharge with or without itching.

Interventions

Provide supportive measures (frequent mouth care, skin care, access to bathroom facilities). Administer antifungal therapy as appropriate. In severe cases, discontinue the drug responsible for the superinfection.

Blood Dyscrasia

Blood dyscrasia is due to bone marrow suppression which can be caused by drugs. This occurs when drugs that can cause cell death (e.g. antineoplastics, antibacterials) are used. Bone marrow cells multiply rapidly and are therefore said to have a rapid turnover. As they go through cell division and multiply so often, they are highly susceptible to any agent that disrupts cell function.

Assessment

Symptoms include fever, chills, sore throat, weakness, back pain, dark urine, decreased haematocrit (anaemia; e.g. sulphonamides and methyldopa), low platelet count (thrombocytopenia; e.g. quinine, heparin, thiazide diuretics), low white blood cell count (leukopaenia; e.g. NSAIDs, clozapine, sulphonamides), and a reduction in all cellular elements of the full blood count (pancytopaenia).

Interventions

Monitor blood counts. The drug treatment should be stopped if bone marrow suppression occurs. In severe cases, discontinue the drug or stop administration until the bone marrow recovers to a safe level. Provide supportive measures (rest, protection from exposure to infections, protection from injury and avoidance of activities that might result in injury or bleeding).

Liver Injury

Oral drugs are absorbed into the bloodstream and passed directly into the liver. This is known as the first-pass effect. This exposes the liver cells (hepatocytes) to the full impact of the drug before it is broken down for circulation throughout the body. Most drugs are metabolized in the liver, so any metabolites that are irritating or toxic will also affect liver integrity, for example from paracetamol overdose.

Assessment

Symptoms may include fever, malaise, nausea, vomiting, jaundice, change in colour of urine or stools, abdominal pain or colic, elevated serum albumin and liver enzymes (e.g. aspartate aminotransferase and alanine aminotransferase), alterations in bilirubin levels and changes in clotting factors (e.g. prothrombin time).

Interventions

Discontinue the drug and notify the prescriber and/or primary caregiver. Offer supportive measures: small, frequent meals; cool environment and rest periods.

Renal Injury

The glomeruli in the kidney have very small capillary networks that filter the blood into the renal tubule. Some drug molecules are just the right size to get plugged into the capillary network, causing acute inflammation and severe renal problems. Some drugs are excreted from the kidney unchanged. They have the potential to directly irritate the renal tubule and alter normal reabsorption and secretion processes. Gentamicin, an antibacterial, is frequently associated with nephrotoxicity.

Assessment
Elevated blood urea nitrogen, elevated creatinine concentration, decreased haematocrit, electrolyte imbalances, fatigue, malaise, oedema, irritability and skin rash may be seen.

Interventions
Notify the prescriber and/or primary caregiver and discontinue the drug as needed. Offer supportive measures, for example diet and fluid restrictions, skin care, electrolyte therapy, rest periods, controlled environment. In severe cases, dialysis may be required for survival.

Poisoning

Poisoning occurs when an overdose of a drug damages multiple body systems, leading to the potential for fatal reactions. Assessment parameters vary with the particular drug. Treatment of drug poisoning also varies, depending on the drug. Where appropriate in this book, specific antidotes or treatments to poisoning are identified (if known). Emergency and life-support measures are often needed in severe cases.

Alterations in Glucose Metabolism

Hypoglycaemia

Some drugs affect the metabolism and use of glucose, causing a low serum blood glucose concentration, or hypoglycaemia. The sulphonylureas are oral antidiabetic agents that have the desired action of lowering blood glucose levels, but which can lower blood glucose too far, causing hypoglycaemia. Other drugs responsible for inducing hypoglycaemia include quinine, propranolol (in combination with strenuous exercise) and pentamidine.

Assessment
Symptoms may include fatigue; drowsiness; hunger; anxiety; headache; cold, clammy skin; shaking and lack of co-ordination (tremulousness); increased heart rate; increased blood pressure; numbness and tingling of the mouth, tongue and/or lips; confusion; and rapid and shallow respirations. In severe cases, seizures and/or coma may occur.

Interventions
Restore glucose, intravenously (IV) or orally if possible. An intramuscular injection of glucagon can also increase blood glucose levels. Provide supportive measures (e.g. environmental control of light and temperature, rest). Institute safety measures as necessary to prevent injury or falls. Offer reassurance to help the patient cope with the experience.

Hyperglycaemia

Some drugs stimulate the breakdown of glycogen or alter metabolism in such a way as to cause high serum glucose levels, or hyperglycaemia. Ephedrine, a drug used to dilate the airways, can break down stored glycogen and cause an elevation of blood glucose by its effects on the sympathetic nervous system. This drug should be used with caution by diabetic patients.

Assessment
Fatigue, increased urination (polyuria), increased thirst (polydipsia), deep respirations (Kussmaul's respirations), restlessness, increased hunger (polyphagia), nausea, hot or flushed skin and odour to breath (acetone or 'pear drops') may be observed.

Interventions
Remove the drug therapy and administer insulin therapy to decrease blood glucose as appropriate.

Electrolyte Imbalances

Hypokalaemia

Some drugs affecting the kidney can cause low serum potassium levels (hypokalaemia) by altering the renal exchange system. For example, loop diuretics and thiazides function by causing the loss of potassium as well as sodium and water. Potassium is essential for the normal functioning of nerves and muscles, particularly cardiac muscle.

Assessment
The normal serum potassium concentration ($[K^+]$) is between 3.5 and 5 mmol/l. When serum $[K^+]$ falls below 3 mmol/l, the symptoms include muscle weakness and cramps, numbness and tingling in the extremities, nausea, vomiting, diarrhoea, decreased bowel sounds, irregular and/or pulse, orthostatic hypotension and disorientation. In severe cases, paralytic ileus (absent bowel sounds, abdominal distension) and cardiac arrest may occur.

Interventions
Replace serum potassium and carefully monitor serum levels, electrocardiogram (ECG) and patient response. Provide supportive therapy (e.g. safety precautions to prevent injury or falls, orientation of the patient, comfort measures for pain and discomfort).

Hyperkalaemia

Some drugs that affect the kidney, such as angiotensin converting enzyme inhibitors, potassium-sparing diuretics and angiotensin receptor antagonists, can lead to potassium retention and a resultant increase in serum potassium levels (hyperkalaemia). Other drugs that cause cell death or injury, such as many antineoplastic agents, can also cause the cells to release potassium, leading to hyperkalaemia.

Assessment
Hyperkalaemia is classified as mild when the serum $[K^+]$ level is between 5.5 and 6 mmol/l, moderate when serum

[K^+] is 6.1 to 6.9 mmol/l and severe when serum [K^+] level is greater than 7 mmol/l. Symptoms include weakness, muscle cramps, diarrhoea, numbness and tingling, slow heart rate, low blood pressure, decreased urine output and difficulty in breathing. There is a risk of cardiac arrest.

Interventions

The Clinical Resource Efficiency Support Team (CREST) Guidelines should be adhered to (CREST, 2006). Monitor the ECG continuously and measure blood urea, electrolytes and glucose regularly. Any drugs which could be causing the hyperkalaemia should be removed; in some cases, for example digoxin toxicity, it may be desirable to perform haemodialysis. To protect the heart, institute measures to decrease the serum potassium concentration: initially an IV infusion of 10% calcium gluconate and insulin (if blood glucose falls below 15 mmol/l, glucose should be administered with the insulin) and nebulized salbutamol. If these measures fail and serum [K^+] remains ≥7 mmol/l, the excess K^+ can be removed either via dialysis or an enema of calcium polystyrene sulphonate resin. Offer supportive measures to cope with discomfort. The patient should subsequently be placed on a low potassium diet.

Sensory Effects

Ocular Toxicity

The blood vessels in the retina are very tiny and are called 'end arteries'; that is, they stop and do not interconnect with other arteries supplying the same cells. Some drugs are deposited into these tiny arteries, causing inflammation and tissue damage. Chloroquine, a drug used to treat some rheumatoid diseases, can cause retinal damage and even blindness.

Assessment

Blurring of vision, colour vision changes, corneal damage and blindness may be observed.

Interventions

Monitor the patient's vision carefully when the patient is receiving known oculotoxic drugs. Consult with the prescriber and/or primary caregiver and discontinue the drug as appropriate. Provide supportive measures, especially if vision loss is irreversible.

Auditory Damage

Tiny vessels and nerves in the eighth cranial nerve are easily irritated and damaged by certain drugs. The aminoglycoside antibacterials, for example gentamicin; can cause severe damage to the sensory cells in the cochlea and vestibular organ. Aspirin, one of the most commonly used drugs, is often linked to auditory ringing and eighth cranial nerve effects.

Assessment

Dizziness, ringing in the ears (tinnitus), loss of balance and loss of hearing may be observed.

Interventions

Consult with the prescriber to decrease dose or discontinue the drug. If the patient complains of tinnitus the drug should be discontinued immediately. Provide protective measures to prevent falling or injury. Provide supportive measures to cope with drug effects.

Neurological Effects

General Central Nervous System Effects

Although the brain is fairly well protected from many drug effects by the blood–brain barrier, some drugs do affect neurologic functioning, either directly (lipid-soluble drugs are able to diffuse across the blood–brain barrier) or by altering electrolyte or glucose levels. β-blockers, used to treat hypertension, angina, and many other conditions, can cause feelings of anxiety, insomnia and nightmares.

Assessment

Symptoms may include confusion, delirium, insomnia, drowsiness, hyperreflexia or hyporeflexia, bizarre dreams and hallucinations.

Interventions

Provide safety measures to prevent injury. Caution the patient to avoid dangerous situations such as driving a car or operating dangerous machinery. Orientate the patient and provide support. Consult with the prescriber to decrease drug dose or discontinue the drug.

Antimuscarinic ('atropine-like') Effects

Some drugs block the effects of the parasympathetic nervous system by directly or indirectly blocking muscarinic receptors. Atropine, the prototype antimuscarinic drug, provides relief from bradycardia and hypotension following a myocardial infarction, and can be used to decrease bronchial and salivary secretions before surgery and for many other indications. Atropine eye drops constrict the pupil and are used in the treatment of glaucoma. Many other drugs also cause antimuscarinic effects.

Assessment

Dry mouth, altered taste perception, dysphagia, heartburn, constipation, bloating, paralytic ileus, urinary hesitancy and retention, impotence, blurred vision, cycloplegia (paralysis of the ciliary muscle of the eye), photophobia, headache, mental confusion, nasal congestion, palpitations, decreased sweating and dry skin may be seen.

Interventions

Provide ice chips and mouth care to help mouth dryness. Arrange for bowel programme as appropriate. Have the patient empty their bladder before taking the drug to aid urination. Provide safety measures if vision changes occur. Arrange for medication for headache and nasal congestion as appropriate. Advise the patient to avoid hot environments and to take protective measures to prevent falling and to prevent dehydration, which may be caused by exposure to heat owing to decreased sweating.

Parkinsonism

Drugs that directly or indirectly affect dopamine levels in the brain can cause a syndrome that resembles Parkinson's disease. Many of the psychotherapeutic and neuroleptic drugs can cause this effect. In most cases, the effects stop when the drug is withdrawn.

Assessment

Lack of activity, muscular tremors, drooling, changes in gait, rigidity, extreme restlessness or 'jitters' (akathisia) or tardive dyskinesias (repetitive involuntary movements such as lip smacking and tongue protrusion) may be observed.

Interventions

Discontinue the drug if necessary. Provide small, frequent meals if swallowing becomes difficult. Provide safety measures if ambulation becomes a problem. Know that treatment with antimuscarinics or antiparkinson drugs may be recommended if the benefit of the drug outweighs the discomfort of its adverse effects.

Neuroleptic Malignant Syndrome

General anaesthetics and other drugs (e.g. psychotherapeutic drugs) that have direct effects on the central nervous system (CNS) can cause neuroleptic malignant syndrome, a generalized syndrome that includes high fever.

Assessment

Muscle rigidity, hyperthermia, autonomic disturbances, tachycardia and fever may be observed.

Interventions

Discontinue the drug and provide supportive care to lower the body temperature. Bromocriptine and dantrolene will provide some relief. Institute safety precautions as needed.

Teratogenicity

Many drugs that reach the developing embryo or foetus can cause death or congenital defects, including skeletal and limb abnormalities, CNS alterations and heart defects. The exact effects of a drug on the foetus may not be known, for example thalidomide was originally used during pregnancy as an antiemetic to treat morning sickness; however, inadequate safety testing was carried out prior to release and the teratogenic effects of thalidomide were unknown. Many thousands of children were born with severe defects.

In some cases, a predictable syndrome occurs when a drug is given to a pregnant woman. Before any drug is administered to a pregnant patient, the actual benefits should be weighed against the potential risks and the patient should be advised of the possible effects on the baby. All pregnant women should be advised not to self-medicate during the pregnancy.

Interventions

Provide emotional and physical support for dealing with foetal death or birth defects.

Box 3.2 summarizes all of the adverse effects that have been described throughout this chapter.

BOX 3.2 Summary of Adverse Drug Effects

- Extension of primary action
- Occurrence of secondary action
- Classification of hypersensitivity reactions
  - Anaphylactic reactions
  - Cytotoxic reactions
  - Immune complex-mediated reactions
  - Delayed allergic reactions
- Tissue and organ damage
  - Dermatological reactions
  - Stomatitis
  - Superinfections
  - Blood dyscrasia
- Toxicity
  - Liver injury
  - Renal injury
  - Poisoning
- Alterations in glucose metabolism
  - Hypoglycaemia
  - Hyperglycaemia
- Electrolyte imbalances
  - Hypokalaemia
  - Hyperkalaemia
- Sensory effects
  - Ocular toxicity
  - Auditory damage
- Neurological effects
  - General CNS effects
  - Antimuscarinic effects
  - Parkinsonism
  - Neuroleptic malignant syndrome (NMS)
- Teratogenicity

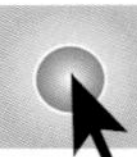

WEB LINKS

Health care providers and patients may want to consult the following Internet sources:

http://bnfc.org The BNF for Children provides UK health care professionals with authoritative and practical information on the selection and clinical use of medicines in children.

http://www.bnf.org.uk The BNF provides UK health care professionals with authoritative and practical information on the selection and clinical use of medicines.

http://www.medicalert.org.uk MedicAlert is a registered charity providing a life-saving identification system for individuals with hidden medical conditions and allergies.

http://www.mhra.gov.uk/mhra/drugsafetyupdate The Commission on Human Medicines and the Medicines Healthcare products Regulatory Authority produce a monthly newsletter on the safety of specific drugs.

http://yellowcard.gov.uk All health care professionals are encouraged to provide details of adverse drug reactions either at this site or using the Yellow Cards located at the back of the British National Formulary.

Points to Remember

- No drug does only what is desired of it. All drugs have adverse effects associated with them, some of which can be used therapeutically, for example codeine, an analgesic, which causes constipation can be used to treat diarrhoea.
- Adverse drug reactions can range from allergic reactions to tissue and cellular damage. The nurse, as the health care provider most associated with drug administration, needs to assess each situation for potential adverse effects and intervene appropriately to minimize those effects.
- Adverse reactions can be classified according to the dose of the drug administered, the time point during drug treatment that the reaction becomes evident and the patient's susceptibility.
- Allergic reactions can occur when a person makes antibodies to a drug or drug protein. If the person is exposed to that drug on another occasion, an immune response may occur. Allergic reactions can be of various types. The exact response should be noted to avoid future confusion in patient care.
- Tissue damage can include skin problems, mucous membrane inflammation, blood dyscrasia, superinfections, liver toxicity, hypoglycaemia or hyperglycaemia, renal toxicity, electrolyte disturbances, various CNS problems (ocular toxicity, auditory damage, antimuscarinic effects, parkinsonism and neuroleptic malignant syndrome), teratogenicity and overdose poisoning.

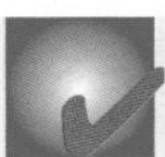

CHECK YOUR UNDERSTANDING

Answers to the questions in this chapter may be found in the answer key in the back of the book.

Multiple Choice

Select the most appropriate answer to the following:

1. An example of a drug allergy is
   a. dry mouth occurring with use of an antihistamine.
   b. increased urination occurring with use of a thiazide diuretic.
   c. hives and difficulty breathing after an injection of penicillin.
   d. skin rash associated with procainamide use.

2. A patient taking an antidiabetic drug has his morning dose and then does not have a chance to eat for several hours. An adverse effect that might be expected from this would be
   a. teratogenic effects.
   b. a skin rash.
   c. anticholinergic effects.
   d. hypoglycaemia.

3. A patient with a severe infection is given gentamicin, the only antibacterial shown to be effective in culture and sensitivity tests. A few hours after the drug is started IV, the patient becomes very restless and develops oedema. Blood tests reveal abnormal electrolytes and elevated blood urea nitrogen. This reaction was most likely caused by
   a. an anaphylactic reaction.
   b. renal toxicity associated with gentamicin.
   c. superinfection related to the antibiotic.
   d. hypoglycaemia.

4. Patients receiving antineoplastic drugs that disrupt cell function often have adverse effects involving cells that turn over rapidly in the body. These cells include
   a. ovarian cells.
   b. liver cells.
   c. cardiac cells.
   d. bone marrow cells.

5. A woman has had repeated bouts of bronchitis throughout the winter and has been taking an

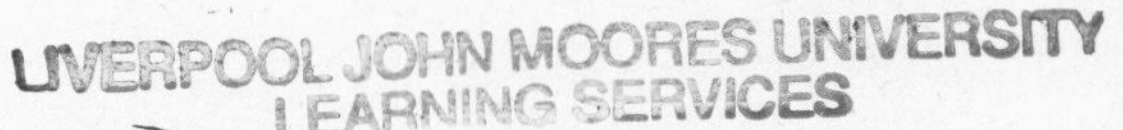

antibacterial. She calls the clinic with complaints of vaginal pain and itching. When she is seen, it is discovered that she has developed a yeast infection. You would explain to her that
a. she should not worry and the infection will disappear without any further treatment.
b. this is called a superinfection, and is commonly seen with some antibacterial use.
c. she has probably developed a sexually transmitted disease related to her lifestyle.
d. she will need to take even more antibacterials to treat this new infection.

6. A patient taking a loop diuretic is at risk of developing hypokalaemia and may experience
a. hypertension, headache and cold and clammy skin.
b. decreased urinary output and yellowing of the sclera.
c. weak pulse, low blood pressure and muscle cramping.
d. constipation.

Extended Matching Questions

Select **all** that apply.

1. A patient is taking a drug that is known to be toxic to the liver. The patient is being discharged to home. What teaching points related to liver toxicity of the drug should the nurse teach the patient to report to the physician?
a. Fever; changes in the colour of urine
b. Changes in the colour of stool; malaise
c. Rapid, deep respirations; increased sweating
d. Dizziness; drowsiness; dry mouth
e. Rash, black or hairy tongue; white spots in the mouth or throat
f. Yellowing of the skin or the whites of the eyes

2. Pregnant women should be advised of the potential risk to the foetus any time they take a drug during pregnancy. What foetal problems can be related to drug exposure *in utero*?
a. Foetal death
b. Nervous system disruption
c. Skeletal and limb abnormalities
d. Cardiac defects
e. Low-set ears
f. Deafness

3. A patient is experiencing a reaction to the penicillin injection that the nurse administered approximately 5 minutes ago. The nurse is concerned that it might be an anaphylactic reaction. What signs and symptoms would validate her suspicion?
a. Rapid heart rate
b. Diaphoresis
c. Constricted pupils
d. Hypotension
e. Rash
f. Patient report of a panic feeling

4. A patient is experiencing a Type IV hypersensitivity reaction to a recent rubella vaccination. Which of the following interventions would be appropriate when caring for this patient?
a. Administration of adrenaline
b. Cool environment
c. Blood transfusion
d. Ice to joints as needed
e. Administration of anti-inflammatory agents
f. Administration of corticosteroids

Matching

Match the adverse drug effect with the appropriate intervention.

1. ____________________ hypoglycaemia
2. ____________________ hyperglycaemia
3. ____________________ hypokalaemia
4. ____________________ superinfection
5. ____________________ muscarinic effects
6. ____________________ parkinsonism

A. Replace serum potassium and carefully monitor serum levels; provide supportive therapy (safety precautions to prevent injury or falls, orient patient, comfort measures for pain and discomfort).
B. Provide ice chips and mouth care to help mouth dryness. Arrange for bowel programme; have the patient urinate before taking the drug; provide safety measures if vision changes occur.
C. Administer insulin therapy to decrease blood glucose as appropriate; provide support to help the patient deal with signs and symptoms (access to bathroom facilities, controlled environment, reassurance, mouth care).
D. Discontinue the drug, if necessary; treat with antimuscarinics or antiparkinson drugs if recommended and if the benefit outweighs the discomfort of adverse effects; provide small, frequent meals if swallowing becomes difficult; provide safety measures.
E. Restore glucose intravenously or orally, if possible; provide supportive measures (skin care, environmental control of light and temperature, rest). Institute safety measures to prevent injury or falls.
F. Provide supportive measures (frequent mouth care, skin care, access to bathroom facilities, small and frequent meals); administer antifungal therapy as appropriate.

Fill in the Blanks

1. Renal injury is a frequent adverse effect associated with __________________.

2. Sulphonylurea antidiabetic drugs may cause __________________, and the patient should be monitored for cool and clammy skin, rapid heart rate, increased blood pressure and rapid and shallow respirations.

3. Retinal damage and even blindness have been associated with the antirheumatoid agent __________________.

4. Dizziness, ringing in the ears, loss of balance and impaired hearing can occur with aspirin therapy and are referred to as __________________.

5. A common adverse effect associated with chemotherapy is __________________, which can lead to increased bleeding, increased risk of infection and fatigue.

6. Patients should be advised to avoid driving or operating machinery, and other safety precautions should be taken if the patient has CNS effects such as __________________.

Bibliography and References

Bennett, P. N., & Brown, M. J. (2008). *Clinical pharmacology* (10th ed.). Edinburgh: Churchill Livingstone.

Clinical Resource Efficiency Support Team. (2006). *CREST guidelines for the treatment of hyperkalaemia in adults*. Available from http://www.crestni.org.uk

Davies, E. C., Green, C. F., Taylor, S., Williamson, P. R. Mottram, D. R., & Pirmohamed, M. (2009). Adverse drug reactions in hospital in-patients: a prospective analysis of 3695 patient-episodes. *PLoS ONE, 4*(2), e4439.

Ferner, R. E., & Butt, T. F. (2008). Adverse drug reactions. *Medicine, 36*(7), 364–368.

Galbraith, A., Bullock, S., Manias, E., Hunt, B., & Richards, A. (1999). *Fundamentals of pharmacology*. Harlow: Addison Wesley Longman Ltd.

Morrison-Griffiths, S., Walley, T. J., Park, B. K., Breckenridge, A. M., & Pirmohamed, M. (2003). Reporting of adverse drug reactions by nurses. *Lancet, 361*, 1347–1348.

Pirmohamed, M., James, S., Meakin, S., Green, C., Scott, A. K., & Walley, T. J., *et al.* (2004). Adverse drug reactions as a cause of admission to hospital: prospective analysis of 18,820 patients. *British Medical Journal, 329*, 15–19.

CHAPTER 4

Nursing Management

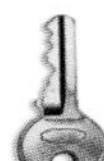

KEY TERMS

assessment
evaluation
intervention
nursing diagnosis
nursing process

LEARNING OBJECTIVES

Upon completion of this chapter, you will be able to:

1. List the responsibilities of the nurse in drug therapy.
2. Explain what is involved in each step of the nursing process as it relates to drug therapy.
3. Describe key points that must be incorporated into the assessment of a patient receiving drugs.
4. Outline the important points that must be assessed and considered before administering a drug, combining knowledge about the drug with knowledge of the patient and the environment.

The delivery of nursing care today is in a constant state of change and sometimes crisis. The population is ageing, resulting in more chronic disease and more complex care issues. The population is also transient, resulting in unstable support systems and fewer at-home care providers and helpers. At the same time, medicine is undergoing a technological boom, including greater use of computed tomography scans, nuclear magnetic resonance imaging scans and experimental drugs. Patients are being discharged earlier from acute care facilities, or they are no longer admitted for procedures that used to be treated in-hospital with follow-up support and monitoring provided. Patients are also becoming more responsible for their own care and receiving medical treatment at home. In addition, the role of nurses is changing, as nurses take on more responsibility by becoming nurse prescribers and nurse practitioners.

The Nursing Process

Although not all nursing theorists completely agree on the process that defines the practice of nursing, most do include certain key elements in the **nursing process**. These elements are the basic components of the decision-making or problem-solving process:

- **Assessment** (gathering information)
- **Nursing diagnosis** (analysing the information gathered to arrive at some conclusions)
- **Interventions** (actions undertaken to meet the patient's needs, such as administration of drugs, education and comfort measures)
- **Evaluation** (determining the effects of the interventions that were performed).

In general, the nursing framework provides an effective method for providing holistic care. With respect to drug therapy, use of the nursing process ensures that the patient receives the best, most efficient, evidence-based care. The steps of the nursing process are outlined in the following sections.

Assessment

The first step of the nursing process is the systematic, organized collection of information about the patient. The nurse is responsible for holistic care, by compiling information about physical, intellectual, emotional, social and environmental factors. This provides the nurse with the facts needed to plan education and discharge programmes, arrange for appropriate consultations and referrals and monitor the physical response to treatment or to disease.

Drug therapy is a complex and important part of health care, and the principles of drug therapy should be incorporated into every patient assessment plan. The particular information that is needed varies with each drug, but the concepts involved are similar.

Three key areas that need to be assessed are the patient's history (past illnesses and the current problem), his or her physical status and the patient's drug regimen including prescribed, over-the-counter (OTC) and herbal medicines.

History

The patient's past experiences and illnesses can influence a drug's effect and multiple drugs can affect each other in previously unknown ways.

Chronic Conditions

Certain conditions, such as renal disease, heart disease, diabetes, and chronic lung disease, may be contraindications to the use of a drug. Or these conditions may require that caution be used when administering a certain drug or that the drug dosage be adjusted.

Drug Use

Prescription drugs, OTC drugs, recreational drugs, alcohol, nicotine, alternative therapies and caffeine may have an impact on a drug's effect. Patients often neglect to mention OTC drugs or alternative therapies, not considering them to be actual drugs or not willing to admit their use to the health care provider. Patients should be asked specifically about OTC drug or alternative therapy use. Patients might also forget to mention prescription drugs that they take all the time, for instance oral contraceptives, as it forms part of their daily routine and they don't think about it. It is a good idea to specifically ask about all types of medications that the patient might use, why the patient takes them and how often the patient takes their drugs.

Allergies

Past exposure to a drug or other allergens can provoke a future reaction or provide a caution for the use of a drug, food or animal product. It is important to describe the particular allergic reaction when noting a drug allergy. In some cases, the reaction is not an allergic response but an actual drug effect.

Level of Education

This information helps the nurse determine the level of explanation required and provides a basis for developing patient education programmes.

Level of Understanding of Disease and Therapy

This information also helps the development of educational information.

Social Supports

Patients are being discharged earlier than ever before and often they need help at home with care and drug therapy. A key aspect of discharge planning involves determining what support, if any, is available to the patient at home. In many situations, it also involves referral to community-based members of the multidisciplinary team.

Physical Assessment

Weight

A patient's weight helps determine whether the recommended drug dosage is appropriate. The recommended dosage is typically based on a 70-kg adult male. Patients who are much lighter or much heavier may need a dosage adjustment.

Age

Patients at the extremes of the age spectrum – children and older adults – often require dosage adjustments based on the functional level of the liver and kidneys and the responsiveness of other organs.

Physical Parameters Related to Disease or Drug Effects

Assessing these factors before drug therapy begins, provides a baseline level to which future assessments can be compared to determine the effects of drug therapy. The specific parameters that need to be assessed depend on the disease process being treated and on the expected therapeutic and adverse effects of the drug therapy. For example, if a patient is being treated for chronic pulmonary disease, the respiratory status and reserve need to be assessed; especially if a drug is being given that has known effects on the respiratory tract. In contrast, a thorough respiratory evaluation would not be warranted in a patient with no known pulmonary disease who is taking a drug with no known effects on the respiratory system. The nurse has the greatest direct and continual contact with the patient and has the best opportunity to detect minute changes that ultimately determine the course of drug therapy – therapeutic success or discontinuation because of adverse or unacceptable responses.

Nursing Diagnosis

Once all the information has been collected, the nurse must organize and analyse the information to arrive at a nursing diagnosis. A nursing diagnosis is simply a statement of the patient's status from a nursing perspective. This statement directs appropriate nursing interventions. A nursing diagnosis shows actual or potential alterations in patient function based on the assessment of the clinical situation. Drug therapy is only a small part of the overall patient situation.

Interventions (Implementation)

The assessment and diagnosis of the patient direct the implementation of specific nursing interventions. Three types of interventions are frequently involved in drug therapy: drug administration, provision of comfort measures and patient/family education and evaluation of the effects of the drug.

Drug Administration

There are seven points to consider in the safe and effective administration of a drug:

1. *Drug:* Know that it is standard nursing practice to ensure that the drug being administered is the correct dose and the correct drug and that it is being given at the correct time and to the correct patient.
2. *Storage:* Be aware that some drugs require specific storage environments (e.g. refrigeration and protection from light).
3. *Route:* Determine the best route of administration; this is frequently established by the formulation of the drug. Nurses can often have an impact in modifying the route to arrive at the most efficient and comfortable method for the patient based on the patient's specific situation.
4. *Dosage:* Calculate the drug dosage appropriately, based on the available drug form, the patient's body weight or surface area or the patient's kidney function.
5. *Preparation:* Know the specific preparation required before administering any drug. For example, liquid drugs may need to be shaken; parenteral drugs may need to be reconstituted or diluted with specific solutions and topical drugs may require specific handling, such as the use of gloves during administration or shaving of a body area before application.
6. *Timing:* Recognize that the administration of one drug may require coordination with the administration of other drugs, foods or physical parameters.
7. *Recording:* The nurse should document the drug, dose, route administered, time given, batch number and expiry date in accordance with the local requirements for recording medication administration.

Comfort Measures

Nurses are in a unique position to help the patient cope with the effects of drug therapy.

Managing Adverse Effects

Interventions can be directed at decreasing the impact of the anticipated adverse effects of a drug and promoting patient safety. Such interventions include environmental control (e.g. temperature and light), safety measures (e.g. avoiding driving, avoiding the sun and using support rails) and physical comfort (e.g. skin care, laxatives and frequent meals).

Lifestyle Adjustment

Some drug effects require that a patient change his or her lifestyle to cope effectively. For example, patients taking diuretics may have to rearrange their day so as to be near toilet facilities when the drug works. In some cases the change in lifestyle that is needed can have a huge impact on the patient and can affect coping and concordance with any medical regimen.

Patient and Family Education

With patients becoming increasingly responsible for their own care, it is essential that they have all of the information necessary to ensure safe and effective drug therapy at home. Key elements that should be included in any drug education programme are the following:

1. *Name, dose and action of drug:* Many patients see more than one health care provider; knowing this information is crucial to ensuring safe and effective drug therapy and avoiding drug–drug interactions.
2. *Timing of administration:* Teach patients when to take the drug with respect to frequency, other drugs and meals.
3. *Special storage and preparation instructions:* Some drugs require particular handling procedures; inform patients how to carry out these requirements.
4. *Specific OTC drugs or alternative therapies to avoid:* Many patients do not consider OTC drugs or herbal or alternative therapies to be 'actual' drugs and may inadvertently take them along with their prescribed medications, causing unwanted or even dangerous drug–drug interactions. Prevent these situations by explaining which drugs or therapies should be avoided.
5. *Special comfort or safety measures:* Teach patients how to cope with anticipated adverse effects to ease anxiety and avoid nonconcordance with drug therapy. Also educate patients about the importance of follow-up tests or evaluation.
6. *Specific points about drug toxicity:* Give patients a list of warning signs of drug toxicity. Advise patients to notify their health care provider if any of these effects occur.
7. *Specific warnings about drug discontinuation:* Some drugs with a small margin of safety and drugs with particular systemic effects cannot be stopped abruptly without dangerous effects. Alert patients who are taking these drugs to this problem and encourage them to call their health care provider immediately if they cannot take their medication for any reason (e.g. illness).

Evaluation

Evaluation is part of the continual process of patient care that leads to changes in assessment, diagnosis and intervention. The patient is continually evaluated for therapeutic response, the occurrence of adverse drug effects and the occurrence of drug–drug, drug–food or drug–alternative therapy interactions. The efficacy of the nursing interventions and the education programme must be evaluated. In some situations, the nurse evaluates the patient simply by reapplying the beginning steps of the nursing process and analysing for change. In some cases of drug therapy, specific therapeutic drug levels also need to be evaluated.

Points to Remember

- The nursing process is a problem-solving one, involving assessment, nursing diagnosis, interventions and evaluation. It is an ongoing, dynamic process that provides safe and efficient care.
- Nursing assessment must include information on the history of past illnesses and the current complaint, as well as a physical examination; this provides a database of baseline information to ensure safe administration of a drug and to evaluate the drug's effectiveness and adverse effects.
- Nursing diagnoses use the data gathered during the assessment to determine actual or potential problems that require specific nursing interventions.
- Nursing interventions should include proper administration of a drug; comfort measures to help the patient cope with the drug effects and patient and family education regarding the drug effects, ways to avoid adverse effects, warning signs to report and any other specific information about the drug that will facilitate patient compliance.
- Evaluation is a continual process that assesses the situation and leads to new diagnoses or interventions as the patient reacts to the drug therapy.
- A nursing care guide and patient education materials can be prepared for each drug being given, using information about a drug's therapeutic effects, adverse effects and special considerations.

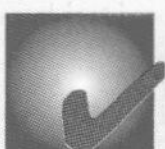

CHECK YOUR UNDERSTANDING

Answers to the questions in this chapter may be found in the answer key in the back of the book.

Multiple Choice

Select the most appropriate response to the following:

1. A patient reports to you that he or she has a drug allergy. In exploring the allergic reaction with the patient, the following might indicate an allergic response:
   a. increased urination.
   b. dry mouth.
   c. rash.
   d. drowsiness.

2. It is important to obtain a medical history from a patient before beginning drug therapy because
   a. many medical conditions alter the pharmacokinetics and pharmacodynamics of a drug.
   b. it is part of the nursing protocol.
   c. a baseline is needed for evaluating drug effects.
   d. it is the first step in the nursing process.

3. A patient receiving an antihistamine complains of dry mouth and nose. An appropriate comfort measure for this patient would be
   a. use of a humidifier and an increase in fluid consumption.
   b. voiding before taking the drug.
   c. avoiding exposure to the sun.
   d. a back rub.

4. When establishing the nursing interventions appropriate for a given patient
   a. the patient should not be actively involved.
   b. the family or other support systems should not be consulted.
   c. education is important only if the patient seems concordant
   d. an evaluation of all of the data accumulated should be incorporated to achieve an effective care plan.

5. The evaluation step of the nursing process
   a. is often not necessary.
   b. is important only in the acute setting.
   c. is a continual process that redirects nursing interventions as needed.
   d. includes making nursing diagnoses.

6. A patient has been through a teaching format for digoxin, a drug used to increase the effectiveness of the myocardial contractions. Which of the following statements would indicate that the teaching was effective?
   a. 'I need to take my pulse every morning before I take my pill'.
   b. 'Sometimes I forget my pills, but I usually make up the missed ones once I remember'.
   c. 'This pill might help my hayfever'.
   d. 'I don't remember the name of it, but it is the white one'.

Extended Matching Questions

Select **all** that apply.

1. A patient is being started on a laxative regimen. Before beginning the regimen, the nurse would perform which of the following assessments?
   a. Liver function test
   b. Abdominal examination
   c. Skin colour and lesion evaluation
   d. Lung auscultation
   e. 24-hour urine
   f. Cardiac assessment

2. The nursing care of a patient receiving drug therapy should include measures to decrease the anticipated adverse effects of the drug. Which of the following measures would a nurse consider to decrease adverse effects?
   a. A positive approach
   b. Environmental temperature control
   c. Safety measures
   d. Skin care
   e. Refrigeration of the drug
   f. Involvement of the family

3. A nurse is preparing to administer a drug to a client for the first time. What questions should the nurse consider before actually administering the drug?
   a. Is this the right patient?
   b. Is this the right drug?
   c. Is there a generic drug available?
   d. Is this the right route for this patient?
   e. Is this the right dose, as ordered?
   f. Did I record this properly?

Complete the List

List the seven points to consider in the safe and effective administration of a drug.

1. ____

2. ____

3. ______________________________

4. ______________________________

5. ______________________________

6. ______________________________

7. ______________________________

Fill in the Blanks

1. The first step of the nursing process, which involves the systematic, organized collection of data about the patient, is called ________________.

2. The continual process that assesses the situation and leads to new diagnoses or interventions as the patient reacts to the drug therapy is called ________________.

3. ________________ use the data gathered during the assessment to determine actual or potential problems that require specific nursing interventions.

4. Inadvertent drug–drug interactions may occur when a patient does not report use of ________________ or ________________ when given a prescription drug.

5. Patients should always be told the name, action and ________________ of each drug being taken.

6. A drug is known to cause dizziness. An important safety warning for the patient taking that drug would be ________________.

Bibliography

Bickley, L. (2005). *Bates' guide to physical examination and history taking* (9th ed.). Philadelphia: Lippincott Williams & Wilkins.

Carpenito, L. J. (2005). *Handbook of nursing diagnoses* (11th ed.). Philadelphia: Lippincott Williams & Wilkins.

Carpenito, L. J. (2005). *Nursing care plans and documentation* (4th ed.). Philadelphia: Lippincott Williams & Wilkins.

Carpenito, L. J. (2005). *Nursing diagnosis: Application in clinical practice* (11th ed.). Philadelphia: Lippincott Williams & Wilkins.

McCloskey, J., & Bulechek, G. (Eds.). (2000). *Nursing interventions classification* (3rd ed.). St. Louis: C. V. Mosby.

Redman, B. (1997). *The practice of patient education* (8th ed.). St. Louis: Mosby-Year Book.

CHAPTER

5

Dosage Calculations

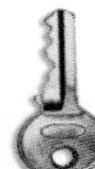

KEY TERMS

body surface area

conversion

metric system

nomogram

ratio and proportion

LEARNING OBJECTIVES

Upon completion of this chapter, you will be able to:

1. Convert within the measuring system when given drug orders and available forms of the drugs.
2. Calculate the correct dose of a drug when given examples of drug orders and available forms of the drugs ordered.
3. Discuss why children require different dosages of drugs than adults.
4. Explain the calculations used to determine a safe paediatric dose of a drug.

To determine the correct dose of a particular drug for a patient, one should take into consideration the patient's gender, weight, age and physical condition, as well as other drugs the patient may be taking. Frequently, the dose that is needed for a patient is not the dose that is available, and it is necessary to convert the dosage form available into the prescribed dosage. Doing the necessary mathematical calculations to determine what should be given is the responsibility of the prescriber who orders the drug, the pharmacist who dispenses the drug and the nurse who administers the drug. This helps to provide for a thorough set of checks on the dosage being given before the patient actually receives the drug. All nurses must ensure that they are familiar with each aspect of a drug label (Figure 5.1). In many institutions, drugs arrive at the patient care area in unit-dose form, prepackaged for each individual patient. The nurse who will administer the drug may come to rely on the prepackaged unit-dose that is sent from the pharmacy and may not even recalculate or recheck the dose to match the order that was written. Always ensure that the five 'rights' of medication administration (Nursing and Midwifery Council, 2008) are adhered to:

1. Right drug?
2. Right route?
3. Right dose?
4. Right time?
5. Right patient?

But mistakes can still happen, and the nurse, as the person who is administering the drug (and usually the last person to protect the patient from medication errors), is legally and professionally responsible for any error that might occur. It is necessary for practicing nurses to know how to convert drug orders into available forms of a drug to ensure that the right patient is getting the right dose of a drug.

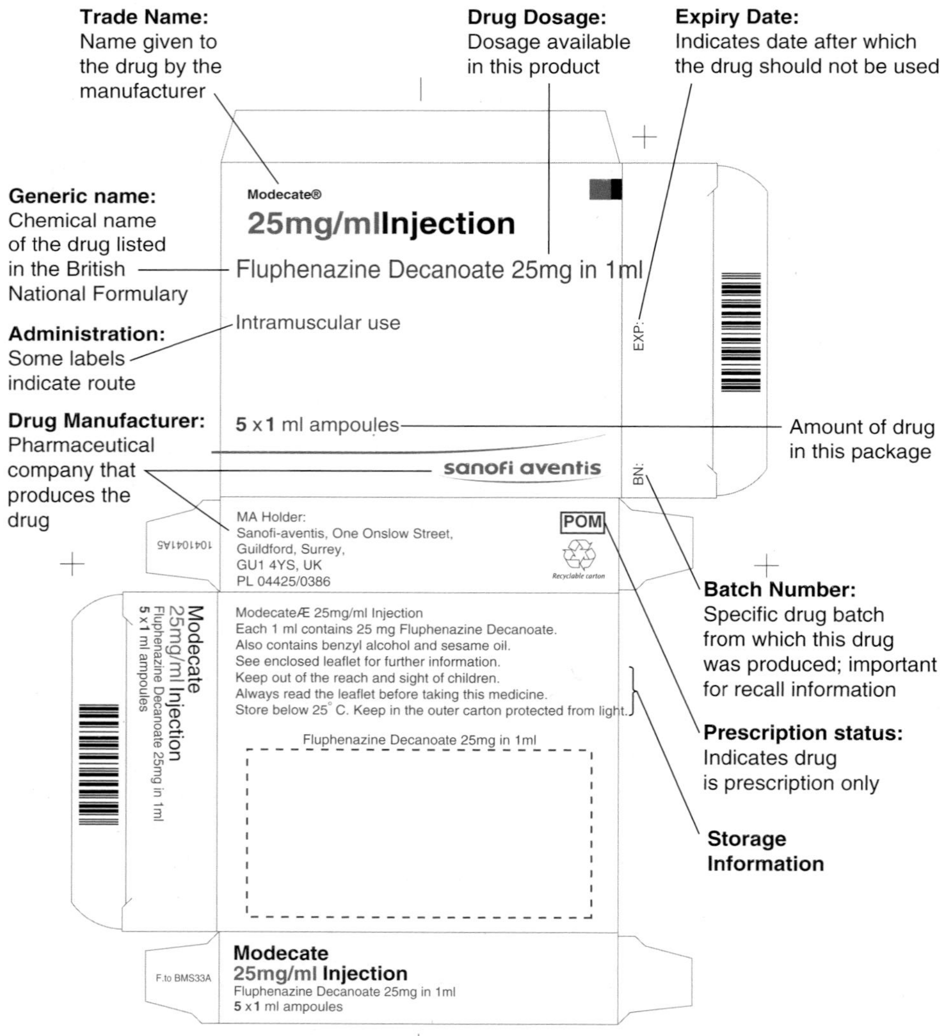

FIGURE 5.1 Reading a drug label (sample drug label courtesy of Sanofi Aventis, Guildford, UK).

Table 5.1 Basic Units of Measure in the Metric System

Solid Measure	Liquid Measure
1 kilogram (kg) = 1000 grams (g)	1 litre (l) = 1000 ml
1 gram (g) = 1000 milligrams (mg)	1 millilitre (ml) = 1000 microlitres (μl)
1 milligram (mg) = 1000 micrograms (μg)	
1 microgram (μg) = 1000 nanograms (ng)	

Measuring Systems

The **metric system** is the system of measure used in drug preparation and delivery. The European Pharmacopoeia established standards requiring that all prescriptions include the metric measure for quantity and strength of drug. The metric system is used worldwide and makes the sharing of knowledge and research information possible. The metric system uses the gram (g) as the basic unit of solid measure and the litre (l) as the basic unit of liquid measure. Table 5.1 lists the standard units of the metric system. It is extremely important to be able to perform **conversions** within this measuring system, for example from grams into milligrams (mg). Some of the examples below will demonstrate this conversion. Box 5.1 illustrates how these conversions are performed. Where appropriate, always include the zero in front of the decimal point, for example 0.75 mg should **not** be written down as .75 mg; the zero should always be present. Likewise, 5 mg should **not** be written down as 5.0 mg. If the decimal point was not noted by the person administering the dose, a patient could receive 10 times too much.

BOX 5.1 CONVERTING BETWEEN DIFFERENT UNITS

As shown in Table 5.1, there are 1000 micrograms (μg) in every gram and 1000 grams in every kilogram. There are also 1000 ml in every l. Note how the units are in multiples of a thousand. You should be able to confidently convert between the units.

Example 1: Convert 650 mg into grams.

Knowing that there are 1000 mg in every 1 g, you should be able to work out that your answer is going to be less than 1 g. In this case, **divide** 650 mg by 1000 to give you the answer as 0.65 g.

Example 2: Convert 2360 g into kg.

Knowing that there are 1000 g in every 1 kg, you should be able to work out that your answer is going to be more than 1 kg. In this case, **divide** 2360 g by 1000 to give you the answer as 2.36 kg.

In examples 1 and 2, the values were converted from smaller units into larger ones, for example from g into kg; and the decimal point is moved to the left. If the conversion is from a larger to a smaller unit, you need to **multiply** your answer by 1000 or move your decimal point to the right three places.

Example 3: Convert 0.075 g into mg.

Knowing that there are 1000 mg in every 1 g, you should be able to work out that your answer is going to be less than 1 g. In this case, **multiply** 0.075 g by 1000 to give you the answer as 75 mg.

The same process is applied when converting between the units of volume.

Example 1: Convert 250 ml into l.

Knowing that there are 1000 ml in every 1 l, you should be able to work out that your answer is going to be less than 1 l. In this case, **divide** 250 ml by 1000 to give you the answer as 0.25 l.

Other Systems

Some drugs are measured in units other than the metric system. These measures may reflect chemical activity or biological equivalence. One of these measures is the unit. A unit usually reflects the biological activity of the drug in 1 ml of solution. The unit is unique for the drug it measures: a unit of heparin would not be comparable with a unit of insulin.

The concentration, or strength, of some medicines can be expressed using other nomenclature:

- *The number of parts (by weight) of the active ingredient (drug) contained in a given volume (ml).* For example, the subcutaneous administration of 1 in 1000 adrenaline during acute anaphylaxis. This represents 1 g of adrenaline contained in 1000 ml of the injection solution.
- *Expressed as a percentage.* This is most commonly used to represent injections of large volume and for topical drugs. Where this percentage relates to a mixture of two solid drugs, this percentage is referred to as weight/weight (w/w). If the solid drug is dissolved in a liquid, the percentage is referred to as weight/volume (w/v), that is weight in g where the volume is 100 ml. Lastly, if the drug is a liquid dispersed in another liquid, this is known as volume/volume (v/v). For example, an intravenous 0.9% saline solution to replace lost fluids. A value of 0.9% represents 0.9 parts in 100, meaning 0.9 g of sodium chloride in 100 ml of the product.
- *Molarity.* This approach is used on a limited number of occasions, for example potassium chloride (KCl) infusions. To use this approach, students need to know that one 'mole' of a drug weighs (in grams) the same as the relative molecular weight of that drug. For example, the molecular weight of KCl is 74.6. Therefore, a one mole solution of KCl infusion contains 74.6 g KCl in 1 l of the solvent.
- In many cases, millimoles (mmol) are used to describe the molarity of a solution, where there are 1000 millimoles in a molar solution. For example, the KCl infusion is available in 20, 27 and 40 mmol/l solutions. Electrolyte values are also given in mmol. To calculate mmol the amount of substance in the blood in mg is divided by

the atomic weight, for example the amount of potassium in blood is 100 mg/l and the atomic weight is 40. Therefore 100 divided by 40 = 2.5 mmol/l.

Calculating Dosage

As mentioned above, because drugs are made available only in certain forms or dosages, it may be necessary to calculate what the patient should be receiving when interpreting a drug order. Frequently, tablets or capsules for oral administration are not available in the exact dose that has been ordered. In these situations, the nurse who is administering the drug must calculate the number of tablets or capsules that should be given to make up the ordered dose. The easiest way to determine this is to set up a **ratio and proportion** equation between the known values and the unknown values. The known value is the amount of drug available in one tablet or capsule; the unknown is the number of tablets or capsules that are needed for the prescribed dose:

$$\frac{\text{amount of drug available}}{\text{one tablet or capsule}} = \frac{\text{amount of drug prescribed}}{\text{number of tablets or capsules to give}}$$

This is more easily explained by working through an example. An order is written for 400 mg of paracetamol. The tablets that are available each contain 200 mg of paracetamol. How many tablets should be given? First, set up the equation given above where Y is the unknown number of tablets:

$$\frac{200\,\text{mg}}{1\,\text{tablet}} = \frac{400\,\text{mg}}{Y}$$

By cross-multiplying the ratio:

$$200\text{ mg} \times Y = 400\text{ mg} \times 1\,(\text{tablet})$$

Rearrange and cancel units and numbers:

$$Y = \frac{400\,\text{mg} \times 1\,\text{tablet}}{200\,\text{mg}}$$

Y = **2 tablets should be administered orally.**

Try another example. An order is written for 0.05 g spironolactone to be given orally. The spironolactone is available in 25 mg tablets. How many tablets would you have to give? First, you will need to convert the grams into milligrams. Remember when converting from a larger unit to a smaller unit, you will need to multiply by 1000 (see Box 5.1).

To convert 0.05 g into mg:

$$= 0.05 \times 1000\text{ mg}$$

$$= 50\text{ mg}$$

Therefore, 50 mg is the same as 0.05 g and the order has now been converted into the same unit as the available tablets. Now solve for the number of tablets that you will need.

$$\frac{25\text{ mg}}{1\text{ tablet}} = \frac{50\text{ mg}}{Y}$$

$$25\text{ mg} \times Y = 50\text{ mg} \times 1\,(\text{tablet})$$

$$Y = \frac{50\text{ mg} \times 1\text{ tablet}}{25\text{ mg}}$$

Y = **2 tablets should be administered orally**

Some tablets come with score markings that allow them to be cut. However, many tablets today come in a matrix system that allows for slow and steady release of the active drug. These drugs cannot be cut, crushed or chewed. Some drugs are enteric-coated to prevent them dissolving in the stomach, for example aspirin. In addition, neither capsules nor tablets that are designated as having delayed or sustained release should be cut. If the only way to deliver the correct dose to a patient is by cutting one of these preparations, consult the pharmacist to see if the drug is available in a smaller strength. Alternatively, a different drug or a different approach to treating the patient should be tried.

Other oral drugs come in liquid preparations. Many of the drugs used in paediatrics and for adults who might have difficulty in swallowing a pill or tablet are prepared in a liquid form. Some drugs that do not come in a standard liquid form can be prepared as a liquid by the pharmacist. If the patient is unable to swallow a tablet or capsule, check for other available forms and consult with the pharmacist about the possibility of preparing the drug in a liquid as a suspension or a solution. The same principle used to determine the number of tablets needed to arrive at a prescribed dose can be used to determine the volume of liquid that will be required to administer the prescribed dose. The ratio on the left of the equation shows the known equivalents, and the ratio on the right side contains the unknown. The phrase 'amount of drug' must appear in the numerator (top) of both ratios, and the volume to administer is the unknown (Y).

$$\frac{\text{amount of drug available}}{\text{volume available}} = \frac{\text{amount of drug prescribed}}{\text{volume to administer}}$$

Try this example: An order has been written for 200 mg ampicillin. The bottle states that the solution contains 125 mg/5 ml. How much of the liquid should you give?

$$\frac{125\,\text{mg}}{5\,\text{ml}} = \frac{200\,\text{mg}}{Y}$$

By cross-multiplying the ratio:

$$125\,\text{mg} \times Y = 200\,\text{mg} \times 5\,\text{ml}$$

Rearrange and cancel units and numbers:

$$Y = \frac{200\,\text{mg} \times 5\,\text{ml}}{125\,\text{mg}}$$

Y = **8 ml of ampicillin will be administered orally**

Tailoring Drug Doses to Individual Patients

Drug doses can be calculated using the patient's body weight, for example cytotoxic drugs used in chemotherapy. To calculate a drug dose, multiply the body weight of the patient by the drug dose required per kg body weight. For example, a patient weighing 65 kg requires a dose of 150 μg/kg:

$$\frac{\text{body}}{\text{weight}} \times \frac{\text{amount/kg}}{\text{body weight}} = \text{amount administered}$$

$$65\,\text{kg} \times 150\,\mu\text{g} = 9750\,\mu\text{g}$$

$$= \mathbf{9.75\,mg}$$

Alternatively, the dose can be calculated from the patient's **body surface area** (BSA); a more accurate representation of an individual's metabolic processes than body weight. The BSA is calculated using a **nomogram.** A nomogram uses the patient's body weight and height to calculate the BSA and is especially useful when calculating certain drug doses for paediatric patients (Figure 5.2) and patients receiving particular antineoplastic drugs. Using a ruler, a line is drawn between the patient's body weight and height – where the line crosses the central scale, this is the patient's BSA.

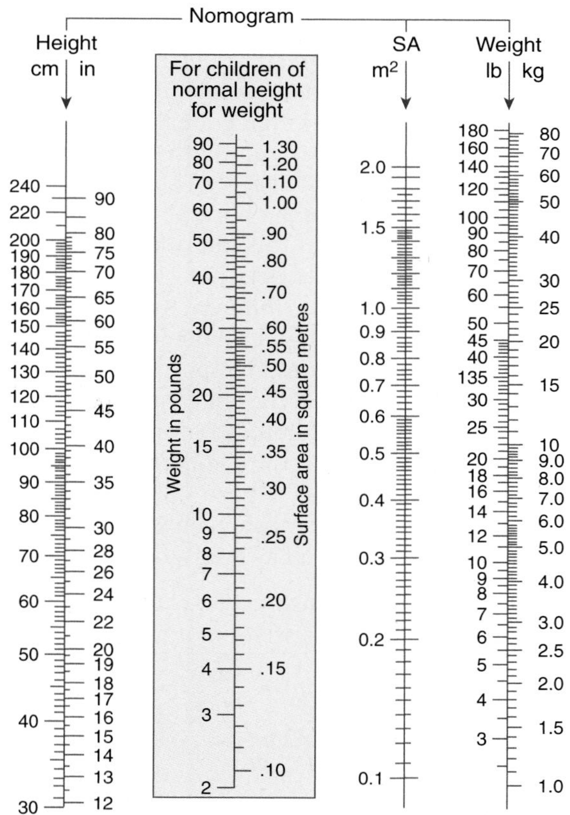

FIGURE 5.2 The West nomogram for calculating body surface area (BSA). Draw a straight line connecting the child's height (left scale) to the child's weight (right scale). The BSA value, which is calculated in square metres, is found at the point where the line intersects the SA column. Normal values are shown in the box.

Methotrexate is administered orally at a dose of 15 mg/m^2. If a patient's BSA is 2.1 m^2, what dose would you administer?

$$\frac{\text{surface}}{\text{area}} \times \frac{\text{amount/m}^2}{\text{surface area}} = \text{amount administered}$$

$$2.1\,\text{m}^2 \times 15\,\text{mg/m}^2 = \mathbf{31.5\ mg\ of\ methotrexate}$$

Practice your calculation skills regularly to make sure that you can figure out the dose of a drug to give. Periodically throughout this text you will find a 'Focus on Calculations' box to help you refresh your dosage calculation skills as they apply to the drugs being discussed.

Parenteral Drugs

All drugs administered parenterally (i.e. either by intradermal, subcutaneous, intramuscular or intravenous injection) must be administered in liquid form. The person administering the drug needs to calculate the volume of liquid that must be given to administer the prescribed dose. The same formula can be used for this determination that was used for determining the dose of an oral liquid drug:

$$\frac{\text{amount of drug available}}{\text{volume available}} = \frac{\text{amount of drug prescribed}}{\text{volume of administer}}$$

Try this example: an order has been written for 75 mg pethidine to be given intramuscularly. The vial states that it contains 1 ml of pethidine at 50 mg/ml. Set up the equation just as before:

$$\frac{50\text{ mg}}{1\text{ ml}} = \frac{75\text{ mg}}{Y}$$

$$50\text{ mg} \times Y = 75\text{ mg} \times 1\text{ ml}$$

$$Y = \frac{75\text{ mg} \times 1\text{ ml}}{50\text{ mg}}$$

Y = **1.5 ml of pethidine will be delivered by intramuscular injection**

Intravenous Solutions

Intravenous (IV) solutions are used to deliver a prescribed amount of fluid, electrolytes, vitamins, nutrients or drugs directly into the bloodstream, either as a single dose or as an infusion. Single doses can be calculated using the equations described above. For infusions, although most hospitals now use electronically monitored delivery systems, it is still important to be able to determine the amount of an IV solution that should be given using standard calculations.

Infusions can be administered under the influence of gravity or using an infusion pump. The rate of flow using a gravity-fed system will depend upon whether either a drug/clear fluid or blood/blood components are delivered: clear solutions are delivered at 20 drops/ml, blood/blood components at 15 drops/ml and paediatric giving sets (burettes) are delivered at 60 drops/ml. It is important to check these rates against the information provided with each giving set.

Information on the amount of drug to infuse and the length of time the infusion is to take are required when using the gravity-fed system.

The following equation is used to determine how many drops of fluid to deliver per minute:

$$\text{drops/minute} = \frac{\text{ml of solution prescribed per h} \times \text{drops delivered per ml}}{\text{60 min/1 h}}$$

That is, the number of drops per minute, or the rate that you will set by adjusting the valve on the IV tubing, is equal to the amount of solution that has been prescribed per hour times the number of drops delivered per millilitre (ml) divided by 60 minutes in an hour.

Try the following example: an order has been written for a patient to receive 400 ml of 5% (w/v) glucose over a period of 4 hours. Calculate how fast the delivery should be. Note that this is a clear solution and therefore should be delivered at 20 drops/ml.

Using the above equation:

$$Y = \frac{400\,\text{ml/4 h} \times 20\,\text{drops/ml}}{60\,\text{min/h}}$$

Simplify:

$$Y = \frac{100\,\text{ml/1 h} \times 20\,\text{drops/ml}}{60\,\text{min/h}}$$

$$Y = \frac{2000\,\text{drops/h}}{60\,\text{min/h}}$$

$$Y = 33.33\,\text{rep.}$$

$$= \mathbf{33\ drops/min}\ \text{(to the nearest whole number)}$$

If a patient has an order to be given an IV drug, the same principle can be used to calculate the speed of the delivery. For example, an order is written for a patient to receive 75 ml of an antibacterial over 30 min. The IV set should deliver the drug at 20 drops/ml. Calculate how fast the delivery should be.

$$Y = \frac{75\,\text{ml/0.5 h} \times 20\,\text{drops/ml}}{60\,\text{min/h}}$$

$$Y = \frac{150\,\text{ml/1 h} \times 20\,\text{drops/ml}}{60\,\text{min/h}}$$

$$Y = \frac{3000\,\text{drops/h}}{60\,\text{min/h}}$$

$$Y = \mathbf{50\ drops/min}$$

If using an infusion pump, the flow rate in ml/h must be calculated. To calculate the flow rate, the prescribed volume in ml is divided by the duration of the infusion (in hours).

$$\text{flow rate} = \frac{\text{total volume (in ml)}}{\text{duration (h)}}$$

If a volume of 500 ml is to be delivered over 4 hours, calculate the flow rate using the above equation.

$$\text{flow rate} = \frac{500\,\text{ml}}{4\,\text{h}}$$

$$\text{flow rate} = \mathbf{125\ ml/h}$$

Paediatric Considerations

For most drugs, children require dosages different from those given to adults. The 'standard' drug dosage that is listed on package inserts and in many references refers to the dose that has been found to be most effective in the adult male. A child's body may handle a drug differently in all areas of pharmacokinetics: absorption, distribution, metabolism and excretion. The responses of the child's organs to the effects of the drug may also vary because of the immaturity of the organs. Most of the time a child requires a smaller dose of a drug to achieve the comparable critical concentration. On rare occasions, a child may require a higher dose of a drug.

For ethical reasons, drug research *per se* is not done on children. Over time, however, enough information can be accumulated from experience with the drug to have a recommended paediatric dosage. The British National Formulary (BNF) used in the clinical setting will have the paediatric dose listed if this information is available. Where the dose for children is not stated, prescribers should consult the ***BNF for Children***. Sometimes there is no recommended dosage but a particular drug is needed for a child. In these situations, the appropriate dose can be determined using either (1) the child's exact body weight (as described above for adults), (2) ideal body weight for age as listed in the BNF, (3) using a nomogram specifically for infants and children (see Figure 5.2) or (4) BSA based on the adult dose. The latter approach is based on knowledge that the average BSA of a 70-kg adult is 1.8 m^2:

$$\text{approximate dose} = \frac{\text{surface area of patient in m}^2}{1.8\,\text{m}^2} \times \text{adult dose}$$

Points to Remember

- The metric system is used in drug preparation and delivery.
- The European Pharmacopoeia requires that all prescriptions include the metric measure for quantity and strength of drug. All drugs are dispensed in the metric system.

- It is important to know how to convert dosages within the metric system. The method of ratio and proportion, which uses basic principles of algebra to find an unknown, is the easiest method of converting doses within systems.
- Children require different dosages of most drugs from those of adults because of the way their bodies handle drugs and the way that drugs affect their tissues and organs.
- The dose given to a child should be calculated according to either the recommended dose for their age, their body weight or by using a nomogram to calculate their BSA.

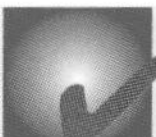

CHECK YOUR UNDERSTANDING

Answers to the questions in this chapter may be found in the answer key in the back of the book.

Multiple Choice

Select the most appropriate response to the following.

1. Digoxin 0.125 mg is ordered for a patient who is having difficulty swallowing. The bottle of digoxin elixir reads 0.05 mg/2 ml. How much would you give?
   a. 5 ml
   b. 0.5 ml
   c. 1.5 ml
   d. 1 ml

2. An order is written for 250 mg ampicillin orally. The drug is supplied in liquid form as 125 mg/5 ml. How much of the liquid should be given?
   a. 12.5 ml
   b. 10 ml
   c. 7.5 ml
   d. 5 ml

3. An order is written for 1000 ml of normal saline to be administered intravenously over 10 hours. What is the IV flow rate?
   a. 50 ml/h at 20 drops/ml
   b. 50 ml/h at 15 drops/ml
   c. 100 ml/h at 20 drops/ml
   d. 100 ml/h at 15 drops/ml

4. Capecitabine is administered orally to adults at a dose of 1.25 mg/m^2. If a patient has a surface area of 1.84 m^2, what dose of capecitabine would be needed?
   a. 230 mg
   b. 23 mg
   c. 2.3 mg
   d. 0.23 mg

5. A patient needs to take 0.75 g tetracycline orally. The drug comes in 250 mg tablets. How many tablets should the patient take?
   a. 2 tablets
   b. 3 tablets
   c. 4 tablets
   d. 30 tablets

6. Aminophylline is supplied in a 500 mg/2.5 ml solution. How much would be given if an order were written for 100 mg aminophylline IV?
   a. 5 ml
   b. 1.5 ml
   c. 2.5 ml
   d. 0.5 ml

Complete the Following Problems

1. Change to equivalents within the system:
   a. 100 mg = ______g
   b. 1500 g = ______kg
   c. 1l = ______ml
   d. 500 ml = ______l

2. Ordered: 6.5 mg. Available: 10 mg/ml. Dose administered: ______ml.

3. Ordered: 0.4 mg. Available: 1.2 mg/2 ml. Dose administered: ______ml.

4. Ordered: 80 mg. Available: 50 mg/ml. Dose administered: ______ml.

5. Ordered: 250 mg. Available: 50 mg/10 ml. Dose administered: ______ml.

Bibliography and References

British Medical Association and Royal Pharmaceutical Society of Great Britain. (2008). *British National Formulary*. London: BMJ & RPS Publishing. *This publication is updated biannually: it is imperative that the most recent edition is consulted.*

British Medical Association and Royal Pharmaceutical Society of Great Britain. (2008). *British National Formulary for Children*. London: BMJ & RPS Publishing. *This publication is updated annually: it is imperative that the most recent edition is consulted.*

Downie, G., Mackenzie, J., & Williams, A. (2006). *Calculating drug doses safely: A handbook for nurses and midwives*. London: Churchill Livingstone.

Nursing and Midwifery Council. (2008). *Standards for medicines management*. Available from http://www.nmc-uk.org/

Scott, W. N., & McGrath, D. (2009). *Dosage calculations made incredibly easy*. Philadelphia: Lippincott Williams & Wilkins.

PART II

Chemotherapeutic Agents

CHAPTER 6

Introduction to Cell Physiology

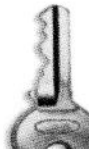

KEY TERMS

active transport
cell cycle
cytoplasm
diffusion
endocytosis
exocytosis
facilitated diffusion
lysosomes
mitochondria
nucleus
organelles
osmosis
phospholipids
plasma membrane
receptor
ribosomes
vesicular transport

LEARNING OBJECTIVES

Upon completion of this chapter, you will be able to:

1. Identify the parts of the human cell.
2. Describe the role of each organelle found within the cell cytoplasm.
3. Explain the unique properties of the plasma membrane.
4. Describe three processes used by the cell to move things across the plasma membrane.
5. Outline the cell cycle, including the activities going on within the cell in each phase.

Chemotherapeutic drugs are used to destroy both organisms that invade the body (bacteria, viruses, parasites, protozoa, fungi) and abnormal cells within the body (neoplasms, cancers). This group of drugs affect cells by (1) altering cellular function or disrupting cellular integrity, causing cell death, or (2) preventing cellular reproduction, eventually leading to cell death. To understand the actions and the adverse effects caused by chemotherapeutic agents, it is important to understand the basic functioning of the cell.

The Cell

The cell is the basic structural unit of the body. The cells that make up living organisms, which are arranged into tissues and organs, all have the same basic structure. Each cell has a nucleus (apart from red blood cells, which do not possess a nucleus), plasma membrane and cytoplasm, which contains a variety of organelles (Figure 6.1).

Cell Nucleus

The **nucleus** of a cell contains all of the genetic material necessary for cell reproduction and for regulation of cellular production of proteins. The nucleus contains genes, or sequences of deoxyribonucleic acid (DNA), that control basic cell functions. Each cell is 'programmed' by the genes for the production of specific proteins that allow the cell to carry out its function, maintain cell homeostasis or stability and promote cell division. The nucleus is surrounded by its own membrane and remains distinct from the rest of the cytoplasm. A small spherical mass, called the nucleolus, is located within the nucleus. Within this mass are dense fibres and proteins that will eventually become **ribosomes**, the site of protein synthesis within the cell.

Protein synthesis is the formation of proteins from DNA and ribonucleic acid (RNA). The first step in the process is known as *transcription* where the genetic information is transferred from DNA to messenger RNA (mRNA, a class of RNA) in the nucleus. The mRNA then passes out of the nucleus and into the cytoplasm where it becomes bound to a ribosome. The ribosome contains the enzymes and other components required for translating the mRNA code into protein.

Plasma Membrane

The cell is surrounded by a thin barrier called the **plasma membrane** separating the intracellular fluid from the extracellular fluid. The membrane is essential for cellular integrity and is equipped with many mechanisms for maintaining cell homeostasis.

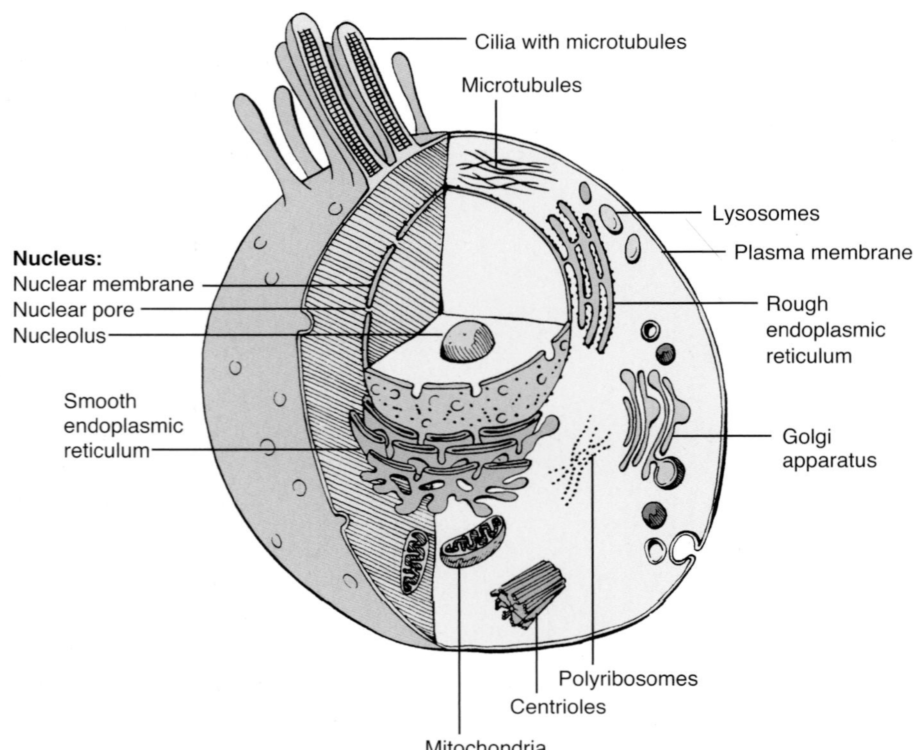

FIGURE 6.1 General structure of a cell and the location of its organelles.

Lipid Bilayer

The plasma membrane is composed of a double layer or bilayer of lipid molecules. The lipid bilayer is constructed mainly from **phospholipids**, consisting of lipids and proteins, but it also contains other lipids such as glycolipids and cholesterol. Phospholipid molecules have a polar head which is hydrophilic (water-loving) and a nonpolar tail which is hydrophobic (water-hating). These molecules line up with their polar regions pointing towards the interior or exterior of the cell and their nonpolar region lying within the plasma membrane to avoid water. These properties allow the membrane to act as a selective barrier, keeping the cytoplasm within the cell and regulating what can enter the cell (Figure 6.2).

Receptor Sites

Embedded in the lipid bilayer membrane are a series of peripheral proteins with several functions. As discussed in Chapter 2, one type of protein located on the plasma membrane is known as a **receptor**. Specific chemicals, such as hormones and chemical transmitters, outside the cell bind to these receptor proteins to stimulate a reaction within the cell. For example in skeletal muscle contraction, the neurotransmitter acetylcholine is released from neurons and binds to receptors on the muscle cell membrane, ultimately causing muscle contraction. Receptor sites are important in the functioning of all cell types and play a very important role in clinical pharmacology.

Identifying Markers

Other surface proteins are surface antigens or genetically determined identifying markers. These proteins include the major histocompatibility complex (MHC) proteins or human leukocyte antigens that the body uses to identify a cell as a self-cell (i.e. a cell belonging to that individual).

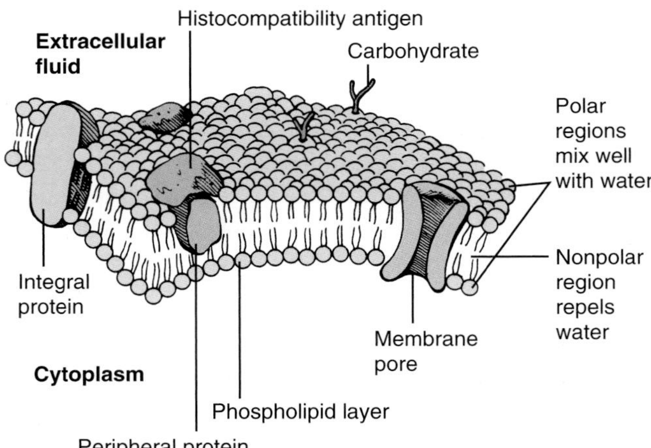

FIGURE 6.2 Structure of the lipid bilayer of the plasma membrane.

The body's immune system recognizes these proteins and acts to protect self-cells and to destroy nonself-cells. When an organ is transplanted from one person to another, every effort is made to match as many MHC proteins as possible to reduce the chance that the 'new' body rejects the transplanted organ.

Histocompatibility antigens can be changed in several ways: by cell injury, with viral invasion of a cell, with age, and so on. If the markers are altered, the body's immune system reacts to the change and can ignore it, allowing neoplasms to grow and develop. The immune system may also attack the cell, leading to many of the problems associated with autoimmune disorders and chronic inflammatory conditions.

Channels

Channels or pores within the plasma membrane are made by proteins in the plasma membrane that allow the passage of small substances in or out of the cell. Specific channels have been identified for sodium, potassium, calcium, chloride, bicarbonate, glucose and water. Other channels may also exist. Some drugs are designed to affect certain channels specifically. For example calcium channel blockers prevent the movement of calcium into a cell through calcium channels thus decreasing excitability in muscle cells. These drugs are used for cardiac arrhythmias, for example.

Cytoplasm

The cell **cytoplasm** is found within the plasma membrane. This complex area contains many **organelles** (structures with specific functions) and is the site of activities of cellular metabolism and special cellular functions. The organelles within the cytoplasm include mitochondria, endoplasmic reticulum (ER), free ribosomes, Golgi apparatus and lysosomes.

Mitochondria

The **mitochondria** are membrane-bound organelles within each cell that produce energy in the form of adenosine triphosphate (ATP), allowing the cell to carry out essential processes. The mitochondria can take carbohydrates, fats and proteins from the cytoplasm and make ATP via the Krebs cycle, which depends on oxygen. Cells use the ATP to maintain homeostasis, produce proteins and carry out specific functions. If oxygen is not available, lactic acid builds up as a by-product of cellular respiration. Lactic acid leaves the cell and is transported to the liver for conversion into glycogen and carbon dioxide.

Mitochondria are abundant in cell types that are very active and consume energy. For example, cardiac muscle cells, which must work continuously to keep the heart contracting, contain a large number of mitochondria. Mitochondria can also reproduce if the level of activity within a cell changes.

Milk-producing cells in breast tissue, which are normally quite dormant, contain very few mitochondria. However, if a woman is lactating, the mitochondria become more abundant to meet the demands of the milk-producing cells.

Endoplasmic Reticulum

Much of the cytoplasm of a cell is made up of a fine network of interconnected tubes which forms the ER. There are two types of ER: rough ER and smooth ER. The rough ER is continuous with the nuclear membrane, and the external surface is studded with the ribosomes responsible for the production of proteins. Other free-floating ribosomes exist throughout the cytoplasm and produce proteins that are important to the structure of the cell and some of the enzymes necessary for cellular activity. The rough ER is also responsible for the manufacture of the phospholipids and proteins that make up the plasma membranes.

The smooth ER is continuous with the rough ER. Integrated into the membrane of the smooth ER are enzyme molecules important in a number of reactions including the metabolism of lipids, synthesis of steroid hormones and the detoxification of drugs.

Golgi Apparatus

The Golgi apparatus is a series of flattened sacs whose major function is to process and package the proteins and lipids manufactured by the rough ER into vesicles for transport to the plasma membrane and excretion from the cell. In addition, the Golgi apparatus also packages digestive enzymes into lysosomes until they are needed.

Lysosomes

Lysosomes are membrane-covered organelles that contain specific digestive enzymes that can break down proteins, nucleic acids, carbohydrates and lipids. These organelles form a membrane around any substance that needs to be digested and secrete digestive enzymes directly into the isolated area, protecting the rest of the cell from injury. The lysosomes are responsible for digesting worn or damaged sections of a cell, which they accomplish by encapsulating the area and self-digesting it. If a cell dies and the membrane ruptures, the release of lysosomes causes the cell to self-destruct. Cells which carry out phagocytosis (the destruction of viruses and bacteria) have large numbers of lysosomes.

Homeostasis

The main goal of a cell is to maintain homeostasis, which means keeping the cytoplasm stable within the plasma membrane. Every cell is bathed in an extracellular fluid known as the interstitial fluid (fluid surrounding the cells). The interstitial fluid is derived from blood and contains a range of components including sugars, amino acids, vitamins, neurotransmitters and waste products. Each cell takes what they require in order to stay alive. For a cell to produce the energy needed to carry out cellular metabolism and other processes, the cell must have the means of obtaining necessary elements from the interstitial fluid. In addition, it must have a way of disposing of waste products that could be toxic to its cytoplasm.

The plasma membrane is selectively permeable, that is allows some molecules to cross the membrane (e.g. those which are lipid-soluble), but not others; therefore, a number of different mechanisms exist by which molecules can cross the membrane using (1) passive transport, (2) active (energy-requiring) transport and (3) vesicular transport.

Passive Transport

Passive transport happens without the expenditure of energy and can occur across any semipermeable membrane. There are four types of passive transport: diffusion, facilitated diffusion, osmosis and filtration.

Diffusion

Diffusion is the movement of a substance from a region of higher concentration to a region of lower concentration. The difference between the concentrations of the substance in the two regions is called the *concentration gradient* of the substance. The greater the concentration gradient, the faster the substance moves. Small lipid-soluble substances and materials with no ionic charge move most freely across the membrane. Lipid-soluble substances such as oxygen, carbon dioxide and fats diffuse directly through the lipid portion of the membrane. Other substances, for example the ions sodium and potassium, move through channels or pores in the plasma membrane (Figure 6.3).

Some molecules, for example glucose, are too large to pass through the channels and are too polar (charged) to dissolve into the lipid bilayer. These molecules attach to a protein molecule, called a transporter, to diffuse across the membrane. This form of diffusion is known as **facilitated diffusion**. There are a finite number of carriers present in the cell membrane; therefore, the number of molecules that can be transported will be limited by the number of carriers in the membrane.

Osmosis

Osmosis, a special form of diffusion, is the movement of a solvent, for example water, across a semipermeable membrane from an area that is low in dissolved solutes (i.e. ions) to one that is high in dissolved solutes. The water attempts to equalize the dilution of the solutes. This diffusion of water across a plasma membrane from an area of high concentration (of water) to an area of low concentration (of water) creates pressure on the plasma membrane, called *osmotic pressure*. The greater the concentration of solutes in the solution to which the water is flowing, the higher the osmotic pressure.

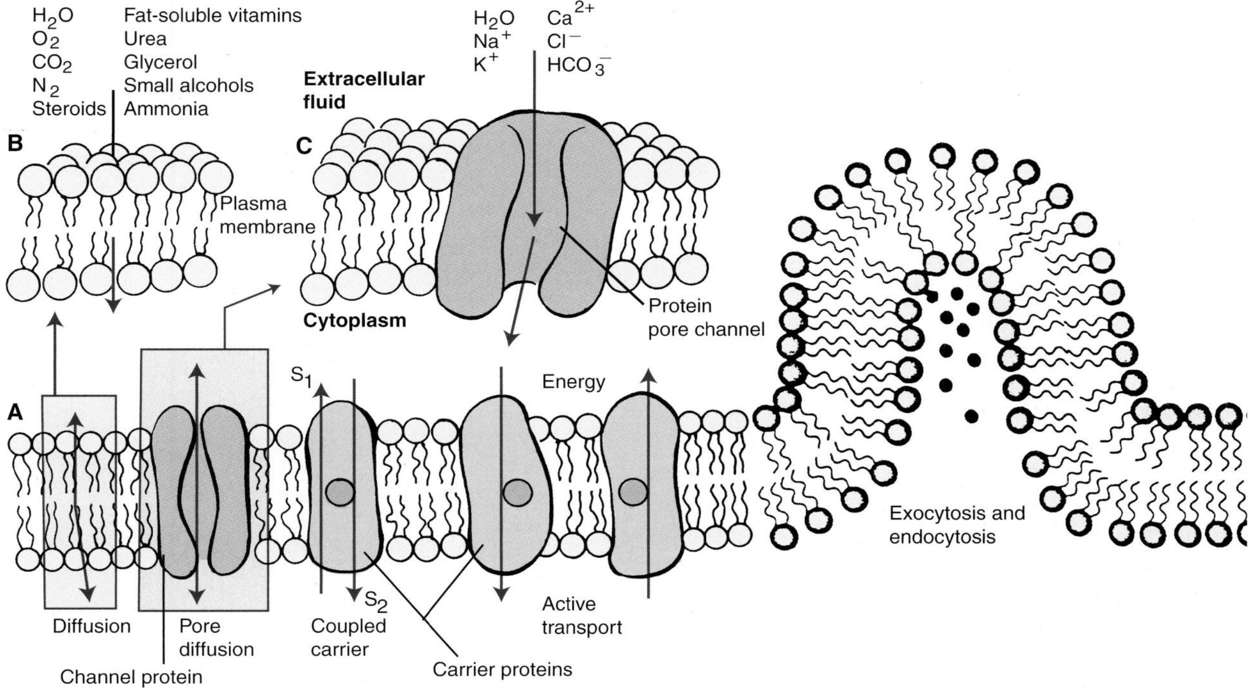

FIGURE 6.3 Schematic representation of transport across a cell membrane **(A)**, which includes *diffusion* through the cell membrane **(B)** and *pore diffusion* through a protein channel **(C)**.

A fluid that contains the same concentration of solutes as human plasma is called an *isotonic* solution. A fluid that contains a higher concentration of solutes than human plasma is a *hypertonic* solution, and it draws water from cells. A fluid that contains a lower concentration of solutes than human plasma is *hypotonic*; it causes water to move into cells. If a human red blood cell, which has a cytoplasm that is isotonic with human plasma, is placed into a hypertonic solution, it shrinks and shrivels because the water inside the cell diffuses out of the cell into the solution. If the same cell is placed into a hypotonic solution, the cell swells and bursts because water moves from the solution into the cell (Figure 6.4).

Filtration

Filtration is also a passive process and combines diffusion and osmosis; however, with filtration there is a pressure gradient for diffusion rather than a concentration gradient. In filtration, the pressure gradient pushes a solute-containing fluid (or filtrate) from a higher pressure area to a lower pressure area. A typical example of filtration is in the kidney, where filtration provides the fluid excreted as urine.

Active Transport

When a substance (molecule) is too large to pass through channels, incapable of dissolving into the lipid membrane or unable to move down the concentration gradient, the cell must use energy in the form of ATP to transport the molecule across the membrane. The two major mechanisms of active membrane transport are **active transport** and **vesicular transport**. When a cell is deprived of oxygen because of a blood supply problem or insufficient oxygenation of the blood, systems of active transport begin to fail, placing the cell's integrity in jeopardy.

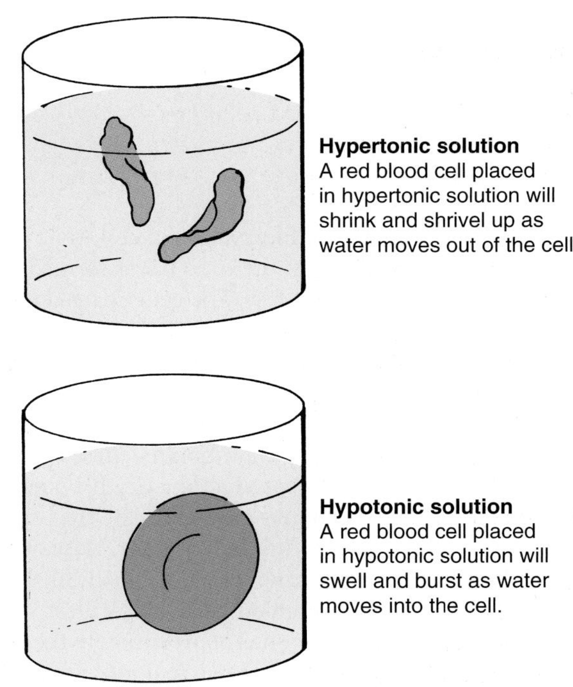

FIGURE 6.4 Red blood cell response to hypertonic and hypotonic solutions.

One of the best known systems of active transport is the sodium–potassium (Na^+/K^+-ATPase) pump. Cells use active transport to maintain higher levels of potassium in the cytoplasm compared with the extracellular fluid and higher levels of sodium in the extracellular fluid compared with the cytoplasm. This allows the cell to maintain an electrical charge on the plasma membrane, causing cells to have a charge across their plasma membrane. Some drugs use energy to move into cells by active transport. Drugs are frequently bonded with a carrier when they are moved into the cell. Cells in the kidney use active transport to excrete drugs from the body as well as to maintain electrolyte and acid–base balance.

Vesicular Transport

Vesicular transport uses vesicles to transport molecules across the membrane. **Endocytosis** uses vesicles to incorporate material into the plasma. Here the plasma membrane gradually engulfs the molecule to be transported until a vesicle is formed. The vesicle is then pinched off and moves into the cytoplasm where the contents are digested.

Receptor-mediated endocytosis, a form of endocytosis, refers to the engulfing of specific substances that have bound to a receptor site on the plasma membrane. This process allows cells to absorb nutrients, enzymes and other materials. Phagocytosis is a similar process allowing the cells such as neutrophils and macrophages, to engulf a bacterium or a foreign protein and destroy it within the cell using the digestive enzymes in the lysosome.

Exocytosis is the opposite of endocytosis. This property allows a cell to move a substance to the plasma membrane and then secrete the substance outside the cell. Hormones, neurotransmitters, enzymes and other substances that are produced within a cell are excreted from the cell by this process (Figure 6.5).

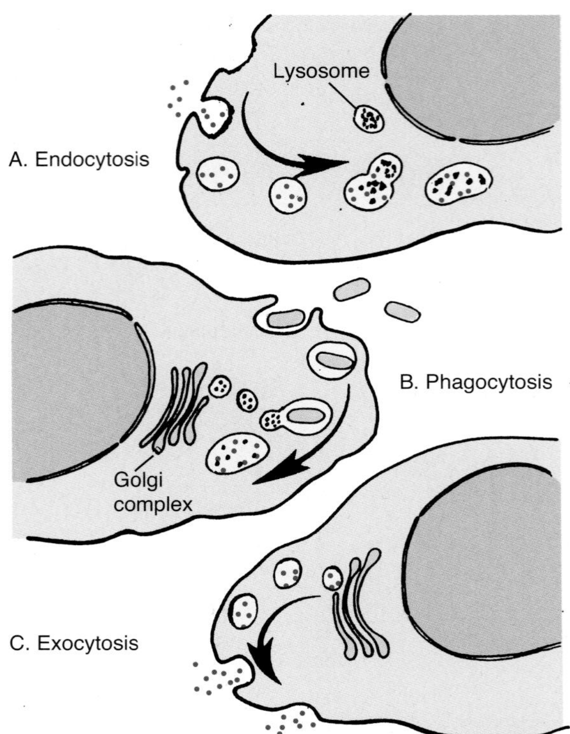

FIGURE 6.5 Schematic representation of endocytosis and exocytosis. Endocytosis **(A)** is the movement of nutrients and needed substances into the cell through specific receptors on the cell surface. Phagocytosis **(B)** involves the destruction of engulfed proteins or bacteria. Exocytosis **(C)** is the movement of substances (waste products, hormones, neurotransmitters) out of the cell.

Cell Cycle

The **cell cycle** relates to the life cycle of a cell, that is the changes a cell undergoes from the time it was formed until the time it reproduces (Figure 6.6). The genetic makeup of a particular cell determines the rate at which that cell can multiply. Some cells reproduce very quickly (e.g. the cells lining the gastrointestinal tract have a generation time of 72 hours), and some reproduce very slowly (e.g. the cells found in breast tissue with a generation time of a few months). In some cases, certain factors influence cell reproduction. Erythropoietin, a hormone produced by the kidney, can stimulate the production of new red blood cells. Active leukocytes release chemicals that stimulate the production of white blood cells when the body needs more white blood cells. Regardless of the rate of reproduction, each cell has approximately the same life cycle. The cell cycle consists of two major phases: interphase when the cell grows and performs its routine activities, and the mitotic phase (M) when the cell divides.

Interphase is the time from cell formation to cell division and represents the preparations the cell undertakes prior to **mitosis**, the production of two identical daughter cells. Interphase is divided into the subphases G_1, S and G_2 (where

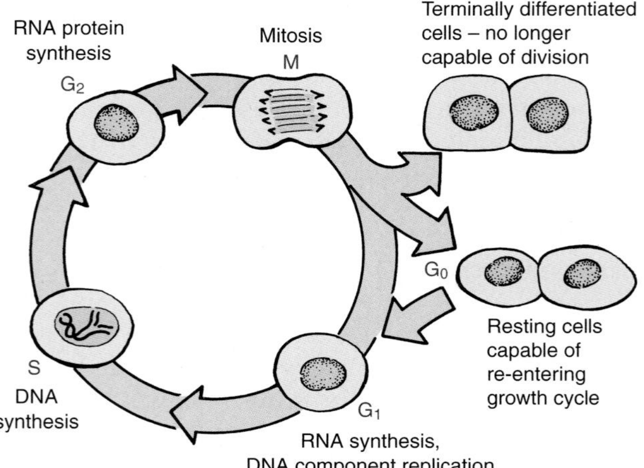

FIGURE 6.6 Diagram of the cell cycle, showing G_0, G_1, S, G_2 and M phases.

G refers to gaps or growth). In the G_1 phase the cells are actively synthesizing new proteins and undergoing a period of rapid growth. It is the length of this phase that varies widely between cell types (see above). As the cells reach the end of G_1, the cells are prepared for cell division and have synthesized the substances required for DNA replication.

The next phase is the S (synthetic) phase where the DNA replicates ensuring that the two new cells, or daughter cells, formed after cell division, will contain identical copies of the genetic material of the parent cell. After the cellular DNA has doubled in preparation for replication, the G_2 phase begins. During this phase, the cell produces all the substances that are required for cell division such as the mitotic spindles.

After the cell has produced all the substances necessary for the formation of new daughter cells, it undergoes cell division. This occurs during the M phase of the cell cycle where the cell divides to form two identical daughter cells. Cells that are not actively dividing are said to be in the G_0 phase. These cells can re-enter the cell cycle in response to extracellular signals such as growth factors and hormones.

A basic understanding of the steps involved in the cell cycle is important in the targeted use of antineoplastic agents to treat cancerous cells which divide continuously and uncontrollably. Many of the antineoplastic agents target specific stages of the life cycle, for example during the S phase when the DNA material is replicated or in cell division in M phase.

Clinical Significance of Cell Physiology

Knowledge of the basic structure and function of the cell may help in understanding the therapeutic and toxic effects of the various classes of chemotherapeutic agents. Drugs may alter the plasma membrane, causing the cell to rupture and die. Alternatively, drugs may deprive the cell of certain nutrients, altering the proteins that the cell produces and interfering with normal cell functioning and cell division (e.g. some antineoplastic agents target specific stages of the cell cycle). Because most chemotherapeutic agents do not possess complete selective toxicity (the ability to target particular cells, for example bacteria and not human cells), they also affect the normal cells of patients to some extent.

Points to Remember

- The cell is the basic structural unit of all living organisms.
- The cell is composed of a nucleus (with the exception of red blood cells) which contains genetic material and controls the production of proteins by the cell; a cytoplasm, which contains various organelles important to cell function; and a plasma membrane, which separates the inside of the cell from the outside environment.
- The plasma membrane functions as a fluid barrier made of lipids and proteins. The arrangement of the lipoprotein membrane controls what enters and leaves the cell.
- Proteins on the plasma membrane surface can act either as receptor sites for specific substances or as histocompatibility markers that identify the cell as a self-cell.
- Channels or pores in the plasma membrane allow for easier movement of specific substances needed by the cell for normal functioning.
- Mitochondria are membrane-bound organelles that produce energy in the form of ATP for use by cells.
- Ribosomes are sites of protein synthesis within the cell cytoplasm. The specific proteins produced by a cell are determined by the genetic material within the cell nucleus.
- The Golgi apparatus packages particular substances for removal from the cell (e.g. hormones, enzymes).
- Lysosomes are membrane-bound packets of digestive enzymes located in the cell cytoplasm. These enzymes are responsible for destroying injured or nonfunctioning parts of the cell, invading micro-organisms and for cellular disintegration when the cell dies.
- Cells maintain homeostasis by regulating the movement of solutes and water into and out of the cell.
- Diffusion, which does not require energy, is the movement of solutes from a region of high concentration to a region of lower concentration across a concentration gradient.
- Osmosis, which like diffusion, does not require energy, is the movement of water from an area low in solutes to an area high in solutes. Osmosis exerts a pressure against the plasma membrane that is called osmotic pressure.
- Active transport, an energy-requiring process, is the movement of particular substances against a concentration gradient, that is from an area of low concentration to an area of high concentration. Active transport is important in maintaining cell homeostasis.
- Endocytosis is the process of moving substances into a cell by extending the plasma membrane around the substance and engulfing it. Receptor-mediated endocytosis refers to the engulfing of necessary materials, and phagocytosis refers to the engulfing and destroying of bacteria or other proteins by white blood cells.
- Exocytosis is the process of removing substances from a cell by moving them towards the plasma membrane and then changing the plasma membrane to allow passage of the substance out of the cell.
- Cells replicate at differing rates depending on the genetic programming of the cell. All cells go through a

life cycle consisting of the following phases: G_1, which involves the production of proteins for DNA replication; S, which involves the replication of DNA; G_2, which involves manufacture of the materials needed for mitotic spindle production; and M, the mitotic phase, in which the cell splits to form two identical daughter cells. G_0 is the resting phase before the cells enter mitosis.

- Chemotherapeutic drugs act on cells to cause cell death or alteration. All properties of the drug that affect cells should be considered when administering a chemotherapeutic agent.

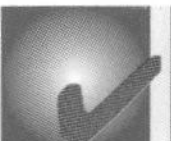

CHECK YOUR UNDERSTANDING

Multiple Choice

Answers to the questions in this chapter may be found in the answer key in the back of the book.

Select the best answer to the following.

1. The basic unit of human structure is the
   a. mitochondria.
   b. nucleus.
   c. nucleolus.
   d. cell.

2. The plasma membrane is composed of
   a. a phospholipid structure.
   b. channels of protein.
   c. a cholesterol-based membrane.
   d. Golgi apparatus

3. The ribosomes are important sites for
   a. digestion of nutrients.
   b. excretion of waste products.
   c. production of proteins.
   d. hormone receptors.

4. A human cell placed in sea water will
   a. burst from water entering the cell.
   b. shrivel and die from water leaving the cell.
   c. not be affected in any way.
   d. break apart from the salt effect.

5. The sodium–potassium pump maintains a negative charge on the plasma membrane by
   a. osmosis.
   b. diffusion.
   c. active transport.
   d. facilitated diffusion.

6. Most cells progress through basically the same cell cycle, including
   a. two phases.
   b. four active phases and a rest phase.
   c. three periods of rest and a dividing phase.
   d. four active phases.

Extended Matching Questions

Select all that apply.

1. The amount of time that a cell takes to progress through the cell cycle is determined by which of the following?
   a. The acidity of the environment
   b. The genetic makeup of the cell
   c. The location of the cell in the body
   d. The number of ribosomes in the cell
   e. The cell response to contact inhibition
   f. The availability of nutrients and oxygen

2. Some substances will pass into the human cell by simple diffusion. Which of the following substances diffuse into the cell?
   a. Calcium
   b. Nitrogen
   c. Sodium
   d. Carbon dioxide
   e. Oxygen
   f. Potassium

3. Some substances require a channel or pore to enter the plasma membrane. Which of the following substances use a channel to enter the cell?
   a. Calcium
   b. Urea
   c. Fat-soluble vitamins
   d. Sodium
   e. Oxygen
   f. Potassium

Matching

Match the phase of the cell cycle with the cell activity during that phase.

1. ________________ G_0 phase
2. ________________ G_1 phase
3. ________________ S phase

4. ________________________ G_2 phase
5. ________________________ M phase

A. Cell splits to form two identical daughter cells
B. Synthesis of DNA
C. Manufacture of substances needed to form mitotic spindles
D. Synthesis of substances needed for DNA production
E. Cells that have ceased dividing

Bibliography

Ganong, W. (2005). *Review of medical physiology* (22nd ed.). New York: McGraw-Hill.
Guyton, A., & Hall, J. (2005). *Textbook of medical physiology* (11th ed.). Philadelphia: W. B. Saunders.
Marieb, E. N., & Hoehn, K. (2009). *Human anatomy & histology* (8th ed.). San Francisco: Pearson.
Porth, C. M., & Matfin, G. (2008). *Pathophysiology: Concepts of altered health states* (8th ed.). Philadelphia: Lippincott Williams & Wilkins.

CHAPTER 7

Antimicrobial Agents

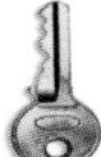

KEY TERMS

culture
normal flora
prophylaxis
resistance
sensitivity testing
spectrum
superinfection

LEARNING OBJECTIVES

Upon completion of this chapter, you will be able to:

1. Explain what is meant by selective toxicity.
2. Differentiate between broad-spectrum and narrow-spectrum drugs.
3. Define bacterial resistance to antibacterials.
4. Explain three ways to minimize bacterial resistance.
5. Describe three common adverse reactions associated with the use of antimicrobials.

Antimicrobial agents are drugs that are designed to act selectively on foreign organisms that have invaded and infected a host. Ideally, these drugs would *only* be toxic to the infecting organisms and would have no effect on the host cells. In other words, they would possess selective toxicity – the ability to affect certain proteins or enzyme systems that are used by the infecting organism but not by human cells. Although human cells are different from the cells of invading organisms, some aspects are similar and no antimicrobial drug has yet been developed that does not affect the host in some way.

This chapter focuses on the principles involved in the use of antimicrobial therapy. The following chapters discuss specific drug categories used to treat particular infections:

- antibacterials to treat bacterial infections;
- antivirals to treat viral infections;
- antifungals to treat fungal infections;
- antiprotozoals to treat infections caused by specific protozoa, including malaria;
- anthelmintics to treat infections caused by worms.

Antimicrobial Therapy

For centuries, people used various naturally occurring chemicals to treat disease. Often this was a random act that proved beneficial. For instance, the ancient Chinese found that applying mouldy soybean curds to boils and infected wounds helped eliminate infection or promote healing. Their use of moulds was a precursor to the use of penicillins today.

The use of drugs to treat systemic infections is a relatively new concept. The first drugs used to treat systemic infections were developed in the 1920s. Paul Ehrlich was the first scientist to work on developing a synthetic chemical that would be effective only against infection-causing cells, not human cells. His research led the way for scientific investigation into antibacterial agents. In the late 1920s, Alexander Fleming discovered penicillin in a mould sample; and in 1935, the sulphonamides were introduced. Since then, the number of antibacterials available for use has grown significantly. However, many of the organisms that these drugs were designed to treat are rapidly learning to resist the actions of antibacterials and other antimicrobial agents, so much work remains to deal with these emergent strains.

Mechanisms of Action

Antimicrobial agents may act on the cells of the invading organisms in several different ways. Their goal is interference with the normal function of the invading organism to prevent it from reproducing and to cause cell death without affecting host cells. Various mechanisms of action are briefly described here. The specific mechanism of action for each drug class is discussed in the chapters that follow.

- Some antibacterials interfere with biosynthesis of the bacterial cell wall. For example, penicillins inhibit bacterial cell wall synthesis causing the bacteria to lyse. The penicillins exhibit selective toxicity because human cells do not have cell walls.
- Many antibacterials interfere with the steps involved in protein synthesis, a necessary function to maintain the cell and allow for cell division. The aminoglycosides, macrolides and chloramphenicol work in this way.
- Some antimicrobials prevent the micro-organisms from using substances essential to their growth and development, leading to an inability to divide and eventually to cell death. The sulphonamides, antituberculosis drugs and trimethoprim work in this way.
- Some antimicrobials interfere with DNA synthesis in the cell, leading to an inability to divide and cell death. The quinolones work in this way.
- Other antimicrobials alter the permeability of the cell membrane to allow essential cellular components to leak out, causing cell death. Some antibiotics, antifungals and antiprotozoal drugs work in this manner. These different methods appear in Figure 7.1.

Human Immune Response

The immune response (see Chapter 14) involves a complex interaction between chemical mediators, leukocytes, lymphocytes, antibodies and locally released enzymes and chemicals to manage invading organisms. However, if a person is immunocompromised for any reason (e.g. malnutrition, age, acquired immune deficiency syndrome [AIDS], diseases such as leukaemia, use of immunosuppressant drugs), the immune system may be incapable of dealing effectively with the invading organisms. It is difficult to treat any infection in such patients because these patients do not have the immune response in place to deal with even a few invading organisms. Immunocompromised patients present a real challenge to health care providers. In helping these people cope with infections, prevention of infection and proper nutrition are often as important as drug therapy.

Resistance

As antimicrobials act on specific enzyme systems or biological processes, many micro-organisms that do not use that system or process are not affected by a particular antimicrobial drug. These organisms are said to have a natural or intrinsic **resistance** to that drug. When prescribing a drug for treatment of an infection, this innate resistance should be anticipated. The selected drug should be one that is known to affect the specific micro-organism that is causing the infection.

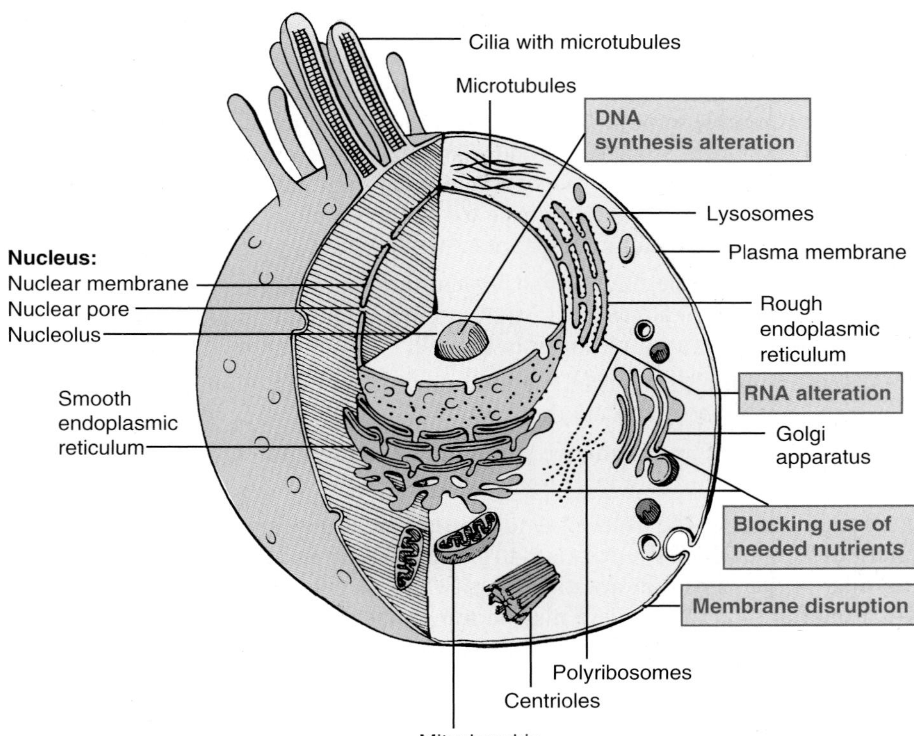

FIGURE 7.1 Antimicrobials can affect cells by disrupting the p membrane, interfering with DNA synthesis, altering RNA, or blocking the use of essential nutrients.

Since the introduction of antimicrobial drugs, micro-organisms that were once very sensitive to the effects of particular drugs have begun to develop acquired resistance to these drugs (Box 7.1). This can result in a serious clinical problem. The emergence of resistant strains of bacteria and other organisms poses a threat: antimicrobial drugs may no longer control potentially life-threatening diseases and uncontrollable epidemics may occur.

Acquiring Resistance

Micro-organisms develop resistance in a number of ways, and once having developed genes for resistance can then

BOX 7.1 Bacterial Resistance to Antibacterial Agents

Staphylococcus aureus (*S. aureus*) is one of the types of bacteria found on skin and mucosa linings. These bacteria are only problematic on entry to the body, for example via a wound, urinary catheters or intravenous (IV) lines. The bacteria can then lead to wound infections, urinary tract infections, septicaemia and even death. Many strains of *S. aureus* are sensitive to a number of different antibacterials; however, some strains are resistant to the antibacterial, meticillin. This strain is known as meticillin-resistant *S. aureus* or MRSA and is of concern to the National Health Service. MRSA infections can spread rapidly among older patients, those with open wounds or immunocompromised patients. A number of initiatives to reduce the spread of MRSA among hospital patients are now in place, including the 'clean **your** hands' campaign established in 2004 by the National Patient Safety Agency. This campaign has been adopted by all National Health Service acute trusts and primary care, mental health and ambulance trusts.

Of great concern is that the MRSA strain is now becoming resistant to other antibacterials. Depending on the nature of the infection, for example urinary tract or soft tissue infection, or septicaemia; there are some antibacterials that can successfully eradicate the infection. Vancomycin, a glycopeptide antibiotic, is one used if the infection is resistant to other antibacterials. However, there are reports on some strains exhibiting resistance to vancomycin.

Clostridium difficile bacteria reside in the colon of approximately 5% of healthy adults and up to 20% of elderly patients in long-term care. Normally the bacteria do not cause any disturbance to health but in some patients who have been treated with a broad-spectrum antibacterial, the normal colonic flora is disrupted allowing *C. difficile* to multiply and release inflammatory toxins. These toxins cause pseudomembranous colitis, characterized by inflammation of the mucosal lining of the colon and diarrhoea. Some debilitated patients who have not been treated with an antibacterial are also susceptible.

C. difficile is transmitted by the faecal–oral route and is usually acquired in a hospital or residential care setting. Between July and September 2008 there were 7061 cases recorded in patients aged 65 years and above (Health Protection Agency, 2008). The Department of Health has set the National Health Service the target of reducing *C. difficile* rates by 30% by 2010/2011. However, *C. difficile* is also becoming more resistant to antibacterials including penicillin, imipenem and metronidazole (Health Protection Agency, 2008) making the infection increasingly difficult to manage.

transfer these genes to other bacteria. Mechanisms of resistance include the following:

- Producing an enzyme that deactivates the antimicrobial drug; for example some strains of bacteria that were once controlled by penicillin now produce an enzyme called penicillinase, which inactivates penicillin before it can affect the bacteria. This occurrence led to the development of new drugs that are resistant to penicillinase.
- Changing cellular permeability to prevent the drug from entering the cell or altering transport systems to exclude the drug from active transport into the cell.
- Altering binding sites on cell membranes or ribosomes, which then no longer accept the drug.
- Development of an alternative pathway to the one the antimicrobial drug uses as a target.

Most commonly, the development of resistance depends on the degree to which the drug acts to eliminate the invading micro-organisms that are most sensitive to its effects. The bacterial cells that remain may be somewhat innately resistant to the effects of the drug and, with time, these cells can form the majority in the population. These cells differ from the general population of the species because of slight variations in their biochemical processes. The drug does not cause a mutation of these cells; it simply allows the somewhat different cells to become the majority or dominant group after elimination of the sensitive cells. Other microbes may develop resistance through actual genetic mutation: a mutant cell survives the effects of an antibacterial and divides, forming a new colony of resistant microbes with a genetic composition that provides resistance to the antibacterial agent. Drug resistance is commonly spread through the sharing of resistance genes between bacteria.

Preventing Resistance

The emergence of resistant strains of micro-organisms is an increasingly serious public health problem and health care providers must work together to prevent the emergence of resistant pathogens. Exposure to an antimicrobial agent can lead to the development of resistance, so it is important to limit the use of antimicrobial agents for the treatment of specific pathogens known to be sensitive to the drug being used.

Drug dosage is important in preventing the development of resistance. Doses should be high enough and the duration of drug therapy should be long enough to eradicate even slightly resistant micro-organisms. The recommended dosage for a specific antimicrobial agent takes this issue into account. Around-the-clock dosing eliminates the peaks and troughs in drug concentration and helps maintain a constant therapeutic level to prevent the emergence of resistant microbes during times of low concentration. The duration of drug use is critical to ensure that the micro-organisms are completely, not partially, eliminated and are not given the chance to grow and develop resistant strains. Many people stop taking a drug once they start to feel better and then keep the remaining tablets or medicine to treat themselves at some time in the future when they do not feel well. This practice favours the emergence of resistant strains. See Box 7.2 for tips on patient education.

> **BOX 7.2** FOCUS ON **CLINICAL SKILLS**
>
> ***Teaching Patients***
>
> When teaching patients who are prescribed an antimicrobial agent, it is important to always include some general points:
>
> - This drug is prescribed for treating the particular infection that you have now. Do not use this drug to treat other infections.
> - This drug needs to be taken as prescribed – for the correct number of times each day and for the full number of days. Do not stop taking the drug even if you start to feel better. You must take the drug for the full number of treatment days to assure that the infection has cleared.

Health care providers should also be cautious about the indiscriminate use of antimicrobials. Antibacterials are not effective in the treatment of viral infections or illnesses such as the common cold. However, many patients demand prescriptions for these drugs when they visit practitioners because they are convinced that they need to take something to get better. Health care providers who prescribe antibacterials without knowing the causative organism and which drugs might be appropriate are promoting the emergence of resistant strains of micro-organisms. With many serious illnesses, including pneumonias for which the causative organism is suspected, antibacterial therapy may be started as soon as a culture is taken and before the results are known. Health care providers also tend to try newly introduced, more powerful drugs when a more established drug may be just as effective. Use of a powerful drug in this way leads to the rapid emergence of resistant strains to that drug, perhaps limiting its potential usefulness when it might be truly necessary.

Treatment of Systemic Infections

Many infections that once led to lengthy, organ-damaging, or even fatal illnesses are now managed quickly and efficiently with the use of systemic antimicrobial agents. Before the introduction of penicillin to treat streptococcal infections, many people developed rheumatic fever with serious cardiac complications. Today, rheumatic fever and the resultant cardiac valve defects are seen less frequently. Several factors should be considered before beginning one of these chemotherapeutic regimens to ensure that the patient obtains the greatest benefit possible with the fewest adverse effects. These factors include identification of the correct pathogen and selection of a drug that is most likely to (1) cause the least complications for that particular patient and (2) be most effective against the pathogen involved.

Identification of the Pathogen

Identification of the infecting pathogen is achieved by **culture** and **sensitivity testing** of a sample from the infected area. Bacterial cultures are performed in a laboratory, where a swab of infected tissue is allowed to grow on an agar plate. Staining and other techniques and microscopic examination are used to identify the offending organisms. When investigators search for parasitic sources of infection, blood and stool samples can be examined for ova and parasites. Microscopic examination of other samples is also used to detect fungal and protozoal infections. The correct identification of the organism causing the infection is an important first step in determining which antimicrobial drug should be used.

Sensitivity of the Pathogen

Antimicrobials are either described as broad or narrow **spectrum** agents. Broad spectrum agents are effective against a wide range of micro-organisms whereas narrow spectrum agents are only effective against specific micro-organisms. In many situations, health care providers use a broad-spectrum antimicrobial agent that is most likely to be effective in treating an infection with certain presenting signs and symptoms. In other cases of severe infection, a broad-spectrum antibacterial is started after a culture is taken but before the exact causative organism has been identified. Again, experience influences selection of the drug, based on the presenting signs and symptoms. In many cases, it is necessary to perform sensitivity testing on the cultured microbes. Sensitivity testing shows which drugs are capable of controlling the particular micro-organism. This testing is especially important with micro-organisms that have known resistant strains. In these cases, culture and sensitivity testing identify the causal pathogen and the most appropriate drug for treating the infection.

Combination Therapy

In some situations, a combination of two or more types of drugs effectively treats the infection. When the offending pathogen is known, combination drugs may be effective in interfering with its cellular structure in different areas or developmental phases.

Combination therapy may be used for several reasons:

- Combination therapy may allow the health care provider to use a smaller dosage of each drug, leading to fewer adverse effects but still having a therapeutic impact on the pathogen.
- Some drugs are synergistic, which means that they are more powerful when given in combination than when used alone.
- Many microbial infections are caused by more than one organism, and each pathogen may react to a different antimicrobial agent.
- Sometimes, the combined effects of the different drugs delay the emergence of resistant strains. This is important in the treatment of tuberculosis (a mycobacterial infection), malaria (a protozoal infection), HIV (a viral infection) and some bacterial infections. However, resistant strains seem more likely to emerge when fixed combinations are used over time, at least in some cases. Individualizing the combination seems to be more effective in destroying the pathogen without allowing time for the emergence of strains that are resistant to the drugs. The effectiveness of multiple drug therapy is reliant upon the patient taking the combination of drugs at the correct times and dosages for extended periods, otherwise resistance can develop.

Adverse Reactions to Antimicrobial Therapy

Because antimicrobial agents affect invading micro-organisms, it is always possible that the host cells will also be damaged (Box 7.3). The most commonly encountered adverse effects associated with the use of antimicrobial agents are direct toxic effects on the kidney, gastrointestinal (GI) tract and nervous system. Hypersensitivity reactions and superinfections can also occur.

Kidney Damage

Kidney damage occurs most frequently with antimicrobial drugs that are metabolized by the kidney and then eliminated in the urine. Such drugs, which have a direct toxic effect on

BOX 7.3 Serious Adverse Effects of Antimicrobial Treatment

Chloramphenicol, a potent broad-spectrum antibacterial, inhibits bacterial protein synthesis in susceptible bacteria. There are a number of potential toxic side-effects associated with chloramphenicol; therefore its use is limited to life-threatening infections for which no other antibacterial is effective. Chloramphenicol produces 'grey syndrome' in neonates and premature babies, which is characterized by abdominal distension, pallid cyanosis, irregular respirations, circulatory collapse and even death. In addition, the drug may cause bone marrow depression, including aplastic anaemia that can result in death. These effects are not seen with use of the ophthalmic and otic forms of the drug. Although the use of chloramphenicol is limited, it has stayed in use to treat serious infections caused by bacteria that are not sensitive to any other antibacterial agent. It is available in oral, IV, ophthalmic and otic forms.

BOX 7.4 Severe Gastrointestinal Toxicity Resulting From Antimicrobial Treatment

Meropenem, an IV antibacterial, inhibits the synthesis of bacterial cell walls in susceptible bacteria. It is used to treat intra-abdominal infections and some cases of meningitis caused by susceptible bacteria. Meropenem almost always causes very uncomfortable GI effects; and use of this drug has been associated with pseudomembranous colitis. It also results in headache, rash and other hypersensitivity reactions and superinfections. It is used only in those infections with proven sensitivity to meropenem and reduced sensitivity to less toxic antibiotics.

the fragile cells in the kidney, can cause conditions ranging from renal dysfunction, for example nephritis, to renal failure. When patients are taking these drugs (e.g. the aminoglycosides), they should be monitored closely for any sign of renal dysfunction and the drug levels monitored in the patient's blood. To prevent any accumulation of the drug in the kidney, patients should be well hydrated throughout the course of the drug therapy.

Gastrointestinal Toxicity

GI toxicity is very common with many of the antimicrobials. Many of these agents have direct toxic effects on the cells lining the GI tract, causing nausea, vomiting or diarrhoea, and such effects are sometimes severe (Box 7.4). The death of micro-organisms releases chemicals and toxins into the body, which can stimulate the vomiting centre in the medulla and induce nausea and vomiting.

In addition, some antimicrobials are toxic to the liver. These drugs can cause hepatitis (inflammation of the liver) and even liver failure. When patients are taking drugs known to be toxic to the liver (e.g. many of the cephalosporins), they should be monitored closely and should stop taking the drug at any sign of liver dysfunction.

Neurotoxicity

Some antimicrobials can damage or interfere with the function of nerve tissue. For example, the aminoglycoside antibacterials collect in the eighth cranial nerve and can cause dizziness, vertigo and loss of hearing. Chloroquine, which is used to treat malaria and some rheumatoid disorders, can accumulate in the retina and optic nerve and cause retinal damage and visual disturbances. Other antimicrobials can cause dizziness, drowsiness, lethargy, changes in reflexes and even hallucinations when they irritate specific nerve tissues.

Hypersensitivity Reactions

Allergic or hypersensitivity reactions have been reported with many antimicrobial agents. Most of these agents, which are protein bound for transfer through the circulation, are able to induce antibody formation in susceptible people. With the next exposure to the drug, immediate or delayed allergic responses may occur. Some of these drugs have demonstrated cross-sensitivity (e.g. penicillins, cephalosporins), and care must be taken to obtain a complete patient history before administering one of these drugs. It is important to determine what the allergic reaction was and when the patient experienced it (e.g. after first use of drug, after years of use). Some patients report having a drug allergy, but closer investigation indicates that their reaction actually constituted an anticipated effect or a known adverse effect to the drug. Proper interpretation of this information is important to allow treatment of a patient with a drug to which the patient reported a supposed allergic reaction but which would be very effective against a known pathogen.

Superinfections

One disadvantage of the use of antimicrobials, especially broad-spectrum antibacterials, is destruction of the **normal flora**, the micro-organisms always present in the human body that can prove beneficial to the host. The normal flora does not have any harmful effects as long as they remain in their correct location. When the normal flora is destroyed, opportunistic pathogens that were kept in check by the 'normal' bacteria have the opportunity to invade tissues and cause infections. These opportunistic infections are called **superinfections**. Common superinfections include vaginal or GI yeast infections caused by *Candida albicans*, which are associated with antibacterial therapy, *C. difficile* causing GI infection and infections caused by *Proteus* and *Pseudomonas* throughout the body, which are a result of broad-spectrum antibacterial use. Patients receiving drugs known to induce superinfections should be monitored closely and the appropriate treatment for any superinfection started as soon as possible.

Prophylaxis

Sometimes it is clinically useful to use antimicrobials as a means of **prophylaxis**, to prevent infections before they occur. For example, when patients anticipate travelling to an area where malaria is endemic, they may begin taking antimalarial drugs before the journey and during the trip. Patients who are undergoing GI or genitourinary surgery, which might introduce bacteria from those areas into the system, often have antibacterials ordered immediately after the surgery and periodically thereafter, as appropriate, to prevent infection. Management of patients with pancreatitis are also given broad-spectrum antibacterials to reduce the risk of complications arising from infections. Individuals who have had their spleens removed are at increased risk of infections and are prescribed penicillin long-term.

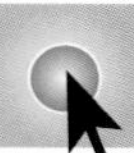

WEB LINKS

Health care providers and patients may want to consult the following Internet sources:

http://bnfc.org The BNF for Children provides UK health care professionals with authoritative and practical information on the selection and clinical use of medicines for children.

http://cks.library.nhs.uk The National Health Service Clinical Knowledge Summaries provides evidence-based practical information on the common conditions observed in primary care.

http://www.bnf.org.uk The BNF provides UK health care professionals with authoritative and practical information on the selection and clinical use of medicines.

http://www.his.org.uk The Hospital Infection Society provides information on the prevention and control of hospital and other health care associated infections.

http://www.hpa.org.uk The Health Protection Agency provides support and advice on public health issues to the National Health Service and other authorities.

http://www.nhsdirect.nhs.uk The National Health Service Direct service provides patients with information and advice about health, illness and health services.

http://www.npsa.nhs.uk The National Patient Safety Agency is part of the Department of Health and is responsible for improving patient care.

Points to Remember

- Antimicrobials are drugs designed to act on foreign organisms that have invaded and infected the human host with selective toxicity. This means that they affect biological systems or structures that are found in the invading organisms but not in the host.
- The goal of antimicrobial therapy is to interfere with the normal function of invading organisms to prevent them from reproducing and to promote cell death with limited negative effects on the host cells. The infection should be eradicated with the least toxicity to the host and the least likelihood for development of resistance.
- Antimicrobials can work by altering the cell membrane of the pathogen, by interfering with protein synthesis, or by interfering with the ability of the pathogen to obtain required nutrients.
- Antimicrobials also work to kill invading organisms or to prevent them from reproducing, thus depleting the size of the invasion to one that can be dealt with by the human immune system.
- Pathogens can have innate resistance or develop resistance to the effects of antimicrobials over time when (1) mutant organisms that do not respond to the antimicrobial become the majority of the pathogen population or (2) the pathogen develops enzymes to block the antimicrobials or alternative routes to obtain nutrients or maintain the cell membrane.
- An important aspect of clinical care involving antimicrobial drugs is preventing or delaying the development of resistance. This can be done by ensuring that the particular antimicrobial agent is the drug of choice for the specific pathogen involved and that it is given in high enough doses for sufficiently long periods to rid the body of the pathogen.
- Culture and sensitivity testing of a suspected infection ensures that the correct drug is used to treat the infection effectively. Culture and sensitivity testing should be performed before an antimicrobial agent is prescribed except in life-threatening infections such as meningitis or pneumonia for example.
- Antimicrobials can have several adverse effects on the human host, including renal toxicity, multiple GI effects, neurotoxicity, hypersensitivity reactions and superinfections.
- Some antimicrobials are used as a means of prophylaxis when patients expect to be in situations that will expose them to a known pathogen, such as travel to an area where malaria is endemic, or oral or invasive GI surgery.

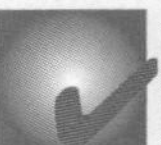

CHECK YOUR UNDERSTANDING

Answers to the questions in this chapter may be found in the answer key in the back of the book.

Multiple Choice

Select the most appropriate response to the following.

1. Spectrum of activity of an antimicrobial indicates the
   a. acidity of the environment in which they are most effective.
   b. cell membrane type that the antimicrobial affects.
   c. antimicrobial's effectiveness against different invading organisms.
   d. resistance factor that bacteria have developed to this antimicrobial.

2. The emergence of resistant strains of microbes is a serious public health problem. Health care providers can work to prevent the emergence of resistant strains by
   a. encouraging the patient to stop the antimicrobial as soon as the symptoms are resolved, to prevent over-exposure to the drug.
   b. encouraging the use of antimicrobial when patients feel they will help.
   c. limiting the use of antimicrobial agents to the treatment of specific pathogens known to be sensitive to the drug being used.
   d. using the most powerful drug available to treat an infection, to ensure eradication of the microbe.

3. Sensitivity testing of a culture shows the
   a. drugs that are capable of controlling that particular micro-organism.
   b. patient's potential for allergic reactions to a drug.
   c. offending micro-organism.
   d. immune reaction to the infecting organism.

4. GI toxicity is a very common adverse effect seen with antimicrobial therapy. A patient experiencing GI toxicity might complain of
   a. elevated blood urea nitrogen.
   b. difficulty breathing.
   c. nausea, vomiting or diarrhoea.
   d. yellowish skin or sclera.

5. Superinfections can occur when antimicrobial agents destroy the normal flora of the body. *Candida* infections are commonly associated with antibiotic use. A patient with this type of superinfection would exhibit
   a. difficulty breathing.
   b. vaginal discharge or white patches in the mouth.
   c. pale complexion.
   d. dark lesions on the skin.

6. An example of an antimicrobial used as a means of prophylaxis would be
   a. amoxicillin used to treat tonsillitis.
   b. penicillin used to treat an abscess.
   c. an antimicrobial used before and during travel to an area where malaria is endemic.
   d. norfloxacin used to treat a urinary tract infection.

7. An important characteristic of any antimicrobial drug is
   a. a broad spectrum of activity.
   b. a narrow spectrum of activity.
   c. resistance.
   d. selective toxicity.

Extended Matching Questions

Select **all** that apply.

1. Bacterial resistance to an antibacterial could be the result of which of the following?
   a. Natural or intrinsic properties of the bacteria
   b. Changes in cellular permeability or cellular transport systems
   c. The production of chemicals that antagonize the drug
   d. Initial exposure to the antibacterial
   e. Combination of too many antibacterial agents for one infection
   f. Narrow spectrum of activity

2. Antimicrobial drugs destroy cells that have invaded the body. They do not specifically destroy only the cells of the invader, and because of this, many adverse effects can be anticipated when an antimicrobial is used. Which of the following adverse effects are often associated with antimicrobial use?
   a. Superinfections
   b. Hypotension
   c. Renal toxicity
   d. Diarrhoea
   e. Loss of hearing
   f. Constipation

Definitions

1. Culture ______________________________

____

2. Prophylaxis ___________________________

____

3. Resistance ______________________________
____

4. Selective toxicity _________________________
____

5. Sensitivity testing ________________________
____

6. Spectrum _______________________________
____

Bibliography and References

British Medical Association and Royal Pharmaceutical Society of Great Britain. (2008). *British National Formulary*. London: BMJ & RPS Publishing. *This publication is updated biannually: it is imperative that the most recent edition is consulted.*

British Medical Association and Royal Pharmaceutical Society of Great Britain. (2008). *British National Formulary for Children*. London: BMJ & RPS Publishing. *This publication is updated annually: it is imperative that the most recent edition is consulted.*

Brunton, L., Lazo, J. S., Parker, K., Goodman, L. S., & Gilman, A. G. (2005). *Goodman and Gilman's the pharmacological basis of therapeutics* (11th ed.). London: McGraw-Hill.

Coia, J. E. Duckworth, G. J., Edwards, D. I., Farrington, M., Fry, C., Humphreys, H., et al., Joint Working Party of the British Society of Antimicrobial Chemotherapy; Hospital Infection Society; Infection Control Nurses Association. (2006). Guidelines for the control and prevention of meticillin-resistant *Staphylococcus aureus* (MRSA) in healthcare facilities. *Journal of Hospital Infection, 63S*, S1–S44.

Health Protection Agency. (2008). Antimicrobial resistance and prescribing in England, Wales and Northern Ireland, 2008. Available from http://www.hpa.org.uk

Howland, R. D., & Mycek, M. J. (2005). *Pharmacology* (3rd ed.). Philadelphia: Lippincott Williams & Wilkins.

Livermore, D. M. (2005). Minimising antibiotic resistance. *Lancet Infectious Diseases, 5*, 450–459.

National Institute for Health and Clinical Excellence. (2003). Infection control: Prevention of healthcare-associated infections in primary and community care. Available from http://www.nice.org.uk

Porth, C. M., & Matfin, G. (2008). *Pathophysiology: Concepts of altered health states* (8th ed.). Philadelphia: Lippincott Williams & Wilkins.

Rang, H. P., Dale, M. M., Ritter, J. M., & Flower, R. J. (2007). *Rang and Dale's pharmacology* (6th ed.). Philadelphia: Churchill Livingstone.

Royal College of Nursing. (2005). Methicillin-resistant *Staphylococcus aureus* (MRSA): Guidance for nursing staff. Available from: http://www.rcn.org.uk/

Simonsen, T., Aarbakke, J., Kay, I., Coleman, I., Sinnott, P., & Lysaa, R. (2006). *Illustrated pharmacology for nurses*. London: Hodder Arnold.

CHAPTER

8

Antibacterial Agents

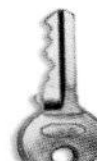

KEY TERMS

aerobic bacteria
anaerobic bacteria
antibacterial
antibiotic
bactericidal
bacteriostatic
Gram-negative
Gram-positive
prophylaxis
superinfections
synergy

LEARNING OBJECTIVES

Upon completion of this chapter, you will be able to:

1. Explain how an antibacterial is selected for use in a particular clinical situation.
2. Differentiate between bactericidal and bacteriostatic drugs.
3. Describe the therapeutic actions, indications, pharmacokinetics, contraindications, most common adverse reactions and important drug–drug interactions associated with each class of antibacterials.
4. Discuss the use of antibacterials across the lifespan.
5. Compare and contrast the key drugs for each class of antibacterials with the other drugs in that class.
6. Outline the nursing considerations for patients receiving each class of antibacterial.

PENICILLINS

amoxicillin
ampicillin
benzylpenicillin (penicillin G)
co-amoxiclav
co-fluampicil
phenoxymethylpenicillin (penicillin V)
piperacillin
pivmecillinam
ticarcillin

PENICILLINASE-RESISTANT ANTIBACTERIALS

flucloxacillin
temocillin

CEPHALOSPORINS

cefaclor
cefadroxil
cefalexin
cefixime
cefotaxime
cefpodoxime
cefradine
ceftazidime
ceftriaxone
cefuroxime

OTHER β-LACTAM ANTIBACTERIALS

aztreonam
ertapenem
imipenem with cilastatin
meropenem

QUINOLONES

ciprofloxacin
levofloxacin
moxifloxacin
nalidixic acid
norfloxacin
ofloxacin

SULPHONAMIDES

co-trimoxazole
sulfadiazine
trimethoprim

AMINOGLYCOSIDES

amikacin
gentamicin
neomycin
netilmicin
tobramycin

MACROLIDES

azithromycin
clarithromycin
erythromycin
telithromycin

LINCOSAMIDES

clindamycin

TETRACYCLINES

demeclocycline
doxycycline
lymecycline
minocycline
oxytetracycline
tetracycline
tigecycline

OTHER ANTIBACTERIALS

chloramphenicol
colistin
daptomycin
linezolid
metronidazole *(Chapter 11)*
quinupristin with dalfopristin
sodium fusidate
teicoplanin
tinidazole *(Chapter 11)*
vancomycin

ANTIMYCOBACTERIAL ANTIBACTERIALS

Antituberculosis Drugs

capreomycin
cycloserine
ethambutol
isoniazid
pyrazinamide
rifabutin
rifampicin
streptomycin

Leprostatic Drugs

dapsone
clofazimine

Antibacterials are chemicals that inhibit specific bacteria and are used to treat a wide variety of systemic and topical infections. The antibacterials used today vary in their effectiveness against invading organisms; that is, the spectrum of activity varies. Some are so selective in their action that they are effective against only a few micro-organisms with a very specific metabolic pathway or enzyme. These drugs are said to have a narrow spectrum of activity. Other drugs interfere with biochemical reactions present in many different kinds of micro-organisms, making them useful in the treatment of a wide variety of infections. Such drugs are said to have a broad spectrum of activity.

Some antibacterials, known as **bactericidal**, cause the death of the cells the micro-organisms have infected. Other antibacterials interfere with the ability of the cells to reproduce or divide and are said to be **bacteriostatic**. Bacteriostatic agents, therefore, rely on a person's immune system to deal with the infection. Several drugs are both bactericidal and bacteriostatic, often depending on the concentration of the drug used. Many of the adverse effects noted with the use of antibacterials are associated with the aggressive properties of the drugs and their effect on the cells of the host as well as those of the micro-organism.

Antibacterials are made in three ways: by living micro-organisms, by synthetic manufacture and, in some cases, through genetic engineering. Antibacterials produced by micro-organisms are known as **antibiotics**, for example penicillin, streptomycin and vancomycin. Discussed in this chapter are the major classes of antibacterials: penicillins and penicillinase-resistant drugs, cephalosporins, monobactams, quinolones, sulphonamides, aminoglycosides, macrolides, lincosamides, tetracyclines and the disease-specific antimycobacterials, including antitubercular and leprostatic drugs.

Bacteria and Antibacterials

Bacteria can invade the human body through many routes, for example respiratory tract, gastrointestinal (GI) tract and skin. Once bacteria invade, the body becomes the host for the bacteria, supplying nutrients and enzymes that the bacteria require for reproduction. Unchallenged, the invading bacteria multiply and further invade tissue.

The human immune response is activated when bacteria invade. Many of the signs and symptoms of an infection are related to the immune response as the body tries to rid itself of the foreign cells. Fever, lethargy and the classic signs of inflammation (i.e. redness, swelling, heat and pain) all indicate that the body is responding to an invader.

The goal of antibacterial therapy is to decrease the population of invading bacteria to a point at which the human immune system can effectively deal with the invader. To determine which antibacterial will effectively treat a specific infection, the causative organism must be identified. Culture and sensitivity testing are performed to identify the invading bacterial species by growing it in the laboratory and then determining the antibacterial to which that particular organism is most sensitive (i.e. which antibacterial best kills or controls the bacteria). Antibacterials have been developed to interfere with specific proteins or enzyme systems, so they are effective only against the bacteria that use those proteins or enzymes.

Gram-positive bacteria are those whose cell wall retains a stain, known as Gram's stain, and resist removal of the stain with alcohol during culture and sensitivity testing. Gram-positive bacteria are commonly associated with infections of the respiratory tract and soft tissues. An example of a Gram-positive bacterium is *Streptococcus pneumoniae*, a common cause of pneumonia. In contrast, the cell walls of **Gram-negative** bacteria lose their staining with alcohol. These bacteria are frequently associated with infections of the genitourinary (GU) or GI tract. An example of a Gram-negative bacterium is *Escherichia coli*, a common cause of cystitis and diarrhoea. **Aerobic bacteria** depend on oxygen for survival, whereas **anaerobic bacteria** (e.g. those bacteria associated with gangrene) do not require oxygen.

If culture and sensitivity testing are not possible, either because the source of the infection is not identifiable or because the patient is too ill to wait for test results to determine the best treatment, clinicians administer an antibacterial with a broad spectrum of activity against a wide range of bacteria. These drugs can be given at the beginning of treatment until the exact organism and its sensitivity are established. These antibacterials have such a wide range of effects that they are frequently associated with adverse effects.

In choosing an antibacterial, clinicians also look for a drug with selective toxicity or the ability to strike foreign cells with little or no effect on human cells. Human cells have many of the same properties as bacterial cells and can be affected in much the same way, so damage may occur to the human cells as well as the bacterial cells. There is no perfect antibacterial that is without effect on the human host, and this factor should be considered in antibacterial selection. Various antibacterials have adverse effects that can be anticipated and may be contraindicated in some patients, such as those who are immunocompromised, with severe GI disease, or who are debilitated. The antibacterial of choice is one that affects the causative organism and leads to the fewest adverse effects for the patient involved. See Box 8.1 for the effects of antibacterials across the lifespan.

Antibacterials can be given in combination to promote **synergy**, so that their combined effect is greater than their

BOX 8.1 **DRUG THERAPY ACROSS THE LIFESPAN**

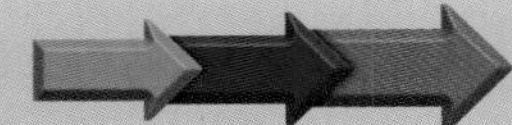

Antibacterials

CHILDREN

Feverish illness is the most common presenting illness in young children but most cases are due to viral infections and are self-limiting. The National Institute for Health and Clinical Excellence therefore recommends that oral antibacterials should not be prescribed to children with fever without an apparent source (National Collaborating Centre for Women's and Children's Health, 2007). Antibacterial treatment of ear infections (otitis media), another common paediatric problem, is controversial. Many ear infections are caused by viruses, and antibacterial treatment should only be used if there is no improvement within 3 days. Ongoing research suggests that judicious use of decongestants and anti-inflammatories to treat otitis media may be just as successful as the use of antibacterials without the risk of development of resistant bacterial strains.

Some antibacterials do not have proven safety and efficacy in paediatric use; therefore, caution should be used when giving them to children. For example, the quinolones are associated with damage to developing cartilage in animals, and it is suggested that these antibacterials should be used only if there is a specific need. Paediatric dosages of antibacterials should be double-checked to make sure that the child receives the correct dose, thereby improving the chance of eradicating the infection and decreasing the risk of adverse effects.

Children are very sensitive to the GI and central nervous system (CNS) effects of most antibacterials, and more severe reactions can be expected when these drugs are used in children. It is important to monitor the hydration and nutritional status of children who are adversely affected by drug-induced diarrhoea, anorexia, nausea and vomiting. Superinfections can be a problem for small children as well. For example, thrush (oral candidiasis) is a common superinfection that makes eating and drinking difficult.

When administering any drug to children, always consult the most recent edition of the British National Formulary for Children.

ADULTS

Many adults believe that antibacterials are a cure-all for any discomfort and fever. It is very important to explain that antibacterials are only useful against specific bacteria and will not clear nonbacterial infections, for example viral infections.

Adults need to be cautioned to take the entire course of the medication as prescribed. Even though their symptoms may have resolved, the infection may not have been cleared completely. If infections re-occur, they are much harder to treat a second time. Unused antibacterials should not be stored for future infections or for sharing with symptomatic friends.

Pregnant and/or women who are breast-feeding should not take antibacterials unless the benefit clearly outweighs the potential risk to the foetus or neonate. Tetracyclines, for example, are associated with pitting of enamel in developing teeth and of calcium deposits in growing bones. These drugs can cause serious problems for neonates. Women of childbearing age should be advised to use barrier contraceptives (rather than oral contraceptives) if antibacterials are used. Many antibacterials interfere with the effectiveness of oral contraceptives and unplanned pregnancies can occur.

OLDER ADULTS

In many instances, older adults do not present with the same signs and symptoms of infections as other patients. Therefore assessing the problem and obtaining appropriate specimens for culture is especially important with this population.

Older patients may be more susceptible to the adverse effects associated with antibacterial therapy. Their hydration and nutritional status should be monitored closely, as should the need for safety precautions if CNS effects occur. If hepatic or renal dysfunction is expected (particularly in older patients, those who are alcohol dependent, and those taking other hepatotoxic or nephrotoxic drugs), the dosage may need to be lowered and the patient should be monitored more frequently.

Older patients also need to be cautioned to complete the full course of drug therapy, even when they feel better, and not to save pills for self-medication at a future time.

individual effect. Use of synergistic antibacterials allows the patient to take a lower dose of each antibacterial to achieve the desired effect. Another possible benefit of combined therapy is that a lower dose of one of the antibacterials can be used, which helps reduce the adverse effects of that particular drug and makes it more useful in certain clinical situations. Alternatively, one drug may 'help' the effectiveness of another. For example, clavulanic acid protects certain β-lactam antibacterials from breakdown in the presence of penicillinase enzymes. A combination of amoxicillin and clavulanic acid is commonly used to allow the amoxicillin to remain effective against certain strains of resistant bacteria. The theory behind the combination of ticarcillin and clavulanic acid is similar.

In some situations, antibacterials are used as **prophylaxis**, to prevent potential infection. Patients placed at risk of specific infections (e.g. patients undergoing GI surgical procedures, which may introduce GI bacteria into the bloodstream or peritoneum), may be given antibacterials before they are exposed to the bacteria. Usually a large, single dose of an antibacterial is given to destroy any bacteria that enter the host immediately and thereby prevent a serious infection.

Bacteria and Resistance to Antibacterials

Bacteria have survived for hundreds of years because they can adapt to their environment. They do this by altering their cell wall or enzyme systems to become resistant (i.e. protect themselves from) to unfavourable conditions or situations. Many species of bacteria have developed resistance to certain antibacterials (Box 8.2). For example, bacteria that were once very sensitive to penicillin have developed an enzyme called penicillinase, which effectively inactivates many of the penicillin-type drugs. New drugs had to be developed to effectively treat infections involving these once-controlled bacteria. Since these newer drugs are resistant to penicillinase, they can no longer be inactivated by the bacteria. Other drugs have been developed specifically to treat resistant infections. It is very important to use these drugs only when the identity and sensitivity of the offending bacterium have been established.

BOX 8.2 Development of Resistance to Antibacterials

The inappropriate use of antibacterials, either from using an antibacterial to treat a viral infection, the use of a broad-spectrum antibacterial to treat a specific infection, or from poor concordance to the drug regimen, has led to the development of bacterial resistance to antibacterials. In particular, meticillin-resistant *Staphylococcus aureus* (MRSA) and glycopeptide-resistant *S. aureus* are of particular importance and linked to hospital-acquired infections.

Resistance to antibacterials can develop by the following mechanisms (Hawkey, 1998):

1. the antibacterial is destroyed by enzymes produced by the bacteria, for example resistance to penicillin;
2. the bacterial cell wall prevents the antibacterial from entering or the drug is rapidly removed from the cell by an efflux pump making the target for the antibacterial inaccessible, for example resistance to tetracycline;
3. the bacteria modify the structure of the drug binding site so the antibacterial drug cannot bind, for example resistance to aminoglycosides;
4. the bacteria may develop alternative metabolic pathways using enzymes not affected by the drug, for example meticillin-resistance in MRSA.

Several new antibacterials have been developed to target antibacterial-resistant infections. These drugs should only be used where the bacterium is clearly identified as being resistant to other antibacterials and sensitive to these. Indiscriminate use of these new drugs can lead to the development of more invasive and resistant strains.

- The glycopeptides, *vancomycin* and *teicoplanin*, are used to inhibit protein synthesis in Gram-positive bacteria. Teicoplanin has greater activity against Gram-positive bacteria than vancomycin. Both are used to treat MRSA. There are reports, however, of increasing resistance in *S. aureus* to both glycopeptides. They are both used to treat peritonitis arising from dialysis, and vancomycin is also used to treat pseudomembranous colitis. (Pseudomembranous colitis can develop up to a month after a course of antibacterial treatment is completed and occurs when the normal intestinal flora is disturbed. It is characterized by diarrhoea. The causative agent is *Clostridium difficile*).
- *Quinupristin with dalfopristin* is available in combination form. They work synergistically to inhibit protein synthesis in specific Gram-positive bacteria involved in serious infections. This combination is reserved for treating infections which have not responded to other antibacterials, for example MRSA. It is also effective in treating vancomycin-resistant enterococci (VRE). The drug also seems to be active against penicillin-resistant pneumococcus.
- *Linezolid* is the first member of a new class of antibacterials known as the oxalizidonones that also inhibit protein synthesis in sensitive bacteria. This antibacterial is indicated specifically for treatment of infections caused by VRE and MRSA bacterial strains. It is also effective against other Gram-positive strains such as *S. pneumoniae.* Linezolid is also a monoamine oxidase inhibitor and patients should be warned of the dangers of consuming tyramine-rich foods with this antibacterial (see Chapter 20).
- The cyclic lipopeptide antibacterial, *daptomycin*, binds to bacterial cell membranes, causing rapid membrane potential depolarization. This leads to the inhibition of protein, DNA and RNA synthesis, resulting in bacterial

BOX 8.3 FOCUS ON THE **EVIDENCE**

Using Antibacterials Properly

In an effort to reduce the inappropriate use of antibacterials, the Department of Health launched a public campaign in 2008 to highlight when it is appropriate to use antibacterials. Nurses can play an important role by including some of the following points about the risks and dangers of antibacterial abuse in the patient education plan (Royal College of Nursing, 2005):

- Explain clearly that a particular antibacterial is effective against only certain bacteria and that a culture needs to be taken to identify the bacteria. They are effective against only certain bacteria; they are not effective against viruses (such as cold germs) or other bacteria.
- Explain that bacteria can develop resistant strains that will not be affected by antibacterials in the future, so use of antibacterials now may make them less effective in situations in which they are really necessary.
- Ensure that patients understand the importance of taking the full course of medication as prescribed, even if they feel better. Stopping an antibacterial midway through a regimen often leads to the development of resistant bacteria. Using all of the medication will also prevent patients' saving unused medication to self-treat future infections or to share with other family members.
- Common effects of these drugs include stomach upset, diarrhoea, changes in taste and in the colour of the tongue. Small, frequent meals may help. It is important to try to maintain good nutrition. These effects should go away when the drug is stopped.
- Tell patients that allergies may develop with repeated exposures to certain antibacterials. In addition, explain to patients that saving antibacterials to take later, when they think they need them again, may lead to earlier development of an allergy, which will negate important tests that could identify the bacteria making them sick.
- Offer other medications, such as antihistamines or decongestants, where appropriate. Explain that viral infections do not respond to antibacterials.

The publicity that many emergent resistant strains of bacteria have received in recent years may help to get the message across to patients about the need to take the full course of an antibacterial and to use antibacterials only when appropriate.

cell death. Daptomycin is approved for treating complicated skin and skin structure infections caused by susceptible Gram-positive bacteria, including MRSA. Patients should be monitored for myopathies.

The longer an antibacterial has been in use, the greater the chance that the bacteria will develop into a resistant strain. Efforts to control the emergence of resistant strains involve intensive education programmes that advocate the use of antibacterials only when necessary and effective and not for treatment of viral infections such as the common cold (Box 8.3).

In addition, the use of antibacterials may result in the development of **superinfections** or overgrowth of resistant pathogens, such as bacteria, fungi, or yeasts, because antibacterials (particularly broad-spectrum agents) destroy bacteria in the flora that normally work to prevent opportunistic infections. When 'normal' bacteria are destroyed or greatly reduced in number, there is nothing to prevent the invaders from occupying the host. In most cases the superinfection is an irritating adverse effect (e.g. vaginal yeast infection, candidiasis, diarrhoea), but in some cases, the superinfection can be more severe than the infection originally being treated. Treatment of the superinfection leads to new adverse effects and the potential for different superinfections. A vicious cycle of treatment and resistance can result.

Penicillins and Penicillinase-Resistant Antibacterials

Penicillin was the first antibacterial introduced for clinical use. Sir Alexander Fleming used *Penicillium* moulds to produce the original penicillin in 1928. Subsequent versions of penicillin were developed to decrease the adverse effects of the drug and to modify it to act on resistant bacteria. Each chemical version of penicillin contains a characteristic β-lactam ring. Other classes of antibacterials, the cephalosporins and monobactams, also contain a β-lactam ring within their structure. Collectively they are known as the β-lactam antibacterials.

With the prolonged use of penicillin, more and more bacterial species have synthesized the enzyme β-lactamase (penicillinase) to counteract the effects of penicillin. Beta-lactamase targets the β-lactam ring, breaking the structure and inactivating the antibacterial. Researchers have developed a group of drugs with a resistance to penicillinase, which allows them to remain effective against bacteria that are now resistant to the penicillins, the *penicillinase-resistant* antibacterials (Table 8.1).

The selection of antibacterial will depend on the sensitivity of the bacteria causing the infection, the desired and available routes and the individual patient, for example age, hypersensitivity to the antibacterial and others.

Therapeutic Actions and Indications

The β-lactam antibacterials, including penicillins and penicillinase-resistant antibacterials, produce their bactericidal effects by interfering with the ability of susceptible bacteria to build their cell walls when they are dividing (Figure 8.1). These drugs prevent the bacteria from biosynthesizing the framework of the cell wall, and the bacteria with weakened cell walls swell and then burst from increased osmotic pressure within the cell. These antibacterials can also activate autolytic enzymes in the bacterial cell wall leading to lysis. This toxicity is bacteria selective because human cells do not possess a cell wall.

Table 8.1 DRUGS IN FOCUS

Penicillins

Drug Name	Available Forms	Usual Indications
amoxicillin	Oral, IV, IM	Broad spectrum of uses for adults and children, including oral infections, urinary tract infections (UTIs), endocarditis and *Helicobacter pylori*
ampicillin	Oral, IV, IM	As for amoxicillin, plus otitis media, chronic bronchitis and *H. influenzae* infections
benzylpenicillin (penicillin G)	IV, IM	Used to treat streptococcal, gonoccocal, enterococcal (endocarditis), meningococcal, clostridium (gangrene) and oropharyngeal infections; Lyme disease
co-amoxiclav	Oral, IV	Combination of amoxicillin and clavulanic acid (a β-lactamase inhibitor). Used to treat β-lactamase resistant strains otherwise sensitive to amoxicillin
co-fluampicil	Oral, IV, IM	Combination of flucoxacillin and ampicillin. Used to treat β-lactamase producing staphylococcal bacteria
phenoxymethylpenicillin (penicillin V)	Oral	Mainly used to treat respiratory tract infections in children and streptococcal tonsillitis
piperacillin	IV	Combination of piperacillin and the β-lactamase inhibitor tazobactam. Treatment of respiratory tract infections, UTIs, septicaemia and skin infections
pivmecillinam	Oral	Infections caused by *E. coli*, klebsiella, enterobacter and salmonellae bacteria
ticarcillin	IV	Severe infections caused by *Pseudomonas aeuroginosa, Proteus* and *Bacteroides fragilis* bacteria
Penicillinase-resistant penicillins		
flucloxacillin	Oral, IV, IM	Penicillin-resistant staphylococci infections
temocillin	IV, IM	Penicillin-resistant infections

The penicillins mainly affect Gram-positive bacteria, but also some Gram-negative bacteria. They are indicated for the treatment of streptococcal infections, including pharyngitis, tonsillitis, scarlet fever and endocarditis; pneumococcal infections; staphylococcal infections (many staphylococci are now resistant to penicillins); fusospirochetal infections; rat bite fever; diphtheria; anthrax; syphilis and uncomplicated gonococcal infections. At high doses, these drugs are also used to treat meningococcal meningitis. Box 8.4 provides calculation practice using phenoxymethylpenicillin to treat tonsillitis.

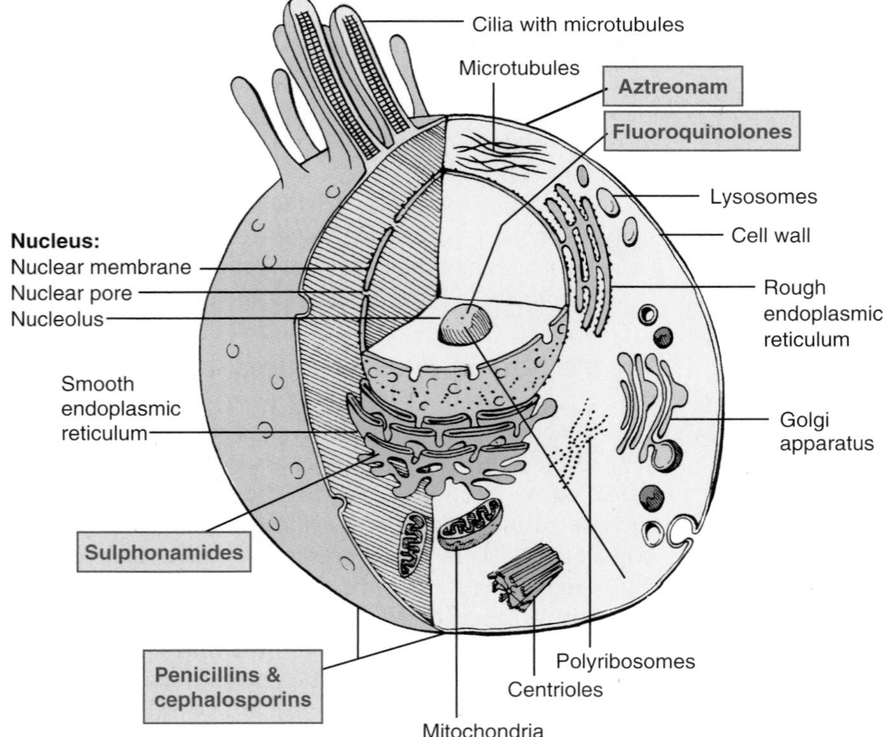

Figure 8.1 Sites of cellular action of aztreonam, penicillins, sulphonamides, fluoroquinolones and cephalosporins. Aztreonam alters cell membranes to allow leakage of intracellular substances and causes cell death. Penicillins prevent bacteria from building their cells during division. Sulphonamides inhibit folic acid synthesis for RNA and DNA production. Cephalosporins cause bacteria to build weak cell walls when dividing. Fluoroquinolones interfere with the DNA enzymes needed for growth and reproduction.

BOX 8.4 FOCUS ON CALCULATIONS

Your patient is a 12-kg child with a severe case of tonsillitis. An order is written for phenoxymethylpenicillin at 12.5 mg/kg/6 hours orally. The drug comes in an oral suspension 125 mg/ml. What should you administer at each dose?

The order is for 12.5 mg/kg, so 12.5 mg/kg × 12 kg = 150 mg. The available form is 125 mg/5 ml. Using the formula:

$$\frac{\text{amount of drug available}}{\text{volume available}} = \frac{\text{amount of drug prescribed}}{\text{volume to administer}}$$

$$\frac{125\text{ mg}}{150\text{ mg}} = \frac{5\text{ ml}}{Y}$$

By cross-multiplying the ratio:

$$125\text{ mg} \times Y = 150\text{ mg} \times 5\text{ ml}$$

Rearrange and cancel units and numbers:

$$Y = \frac{150\text{ mg} \times 5\text{ ml}}{125\text{ mg}}$$

Y = 6 ml of phenoxymethylpenicillin will be administered orally

Pharmacokinetics

The penicillins are absorbed from the GI tract at different rates and to varying extents, for example the antipseudomonal antibacterial piperacillin is so poorly absorbed from the GI tract, that it must be given parenterally. They are sensitive to gastric acid levels in the stomach and should be taken on an empty stomach to ensure adequate absorption. Once absorbed, the penicillins are widely distributed around the body apart from the CNS. The penicillins can only cross the blood–brain barrier if the meninges are inflamed, as in meningitis. Penicillins are rapidly excreted unchanged in the urine, making renal function an important factor in safe use of the drug.

Penicillins can cross the placenta and also enter breast milk but are considered safe for use in pregnancy and breast-feeding.

Contraindications and Cautions

These drugs are contraindicated in patients with allergies to penicillin or cephalosporins or other allergens. Penicillin sensitivity tests are available if the patient's history of allergy is unclear and a penicillin is the drug of choice. Caution should be exercised in patients with a history of allergies or renal impairment (a reduced dose may be necessary if excretion is reduced).

Adverse Effects

The major adverse effects of penicillin therapy involve the GI tract. Common adverse effects include nausea, vomiting and diarrhoea. These effects are primarily related to the loss of bacteria from the normal flora. Pain and inflammation at the injection site can occur with injectable forms of the drugs. Hypersensitivity reactions occur in up to 10% of patients and may include rash, urticaria, fever, wheezing and anaphylaxis that can progress to anaphylactic shock and death.

Clinically Important Drug–Drug Interactions

When penicillins and penicillinase-resistant antibacterials are taken concurrently with probenecid or sulfinpyrazone, the excretion of the antibacterial will be reduced leading to increased concentrations of antibacterial in the plasma.

Always consult a current copy of the British National Formulary for further guidance.

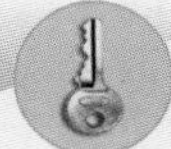

Key Drug Summary: *Amoxicillin*

Indications: Treatment of infections caused by susceptible strains of bacteria, postexposure prophylaxis for anthrax, prophylaxis of endocarditis, treatment of *Helicobacter* infections as part of combination therapy

Actions: Inhibits synthesis of the cell wall in susceptible bacteria, causing cell death

Pharmacokinetics:

Route	Onset	Peak	Duration
Oral	Varies	1 h	6–8 h
IM	Varies	30–60 min	6–8 h
IV	Immediate	10–20 min	6–8 h

$T_{1/2}$: 1–1.4 hours; excreted unchanged in the urine

Adverse effects: Nausea, vomiting, diarrhoea, bone marrow suppression, rash, fever

General Guidance for Patients Receiving Antibacterials

Regardless of the class of antibacterial prescribed, the following points apply to all cases:

- Check the culture and sensitivity reports *to ensure that this is the drug of choice for this patient.*
- Establish which other drug(s) the patient is currently taking, if any *to avoid potential drug–drug interactions*. This includes prescription drugs, over-the-counter products and herbal treatments.
- Ensure that the patient receives the full course of antibacterials as prescribed, divided where

necessary, *to increase effectiveness and decrease the risk for development of resistant strains of bacteria.*

- Encourage patient to maintain fluid intake and nutrition (very important) even though nausea, vomiting and diarrhoea may occur. Provide small, frequent meals as tolerated; and frequent mouth care *to relieve discomfort.*
- Ensure that the patient is instructed about the appropriate dosage regimen and possible adverse effects *to enhance patient knowledge of drug therapy and to promote concordance.*

Nursing Considerations for Patients Receiving Penicillins and Penicillinase-Resistant Antibacterials

Assessment: History and Examination

Screen for the following, *which are possible contraindications or cautions for use of the drug*: known allergy to any cephalosporins, penicillins or other allergens *because cross-sensitivity often occurs* (obtain specific information about the nature and occurrence of allergic reactions) and history of renal disease *that could interfere with excretion of the drug.*

Physical assessment should be performed *to establish baseline data for evaluating the effectiveness of the drug and the occurrence of any adverse effects associated with drug therapy.* Perform culture and sensitivity tests at the site of infection *to ensure that this is the drug of choice for this patient.* Examine the skin and mucous membranes for any rashes *to provide a baseline for possible adverse effects.* Note respiratory rate and adventitious sounds *to provide a baseline for the occurrence of hypersensitivity reactions.* Examine the abdomen *to monitor for adverse effects.* Assess the status of renal functioning and to determine any dosage alterations. Examine injection sites *to provide a baseline for determining adverse reactions.*

Nursing Diagnoses

The patient receiving a penicillin may have the following nursing diagnoses related to drug therapy:

- Acute pain related to GI effects of drug
- Imbalanced nutrition: less than body requirements related to multiple GI effects of the drug or to superinfections
- Deficient knowledge regarding drug therapy

Implementation With Rationale

- Monitor vital signs, for example temperature and pulse.
- Monitor electrolyte levels *as some penicillin preparations contain high levels of sodium and potassium salts.* The nurse should monitor for hyperkalaemia and hypernatraemia prior to and during therapy.
- Monitor renal function tests before and periodically during therapy *to arrange for dosage reduction as needed.*
- A complete blood count may be required to assess bone marrow function.
- Explain storage requirements for suspensions and the importance of completing the prescribed therapeutic course even if signs and symptoms have disappeared *to increase the effectiveness of the drug and decrease the risk of developing resistant strains.*
- Monitor the site of infection and presenting signs and symptoms (e.g. fever, lethargy) throughout the course of drug therapy. *Failure of these signs and symptoms to resolve may indicate the need to re-culture the site.*
- Patients should complete drug course even if all signs and symptoms have resolved.
- Discontinue drug immediately if hypersensitivity occurs to prevent potential fatal reactions.
- Monitor the patient for any signs of superinfection *to arrange for treatment if superinfections occur.*
- Monitor injection sites regularly and *provide warm compresses and gentle massage to injection sites if painful or swollen.* If signs of phlebitis occur, remove the IV line and reinsert it in a different vein to continue the drug regimen.
- The patient should report difficulty in breathing, severe headache, severe diarrhoea, dizziness, weakness, mouth sores and vaginal itching or sores to a health care provider.

Evaluation

- Monitor patient response to the drug (resolution of bacterial infection).
- Monitor for adverse effects (GI effects, local irritation, phlebitis at injection and IV sites, and superinfections).
- Evaluate the effectiveness of the teaching plan (patient can name the drug, dosage, possible adverse effects to expect, and specific measures to help avoid adverse effects).

- Monitor the effectiveness of comfort and safety measures and concordance with the regimen (Critical Thinking Scenario 8-1)

Cephalosporins

First introduced in the 1960s, the cephalosporins are similar to the penicillins in structure (they have the same β-lactam ring) and activity. The cephalosporins inhibit bacterial cell wall synthesis and are, therefore, bactericidal. Four generations of cephalosporins have been developed, each group with its own spectrum of activity (Table 8.2). Each subsequent generation of cephalosporins has increased effectiveness against Gram-negative bacteria and reduced effectiveness against Gram-positive bacteria.

First-generation cephalosporins are largely effective against the same Gram-positive bacteria that are affected by benzylpenicillin, as well as the Gram-negative bacteria *Proteus mirabilis, E. coli* and *Klebsiella pneumoniae*.

Second-generation cephalosporins are effective against those strains, as well as *Haemophilus influenzae, Enterobacter aerogenes* and *Neisseria* species.

Third-generation cephalosporins have relatively weak action against Gram-positive bacteria but are more potent against the Gram-negative bacilli as well as *Serratia marcescens.*

Fourth-generation cephalosporins are currently in development. The first drug of this group, cefepime, is active against Gram-negative and Gram-positive organisms, including cephalosporin-resistant staphylococci and *P. aeruginosa.* This antibacterial is not currently licensed in the United Kingdom.

Therapeutic Actions and Indications

The cephalosporins are bactericidal and in susceptible species, these agents interfere with the cell wall-building ability of bacteria when they divide. Bacteria with weakened cell walls swell and burst as a result of the osmotic pressure within the cell (see Figure 8.1).

Cephalosporins are indicated for the treatment of infections caused by susceptible bacteria. Selection of an antibacterial from this class depends on the sensitivity of the involved organism and the route of choice, and sometimes the cost involved. Before therapy begins, a culture and sensitivity test should always be performed to evaluate the causative organism and appropriate sensitivity to the antibacterial being used. It is important to reserve cephalosporins for appropriate situations because cephalosporin-resistant bacteria are appearing in increasing numbers. Many of the cephalosporins require parenteral administration and are therefore often reserved for hospitalized patients with severe infections.

Table 8.2 DRUGS IN FOCUS

Cephalosporins

Drug Name	Available Forms	Usual Indications
First-Generation		
cefadroxil	Oral	Less active against *H. influenzae* than cefaclor. Indicated for respiratory tract infections, skin and soft tissue infections, UTIs and otitis media
cefalexin	Oral	Indicated for respiratory tract infections, skin and soft tissue infections, UTIs and otitis media
cefradine	Oral, IV, IM	Indicated for respiratory tract infections, skin and soft tissue infections, UTIs and otitis media; useful in situations where a switch from parenteral to oral route is expected (e.g. preoperative prophylaxis followed by oral postoperative prophylaxis)
Second-Generation		
cefaclor	Oral	Active against *H. influenzae.* Indicated for respiratory tract infections, skin and soft tissue infections, UTIs and otitis media
cefuroxime	Oral, IV, IM	Wide range of infections, as listed for the first-generation drugs; also used to treat Lyme disease and in surgical prophylaxis. Active against *H. influenzae* and *Neisseria gonorrhoeae*
cefixime	Oral	Licensed to treat a wide range of acute infections, including those listed for cefaclor. Unlicensed treatment of gonorrhoea
Third-Generation		
cefotaxime	IV, IM	As for cefaclor, plus surgical prophylaxis; gonorrhoea, *Haemophilus* epiglottitis and meningitis
cefpodoxime	Oral	Respiratory infections, UTIs, gonorrhoea, skin and soft tissue infections
ceftazidime	IV, IM	As for cefaclor. Demonstrates good activity against *Pseudomonas* and other Gram-negative bacteria
ceftriaxone	IV, IM	Serious infections including septicaemia, gonorrhoea, pneumonia and meningitis; and also surgical prophylaxis. Unlicensed for meningococcal prophylaxis

Pharmacokinetics

The following cephalosporins are well absorbed from the GI tract: first-generation drugs cefadroxil, cefalexin, cefradine; second-generation drugs cefaclor and cefuroxime; third-generation drugs cefpodoxime, cefprozil and cefixime and fourth-generation cefepime. The others are absorbed well after intramuscular (IM) injection or intravenous (IV) administration.

Most of the cephalosporins are excreted unchanged in the urine. Patients with renal impairment will require a reduced dose. The cephalosporins are not known to be harmful during pregnancy and can be used safely. They can enter breast milk and are present in low concentrations; however, it is advised to avoid only cefixime during lactation.

Contraindications and Cautions

These drugs should not be used in patients with known allergies to cephalosporins or penicillins *because cross-sensitivity is common in approximately 10% of patients.* In addition, caution must be used in patients with renal failure because *these drugs can be nephrotoxic.*

Adverse Effects

The most common adverse effects of the cephalosporins involve the GI tract and include nausea, vomiting, diarrhoea and abdominal pain. Pseudomembranous colitis, a potentially dangerous disorder, has also been reported with higher doses of cephalosporins. A particular drug should be discontinued immediately at any sign of violent, bloody diarrhoea or abdominal pain.

CNS symptoms include headache, confusion and dizziness. Nephrotoxicity is also associated with the use of cephalosporins, most particularly in patients who have a predisposing renal insufficiency. Other adverse effects include rashes and other allergic reactions, and blood disorders. Superinfections, including *Candida*, are more likely to occur with the cephalosporins and can occur because of the death of protective bacteria of the normal flora. Patients receiving parenteral cephalosporins should also be monitored for the possibility of phlebitis with IV administration or local abscess at the site of an IM injection.

Clinically Important Drug–Drug Interactions

The concurrent administration of cephalosporins with aminoglycosides increases the risk of nephrotoxicity. Patients who receive this combination should have serum blood urea nitrogen and creatinine levels frequently monitored. Probenecid can block the secretion of cephalosporins by the kidney and should not be prescribed concurrently.

Patients who receive oral anticoagulants in addition to cephalosporins may experience increased bleeding. They should be taught how to monitor for blood loss (e.g. bleeding gums, bruising easily) and should be aware that the dose of the oral anticoagulant may need to be reduced.

Always consult a current copy of the British National Formulary for further guidance.

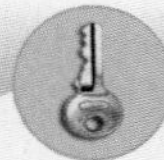

Key Drug Summary: Cefaclor

Indications: Treatment of respiratory, dermatological, urinary tract and middle ear infections caused by susceptible strains of bacteria. Effective against *H. influenzae.*

Actions: Inhibits the synthesis of bacterial cell walls, causing cell death in susceptible bacteria

Pharmacokinetics:

Route	Peak	Duration
Oral	30–60 min	8–10 h

$T_{1/2}$: 30–60 minutes; excreted unchanged in the urine

Adverse effects: Nausea, vomiting, diarrhoea, rash, superinfection, bone marrow depression, risk of pseudomembranous colitis

Nursing Considerations for Patients Receiving Cephalosporins

Assessment: History and Examination

Screen for the following, *which are possible contraindications or cautions for use of the drug*: known allergy to any cephalosporin, penicillin or any other allergens *because cross-sensitivity often occurs* (obtain specific information about the nature and occurrence of the allergic reactions); history of renal disease, *which could exacerbate nephrotoxicity related to the cephalosporin* and current pregnancy or lactation status.

Physical assessment should be performed *to establish baseline data for assessing the effectiveness of the drug and the occurrence of any adverse effects associated with drug therapy*. Perform culture and sensitivity tests at the site of infection. Examine skin for any rash or lesions *for possible adverse effects*. Note respiratory status, including rate, depth and adventitious sounds. Check renal function test results *to assess the status of renal functioning and to detect the possible need to alter dosage.*

Nursing Diagnoses

Patients receiving a cephalosporin may have the following nursing diagnoses related to drug therapy:

- Acute pain related to GI and CNS effects of drug
- Risk of infection related to repeated injections
- Deficient fluid volume and imbalanced nutrition: less than body requirements related to diarrhoea
- Deficient knowledge regarding drug therapy
- Observe for any bleeding as the cephalosporins may reduce prothrombin levels through the interference with vitamin K metabolism.

Implementation With Rationale

- Monitor renal function test values before and periodically during therapy *to arrange for appropriate dosage reduction as needed.*
- Monitor the site of infection and presenting signs and symptoms (e.g. fever, lethargy) throughout the course of drug therapy. *Failure of these signs and symptoms to resolve may indicate the need to re-culture the site.* Patients should complete drug course even if all signs and symptoms have resolved.
- Monitor patient for any signs of superinfection *to arrange for treatment if superinfection occurs.*
- If CNS effects occur, initiate appropriate safety measures *to protect the patient from injury.*

The patient should:

- Take safety precautions, including changing position slowly and avoiding driving and hazardous tasks, if CNS effects occur.
- Report difficulty in breathing, severe headache, severe diarrhoea, dizziness or weakness to the health care provider.

Evaluation

- Monitor for adverse effects (orientation and affect, renal toxicity, hepatic dysfunction, GI effects and local irritation, including phlebitis at injection and IV sites).
- Additional information is listed under Nursing Considerations for Patients Receiving Penicillins and Penicillinase-Resistant Antibacterials.

Other β-Lactam Antibacterials

Other β-lactam antibacterials include the monobactam, aztreonam; and the carbapenems, ertapenem, imipenem and meropenem.

The structure of aztreonam is unique among the antibacterials, and it is also resistant to most β-lactamases. Aztreonam is effective against Gram-negative enterobacteria and has no effect on Gram-positive or anaerobic bacteria. The drug is regarded as a safer alternative for treating infections caused by susceptible bacteria in patients who may be allergic to penicillins or cephalosporins. Aztreonam is absorbed well after IM injection, reaching peak effect levels in 1 to 1.5 hours. Its half-life is 1.5 to 2 hours and it is excreted unchanged in the urine. Aztreonam can cross the placenta and also enter breast milk and should therefore be avoided during pregnancy and lactation.

The carbapenems have a broader spectrum of activity than the other β-lactam antibacterials (Table 8.3). Imipenem is not absorbed orally and must be given parenterally. It is inactivated by dipeptidase enzymes found in the renal tubules and is therefore combined with cilastatin, a dipeptidase inhibitor, to prevent breakdown. Its half-life is 1 hour and it is excreted mostly unchanged in the urine. Meropenem is similar in activity to imipenem. It is insensitive to renal tubular dipeptidases and does not need to be administered with cilastatin.

Table 8.3 DRUGS IN FOCUS

Other β-Lactam Antibiotics

Drug Name	Available Forms	Usual Indications
aztreonam	IV, IM	Treatment of Gram-negative infections including *E. coli, Serratia, Proteus, Salmonella, Providencia, Pseudomonas, Haemophilus, Neisseria* and *Klebsiella.* Some strains of *Enterobacter* and *Citrobacter* spp. are resistant. Often used as an alternative to penicillin
ertapenem	IV	Similar spectrum of activity to imipenem but inactive against *Acinetobacter* or *P. aeruginosa*
imipenem with cilastatin	IV, IM	Effective against many aerobic and anaerobic Gram-positive and Gram-negative bacteria including *Enterococcus, Listeria, Citrobacter, Enterobacter* spp., *E. coli, Klebsiella, Proteus, Salmonella, Haemophilus, Neisseria* and *Serratia.* Used to treat septicaemia and as surgical prophylaxis
meropenem	IV	Bacterial sensitivity as for imipenem. Also used to treat hospital-acquired infections and meningitis

Ertapenem has a similar spectrum of activity to the other carbapenems except that it is not active against *Pseudomonas* and *Acinetobacter*. Its effectiveness against a wide range of bacteria may help to slow the emergence of resistant strains previously sensitive only to well-established antibacterials and may also provide successful treatment of some infections that are resistant to regularly used antibacterials.

Therapeutic Actions and Indications

Aztreonam disrupts bacterial cell wall synthesis, which promotes leakage of cellular contents and cell death in susceptible bacteria (see Figure 8.1). The drug is indicated for the treatment of urinary tract, skin, intra-abdominal and gynaecological (gonococci) infections, as well as septicaemia caused by susceptible bacteria (see Table 8.3).

The carbapenems also interfere with cell wall synthesis and are active against a broad spectrum of aerobic and anaerobic Gram-positive and Gram-negative bacteria. These antibacterials are used to treat a similar range of infections as aztreonam, as well as prophylaxis prior to surgery.

Contraindications and Cautions

Aztreonam is contraindicated with any known allergy to aztreonam. Caution should be used in patients with a history of acute allergic reaction to penicillins or cephalosporins *because of the possibility of cross-reactivity (although reduced compared to other β-lactam antibacterials)*; in those with renal or hepatic dysfunction *that could interfere with the clearance and excretion of the drug* and in pregnant and lactating women *because of potential adverse effects on the foetus or neonate*.

The carbapenems are contraindicated with any known allergy to one of the carbapenems. Caution should be used in patients with sensitivity to β-lactam antibacterials; those with renal or hepatic impairment; those with a history of seizures and in pregnant and lactating women.

Adverse Effects

The adverse effects associated with the use of aztreonam are relatively mild. Local GI effects include nausea, GI upset, vomiting and diarrhoea. Hepatic enzyme elevations related to direct drug effects on the liver may also occur. Other effects include inflammation, phlebitis and discomfort at injection sites, as well as the potential for allergic response.

The adverse effects associated with the carbapenems are similar to those with other β-lactam antibacterials. There is a risk of seizures with high doses of imipenem and ertapenem.

Always consult a current copy of the British National Formulary for further guidance.

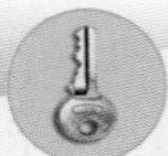

Key Drug Summary: Aztreonam

Indications: Treatment of lower respiratory, dermatological, urinary tract, intra-abdominal and gynaecological infections caused by susceptible strains of Gram-negative bacteria

Actions: Interferes with bacterial cell wall synthesis, causing cell death in susceptible Gram-negative bacteria; ineffective against Gram-positive or anaerobic bacteria

Pharmacokinetics:

Route	Onset	Peak	Duration
IM	Varies	60–90 min	6–8 h
IV	Immediate	30 min	6–8 h

$T_{1/2}$: 1.5–2 hours; excreted unchanged in the urine

Adverse effects: Nausea, vomiting, diarrhoea, rash, superinfection, hypersensitivity reactions, local discomfort at injection sites

Nursing Considerations for Patients Receiving Monobactam Antibacterials

Assessment: History and Examination

Screen for the following, *which are possible contraindications or cautions for use of the drug*: known allergy to monobactam antibacterials (obtain specific information about the nature and occurrence of allergic reactions); history of acute allergic reactions to penicillins or cephalosporins; history of liver or kidney disease *that could interfere with clearance and excretion of the drug*; history of seizures *that could be exacerbated by the carbapenems* and current pregnancy or lactation status *because of potential adverse effects on the foetus or infant.*

Physical assessment should be performed *to establish baseline data for assessing the effectiveness of the drug and the occurrence of any adverse effects associated with drug therapy.* Obtain specimens for culture and sensitivity tests from the site of infection *to ensure that this is the most appropriate drug for this patient.* Monitor temperature *to detect infection.* Abdominal examination should be performed and liver and kidney function tests should be done *to determine any needed alteration in dosage.*

Nursing Diagnoses

The patient receiving monobactams may have the following nursing diagnoses related to drug therapy:

- Acute pain related to GI and local effects of drug
- Deficient knowledge regarding drug therapy
- Deficient fluid volume (due to diarrhoea)

Implementation With Rationale

- Monitor hepatic and renal function tests before therapy *to arrange to reduce dosage as needed.*
- Monitor the site of infection and presenting signs and symptoms (e.g. fever, lethargy) throughout the course of drug therapy. *Failure of drug therapy to resolve these signs and symptoms may indicate the need to re-culture the site.*
- Ensure ready access to bathroom facilities *to assist patients with problems associated with diarrhoea.*
- Discuss with the patient the route of administration and possible side-effects *to enhance patient knowledge about drug therapy and to promote concordance.* The drug can be given only IV or IM, so the patient will not be responsible for administering the drug.
- The patient should report difficulty in breathing, severe diarrhoea, or mouth or vaginal sores to a health care provider.

Evaluation

- Monitor for adverse effects (orientation and affect, GI effects and local inflammation).
- Additional information is listed under Nursing Considerations for Patients Receiving Penicillins and Penicillinase-Resistant Antibacterials.

Quinolones (and Fluoroquinolones)

The quinolones (Table 8.4) are a relatively new class of antibacterials with a broad spectrum of activity. These drugs, which are all made synthetically, are associated with relatively mild adverse reactions. Nalidixic acid was the first quinolone to be introduced. Since then, fluorinated forms of quinolones, the fluoroquinolones, have also been introduced: ciprofloxacin, levofloxacin, ofloxacin, norfloxacin and moxifloxacin. The most widely used fluoroquinolone is ciprofloxacin, which is effective against a wide spectrum of Gram-negative and some Gram-positive bacteria.

Therapeutic Actions and Indications

The quinolones enter the bacterial cell by passive diffusion. Once inside, they inhibit the action of the DNA enzyme, DNA gyrase (topoisomerase II and IV). DNA gyrase is vital for the 'supercoiling' of bacterial DNA in replication (see Figure 8.1). The quinolones prevent supercoiling from occurring and thus bacterial replication; cell death follows.

Misuse of these drugs in the short time that this class has been available has led to the existence of resistant strains of bacteria. For example, *S. aureus* and *P. aeruginosa* are becoming increasingly resistant to the quinolones. Infected tissue should be cultured to determine the exact bacterial cause and sensitivity.

The quinolones are indicated for treating infections caused by susceptible strains of Gram-negative bacteria, including *E. coli, P. mirabilis, K. pneumoniae, Enterobacter cloacae, Proteus vulgaris, Proteus rettgeri, Morganella morganii, Moraxella catarrhalis, H. influenzae, H. parainfluenzae, P. aeruginosa, Citrobacter freundii, S. aureus, Staphylococcus*

Table 8.4 DRUGS IN FOCUS

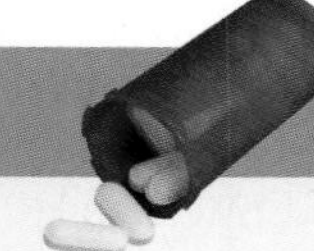

Quinolones and Fluoroquinolones

Drug Name	Available Forms	Usual Indications
ciprofloxacin	Oral, IV, topical	Treatment of infections caused by a wide spectrum of Gram-negative (and some Gram-positive) bacteria, including respiratory tract infections, UTIs, gonorrhoea, prostatitis, meningitis, typhoid, anthrax and surgical prophylaxis. Also available as an ophthalmic and otic (unlicensed) agent.
levofloxacin	Oral, IV, topical	Treatment of respiratory, urinary tract, skin and soft tissue and sinus infections caused by susceptible Gram-negative and Gram-positive bacteria. Second-line treatment of community-acquired pneumonia. Also available as an ophthalmic agent.
moxifloxacin	Oral	Greater activity against Gram-positive than Gram-negative bacteria. Treatment of adults with sinusitis and second-line treatment of bronchitis or community-acquired pneumonia
nalidixic acid	Oral	Treatment of UTIs
norfloxacin	Oral	Treatment of various UTIs, including recurrent UTIs; and chronic prostatitis
ofloxacin	Oral, IV, topical	Treatment of respiratory, skin and soft tissue and urinary tract infections; chronic prostatitis, gonorrhoea, Chlamydia, septicaemia and pelvic inflammatory disease. Also available as an ophthalmic and otic (unlicensed) agent.

epidermidis, some *Neisseria gonorrhoeae* and group D streptococci. These infections frequently include urinary tract, respiratory tract and skin infections. There is also some, but limited, activity against some Gram-positive bacteria, for example ciprofloxacin and *S. pneumoniae*.

Pharmacokinetics

The quinolones are well absorbed from the GI tract and distributed widely around the body. They are excreted in the urine and so caution should be used in patients with renal impairment, which could interfere with excretion of the drugs. The quinolones can cross the placenta and effect cartilage formation in the developing foetus. The quinolones can also enter breast milk. An alternative antibacterial should therefore be used during pregnancy and lactation.

Contraindications and Cautions

Quinolones are contraindicated in patients with known allergy to any quinolone drug and in pregnant or lactating women *because these drugs have known effects on the foetus and neonate*. These drugs have been associated with lesions in developing cartilage (arthropathy) and are therefore not recommended for use in children and adolescents. Moxifloxacin is contraindicated in patients with hepatic dysfunction or a history of myocardial problems, including long QT-interval and arrhythmias. Caution should be used in the presence of renal dysfunction, *which could interfere with drug excretion*; seizures and myasthenia gravis, *which could be exacerbated*. Seizures can be precipitated by the concurrent use of nonsteroidal anti-inflammatory drugs (NSAIDs). Patients who are glucose-6-phosphate deficient may develop haemolytic anaemia with nalidixic acid.

Adverse Effects

Several adverse effects are associated with quinolones. The most common CNS effects are headache, dizziness and insomnia. GI effects include nausea, vomiting, dyspepsia, diarrhoea and abdominal pain, related to direct drug effects on the GI tract.

Immunological effects include bone marrow depression, which may be related to drug effects on the cells of the bone marrow that rapidly turn over. Other adverse effects include fever, rash and photosensitivity, a potentially serious adverse effect that can cause severe skin reactions. Patients should be advised to avoid sun and ultraviolet light exposure and to use protective clothing and sunscreens.

Clinically Important Drug–Drug Interactions

When quinolones are taken concurrently with iron salts, sucralfate, mineral supplements, or antacids, the absorption and therefore therapeutic effect of the antibacterial is decreased. If this drug combination is necessary, administration of the two agents should be separated by at least 4 hours.

If quinolones are taken with drugs that increase the QT interval or cause torsades de pointes (quinidine, procainamide, amiodarone, disopyramide, erythromycin, pentamidine, tricyclic antidepressants, antihistamines, antimalarials, antipsychotics, atomoxetine, β-blockers), severe to fatal cardiac reactions are possible. These combinations should be avoided; if they must be used, patients should be hospitalized with continual cardiac monitoring.

Combining quinolones with theophylline leads to increased theophylline levels because the two drugs use similar metabolic pathways. The theophylline dose should be reduced, and serum theophylline levels should be monitored carefully. In addition, when quinolones are combined with NSAIDs, an increased risk of seizures is possible, especially those who have a history of seizures or CNS problems. If this combination is necessary, patients should be monitored closely.

Always consult a current copy of the British National Formulary for further guidance.

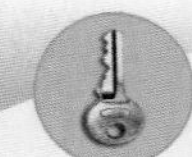

Key Drug Summary: *Ciprofloxacin*

Indications: Treatment of respiratory, dermatological, urinary tract, ear, eye, bone and joint infections; treatment after anthrax exposure, typhoid fever

Actions: Interferes with DNA replication in susceptible Gram-negative (less active against Gram-positive) bacteria, preventing cell reproduction

Pharmacokinetics:

Route	Onset	Peak	Duration
Oral	Varies	60–90 min	4–5 h
IV	10 min	30 min	4–5 h

$T_{1/2}$: 3.5–4 hours; partly metabolized in the liver and partly excreted in the urine

Adverse effects: Headache, dizziness, hypotension, nausea, vomiting, diarrhoea, flatulence, fever, rash

Nursing Considerations for Patients Receiving Quinolones

Assessment: History and Examination

Screen for the following, *which are possible contraindications or cautions for use of the drug*: known allergy to any quinolone (obtain specific information about the nature and occurrence of allergic reactions); history of renal disease, *which could interfere with excretion of the drug*; history of cardiac arrhythmias, seizures and myasthenia gravis and current pregnancy or lactation status *because of potential adverse effects on the foetus or infant.*

Physical assessment should *establish baseline data for assessing the effectiveness of the drug and the occurrence of any adverse effects associated with drug therapy*. Perform culture and sensitivity tests at the site of infection. Examine the skin for any rash or lesions *to provide a baseline for possible adverse effects*. Assess orientation, affect and reflexes *to establish a baseline for any CNS effects of the drug*. Perform renal function tests *to evaluate the status of renal functioning and to assess necessary changes in dosage*.

Nursing Diagnoses

The patient receiving a quinolone may have the following nursing diagnoses related to drug therapy:

- Acute pain related to GI, CNS, skin effects of drug
- Deficient fluid volume and imbalanced nutrition: less than body requirements, related to GI effects of drug
- Deficient knowledge regarding drug therapy

Implementation With Rationale

- Monitor renal function tests before initiating therapy *to appropriately arrange for dosage reduction if necessary*.
- Monitor the site of infection and presenting signs and symptoms (e.g. fever, lethargy, urinary tract signs and symptoms) throughout the course of drug therapy. *Failure of these signs and symptoms to resolve may indicate the need to re-culture the site.*
- Patients should complete drug course even if all signs and symptoms have resolved.
- Implement safety measures *to protect patient from injury if CNS effects occur.*

The patient should:

- Take safety precautions, including changing position slowly and avoiding driving and hazardous tasks, if CNS effects occur.
- Avoid ultraviolet light and sun exposure, using protective clothing and sunscreens.
- Report difficulty in breathing, severe headache, severe diarrhoea, severe skin rash, fainting and heart palpitations to the health care provider.

Evaluation

- Monitor for adverse effects (orientation and affect, GI effects and photosensitivity).
- Additional information is listed under Nursing Considerations for Patients Receiving Penicillins and Penicillinase-Resistant Antibacterials.

Sulphonamides

The sulphonamides (Table 8.5) inhibit folic acid synthesis. Folic acid is necessary for the synthesis of purine and pyrimidines, which are precursors of RNA and DNA. For cells to grow and reproduce, they require folic acid. Humans cannot synthesize folic acid and depend on folate obtained in their diet. Bacteria are impermeable to folic acid and must synthesize it inside the cell.

The emergence of resistant bacterial strains and the development of newer antibacterials have meant the sulphonamides are not used as much any more. However, they remain an inexpensive and effective treatment for urinary and respiratory tract infections, especially in developing countries and when cost is an issue.

Co-trimoxazole is a combined preparation of the sulphonamides trimethoprim and sulfamethoxazole. Co-trimoxazole is limited to the treatment of pneumonia caused by *Pneumocystis jiroveci* (*P. carinii*), which is a serious problem in immunocompromised patients (e.g. those with AIDS). Although also effective in the treatment of otitis media, bronchitis and urinary tract infections, this

Table 8.5 DRUGS IN FOCUS

Sulphonamides

Drug Name	Available Forms	Usual Indications
co-trimoxazole	Oral, IV	Combined preparation of sulfamethoxazole and trimethoprim. Treatment of choice in *Pneumocystis jiroveci* (*P. carinii*), *toxoplasmosis* and nocardiasis. Must be strong evidence to suggest use in otitis media, bronchitis and urinary tract infections
sulfadiazine	Oral, topical	Prevention of reoccurrence of rheumatic fever. Used topically to treat and prevent infections in burns and to treat leg ulcers
trimethoprim	Oral	Treatment of UTIs, bronchitis and pneumocystis pneumonia

combination can only be used to treat these infections if other antibacterials are inappropriate.

Therapeutic Actions and Indications

The sulphonamides inhibit folic acid synthesis in bacteria. Para-aminobenzoic acid (PABA) is a precursor of folic acid and is converted into dihydropteroate by the enzyme dihydropteroate synthetase. The sulphonamides are structural analogues of PABA and compete with PABA to prevent the synthesis of dihydropteroate. Dihydropteroate is converted into dihydrofolate and then tetrahydrofolate by the enzyme dihydrofolate reductase. It is this reductase enzyme that is the target of trimethoprim. The sulphonamides therefore target two stages of the folic acid synthesis pathway and susceptible bacteria are unable to produce their own RNA and DNA (see Figure 8.1). As a result bacterial growth is prevented; the sulphonamides are thus bacteriostatic.

Susceptible bacteria include Gram-negative and Gram-positive bacteria such as *C. trachomatis, Nocardia* and some strains of *H. influenzae, E. coli* and *P. mirabilis*. The usual indications of the sulphonamides are listed in Table 8.5.

Pharmacokinetics

The sulphonamides are well absorbed from the GI tract and widely distributed in the tissues. Some metabolism occurs in the liver; the remaining drug is excreted unchanged via the kidneys. The half-lives of sulfadiazine, co-trimoxazole and trimethoprim are 10, 7–12, and 10 hours respectively. The sulphonamides are teratogenic; they are also distributed into breast milk and should not be used during pregnancy or lactation.

Contraindications and Cautions

The sulphonamides are contraindicated with any known allergy to any sulphonamide or a history of porphyria or blood disorders. They are also contraindicated during pregnancy *because the drugs can cause birth defects*; and during lactation *because of a risk of kernicterus (CNS damage) in the infant.* Caution should be used in patients with renal or hepatic disease or a history of kidney stones *because of the possibility of increased toxic effects of the drugs*, and asthma *because of potential worsening of symptoms*.

Adverse Effects

Adverse effects associated with sulphonamides include GI effects such as nausea, vomiting and diarrhoea. Less common effects include anorexia, glossitis, stomatitis and hepatic injury. Renal effects are related to the filtration of the drug in the glomerulus and include crystalluria, which can progress to nephritis and hyperkalaemia. CNS effects include headache, vertigo, ataxia, convulsions and depression. Bone marrow depression may occur and is related to drug effects on the cells that turn over rapidly in the bone marrow.

Dermatological effects include photosensitivity and rash related to direct effects on the dermal cells. A wide range of hypersensitivity reactions may also occur.

Clinically Important Drug–Drug Interactions

Concomitant administration of sulphonamides with amiodarone, methenamine, coumarins, pyrimethamine, clozapine, and the cytotoxics mercaptopurine, azathioprine and methotrexate; should be avoided. There is an increased risk of nephrotoxicity when sulphonamides are taken with ciclosporin. If this combination is essential, the patient should be monitored closely and the sulphonamide stopped at any sign of renal dysfunction.

Always consult a current copy of the British National Formulary for further guidance.

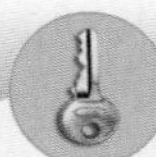

Key Drug Summary: Co-trimoxazole

Indications: Treatment of *Pneumocystis jiroveci* (*P. carinii*) pneumonia, *toxoplasmosis* and *nocardiasis*

Actions: Blocks PABA and dihydrofolate reductase, two essential components of the folic acid synthesis pathway in susceptible Gram-negative and Gram-positive bacteria

Pharmacokinetics:

Route	Onset	Peak
Oral	Varies	1.5–6 h
IV	30 min	60–90 min

$T_{1/2}$: 7–12 hours; metabolized in the liver, excreted in the urine

Adverse effects: Nausea, vomiting, diarrhoea, nephritis, bone marrow suppression, Stevens–Johnson syndrome, rash, photophobia

Nursing Considerations for Patients Receiving Sulphonamides

Assessment: History and Examination

The approach for patients receiving sulphonamide antibacterials is the same as for Nursing Considerations for Patients Receiving Penicillins and Penicillinase-Resistant Antibacterials.

Nursing Diagnoses

In addition to the nursing diagnoses related to patients receiving penicillins and penicllinase-resistant antibacterials, the patient may also experience disturbed sensory perception related to the CNS effects of the drugs.

Implementation With Rationale

- Monitor renal function tests before and periodically during therapy *to arrange for a dosage reduction as necessary.*
- Administer the oral drug on an empty stomach 1 hour before or 2 hours after meals with a full glass of water *to promote adequate absorption of the drug.*
- Discontinue the drug immediately if hypersensitivity reactions occur *to prevent potentially fatal reactions.*
- Monitor full blood count and urinalysis test results before and periodically during therapy *to check for adverse effects.*
- Instruct the patient about the appropriate dosage regimen, the proper way to take the drug (on an empty stomach with a full glass of water), and possible adverse effects, *to enhance patient knowledge about drug therapy and to promote concordance.*

The patient should:

- Avoid driving or operating dangerous machinery because dizziness, lethargy and ataxia may occur.
- Report to a health care provider any difficulty in breathing, rash, ringing in the ears, fever, sore throat or blood in the urine.

Evaluation

- Monitor for adverse effects (GI effects, CNS effects, rash and crystalluria).
- Additional information is listed under Nursing Considerations for Patients Receiving Penicillins and Penicillinase-Resistant Antibacterials.

Aminoglycosides

The aminoglycosides (Table 8.6) are used to treat serious infections usually caused by Gram-negative aerobic bacilli, but also some Gram-positive bacilli. These drugs have potentially serious adverse effects and the problem of increasing resistance.

Therapeutic Actions and Indications

The aminoglycosides are bactericidal. They inhibit protein synthesis in susceptible strains of bacteria by causing the bacteria's ribosomes to misread the amino acid code on the messenger RNA. The proteins produced will have an incorrect amino acid sequence and in turn this leads to loss of functional integrity of the bacterial cell membrane, causing cell death (Figure 8.2). These drugs are used to treat serious infections caused by susceptible strains of Gram-negative bacteria, including *Pseudomonas aeruginosa, E. coli, Proteus* species, the *Klebsiella-Enterobacter-Serratia* group and *Staphylococcus* species such as *S. aureus*. Aminoglycosides are indicated for the treatment of serious infections that are susceptible to penicillin when penicillin is contraindicated. In appropriate clinical situations where infection is severe, they can be used before culture and sensitivity tests have been completed.

Pharmacokinetics

The aminoglycosides are poorly absorbed from the GI tract and are therefore administered either by IM injection or IV infusion. They are not able to cross the blood–brain barrier unless the meninges are inflamed. The aminoglycosides can cross the placenta and should only be used during pregnancy if essential. No information is available of the risk to breast-fed infants and should therefore be used with caution.

Aminoglycosides are excreted unchanged in the urine and have an average half-life of 2 to 3 hours. Renal function should be tested regularly in patients with impaired renal

Table 8.6 DRUGS IN FOCUS

Aminoglycosides

Drug Name	Available Forms	Usual Indications
amikacin	IV, IM	Treatment of serious gentamicin-resistant Gram-negative infections
gentamicin	IV, IM, intrathecal, topical	Treatment of Pseudomonas infections and a wide variety of Gram-negative infections, including septicaemia, meningitis; as adjunct treatment in endocarditis and pyelonephritis
neomycin	Topical	Suppression of GI normal flora preoperatively; treatment of hepatic failure; topical treatment of skin infections
netilmicin	IV, IM	Treatment of serious gentamicin-resistant Gram-negative infections
tobramycin	IV, IM, nebulizer	Similar indications as gentamicin. More active against *P. aeruginosa* than gentamicin

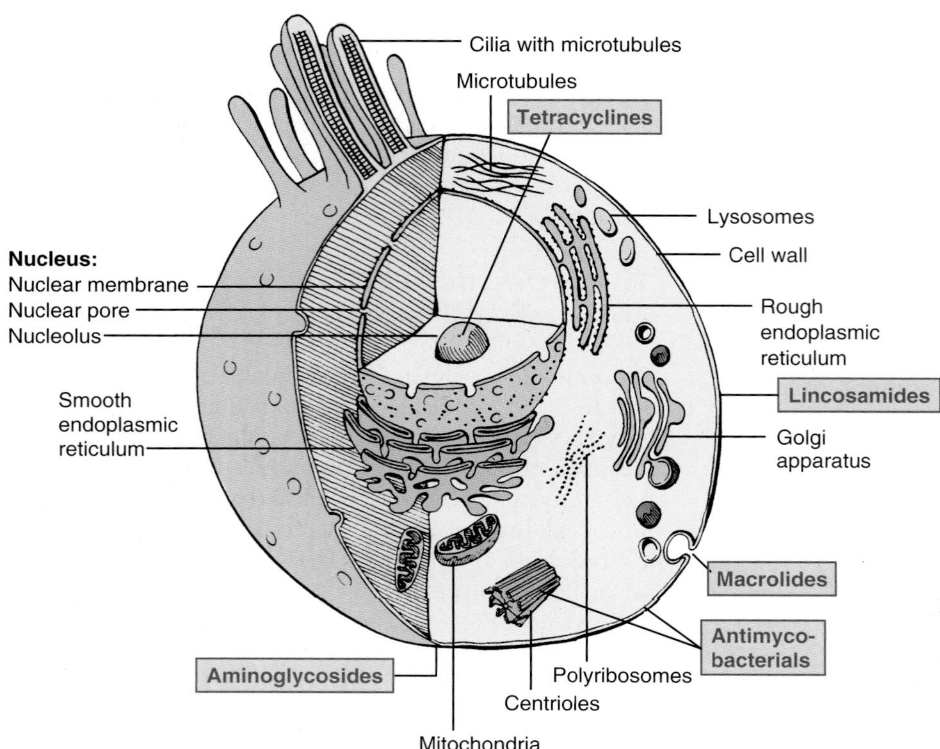

FIGURE 8.2 Sites of cellular action of aminoglycosides, lincosamides, tetracyclines, macrolides and antimycobacterials. Aminoglycosides disrupt the cell membrane. Lincosamides change protein function and prevent cell division or cause cell death. Macrolides disrupt protein function by preventing cell division. Tetracyclines inhibit protein synthesis, thereby preventing reproduction. Antimycobacterial drugs affect mycobacteria in three ways: They (1) affect the mycolic coat of the bacteria, (2) alter DNA and RNA, and (3) prevent cell division.

function as these drugs depend on the kidney for excretion and can be toxic to the kidney.

Contraindications and Cautions

Aminoglycosides are contraindicated in the following conditions: known allergy to any of the aminoglycosides; and myasthenia gravis *which is often exacerbated by the effects of a particular aminoglycoside on the nervous system*. These drugs should be used with caution in: renal disease *that could be exacerbated by the toxic effects of aminoglycoside and could interfere with drug excretion, leading to higher toxicity*; pre-existing hearing loss, *which could be intensified by toxic drug effects on the auditory nerve*; pregnancy *because aminoglycosides could cause adverse effects to the foetus*; and lactation *because the effects of aminoglycosides on neonates are unknown*.

Adverse Effects

The many serious adverse effects associated with aminoglycosides are dose-dependent and can be seen at therapeutic concentrations. CNS effects include ototoxicity, possibly leading to irreversible deafness; and vestibular damage resulting from drug effects on the vestibular organ.

Renal toxicity is caused by direct damage to the kidney tubules. The risk of damage increases in patients with renal dysfunction, low urine outputs or concurrent use of other nephrotoxic drugs. Bone marrow depression may result from direct drug effects on the rapidly dividing cells in the bone marrow, leading, for example, to immune suppression and resultant superinfections. Haemolytic anaemia has also been reported. GI effects include nausea, vomiting and diarrhoea (neomycin).

Clinically Important Drug–Drug Interactions

If aminoglycosides are taken in combination with loop diuretics, the incidence of ototoxicity increases. This combination should be avoided if at all possible. There is an increased risk of nephrotoxicity with some of the other antibacterials, antifungals, ciclosporin, cytotoxics and tacrolimus.

If these antibacterials are given with nondepolarizing muscle relaxants or suxamethonium, increased neuromuscular blockade with paralysis is possible. If a patient has been receiving an aminoglycoside and now requires surgery, the aminoglycoside should be indicated prominently on the chart.

In addition, most aminoglycosides have a synergistic bactericidal effect when given with penicillins; and in certain conditions, this synergism is used therapeutically to increase the effectiveness of treatment.

Always consult a current copy of the British National Formulary for further guidance.

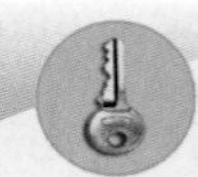

Key Drug Summary: *Gentamicin*

Indications: Treatment of *Pseudomonas* infections and a wide variety of Gram-negative infections, including septicaemia, meningitis; and as adjunct treatment in endocarditis and pyelonephritis

Actions: Inhibits protein synthesis in susceptible strains of Gram-negative bacteria, disrupting functional integrity of the cell membrane and causing cell death

Pharmacokinetics:

Route	Onset	Peak
IM, IV	Rapid	30–90 min

$T_{1/2}$: 2–3 hours; excreted unchanged in the urine

Adverse effects: Vestibular and auditory damage, risk of nephrotoxicity, nausea, vomiting, rash, stomatitis, blood disorders

Nursing Considerations for Patients Receiving Aminoglycosides

Assessment: History and Examination

Screen for the following *which are possible contraindications or cautions for use of the drug*: known allergy to any aminoglycoside (obtain specific information about the nature and occurrence of allergic reactions); history of renal or hepatic disease; pre-existing hearing loss; myasthenia gravis and current pregnancy or lactation status.

Physical assessment should be performed *to establish baseline data for assessing the effectiveness of the drug and the occurrence of any adverse effects associated with drug therapy*. Perform culture and sensitivity tests at the site of infection. Conduct orientation and reflex assessment as well as auditory testing *to evaluate any CNS effects of the drug*. Also assess vital signs: respiratory rate and adventitious sounds *to monitor for signs of infection or hypersensitivity reactions*; temperature *to assess for signs and symptoms of infection*; blood pressure *to monitor for cardiovascular effects of the drug*. Renal and hepatic function tests should be done *to determine baseline function of these organs and, possibly, the need to adjust dosage*.

Nursing Diagnoses

Patients who receive aminoglycosides may have the following nursing diagnoses related to drug therapy:

- Acute pain related to GI, CNS effects of drug
- Disturbed sensory perception (auditory) related to CNS effects of drug
- Risk of infection related to bone marrow suppression
- Excess fluid volume related to nephrotoxicity
- Deficient knowledge regarding drug therapy

Implementation With Rationale

- Monitor the site of infection and presenting signs and symptoms (e.g. fever, lethargy) throughout the course of drug therapy. *Failure of these signs and symptoms to resolve may indicate the need to re-culture the site.* Patients should complete drug course even if all signs and symptoms have resolved.
- Monitor the patient regularly for signs of nephrotoxicity, neurotoxicity and bone marrow suppression *to effectively arrange for discontinuation of drug or decreased dosage, as appropriate, if any of these toxicities occurs.*
- Monitor baseline audiometry and vestibular function prior to administration and throughout therapy. Hearing loss may occur after therapy has been completed.
- Provide safety measures *to protect the patient if CNS effects, such as imbalance occur*.
- Ensure that the patient is hydrated at all times during drug therapy *to minimize renal toxicity from drug exposure*.

The patient should:

- Take safety precautions, such as changing position slowly and avoiding driving and hazardous tasks, if CNS effects occur.
- Report difficulty in breathing, severe headache, loss of hearing or ringing in the ears or changes in urine output to the health care provider immediately.

Evaluation

- Monitor for adverse effects (orientation and affect, hearing changes, bone marrow suppression, renal toxicity, hepatic dysfunction and GI effects).
- Additional information is listed under Nursing Considerations for Patients Receiving Penicillins and Penicillinase-Resistant Antibacterials.

Macrolides

The macrolides also interfere with protein synthesis in susceptible bacteria. The macrolides include azithromycin, clarithromycin, erythromycin and telithromycin (Table 8.7).

The first macrolide to be developed was erythromycin. With a similar spectrum of antibacterial activity as penicillin, erythromycin has proved to be a useful alternative for patients who are allergic to penicillins. Effective against Gram-positive bacteria, it is the drug of choice for the treatment of Legionnaire's disease, infections caused by *Corynebacterium diphtheriae, U. urealyticum*, syphilis, mycoplasmal pneumonias and chlamydial infections. Pharmacokinetic details are provided in the Key Drug Summary for erythromycin.

Azithromycin is less effective against Gram-positive bacteria than erythromycin. However, it is more effective against some Gram-negative bacteria including *H. influenzae* and *N. gonorrhoeae*. Absorption from the GI tract is rapid and it is widely distributed around the body. It is mainly excreted unchanged in bile and faeces. The half-life of azithromycin is 68 hours, meaning it can be administered once a day.

Clarithromycin has a similar antibacterial spectrum as erythromycin but is more effective against *H. influenzae* than erythromycin. In addition, it is effective against mycobacteria. Readily absorbed from the GI tract, clarithromycin is metabolized in the liver for excretion in the urine.

Telithromycin is a derivative of erythromycin with a similar antibacterial spectrum. It is also effective in the treatment of erythromycin-resistant strains of *S. pneumoniae*. The majority of the dose is metabolized by the liver and the remainder is excreted unchanged in the faeces and urine.

Therapeutic Actions and Indications

The macrolides, which may be bactericidal or bacteriostatic, exert their effect by inhibiting the binding of transfer RNA to the ribosome. This prevents the addition of new amino acids to peptide chains (see Figure 8.2). This action can prevent the cell from dividing or cause cell death, depending on the sensitivity of the bacteria and the concentration of the drug.

Macrolides are indicated for treatment of the following conditions: acute infections caused by susceptible strains of *S. pneumoniae, Mycoplasma pneumoniae, Listeria monocytogenes*, and *Legionella pneumophila*; infections caused by group A β-haemolytic streptococci; pelvic inflammatory disease caused by *N. gonorrhoeae*; upper respiratory tract infections caused by *H. influenzae* (with sulphonamides); infections caused by *C. diphtheriae* and *Corynebacterium minutissimum* (with antitoxin); intestinal amoebiasis; and infections caused by *Chlamydia trachomatis*. Topical macrolides are indicated for the treatment of acne vulgaris.

Contraindications and Cautions

Macrolides are contraindicated in patients with a known allergy to any macrolide *because cross-sensitivity occurs*; hepatic dysfunction (azithromycin) or myasthenia gravis (telithromycin). Caution should be used in patients with hepatic dysfunction *that could alter the metabolism of the drug*; in those with renal disease *that could interfere with the excretion of some of the drug*; those predisposed to long QT intervals *because of the risk of cardiac arrhythmias*; in pregnant or lactating women *because of potential adverse effects on the developing foetus or neonate*. With the exception of erythromycin, the macrolides should only be used during pregnancy and lactation if the benefit clearly outweighs the risk to the foetus or neonate or alternative antibacterials are unavailable.

Adverse Effects

Relatively few adverse effects are associated with the macrolides. The most frequent ones involve the direct

Table 8.7 DRUGS IN FOCUS

Macrolides

Drug Name	Available Forms	Usual Indications
azithromycin	Oral	Treatment of mild to moderate respiratory infections, skin and soft-tissue infections, Chlamydia, urethritis and otitis media. Prophylactic treatment of endocarditis in children (unlicensed) and streptococcal infections
clarithromycin	Oral, IV	Treatment of various respiratory, skin and soft tissue infections and otitis media. Also used to eradicate *H. pylori*
erythromycin	Oral, IV	For use by patients allergic to penicillin. Treatment of respiratory, oral and skin infections. Also nonspecific urethritis, campylobacter enteritis, syphilis and chronic prostatitis
telithromycin	Oral	Reserved for the treatment of respiratory infections where standard treatment with β-lactam antibiotics is inappropriate

effect of the drugs on the GI tract and include abdominal cramping, diarrhoea, vomiting and pseudomembranous colitis. Rare neurological effects include symptoms such as confusion and abnormal thinking. Hypersensitivity reactions ranging from rash to Stevens–Johnson syndrome can occur.

Clinically Important Drug–Drug Interactions

Increased serum levels of some antiarrhythmics, other antibacterials, antihistamines, antivirals, coumarins, carbamazepine, ciclosporin, digoxin, phenytoin, midazolam, buspirone, felodipine, verapamil, diuretics, statins and theophylline occur when taken concurrently with macrolides, reportedly as a result of metabolic changes in the liver. There is also an increased risk of ventricular arrhythmias when ivabradine, moxifloxacin and antipsychotics are administered concurrently with macrolides.

Always consult a current copy of the British National Formulary for further guidance.

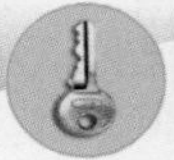

Key Drug Summary: *Erythromycin*

Indications: Treatment of respiratory, oral, dermatological, GU and GI infections caused by susceptible strains of bacteria

Actions: Inhibits protein synthesis; can be bacteriostatic or bactericidal

Pharmacokinetics:

Route	Onset	Peak
Oral	1–2 h	1–4 h
IV	Rapid	1 h

$T_{1/2}$: 1.6 hours; concentrated in the liver and excreted in bile and faeces

Adverse effects: Abdominal cramping, vomiting, diarrhoea (including pseudomembranous colitis), cholestatic jaundice, rash, Stevens–Johnson syndrome, reversible hearing loss (higher doses)

Clinically Important Drug–Food Interactions

Food in the stomach decreases the absorption of oral macrolides. Therefore the antibacterial should be given on an empty stomach, 1 hour before or at least 2 to 3 hours after meals. A macrolide should be taken with a full glass of water.

Nursing Considerations for Patients Receiving Macrolides

Assessment: History and Examination

The approach for patients receiving a macrolide antibacterial is the same as for quinolones.

Nursing Diagnoses

The patient receiving a macrolide may have the following nursing diagnoses related to drug therapy:

- Acute pain related to GI or CNS effects of the drug
- Risk of infection related to potential for superinfections
- Deficient knowledge regarding drug therapy

Implementation With Rationale

- Monitor hepatic and renal function tests before therapy begins *to arrange reduction in dosage as needed.*
- Monitor the site of infection and presenting signs and symptoms (e.g. fever, lethargy, urinary tract signs and symptoms) throughout the course of drug therapy. *Failure of these signs and symptoms to resolve may indicate the need to re-culture the site.* Patients should complete drug course even if all signs and symptoms have resolved.
- Ensure ready access to bathroom facilities *to assist patients with problems associated with diarrhoea.*
- Arrange for appropriate treatment of superinfections as needed *to decrease severity of infection and complications.*

The patient should:

- Report difficulty in breathing, severe headache, severe diarrhoea, severe skin rash, and mouth or vaginal sores to a health care provider.

Evaluation

- Monitor for adverse effects (GI effects, rashes and superinfections).
- Additional information is listed under Nursing Considerations for Patients Receiving Penicillins and Penicillinase-Resistant Antibacterials.

Lincosamides

The lincosamides are similar to the macrolides: they act at almost the same site in bacterial protein synthesis and are effective against similar strains of bacteria (Figure 8.2).

Clindamycin, the only drug currently used in this class, is reserved for severe infections caused by streptococci and staphylococci bacteria. It is also active against some anaerobic strains, including *Bacteroides fragilis* associated with abdominal sepsis.

Clindamycin is rapidly absorbed from the GI tract or from IM injections and distributed widely, including in bone. Clindamycin is metabolized in the liver and excreted in urine and bile. Caution must be applied to patients with hepatic or renal impairment, which could interfere with the metabolism and excretion of the drug. The drug is not known to be harmful during pregnancy, but should be used with caution whilst breast-feeding. GI reactions, which are often severe, limit the usefulness of clindamycin. Severe pseudomembranous colitis has occurred as a result of treatment. However, for a serious infection caused by a susceptible bacterium, clindamycin may be the drug of choice.

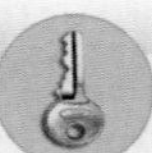

Key Drug Summary: *Clindamycin*

Indications: Treatment of serious infections caused by susceptible strains of bacteria including some anaerobes; useful in septicaemia and chronic bone and joint infections

Actions: Inhibits protein synthesis in susceptible bacteria, causing cell death

Pharmacokinetics:

Route	Onset	Peak	Duration
Oral	Varies	1–2 h	8–12 h
IM	20–30 min	1–3 h	8–12 h
IV	Immediate	Minutes	8–12 h

$T_{1/2}$: 2–3 hours; metabolized in the liver, excreted in the urine and faeces

Adverse effects: Nausea, vomiting, diarrhoea, pseudomembranous colitis, bone marrow suppression, hypotension, rash, urticaria, Stevens–Johnson syndrome, pain on injection, abscess at IM injection site

Tetracyclines

The tetracyclines (Table 8.8) were developed as semisynthetic antibacterials based on the structure of a common soil mould. The tetracyclines inhibit protein synthesis in susceptible bacteria in a similar mechanism to the macrolides. They are active against a wide range of Gram-positive and Gram-negative strains and can be used when penicillin is contraindicated. However, widespread resistance to the tetracyclines has limited their use in recent years.

The characteristics of the individual tetracyclines are very similar and can be related to those of the Key Drug for tetracycline.

Tigecycline, a glycylcycline, is structurally related to the tetracyclines. This antibacterial also inhibits protein translation on ribosomes of certain bacteria. Importantly, it is effective against MRSA and vancomycin-resistant enterococci. It is therefore reserved for the treatment of complicated skin and soft tissue infections and intra-abdominal infections caused by susceptible bacteria.

Therapeutic Actions and Indications

The tetracyclines inhibit protein synthesis in susceptible bacteria, leading to the inability of the bacteria to multiply (see Figure 8.2). Tetracyclines, which are effective against a wide range of bacteria, are indicated for treatment of infections caused by *rickettsiae, M. pneumoniae, Borrelia recurrentis, H. influenzae, Haemophilus ducreyi,*

Table 8.8 DRUGS IN FOCUS

Tetracyclines

Drug Name	Available Forms	Usual Indications
demeclocycline	Oral	As for tetracycline plus the treatment of inappropriate antidiuretic hormone secretion
doxycycline	Oral	Treatment of a wide variety of infections, including traveller's diarrhoea and sexually transmitted diseases; periodontal disease, acne and sinusitis. Also used in the prophylaxis and treatment of malaria and anthrax (unlicensed).
lymecycline	Oral	As for tetracycline
minocycline	Oral	As for tetracycline plus treatment of meningococcal carriers
oxytetracycline	Oral	As for tetracycline
tetracycline	Oral	Treatment of a wide variety of infections, including acne vulgaris, rosacea and minor skin infections caused by susceptible organisms; infections caused by *Chlamydia trachomatis*, rickettsia and spirochaetes
tigecycline	IV	Reserved for complicated skin, soft tissue and abdominal infections

Pasteurella pestis, Pasteurella tularensis, Bartonella bacilliformis, Bacteroides species, *Vibrio* comma, *Vibrio fetus, Brucella* species, *E. coli, E. aerogenes, Shigella* species, *Acinetobacter calcoaceticus, Klebsiella* species, *Diplococcus pneumoniae* and *S. aureus*; against agents that cause psittacosis, ornithosis, lymphogranuloma venereum and granuloma inguinale; when penicillin is contraindicated in susceptible infections; and for treatment of acne and uncomplicated GU infections caused by *C. trachomatis.* Some of the tetracyclines are also used as adjuncts in the treatment of certain protozoal infections.

Pharmacokinetics

Tetracyclines are absorbed adequately, but not completely, from the GI tract. Any drug remaining in the GI tract can affect the normal flora and cause diarrhoea. Their absorption is affected by iron, calcium, aluminium and antacids in the stomach. Tetracyclines are concentrated in the liver and excreted unchanged in the urine, with half-lives ranging from 12 to 25 hours.

Contraindications and Cautions

Tetracyclines are contraindicated in patients with known allergy to tetracyclines; during pregnancy and lactation and to children younger than 12 years *because they can permanently discolour and damage enamel in developing teeth.* They can also promote calcium complex formations in bone, leading to decreased bone growth.

Tetracyclines should be used with caution in patients with hepatic or renal dysfunction *because they are concentrated in the bile and excreted in the urine*; and myasthenia gravis *because they can cause further muscle weakness.*

Adverse Effects

The major adverse effects of tetracycline therapy involve direct irritation of the GI tract and include nausea, vomiting, diarrhoea (including pseudomembranous colitis), oesophageal irritation and dysphagia. Tetracyclines can accumulate in teeth and bones, weakening the structure and causing staining and pitting of teeth and bones. Less frequent effects include hepatotoxicity, photosensitivity, rash and haematological effects, such as haemolytic anaemia and bone marrow depression. Superinfections, including yeast infections, occur when bacteria of the normal flora are destroyed. Hypersensitivity reactions reportedly range from urticaria to anaphylaxis.

Clinically Important Drug–Drug Interactions

The most significant drug interactions occur between tetracyclines and anticoagulants, ciclosporin and retinoids. When oral contraceptives are taken with tetracyclines, the effectiveness of the contraceptives decreases. Although the risk is probably small, patients who take oral contraceptives should be advised to use an additional form of birth control while receiving a tetracycline.

Decreased absorption of tetracyclines results from oral combinations with calcium (including those in dairy products), magnesium, zinc, aluminium or bismuth salts (present in antacids), iron and ACE inhibitors. Tetracyclines should therefore be given on an empty stomach 1 hour before or 2 to 3 hours after any meal or other medication.

Always consult a current copy of the British National Formulary for further guidance.

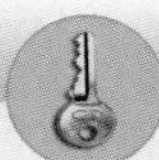

Key Drug Summary: *Tetracycline*

Indications: Treatment of various infections caused by susceptible strains of bacteria, acne, when penicillin is contraindicated for eradication of susceptible organisms

Actions: Inhibits protein synthesis in susceptible bacteria, preventing cell replication

Pharmacokinetics:

Route	Onset	Peak
Oral	Varies	2–4 h

$T_{1/2}$: 6–12 hours; excreted unchanged in the urine

Adverse effects: Nausea, vomiting, diarrhoea, discolouration and inadequate calcification of primary teeth of foetus when used in pregnant women or of secondary teeth when used in children, bone marrow suppression, photosensitivity, superinfections, rash

Nursing Considerations for Patients Receiving Tetracyclines

Assessment: History and Examination

Screen for the following, *which are possible contraindications or cautions for use of the drug*: known allergy to any tetracycline or to tartrazine found in certain oral preparations *because cross-sensitivity often occurs* (obtain specific information about the nature and occurrence of allergic reactions); any history of renal or hepatic disease *that could interfere with metabolism and excretion of the drug and lead to increased toxicity*; current pregnancy or lactation status and age.

Physical examination should be performed *to establish baseline data for assessing the effectiveness of the drug and the occurrence of any adverse effects associated with drug therapy*. Perform culture and sensitivity tests at the site of infection *to ensure that this is the appropriate drug for this patient*. Conduct examination of the skin for any rash or lesions *to provide a baseline for possible adverse effects*. Note respiratory status *to provide a baseline for the occurrence of hypersensitivity reactions*. Evaluate renal and liver function test reports *to assess the status of renal and liver functioning, which helps to determine any needed changes in dosage.*

Nursing Diagnoses

The patient receiving a tetracycline may have the following nursing diagnoses related to drug therapy:

- Diarrhoea related to drug effects
- Imbalanced nutrition: less than body requirements related to GI effects and superinfections
- Impaired skin integrity related to rash and photosensitivity
- Deficient knowledge regarding drug therapy

Implementation With Rationale

- Monitor renal and liver function test results before and periodically during therapy *to arrange for a dosage reduction as needed.*
- The oral drug should be taken on an empty stomach 1 hour before or 2–3 hours after meals with a full glass of water. Concomitant use of antacids or salts should be avoided because they interfere with drug absorption. *These precautions will increase drug effectiveness and decrease development of resistant strains of bacteria.*
- Discontinue the drug immediately if hypersensitivity reactions occur *to avoid the possibility of severe reactions.*
- Monitor for signs of superinfections *to arrange for treatment as appropriate.*
- Encourage the patient to apply sunscreen and wear clothing *to protect exposed skin from skin rashes and sunburn associated with photosensitivity reactions.*

The patient should:

- Use a barrier contraceptive method because oral contraceptives may not be effective while a tetracycline is being used.
- Know that superinfections may occur. Appropriate treatment can be arranged through the health care provider.
- Use sunscreens and protective clothing if sensitivity to the sun occurs.
- Know when to report dangerous adverse effects to the health care provider, such as difficulty in breathing, rash, itching, watery diarrhoea, cramps, or changes in colour of urine or stool.

Evaluation

- Monitor for adverse effects (GI effects, rash and superinfections).
- Additional information is listed under Nursing Considerations for Patients Receiving Penicillins and Penicillinase-Resistant Antibacterials.
- For related data, see Critical Thinking Scenario 8-1.

Additional Antibacterials

Chloramphenicol has a broad spectrum of activity against aerobic and anaerobic bacteria and is a potent inhibitor of bacterial protein synthesis. Against most bacteria, chloramphenicol is bacteriostatic, but bactericidal against *H. influenzae, N. meningitides* and *S. pneumoniae.* Chloramphenicol can significantly reduce bone marrow function leading to reversible and irreversible aplastic anaemia in some individuals, and is therefore restricted to treatment of serious infections such as septicaemia and meningitis. Chloramphenicol can also be used topically to treat ear and eye infections. Chloramphenicol should not be used during pregnancy or whilst breast-feeding because of the potential for 'grey baby' syndrome where cyanosis and circulatory collapse can occur.

The polymyxin antibacterial, colistin, disrupts the bacterial cell membrane of a range of Gram-negative bacteria including *K. pneumoniae* and *P. aeruginosa*. Colistin is used to sterilize the bowel of neutropaenic patients and by cystic fibrosis patients to treat respiratory tract infections. Colistin is associated with neuro- and nephrotoxicity.

Sodium fusidate is a narrow-spectrum steroid antibacterial, targeting mainly Gram-positive bacteria. It is mainly used to treat penicillin-resistant staphylococci. Well absorbed from the GI tract, sodium fusidate is widely distributed around the body and is concentrated in bone, making it useful for treating osteomyelitis. Sodium fusidate is usually prescribed in combination with another antistaphylococcal antibacterial to prevent resistance. Also available as a topical agent to treat staphylococcal skin and eye infections.

Antimycobacterial Antibacterials

Mycobacteria, the group of bacteria that contain the pathogens that cause tuberculosis and leprosy, are classified on the basis of their ability to hold a stain even in the presence of a 'destaining' agent such as acid. They are called 'acid-fast' bacteria because of this property. The mycobacteria have an outer coat of mycolic acid that protects them from many disinfectants and allows them to survive for long periods in the environment. These slow-growing bacteria may need to be treated for several years before they can be eradicated.

Mycobacteria cause serious infectious diseases. The bacterium *Mycobacterium tuberculosis* causes tuberculosis, the leading cause of death from infectious disease in the world. For several years the disease was thought to be under control, but with the increasing number of people with compromised immune systems and the emergence of resistant bacterial strains, tuberculosis is once again on the rise.

Mycobacterium leprae causes leprosy, also known as Hansen's disease, which is characterized by disfiguring skin lesions and destructive effects on the respiratory tract. Leprosy is also a worldwide health problem; it is infectious when the mycobacteria invade the skin or respiratory tract of susceptible individuals. *Mycobacterium avium-intracellulare*, which causes mycobacterium avium complex (MAC), is seen in patients with AIDS or in other patients who are severely immunocompromised. Rifabutin is the most effective prophylactic drug against MAC.

Antituberculosis Drugs

Tuberculosis can lead to serious damage in the lungs, the GU tract, bones and the meninges. *M. tuberculosis* grows very slowly and therefore the period of treatment can range from 6 months to 2 years. Mycobacteria are intracellular and require the drugs to cross the cell membrane to exert their action.

Tuberculosis is usually treated into two stages: an *initial phase* lasting 2 months and a *continuation phase* lasting 4 months. In the initial phase the aim is to reduce the number of bacteria as quickly as possible using a combination of four drugs:

- isoniazid – inhibits the synthesis of mycolic acid present in the cell wall of the bacterium. An important note is that some patients will metabolize isoniazid more quickly than others, so-called fast and slow acetylators. Patients who are fast acetylators may require higher doses of isoniazid
- rifampicin – inhibits protein synthesis
- pyrazinamide – bactericidal action on dividing mycobacterium via an unknown mechanism
- ethambutol – bacteriostatic action via an unknown mechanism

The continuation phase uses a combination of isoniazid and rifampicin and can extend beyond the proposed 4-month period if the organisms are resistant to the proposed drug combinations. Capreomycin, cycloserine and streptomycin can be used in combination with other drugs if drug-resistance occurs.

Using the drugs in combination helps to decrease the emergence of resistant strains and to affect the bacteria at various phases during their long and slow life cycle. (See Table 8.9 for a listing of all the antituberculosis drugs.)

Leprostatic Drugs

There are currently three antibacterials used as first-line treatment of leprosy, clofazimine, dapsone and rifampicin (Table 8.9). Dapsone was the mainstay of leprosy treatment for many years, until clofazimine and rifampicin were introduced in the 1960s. Similar to the sulphonamides, dapsone inhibits folate synthesis in susceptible bacteria. In addition to its use in leprosy, dapsone is used to treat *P. jiroveci* (*P. carinii*) pneumonia in AIDS patients. Clofazimine is thought to target DNA and bacterium replication.

The hypnotic drug thalidomide can also be used (unlicensed indication) to treat a condition that occurs after treatment for leprosy (Box 8.5).

Therapeutic Actions and Indications

Most of the antimycobacterial agents act on the DNA of the bacteria, leading to a lack of growth and eventually to bacterial death (see Figure 8.2). Isoniazid specifically affects the mycolic acid coat around the bacterium. Although many of the antimycobacterial agents are effective against other species of susceptible bacteria, their primary indications are in the treatment of tuberculosis or leprosy (as previously indicated). The antituberculosis drugs are always used in combination to affect the bacteria at various stages and to help to decrease the emergence of resistant strains.

BOX 8.5 New Indication for Thalidomide

In the 1950s, the drug thalidomide became internationally known because, when given to women during pregnancy to help them sleep and to prevent morning sickness, it caused serious foetal abnormalities (e.g. lack of limbs, defective limbs). This tragedy led to the recall of thalidomide and the establishment of more stringent standards for drug testing and labelling. This controversial drug can now be used for the treatment of erythema nodosum leprosum, a painful inflammatory condition related to an immune reaction to dead bacteria that occurs after treatment for leprosy. It can also be used in the treatment of refractory myeloma. Thalidomide should never be given to women of childbearing age.

Table 8.9 DRUGS IN FOCUS

Antimycobacterial Drugs

Drug Name	Usual Indications
Antituberculosis Drugs	
capreomycin	Second-line drug for treatment of *Mycobacterium tuberculosis*
cycloserine	Second-line drug for treatment of *M. tuberculosis*
ethambutol	Used in combination with other antimycobacterial drugs to treat the initial phase of *M. tuberculosis*
isoniazid	Used in combination with other antimycobacterial drugs to treat the initial phase of *M. tuberculosis*; also used to treat the continuation phase with rifampicin
pyrazinamide	Used in combination with other antimycobacterial drugs to treat the initial phase of *M. tuberculosis*
rifabutin	Prophylaxis of Mycobacterium avium complex (MAC) in patients with advanced HIV infection; used in combination with other drugs to treat nontuberculous mycobacterial disease and pulmonary tuberculosis
rifampicin	Used in combination with other antimycobacterial drugs to treat the initial phase of *M. tuberculosis*; also used to treat the continuation phase with isoniazid. Treatment of brucellosis, legionnaire's disease, leprosy, endocarditis and staphylococcal infections
streptomycin	Used in combination to treat *M. tuberculosis*, brucellosis and enterococcal endocarditis
Leprostatic Drugs	
clofazimine	Treatment of leprosy
dapsone	Treatment of leprosy, *P. jiroveci* (*P. carinii*) pneumonia in AIDS patients and dermatitis herpetiformis

Pharmacokinetics

The antimycobacterial agents are generally well absorbed from the GI tract, metabolized in the liver and excreted in the urine. Caution should be used in patients with hepatic or renal dysfunction, which could interfere with the metabolism and excretion of the drugs. These drugs can cross the placenta and enter breast milk; but if an antituberculosis regimen is necessary during pregnancy and breast-feeding, the combination of isoniazid, ethambutol, pyrazinamide and rifampicin is considered the safest.

Contraindications and Cautions

Antimycobacterial drugs are contraindicated for patients with any known allergy to these agents; in those with severe renal or hepatic failure, *which could interfere with the metabolism or excretion of the drug*; in those with severe CNS dysfunction, *which could be exacerbated by the actions of the drug*; and ethambutol should not be used by patients with optic neuritis.

Adverse Effects

CNS effects, such as neuritis, dizziness, headache, malaise, drowsiness and hallucinations, are often reported and are related to direct effects of the drugs on neurons. These drugs are also irritating to the GI tract, causing nausea, vomiting, anorexia, stomach upset and abdominal pain. Rifampicin and rifabutin cause discolouration of body fluids (urine, sweat and tears are tinged orange-red). As with other antibacterials, there is always a possibility of hypersensitivity reactions, and the patient should be monitored on a regular basis.

Clinically Important Drug–Drug Interactions

Rifampicin, pyrazinamide and isozianid are associated with liver toxicity and when used in combination, the risk of liver toxicity increases. Patients liver function should be checked prior to treatment and monitored closely thereafter.

Isoniazid can increase the plasma concentration of antiepileptic drugs and increase the risk of toxicity. Increased metabolism and decreased drug effectiveness occur as a result of administration of antiarrhythmics, antibacterials, antipsychotics, antivirals, β-blockers, corticosteroids, oral contraceptives, oral anticoagulants, oral antidiabetic agents, cytotoxics, diuretics, theophylline, antiepileptics, calcium channel blockers, ciclosporin or antifungals in combination with rifampicin or rifabutin. Patients who are taking these drug combinations should be monitored closely and dosage adjustments made as needed.

Always consult a current copy of the British National Formulary for further guidance.

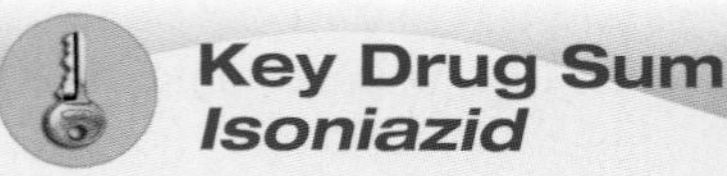

Indications: Treatment of tuberculosis as part of combination therapy; prophylactic treatment of household members of recently diagnosed tuberculars

Actions: Inhibits the synthesis of mycolic acid in actively growing tubercle bacilli

Pharmacokinetics:

Route	Onset	Peak	Duration
Oral	Varies	1–2 h	24 h
IM	Varies	60–90 min	24 h
IV	30 min	1 h	24 h

$T_{1/2}$: 1–4 hours (reflects rate of acetylation); partly metabolized in the liver, excreted in the urine

Adverse effects: Peripheral neuropathies, nausea, vomiting, hepatitis, bone marrow suppression, fever, gynaecomastia, lupus syndrome

Nursing Considerations for Patients Receiving Antimycobacterial Antibacterials

Assessment: History and Examination

Screen for the following, *which are possible contraindications or cautions for use of the drug*: known allergy to any antimycobacterial drug (obtain specific information about the nature and occurrence of allergic reactions); history of renal or hepatic disease, *which could interfere with metabolism and excretion of the drug and lead to toxicity*; history of CNS dysfunction, including epilepsy and neuritis, *which could be exacerbated by adverse drug effects*; and current pregnancy status.

Physical examination should be performed *to establish baseline data for assessing the effectiveness of the drug and the occurrence of any adverse effects associated with drug therapy.* Obtain specimens for culture and sensitivity testing *to establish the sensitivity of the organism being treated.* Examine skin for any rash or lesions *to provide a baseline for possible adverse effects.* Evaluate CNS for orientation, affect and reflexes *to establish a baseline and to monitor for adverse effects.* Note respiratory rate and adventitious sounds *to provide a baseline for the occurrence of hypersensitivity reactions.* Evaluate renal and liver function tests *to assess the status of renal and liver functioning so as to determine any necessary dosage alterations.*

Nursing Diagnoses

The patient receiving an antimycobacterial drug may have the following nursing diagnoses related to drug therapy:

- Imbalanced nutrition: less than body requirements, related to GI effects
- Disturbed sensory perception (kinaesthetic) related to CNS effects of the drug
- Acute pain related to GI effects of drug
- Deficient knowledge regarding drug therapy

Implementation With Rationale

- Monitor renal and liver function test results before and periodically during therapy *to arrange for dosage reduction as needed.*
- These drugs are taken for years and often in combination. Periodic medical evaluation and re-teaching are often essential to ensure concordance.
- Discontinue the drug immediately if hypersensitivity reactions occur *to avert potentially serious reactions.*
- Encourage the patient to eat small, frequent meals as tolerated; perform frequent mouth care; and drink adequate fluids *to ensure adequate nutrition and hydration.* Monitor nutrition if GI effects become a problem.
- Ensure that the patient is instructed about the appropriate dosage regimen, use of drug combinations, and possible adverse effects *to enhance patient knowledge about drug therapy and to promote concordance.*

The patient should:

- Use barrier contraceptives and understand that oral contraceptives may not be effective if antimycobacterial drugs are being used.
- Understand that normally some of these drugs impart an orange stain to body fluids. If this occurs, the fluids may stain clothing and tears may stain contact lenses.
- Report difficulty in breathing, hallucinations, numbness and tingling, worsening of condition, fever and chills, or changes in colour of urine or stool to a health care provider.

Evaluation

- Monitor patient response to the drug (resolution of mycobacterial infection).
- Monitor for adverse effects (GI effects, CNS changes and hypersensitivity reactions).
- Evaluate the effectiveness of the teaching plan (patient can name the drug, dosage, possible adverse effects to expect, and specific measures to help avoid adverse effects).
- Monitor the effectiveness of comfort and safety measures and concordance with the regimen.

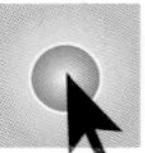

WEB LINKS

Health care providers and patients may want to consult the following Internet sources:

http://bnfc.org The BNF for Children provides UK health care professionals with authoritative and practical information on the selection and clinical use of medicines in children.

http://cks.library.nhs.uk The National Health Service Clinical Knowledge Summaries provides evidence-based practical information on the common conditions observed in primary care.

http://www.bnf.org.uk The BNF provides UK health care professionals with authoritative and practical information on the selection and clinical use of medicines.

http://www.hpa.org.uk The Health Protection Agency provides guidance, advice and the latest antimicrobial resistance data.

http://www.nhsdirect.nhs.uk The National Health Service Direct service provides patients with information and advice about health, illness and health services.

http://www.nice.org.uk The National Institute for Health and Clinical Excellence provides guidance on public health, new and existing treatments within the NHS and also information on the most appropriate care for patients.

http://www.who.int The World Health Organisation provides information on the treatment of many infectious diseases including tuberculosis and leprosy.

Points to Remember

- Antibacterials work by disrupting protein or enzyme systems within a bacterium, causing cell death (bactericidal) or preventing multiplication (bacteriostatic).
- The proteins or enzyme systems affected by antibacterials are more likely to be found or used in bacteria than in human cells.
- The goal of antibacterial therapy is to reduce the number of invading bacteria so that the normal immune system can deal with the infection.
- The primary therapeutic use of each antibacterial is determined by the bacterial species that are sensitive to that drug, the clinical condition of the patient receiving the drug, and the benefit-to-risk ratio for the patient.
- The longer an antibacterial has been available, the more likely it is that mutant bacterial strains resistant to the mechanisms of antibacterial activity will have developed.
- The most common adverse effects of antibacterial therapy involve the GI tract (nausea, vomiting, diarrhoea, anorexia, abdominal pain) and superinfections (invasion of the body by normally occurring micro-organisms that are usually restricted by the normal flora).
- To prevent or contain the growing threat of drug-resistant strains of bacteria, it is very important to use antibacterials cautiously, to complete the full course of an antibacterial prescription and to avoid saving antibacterials for self-medication in the future. A patient and family teaching programme should address these issues, as well as the proper dosing procedure for the drug (even if the patient feels better) and the importance of keeping a record of any reactions to antibacterials.

CRITICAL THINKING SCENARIO 8-1

Antibacterials and Oral Contraceptives

The Situation

Lindsay, a 27-year-old female, attends her local walk-in centre with symptoms of severe sinusitis and complains of head pressure, difficulty in sleeping, fever and muscle aches and pains. A swab is taken and a culture carried out. The next day the culture and sensitivity report identifies the infecting organism as a strain of *Klebsiella* that is sensitive to tetracycline. Lindsay returns to the clinic to collect a prescription for doxycycline. Whilst talking to the nurse, Lindsay informs her that she is currently taking the oral contraceptive pill as a form of birth control.

Critical Thinking

- How do tetracyclines and some other antibacterials and oral contraceptives interact? What are the possible consequences of continuing to take oral contraceptives during a pregnancy?
- What nursing interventions are appropriate for Lindsay?
- What teaching points should be stressed? Think about the problems that an unplanned pregnancy might cause.
- How can you help Lindsay to cope with her infection and her drug regimen?

Discussion

Several antibacterials, including doxycycline, are known to lead to the failure of oral contraceptives as evidenced by breakthrough bleeding and unplanned pregnancy. Although the exact way in which these drugs interact is not completely understood, it is thought that the antibacterials destroy certain bacteria in the normal flora of the GI tract. These bacteria are necessary for the breakdown and eventual absorption of the female hormones contained in the contraceptives. The 7 days of antibacterial treatment together with the time necessary for rebuilding the normal flora can be long enough for the hypothalamus to lose the negative feedback signal provided by the contraceptives that prevents ovulation and preparation of the uterus. Sensing the low hormone levels, the hypothalamus releases gonadotropin-releasing hormone, which leads to the release of follicle-stimulating hormone and luteinizing hormone, with subsequent ovulation.

Lindsay should be encouraged to use a barrier form of birth control during the course of her antibacterial use and to read all of the literature that comes with oral contraceptives as well as patient teaching information that should be provided with the antibacterial.

The nurse should stress the importance of a good diet, which will ensure that her body has the components she will need to fight this infection and to heal and to ward off other infections, as well as the importance of adequate rest and exercise.

Nursing Care Guide for Lindsay: Doxycycline

Assessment: History and Examination

- Allergy to any tetracycline
- Hepatic or renal dysfunction
- Pregnancy or lactation
- Concurrent use of oral contraceptives, antacids, iron products, digoxin or penicillins
- General: site of infection, culture and sensitivity
- Respiratory: respiratory rate and depth, adventitious sounds
- GI: liver evaluation, bowel sounds, usual output

Nursing Diagnoses

- Acute pain related to GI effects, superinfections
- Imbalanced nutrition, less than body requirements related to GI effects
- Potential for injury related to CNS effects
- Deficient knowledge regarding drug therapy

Implementation

- Perform culture and sensitivity tests before beginning therapy.
- Do not administer with antacids, milk or iron products.
- Monitor for and provide hygiene measures and treatment if superinfections occur.
- Monitor nutritional status and fluid intake.
- Provide ready access to bathroom facilities if diarrhoea is a problem.
- Provide support and reassurance for dealing with the drug effects and infection.
- Provide patient teaching regarding drug name, dosage, adverse effects, precautions, warnings to report, and drugs that might cause a drug–drug interaction, including the need to use a barrier contraceptive if using oral contraceptives.

(continued)

Antibacterials and Oral Contraceptives *(continued)*

Evaluation

- Evaluate drug effects: resolution of bacterial infections.
- Monitor for adverse effects: GI effects, superinfections and CNS effects.
- Monitor for drug–drug interactions: lack of effectiveness of oral contraceptives, lack of antibacterial effect with antacids or iron.
- Evaluate effectiveness of patient teaching programme.
- Evaluate effectiveness of comfort and safety measures.

Patient Teaching for Lindsay

- ☐ Doxycycline is an antibacterial that is specific for your infection. You should take it throughout the day for best results.
- ☐ Do not take this drug with dairy products, iron preparations or antacids.
- ☐ Take the full course of this antibacterial. Do not stop taking it even if you feel better.
- ☐ Oral contraceptives may become ineffective while you are taking this drug. If you rely on oral contraceptives for birth control, use a barrier contraceptive whilst taking this drug.
- ☐ You may experience stomach upset or diarrhoea.
- ☐ You may develop other infections in your mouth or vagina. If this occurs, consult with your health care provider for appropriate treatment.
- ☐ Tell any health care provider who is caring for you that you are taking this drug.
- ☐ Keep this, and all medications, out of the reach of children and pets.
- ☐ Report any of the following to your health care provider: changes in colour of urine or stool, severe cramps, difficulty in breathing, rash or itching, yellowing of the skin or eyes.

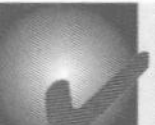

CHECK YOUR UNDERSTANDING

Answers to the questions in this chapter may be found in the answer key in the back of the book.

Multiple Choice

Select the most appropriate answer to the following.

1. A bacteriostatic substance is one that
   a. directly kills any bacteria it comes in contact with.
   b. directly kills any bacteria that are sensitive to the substance.
   c. prevents the growth of any bacteria.
   d. prevents the growth of specific bacteria that are sensitive to the substance.

2. Gram-negative bacteria
   a. are mostly found in the respiratory tract.
   b. are mostly associated with soft tissue infections.
   c. are mostly found in the GI and GU tracts.
   d. accept a positive stain when tested.

3. Antibacterials that are used together to increase their effectiveness and limit the associated adverse effects are said to be
   a. broad spectrum.
   b. synergistic.
   c. bactericidal.
   d. anaerobic.

4. An aminoglycoside antibacterial might be the drug of choice in treating
   a. serious infections caused by susceptible strains of Gram-negative bacteria.
   b. otitis media in an infant.
   c. cystitis in a woman who is 4 months pregnant.
   d. suspected pneumonia before the culture results are available.

5. Which of the following is not a caution for the use of cephalosporins?
   a. Allergy to penicillin
   b. Renal failure
   c. Allergy to aspirin
   d. Concurrent treatment with aminoglycosides

6. The quinolones are
   a. found freely in nature.
   b. associated with severe adverse reactions.
   c. widely used to treat Gram-positive infections.
   d. broad-spectrum antibacterials with few associated adverse effects.

7. Ciprofloxacin, a widely used antibacterial, is an example of
   a. a penicillin.
   b. a quinolone.
   c. an aminoglycoside.
   d. a macrolide antibacterial.

8. A patient receiving a quinolone should be cautioned to anticipate
   a. increased salivation.
   b. constipation.
   c. photosensitivity.
   d. cough.

9. The goal of antibacterial therapy is to
   a. eradicate all bacteria from the system.
   b. suppress resistant strains of bacteria.
   c. reduce the number of invading bacteria so that the immune system can deal with the infection.
   d. stop the drug as soon as the patient feels better.

10. The penicillins
   a. are bacteriostatic.
   b. are bactericidal, interfering with bacteria cell walls.
   c. are effective only if given intravenously.
   d. do not produce cross-sensitivity within their class.

Extended Matching Questions

Select **all** that apply

1. A young woman is found to have a soft tissue infection that is most responsive to tetracycline. Your teaching plan for this woman should include which of the following points?
   a. Tetracycline can cause grey baby syndrome.
   b. Do not use this drug if you are pregnant, because it can cause tooth and bone defects in the foetus.
   c. Tetracycline can cause severe acne.
   d. You should use a barrier contraceptive because tetracycline can make oral contraceptive ineffective.
   e. This drug should be taken in the middle of a meal to decrease GI upset.
   f. You may experience a vaginal yeast infection as a result of this drug therapy.

2. In general, all patients receiving antibacterials should receive teaching that includes which of the following points?
   a. The need to complete the full course of drug therapy
   b. The possibility of oral contraceptive failure
   c. When to take the drug related to food and other drugs
   d. The need for screening blood tests
   e. Advisability of saving any leftover medication for future use
   f. How to detect superinfections and what to do if they occur

True or False

Indicate whether the following statements are true (T) or false (F).

_____ 1. Aerobic bacteria depend on oxygen for survival.

_____ 2. Bactericidal refers to a substance that prevents the replication of bacteria.

_____ 3. Bacteriostatic refers to a drug that causes the death of bacteria.

_____ 4. Anaerobic bacteria survive without oxygen.

_____ 5. Gram-negative refers to bacteria that take a positive stain and are frequently associated with infections of the respiratory tract and soft tissues.

_____ 6. An antibacterial is a chemical that inhibits the growth of specific bacteria or causes the death of susceptible bacteria.

_____ 7. Antibacterials usually eradicate all of the bacteria that have entered the body.

_____ 8. Synergistic drugs are drugs that work together to increase a drug's effectiveness.

Matching

Match the following antibacterials with the correct class (each class may be used more than once).

1. ____________________ minocycline
2. ____________________ flucloxacillin
3. ____________________ capreomycin
4. ____________________ amikacin
5. ____________________ cefuroxime
6. ____________________ erythromycin
7. ____________________ norfloxacin
8. ____________________ clindamycin
9. ____________________ ampicillin
10. ____________________ levofloxacin
11. ____________________ gentamicin
12. ____________________ dapsone

A. Aminoglycosides
B. Cephalosporins
C. Quinolones

D. Lincosamides
E. Penicillins
F. Sulphonamides
G. Tetracyclines
H. Leprostatic
I. Antimycobacterials
J. Macrolides
K. Penicillinase-resistant antibacterials

Bibliography and References

British Medical Association and Royal Pharmaceutical Society of Great Britain. (2008). *British National Formulary*. London: BMJ & RPS Publishing. *This publication is updated biannually: it is imperative that the most recent edition is consulted.*

British Medical Association and Royal Pharmaceutical Society of Great Britain. (2008). *British National Formulary for Children*. London: BMJ & RPS Publishing. *This publication is updated annually: it is imperative that the most recent edition is consulted.*

Brunton, L., Lazo, J. S., Parker, K., Goodman, L. S., & Gilman, A. G. (2005). *Goodman and Gilman's the pharmacological basis of therapeutics* (11th ed.). London: McGraw-Hill.

Gruchalla, R. S., & Pirmohamed, M. (2006). Antibacterial allergy. *New England Journal of Medicine, 354*(6), 601–609.

Grundmann, H., Aires-de-Sousa, M., Boyce, J., & Tiemersma, E. (2006). Emergence and resurgence of meticillin-resistant *Staphylococcus aureus* as a public-health threat. *Lancet, 368*(9538), 874–885.

Hawkey, P. M. (1998). The origins and molecular basis of antibiotic resistance. *British Medical Journal, 317*, 657–660.

Howland, R. D., & Mycek, M. J. (2005). *Pharmacology* (3rd ed.). Philadelphia: Lippincott Williams & Wilkins.

National Collaborating Centre for Women's and Children's Health. (2007). *Feverish illness in children. Assessment and initial management in children younger that 5 years*. Available from http://guidance.nice.org.uk/CG47

National Collaborating Centre for Women's and Children's Health. (2007). Urinary tract infection in children: diagnosis, treatment and long-term management. Available from http://guidance.nice.org.uk/CG54

Porth, C. M. (2004). *Pathophysiology: Concepts of altered health states* (7th ed.). Philadelphia: Lippincott Williams & Wilkins.

Rang, H. P., Dale, M. M., Ritter, J. M., & Flower, R. J. (2007). *Rang and Dale's pharmacology* (6th ed.). Philadelphia: Churchill Livingstone.

Royal College of Nursing. (2005). *Good practice in infection prevention and control. Guidance for nursing staff*. Available from http://www.rcn.org.uk

Royal College of Nursing. (2005). *Methicillin-resistant* Staphylococcus aureus. *Guidance for nursing staff*. Available from http://www.rcn.org.uk

Simonsen, T., Aarbakke, J., Kay, I., Coleman, I., Sinnott, P., & Lysaa, R. (2006). *Illustrated pharmacology for nurses*. London: Hodder Arnold.

CHAPTER 9

Antiviral Agents

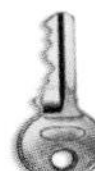

KEY TERMS

acquired immunodeficiency syndrome (AIDS)

AIDS-related complex (ARC)

cytomegalovirus (CMV)

helper T cell

herpesvirus

human immunodeficiency virus (HIV)

influenza A

interferons

non-nucleoside reverse transcriptase inhibitors

nucleoside reverse transcriptase inhibitors

protease inhibitors

virus

virion

LEARNING OBJECTIVES

Upon completion of this chapter, you will be able to:

1. Discuss problems with treating viral infections in humans and the use of antivirals across the lifespan.
2. Describe characteristics of common viruses and the resultant clinical presentations of viral infections including a respiratory viral infection, a herpes infection, CMV, HIV/AIDS, hepatitis B.
3. Describe the therapeutic actions, indications, pharmacokinetics, contraindications, most common adverse reactions, and important drug–drug interactions associated with each antiviral class.
4. Compare and contrast the key drugs for each class of antivirals with the other drugs within that class.
5. Outline the nursing considerations for patients receiving each class of antiviral agent.

AGENTS FOR INFLUENZA A AND RESPIRATORY VIRUSES

oseltamivir
palivizumab
ribavirin
zanamivir

AGENTS FOR HERPES AND CYTOMEGALOVIRUS

aciclovir
cidofovir
famciclovir
foscarnet
ganciclovir
inosine pranobex
valaciclovir
valganciclovir

AGENTS FOR HIV AND AIDS

Nucleoside Reverse Transcriptase Inhibitors

abacavir
didanosine
emtricitabine
lamivudine
stavudine
tenofovir
zidovudine

Non-Nucleoside Reverse Transcriptase Inhibitors
efavirenz
nevirapine

Protease Inhibitors
amprenavir
atazanavir
darunavir
fosamprenavir
indinavir
lopinavir
nelfinavir
ritonavir
saquinavir
tipranavir

Other antiretrovirals
enfuvirtide

AGENTS FOR HEPATITIS B

adefovir
entecavir
interferon alfa
peginterferon α-2a
telbivudine

LOCALLY ACTIVE ANTIVIRAL AGENTS

idoxuridine
imiquimod
penciclovir

Viruses cause a variety of conditions, ranging from warts, the common cold and influenza, to diseases such as chickenpox and measles. Viruses have a simple structure. A single virus particle or **virion** is composed of a piece of either DNA or RNA inside a protein coat which encloses the nucleic acid. Some virions are also surrounded by a lipid envelope. To carry out any metabolic processes, including replication, a virus must enter a cell. For a virus to infect a host cell, specific molecules on the viral surface must bind to molecules on the plasma membrane of the host cell. Once a virus has injected its DNA or RNA into the host cell, that cell is altered, that is, it is "programmed" to control the metabolic processes that the virus needs to survive. The virus, including the protein coat, replicates in the host cell (Figure 9.1). When the host cell can no longer carry out its own metabolic functions because of the viral invader, the host cell dies and releases the new viruses into the body to invade other cells.

As viruses are contained inside human cells while they are in the body, it has proved difficult to develop effective drugs that destroy a virus without harming the human host. **Interferons** (see Chapter 14) are released by the host in response to viral invasion of a cell and prevent the replication of that particular virus. Genetic engineering has

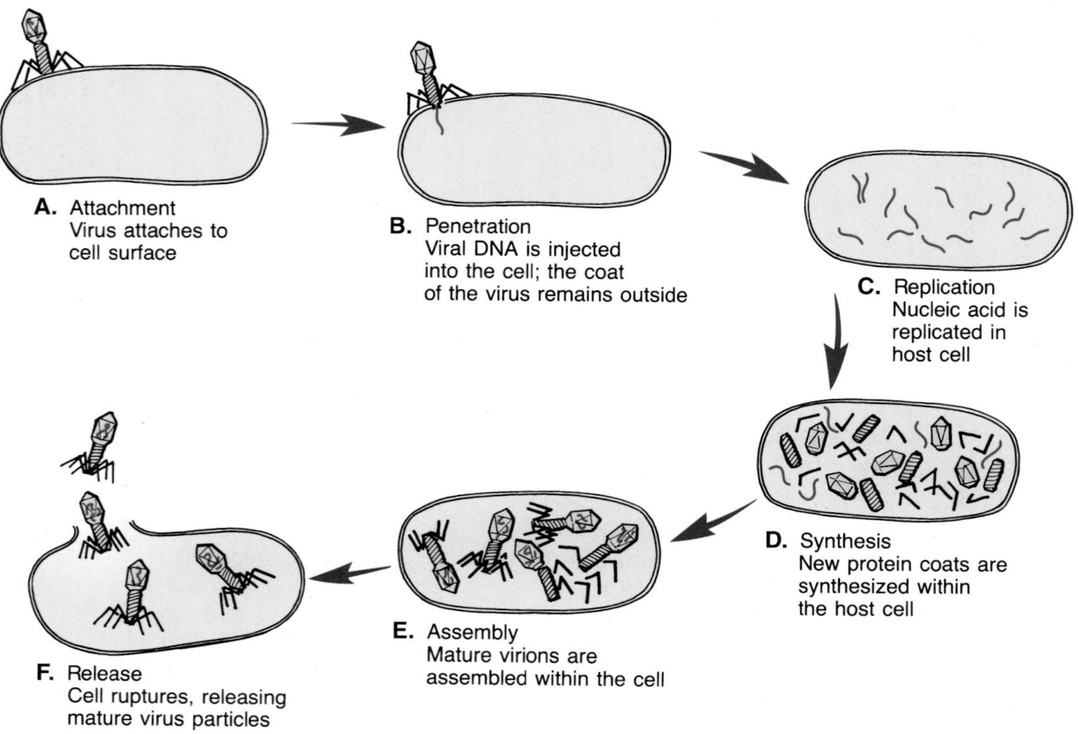

FIGURE 9.1 The stages in the replication cycle of a virus.

BOX 9.1 DRUG THERAPY ACROSS THE LIFESPAN

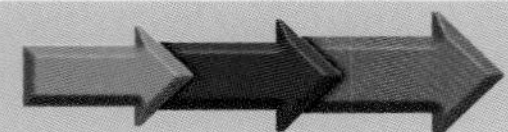

Antivirals

CHILDREN

Children are very sensitive to the effects of most antiviral drugs, and more severe reactions can be expected when these drugs are used in children. Many of these drugs do not have proven safety and efficacy in children, and, therefore, symptomatic control of viral infections is preferred, for example, antihistamines, paracetamol. Antivirals are recommended to treat viral infections of children who are systemically compromised or at risk (e.g. severe cardiorespiratory disease, babies under 4 weeks of age). Antivirals are also advised in cases where herpes simplex virus has affected the eyes and/or ears which places the patient at risk of developing secondary encephalitis.

The drugs used in the treatment of AIDS are frequently used in children even when no scientific data are available. This need relates to the seriousness of the disease. Dosage should be lowered according to body weight, and children must be monitored very closely for adverse effects on kidneys, bone marrow and liver.

When administering any drug to children, always consult the most recent edition of the British National Formulary for Children.

ADULTS

Adults need to know that these drugs are specific for the treatment of viral infections. The inappropriate use of antibacterials to treat such infections can lead to the development of resistant strains and superinfections that can cause additional problems.

Patients with HIV infection who are taking antiviral medications need to be taught that these drugs do not cure the disease, that opportunistic infections can still occur, and that precautions to prevent transmission of the disease need to be taken.

For pregnant women, antiviral treatment for HIV could be toxic to the foetus; however, continuing treatment can reduce the rate at which the disease develops in the mother and can also prevent transmission from the mother to the baby. Women with HIV infection are advised not to breast feed, to protect the neonate from the virus. Other antiviral agents should not be used unless the benefit clearly outweighs the potential risk to the foetus or neonate.

OLDER ADULTS

Older patients may be more susceptible to the adverse effects associated with these drugs; they should be monitored closely. Patients with hepatic dysfunction are at increased risk of worsening hepatic problems and toxic effects of those drugs that are metabolized by the liver. Drugs that are excreted unchanged in the urine can be especially toxic to patients who have renal dysfunction. If hepatic or renal dysfunction is expected (elderly patients, alcohol abuse, concomitant use of other hepatotoxic or nephrotoxic drugs), the dosage may need to be lowered and the patient should be monitored more frequently.

BOX 9.2 CONSIDERATIONS FOR DRUG THERAPY

Alternative Therapies and Antiviral Drugs

An increasing number of people use alternative therapies as part of their daily regime. St. John's wort is one of the more popular alternative therapies sold today. This herb has been used as an anti-inflammatory agent, an antidepressant, diuretic and treatment for gastritis and insomnia. However, St. John's wort is known to interact with many prescription drugs. When taken with St. John's wort, the protease inhibitors used in treating HIV were found to have decreased serum levels, leading to possible treatment failure. St. John's wort induces the cytochrome P450 liver enzyme system, therefore there is a possibility that it could increase the metabolism of many other antiviral drugs metabolized by that system and cause treatment failures with those drugs.

Patients may be reluctant to discuss their use of alternative therapies with health care providers, mainly because they want to maintain control over that aspect of their medical regimen or because they believe that the health care provider would not approve of their use. When a patient is prescribed an antiviral agent, it is imperative to ask specifically about the use of herbal or alternative medicines. Explain to the patient that antiviral drugs may interact with some herbal medicines and that it is important to try to avoid any adverse effects or drug failures.

enabled pharmaceutical companies to generate interferons to target particular viruses. Other drugs that are used in treating viral infections have been effective against a limited number of viruses. Viruses that respond to some antiviral therapy include influenza A and B, and some respiratory viruses, herpesviruses, cytomegalovirus (CMV), the human immunodeficiency virus (HIV) that causes acquired immune deficiency syndrome (AIDS), hepatitis B and some viruses that cause warts and certain eye infections. Box 9.1 discusses the use of antivirals across the lifespan. Some viruses, for example, the rhinovirus which causes the common cold; are self-limiting and do not require medical intervention in immunocompromised patients.

Patients need to be cautioned against using certain alternative therapies, for example St. John's wort or garlic supplements; while taking antiviral medication (Box 9.2).

Agents for Influenza A and Respiratory Viruses

Influenza A and other respiratory viruses, including influenza B, invade the respiratory tract and cause the signs and symptoms of respiratory influenza, for example sore throat, fever, cough and headache. For patients in at-risk groups (e.g. patients with chronic respiratory, heart, renal, liver or neurological disease; diabetic or immunocompromised patients and those over the age of 65 years; NICE, 2008) an influenza infection can lead to secondary infections including pneumonia and bronchitis and prove fatal. The most effective approach is to reduce the opportunity for infection, either by minimising contact with individuals with the virus or by immunised against the virus in the annual vaccination programme. Vaccination is the most effective way of preventing influenza (NICE, 2008).

The respiratory syncytial virus (RSV), an 'influenza-like' illness, causes the common cold; in infants this virus can infect the lower respiratory tract causing bronchiolitis and pneumonia.

Oseltamivir is effective in the treatment of uncomplicated influenza A and B infections that have been symptomatic for less than 2 days. This drug inhibits the influenza A and B viral enzyme neuraminidase, reducing the ability of the virus to release new virions. Treatment must be started within 48 hours of the onset of symptoms (NICE, 2008). Only patients who are at-risk should be prescribed oseltamivir. It is readily absorbed from the gastrointestinal (GI) tract, extensively metabolized in the liver, and excreted in the urine with a half-life of 1 to 3 hours. The dosage should be reduced and the patient closely monitored if there is renal dysfunction. Oseltamivir should only be used during pregnancy and lactation if the benefits clearly outweigh the risks to the foetus or neonate.

Zanamivir is used as an alternative to treat influenza A and B infections. Treatment should also be started within 48 hours of symptom onset and within 36 hours for children (NICE, 2008). Zanamivir must be delivered by a *Diskhaler* device because it is poorly absorbed after oral administration. It is absorbed across the respiratory epithelium and excreted unchanged in the urine with a half-life of 2.6 to 5 hours. Zanamivir has the same mechanism of action as oseltamivir and should be used cautiously in patients with asthma or other chronic pulmonary disease because there is a risk of bronchospasm. It should be used during pregnancy and lactation only if the benefits clearly outweigh the risks to the foetus or neonate.

Palivizumab is a monoclonal antibody used for the prophylaxis of RSV in at-risk children, for example immune deficiency, congenital heart disease and premature infants. Palivizumab should only be prescribed under specialist supervision. Delivery is via intramuscular injection and the drug has a half-life of 20 days.

Ribavirin is effective in the treatment of children with bronchiolitis caused by RSV and is also used with interferon-α to treat chronic hepatitis C infection. Ribavirin can be administered orally or by inhalation in the treatment of bronchiolitis. It is absorbed well through the respiratory tract and across the GI tract. Some of the dose is metabolized by the liver; the remainder is excreted unchanged in the urine. Ribavarin has a half-life of 9.5 hours. It is teratogenic and women of childbearing age should be advised to use barrier contraceptives during treatment and for 4 months after treatment. This is extended to 7 months for men receiving the drug. Women who are breast feeding should also avoid ribavirin.

Therapeutic Actions and Indications

The mechanisms of actions and indications of these drugs are listed in Table 9.1. All four drugs reduce the severity of infection in at-risk individuals. Oseltamivir and zanamivir are both neuraminidase inhibitors. Neuraminidase plays an important role in the release of newly replicated virus particles from the infected cell; these drugs prevent the release of viral particles and therefore reduce the viral load (Figure 9.2). In simplistic terms, palivizumab neutralizes the activity of RSV strains. Ribavirin is phosphorylated but its mode of action is still unclear; it may act at several sites, including cellular enzymes, to disrupt viral nucleic acid synthesis.

Contraindications and Cautions

Ribavirin is contraindicated in pregnancy and breastfeeding. The oral form of ribavirin is also contraindicated

Table 9.1 DRUGS IN FOCUS

Influenza A and Respiratory Virus Drugs

Drug Name	Actions	Usual Indications
oseltamivir	Neuraminidase inhibitor	Treatment of uncomplicated influenza infections in at-risk patients. Not for postexposure prophylactic use unless the patient is at-risk and living in long-term residential or nursing homes – this should only be carried out if it is clear that there is an outbreak of influenza in the community (NICE, 2008). Can be used to treat avian flu
palivizumab	A monoclonal antibody that neutralizes the activity of respiratory syncytial virus (RSV)	Preventive treatment of respiratory syncytial viral infection in at-risk children, *e.g.* congenital heart disease or pulmonary hypertension
ribavirin	Mode of action is unclear; may inhibit cellular enzymes, to interfere with viral nucleic acid synthesis.	Treatment of bronchiolitis associated with RSV infection; chronic hepatitis C in patients who relapse after interferon-α therapy
zanamivir	Neuraminidase inhibitor	Refer to oseltamivir

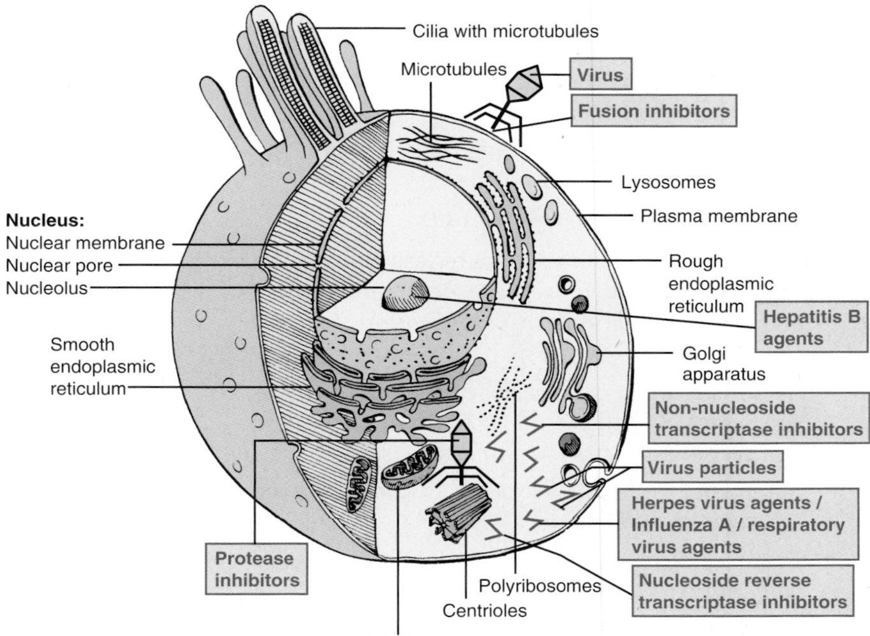

FIGURE 9.2 Agents for influenza A and respiratory viruses prevent release of viral particles. Herpes virus agents alter viral DNA production. Agents that attempt to control HIV and AIDS work in the following ways: nucleoside and non-nucleoside reverse transcriptase inhibitors block the transfer of information that allows viral replication; protease inhibitors block protease within the virus, leading to immature, non-infective virus particles; fusion inhibitors prevent the virus from fusing with the cellular membrane, thereby preventing the HIV-1 virus from entering the cell. Antihepatitis B agents block DNA formation, preventing the formation of new viruses.

in severe cardiac disease, haemoglobinopathies, hepatic dysfunction, autoimmune disease and severe psychiatric conditions. Caution should be used when giving these antiviral agents to patients with a known allergy; to pregnant or lactating women; to patients with asthma or chronic pulmonary disease or to patients with renal or liver disease, *which could alter metabolism and excretion of the drug.*

Adverse Effects

Use of either oseltamivir or zanamivir is associated with various adverse effects including GI disturbances, headache, light-headedness, dizziness, insomnia, rash and hypersensitivity reactions. Palivizumab can cause fever, nervousness and reactions at the injection-site. The side-effects associated with ribavirin are dependent upon the formulation. The inhaled form of ribavirin can cause weakened ventilation, bacterial pneumonia and pneumothorax. The oral formulation can cause a range of adverse effects including haemolytic anaemia, GI disturbances, pulmonary embolism, palpitations and peripheral oedema. The complete list of adverse effects is detailed in the latest version of the British National Formulary.

Clinically Important Drug–Drug Interactions

Patients receiving ribavirin should not take other antivirals at the same time.

Always consult a current copy of the British National Formulary for further guidance.

Nursing Considerations for Patients Receiving Influenza A and Respiratory Virus Drugs

Assessment: History and Examination

Patients who receive respiratory antiviral agents should be assessed for the following conditions, *which are either contraindications to the use of these drugs or necessitate precautionary measures*: known history of allergy to antivirals; history of asthma or chronic pulmonary disease *because zanamivir may cause bronchospasm*; history of liver or renal dysfunction *that might interfere with drug metabolism and excretion*; and current pregnancy or lactation status. Establish if patient is currently taking other medications or herbal therapies which may potentially interact with the antiviral drug.

Physical assessment should be performed to *establish baseline data for evaluating the effectiveness of the drug and the occurrence of any adverse effects associated with drug therapy.* Include screening for orientation and reflexes *to evaluate any central nervous system (CNS) effects of the drug*; and vital signs (respiratory rate, heart sounds, temperature) *to assess for signs and symptoms of the viral infection.*

Nursing Diagnoses

The patient receiving a respiratory antiviral drug may have the following nursing diagnoses related to drug therapy:

- Acute pain related to GI or CNS effects of drug
- Disturbed sensory perception (kinaesthetic) related to CNS effects of drug
- Deficient knowledge regarding drug therapy

Implementation With Rationale

- Start drug regimen as soon after exposure to the virus as possible *to achieve best effectiveness and decrease the risk of complications of viral infection.*
- Administer influenza A vaccine before the 'flu' season begins, if at all possible, *to prevent the disease and decrease the risk of complications.*
- Administer the full course of the drug *to obtain the full beneficial effects.*
- Ensure patient maintains fluid intake *to prevent dehydration.*
- Treat the symptoms (fever, aching muscles, sore throat) as necessary, for example, a nonsteroidal anti-inflammatory drug or paracetamol.
- Provide safety provisions if CNS effects occur *to protect the patient from injury.*
- Reassure and instruct the patient about the appropriate dosage scheduling regimen; safety precautions, including changing position slowly and avoiding driving and hazardous tasks *to enhance patient knowledge about drug therapy and to promote concordance.*

Evaluation

- Monitor patient response to the drug (prevention of respiratory flu-like symptoms; alleviation of flu-like symptoms).
- Monitor for adverse effects.
- Evaluate the effectiveness of the teaching plan (patient can name the drug, dosage, possible adverse effects to watch for, and specific measures to help avoid adverse effects).
- Monitor the effectiveness of comfort and safety measures and concordance with the regimen.

Agents for Herpes and Cytomegalovirus

Herpesviruses account for a broad range of conditions, including cold sores, encephalitis, chickenpox and genital infections. The most common herpesviruses are herpes simplex and varicella-zoster (chickenpox-shingles). **Cytomegalovirus (CMV)** can affect the eye, respiratory tract and liver; and although slightly different from the herpesvirus, responds to many of the same drugs. A number of antiviral drugs are used to combat these infections and their indications are listed in Table 9.2.

Aciclovir is specific for herpes virus infections. It is excreted unchanged in the urine and therefore must be used cautiously in the presence of renal impairment. Aciclovir should be used with caution during pregnancy and lactation.

Cidofovir is associated with severe renal toxicity and neutropaenia; both renal function and neutrophil levels should be assessed before administering the drug. Cidofovir is mainly excreted unchanged in the urine and must be given with probenecid and intravenous fluids to increase renal clearance of the drug. The dosage must be adjusted according to renal function and creatinine clearance. There is little information available on the use of cidofovir by children and should be used cautiously by children with AIDS because of potential carcinogenic effects and effects on fertility. If no other treatment option is available, monitor the child very closely.

Famciclovir is most effective in treating herpes infections. It is well absorbed from the GI tract, reaching peak levels in about 1 hour. Famciclovir is metabolized in the liver to the active compound penciclovir and excreted in the urine.

Foscarnet can be toxic to the kidneys and is reserved for treatment of CMV retinitis and for mucocutaneous aciclovir-resistant herpes simplex infections in immunocompromised patients. About 90% of foscarnet is excreted unchanged in the urine, so it should be used cautiously and at reduced dosage in patients with renal impairment. Foscarnet can accumulate in bone where it chelates the divalent ions calcium and magnesium leading to deficiencies in both electrolytes – patients should have their electrolyte levels monitored regularly to reduce the risk of cardiovascular disturbances and paraesthesia (tingling or numbing of the skin).

Ganciclovir is more active against CMV infections than aciclovir. However, it is more toxic causing bone marrow suppression, and is also thought to be a potential carcinogen and teratogen. Health care professionals should take care when preparing and administering the drug. Ganciclovir is primarily excreted unchanged in the urine.

Valganciclovir is the oral prodrug of ganciclovir; therefore the same caution should be applied with this drug. It is rapidly metabolized in the liver to ganciclovir and primarily excreted unchanged in the urine as ganciclovir.

Inosine pranobex is rapidly absorbed from the GI tract and metabolized by the liver and the metabolites excreted in the urine. The dose is adjusted according to the indication.

Valaciclovir is rapidly absorbed from the GI tract and metabolized in the liver to aciclovir. Excretion occurs through the urine mostly as aciclovir, so caution should be used in patients with renal impairment.

Therapeutic Actions and Indications

Most of these drugs are activated inside infected cells by conversion to their phosphorylated forms. In this

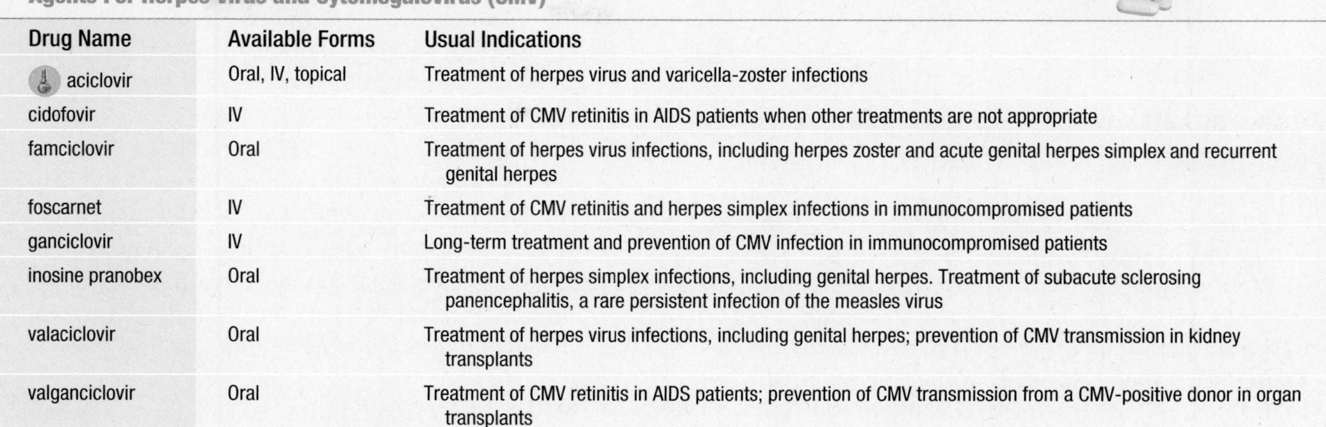

Table 9.2 DRUGS IN FOCUS

Agents For Herpes Virus and Cytomegalovirus (CMV)

Drug Name	Available Forms	Usual Indications
aciclovir	Oral, IV, topical	Treatment of herpes virus and varicella-zoster infections
cidofovir	IV	Treatment of CMV retinitis in AIDS patients when other treatments are not appropriate
famciclovir	Oral	Treatment of herpes virus infections, including herpes zoster and acute genital herpes simplex and recurrent genital herpes
foscarnet	IV	Treatment of CMV retinitis and herpes simplex infections in immunocompromised patients
ganciclovir	IV	Long-term treatment and prevention of CMV infection in immunocompromised patients
inosine pranobex	Oral	Treatment of herpes simplex infections, including genital herpes. Treatment of subacute sclerosing panencephalitis, a rare persistent infection of the measles virus
valaciclovir	Oral	Treatment of herpes virus infections, including genital herpes; prevention of CMV transmission in kidney transplants
valganciclovir	Oral	Treatment of CMV retinitis in AIDS patients; prevention of CMV transmission from a CMV-positive donor in organ transplants

form they inhibit the action of viral DNA polymerase to prevent the DNA chains from extending into effective DNA chains, thereby inhibiting DNA synthesis and replication. Ganciclovir (and valganciclovir) can also be incorporated into viral DNA to prevent replication (see Figure 9.2). These drugs have little effect on uninfected cells because they are less able to convert the drugs into their phosphorylated form. The mechanism of action of inosine pranobex is not clear.

Research has shown that they are very effective in immunocompromised individuals, such as patients with AIDS, those taking immunosuppressants and those with multiple infections.

Contraindications and Cautions

Of the agents described here, only aciclovir, foscarnet and valaciclovir can be used with caution during pregnancy; the other drugs are contraindicated in pregnancy. Aciclovir and valaciclovir can also be used with caution during lactation; the remaining drugs are contraindicated. They should not be used by patients with known allergies to antiviral agents or renal disease, *which could interfere with excretion of the drug.*

Adverse Effects

The adverse effects most commonly observed include nausea and vomiting, headache, drowsiness, rash and hair loss (cidofovir, ganciclovir and valganciclovir). Rash, inflammation and burning often occur at sites of IV injection and topical application. Bone marrow suppression, renal dysfunction and renal failure have also been reported. Patients taking cidofovir should have regular ophthalmological examinations to monitor for iritis (inflammation of the iris) and uveitis (inflammation of the uveal tract).

Clinically Important Drug–Drug Interactions

The risk of nephrotoxicity increases when agents indicated for the treatment of herpes and CMV are used in combination with other nephrotoxic drugs. The risk of bone marrow suppression also rises when ganciclovir and valganciclovir are given with other myelosuppressants.

Always consult a current copy of the British National Formulary for further guidance.

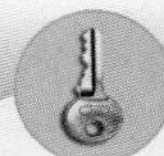

Key Drug Summary: *Aciclovir*

Indications: Treatment of herpes simplex virus (HSV) 1 and 2 infections; prophylactic treatment of HSV in immunocompromised patients; treatment of severe genital HSV infections; treatment of HSV encephalitis; acute treatment of shingles and chickenpox; topically for the treatment of genital herpes infections and cold sores (herpes labialis)

Actions: Inhibits viral DNA replication

Pharmacokinetics:

Route	Onset	Peak	Duration
Oral	Varies	1.5–2 h	Not known
IV	Immediate	1 h	8 h
Topical	Not generally absorbed systemically		

$T_{1/2}$: 2–3 hours (up to 20 hours in renal impairment); excreted unchanged in the urine

Adverse effects: Headache, diarrhoea, abdominal pain, nausea, vomiting, rash, urticaria (hives), pruritis (itching), photosensitivity, fatigue

Nursing Considerations for Patients Receiving Agents for Herpesvirus and Cytomegalovirus

Assessment: History and Examination

Patients receiving DNA-active antiviral agents should be assessed for the following conditions, *which are cautions or contraindications to the use of these drugs*: any history of allergy to antivirals; hepatic or renal dysfunction *that might interfere with the metabolism and excretion of the drug*; and pregnancy or lactation. Establish if patient is currently taking other medications or herbal therapies which may potentially interact with the antiviral drug.

Physical assessment should *be performed to establish baseline data for assessing the effectiveness of the DNA-active antiviral drug and the occurrence of any adverse effects associated with drug therapy.* Assess orientation *to evaluate any CNS effects of the drug.* Examine skin (colour, temperature and lesions) *to monitor the effectiveness of the drug.* Evaluate renal function tests *to determine baseline function of the kidneys.* Complete a full blood count with differential *to monitor bone marrow activity and evaluate toxic effects.*

Nursing Diagnoses

The patient receiving a DNA-active antiviral agent may have the following nursing diagnoses related to drug therapy:

- Acute pain related to GI, CNS or local effects of drug
- Disturbed sensory perception (kinaesthetic) related to CNS effects of drug
- Deficient knowledge regarding drug therapy

Implementation With Rationale

- Ensure good hydration *to decrease the toxic effects on the kidneys.*
- Administer the drug as soon as possible after the diagnosis has been made *to improve effectiveness of the antiviral activity.*
- Ensure that the patient takes the complete course of the drug regimen *to improve effectiveness and decrease the risk of the emergence of resistant viruses.*
- Wear protective gloves when applying the drug topically *to decrease risk of exposure to the drug and inadvertent absorption.*
- Provide safety precautions if CNS effects occur (e.g. orientation, assistance) *to protect the patient from injury.*
- Warn the patient that GI upset, nausea and vomiting can occur *to increase awareness of the importance of maintaining a good level of nutrition.*
- Full blood count with differential to monitor patients for anaemia, thrombocytopaenia and neutropaenia *to detect bone marrow suppression.*
- Where the patients history suggests potential problems, monitor renal function (plasma creatinine, urea and electrolytes) periodically during treatment *to detect and respond to renal toxicity as soon as possible.*
- Monitor liver function (plasma alanine transaminase and aspartate transaminase) during treatment *to detect and respond to hepatic toxicity as soon as possible.*
- Provide the patient with instructions about the drug *to enhance patient knowledge about drug therapy and to promote concordance.*

The patient should:

- Avoid sexual intercourse if genital herpes is being treated because these drugs do not cure the disease.
- Wear protective gloves when applying topical agents.
- Avoid driving and hazardous tasks if dizziness or drowsiness occurs.

Evaluation

- Monitor patient response to the drug (alleviation of signs and symptoms of herpes or CMV infection).
- Monitor for adverse effects (orientation, GI upset and renal function).
- Evaluate the effectiveness of the teaching plan (patient can name the drug, dosage, possible adverse effects to watch for, and specific measures to help avoid adverse effects).
- Monitor the effectiveness of comfort and safety measures and concordance with the regimen.

Agents for HIV and AIDS

According to the World Health Organisation (2007), 33 million people worldwide were infected with the **human immunodeficiency virus (HIV)**. In the United Kingdom there were an estimated 77,400 people living with HIV at the end of 2007 (Health Protection Agency, 2008). Worryingly, over a quarter of these individuals were unaware of their infection and therefore sought treatment at a late stage in the progression of the infection. A late diagnosis leads to a delay in receiving antiretroviral therapy, giving the virus opportunity to mutate. (See Box 9.3 for public education information regarding AIDS.)

There are two forms of the virus: HIV-1 and HIV-2; the HIV-1 form is prevalent around the world whereas the HIV-2 form is confined to specific African regions. The HIV-1 form mutates at a very high rate producing new variant forms of the virus making it difficult to treat.

HIV is a RNA retrovirus which mainly targets the **helper T cells** (also known as $CD4^+$ T cells) within the immune system. Macrophages and dendritic cells expressing the CD4 molecule are also targeted. The virus binds to specific receptors, including the CD4 molecule, on the surface of the helper T cells. Once the virus enters the helper T cell the enzyme reverse transcriptase converts the viral single-stranded RNA molecule into a double-stranded DNA molecule. The DNA molecule is then transported into the host cell nucleus and integrated into the host cells' DNA by the enzyme integrase. The virus can then lie dormant for between 10 and 15 years. When the infected cell is activated, for example during an infection; the host cell's DNA is transcribed into viral RNA from which viral proteins and enzymes are translated. The viral proteins are then broken into smaller proteins by a protease enzyme. The shorter proteins are re-packaged together with the viral RNA to form new viral particles. When the cell ruptures, many viral particles are released to attack other helper T cells.

The end result is that the number of helper T cells decreases from the direct killing of infected cells by the virus and also through the targeted killing of infected helper T cells by the cytotoxic T lymphocytes which recognize infected cells. As the number of helper T cells decrease the immune system loses an important monitor that propels the immune reaction into full force when the body is invaded.

Loss of T-cell function causes **acquired immunodeficiency syndrome (AIDS)** or **AIDS-related complex (ARC)**, diseases that are characterized by the emergence of a variety of opportunistic infections (e.g. oral candidiasis, cytomegalovirus or herpes simplex infections) and cancers that occur when the immune system is depressed and unable to function properly. The HIV mutates over time, presenting a slightly different configuration with each new generation. Treatment of AIDS and ARC has been difficult for several reasons: (1) the length of time the virus can remain dormant within the T cells (i.e. months to years), (2) the high rate of mutation of

BOX 9.3 FOCUS ON THE **EVIDENCE**

Public Education about AIDS

When AIDS was first diagnosed in the early 1980s, it was found in a certain population in New York City. The people in this group tended to be homosexuals, intravenous drug users and homeless people with poor hygiene and nutrition habits. Originally, a number of health care practitioners thought that the disease was a syndrome of opportunistic infections that occurred in a population with repeated exposure to infections that naturally deplete the immune system. It was not until several years later that the human immunodeficiency virus (HIV) was identified. Since then, it has been discovered that HIV infection is rampant in many African countries. As scientists have learned, HIV is not particular about the body it invades and once introduced into a body, it infects T cells and causes HIV infection.

HIV is transmitted via infected body fluids in several ways:

- Unprotected heterosexual or homosexual intercourse. Using a condom during sexual intercourse is the most effective way of reducing transmission of the virus and other sexually transmitted diseases.
- Through the sharing of contaminated needles and syringes between intravenous drug users or from contaminated needles used for tattoos or body piercings.
- Receipt of infected blood or blood products from a transfusion (this risk is minimal in the developed world where blood donations are screened for HIV). Contaminated medical equipment used in procedures can also transmit the virus.
- There is a risk of maternal/foetal transmission. The risks can be minimised by antiretroviral drug treatment during the pregnancy and delivery via Caesarean section to avoid the mothers' blood coming into contact with the baby. The baby may also be given antiretroviral therapy following birth. It is also recommended that the baby is bottle-fed rather than breastfed to reduce transmission through breast milk (John-Stewart *et al.*, 2004).
- Although rare, there have been cases of health care workers infected via needle stick injuries or blood splashes. Health care workers should always ensure they use and dispose of contaminated sharps safely and follow local guidelines in cleaning areas and disposing of contaminated waste.

The evidence shows that when a patient is diagnosed with HIV infection, the nurse faces a tremendous challenge for patient education and support. The patient and any significant others should be counselled about the risks of transmission and reassured about ways in which the virus is not transmitted (Chippindale & French, 2001). They will need to learn about drug protocols, T-cell levels, adverse drug effects and anticipated progress of the disease. They will also need consistent support: many communities have AIDS support groups and other resources that can be very helpful; the nurse can direct the patient to these resources as appropriate.

The combinations of drugs used today and the constant development of more drugs makes the disease less of a death sentence than it was in the past. The result, however, is that many people must take a large number of pills each day, which can place patient compliance to drug treatment at risk. Many people today do live for long periods with HIV infection. An AIDS vaccine is currently being studied and offers hope for preventing this disease in the future.

the virus, and (3) the adverse effects of many potent drugs, which may include further depression of the immune system. The types of antiviral agents that are used to treat HIV infections are the nucleoside reverse transcriptase inhibitors, the non-nucleoside reverse transcriptase inhibitors, the protease inhibitors and a new class of drugs called fusion inhibitors (Table 9.3) – each drug class targets a different stage of the life cycle of the virus and results in viral death or inactivation (see Figure 9.2). Collectively these drugs are known as antiretroviral agents. At present, a combination of several different antiretroviral drugs is used to attack the virus at various points in its life cycle to achieve maximum effectiveness with the least amount of toxicity. This approach will also reduce the number of mutant virions that are formed and spread to noninfected cells. The combination therapy is referred to as HAART (**h**ighly **a**ctive **a**nti**r**etroviral **t**herapy) and includes two nucleoside reverse transcriptase inhibitors with either a protease inhibitor or a non-nucleoside reverse transcriptase inhibitor.

Nucleoside Reverse Transcriptase Inhibitors

Nucleoside reverse transcriptase inhibitors are nucleoside analogues that interfere with HIV replication by inhibiting reverse transcriptase, the enzyme responsible for converting the viral RNA molecule into a DNA molecule (see above), leading to viral death. The drugs belonging to this class are listed in Table 9.3. All the nucleoside reverse transcriptase

Table 9.3 DRUGS IN FOCUS

HIV and AIDS Drugs

Drug Name	Usual Indications
Nucleoside Reverse Transcriptase Inhibitors	
abacavir	Combination therapy for the treatment of adults and children with HIV
didanosine (ddI, DDI)	Treatment of infections in adults and children with HIV as part of combination therapy
emtricitabine	Combination therapy for the treatment of adults and children with HIV
lamivudine (3TC)	With other antiretroviral agents for the treatment of adults and children with HIV; also the treatment of chronic hepatitis B
stavudine (d4T)	Treatment of adults and children with HIV in combination with other antiretroviral agents
tenofovir	Treatment of adults with HIV infection in combination with other antiretroviral drugs
zidovudine (AZT)	Treatment of symptomatic HIV in adults and children as part of combination therapy; prevention of maternal/foetal transmission of HIV
Non-Nucleoside Reverse Transcriptase Inhibitors	
efavirenz	Treatment of adults and children with HIV in combination with other antiretroviral agents
nevirapine	Treatment of adults and children with progressive or advanced HIV infection in combination with at least two other antiretroviral agents
Protease Inhibitors	
amprenavir	HIV treatment in combination with other antiretroviral agents in adults and children who have been treated with other protease inhibitors
atazanavir	As for amprenavir
darunavir	Combination therapy of adults with HIV infection unresponsive to other protease inhibitors
fosamprenavir	Part of combination therapy for the treatment of HIV in adults
indinavir	Treatment of adults with HIV as part of combination therapy with nucleotide reverse transcriptase inhibitors
lopinavir	Treatment of adults and children with HIV in combination with ritonavir
nelfinavir	Combination therapy for the treatment of adults and children with HIV
ritonavir	Part of combination therapy with nucleotide reverse transcriptase inhibitors for the treatment of adults and children with HIV
saquinavir	Treatment of adults with HIV as part of combination therapy
tipranavir	Treatment of adults with HIV in combination with ritonavir
Fusion Inhibitor	
enfuvirtide	Part of combination therapy in treatment of HIV patients with evidence of HIV replication despite antiretroviral therapy

inhibitors are used in combination with other antiretroviral therapy (Box 9.4 discusses the use of combination drugs). Resistance can occur with all the drugs in this class and they should be combined with antiretroviral drugs from other classes.

Abacavir is used in combination therapy in adults and children. After rapid GI absorption, abacavir is metabolized in the liver and excreted in urine. Serious-to-fatal hypersensitivity reactions have occurred with this drug, and it must be stopped immediately at any sign of a hypersensitivity reaction (fever, chills, rash, fatigue, GI upset, flu-like symptoms). These symptoms usually occur in the first 6 weeks of treatment.

Didanosine is used to treat advanced infections in adults and children. It is rapidly destroyed in an acid environment and therefore must be taken in a buffered form. Didanosine undergoes intracellular metabolism to form the active metabolite. Peak levels are reached within 1 hour with a plasma half-life of 1.5 hours. Serious pancreatitis, hepatomegaly and peripheral neuropathy have been reported with this drug. The treatment should be suspended if serum lipase levels increase or if symptoms of pancreatitis develop.

Emtricitabine is also used in combination with other antiretroviral drugs. It is extensively absorbed from the GI tract and has a plasma half-life of 10 hours. Emtricitabine is mostly excreted unchanged in the urine. The side-effects of emtricitabine are similar to those observed with other nucleoside reverse transcriptase inhibitors and include abnormal dreams, pruritus and hyperpigmentation.

Lamivudine is recommended for the treatment of HIV and chronic hepatitis B. After rapid GI absorption, lamivudine is excreted primarily unchanged in the urine, with a half-life of 5 to 7 hours.

Stavudine is also rapidly absorbed from the GI tract, reaching peak levels in 1 hour. The half-life of stavudine is 1.5 hours and most of the drug is excreted unchanged in the urine, making it important to reduce dosage and monitor patients carefully in the presence of renal dysfunction. Stavudine should be used with caution by patients with a history of peripheral neuropathy or pancreatitis.

Tenofovir is used only in combination with other antiretroviral agents. It is rapidly absorbed from the GI tract, reaching peak levels in 1 to 2 hours. Its pathway of metabolism is unknown, but it is excreted in the urine. Severe hepatomegaly with steatosis has been reported with tenofovir, so it must be used with great caution in any patient with hepatic impairment. Tenofovir can cause polyuria and renal failure and treatment should be interrupted if renal function declines. Patients should also be alerted that the drug may cause changes in body fat distribution, with loss of fat from arms, legs and face and deposition of fat on the trunk, neck and breasts.

Zidovudine was one of the first drugs found to be effective in the treatment of AIDS. It is used to treat symptomatic disease in adults and children and to prevent maternal transmission of HIV. It is rapidly absorbed from the GI tract, with peak levels occurring within 30 to 75 minutes. Zidovudine is metabolized in the liver and excreted in the urine, with a plasma half-life of 1 hour. Patients with marked renal or hepatic impairment may require lower doses because of the role of these organs in metabolism and excretion. Severe bone marrow suppression has occurred with this drug, which must be used very cautiously in patients with compromised bone marrow function. Zidovudine has been used safely during pregnancy.

Pharmacokinetics

Pharmacokinetic details of each of the nucleoside reverse transcriptase inhibitors are described above. Where the half-life is given, the value refers to the plasma half-life rather than the intracellular half-life of the drug which is longer. Zidovudine is the only agent that has been proven to be safe when used during pregnancy. Of the other agents, there have been no adequate studies in pregnancy, so use should be limited to situations in which the benefits clearly outweigh any risks.

BOX 9.4 Fixed Combination Drugs for Treatment of HIV Infection

Patients who are taking combination drug therapy for HIV infection may have to take a very large number of pills each day. Keeping track of these pills and swallowing such a large number each day can be an overwhelming task. In an effort to improve patient concordance and make it easier for some of these patients, some anti-HIV agents are now available in combination products (the drug names given below are trade names). However, because these are fixed combinations of drugs, they may not be the drug of choice for patients who require a dosage reduction owing to renal impairment or adverse effects that limit dose tolerance. Patients should be stabilized on each antiretroviral individually before being switched to the combination form.

- *Combivir* is a combination of 150 mg lamivudine and 300 mg zidovudine. The patient takes one tablet, twice a day.
- *Trizivir* combines 300 mg abacavir, 150 mg lamivudine and 300 mg zidovudine. The patient takes one tablet, twice a day. Patients taking *Trizivir* should be warned at the time the prescription is filled about the potentially serious hypersensitivity reactions associated with abacavir.
- *Kivexa* is a combination of 600 mg abacavir with 300 mg lamivudine and is taken as one tablet once a day.
- *Truvada* (200 mg emtricitabine plus 245 mg tenofovir) is also a once-a-day tablet.

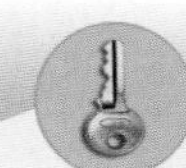

Key Drug Summary: *Zidovudine*

Indications: Management of adults with symptomatic HIV infection in combination with other antiretrovirals; prevention of maternal–foetal HIV transmission

Actions: A thymidine analogue that is converted by cellular enzymes into the active triphosphate form. The active drug inhibits HIV reverse transcriptase, the enzyme used to convert the viral RNA into a double-stranded DNA molecule. The virus is unable to integrate into the host cells' DNA and cannot replicate.

Pharmacokinetics:

Route	Onset	Peak
Oral	Varies	30–90 min
IV	Rapid	End of infusion

$T_{1/2}$: 1 hour; metabolized in the liver and excreted in the urine

Adverse effects: Headache, insomnia, dizziness, nausea, diarrhoea, fever, rash, liver damage, bone marrow suppression, taste disturbances, chest pain, 'flu-like' symptoms, paraesthesia (tingling of the skin), neuropathy, CNS disturbances, myopathy, gynaecomastia, increased urination, sweating, pruritus, pigmentation

Non-Nucleoside Reverse Transcriptase Inhibitors

The **non-nucleoside reverse transcriptase inhibitors** bind directly to HIV reverse transcriptase causing a structural change in the enzyme molecule. Enzyme inhibition blocks both RNA- and DNA-dependent DNA polymerase activities and prevents the transfer of information that would allow the virus to replicate and survive. *Efavirenz* and *nevirapine* both belong to this group of antiretroviral drugs and inhibit the HIV-1 form of the virus rather than HIV-2. The indications are listed in Table 9.3.

Pharmacokinetics

Both drugs are rapidly absorbed from the GI tract and extensively metabolized by cytochrome P450 enzymes in the liver. They both induce the liver enzymes responsible for their own metabolism. This is known as autoinduction which decreases the half-life of the drug over the duration of drug treatment as the rate of metabolism is increased (refer to Chapter 2). The metabolites are excreted in the urine and faeces (efavirenz). Both drugs should be used with caution by patients with chronic hepatitis B or C or hepatic dysfunction because of increased risk of hepatic side-effects. Efavirenz has a half-life of 52–76 hours (initial dose) to 40–55 hours (subsequent doses). The half-life of nevirapine is detailed below.

The use of efavirenz and nevirapine in pregnancy should be limited to situations in which the benefits clearly outweigh any risks. Neither drug should be used during breast-feeding.

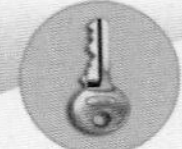

Key Drug Summary: *Nevirapine*

Indications: Treatment of HIV-1 infected patients who have experienced clinical or immunologic deterioration, in combination with at least two other antiretrovirals

Actions: Binds to HIV-1 reverse transcriptase and blocks replication of the HIV by changing the structure of the HIV enzyme

Pharmacokinetics:

Route	Onset	Peak
Oral	Rapid	4 h

$T_{1/2}$: 45 hours, then 25–30 hours; metabolized in the liver and excreted in the urine

Adverse effects: Headache, nausea, vomiting, rash (including Stevens–Johnson syndrome), hepatotoxicity, chills, fever

Protease Inhibitors

The **protease inhibitors** block protease activity within the HIV virus. Protease is the enzyme responsible for the conversion of precursor viral polyproteins into functional proteins and is essential for the final assembly of the HIV virions. Without protease, an HIV particle is immature and noninfective. The protease inhibitors that are available for use and their indications are listed in Table 9.3. Protease inhibitors should be used with caution in diabetic patients because these drugs can cause hyperglycaemia; and haemophiliacs because there is an increased risk of bleeding.

Amprenavir is rapidly absorbed from the GI tract, reaching peak levels within 1 hour. After undergoing metabolism in the liver, amprenavir is excreted mainly in the faeces with a half-life of 7.1 to 10.6 hours. During the second week of therapy a rash may appear. Treatment should be stopped if the rash is severe and associated with systemic symptoms.

The absorption of *atazanivir* from the GI tract is improved when the drug is taken with food. After metabolism in the liver, it is excreted in the urine and faeces with a half-life of about 7 hours.

The presence of food also increases the bioavailability of *darunavir*. Darunavir is metabolized in the liver; some of the metabolites also possess some antiretroviral activity. The majority of the drug is excreted in the faeces, partly as metabolites and the remainder as unchanged drug. The half-life is approximately 15 hours.

Fosamprenavir, a pro-drug of amprenavir, is hydrolyzed by the epithelial cells lining the GI tract to the active drug. Peak plasma levels of amprenavir are reached in 1.5 to 4 hours. This drug is metabolized and excreted by the same mechanism as amprenavir.

Indinavir is rapidly absorbed from the GI tract, reaching peak levels in 0.8 hours. Indinavir is metabolized in the liver by the cytochrome P450 system and excreted mainly in the faeces with a half-life of 1.8 hours. Patients with renal impairment are at risk of increased toxic effects, and the dosage may need to be reduced.

Lopinavir is used as a fixed combination drug that combines lopinavir and ritonavir. The ritonavir inhibits the metabolism of lopinavir, leading to increased lopinavir serum levels and effectiveness. It is readily absorbed from the GI tract and undergoes extensive hepatic metabolism by the cytochrome P450 system. Lopinavir is excreted in urine and faeces. Patients with pancreatitis should use lopinavir with caution. Treatment should be discontinued if serum lipase levels increase and pancreatitis is diagnosed.

Nelfinavir is well absorbed from the GI tract, reaching peak levels in 2 to 4 hours. Nelfinavir is metabolized in the liver by the CYP450 system, and caution must be used in patients with any hepatic dysfunction. It is primarily excreted in the faeces, with a half-life of 3.5 to 5 hours.

Ritonavir is rapidly absorbed from the GI tract, reaching peak levels in 2 to 4 hours. Ritonavir undergoes extensive metabolism in the liver and is excreted mainly in the faeces. Many potentially serious toxic effects can occur when ritonavir is taken with a number of drugs including antifungals, antibacterials and hypnotics, because of the activity of ritonavir in the liver. The same cautions apply to ritonavir as for lopinavir.

Saquinavir is poorly absorbed from the GI tract and undergoes first-pass metabolism in the liver. As a result the bioavailability is low; different formulations can boost the bioavailability. It is primarily excreted in the faeces with a short half-life. Saquinavir should not be taken with garlic supplements – garlic is known to decrease plasma concentrations of saquinavir.

Tipranavir is slowly absorbed, reaching peak levels in 2.9 hours. It is metabolized in the liver with a half-life of 4.8 to 6 hours; excretion is through urine and faeces. When given with ritonavir, metabolism of tipranavir is significantly reduced and it is mainly excreted as the unchanged drug. Tipranavir interacts with many other drugs, and its use must be carefully monitored based on other drugs in the overall drug regimen. Patients receiving tipranavir must have liver function monitored regularly because of the possibility of potentially fatal hepatotoxicity.

Pharmacokinetics

All the drugs in this group are metabolized by the liver enzyme systems, increasing the potential for interactions with other drugs. Furthermore, because of the extensive hepatic metabolism these drugs undergo, caution must be used with any patient with hepatic dysfunction.

These drugs can be used during pregnancy in situations in which the benefits clearly outweigh any risks. Women are advised not to breast-feed if taking any of these drugs.

Fusion Inhibitors

A new class of drugs, called fusion inhibitors, was first introduced in 2003. Fusion inhibitors prevent the fusion of the virus with the human cellular membrane, which prevents the virus from entering the cell. This agent acts at a different site than other HIV antiretrovirals and is used in combination with drugs from the other classes to target the virus at many points.

Enfuvirtide is used in combination with other antiretroviral agents where there is evidence of HIV-1 replication, despite ongoing antiretroviral therapy, that is resistance; or when patients are unable to take other antiviral therapies. It is given by subcutaneous injection and peaks in effect in 4 to 8 hours. The pathways for metabolism and excretion are not clear. The half-life of enfuvirtide is 3.2 to 4.4 hours. The drug has been associated with pancreatitis, anorexia, anxiety, peripheral neuropathy, pneumonia and injection site reactions.

Contraindications and Cautions for Antiretroviral Agents

There are no true contraindications to the use of these drugs because they are used in the treatment of a potentially fatal disease with no known cure. All the antiretroviral drugs are contraindicated in breast-feeding, but note that women are advised not to breast-feed to reduce the risk of virus transmission in breast milk. In pregnancy, zidovudine is the drug of choice *to block maternal transmission of the virus.* Caution should be used with known allergies to any of these drugs; with hepatic or renal dysfunction, *which could lead to increased drug levels and toxicity*; and in patients with chronic hepatitis B or C *who are at greater risk of side-effects.*

Adverse Effects Associated with Antiretroviral Agents

The adverse effects reported with the use of these drugs are often indistinguishable from the effects of the ongoing disease process. Adverse effects that are most often reported include the CNS effects of headache, dizziness, and myalgia; GI upset, including nausea, vomiting, and diarrhoea; hepatic toxicity related to direct drug effects on the liver; fever and 'flu-like' symptoms; rash; and bone marrow depression, including agranulocytosis and anaemia. Other serious adverse effects associated with each antiretroviral class are described below.

Nucleoside reverse transcriptase inhibitors – are associated with hepatic necrosis and subsequent lactic acidosis. This can be fatal and patients with hepatic impairment should be closely monitored. Other adverse effects include lipodystrophy syndrome where body fat is redistributed in a similar manner described in Chapter 35; and the patient's metabolism changes causing hyperglycaemia and elevated lipid levels.

Non-nucleoside reverse transcriptase inhibitors – rashes are common with this group, including the potentially fatal Stevens–Johnson syndrome.

Protease inhibitors – these drugs are also associated with lipodystrophy syndrome.

Fusion inhibitors – hypersensitivity reactions are common with enfuvirtide.

Clinically Important Drug–Drug Interactions

Nucleoside reverse transcriptase inhibitors – stavudine and tenofovir can cause large increases in the serum level of didanosine. If both of these drugs are given, tenofovir should be given 2 hours before or 1 hour after didanosine. If zidovudine is given together with other nephrotoxic and myelosuppressive drugs, there is an increased risk of toxicitiy.

Non-nucleoside reverse transcriptase inhibitors – nevirapine and indinavir interact to cause severe toxicity. If these two drugs are given in combination, the dosages should be adjusted and the patient should be monitored closely. Efavirenz and nevirapine can reduce the plasma concentration of protease inhibitors.

Protease inhibitors – if nelfinavir is combined with amiodarone, pimozide, rifampicin or midazolam, severe toxic effects and life-threatening arrhythmias may occur. Such combinations should be avoided. Tipranavir has been shown to interact with many other drugs.

Always consult a current copy of the British National Formulary for further guidance.

Nursing Considerations for Patients Receiving Agents for HIV and AIDS

Assessment: History and Examination

Screen for the following conditions, *which are cautions or contraindications to the use of these drugs*: any history of allergy to antiretrovirals; renal or hepatic dysfunction *that might interfere with the metabolism and excretion of the drug*; and pregnancy or lactation. Establish if patient is currently taking other medications or herbal therapies which may potentially interact with the antiviral drug.

Physical assessment should be performed *to establish baseline data for assessing the effectiveness of the drug and the occurrence of any adverse effects associated with drug therapy.* Perform assessment of orientation and reflex *to evaluate any CNS effects of the drug.* Check temperature *to monitor for infections.* Evaluate hepatic and renal function tests *to determine baseline function of the kidneys and liver.* Check results of a full blood count with differential *to monitor bone marrow activity* and T-cell number *to indicate effectiveness of the drugs.*

Nursing Diagnoses

The patient receiving drugs for HIV and AIDS may have the following nursing diagnoses related to drug therapy:

- Acute pain related to GI, CNS or dermatological effects of the drugs
- Disturbed sensory perception (kinaesthetic) related to CNS effects of the drugs
- Imbalanced nutrition: less than body requirements, related to GI effects of the drugs
- Deficient knowledge regarding drug therapy

Implementation With Rationale

- Monitor renal and hepatic function before and periodically during therapy *to detect renal or hepatic function changes and arrange to reduce dosage or provide treatment as needed.*
- Ensure that the patient takes the complete course of the drug regimen and takes all drugs included in a particular combination *to improve effectiveness of the drug and decrease the risk of emergence of resistant viral strains.*
- Administer drug around the clock, if indicated, *to provide the critical concentration needed for the drug to be effective.*
- Monitor nutritional status if GI effects are severe, and *take appropriate action to maintain nutrition.*
- Stop drug if severe rash occurs, especially if accompanied by blisters and fever *to avert potentially serious reactions.*
- Provide safety precautions (e.g. orientation, assistance) if CNS effects occur, *to protect patient from injury.*
- Teach the patient about the drugs prescribed *to enhance patient knowledge about drug therapy and to promote concordance.* Include as a teaching point the fact that these drugs do not cure

the disease, so appropriate precautions should still be taken *to prevent transmission.*

The patient should:

- Understand the need to take the drug treatment as prescribed to reduce viral mutation and to slow disease progression.
- Have periodic blood tests (full blood count with differential) to monitor the effectiveness and toxicity of the drug.
- Realise that GI upset, nausea and vomiting may occur but that efforts must be taken to maintain adequate nutrition.
- Avoid driving and hazardous tasks if dizziness or drowsiness occurs.
- Report extreme fatigue, severe headache, difficulty in breathing, or severe rash to a health care provider.

Evaluation

- Monitor patient response to the drug (alleviation of signs and symptoms of AIDS or ARC and maintenance of T-cell levels).
- Monitor for adverse effects (orientation and affect, GI upset, renal and hepatic function, skin, levels of blood components).
- Evaluate the effectiveness of the teaching plan (patient can name the drug, dosage, possible adverse effects to watch for, and specific measures to help avoid adverse effects).
- Ensure that the patient can clearly explain the main modes of HIV transmission and ways to reduce further spread.
- Monitor the effectiveness of comfort and safety measures and concordance with the regimen (see Critical Thinking Scenario 9-1).

Drugs Used to Treat Hepatitis

Some viruses target the liver to cause viral hepatitis; these include hepatitis A, B and C. Hepatitis A is transmitted by the faecal–oral route via contaminated food or drinks and can range from mild to severe. Hepatitis B is a more serious to potentially fatal viral infection of the liver. The hepatitis B virus can be spread by blood or blood products, sexual contact, or contaminated needles or instruments. Health care workers are at especially high risk for encountering hepatitis B due to needle stick injuries. Hepatitis B has a higher mortality than other types of hepatitis and also brings with it the possibility of developing a chronic condition or becoming a carrier. Hepatitis C can also be transmitted via infected blood and the same precautions against hepatitis B should be applied to hepatitis C. This form of the virus can result in severe liver damage. Vaccinations against both hepatitis A and B are available.

Hepatitis B can be treated with either of the two interferons, peginterferon α-2a or interferon-α (see Chapter 16, Immune Modulators). Either interferon can be used in the initial treatment; however, peginterferon α-2a is preferable. Adefovir, entecavir and telbivudine are new drugs used to specifically treat chronic hepatitis B. Hepatitis C can be treated with a combination of ribavirin and peginterferon.

Therapeutic Actions and Indications

Adefovir, entecavir and telbivudine are indicated for the treatment of adults with chronic hepatitis B who have evidence of active viral replication and either evidence of persistent elevations in serum aminotransferases or histologically active disease. These antiviral drugs decrease the viral load by specific inhibition of reverse transcriptase in the hepatitis B virus, preventing viral DNA synthesis and thereby viral replication (Table 9.4).

Table 9.4 DRUGS IN FOCUS

Hepatitis B Drugs

Drug Name	Usual Indications
adefovir	Treatment of hepatitis B with either evidence of active viral replication and persistent elevations in liver enzymes or decompensated liver disease
entecavir	Treatment of chronic hepatitis B with compensated liver disease, evidence of active viral replication and persistent liver enzyme elevations
telbivudine	As for entecavir

Pharmacokinetics

These drugs are rapidly absorbed from the GI tract with peak effects occurring in 0.5 to 4 (adefovir), 0.5 to 1.5 (entecavir), and 3 hours (telbivudine). Each drug is eliminated by the kidneys. The half-lives of adefovir, entecavir and telbivudine are 7.5, 128 to 149 and 30 to 53 hours, respectively. None of these drugs should be used during pregnancy unless the potential benefits outweigh the risk and should also be avoided whilst breast-feeding.

Contraindications and Cautions

These drugs are contraindicated with any known allergy to the drugs and with lactation, because of potential toxicity to the nursing baby. Caution should be used with renal impairment, pregnancy and severe liver disease.

Adverse Effects

The adverse effects most frequently seen with these drugs are headache, dizziness, nausea, diarrhoea and elevated liver enzymes. Severe hepatomegaly (an enlarged liver) with steatosis (an accumulation of fat in the hepatocytes), sometimes fatal, has been reported with adefovir use. Lactic acidosis and renal impairment have also been reported. There is a risk that hepatitis B exacerbation could occur when the drugs are stopped.

Clinically Important Drug–Drug Interactions

There is an increased risk of renal toxicity if these drugs are taken with other nephrotoxic drugs. If such a combination is used, the patient should be closely monitored and the evaluation of risks versus benefits may need to be made if renal function begins to deteriorate.

Always consult a current copy of the British National Formulary for further guidance.

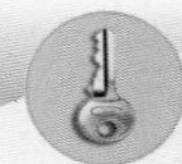

Key Drug Summary: *Adefovir*

Indications: Treatment of chronic hepatitis B in adults with evidence of active viral replication and either evidence of persistent elevations in the enzymes alanine transaminase (ALT) or aspartate aminotransferase (AST), or histologically active disease

Actions: Inhibits hepatitis B virus reverse transcriptase, causes DNA chain termination and blocks viral replication

Pharmacokinetics:

Route	Onset	Peak	Duration
Oral	Rapid	0.6–4 h	Unknown

$T_{1/2}$: 7.5 hours; excreted in the urine

Adverse effects: Headache, loss of strength, nausea, dyspepsia, abdominal pain, severe-to-fatal hepatomegaly with steatosis, nephrotoxicity, lactic acidosis, hypophosphataemia, exacerbation of hepatitis B when discontinued

Nursing Considerations for Patients Receiving Agents for Hepatitis B

Assessment: History and Examination

Patients receiving agents to treat hepatitis B should be assessed for the following conditions, *which are cautions or contraindications to the use of these drugs*: any history of allergy to adefovir, entecavir or telbivudine; renal dysfunction, *which could be exacerbated by the nephrotoxic effects of these drugs;* severe liver impairment, *which could exacerbate the liver toxicity of these drugs*; and pregnancy and lactation, *because of the potential adverse effects of these drugs on the foetus or baby.*

Physical assessment should be performed *to establish baseline data for assessing the effectiveness of these drugs and the occurrence of any adverse effects associated with drug toxicity.* Assess body temperature *to monitor underlying disease*, and muscle strength *to assess for CNS changes.* Evaluate renal and liver function tests *to monitor for developing toxicity and for drug effectiveness.*

Nursing Diagnoses

The patient receiving an agent for chronic hepatitis B may have the following nursing diagnoses related to drug therapy:

- Acute pain related to CNS and GI effects of the drug
- Imbalanced nutrition: less than body requirements related to the GI effects of the drug
- Deficient knowledge regarding drug therapy

Implementation With Rationale

- Monitor renal and hepatic function prior to and periodically during therapy *to detect renal or*

Table 9.5 DRUGS IN FOCUS

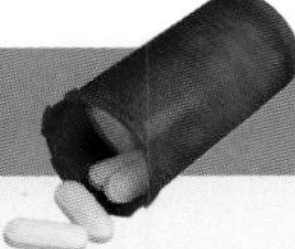

Locally Active Antiviral Agents

Drug Name	Usual Indications
idoxuridine	Local treatment of herpes simplex and hepatitis zoster infection (of little therapeutic value)
imiquimod	Local treatment of genital and perianal warts
penciclovir	Local treatment of herpes labialis (cold sores) on the face and lips

hepatic function changes and arrange to reduce dosage or provide treatment as needed.

- Withdraw the drug and monitor the patient if patient develops signs of lactic acidosis or hepatotoxicity, *because these adverse effects can be life threatening.*
- Caution patient to not run out of this drug, but to take it continually *because acute exacerbation of hepatitis B can occur when the drug is stopped.*
- Advise women of childbearing age to use barrier contraceptives *because of the potential adverse effects of this drug on the foetus.*
- Advise women who are breast-feeding to find another method of feeding the baby while using the drug, *because of the potential toxic effects on the baby.*
- Advise patients that these drugs do not cure the disease and there is still a risk of transferring the disease, *so the patient should continue to take appropriate steps to prevent transmission of hepatitis B.*
- Teach the patient about the drug prescribed, *to enhance patient knowledge about drug therapy and to promote concordance.*

The patient should:

- Monitor serological markers for hepatitis B every 6 months.
- Have regular blood tests to monitor renal function (plasma creatinine, urea and electrolyes) and liver function (plasma alanine transaminase and aspartate transaminase).
- Take precautions to avoid running out of the drug, because the drug must be taken continually.
- Realise that GI upset, with nausea and diarrhoea, is common with this drug.
- Report severe weakness, muscle pain and yellowing of the eyes or skin and difficulty in breathing.

Evaluation

- Monitor patient response to the drug (decreased viral load of hepatitis B).
- Monitor for adverse effects (liver or renal dysfunction, headache, nausea, diarrhoea).
- Evaluate the effectiveness of the teaching plan (patient can name the drug, dosage, possible adverse effects to watch for, and specific measures to avoid adverse effects).
- Monitor the effectiveness of comfort and safety measures and compliance with the drug regimen.

Locally Active Antiviral Agents

Some antiviral agents are given locally to treat local viral infections. These agents include idoxuridine, imiquimod and penciclovir (see also Table 9.5). Box 9.5 describes how to apply these topical drugs.

Therapeutic Actions and Indications

These antiviral agents act on viruses by interfering with normal viral replication and metabolic processes. They are indicated for specific, local viral infections.

Contraindications and Cautions

Locally active antiviral drugs are not absorbed systemically, but caution should be used in patients with known allergic reactions to any topical drugs.

Adverse Effects

As these drugs are not absorbed systemically, the adverse effects most commonly reported are local burning, stinging and discomfort. These effects usually occur at the time of administration and pass with time.

BOX 9.5

FOCUS ON CLINICAL SKILLS

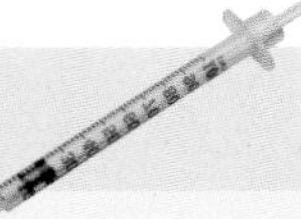

Before applying a topical drug, it is important to remember that these drugs are intended for topical, not systemic use.

1. Assess the affected area and make sure that there are no open lesions or abrasions that could allow for systemic absorption of the drug.
2. Clean the area to be treated and pat dry.
3. Always clean any old drug from the site before applying a new dose.
4. Apply the drug using gloves or an applicator to prevent exposure to the drug and cross-contamination.
5. Make sure that the drug is applied only to affected areas and not spread to a wider area.

Nursing Considerations for Patients Receiving Locally Active Antiviral Agents

Assessment: History and Examination

Patients receiving locally active antiviral agents should be assessed for any history of allergy to antivirals. Physical assessment should be performed *to ensure patient is not systemically unwell and to establish baseline data for evaluating the effectiveness of the drug and the occurrence of any adverse effects associated with drug therapy*, including inflammation at the site of infection.

Nursing Diagnoses

The patient receiving locally active antiviral drugs may have the following nursing diagnoses related to drug therapy:

- Acute pain related to local effects of drug
- Deficient knowledge regarding drug therapy

Implementation With Rationale

- Ensure proper administration of the drug *to improve effectiveness and decrease risk of adverse effects.*
- Stop the drug if severe local reaction occurs or if open lesions occur near the site of administration *to prevent systemic absorption.*
- Teach the patient about the drug being used *to enhance patient knowledge about drug therapy and to promote concordance.* Include as a teaching point the fact that these drugs do not cure the disease but should alleviate discomfort and prevent damage to healthy tissues. Encourage the patient to report severe local reaction or discomfort.

Evaluation

- Monitor patient response to the drug (alleviation of signs and symptoms of viral infection).
- Monitor for adverse effects (local irritation and discomfort).
- Evaluate the effectiveness of the teaching plan (patient can name the drug, the dosage, proper administration technique, and adverse effects to watch for and report to a health care provider).
- Monitor the effectiveness of comfort and safety measures and concordance with the regimen.

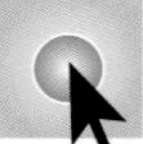

WEB LINKS

Health care providers and patients may want to consult the following Internet sources:

http://bnfc.org The BNF for Children provides UK health care professionals with authoritative and practical information on the selection and clinical use of medicines in children.

http://cks.library.nhs.uk The National Health Service Clinical Knowledge Summaries provides evidence-based practical information on the common conditions observed in primary care.

http://www.aidsinfo.nih.gov This site of the US National Institutes of Health provides extensive information on a number of topics including treatment regimes, drugs used, clinical trials and vaccines.

http://www.bashh.org The British Association for Sexual Health and HIV is for health care professionals to promote the study, diagnosis and treatment of sexually transmitted infections and HIV.

http://www.bhiva.org The British HIV Association provides advice on all aspects of HIV care. Provides many useful guidelines on issues such as the management of HIV infection in pregnant women, HIV-associated malignancies and treatment with antiretroviral therapy.

http://www.bnf.org.uk The BNF provides UK health care professionals with authoritative and practical information on the selection and clinical use of medicines.

http://www.hpa.org.uk The Health Protection Agency provides information on influenza including pandemic and avian influenza.

http://www.nhsdirect.nhs.uk The National Health Service Direct service provides patients with information and advice about health, illness and health services.

http://www.tht.org.uk The Terence Higgins Trust can provide information to health care professionals and the public on HIV, AIDS and sexual health.

Points to Remember

- Viruses are particles of DNA or RNA surrounded by a protein coat that survive by injecting their own DNA or RNA into a healthy cell and taking over its functioning.
- Because viruses are contained within human cells, it has been difficult to develop drugs that are effective antivirals and yet do not destroy human cells. Antiviral agents are available that are effective against only a few types of viruses.
- Influenza A and respiratory viruses cause the signs and symptoms of the common cold or 'flu'. The drugs that are available to prevent the replication of these viruses are used for prophylaxis against these diseases during peak seasons for at-risk patients. However, most cold and 'flu' viruses are self-limiting and require no intervention.
- Herpesviruses and CMV are DNA viruses that cause a multitude of problems, including cold sores, chicken pox, encephalitis, infections of the eye and liver, and genital herpes.
- Helper T cells are essential for maintaining a vigilant, effective immune system. When these cells are decreased in number or effectiveness, opportunistic infections occur. AIDS and ARC are syndromes of opportunistic infections that occur when the immune system is depressed.
- HIV, which specifically attacks helper T cells, may remain dormant in T cells for long periods and has been known to mutate easily.
- Antiretroviral agents that are effective against HIV and AIDS include reverse transcriptase inhibitors, protease inhibitors, nucleosides, and fusion inhibitors, all of which affect the way the virus communicates, replicates, or matures within the cell. They are given in combination to most effectively destroy the HIV virus and prevent mutation.
- Some antivirals are available only for the local treatment of viral infections, including warts and eye infections. These drugs are not absorbed systemically.

CRITICAL THINKING SCENARIO 9-1

Antiviral Agents for HIV and AIDS

The Situation

Harry is a 34-year-old who was diagnosed with AIDS, having had a positive HIV test 3 years ago. Although his helper T-cell count had been stabilized with treatment with zidovudine and efavirenz, it recently dropped remarkably. He presents with numerous opportunistic infections. Harry admits that he has been under tremendous stress at work and home in the past few weeks. He begins a combination regimen of lamivudine, zidovudine, ritonavir and zalcitabine.

Critical Thinking

- What are the important nursing implications in this case?
- What role would stress play in the progression of this disease?
- What specific issues should be discussed?
- What other clinical implications should be considered?

Discussion

Combination therapy with antiretrovirals has been found to be effective in decreasing some of the morbidity and mortality associated with HIV and AIDS. However, this treatment does not cure the disease. Harry needs to understand that opportunistic infections can still occur and therefore should be educated on ways to reduce the risk of infections, for example effective hand washing, avoiding contact with people with colds. Regular medical help should be sought particularly if early symptoms of infection develop such as fever, sore throat and cough. He also needs to understand that these drugs do not decrease the risk of transmitting HIV by sexual contact or through blood contamination and he should be encouraged to take appropriate precautions.

It is important to make a dosing schedule for Harry, or even to prepare a weekly drug box, to ensure that all medications are taken as indicated. Harry should also receive interventions to help him decrease his stress, because activation of the sympathetic nervous system during periods of stress depresses the immune system. Further depression of his immune system could accelerate the development of opportunistic infections and decrease the effectiveness of his antiretroviral drugs. Measures that could be used to decrease stress should be discussed and tried with Harry.

Discussing the adverse effects that Harry may experience is important because GI upset and discomfort may occur while he is taking all of these anti-HIV/AIDS medications. Small, frequent meals may help alleviate

(continued)

Antiviral Agents for HIV and AIDS *(continued)*

the discomfort. It is important that every effort is made to maintain Harry's nutritional status, and referral to a dietician may be necessary if GI effects are severe. Harry may also experience dizziness, fatigue and confusion, which could cause more problems for him at work and may necessitate changes in his workload. As some of the prescribed drugs must be taken around the clock, provisions may be needed to allow Harry to take his drugs on time throughout the day. For example, he may need to wear an alarm wristwatch, establish planned breaks in his schedule at dosing times, or devise other ways to follow his drug regimen without interfering with his work schedule. The adverse effects and inconvenience of taking this many drugs may add to his stress. It is important that health care providers work consistently with him to help him to manage his disease and treatment as effectively as possible. Harry should be given access to counselling services to assist him in managing a chronic illness.

Nursing Care Guide for Harry: Antiviral Agents for HIV and AIDS

Assessment: History and Examination

- Allergies to any of these drugs
- Bone marrow depression
- Renal or liver dysfunction
- Skin: colour, lesions, texture
- CNS: affect, reflexes, orientation
- GI: abdominal and liver evaluation
- Respiratory: breath sounds, chest X-ray
- Haematological: full blood count and differential; viral load; T-cell levels; hepatitis B status; hepatitis C antibody; renal and hepatic function tests

Nursing Diagnoses

- Acute pain related to GI, CNS, skin effects
- Disturbed sensory perception (kinaesthetic) related to CNS effects
- Imbalanced nutrition: less than body requirements related to GI effects
- Deficient knowledge regarding drug therapy

Implementation

- Monitor full blood count before and during therapy.
- Provide comfort and implement safety measures: assistance, temperature control, lighting control and mouth care.
- Provide small, frequent meals and monitor nutritional status.
- Monitor for opportunistic infections and arrange treatment as indicated.
- Provide support and reassurance for dealing with drug effects and discomfort.
- Provide patient teaching regarding drug name, dosage, adverse effects, warnings, precautions, use of OTC or herbal remedies, and signs to report. Patient must understand how these drugs should be taken, for example, some nucleoside reverse transcriptase inhibitors should be taken on an empty stomach and with water.

Evaluation

- Evaluate drug effects: relief of signs and symptoms of AIDS and ARC; stabilization of T-cell levels.
- Monitor for adverse effects: GI alterations, dizziness, confusion, headache, fever.
- Monitor for drug-drug interactions as indicated for each drug.
- Evaluate effectiveness of patient teaching plan.
- Evaluate effectiveness of comfort and safety measures.

Patient Teaching for Harry

A combination of antiretroviral drugs has been prescribed to treat your HIV infection. These drugs work in combination to stop the replication of HIV, to control AIDS, and to maintain the functioning of your immune system. A schedule will be plotted out to show exactly when to take each of the drugs. It is very important that you take all of the drugs and that you stick to this schedule to ensure that the drugs can be effective and won't encourage the development of resistant strains of the virus.

These drugs are not a cure for HIV, AIDS or AIDS-related complex (ARC). Opportunistic infections may occur, and regular medical follow-ups should be sought to deal with the disease.

These drugs do not reduce the risk of transmission of HIV to others by sexual contact or by blood contamination; use appropriate precautions.

Common effects of these drugs include the following:

- ☐ *Dizziness, weakness and loss of feeling*: change positions slowly. If you feel drowsy, avoid driving and dangerous activities.
- ☐ *Headache, fever, muscle aches*: analgesics may be ordered to alleviate this discomfort. Consult your health care provider.

Antiviral Agents for HIV and AIDS *(continued)*

- ☐ *Nausea, loss of appetite, change in taste*: small, frequent meals may help. It is important to try to maintain a balanced diet. Consult your health care provider if this becomes a severe problem.
- ☐ Seek early medical advice if you feel unwell. Report any of the following to your health care provider: fever, cough, excessive fatigue, lethargy, severe headache, difficulty in breathing or skin rash.
- ☐ Avoid over-the-counter medications and herbal therapies; many of them interact with your drugs and may make them ineffective. If you feel that you need one of these, check with your health care provider first.
- ☐ Schedule regular medical evaluations, including blood tests, which are needed to monitor the effects of these drugs on your body and to adjust dosages as needed.
- ☐ Tell any doctor, nurse or other health care provider of your condition and that you are taking these drugs.
- ☐ Keep these drugs and all medications out of the reach of children. Do not share these drugs with other people.

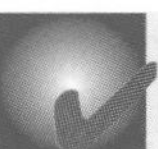

CHECK YOUR UNDERSTANDING

Answers to the questions in this chapter may be found in the answer key in the back of the book.

Multiple Choice

Select the most appropriate answer to the following.

1. Viruses are known to cause
   a. tuberculosis.
   b. leprosy.
   c. the common cold.
   d. gonorrhoea.

2. Herpesviruses cause a broad range of conditions but have not been identified as the causative agent in
   a. cold sores.
   b. shingles.
   c. genital infections.
   d. leprosy.

3. An important teaching point for the patient receiving an agent to treat herpesvirus or CMV would be the following:
   a. stop taking the drug as soon as the lesions have disappeared.
   b. sexual intercourse is fine – as long as you are taking the drug, you are not contagious.
   c. drink plenty of fluids to decrease the drug's toxic effects on the kidneys.
   d. there are no associated GI adverse effects.

4. HIV (human immunodeficiency virus) attacks
   a. antibodies.
   b. helper T cells.
   c. suppressor T cells.
   d. cytotoxic T cells.

5. Nursing interventions for the patient receiving antiretroviral drugs for the treatment of HIV probably would include
   a. monitoring renal and hepatic function periodically during therapy.
   b. administering the drugs just once a day to increase drug effectiveness.
   c. encouraging the patient to avoid eating if GI upset is severe.
   d. stopping the drugs and notifying the prescriber if severe rash occurs.

6. Locally active antiviral agents can be used to treat
   a. HIV infection.
   b. herpes simplex, keratitis and warts.
   c. RSV.
   d. CMV systemic infections.

Extended Matching Questions

Select **all** that apply.

1. When explaining to a patient the reasoning behind using combination therapy in the treatment of HIV, the nurse would include which of the following points?
   a. The virus can remain dormant within the T cell for a very long time; they can mutate whilst in the T cell.
   b. Adverse effects of many of the drugs used to treat this virus include immune depression, so the disease could become worse.

c. The drugs are cheaper if used in combination.
d. The virus slowly mutates with each generation.
e. Attacking the virus at many points in its life cycle has been shown to be most effective.
f. Research has shown that using only one type of drug that targeted only one point in the virus life cycle led to more mutations and more difficulty in controlling the disease.

2. Appropriate nursing diagnoses related to the drug therapy for a patient receiving combination antiviral therapy for the treatment of HIV infection would include
   a. Disturbed sensory perception (kinaesthetic) related to the CNS effects of the drugs.
   b. Imbalanced nutrition: more than body requirements related to appetite stimulation.
   c. Congestive heart failure related to cardiac effects of the drugs.
   d. Adrenal insufficiency related to endocrine effects of the drugs.
   e. Acute pain related to GI, CNS or dermatologic effects of the drugs.
   f. Deficient knowledge regarding drug therapy.

Fill in the Blanks

1. A *Diskhaler* is used to deliver_____________ to treat uncomplicated influenza A infections in adults and children.

2. Children with respiratory syncytial virus (RSV) often respond very well to treatment with_____________.

3. _____________ is available only in intravenous (IV) form and is very toxic to the renal system. It is effective in treating CMV retinitis and herpes simplex infections in immunocompromised patients.

4. Herpes zoster and recurrent genital herpes are often treated with the oral agents _____________.

5. A very commonly used drug for the treatment of herpes infections is _____________.

6. One of the first drugs approved for treating HIV infections that is still used frequently in combination therapy is _____________, also known as AZT.

7. A topical drug that is applied locally for the treatment of cold sores is_____________.

Bibliography and References

British HIV Association. (2008). *Treatment of HIV-1 infected adults with antiretroviral therapy 2008.* Available from http://www.bhiva.org

British Medical Association and Royal Pharmaceutical Society of Great Britain. (2008). *British National Formulary*. London: BMJ & RPS Publishing. *This publication is updated biannually: it is imperative that the most recent edition is consulted.*

British Medical Association and Royal Pharmaceutical Society of Great Britain. (2008). *British National Formulary for Children*. London: BMJ & RPS Publishing. *This publication is updated annually: it is imperative that the most recent edition is consulted.*

Brunton, L., Lazo, J. S., Parker, K., Goodman, L. S., & Gilman, A. G. (2005). *Goodman and Gilman's the pharmacological basis of therapeutics* (11th ed.). London: McGraw-Hill.

Chippindale, S., & French, L. (2001). ABC of AIDS: HIV counselling and the psychosocial management of patients with HIV or AIDS. *British Medical Journal, 322*, 1533–1535.

Howland, R. D., & Mycek, M. J. (2005). *Pharmacology* (3rd ed.). Philadelphia: Lippincott Williams & Wilkins.

Health Protection Agency. (2008). *HIV in the United Kingdom. 2008 Report*. Available from http://www.hpa.org.uk

NICE. (2006). *Hepatitis B (chronic) – adefovir dipivoxil and pegylated interferon alpha-2a*. Available from http://www.nice.org.uk

NICE. (2008). *Oseltamivir, amantadine (review) and zanamivir for the prophylaxis of influenza*. Available from http://www.nice.org.uk

John-Stewart, G., Mbori-Ngacha, D., Ekpini, R., Janoff, E. N., Nkengasong, J., Read, J. S., et al. (2004). Breast-feeding and Transmission of HIV-1. *Journal of Acquired Immune Deficiency Syndrome, 35*(2), 196–202.

Porth, C. M., & Matfin, G. (2008). *Pathophysiology: Concepts of altered health states* (8th ed.). Philadelphia: Lippincott Williams & Wilkins.

Rang, H. P., Dale, M. M., Ritter, J. M., & Flower, R. J. (2007). *Rang and Dale's pharmacology* (6th ed.). Philadelphia: Churchill Livingstone.

Simonsen, T., Aarbakke, J., Kay, I., Coleman, I., Sinnott, P., & Lysaa, R. (2006). *Illustrated pharmacology for nurses.* London: Hodder Arnold

The Antiretroviral Therapy Cohort Collaboration. (2006). HIV treatment response and prognosis in Europe and North America in the first decade of highly active antiretroviral therapy: A collaborative analysis. *Lancet, 368*, 451–458.

UK Chief Medical Officers' Expert Advisory Group on AIDS. (2004). *HIV post-exposure prophylaxis*. Available from http://www.dh.gov.uk

Weller, I. V. D., & Williams, I. G. (2001). ABC of AIDS: Treatment of infection. *British Medical Journal, 322*(7298), 1350–1354

Weller, I. V. D., & Williams, I. G. (2001). ABC of AIDS: Antiretroviral drugs. *British Medical Journal, 322*(7299), 1410–1412.

CHAPTER
10

Antifungal Agents

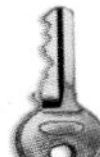

KEY TERMS

azoles
Candida
ergosterol
fungus
mycosis
tinea
yeast

LEARNING OBJECTIVES

Upon completion of this chapter, you will be able to:

1. Describe the characteristics of fungi and fungal infections.
2. Describe the therapeutic actions, indications, pharmacokinetics, contraindications, most common adverse reactions and important drug–drug interactions associated with systemic and topical antifungals.
3. Compare and contrast the key drugs for systemic and topical antifungals with the other drugs in each class.
4. Discuss the impact of using antifungals across the lifespan.
5. Outline the nursing considerations for patients receiving a systemic or topical antifungal.

SYSTEMIC ANTIFUNGALS

amphotericin
caspofungin
fluconazole
flucytosine
griseofulvin
itraconazole
ketoconazole
nystatin
posaconazole
terbinafine
voriconazole

TOPICAL ANTIFUNGALS

amorolfine
benzoic acid
clotrimazole
econazole
griseofulvin
ketoconazole
miconazole
nystatin
salicylic acid
sulconazole
terbinafine
tioconazole
tolnaftate
undecyclenic acid

Fungal infections in humans range from conditions such as 'athlete's foot' to potentially fatal systemic infections. An infection caused by a **fungus** is called a **mycosis**. Fungi differ from bacteria in that fungi are eukaryotic, like human cells, but fungi have cell walls (like most bacteria). The components of the cell wall; however, differ from bacterial cell walls. Fungal cell walls are made up of chitin and various polysaccharides and a cell membrane that contains **ergosterol**, whereas bacterial cell walls contain peptidoglycan. You will remember that human cells do not have cell walls. The composition of the fungal cell wall means that many antibacterial agents are ineffective against fungal infections and conversely antifungal agents are ineffective in treating bacterial infections.

There are two main types of fungi, moulds and yeasts. Fungi are responsible for opportunistic infections. This means that fungi are generally not a problem for humans unless there is some change in conditions which allows them to cause infection, for example wet, damp feet are the ideal environment for athlete's foot (tinea pedis); taking antibacterials can cause changes in the normal flora of the mouth, vagina or gastrointestinal (GI) tract and fungal infections can take hold. When the body's defences are intact then it is unlikely that fungi will cause infection.

The incidence of fungal infections has increased with the rising number of immunocompromised individuals, for example patients with acquired immune deficiency syndrome (AIDS) and AIDS-related complex (ARC), those taking immunosuppressant drugs and those who have undergone transplantation surgery or cancer treatment (Box 10.1). For example, ***Candida***, a fungus that is normally found on mucous membranes in healthy individuals, can cause **yeast** infections or 'thrush' of the GI tract and vagina in people whose immune system is compromised in some way.

Systemic Antifungals

The drugs used to treat systemic fungal infections (Table 10.1) can be toxic to the host and are not used indiscriminately. It is important to get a culture of the fungus causing the infection to ensure that the right drug is selected so that the patient is not put at additional risk from the toxic adverse effects associated with these drugs.

Amphotericin is available in intravenous (IV) form and as lozenges to treat oral and perioral fungal infections. This drug is indicated for a number of advanced and progressive systemic fungal infections (see Table 10.1). This is a potent drug with a number of adverse effects including renal toxicity. Use is reserved for progressive, potentially fatal infections unresponsive to other antifungals such as fungal septicaemia due to *Candida* or other species. The metabolism of amphotericin is not fully understood but it is excreted in the urine, with an initial half-life of 24 hours and then a 15-day half-life. Amphotericin should be avoided during pregnancy unless the potential benefit to the mother outweighs the risk to the foetus. No information is available on risks to the neonate through breast-feeding.

BOX 10.1 DRUG THERAPY ACROSS THE LIFESPAN

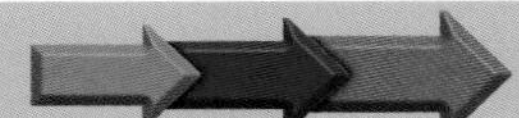

Antifungal Agents

CHILDREN

Children are very sensitive to the effects of most antifungal drugs and more severe reactions can be expected when these drugs are used in children. The systemic antifungals (excluding posaconazole) have established paediatric doses. Itraconazole is associated with liver damage and should not be used in children with liver dysfunction.

Topical agents should not be used over open wounds that would increase the risk of systemic absorption and toxicity. Occlusive dressings including tight nappies, should be avoided over the affected areas.

When administering any drug to children, always consult the most recent edition of the British National Formulary for Children.

ADULTS

These drugs can be very toxic to the body and their use should be reserved for situations in which the causative organism has been identified. Over-the-counter (OTC) topical preparations are widely used, and patients should be cautioned to follow the instructions and to report continued problems to their health care provider. Topical agents should not be used over open wounds that would increase the risk of systemic absorption.

Pregnant and lactating women should not use these drugs unless the benefit clearly outweighs the potential risk to the foetus or neonate. Women of childbearing age should be advised to use barrier contraceptives, both during treatment and for a period of time after treatment has ceased. A severe fungal infection may threaten the life of the mother and/or foetus; in these situations, the potential risk of treatment should be carefully explained.

OLDER ADULTS

Older patients may be more susceptible to the adverse effects associated with these drugs and should be monitored closely. Patients with hepatic dysfunction are at an increased risk of worsening hepatic problems and toxic effects of many of these drugs (caspofungin, fluconazole, griseofulvin, itraconazole, ketoconazole, terbinafine, voriconazole). If hepatic dysfunction is expected (age, alcohol abuse, use of other hepatotoxic drugs), the dosage may need to be lowered and the patient monitored more frequently.

Other agents are associated with renal toxicity (amphotericin, flucytosine, fluconazole, itraconazole, terbinafine, voriconazole) and should be used cautiously in patients with renal impairment. Patients at risk of renal toxicity should be monitored carefully via renal function tests.

Table 10.1 DRUGS IN FOCUS

Systemic Antifungals

Drug Name	Usual Indications
amphotericin	Treatment of aspergillosis, cryptococcal meningitis, disseminated cryptococcosis, blastomycosis, coccidioidomycosis, histoplasmosis, mucormycosis, and severe invasive *Candida*
caspofungin	Treatment of invasive aspergillosis in patients who are refractory or intolerant to other therapies, invasive candidiasis
fluconazole	Treatment of candidiasis, cryptococcal meningitis, other systemic fungal infections; prophylaxis for reducing the incidence of fungal infections in immunocompromised patients
flucytosine	Treatment of candidiasis, cryptococcosis
griseofulvin	Treatment of dermatophytoses where topical therapy has failed
itraconazole	Treatment of onchomycosis, cryptococcosis, histoplasmosis, and aspergillosis, candidiasis, pityriasis versicolor, tinea corporis, tinea cruris, tinea pedis, tinea manuum; and prophylaxis in patients undergoing bone marrow transplants
ketoconazole	Treatment of blastomycosis, coccidioidomycosis, histoplasmosis and paracoccidiodomycosis; skin, hair and mucosal mycoses that cannot be treated with other antifungals
nystatin	Treatment of candidiasis; vaginal, skin or oral infection
posaconazole	Treatment of invasive aspergillosis, fusariosis, chromoblastomycosis, mycetoma, coccidioidomycosis; oropharyngeal candidiasis; prophylaxis in patients undergoing bone marrow transplants or receiving chemotherapy
terbinafine	Treatment of onychomycosis of the fingernail or toenail and ringworm infections (tinea pedis, cruris and corporis)
voriconazole	Treatment of invasive aspergillosis; treatment of serious fungal infections caused by *Scedosporium apiospermum, Fusarium* species, or resistant *Candida* species

Caspofungin, available for IV use, is approved for the treatment of invasive aspergillosis and invasive candidiasis in patients who are unresponsive to other treatments. This drug can cause hepatic dysfunction; reduced doses must be used if a patient has moderate hepatic impairment. Caspofungin is slowly metabolized in the liver with half-lives of 9 to 11 hours and then 40 to 50 hours. It is bound to plasma proteins, widely distributed throughout the body and excreted via urine and faeces. Concurrent use of ciclosporin is contraindicated unless the benefit clearly outweighs the risk of hepatic injury. Caspofungin should be avoided during pregnancy and whilst breast-feeding unless essential.

Flucytosine, available in IV form and also as an oral form (on a named-patient basis only, i.e. the oral form isn't currently licensed; however, the drug can be prescribed if the clinician believes the patient has a specific need), is a less toxic drug used either alone or with amphotericin in the treatment of systemic infections caused by *Candida* or *Cryptococcus*. It is well absorbed from the GI tract, with peak levels occurring in 2 hours. Most of the drug is excreted unchanged in the urine, and a small amount in the faeces. As the drug is excreted primarily in the urine, extreme caution is needed in the presence of renal impairment because drug accumulation and toxicity can occur. There is potential for adverse reactions in the foetus or neonate and flucytosine should be used during pregnancy only if the benefits clearly outweigh the risks, and avoided during lactation.

Griseofulvin is used orally to treat mycotic infections of the skin, scalp and nails where topical antifungal treatment has proved ineffective. This drug concentrates in keratin precursor cells and prevents fungal growth in newly formed cells. Absorption of griseofulvin can be variable depending on particle size, leading to variation in plasma levels. Peak concentrations are reached in ~4 hours. Griseofulvin is metabolized by the liver and mainly excreted via urine. Pregnant women should avoid the drug and women planning to become pregnant should use effective contraceptive during and at least 1 month after treatment. Men should also avoid trying to father a child during and at least 6 months after treatment. No information is available on the risks to neonates through breast milk. Griseofulvin should be used with caution with driving as performance of skilled tasks may be impaired.

Nystatin is used orally for the treatment of intestinal candidiasis. In addition, it is available in a number of topical preparations – oral suspension, cream and ointment – for the treatment of oral candidiasis, vaginal candidiasis and cutaneous infections caused by *Candida* species. It is not absorbed from the GI tract and passes unchanged in faeces. It is not known whether nystatin crosses the placenta or enters breast milk, so it should not be used during pregnancy or lactation unless the benefits clearly outweigh the potential risks.

The 'Azoles'

The **azoles** are newer drugs used to treat systemic fungal infections. Although they are less toxic than amphotericin, they may be less effective in very severe and progressive infections. The azoles inhibit the cytochrome P450 3A enzyme which converts lanosterol to ergosterol, a key sterol in the cell membrane of fungi. This inhibits fungal cell division.

Ketoconazole is used orally to treat many of the same mycoses as amphotericin; and also topically in shampoo to reduce the scaling associated with dandruff and as a cream to treat topical mycoses. Ketoconazole is absorbed rapidly from the GI tract, with peak levels occurring within 1 to 3 hours. It is extensively metabolized in the liver and excreted via faeces and urine. Ketoconazole strongly inhibits the cytochrome P450 enzyme system in the liver and is associated with the inhibition of steroid biosynthesis, including testosterone and cortisol. Therefore ketoconazole is not suitable for patients with adrenocortical insufficiency. Inhibition of liver enzyme systems also leads to many drug–drug interactions. Ketoconazole has been associated with severe hepatic toxicity and should only be used when the potential benefits to the patient outweigh the risk of hepatic damage. Ketoconazole has teratogenic effects in animal studies and can enter breast milk and is not recommended for use in pregnancy or breast-feeding.

Fluconazole is available in oral and IV preparations. Seriously ill patients can be treated with the IV form and switched to the oral form as their condition improves. Fluconazole is not associated with the endocrine problems observed with ketoconazole and is used to treat candidiasis and other systemic fungal infections. As fluconazole can reach high concentrations in cerebrospinal fluid it is effective in treating cryptococcal meningitis. This drug has also been used successfully as a prophylactic agent for reducing the incidence of fungal infections in bone marrow transplant recipients and immunocompromised patients. Peak levels after oral administration occur within 1 to 2 hours. Most of the drug is excreted unchanged in the urine, making use with renal dysfunction difficult. Fluconazole also strongly inhibits some of the liver cytochrome P450 enzymes and may be associated with drug–drug interactions. This drug should be avoided during pregnancy but can be used with caution whilst breast-feeding.

Itraconazole is an oral agent used for the treatment of assorted systemic mycoses. This drug, which has been associated with hepatic failure, should not be used in patients with hepatic failure and should be used with caution in those with hepatic impairment. There are also some reports of cardiac failure in patients with cardiac disease. Itraconazole is slowly absorbed from the GI tract and absorption is reduced in patients with AIDS or neutropaenia (a low number of neutrophils). Itraconazole is extensively metabolized in the liver by cytochrome P450 enzymes and excreted in the urine and faeces. In pregnancy, itraconazole should only be used in life-threatening situations. Nonpregnant females are advised to use effective contraception during treatment and until the next menstrual period following treatment. Breast-feeding mothers should also avoid using itraconazole.

Posaconazole is a triazole antifungal and inhibits ergosterol synthesis in cell membranes of sensitive fungi. Taken orally, posaconazole is absorbed slowly and only a small amount is metabolized. The majority of the dose is eliminated unchanged via the faeces. Posaconazole should not be used during pregnancy unless the potential benefit outweighs the risk to the foetus. The manufacturers recommend the use of barrier contraceptives during treatment. Breast-feeding mothers should avoid using this drug.

Voriconazole is available in oral and IV forms, making it useful for starting in a serious infection and switching to an oral form when the patient is able to take oral medications. Voriconazole should not be used by patients with a history of long QT syndrome or with any other drugs that prolong the QT interval. Concomitant use with ergot alkaloids can cause ergotism, including diarrhoea, vomiting and CNS effects (including hallucinations). Voriconazole should be avoided during pregnancy unless the potential benefits outweigh the risks. Nonpregnant females are advised to use effective contraception during treatment. Voriconazole should be avoided whilst breast-feeding.

Terbinafine is a similar drug that blocks the formation of ergosterol. Terbinafine is available as an oral drug for the treatment of onychomycosis of the toenails or fingernails. It is rapidly absorbed from the GI tract and accumulates in skin, nails, hair and adipose tissue. Terbinafine is extensively metabolized in the liver and mainly excreted in the urine. This drug should be avoided during pregnancy (unless the potential benefits outweigh the risks) and breast-feeding.

Therapeutic Actions and Indications

The systemic antifungal drugs listed above work by either (1) impairing ergosterol synthesis in the fungal cell membrane and therefore inhibiting cell division (Figure 10.1); (2) increasing cellular permeability; (3) inhibition of DNA synthesis; or (4) disruption of the mitotic spindle structure and therefore cell division.

Contraindications and Cautions

Caution should be used when systemic antifungal agents are administered to anyone with a known allergy; during pregnancy and lactation; or to patients with renal or liver disease, *which could either alter drug metabolism and excretion or worsen as a result of the actions of the drug.* Patients taking either high doses or an extended course of fluconazole, itraconazole or ketoconazole should have their liver function monitored and treatment should be discontinued if signs of hepatic disease become apparent. Itraconazole and posaconazole should be used with caution by patients with a history of cardiac problems, including arrhythmias and long QT interval.

Adverse Effects

Adverse effects frequently encountered with the use of systemic antifungal agents include CNS effects, such as headache, dizziness, fever, shaking, chills and malaise. GI effects include nausea, vomiting, dyspepsia and anorexia.

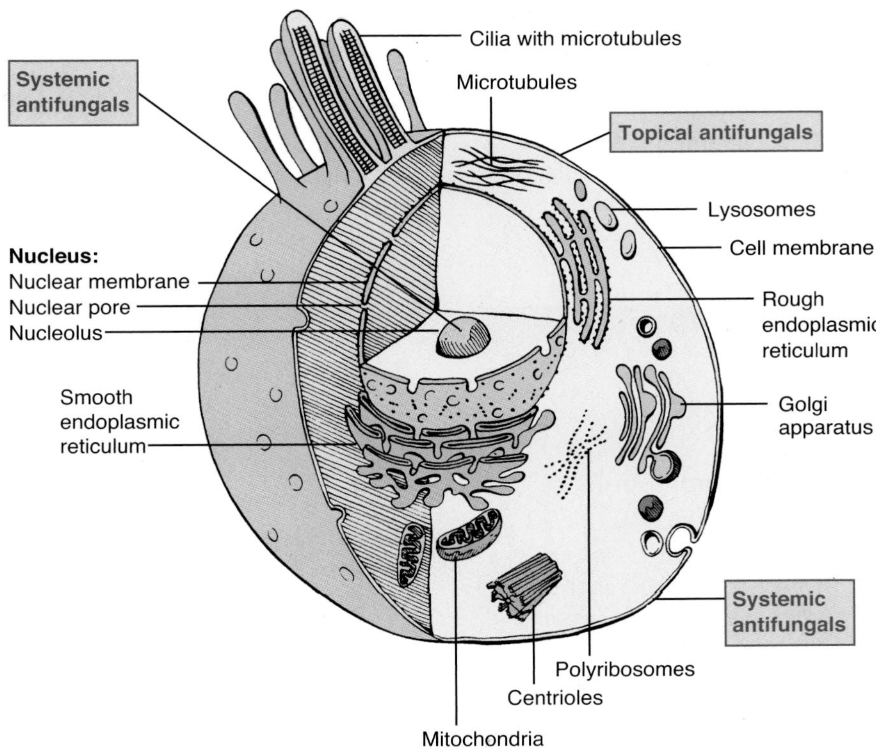

FIGURE 10.1 Sites of action of antifungal agents.

Hepatic dysfunction, which is seen more often with ketoconazole and itraconazole, is associated with the toxic effects of the drug on the liver. Dermatological effects, such as rash and pruritus associated with local irritation, may occur. Renal dysfunction, which is more often seen with amphotericin, is probably related to the drug effects on cell membranes. Several of the azole drugs can also cause Stevens-Johnson syndrome, a serious condition involving blistering of the skin, eyes, mouth and genitalia and fever.

Clinically Important Drug–Drug Interactions

Patients who receive amphotericin should not take other nephrotoxic drugs, ciclosporin, antibacterials or corticosteroids unless absolutely necessary *because of the increased risk of severe renal toxicity.*

The azole family of antifungal drugs can cause increased serum levels of a range of drugs including: antidepressants, antiepileptics, antipsychotics, anxiolytics and hypnotics, calcium channel blockers, ergot alkaloids, ciclosporin, oral hypoglycaemics and oral anticoagulants. Toxicity may occur *because the azoles inhibit the CYP450 liver enzyme system needed for metabolism of these drugs.* If these combinations cannot be avoided, patients should be closely monitored and dosage adjustments made.

The azoles have also been associated with potentially severe cardiovascular events when taken with antiarrhythmics, lipid-lowering drugs and antipsychotics, and use of these drugs in combination with azoles should be avoided.

Always consult a current copy of the British National Formulary for further guidance.

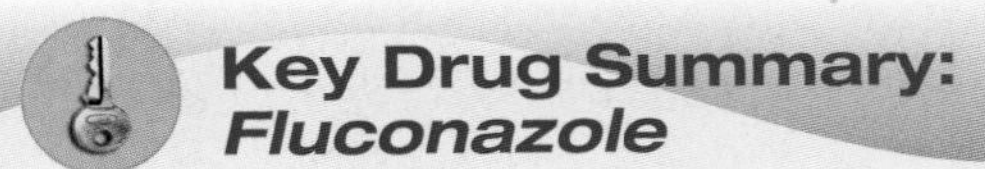

Key Drug Summary: *Fluconazole*

Indications: Treatment of oropharyngeal, oesophageal and vaginal candidiasis; cryptococcal meningitis; systemic fungal infections; prophylaxis to decrease incidence of candidiasis in bone marrow transplants

Actions: Binds to sterols in the fungal cell membrane, changing membrane permeability; fungicidal or fungistatic depending on concentration of drug and organism

Pharmacokinetics:

Route	Onset	Peak	Duration
Oral	Slow	1–2 h	2–4 d
IV	Rapid	1 h	2–4 d

$T_{1/2}$: 30 hours; metabolized in the liver and excreted in the urine

Adverse effects: Headache, nausea, vomiting, diarrhoea, abdominal pain, flatulence, rash. Rare adverse effects include hypersensitivity reactions, anaphylaxis and Stevens-Johnson syndrome

Nursing Considerations for Patients Receiving Systemic Antifungals

Assessment: History and Examination

Screen for the following, *which are cautions or contraindications for the use of these drugs:* history of allergy to antifungals; history of liver or renal dysfunction *that might interfere with metabolism and excretion of the drug;* and pregnancy or lactation. Establish if patient is currently taking other medications or herbal therapies which may potentially interact with the antifungal drug.

Physical assessment should be performed *to establish baseline data for assessing the effectiveness of the drug and the occurrence of any adverse effects associated with drug therapy.* Perform a scraping of the infected area *to make an accurate determination of the type and responsiveness of the fungus.* Examine the skin for colour and lesions *to check for dermatological effects of the drug.* Evaluate renal and hepatic function *to determine baseline function of these organs, to assess possible toxicity during drug therapy.*

Nursing Diagnoses

The patient receiving a systemic antifungal drug may have the following nursing diagnoses related to drug therapy:

- Acute pain related to GI, CNS and local effects of drug
- GI disturbances due to drug administration
- Deficient knowledge regarding drug therapy

Implementation With Rationale

- Arrange for appropriate culture and sensitivity tests before beginning therapy *to ensure that the appropriate drug is being used.* With serious systemic infections, treatment may begin before test results are known.
- Administer the entire course of the drug *to get the full beneficial effects;* this may take as long as 6 months for some chronic infections.
- Amphotericin and caspofungin can cause pain and thrombophlebitis at IV injection sites. Treat appropriately and restart IV at another site if phlebitis occurs. Anaphylaxis may occur with an IV infusion of amphotericin. A test dose of amphotericin should be given prior to infusion and the patient observed for at least 30 minutes after the test dose (BNF, 2008).
- Monitor renal and hepatic function before and periodically during treatment *and arrange to stop drug if signs of organ failure occur.*
- Provide comfort and safety provisions if CNS effects occur; for example assistance with mobility for dizziness and weakness, analgesics for headache, antipyretics for fever and chills, temperature regulation for fever.
- Provide small, frequent, nutritious meals if GI upset is severe. Monitor nutritional status and arrange a dietary consultation as needed *to ensure nutritional status.* GI upset may be decreased by taking an oral drug with food.
- Provide patient instruction *to enhance patient knowledge about drug therapy and to promote concordance.*

The patient should:

- Follow the appropriate dosage regimen.
- Take safety precautions, including changing position slowly and avoiding driving and hazardous tasks (with griseofulvin), if CNS effects occur.
- Report to a health care provider any of the following: sore throat, unusual bruising and bleeding which could indicate blood dyscrasias; and anorexia, nausea, vomiting, fatigue, abdominal pain or dark urine which could indicate hepatic toxicity. Severe local irritation associated with local application of an antifungal could indicate a sensitivity reaction and worsening of the infection.

Evaluation

- Monitor patient response to the drug (resolution of fungal infection).
- Monitor for adverse effects (orientation, nutritional state, skin colour and lesions, renal and hepatic function).
- Evaluate the effectiveness of the teaching plan (patient can name the drug, dosage, possible adverse effects to watch for, and specific measures to help avoid adverse effects).
- Monitor the effectiveness of comfort and safety measures and compliance with the regimen (see Critical Thinking Scenario 10-1).

Topical Antifungals

Some antifungal drugs are available only in topical forms and treat a variety of mycoses of the skin and mucous membranes. Fungi that cause these infections are called *dermatophytes*. These diseases include a variety of **tinea** infections, often referred to as ringworm, although the causal organism is a fungus, not a worm. Types of tinea include the body (tinea corporis), athlete's foot (tinea pedis), groin (tinea cruris), scalp (tinea capitis), nail (tinea unguiumm). Other infections include yeast infections of the mouth and vagina, often caused by *Candida*. Some of the antifungal drugs listed as systemic antifungals can also be used topically (see Table 10.2).

Therapeutic Actions and Indications

Topical antifungal drugs alter the cell permeability of the fungus, preventing replication and fungal death (see Figure 10.1). They are indicated only for local treatment of mycoses, including tinea infections. They are not indicated for use near open lesions or wounds because of the increased risk of systemic absorption.

Contraindications and Cautions

These drugs are not usually absorbed systemically; therefore contraindications are limited to known allergy to any of these drugs.

Adverse Effects

When these drugs are applied locally as a cream, lotion, or spray, local effects include irritation, burning, erythema and itching. Adverse effects include nausea, vomiting and diarrhoea when these drugs are taken in lozenge form.

Clinically Important Drug–Drug Interactions

There are no reported drug–drug interactions because these drugs are not generally absorbed systemically.

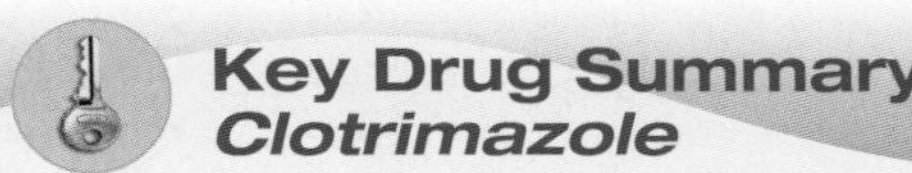

Key Drug Summary: *Clotrimazole*

Indications: Treatment of vaginal candidiasis, tinea pedia, tinea cruris and tinea corporis

Actions: Binds to sterols in the fungal cell wall, and changes the membrane permeability causing intracellular components to leak out of the cell, causing cell death

Pharmacokinetics: Not absorbed systemically; pharmacokinetics are unknown

Adverse effects: Mild burning, redness, urticaria, burning

Table 10.2 DRUGS IN FOCUS

Topical Antifungals

Drug Name	Usual Indications
amorolfine	Treatment of skin and nail infections
benzoic acid	Treatment of tinea infections
clotrimazole	Available OTC for treatment of vaginal *Candida* infections; tinea infections
econazole	Treatment of tinea and vaginal *Candida* infections
griseofulvin	Treatment of tinea pedis; resistant fungal infections
ketoconazole	Treatment of fungal skin infections, systemic or resistant fungal infections, vulval candidiasis
miconazole	Treatment of fungal skin infections, oral and intestinal fungal infections, vaginal candidiasis
nystatin	Treatment of skin infections due to *Candida* species, intestinal and vaginal candidiasis, oral fungal infections
salicyclic acid	Treatment of fungal nail infections, hyperkeratotic skin disorders, acne vulgaris
sulconazole	Treatment of fungal skin infections
terbinafine	Treatment of fungal skin infections
tioconazole	Treatment of tinea unguium
tolnaftate	Available OTC for treatment of tinea pedis
undecyclenic acid	Treatment and prevention of tinea pedis

Dosage/Route for all antifungals: apply topically to affected area once or twice a day.

Nursing Considerations for Patients Receiving Topical Antifungals

Assessment: History and Examination

Patients receiving a topical antifungal agent should be assessed for known allergies to any topical antifungal agent. Physical assessment should be performed *to establish baseline data for assessment of the effectiveness of the drug and the occurrence of any adverse effects associated with drug therapy.* Perform a skin scraping of the affected area *to determine the causative fungus and appropriate medication.* Conduct local evaluation (e.g. colour, temperature, lesions) *to monitor the effectiveness of the drug and to monitor for local adverse effects of the drug.*

Nursing Diagnoses

The patient receiving a topical antifungal drug may have the following nursing diagnoses related to drug therapy:

- Acute pain related to local effects of drug
- Deficient knowledge regarding drug therapy

Implementation With Rationale

- Culture the affected area before beginning therapy *to identify the causative fungus.*
- Ensure that the patient takes the complete course of the drug regimen *to achieve maximum results.*
- Ensure that the patient is using the correct method of administration depending on the route *to improve effectiveness and decrease risk of adverse effects.*
- Vaginal suppositories should be inserted high into the vagina with the patient remaining recumbent for at least 10 to 15 minutes after insertion.
- Topical creams and lotions should be rubbed into the affected area after it has been cleansed with soap and water.
- Stop the drug if a severe rash occurs, especially if it is accompanied by blisters or if local irritation and pain are very severe. *This development may indicate sensitivity to the drug or worsening of the condition being treated.*
- Provide patient instruction *to enhance patient knowledge about drug therapy and to promote concordance.*

The patient should:

- Know the correct method of drug administration.
- Know the length of time necessary to treat the infection adequately.
- Use clean, dry socks when treating athlete's foot, to help eradicate the infection and keep feet clean and dry. Shoes should be worn in communal shower and bathing areas.
- Avoid occlusive dressings because of the risk of increasing systemic absorption. Drugs should not be placed near open wounds or active lesions because these agents are not intended to be absorbed systemically.
- Report severe local irritation, burning or worsening of the infection to a health care provider.

Evaluation

- Monitor patient response to the drug (alleviation of signs and symptoms of the fungal infection).
- Monitor for adverse effects: rash, local irritation and burning.
- Evaluate the effectiveness of the teaching plan (patient can name the drug, dosage, possible adverse effects to watch for, and specific measures to help avoid adverse effects).
- Monitor the effectiveness of comfort and safety measures and compliance with the regimen.

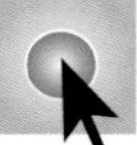

WEB LINKS

Health care providers and patients may want to consult the following Internet sources:

http://bnfc.org The BNF for Children provides UK health care professionals with authoritative and practical information on the selection and clinical use of medicines in children.

http://cks.library.nhs.uk The National Health Service Clinical Knowledge Summaries provides evidence-based practical information on the common conditions observed in primary care.

http://www.bnf.org.uk The BNF provides UK health care professionals with authoritative and practical information on the selection and clinical use of medicines.

http://www.nhsdirect.nhs.uk The National Health Service Direct service provides patients with information and advice about health, illness and health services.

Points to Remember

- A fungus is a eukaryotic organism with a rigid cell wall that contains chitin and polysaccharides and a cell membrane containing ergosterols. Fungi can be single or multicelled.

- Any infection with a fungus is called a mycosis. Systemic fungal infections, which can be life-threatening, are increasing with the rise in the number of immunocompromised patients.
- Systemic antifungals can prevent cell growth, increase cell permeability or prevent replication.
- Some systemic antifungals can be very toxic and patients should be monitored closely while receiving them. Adverse effects may include hepatic and renal failure, Stevens-Johnson syndrome and blood dyscrasias.
- Local fungal infections include vaginal and oral yeast infections (*Candida*) and a variety of tinea infections, including athlete's foot.
- Tinea, a fungal infection, is also known as ringworm.
- Proper administration of topical antifungals improves their effectiveness. They should not be used on or near open wounds or lesions to avoid systemic absorption.
- Topical antifungals can cause serious local irritation, burning and pain. The drug should be stopped if these conditions persist.

CRITICAL THINKING SCENARIO 10-1

Poor Nutrition and Opportunistic Infections

The Situation

Paula, a 19-year-old woman and aspiring model, complains of abdominal pain, difficulty in swallowing, and a very sore throat. The strict diets she has followed for long periods have sometimes amounted to a starvation regime. In the past 18 months, she has received treatment for a variety of bacterial infections (e.g. pneumonia, cystitis) with a series of antibacterials.

Paula appears to be a very thin, extremely pale young woman who looks older than her stated age. Her mouth is moist, and small, white colonies that extend down the pharynx cover the mucosa. A vaginal examination reveals similar colonies. Cultures are performed, and it is determined that she has mucocutaneous candidiasis. Ketoconazole is prescribed and Paula is asked to return in 10 days for follow-up.

Critical Thinking

- What are the effects of taking a variety of antibacterials on the normal flora? Think about the possible cause of the mycosis.
- What happens to the immune system and to the skin and mucous membranes when a person's nutritional status becomes insufficient?
- How does Paula's chosen profession affect her health?
- What are the important nursing implications for Paula?
- Think about how the nurse can work with Paula to ensure some concordance with therapy and a return to a healthy state.

Discussion

Paula's appearance should prompt a complete physical examination before drug therapy is initiated. It is necessary to make baseline observations to evaluate any underlying problems that may exist. Poor nutrition and total starvation result in characteristic deficiencies that predispose individuals to opportunistic infections and prevent their bodies from protecting themselves adequately through inflammatory and immune responses. In this case, the fact that liver changes often occur with poor nutrition is particularly important; such hepatic dysfunction may cause deficient drug metabolism and lead to toxicity. The use of antibacterials has predisposed Paula to opportunistic infections.

An intensive programme of teaching and support should be started for Paula. She needs help accepting her diagnosis and adapting to the drug therapy and nutritional changes that are necessary for the effective treatment of this infection. She should understand the possible causes of her infection (poor nutrition and the loss of normal flora secondary to antibacterial therapy); the specifics of her drug therapy, including timing and administration; and adverse effects and warning signs that should be reported. Paula should be monitored closely for adverse effects and should return for follow-up.

The actual resolution of the fungal infection may occur only after a combination of prolonged drug and nutritional therapy. The required therapy will significantly affect Paula's lifestyle and she will need a great deal of support and encouragement to make the necessary changes and to maintain concordance. A health care provider, such as a nurse whom Paula trusts and with

(continued)

Poor Nutrition and Opportunistic Infections *(continued)*

whom she can regularly discuss her concerns, may be an essential element in helping eradicate the fungal infection. Nutritional counselling or referral to a dietician for thorough nutritional teaching together with referral to a counsellor who specialises in eating disorders may prove beneficial.

Nursing Care Guide for Paula: Antifungal Agents

Assessment: History and Examination

Assess history of allergy to any antifungal drug. Also check history of renal or hepatic dysfunction and pregnancy or breast-feeding status.

Focus the physical examination on the following:

- Local: culture of infected site
- Skin: colour, lesions, texture
- Genitourinary: urinary output
- GI: abdominal, liver evaluation
- Haematological: renal and hepatic function tests

Nursing Diagnoses

- Acute pain related to GI and CNS effects
- Disturbed sensory perception (kinaesthetic) related to CNS effects
- Imbalanced nutrition: less than body requirements related to GI effects and excessive dieting
- Altered body image related to food issues
- Deficient knowledge regarding drug therapy

Implementation

- Culture infection before beginning therapy.
- Provide comfort and implement safety measures. Ensure temperature control, lighting control, mouth care and skin care.
- Provide small, frequent meals and monitor nutritional status.
- Provide support and reassurance for dealing with drug effects and discomfort.
- Provide patient teaching regarding drug name, dosage, adverse effects, precautions and warning signs to report.
- Referral to a dietician and counsellor.

Evaluation

- Evaluate drug effects: relief of signs and symptoms of fungal infection.
- Monitor for adverse effects: GI alterations, pruritis, drowsiness, rash, dizziness, headache, hepatic dysfunction, menstrual disorders. If Paula continues ketoconazole treatment for longer than 10 days her liver function should be monitored before and during treatment.
- Monitor for drug–drug interactions as indicated for each drug.
- Evaluate effectiveness of patient teaching programme and of comfort and safety measures.

Patient Teaching for Paula

- ☐ Ketoconazole is an antifungal drug that works to destroy the fungi that have invaded the body.
- ☐ It is very important to take all of the prescribed medication.
- ☐ Common adverse effects of this drug include:
  - *Headache and weakness* – change positions slowly. An analgesic may be ordered to help alleviate the headache. If you feel drowsy, avoid driving or dangerous activities.
  - *Stomach upset, nausea and vomiting* – small, frequent meals may help. Take the drug with food if appropriate, because this may decrease the GI upset associated with these drugs. Try to maintain adequate nutrition.
- ☐ Report any of the following to your health care provider: severe vomiting, abdominal pain, fever or chills, yellowing of the skin or eyes, dark urine or pale stools, or skin rash.
- ☐ Avoid over-the-counter medications. If you require one of these, check with a health care provider first.
- ☐ Take the full course of your prescription. Never use this drug to self-treat any other infection, and never give this drug to any other person.
- ☐ Tell any doctor, nurse, or other health care provider involved in your care that you are taking this drug.
- ☐ Keep this drug and all medications out of the reach of children.

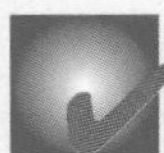

CHECK YOUR UNDERSTANDING

Answers to the questions in this chapter may be found in the answer key in the back of the book.

Multiple Choice

Select the most appropriate answer to the following.

1. A fungus is resistant to antibacterials because
   a. fungal cell walls contain folic acid and vitamin B.
   b. fungal cell walls contain chitin and ergosterol.
   c. fungi does not reproduce by cell division.
   d. antibacterials affect only bacterial cell walls.

2. Amphotericin is associated with potentially serious nephrotoxicity and should not be given concurrently to a patient who is also taking
   a. digoxin.
   b. oral anticoagulants.
   c. phenytoin.
   d. corticosteroids.

3. Fungi that cause infections of the skin and mucous membranes are called
   a. mycoses.
   b. meningeal fungi.
   c. dermatophytes.
   d. worms.

4. A woman with repeated vaginal yeast infections may be advised to obtain
   a. tolnaftate.
   b. amphotericin.
   c. clotrimazole.
   d. salicyclic acid.

5. Care must be taken when using topical antifungal agents to prevent systemic absorption because
   a. the fungus is only on the surface.
   b. these drugs can be toxic when given systemically.
   c. absorption would prevent drug effectiveness.
   d. these drugs can cause serious local burning and pain.

6. A patient with a severe case of athlete's foot is seen with lesions between the toes, which are oozing blood and serum. The patient would be noted to have a good understanding of teaching information if he reported:
   a. 'I must be careful not to change my socks very often because it could pull more skin off of my feet.'
   b. 'I need to apply a thick layer of the antifungal cream between my toes, making sure that all of the lesions are full of cream.'
   c. 'I should keep my feet clean and dry. I should not use the antifungal cream in areas where I have open lesions.'
   d. 'After I apply the cream to my feet, I should cover my feet in plastic wrap for several hours to make sure the drug is absorbed.'

Extended Matching Questions

Select **all** that apply.

1. When administering an antifungal, the nurse would consider which of the following interventions to be appropriate?
   a. Ensuring that a culture of the affected area had been done
   b. Having the patient swallow the lozenge used for oral *Candida* infections
   c. Ensuring that the patient stays flat for at least 1 hour if receiving a vaginal suppository
   d. Monitoring the IV site to prevent phlebitis
   e. Keeping the patient nil-by-mouth if GI upset occurs to prevent vomiting
   f. Providing antipyretics if fever occurs with IV antifungals

2. Teaching a patient who is receiving an oral antifungal drug should include which of the following points?
   a. It is important that you complete the full course of your drug therapy.
   b. You can share this drug with other members of your family if they develop the same symptoms.
   c. If you feel drowsy or dizzy, you should avoid driving or operating dangerous machinery.
   d. If GI upset occurs, try to avoid eating and drinking as much as possible, to ensure that you do not vomit the drug and lose its effectiveness.
   e. You should use over-the-counter drugs to counteract any adverse effects you experience—headache, fever or rash.
   f. Notify your health care provider if you experience yellowing of the skin or eyes, dark urine or light-coloured stools, or fever and chills.

Fill in the Blanks

1. A fungus is a cellular organism with a __________ cell wall that contains chitin and polysaccharides and a cell membrane that contains __________.

2. Any infection with a fungus is called a (n) __________.

3. Systemic antifungals can be very toxic; adverse effects may include__________ and __________ failure.

4. Vaginal and oral yeast infections are often caused by __________ .

5. Athlete's foot is an example of __________ infections.

6. Topical antifungals can be toxic and should not be absorbed __________

7. Topical antifungals should not be used near __________or lesions, which could increase absorption.

8. Topical antifungals can cause serious local __________, __________ and __________.

Bibliography and References

British Medical Association and Royal Pharmaceutical Society of Great Britain (2008). *British National Formulary*. London: BMJ & RPS Publishing. *This publication is updated biannually: it is imperative that the most recent edition is consulted.*

British Medical Association and Royal Pharmaceutical Society of Great Britain (2008). *British National Formulary for Children*. London: BMJ & RPS Publishing. *This publication is updated annually: it is imperative that the most recent edition is consulted.*

Brunton, L., Lazo, J. S., Parker, K., Goodman, L. S., & Gilman, A. G. (2005). *Goodman and Gilman's The Pharmacological Basis of Therapeutics* (11th ed.). London: McGraw-Hill.

Howland, R. D., & Mycek, M. J. (2005). *Pharmacology* (3rd ed.). Philadelphia: Lippincott Williams & Wilkins.

Patterson, T. F. (2005). Advances and challenges in management of invasive mycoses. *Lancet* **366(9490)**: 1013–1025.

Porth, C. M., & Matfin, G. (2008). *Pathophysiology: Concepts of Altered Health States* (8th ed.). Philadelphia: Lippincott Williams & Wilkins.

Rang, H. P., Dale, M. M., Ritter, J. M., & Flower, R. J. (2007). *Rang and Dale's Pharmacology* (6th ed.). Philadelphia: Churchill Livingstone.

Simonsen, T., Aarbakke, J., Kay, I., Coleman, I., Sinnott, P., & Lysaa, R. (2006). *Illustrated Pharmacology for Nurses*. London: Hodder Arnold.

CHAPTER
11

Antiprotozoal Agents

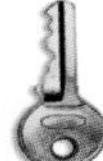

KEY TERMS

amoebiasis
Anopheles mosquito
cinchonism
giardiasis
leishmaniasis
malaria
Plasmodium
Pneumocystis carinii pneumonia (PCP)
protozoa
trichomoniasis
trophozoite
trypanosomiasis

LEARNING OBJECTIVES

Upon completion of this chapter, you will be able to:

1. Outline the life cycle of the protozoan that causes malaria.
2. Describe the therapeutic actions, indications, pharmacokinetics and contraindications associated with drugs used to treat malaria.
3. List the most common adverse reactions and important drug–drug interactions associated with drugs used to treat malaria.
4. Describe other common protozoal infections, including cause and clinical presentation.
5. Compare and contrast the antimalarials with other drugs used to treat protozoal infections.
6. Outline the nursing considerations for patients receiving an antiprotozoal agent.

ANTIMALARIALS

artemether with lumefantrine
chloroquine
doxycycline
mefloquine
primaquine
proguanil
pyrimethamine
quinine

OTHER ANTIPROTOZOALS

atovaquone
co-trimoxazole
diloxanide furoate
mepacrine
metronidazole
pentamidine
sodium stibogluconate
tinidazole

Infections caused by **protozoa** are very common in several parts of the world. In tropical and subtropical areas, where these types of illnesses are most prevalent, many people suffer multiple infestations at the same time. These infections are relatively rare in the United Kingdom, but with people travelling throughout the world in increasing numbers, it is not unusual to find an individual returning home from a trip to Africa, Asia or South America with fully developed protozoal infections. Protozoa thrive in tropical climates, but the warmer temperatures and higher rainfalls associated with climate change are likely to change the geographical incidence of protozoa, and we may see protozoa thriving in areas not previously identified with the protozoa. Protozoa can also survive and reproduce in areas where people live in very crowded and unsanitary conditions.

Protozoa are microscopic, single celled eukaryotic organisms that generally live in water. Some protozoa are parasitic and cause diseases in humans. Protozoa are classified by movement, either via one or more flagellae (tails), cilia (hairlike structures) or amoeboid movement. Some, like the protozoan that causes malaria, are nonmotile.

This chapter focuses on protozoal infections that are caused by insect bites (malaria, trypanosomiasis and leishmaniasis) and on those that result from ingestion or contact with the causal organism (amoebiasis, giardiasis and trichomoniasis). Box 11.1 discusses the use of antiprotozoals for various age groups affected by protozoal infections.

Malaria

Malaria is a parasitic disease that affects over 247 million people each year and kills up to 1 million people every year (WHO, 2009). Even with the introduction of drugs for the treatment of this disease, it remains endemic in many parts of the world. Malaria is spread via the bite of a female ***Anopheles mosquito***, which harbours the protozoal parasite and carries it to humans. The parasite can also be transmitted in contaminated blood transfusions, via contaminated medical equipment or between infected intravenous drug users sharing needles.

Four protozoal parasites, all in the genus ***Plasmodium***, have been identified as causes of malaria:

- *Plasmodium falciparum* is considered to be the most dangerous type of protozoan. Infection with this protozoan results in an acute, rapidly fulminating disease with high fever, pulmonary oedema, jaundice, acute renal failure, haemolytic anaemia and even death.
- *Plasmodium vivax* causes a milder form of the disease, which can cause relapses up to 2 years after infection.
- *Plasmodium malariae* is endemic in many tropical countries and causes very mild signs and symptoms in the population. It can cause more acute disease in travellers to endemic areas.
- *Plasmodium ovale*, which is rarely seen, can also cause relapses up to 2 years after the initial infection.

BOX 11.1 **DRUG THERAPY ACROSS THE LIFESPAN**

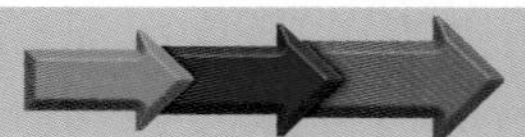

Antiprotozoal Agents

CHILDREN

Children are very sensitive to the effects of most antiprotozoal drugs, and more severe reactions can be expected when these drugs are used in children. However, the dangers of infection resulting from travel to areas endemic with many of these diseases are often much more severe than the potential risks associated with cautious drug use. Some of these drugs do have proven safety in children, including quinidine, artemether with lumefantrine and proguanil with atovaquone. If a child needs to travel to an area with endemic protozoal infections, the Health Protection Agency should be consulted about the safest possible preventative measures.

When administering any drug to children, always consult the most recent edition of the British National Formulary for Children.

ADULTS

Adults should be well advised about the need for prophylaxis against various protozoal infections and the need for immediate treatment if the disease is contracted. It is very helpful to mark calendars as reminders of the days before, during and after exposure on which the drugs should be taken. Due to increasing drug resistance in some species such as the protozoan that causes malaria, nondrug methods of preventing bites should be strongly recommended, for example long-sleeved clothing, insecticide-impregnated mosquito nets and insect repellents.

Pregnant and nursing women should not use these drugs unless the benefit clearly outweighs the potential risk to the foetus or neonate. Women of childbearing age should be advised to use barrier contraceptives if any of these drugs are used. A pregnant woman travelling to an area endemic with protozoal infections should be advised of the serious risks to the foetus associated with both preventive therapy and treatment of acute attacks, as well as the risks associated with contracting the disease.

OLDER ADULTS

Older patients may be more susceptible to the adverse effects associated with these drugs and should be monitored closely. Patients with hepatic dysfunction are at increased risk of worsening hepatic problems and toxic effects of many of these drugs. If hepatic dysfunction is expected (elderly individuals, alcohol abuse, use of other hepatotoxic drugs), the dosage may need to be lowered and the patient monitored more frequently.

Part of the problem with malaria control is that the female mosquito, which is responsible for transmitting the disease, has developed resistance to the insecticides designed to eradicate the mosquito. Widespread efforts at mosquito control were successful for a long period, with fewer cases of malaria seen each year. Because the insecticide-resistant mosquitoes continue to flourish, however, the incidence of malaria is again increasing. In addition, the protozoa that cause malaria have developed strains resistant to the usual antimalarial drugs. This combination of factors has led to a worldwide public health challenge.

Life Cycle of *Plasmodium*

The parasites that cause human malaria spend part of their life in the *Anopheles* mosquito and part in the human host (Figure 11.1). When a mosquito bites a human infected with malaria, it sucks blood infested with trophozoites which are gametocytes, the male and female forms of the plasmodium. These gametocytes fuse in the stomach of the mosquito and produce zygotes that go through several phases before forming sporozoites that make their way to the mosquito's salivary glands. The next person who is bitten by that mosquito is injected with thousands of sporozoites. These sporozoites travel through the bloodstream, where they quickly invade human liver cells (hepatocytes) and thereafter human red blood cells (erythrocytes).

Inside human cells, the organisms undergo asexual cell division and reproduction. The protozoal cell which is going to undertake further division in either hepatocytes or erythrocytes is called a *schizont*. Over a few days or weeks, the schizonts grow and multiply within the hepatocytes to form

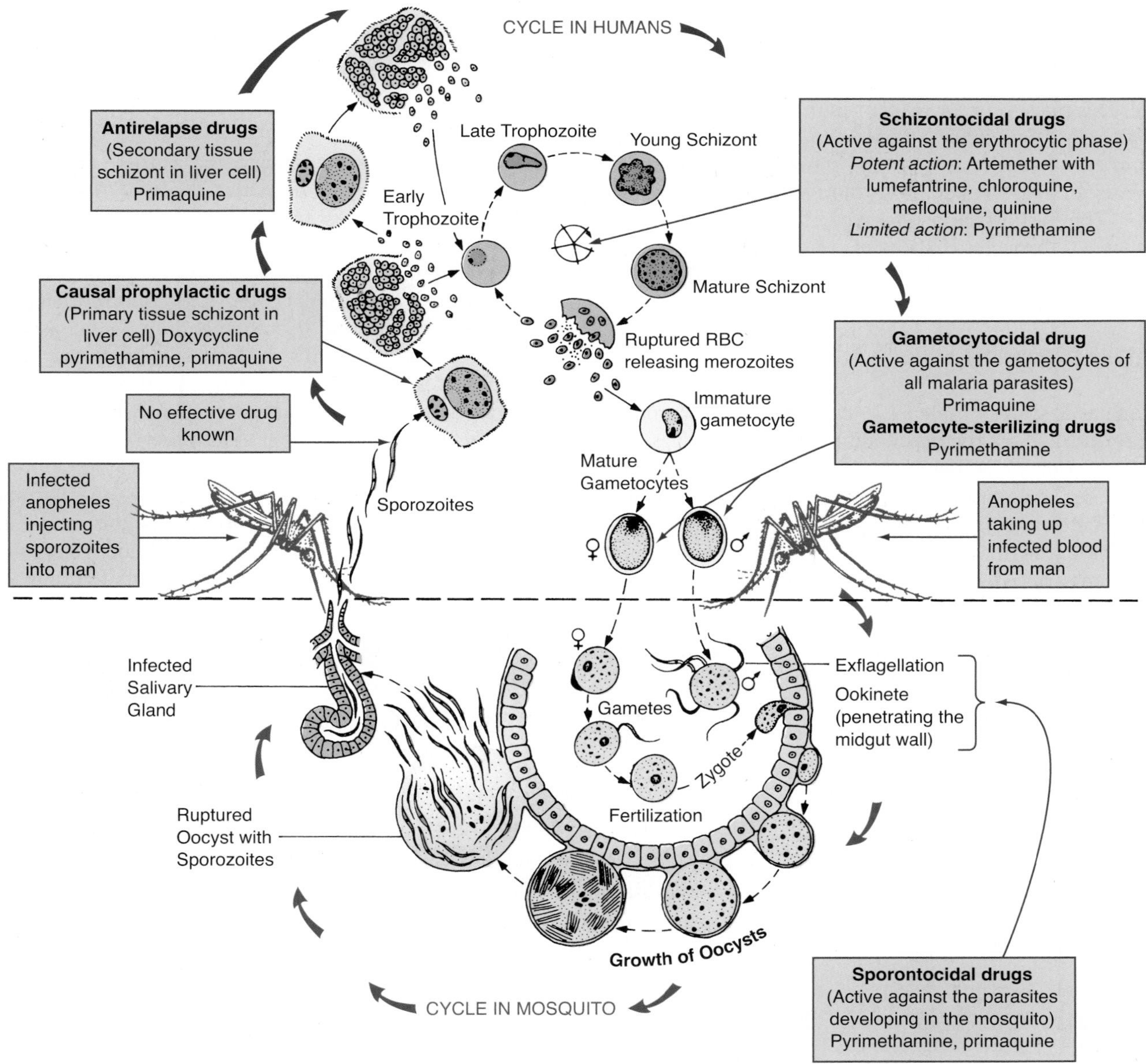

FIGURE 11.1 Types of antimalarial drugs in relation to the stages in the life cycle of *Plasmodium*.

merozoites and within erythrocytes to form *trophozoites*. Merozoites then burst from invaded cells when they rupture because of overexpansion. The merozoites enter the circulation and invade erythrocytes, in which they continue to divide until the erythrocytes also burst, sending more merozoites into the circulation to invade yet more erythrocytes. Some merozoites form trophozites which are taken up by another mosquito and the life cycle in the mosquito begins again.

Eventually, there are a large number of merozoites in the body, as well as many ruptured and invaded erythrocytes. At this point, the acute malarial attack occurs. The rupture of the erythrocytes causes chills and fever related to the pyrogenic effects of the protozoa and the toxic effects of the ruptured erythrocyte and components on the system. This cycle of chills and fever usually occurs about every 72 hours and is characteristic for each species of *Plasmodium*.

With *P. vivax* and *P. ovale* malaria, this cycle may continue for a long period. Many of the schizonts can lie dormant in the liver for several years, before they multiply into merozoites and then invade more erythrocytes, again causing the acute cycle. This may occur for years in an untreated patient.

With *P. falciparum* and *P. malariae* malaria, there are no extrahepatic sites for the schizonts. If the patient survives an acute attack, no prolonged periods of relapse occur. The first attack of this type of malaria can destroy so many erythrocytes that the patient's capillaries become blocked and the circulation to vital organs is interrupted, leading to death.

Antimalarials

Antimalarial drugs (Table 11.1) can be given in combination form to attack the plasmodium at various stages of its life cycle (Box 11.2). Using this approach, it is possible to prevent the acute malarial reaction in individuals who have been infected by the parasite.

Quinine, the first drug found to be effective in the treatment of malaria, is derived from the bark of the Cinchona tree. Quinine is a blood schizonticide, that is these drugs inhibit the growth of *Plasmodium*. Once inside erythrocytes, the malarial parasites digest haemoglobin in their food vacuoles and produce toxic-free radicals and haem. The haem is normally polymerized by the parasites into an inactive compound using the enzyme haem polymerase. The schizonticides prevent the inactivation of haem which kills the parasites via oxidative damage to their membranes. Quinine may lead to a condition called **cinchonism** (nausea, flushed skin, rashes, tinnitus, headache, visual disturbances and abdominal pain), which makes it less desirable than newer, less toxic drugs. Its use is mainly for treating cerebral malaria. Quinine is readily absorbed from the upper small intestine, with peak serum levels occurring within 3 to 8 hours. It is metabolized in the liver and excreted in the urine. Quinine is toxic to the foetus but in malaria treatment the benefits to the mother

BOX 11.2 Combination Drugs Used for Malaria Prevention and Treatment

Combining two different preparations in one drug may increase compliance by reducing the number of pills a patient has to take, and it conforms to the treatment protocol of taking drugs that affect the protozoa at different stages on their life cycle.

- *Artemether with lumefantrine* is indicated for the treatment of acute *P. falciparum* malaria and benign malaria. Artemether is concentrated in erythrocytes infected with the parasite and is thought to irreversibly damage the parasites' cell membrane. Avoid use while breast-feeding.
- *Pyrimethamine with sulfadoxine* is used as an adjunct to quinine in the treatment of *P. falciparum* malaria. There is a risk to the neonate if breast-feeding while taking these drugs.
- *Proguanil with atovaquone* is indicated for the prevention and treatment of *P. falciparum* malaria where resistance to other drugs has been reported. When using this combination as a prophylactic, the amount entering breast milk is too small to prove harmful to the neonate.

Table 11.1 DRUGS IN FOCUS

Antimalarials

Drug Name	Usual Indications
artemether with lumefantrine	Treatment of acute uncomplicated *P. falciparum* infection and benign malaria
chloroquine	Prophylaxis and treatment of *Plasmodium* malaria
doxycycline	Prophylaxis of Plasmodium malaria; adjunct therapy in the treatment of *P. falciparum*
mefloquine	Prophylaxis and treatment of *Plasmodium* malaria (but used less for *P. falciparum* infection)
primaquine	Adjunct therapy in the treatment of *P. vivax* and *P. ovale* infections
proguanil	Prophylaxis of *Plasmodium* malaria
proguanil with atovaquine	Prophylaxis of *P. falciparum* and treatment of acute uncomplicated *P. falciparum* infection and benign malaria
pyrimethamine with sulfadoxone	Used with quinine in the treatment of *P. falciparum*; pyrimethamine used alone in the treatment of toxoplasmosis
quinine	Treatment of *P. falciparum* infections

outweigh the risks. Women of childbearing age who need to take quinine should be advised to use barrier contraceptives. Quinine can affect the rhythm of the heart and should be used with caution in patients with arrhythmias.

Chloroquine is also a schizonticide, acting in the same way as quinine. Chloroquine also prevents digestion of haemoglobin by the parasite, therefore reducing the supply of amino acids required for viability. In many areas of the world, *P. falciparum* protozoa are now resistant to chloroquine so it is not recommended for treatment of *P. falciparum*. When given orally, chloroquine is readily absorbed from the gastrointestinal (GI) tract, with peak serum levels occurring in 3 to 5 hours. The drug is concentrated in infected erythrocytes. Metabolism occurs in the liver and is excreted very slowly in the urine, primarily as unchanged drug. Chloroquine sometimes has serious adverse effects, such as hepatic toxicity, permanent eye damage and blindness; but this is usually at higher doses. Use during pregnancy and lactation should be restricted to situations in which the benefit clearly outweighs the potential risk to the foetus or neonate.

Mefloquine also inhibits the haem polymerase. Mefloquine exists as a mixture of isomers (different structural types) that are absorbed, metabolized and excreted at different rates. The terminal half-life is 13 to 24 days. Metabolism occurs in the liver; therefore, caution should be used in patients with hepatic dysfunction. Where mefloquine is used as treatment, pregnancy should be avoided during and for 3 months after completion of therapy because in preclinical studies mefloquine has demonstrated teratogenicity. However, when used prophylatically, mefloquine is thought suitable for use in pregnancy in areas where there is a high risk of chloroquine-resistant *P. falciparum*. It also crosses into breast milk but the risk to the baby is thought to be minimal.

Primaquine, another very old drug for treating malaria, is thought to disrupt the mitochondria of the plasmodium. It also causes death of gametocytes and exoerythrocytic forms and prevents other forms from reproducing and is therefore especially useful in preventing relapses of *P. vivax* and *P. ovale* infections. Primaquine is readily absorbed and metabolized in the liver. Excretion occurs primarily in the urine. This drug can cause neonatal haemolysis; however, the benefits to the mother either in prophylaxis or treatment, outweigh the risk. Safety for use during breast-feeding has not been established. Primaquine should be taken with food to avoid gastric irritation. This drug should not be given to people with a deficiency in the enzyme glucose-6-phosphate dehydrogenase (G6PD), an enzyme involved in red blood cell metabolism.

Doxycycline is a broad-spectrum antibacterial which acts by inhibiting protein synthesis in sensitive organisms. This antibacterial is used in the prophylaxis and treatment of malaria. Following absorption from the stomach and upper small intestine, 80% to 95% of doxycycline is distributed bound to plasma proteins. Doxycycline is mainly excreted in the faeces. As with all tetracyclines, this drug should be avoided during pregnancy and also while breast-feeding and in young children before the appearance of the second teeth.

Proguanil is an antifolate drug and inhibits dihydrofolate reductase, an important enzyme used by the plasmodium to convert folic acid into folinic acid for DNA synthesis. If the plasmodium is unable to synthesize DNA this eventually leads to an inability to reproduce and cell death. This drug is usually used with chloroquine in malaria prophylaxis or in combination with atovaquone in the treatment of *P. falciparum*. Absorption is slow but complete. Proguanil is also a prodrug and is metabolized in the liver to the active metabolite, cycloguanil. The parent drug and active metabolites are excreted in the urine. Safe for use in pregnancy and breast-feeding but not when given in combination with atovaquone.

Pyrimethamine is also an antifolate drug and is used in combination with sulfadoxine and quinine in the treatment of *P. falciparum* infection. Pyrimethamine is slowly absorbed from the GI tract, metabolized in the liver and has a half-life of 4 days. It usually maintains suppressive concentrations in the body for about 2 weeks. Pyrimethamine should not be used during pregnancy or lactation unless the benefit clearly outweighs the potential risk to the foetus or neonate.

Therapeutic Actions and Indications

The antimalarial agents are effective in interrupting plasmodial reproduction in the erythrocyte stage of the life cycle, as well as in the hepatic and gametocyte stages in some cases (Figures 11.1 and 11.2). The agents used for chemoprophylaxis target the merozoites leaving the liver cells to prevent infection of erythrocytes. Chemoprophylaxis should be started at least 1 week (4 weeks for mefloquine) prior to travel into an endemic area and continued for 4 weeks after leaving (1 week for proguanil hydrochloride with atovaquone).

Contraindications and Cautions

Contraindications to the use of antimalarials are the presence of known allergy to any of these drugs; liver disease or alcoholism, *both because of the parasitic invasion of the liver and because of the need for a functioning liver to metabolize these drugs to avoid toxic levels in the plasma*; and pregnancy and lactation *because the drugs could be toxic to the foetus or infant*. Caution should be used in patients with retinal disease or damage *because many of these drugs can affect the retina and therefore vision, and the likelihood of problems increases if the retina is already damaged*; with psoriasis *because of skin damage*; or with renal dysfunction, *which could reduce excretion of the drug leading to toxic levels*.

Caution should also be taken for patients with G6PD deficiency—which is more likely to occur in people of

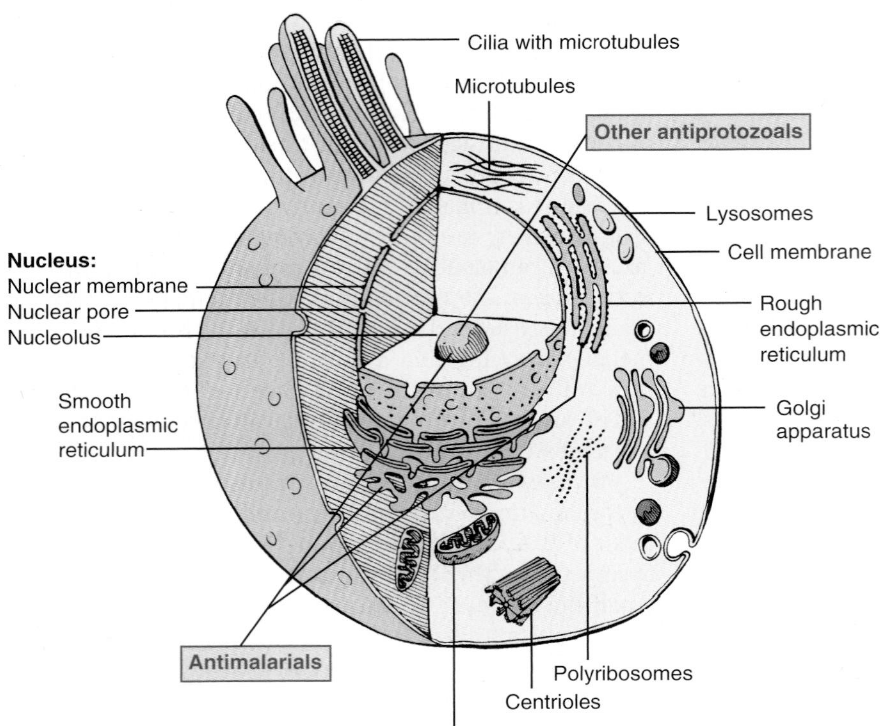

FIGURE 11.2 Sites of action of antimalarials and other antiprotozoals. Antimalarials block protein synthesis and cause cell death. Other antiprotozoals block DNA synthesis, prevent cell reproduction and lead to cell death.

Mediterranean, African or Asian descent. These patients may experience a haemolytic crisis while taking chloroquine, primaquine or quinine. Patients should be questioned about any history of potential G6PD deficiency. If no history is known, the patient should be tested before any of these drugs are prescribed. If testing is not possible and the drugs are needed, the patient should be monitored very closely and informed about the potential need for hospitalization and emergency services.

Adverse Effects

A number of adverse effects are encountered including headache, dizziness, fever, shaking, chills and malaise are associated with central nervous system (CNS) effects of the drugs and immune reaction to the release of the merozoites. Nausea, vomiting, diarrhoea, dyspepsia and anorexia are associated with direct drug effects on the GI tract and effects on CNS control of vomiting related to cell death and protein changes. Hepatic dysfunction is associated with the toxic effects of the drug on the liver and the effects of the disease on the liver. Dermatological effects include rash, pruritus and loss of hair associated with changes in protein synthesis. Visual changes, including possible blindness related to retinal damage and ototoxicity related to additional nerve damage, may occur.

All three combination drugs should be avoided during pregnancy unless the potential benefit to the mother outweighs the risks to the foetus.

Clinically Important Drug–Drug Interactions

The main drug groups where interactions occur are anti-arrhythmics, β-blockers, cardiac glycosides, antibacterials, antidepressants, antipsychotics and cimetidine. There is a risk of ventricular arrhythmias when some of the drugs are combined with antimalarial treatment. There is also a risk of increased plasma drug concentrations if some antimalarials are taken with grapefruit juice which is known to inhibit the metabolism of a number of drugs. Chloroquine and mefloquine should not be taken together because there is an increased risk of convulsions.

If pyrimethamine is combined with other antifolate drugs (e.g. methotrexate, the antibacterial sulphonamides), the mammalian form of dihydrofolate reductase may also be inhibited leading to folate deficiency and megaloblastic anaemia. Folic acid supplements may be necessary.

Always consult a current copy of the British National Formulary for further guidance.

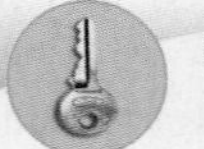

Key Drug Summary: *Chloroquine*

Indications: Treatment and prophylaxis of malaria caused by susceptible strains of *Plasmodia,* that is excluding *P. falciparum* which is resistant to chloroquine. For prophylaxis of malaria, treatment should be started 1 week before arriving in the endemic area and continued for 4 weeks after leaving.

Actions: Inhibits protozoal reproduction by irreversibly damaging the cell membrane of the parasites and also reducing the supply of amino acids required for protein synthesis

Pharmacokinetics:

Route	Onset	Peak	Duration
Oral	Varies	3–5 h	1 week

$T_{1/2}$: 70–120 hours; metabolized in the liver and excreted in the urine

Adverse effects: Visual disturbances including blindness (patients should have their vision checked before and following treatment), headache, convulsions, hypotension, GI disturbances, rashes, pruritis, hair loss.

BOX 11.3 FOCUS ON THE **EVIDENCE**

World Travel and the Spread of Pathogens

Nowadays, people travel to more exotic areas of the world than ever before. People are therefore exposed to more pathogens and are also potentially spreading pathogens to different areas of the world. Pathogens that are endemic in one area of the world, causing mild disease, can be quite devastating in a population that has not previously been exposed to that pathogen.

World health agencies and governments have established guidelines for prophylaxis and treatment of such diseases for travellers. People who are planning to travel out of the country should contact their GP or consult the National Health Service website (see Web Links) for the latest information on what prophylactic measures are required in the area they plan to visit and to learn about potential health hazards in that area. The information is updated frequently; treatment and prophylaxis suggestions are based on current clinical experience in the area and should be consulted regularly.

Patients who have travelled to other areas of the world and who present with any illness should be questioned about where they travelled, what precautions (including prophylactic measures) were taken, and when they first experienced any signs or symptoms of illness. There are a number of Travel Medicine Teams (details given in British National Formulary [BNF]) based around the country who can be consulted about diagnosis and treatment guidelines for any tropical disease that is unfamiliar to a health care provider, as well as what precautions should be used in caring for such patients.

Other Protozoal Infections

Other protozoal infections are encountered in clinical practice include amoebiasis, leishmaniasis, trypanosomiasis, trichomoniasis and giardiasis. These infections, which are caused by single-celled protozoa, are usually associated with unsanitary, crowded conditions and use of poor hygienic practices. Patients travelling to other countries may encounter these infections. (See Box 11.3 for a discussion of travel and tourism helping to spread pathogens.)

Amoebiasis

Amoebiasis, an intestinal infection caused by *Entamoeba histolytica*, is often known as amoebic dysentery. Approximately 500 million people are believed to carry *E. histolytica* in their intestines, and amoebiasis is responsible for up to 100,000 deaths worldwide (Stanley, 2003).

E. histolytica has a two-stage life cycle (Figure 11.3). The organism exists in two stages: (1) a cystic, dormant stage, in which the protozoan can live for long periods outside the body or in the human intestine, and (2) a **trophozoite** stage in the human large intestine. The disease is transmitted while the protozoan is in the cystic stage in faecal matter, from which it can enter water and the ground. It can be passed to other humans who drink the contaminated water or eat food that has been grown in contaminated ground. The cysts are swallowed and pass, unaffected by gastric acid, into the intestine. Some of these cysts are passed in faecal matter, and some of them become trophozoites that grow and reproduce. The trophozoites adhere to the mucosa of the colon, where they penetrate into the intestinal wall, forming erosions. These forms of *Entamoeba* release a chemical that dissolves mucosal cells, and eventually they erode tissue until they enter the vascular system, which carries them throughout the body. The trophozoites commonly lodge in the liver and cause abscesses.

Early signs of amoebiasis include abdominal pain and mild-to-severe diarrhoea alternating with constipation. In the worst cases, if the protozoan is able to invade extraintestinal tissue, it can dissolve the tissue and eventually cause the death of the host. Some individuals can become carriers of the disease without having any overt signs or symptoms. These people seem to be resistant to the intestinal invasion but pass the cysts on in the stool.

Leishmaniasis

Leishmaniasis is a disease caused by a protozoan that is passed from sandflies to humans from dogs and rats. Each year there are 2 million new cases of leishmaniasis (Centers for Disease Control and Prevention, 2008). The sandfly injects an asexual form of this flagellated protozoan, called a promastigote, into the human host, where it is rapidly attacked and digested by human macrophages. Inside the macrophages, the promastigote divides, developing many new forms called amastigotes, which keep dividing and eventually kill the macrophage, releasing the amastigotes into the systemic circulation to infect other macrophages. Thus,

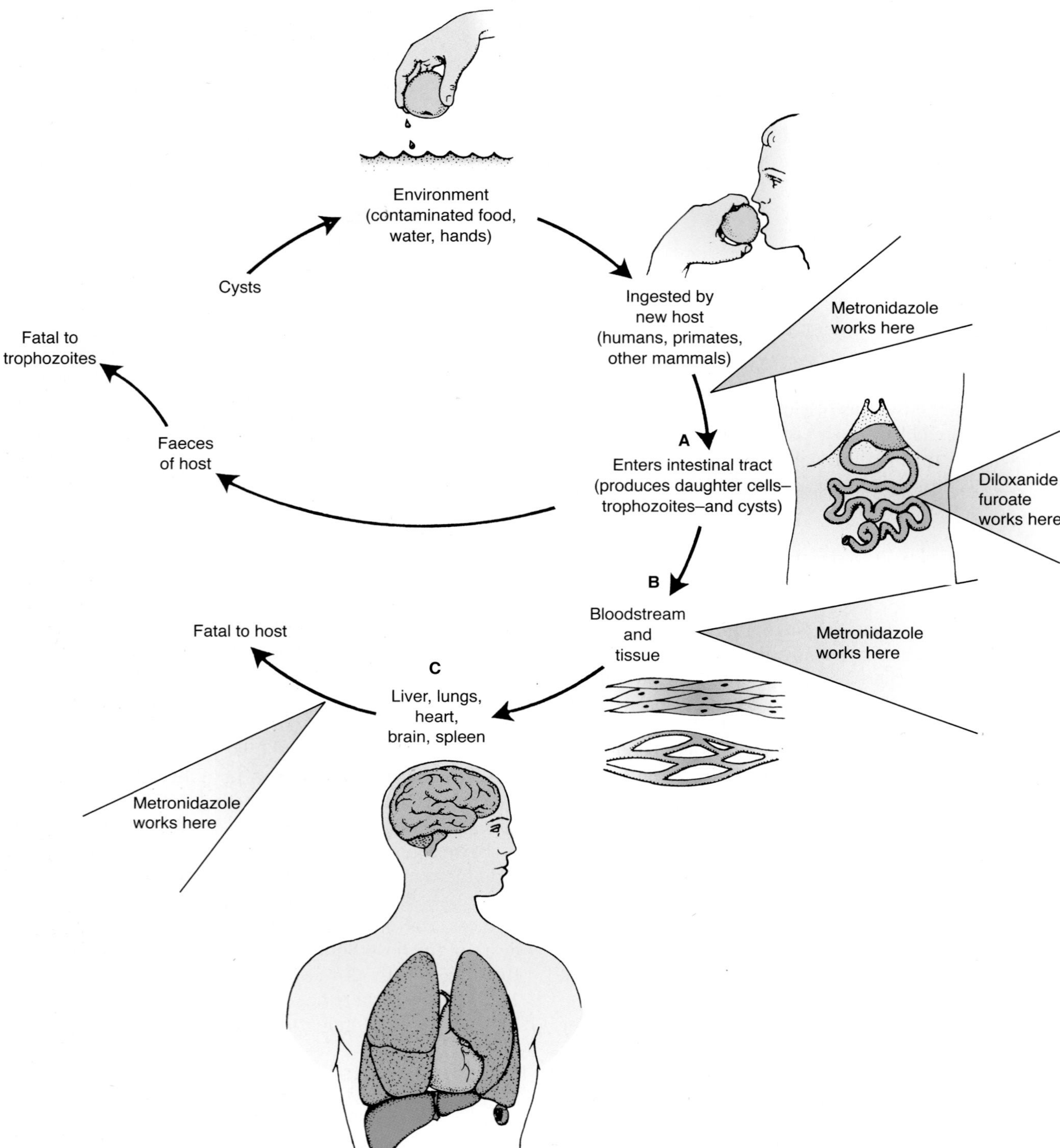

FIGURE 11.3 Life cycle of *Entamoeba histolytica* and the sites of action of metronidazole and diloxanide furoate which are used to treat amoebiasis.

a cyclic pattern of infection is established. These amastigotes can cause serious lesions in the skin, the viscera, or the mucous membranes of the host.

Trypanosomiasis

Trypanosomiasis is caused by infection with *Trypanosoma*. This protozoa is found across sub-Saharan Africa and there are an estimated 50,000 to 70,000 new cases each year (WHO, 2009). Its presence renders large areas of Africa uninhabitable as it affects livestock as well as humans. Two parasitic protozoal species cause very serious and often fatal diseases in humans:

- African sleeping sickness, which is caused by *Trypanosoma brucei gambiense*, is transmitted by the tsetse fly. After the pathogenic organism has lived and grown in human blood, it eventually invades the CNS, leading to encephalopathy, and even death.
- Chagas' disease, which is caused by *Trypanosoma cruzi*, is almost endemic in many South American countries. This protozoan results in a severe cardiomyopathy that accounts for numerous deaths and disabilities in more rural regions.

Trichomoniasis

Trichomoniasis is caused by another flagellated protozoan *Trichomonas vaginalis*. This protozoan is part of the normal flora of the GI tract and/or vagina and is a common cause of vaginitis. This infection is usually spread during sexual intercourse by men who have no signs and symptoms of infection. In women, this protozoan causes reddened, inflamed vaginal mucosa, itching, burning and a yellowish-green discharge with a distinctive odour.

Giardiasis

Giardiasis, which is caused by *Giardia lamblia*, is found worldwide and is the most commonly imported parasite into the United Kingdom with 4,000 to 6,000 cases diagnosed each year. Although the majority of giardiasis cases result from infection during overseas travel, a number of giardiasis cases in the United Kingdom have been associated with contaminated drinking water supplies or swimming pools (Stuart *et al.*, 2003). This protozoan forms cysts, which survive outside the body and allow transmission through contaminated water or food, and trophozoites, which break out of the cysts in the upper small intestine and eventually cause signs and symptoms of disease. Diarrhoea, rotten egg-smelling stools and pale and mucous-filled stools are commonly seen. Some patients experience abdominal pain, weight loss and malnourishment as a result of the invasion of the mucosa.

Pneumocystis carinii Pneumonia

P. carinii (now known as *P. jiroveci*) is similar to protozoa with respect to life cycle, morphology and drug treatment but it is actually a fungus. This fungus does not usually cause illness in humans. However, when an individual's immune system becomes suppressed, because of acquired immune deficiency syndrome (AIDS) or AIDS-related complex, the use of immunosuppressant drugs or advanced age, *P. jiroveci* is able to invade the lungs, leading to severe inflammation and the condition still known as ***Pneumocystis carinii* pneumonia (PCP)**. This disease is the most common opportunistic infection in patients with AIDS.

Toxoplasmosis

Toxoplasmosis is caused by *Toxoplasma gondii*. The gametocytes reside in the GI tract of the cat where large numbers of oocysts are produced and subsequently excreted in faeces. Humans are infected either by inhaling the oocysts or through ingestion of undercooked contaminated meat. Most toxoplasmosis infections are asymptomatic or mild; however, placental transmission of the protozoan can cause severe congenital abnormalities in the foetus.

Other Antiprotozoal Drugs

Drugs that are available specifically for the treatment of these various protozoan infections include some of the antimalarial drugs; for example pyrimethamine is effective in treating toxoplasmosis. Other drugs, including antibacterials, are used for treating these conditions at various stages of the disease (Table 11.2). Other antiprotozoals include the following agents.

- *Atovaquone* is used for the treatment of mild-to-moderate *Pneumocystis* pneumonia. It is slowly absorbed and is highly protein bound in circulation. It is excreted slowly through the faeces in its unchanged form, with a half-life of 36 to 72 hours. Use during pregnancy and lactation should be limited to those situations in which the benefit to the mother clearly outweighs the potential risks to the foetus or neonate. Atovaquone is not recommended for children.
- *Co-trimoxazole* is a combination of trimethoprin and sulfamethoxazole and is the treatment of choice for *Pneumocystis* pneumonia. This combination should be avoided in pregnancy and lactation.
- *Diloxanide furoate* is used to treat asymptomatic patients with *E. histolytica*. This drug is metabolized in intestinal mucosa and excreted in urine. The metabolite diloxanide is readily absorbed and mainly excreted in the urine after metabolism in the liver. Diloxanide should be avoided in pregnancy and lactation.
- *Mepacrine* is an antigiardial drug effective against *G. lamblia* infections. After absorption in the GI tract, mepacrine is widely distributed throughout the body and is known to accumulate in tissues, including the liver, from where it is slowly released. The safety of mepacrine during pregnancy and lactation has not been established.

Table 11.2 DRUGS IN FOCUS

Other Antiprotozoal Agents

Drug Name	Usual Indications
atovaquone	Prevention and treatment of *Pneumocystis* pneumonia
co-trimoxazole	Treatment of *Pneumocystis* pneumonia
diloxanide furoate	Used together with metronidazole or tinidazole in the treatment of acute amoebiasis
mepacrine	Treatment of giardiasis
metronidazole	Treatment of amoebiasis, trichomoniasis, giardiasis
pentamidine	As treatment of mild *Pneumocystis* pneumonia; as a systemic agent in the treatment of leishmaniasis and trypanosomiasis
sodium stibogluconate	Treatment of leishmaniasis
tinidazole	Treatment of trichomoniasis, giardiasis, amoebiasis

- *Metronidazole*, which is used to treat amoebiasis, trichomoniasis and giardiasis, is well absorbed orally, reaching peak levels in 1 to 2 hours. Metronidazole is a prodrug and is activated by susceptible organisms. It is partially metabolized in the liver with a half-life of 7 hours. Most of the drug is excreted unchanged in urine. Metronidazole rapidly crosses the placenta and enters the foetal circulation. It also passes into breast milk. Use during pregnancy and lactation should be avoided.
- *Pentamidine* can be delivered parenterally or by inhalation to treat PCP, leishmaniasis and trypanosomiasis. The mechanism for metabolism is unclear; excretion is mainly via urine. Pentamidine should be avoided during pregnancy and lactation.
- *Sodium stibogluconate* is used to treat leishmaniasis. Sodium stibogluconate should only be used during pregnancy when the benefits to the mother outweigh the risks to the foetus. The amounts present in breast milk are likely to be too small to adversely affect the neonate.
- *Tinidazole* is approved for the treatment of trichomoniasis, giardiasis and amoebiasis. It is rapidly absorbed after oral administration, reaching peak levels within 60 to 90 minutes. It is excreted in the urine with a half-life of 12 to 14 hours. Tinidazole should not be administered during the first trimester of pregnancy. Tinidazole can also enter breast milk and breast-feeding mothers should find an alternative method of feeding their baby during treatment with this drug. It should not be combined with alcohol and should be used cautiously with liver dysfunction.

Therapeutic Actions and Indications

These agents act to inhibit DNA synthesis in susceptible protozoa, leading to the inability to reproduce and subsequent cell death (see Figure 11.2). These drugs are indicated for the treatment of infections caused by susceptible protozoa.

Contraindications and Cautions

Contraindications include the presence of any known allergy or hypersensitivity to any of these drugs and pregnancy (diloxanide) *because drug effects on developing foetal DNA and proteins can cause foetal abnormalities and even death*. Caution should be used in the presence of CNS disease *because of possible exacerbation when the drug affects the CNS*; hepatic and renal impairment *because of possible exacerbation when hepatic or renal drug effects occur*; and lactation, *because these drugs may pass into breast milk and could have severe adverse effects on the infant*.

Always consult a current copy of the British National Formulary for further guidance.

Adverse Effects

Adverse effects that occur with antiprotozoal agents include CNS effects such as headache, dizziness, ataxia and loss of coordination. GI effects include nausea, vomiting, diarrhoea, cramps and changes in liver function.

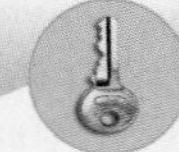

Key Drug Summary: *Metronidazole*

Indications: Acute intestinal amoebiasis, amoebic liver abscess, trichomoniasis, giardiasis and acute infections caused by susceptible strains of anaerobic bacteria

Actions: Inhibits DNA synthesis of specific anaerobes, causing cell death

Pharmacokinetics:

Route	Onset	Peak
Oral	Varies	1–2 h
IV	Rapid	1–2 h

$T_{1/2}$: 7 hours; partially metabolized in the liver and excreted unchanged in the urine

Adverse effects: Headache, dizziness, ataxia, nausea, vomiting, anorexia, metallic taste in the mouth, furred tongue, darkening of the urine. Vomiting is induced if taken with alcohol.

Nursing Considerations for Patients Receiving Antiprotozoal Agents

Assessment: History and Examination

Screen for the following: history of allergy to any of the antimalarials or antiprotozoals; liver dysfunction or alcoholism *that might interfere with metabolism and excretion of the drug*; psoriasis, *which could be exacerbated by an antimalarial drug*; retinal disease *that could increase the visual disturbances associated with some of the antimalarial drugs*; CNS disease *that could be exacerbated*; pregnancy and lactation *because these drugs could affect the foetus and could enter breast milk and be toxic to the infant.* Establish if patient is currently taking other medications or herbal therapies which may potentially interact with the antiprotozoal agent.

Physical assessment should be performed *to establish baseline data for assessment of the effectiveness of the drug and the occurrence of any adverse effects associated with drug therapy*. Perform retinal examination and ophthalmic and auditory screening *to detect cautions for drug use and to evaluate changes that occur as a result of antimalarial therapy*. Conduct an examination of the CNS *to check reflexes and muscle strength to detect cautions for drug use and to evaluate changes that can occur as a result of antiprotozoal therapy.* Assess alcohol intake (for antimalarial agents) and obtain liver function tests *to determine appropriateness of therapy and to monitor for toxicity.* Prepare a blood film and stain *to determine which protozoal species is causing the disease.*

Nursing Diagnoses

Patients receiving an antiprotozoal drug may have the following nursing diagnoses related to drug therapy:

- Acute pain related to GI, CNS and skin effects of drug
- Imbalanced nutrition: less than body requirements related to severe GI effects of drug
- Disturbed sensory perception (kinaesthetic, visual) related to CNS effects
- Skin lesions, colour, temperature related to drug therapy
- Deficient knowledge regarding drug therapy

Implementation With Rationale

- Arrange for blood films to be prepared prior to therapy *to ensure proper drug for susceptible Plasmodium species*. Treatment may begin before test results are known.
- Administer the complete course of the drug *to get the full beneficial effects*. Mark a calendar for prophylactic doses. Use combination therapy as indicated.
- Monitor hepatic function and ophthalmologic examination (antimalarials only) before and periodically during treatment *to effectively arrange to stop the drug if signs of failure or deteriorating vision occur*.
- Provide comfort and safety measures if CNS effects occur (e.g. physical support if dizziness and weakness are present) *to prevent patient injury*. Provide oral hygiene and ready access to bathroom facilities as needed *to cope with GI effects*.
- Provide small, frequent, nutritious meals if GI upset is severe *to ensure adequate nutrition*. Taking the drug with food may also decrease GI upset. Monitor nutritional status.
- Ensure that the patient is instructed concerning the appropriate dosage regimen *to enhance patient knowledge about drug therapy and to promote concordance.*

The patient should:

- Take safety precautions, including changing position slowly and avoiding driving and hazardous tasks, if CNS effects occur.
- Take the drug with meals and try small, frequent meals if GI upset is a problem.
- For antimalarial agents: report blurring of vision, which could indicate retinal damage; loss of hearing or ringing in the ears, which could indicate CNS toxicity; and fever or worsening of condition, which could indicate a resistant strain or noneffective therapy.
- For other antiprotozoal agents: report severe GI problems and interference with nutrition; fever and chills, dizziness, unusual fatigue, or weakness, which may indicate CNS effects (see Critical Thinking Scenario 11-1).

Evaluation

- Monitor patient response to the drug (prevention of malaria, resolution of infection and negative blood samples for parasite).

- Monitor for adverse effects (orientation and affect, nutritional state, rash, hepatic function, and visual and auditory changes).
- Evaluate the effectiveness of the teaching plan (patient can name the drug, dosage, possible adverse effects to watch for, and specific measures to help avoid adverse effects).
- Monitor the effectiveness of comfort and safety measures and concordance with the regimen.

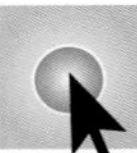

WEB LINKS

Health care providers and patients may want to consult the following Internet sources:

http://bnfc.org The BNF for Children provides UK health care professionals with authoritative and practical information on the selection and clinical use of medicines in children.

http://cks.library.nhs.uk The National Health Service Clinical Knowledge Summaries provides evidence-based practical information on the common conditions observed in primary care.

http://www.bnf.org.uk The BNF provides UK health care professionals with authoritative and practical information on the selection and clinical use of medicines.

http://www.cdc.gov/travel The American Centers for Disease Control and Prevention provides up-to-date and comprehensive information on prophylaxis, diagnosis and treatment of infectious diseases obtained from travelling.

http://www.nhsdirect.nhs.uk The National Health Service Direct service provides patients with information and advice about health, illness and health services.

http://www.who.int/ith The World Health Organization provides information on the main health risks for travellers.

http://www.fitfortravel.nhs.uk The National Health Service provides advice for travellers.

Points to Remember

- A protozoan is a parasitic single celled eukaryotic organism. Its life cycle includes a parasitic phase inside human tissues or cells.
- Malaria, which occurs in many tropical parts of the world, has been spreading in recent years because of resistance to insecticides occurring in the *Anopheles* mosquito.
- Malaria is caused by the *Plasmodium* protozoa, which must go through a cycle in the female *Anopheles* mosquito before being passed to humans by the mosquito bite. Once inside a human, the protozoa invade the hepatocytes and then erythrocytes.
- The characteristic cyclic chills and fever of malaria occur when erythrocytes burst, releasing more protozoa into the bloodstream.
- Malaria is treated with a combination of drugs that attack the protozoan at various stages in its life cycle.
- Amoebiasis is caused by the protozoan *E. histolytica*, which invades human intestinal tissue after being passed to humans through unsanitary food or water.
- Leishmaniasis, a protozoan-caused disease, can result in serious lesions in the mucosa, viscera and skin.
- Trypanosomiasis, which is caused by infection with a *Trypanosoma* parasite, may assume two forms: African sleeping sickness leads to inflammation of the CNS; and Chagas' disease results in serious cardiomyopathy.
- Trichomoniasis is caused by *T. vaginalis*. This common cause of vaginitis results in no signs or symptoms in men but serious vaginal inflammation in women.
- Giardiasis, which is caused by *G. lamblia*, is a commonly diagnosed intestinal parasite. This disease may lead to serious malnutrition when the pathogen invades intestinal mucosa.
- *P. carinii* (renamed *P. jiroveci*) does not usually cause illness in humans unless they become immunosuppressed. *Pneumocystis* pneumonia (PCP) is the most common opportunistic infection seen in AIDS patients.
- Toxoplasmosis, which is caused by *T. gondii*, can cause mild illness in adults who inhale the cysts in the faeces of infected cats or ingest the cysts in undercooked contaminated meat. It can cause severe malformations of the foetus if contracted by pregnant women.
- Patients receiving antiprotozoal agents should be monitored regularly to detect any serious adverse effects, including loss of vision and liver toxicity.

CRITICAL THINKING SCENARIO 11-1

Coping with Amoebiasis

The Situation

Jonathan, a 20-year-old male undergraduate student, reported to the university health centre complaining of severe diarrhoea, abdominal pain and, most recently, blood in his stools. He had a mild fever and appeared to be dehydrated and very tired. The young man, who denied travel outside the country, reported eating most of his meals at the local pizzeria, where he worked in the kitchen each night making pizza.

A stool sample for cysts was obtained and a diagnosis of amoebiasis was made. Metronidazole was prescribed. A public health representative was sent to find the source of the infection, which was the kitchen of the pizza place where Jonathan worked. The kitchen was shut down until all the food, utensils and environment passed health inspection.

Critical Thinking

- What are the important nursing implications for Jonathan? *Think about the usual nutritional state of students.*
- What are the implications for recovery when a patient is potentially malnourished and then has a disease that causes severe diarrhoea, dehydration and potential malnourishment? *Consider how difficult it will be for Jonathan to be a full-time student while trying to cope with the signs and symptoms of his disease, as well as the adverse effects associated with his drug therapy and the need to maintain adequate nutrition to allow some healing and recovery.*
- What potential problems could the added stress of being out of work have for Jonathan? *Consider the physiological impact of stress, as well as the psychological problems of trying to cope with one more stressor.*

Discussion

Jonathan needed a great deal of reassurance and an explanation of his disease. He learned that oral hygiene and small, frequent meals would help alleviate some of his discomfort until the metronidazole could control the amoebiasis and that good hygiene and strict hand washing when the disease is active would help to prevent transmission. He was advised to watch for the occurrence of specific adverse drug effects, such as a possible severe reaction to alcohol (he was advised to avoid alcoholic beverages while taking this drug as alcohol combined with metronidazole causes vomiting); GI upset and a strange metallic taste (the importance of good nutrition to promote healing of the GI tract was stressed); dizziness or light-headedness and a possibility of superinfections.

Jonathan was scheduled for a follow-up examination for stool cysts and nutritional status. Metronidazole was continued until the stool sample came back negative. He needed and received a great deal of support and encouragement because he was far from home and the disease and the drug effects were sometimes difficult to cope with. The effects of stress – decreasing blood flow to the GI tract, for example – can make it more difficult for patients such as Jonathan to recover.

Nursing Care Guide for Jonathan: Metronidazole

Assessment: History and Examination

- Allergies to metronidazole, renal or liver dysfunction
- Concurrent use of barbiturates, oral anticoagulants, alcohol
- Local: culture of stool for accurate diagnosis of infection
- CNS: orientation, affect, vision, reflexes
- Skin: colour, lesions
- GI: abdominal, liver evaluation
- Haematological: full blood count, liver function tests

Nursing Diagnoses

- Acute pain related to GI effects
- Disturbed sensory perception (kinaesthetic, visual) related to CNS effects
- Imbalanced nutrition: less than body requirements related to GI effects
- Deficient knowledge regarding drug therapy

Implementation

- Culture infection before beginning therapy.
- Provide comfort and safety measures: oral hygiene, safety precautions, maintenance of nutrition, treatment of superinfections if they occur.

(continued)

Coping with Amoebiasis *(continued)*

- Provide small, frequent meals and monitor nutritional status.
- Provide support and reassurance for dealing with drug effects and discomfort.
- Provide patient teaching regarding drug name, dosage, adverse effects, precautions, and warning signs to report and hygiene measures to observe.

Evaluation

- Evaluate drug effects: resolution of protozoal infection.
- Monitor for adverse effects: GI alterations, dizziness, confusion, CNS changes, vision loss, hepatic function, superinfections.
- Monitor for drug–drug interactions with oral anticoagulants, alcohol or barbiturates.
- Evaluate effectiveness of patient teaching programme.
- Evaluate effectiveness of comfort and safety measures.

Patient Teaching for Jonathan

You have been prescribed metronidazole to treat your amoebic infection. This antiprotozoal drug acts to destroy the protozoal infection you have contracted. Because it affects specific phases of the protozoal life cycle, it must be taken over a period (5–10 days) to be effective. It is very important to take the entire drug course that has been ordered for you.

- ☐ This drug frequently causes stomach upset. If it causes you to have nausea or vomiting, take the drug with meals or a light snack.
- ☐ Common effects of this drug include the following:
  - *Nausea, vomiting and loss of appetite:* take the drug with food and have small, frequent meals.
  - *Superinfections of the mouth:* these go away when the course of the drug has been completed. If they become uncomfortable, notify your health care provider for an appropriate solution.
  - *Taste disturbances:* frequent mouth care may help. This effect will also go away when the course of the drug is finished.
  - *Intolerance to alcohol (nausea, vomiting, flushing, headache and stomach pain):* avoid alcoholic beverages or products containing alcohol while taking this drug.
- ☐ Report any of the following to your health care provider: skin rash or redness; severe GI upset; and unusual fatigue, clumsiness or weakness.
- ☐ Take the full course of your prescription. Never use this drug to self-treat any other infection or give it to any other person.
- ☐ Tell any doctor, nurse or other health care provider that you are taking this drug.
- ☐ Keep this drug and all medications out of the reach of children.

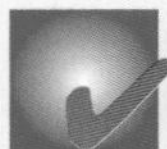

CHECK YOUR UNDERSTANDING

Answers to the questions in this chapter may be found in the answer key in the back of the book.

Multiple Choice

Select the most appropriate answer to the following.

1. Of the following protozoal infections, the one that is not caused by insect bites is
   a. malaria.
   b. trypanosomiasis.
   c. leishmaniasis.
   d. giardiasis.

2. Malaria is caused by the *Plasmodium* protozoan, which depends on
   a. a snail to act as intermediary in the life cycle of the protozoan.
   b. a mosquito and a red blood cell for maturation.
   c. a human liver cell for cell division and reproduction.
   d. stagnant water for maturation.

3. Drugs used to treat malaria are given in combination because
   a. they are less toxic that way.
   b. they are absorbed better if taken together.
   c. mosquitoes are less likely to bite a person who is taking combination drugs.
   d. the drugs can then affect the protozoan at various stages of the life cycle.

4. Which of the following prophylactic measures should a patient travelling to an area of the world where malaria is known to be endemic take?
   a. avoid drinking the water.
   b. begin prophylactic antimalarial therapy before travelling and continue it through the visit and for 4 weeks after the visit.
   c. take a supply of antimalarial drugs in case he or she gets a mosquito bite.
   d. begin prophylactic antimalarial therapy 2 weeks before travelling and stop the drugs on arrival at the destination.

5. Amoebiasis or amoebic dysentery
   a. is seen only in developing countries.
   b. is caused by a protozoan that enters the body through an insect bite.
   c. is caused by a protozoan that can enter the body in the cyst stage in water or food, usually under unsanitary conditions.
   d. has no signs and symptoms to distinguish from normal diarrhoea.

6. Giardiasis
   a. does not respond to drug therapy.
   b. can invade the liver and cause death.
   c. is seen only in areas with no sanitation.
   d. is associated with rotten egg-smelling stool, diarrhoea and mucous-filled stools.

7. PCP (*Pneumocystis* pneumonia) is
   a. a common illness in humans.
   b. responsive to doxycycline.
   c. an opportunistic bacterial infection.
   d. frequently associated with immune suppression and AIDS.

8. Trypanosomiasis may assume two different forms:
   a. African sleeping sickness and Chagas' disease.
   b. elephantiasis and malaria.
   c. dysentery and African sleeping sickness.
   d. malaria and Chagas' disease.

9. A nurse would note that a patient had a good understanding of his antimalarial drug regimen if the patient reported
   a. 'I keep these pills and take them only when I have been bitten by a mosquito'.
   b. 'I will need to take these pills daily for the rest of my life'.
   c. 'I will need to start taking these pills before my trip, the whole time I am on vacation, and for a period of time after I get back home'.
   d. 'I start taking these pills as soon as I arrive at my vacation destination'.

Extended Matching Questions

Select **all** that apply.

1. A mother calls in concerned that her son has been diagnosed with giardiasis. The nurse would respond to the mother's concerns by telling her which of the following?
   a. You should have your son come home immediately so that he can be treated appropriately.
   b. This infection is usually transmitted through food or water.
   c. This is the most common imported protozoal infection seen in this country.
   d. This infection can be treated with oral drugs, and he should be able to get the drugs where his infection was diagnosed.
   e. This is an infection that has to be treated quickly with IV medications.
   f. Encourage your son to get the medicine and to try very hard to eat nutritious food.

Matching

Match the following antiprotozoal drugs with the protozoal infection they are used to treat. Some drugs may be used to treat more than one of the categories of infections.

1. ____________________ primaquine
2. ____________________ atovaquone
3. ____________________ quinine
4. ____________________ pentamidine
5. ____________________ chloroquine
6. ____________________ metronidazole
7. ____________________ co-trimoxazole
8. ____________________ tinidazole

A. Malaria
B. PCP infection
C. Trypanosomiasis and leishmaniasis
D. Trichomoniasis, giardiasis, amoebiasis

Bibliography and References

British Medical Association and Royal Pharmaceutical Society of Great Britain. (2008). *British National Formulary*. London: BMJ & RPS Publishing. *This publication is updated biannually: it is imperative that the most recent edition is consulted.*

British Medical Association and Royal Pharmaceutical Society of Great Britain. (2008). *British National Formulary for Children*. London: BMJ & RPS Publishing. *This publication is updated annually: it is imperative that the most recent edition is consulted.*

Brunton, L., Lazo, J. S., Parker, K., Goodman, L. S., & Gilman, A. G. (2005). *Goodman and Gilman's the pharmacological basis of therapeutics* (11th ed.). London: McGraw-Hill.

Centers for Disease Control & Prevention. (2008). *Leishmania infection*. Available from http://www.cdc.gov

Howland, R. D., & Mycek, M. J. (2005). *Pharmacology* (3rd ed.). Philadelphia: Lippincott Williams & Wilkins.

Lee, G., & Bishop, P. (2006). *Microbiology and infection control for health professionals* (3rd ed.). Australia: Pearson Education.

Porth, C. M., & Matfin, G. (2008). *Pathophysiology: Concepts of altered health states* (8th ed.). Philadelphia: Lippincott Williams & Wilkins.

Rang, H. P., Dale, M. M., Ritter, J. M., & Flower, R. J. (2007). *Rang and Dale's pharmacology* (6th ed.). Philadelphia: Churchill Livingstone.

Simonsen, T., Aarbakke, J., Kay, I., Coleman, I., Sinnott, P., & Lysaa, R. (2006). *Illustrated pharmacology for nurses.* London: Hodder Arnold.

Stanley, S. L. (2003). Amoebiasis. *Lancet, 361*(9362), 1025–1034.

Stuart, J. M., Orr, H. J., Warburton, F. G., Jeyakanth, S., Pugh, C., Harris, I., et al. (2003). Risk factors for sporadic giardiasis: a case control study in southwestern England. *Emerging Infectious Diseases, 9*, 229–233.

CHAPTER 12

Anthelmintic Agents

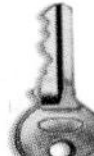

KEY TERMS

cestode
flatworm
fluke
helminth
nematode
roundworm
schistosomiasis
tapeworm
threadworm
trematodes
trichinosis

LEARNING OBJECTIVES

Upon completion of this chapter, you will be able to:

1. List the common helminths that cause disease in humans.
2. Describe the therapeutic actions, indications, pharmacokinetics, contraindications, most common adverse reactions and important drug–drug interactions associated with the anthelmintics.
3. Discuss the use of anthelmintics across the lifespan.
4. Compare and contrast the key drug mebendazole with other anthelmintics.
5. Outline the nursing considerations, including important teaching points to stress, for patients receiving an anthelmintic.

DRUG LIST

albendazole
ivermectin
levamisole
mebendazole
niclosamide
piperazine
praziquantel
tiabendazole

Over 1 billion people throughout the world have helminths (worms) in their gastrointestinal (GI) tract or other tissues, which makes helminthic infections among the most common of all diseases. These infestations are very common in tropical areas, but they are also found in all other countries. Although rare in the United Kingdom, **helminth** infections may be encountered occasionally. With so many people travelling to many parts of the world, it is not uncommon for a traveller to pick up a helminthic infection in another country and inadvertently bring it home, where the worms are able to infect other individuals (Box 12.1).

Helminths range in size from microscopic to many metres in length. The life cycle of helminths can be complex and involves two hosts: a definitive or primary host and an intermediate or secondary host. The intermediate host is the human or animal that harbours the eggs or larvae, whereas the definitive host is the human or animal that harbours the worm until it reaches maturity and reproduces. For example, in the case of the tapeworm, larvae can be lodged in beef, pork or fish tissues (the intermediate hosts) and the ingestion of undercooked or raw meat can cause humans (the definitive host) to have the tapeworm.

Many of the helminths that infect humans live only in the intestinal tract. Other worms exist outside the intestinal tract and can seriously damage the tissues they invade. Their location within healthy tissue can make them more difficult to treat.

Proper diagnosis of a helminthic infection requires a stool examination for ova (eggs) and parasites or segments of parasites. Treatment of a helminthic infection entails the use of an anthelmintic drug. Another important part of therapy for helminthic infections involves the prevention of reinfection or spread of an existing infection. Measures such as thorough hand-washing after use of the toilet; frequent washing of bed linen and underwear in very hot, chlorine-treated water; disinfection of toilets and bathroom areas after each use; and good personal hygiene to wash away ova are important in the effectiveness of drug therapy and prevention of the spread of some types of infection. Other mechanisms of prevention rely on preventing contamination of soil and water by larvae.

The helminths that most commonly infect humans are of two types: the nemathelminths (**nematodes** or **roundworms**), and the platyhelminths (**flatworms**). The platyhelminths can be subdivided into trematodes (**flukes**) and cestodes (**tapeworms**).

BOX 12.1 Managing Threadworm Infections

Threadworm (pinworm) infections are common throughout the world affecting approximately 200 million people. Infestation can be a frightening and traumatic experience for most people, especially if they should see the worm, which grows to approximately 0.5 cm. The most common visualization is eggs on sticky tape applied to the anal region.

Threadworms can spread very rapidly among children, especially school-age children. Once the infestation starts, careful hygiene measures and drug therapy are required to eradicate the disease. After the diagnosis has been made and appropriate drug therapy started, proper hygiene measures are essential. Some suggested hygiene measures that might help to control the infection include the following:

- Keep the child's nails cut short and hands well scrubbed, because reinfection results from the worm's eggs being carried back to the mouth after becoming lodged under the fingernails when the child scratches the pruritic perianal area. Try to get the child to avoid nail biting or putting their fingers in their mouth.
- Give the child a bath in the morning to wash away any ova deposited in the anal area during the night.
- Provide each member of the family with their own towel.
- Change and wash underwear, bed linens and pyjamas every day. Wash clothing and bed linen, which can be a source of infection, in very hot water.
- Disinfect toilet seats daily and the floors of bathrooms and bedrooms periodically.
- Encourage the child to wash hands vigorously after using the toilet.

It is important to reassure patients and families that these types of infections do not necessarily reflect negatively on their hygiene or lifestyle. It takes a co-ordinated effort among medical personnel, families and patients to control a threadworm infestation.

Nematode Infestations

Nematodes, or roundworms, include *Ascaris lumbricoides* (roundworm), *Trichuris trichiura* (whipworm), *Ancylostoma duodenale* (hookworm), *Strongyloides stercoralis*, *Enterobius vermicularis* (threadworm) and *Trichinella spiralis* (pork roundworm). The most commonly reported nematode in the United Kingdom is threadworm (pinworm).

Ascaris lumbricoides (roundworm)

Ascaris are also known as roundworms, the same name given to the whole group of worms belonging to this genus because these worms resemble pale earthworms in terms of diameter and length (between 25 and 35 cm). *Ascaris* infection is the most prevalent helminthic infection worldwide affecting over 1 billion people and occurs wherever sanitation is poor. Although many individuals have no idea that they have this infestation unless they see a worm in their stool, others can become quite ill.

Initially, the individual ingests fertilized roundworm eggs in contaminated food, which hatch in the small intestine, enter the circulation and travel to the lungs, where they may cause cough, fever and other signs of a pulmonary infiltrate, such as asthma and pneumonia. Upon reaching the lungs, the larvae are coughed up and then swallowed.

They make their way back to the small intestine where they grow to adult size (i.e. about as long and as big in diameter as an earthworm) and mate. In the small intestine, the worms can cause abdominal distension and pain. In the most severe cases, obstruction of the pancreatic or bile duct or intestine by masses of worms can occur.

Trichuris trichiura (whipworm)

Trichuris are smaller in length (3–5 cm in length) than *Ascaris* and have a characteristic coiled anterior end which resembles a whip. These worms are common in tropical areas and are contracted by swallowing the infective ova in contaminated food or water. The ova develop into adult worms when they reach the lower small intestine and colon, where they attach themselves to the wall of the caecum, lower ileum, colon and anal canal. When large numbers of whipworms are present, they can cause colic and bloody diarrhoea. In severe cases, whipworm infestation may result in rectal prolapse and anaemia related to excessive blood loss.

Ancylostoma duodenale (hookworm)

Hookworm is estimated to affect approximately 800 million people worldwide. Hookworm larvae penetrate the skin of either the hands or feet and enter the circulation. Once in the circulation, the larvae migrate to the lungs, trachea and pharynx where they are swallowed. Once in the intestine, the larvae develop and the worms attach themselves to the small intestine and suck blood from the walls of the intestine. This damages the intestinal wall and can cause severe anaemia with lethargy, weakness and fatigue. Malabsorption problems may occur as the small intestinal mucosa is affected. Treatment for anaemia and fluid and electrolyte disturbances is an important part of the therapy for this infection.

Strongyloides stercoralis

S. stercoralis are more persistent than most of the other helminths. These helminths penetrate the skin and the female worms burrow into the mucosa and submucosa of the small intestine to lay their eggs. These eggs hatch into larvae that invade other body tissues, including the lungs, brain and blood. In very severe cases, death may occur from pneumonia, meningitis or septicaemia.

Enterobius vermicularis (threadworm)

Threadworms (or pinworms) caused by *E. vermicularis* develop in the small intestine and the adult worms reside in the colon. The female worms lay their eggs or ova around the anus, mostly at night; and cause perianal itching or occasionally vaginal itching. Ova can be detected by pressing sticky tape against the anal area in the morning before bathing. The sticky tape is then pressed against a slide that can be sent to a clinical laboratory for evaluation. Infection with threadworms is the most common helminthic infection among school-age children (Box 12.1).

Trichinella spiralis (pork roundworm)

Trichinosis is the disease caused by ingestion of the encysted larvae of the roundworm, *T. spiralis*, in undercooked pork. The female worms burrow deeply into the intestinal mucosa of the small intestine and deposit larvae in the mucosa. From there, the larvae can enter the lymphatics and the bloodstream for carriage throughout the body. They can penetrate skeletal muscle and can cause an inflammatory reaction in cardiac muscle and in the brain. Facial oedema is also common. Fatal pneumonia, pulmonary embolism, heart failure and encephalitis may occur. The best treatment for trichinosis is prevention. As the larvae are ingested by humans in undercooked pork, pork should always be well cooked.

Platyhelminths: Cestodes and Trematode Infestations

The platyhelminths (flatworms) include the **cestodes** (tapeworms) that live in the human intestine and the **trematodes** (flukes or schistosomes) that invade other tissues as part of their life cycle. Cestodes are segmented flatworms with a head, or scolex, and a variable number of segments that grow from the head; sometimes the worms are several metres long.

Tapeworms

Humans can acquire tapeworms from eating undercooked pork (*Taenia solium*), beef (*Taenia saginata*) or fish (*Diphyllobothrium latum*). Individuals with a tapeworm may experience some abdominal discomfort and distension as well as weight loss because the worm survives on ingested nutrients. A deficiency of vitamin B_{12} may also develop and lead to anaemia. Many infected patients require a great deal of psychological support when they excrete parts of the tapeworm or when the worm comes out the mouth or nose, which may occur occasionally.

Tapeworms in dogs (*Echinococcus granulosus*) or cats (*Echinococcus multilocuraris*) can cause echinococcosis, or hydatid disease. The larvae, or hydatid cysts, can infect many animals including sheep, cattle and wildlife through contaminated land or water. The eggs may be ingested by humans during the handling of an infected animal. Inside the hosts small intestine the eggs hatch and the released embryo can enter the bloodstream and become lodged in various organs in the body, for example the liver, brain or lungs or in the peritoneal cavity. Here the embryo develops into hydatid cysts which contain the larvae of the tapeworm. The hydatid cysts have to be surgically removed. Hydatid disease can be avoided by worming animals regularly.

Filariasis

Filariasis is caused by a tissue-dwelling nematode and affects approximately 120 million people in 73 countries. The worms are transmitted to humans via infected mosquitoes. They develop into adult worms in the lymphatic system causing massive inflammatory reactions. This may lead to severe swelling of the hands, feet, legs, arms, scrotum or breasts; a disfiguring condition called elephantiasis. The worms release microfilariae into the bloodstream which are then taken up when a mosquito bites the infected person. The microfilariae become larvae in the mosquito and undergo part of the life cycle in the mosquito. The mosquito can then go on to infect another person and the life cycle begins again.

Schistosomiasis

Schistosomiasis or bilharziasis (Figure 12.1) affects approximately 200 million people in the world in approximately 76 countries, mainly in tropical settings such as Puerto Rico, islands of the West Indies, Africa, eastern South America, the Philippines, China and Southeast Asia. People who come from or travel to areas of the world where schistosomiasis is endemic should always be investigated for the possibility of infection with such a disease when seen for health care.

Schistosomiasis is caused by a fluke, *Schistosoma* spp., which spends part of its complex life cycle in a certain species of snail. The life cycle of schistosomes is as follows. The eggs, which are excreted in the urine and faeces of infected individuals, hatch in fresh water and infect a certain snail species. Larvae, known as cercariae, develop in the snail, which are released into the freshwater pond or lake. Individuals travelling to areas where *Schistosoma* spp. is endemic should be warned about wading, swimming or bathing in freshwater streams, ponds or lakes. People become infected when they come in contact with the infested water. The larvae burrow through the skin and enter the bloodstream and lymphatics. After they move into the lungs, and later the liver, they mature into adult worms that mate and migrate to the intestines and urinary bladder. The female worms then lay large numbers of eggs, which are expelled in the faeces and urine, and the cycle begins again. Poor sanitation and the presence

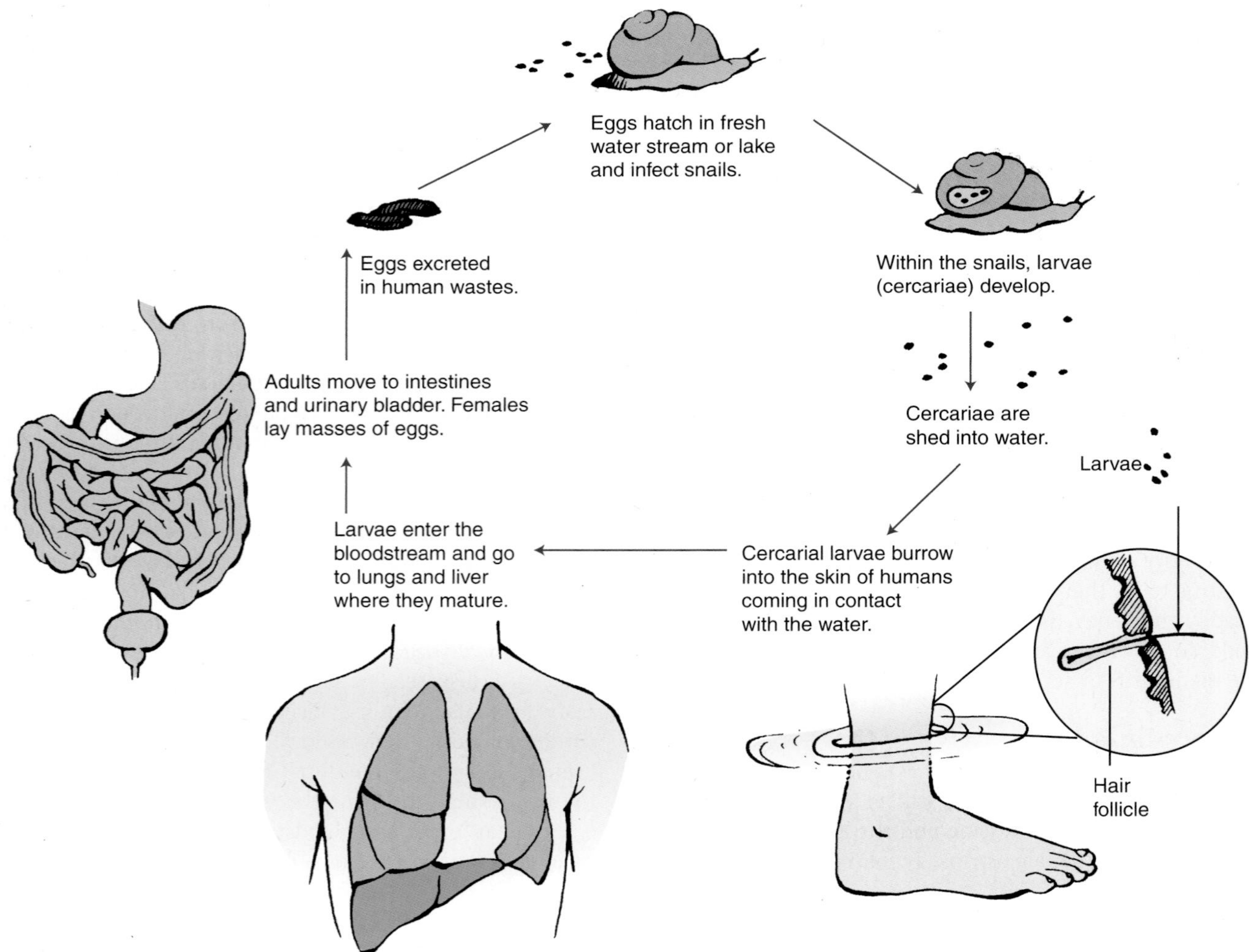

FIGURE 12.1 Life cycle of schistosomes.

of the specific species of snail are responsible for the spread of its infection.

Signs and symptoms of schistosomiasis may include a pruritic rash where the larva attaches to the skin. About 1 or 2 months later, affected individuals may experience fever, chills, headache and other symptoms. Chronic or severe infestation may lead to abdominal pain and diarrhoea, as well as blockage of blood flow to areas of the liver, lungs and central nervous system (CNS). These blockages can lead to liver and spleen enlargement (see Critical Thinking Scenario 12-1). Signs of CNS and cardiac ischaemia can also occur months after infection.

Anthelmintics

The anthelmintic drugs act on metabolic pathways that are present in the invading worm but absent or significantly different in the human host. Refer to Box 12.2 for more information about using anthelmintics with various age groups.

Mebendazole is probably the most commonly used of all of the anthelmintics and is effective against threadworms, roundworms, whipworms and hookworms. It is available in two forms: (1) a chewable tablet and (2) oral suspension. A typical 3-day course can be repeated in 2 weeks if reinfection occurs. The pharmacokinetic details are given under the key drug summary. It should not be used during pregnancy because teratogenic effects have been demonstrated in animal studies and there is a possible risk to the foetus. Lactating women are advised to select another way to feed the baby.

Piperazine can also be used to treat threadworm and roundworm infections. By paralyzing the worm's muscles, the worms are then expelled from the host by peristalsis, the natural movement of the GI tract. Piperazine is contraindicated in patients with either a history of epilepsy or renal or liver impairment. Manufacturers recommend that this drug is not to be used during the first trimester of pregnancy or during breast-feeding. Piperazine is partially metabolized by the liver and excretion is mainly via urine: piperazine can have neurotoxic effects in patients with renal impairment.

Levamisole is the drug of choice in the treatment of common roundworm infections. This drug is available on what is known as a 'named-patient' basis, meaning that the health care provider must approach the pharmaceutical company directly to obtain the drug. This is because the drug has not been licensed yet, either because insufficient clinical trials have been performed or the company has decided not to apply for a product license. This drug blocks the neuromuscular junctions in the worms leading to paralysis of the worms and expulsion in the faeces in a similar manner to piperazine. Levamisole is primarily metabolized by the liver and excreted mainly via urine. The risks during pregnancy or lactation are unknown.

Niclosamide is also available on a named-patient basis. The drug of choice in the treatment of tapeworms, niclosamide disrupts the connection between the worm's scolex (head) and the intestinal wall. Following treatment with a laxative, the tapeworm is then excreted in the faeces. Niclosamide is not significantly absorbed by the GI tract and is excreted via faeces. The risks during pregnancy or lactation are unknown.

Praziquantel is effective in the treatment of a wide variety of schistosomes (flukes) and is available on a named-patient basis. This drug has relatively few adverse effects. The drug is rapidly absorbed from the GI tract and reaches peak plasma levels within 1 to 2 hours. It is extensively metabolized in the liver with a half-life of 0.8 to 3.0 hours. Excretion of praziquantel occurs primarily through the urine. There are no adequate studies regarding the use of this drug during pregnancy, therefore it is recommended that the drug not be used unless the benefit clearly outweighs the potential risk. Praziquantel crosses into breast milk and should not be used during lactation; in addition, the baby should not be nursed for 72 hours after treatment is finished.

Albendazole is effective against cystic disease of the liver, lungs and peritoneum caused by hydatid disease and also

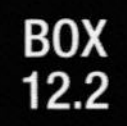

DRUG THERAPY ACROSS THE LIFESPAN

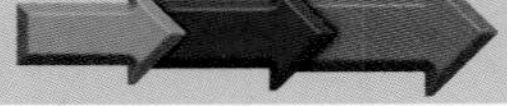

Anthelmintic Agents

CHILDREN

Identification of the suspected worm is important before beginning any drug therapy. Nutritional status and hydration are major concerns with children taking these drugs who develop serious GI effects. The most commonly used anthelmintic, mebendazole, comes as a chewable tablet or oral solution that is convenient for use by children.

When administering any drug to children, always consult the most recent edition of the British National Formulary for Children.

ADULTS

Adults may be somewhat repulsed by the idea that they have a worm infestation and they may be reluctant to discuss the needed lifestyle adjustments and treatment plans. Pregnant and nursing women should not use these drugs unless the benefit clearly outweighs the potential risk to the foetus or neonate. If a severe helminth infestation threatens the mother, some of the drugs can be used as long as the mother is informed of the potential risk.

OLDER ADULTS

Older patients may be more susceptible to the CNS and GI effects of some of these drugs. Their hydration and nutritional status should be monitored carefully.

hookworms. This drug is also available on a named-patient basis and is usually used in conjunction with surgical techniques to remove the cysts. Albendazole can have serious adverse effects on the liver and liver function should be monitored. Poorly absorbed from the GI tract, albendazole reaches peak plasma levels in about 5 hours. It is extensively metabolized in the liver and primarily excreted in urine. Albendazole has been shown to be teratogenic in animal studies and should not be used during pregnancy or lactation. Women of childbearing age should be advised to use barrier contraceptives while taking this drug.

Tiabendazole may be used on a named-patient basis to treat hookworm infections. It is most effective in treating multiple infections. It is readily absorbed from the GI tract, reaching peak levels in 1 to 2 hours. It is completely metabolized in the liver and primarily excreted in the urine. There are no established studies regarding use during pregnancy or lactation, so it is recommended that the drug not be used unless the benefit clearly outweighs the potential risk.

Ivermectin is effective against the filaricide nematodes that cause onchocerciasis, or river blindness, which is found in tropical areas of Africa, Mexico and South America. This drug also causes muscular paralysis in the nematode. It is readily absorbed from the GI tract and reaches peak plasma levels in 4 hours. It is completely metabolized in the liver with a half-life of 16 hours and excreted in the faeces. Ivermectin is not recommended during pregnancy and women of childbearing age should be advised to use barrier contraceptives while taking this drug. Ivermectin crosses into breast milk and the drug should be used with caution during lactation.

Therapeutic Actions and Indications

Anthelmintic agents are indicated for the treatment of infections by certain susceptible worms. The main drug targets are either in interference with metabolic processes or muscle paralysis in particular worms (Figure 12.2). Worms can take up to 3 days to die.

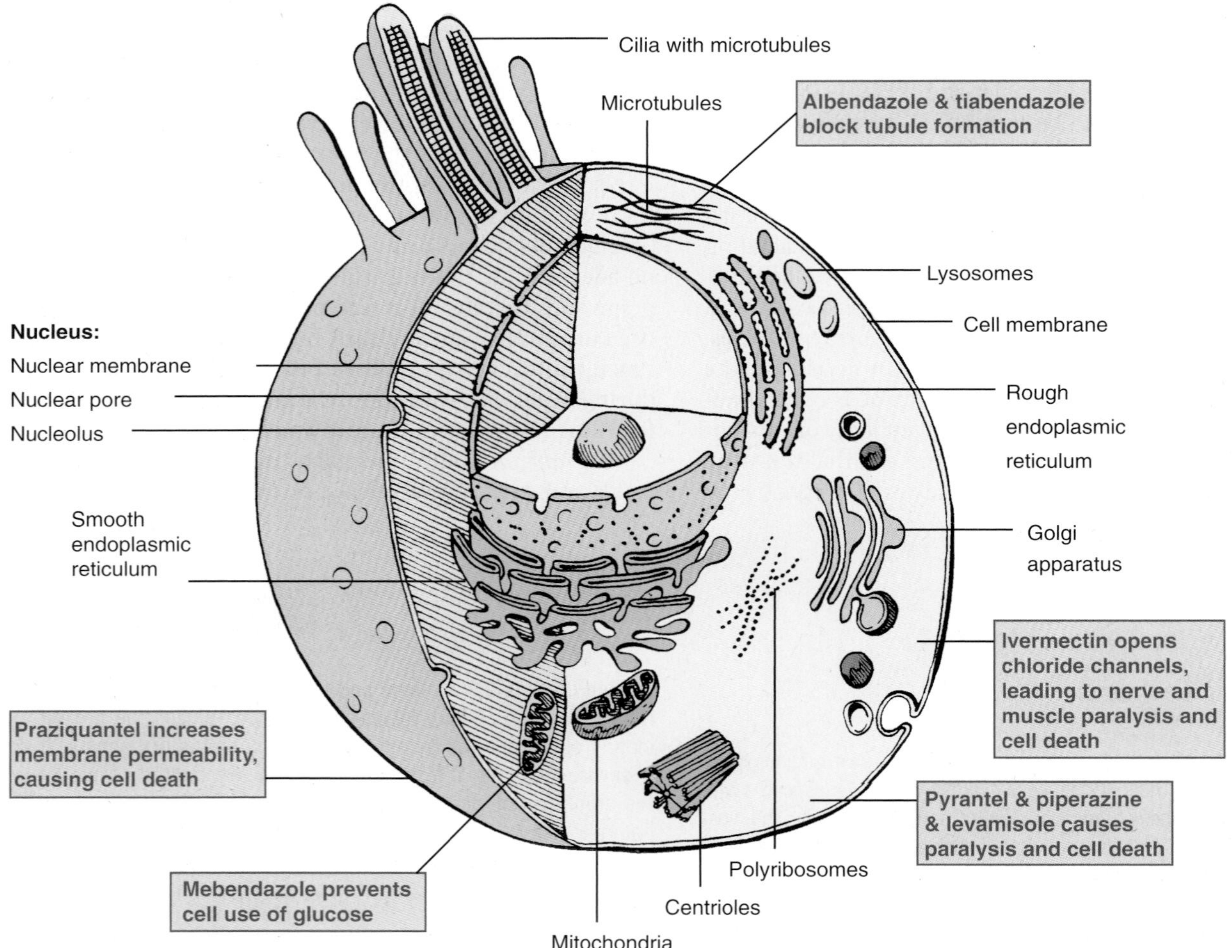

FIGURE 12.2 General structure of a cell, showing the sites of action of the anthelmintic agents. Mebendazole interferes with the ability to use glucose, leading to an inability to reproduce and cell death. Albendazole blocks tubule formation, resulting in cell death. Ivermectin opens chloride channels, leading to nerve and muscle paralysis and cell death. Pyrantel, piperazine and levamisole are neuromuscular polarizing agents that cause paralysis and cell death. Praziquantel increases membrane permeability, leading to an increase in intracellular calcium and muscular paralysis; it may also result in disintegration of the integument. Albendazole and tiabendazole inhibit microtubule formation.

Contraindications and Cautions

Contraindications to the use of anthelmintic drugs include the presence of known allergy to any of these drugs; lactation *because the drugs can enter breast milk and could be toxic to the infant*; and pregnancy (in most cases) *because of reported associated foetal abnormalities or death*. Caution should be used in the presence of renal or hepatic disease *that interferes with the metabolism or excretion of drugs that are absorbed systemically* and in patients with a history of epilepsy.

Adverse Effects

The majority of anthelmintic agents are well-tolerated and associated adverse effects are mild. Adverse effects occasionally encountered with the use of these anthelmintic agents are related to their absorption or direct action in the intestine, including abdominal pain, mild nausea or vomiting. In addition to the effects on the GI tract, piperazine can also cause allergic reactions including fever, urticaria, bronchospasm and rarely Stevens–Johnson syndrome (a serious condition involving blistering of the skin, eyes, mouth and genitalia and fever). Patients taking albendazole should have their liver function monitored.

Clinically Important Drug–Drug Interactions

Combinations of levamisole and warfarin may lead to increased plasma concentrations of warfarin, and patients who take both of these drugs may require frequent monitoring and dosage reduction. The effects of mebendazole may increase if the drug is combined with cimetidine. These combinations should be avoided if at all possible; if they are necessary, patients should be monitored closely for occurrence of adverse effects.

Always consult a current copy of the British National Formulary for further guidance.

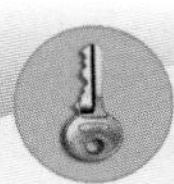

Key Drug Summary: *Mebendazole*

Indications: Treatment of whipworm, threadworm, roundworm and hookworm infections

Actions: Irreversibly blocks glucose uptake by adult and larval forms of susceptible helminths, depleting glycogen stores needed for survival and reproduction, causing the death of the helminth

Pharmacokinetics:

Route	Onset	Peak
Oral	Slow	3–7 h

$T_{1/2}$: 1–2.5 hours; poorly absorbed from the GI tract and undergoes extensive first-pass elimination in the liver; excreted mostly in the faeces

Adverse effects: Rarely transient abdominal pain, diarrhoea, rash

Nursing Considerations for Patients Receiving Anthelmintics

Assessment: History and Examination

Screen for the following: history of allergy to any of the anthelmintics; hepatic or renal dysfunction *that might interfere with the metabolism and excretion of the drug*; pregnancy, *which is a contraindication to the use of some of these agents because of reported effects on the foetus*; and lactation *because these drugs could enter the breast milk and be toxic to the infant*. Establish if patient is currently taking other medications or herbal therapies which may potentially interact with the anthelmintic drug.

Physical assessment should be performed to *establish baseline data for determining the effectiveness of the drug and the occurrence of any adverse effects associated with drug therapy*. Obtain a stool sample to look for ova and parasites *to determine the infecting worm and establish appropriate treatment*. Conduct liver function test prior to treatment with albendazole *to monitor for toxicity*. Examine skin (lesions, colour, temperature and texture) and abdomen, *to evaluate any changes from baseline related to the infection and to monitor for improvement and the possibility of adverse effects*.

Nursing Diagnoses

The patient receiving an anthelmintic drug may have the following nursing diagnoses related to drug therapy:

- Headache, dizziness, nausea, cramps and diarrhoea related to GI or CNS effects of drug (these effects are mainly limited to mebendazole and piperazine)
- GI disturbance due to worm infection
- Weight loss due to beef or pork tapeworm infection
- Anaemia due to hookworm infection
- CNS, liver or abdominal symptoms due to the presence of hydatid cysts
- Disturbed personal identity related to diagnosis and treatment
- Deficient knowledge regarding drug therapy

Implementation With Rationale

- Arrange for analysis of stool sample before beginning therapy *to ensure that the appropriate drug is being used.*
- Administer the complete course of the drug *to obtain the full beneficial effects.* Ensure that chewable tablets are chewed fully. The drug may be taken with food if necessary.
- Monitor hepatic function before and periodically during treatment *to arrange to stop administration of albendazole if signs of liver failure occur.*
- Provide comfort and safety measures if CNS effects occur (e.g. hand rails and assistance with ambulation in the presence of dizziness and weakness) *to protect patient from injury.* Provide ready access to bathroom facilities as needed *to cope with GI effects.*
- Provide small, frequent, nutritious meals if GI upset is severe *to ensure adequate nutrition.* Monitor nutritional status and arrange a dietary consultation as needed. Taking the drug with food may also decrease GI upset.
- Ensure that the patient is instructed about the appropriate dosage regimen and other measures *to enhance patient knowledge about drug therapy and to promote compliance.*

The patient should:

- Take safety precautions, including changing position slowly and avoiding driving and hazardous tasks, if CNS effects occur.
- Take the drug with meals and try small, frequent meals if GI upset is a problem.
- Note the importance of strict hand washing and hygiene measures, including daily laundering of underwear and bed linens, daily disinfection of toilet facilities, and periodic disinfection of bathroom floors.
- Report fever, severe diarrhoea, or aggravation of condition, which could indicate a resistant strain or noneffective therapy, to a health care provider.

Evaluation

- Monitor patient response to the drug (resolution of helminth infestation and improvement in signs and symptoms).
- Monitor for adverse effects (orientation and affect, nutritional state, skin colour and lesions, hepatic and renal function, and abdominal discomfort).
- Evaluate the effectiveness of the teaching plan (patient can name the drug, dosage, possible adverse effects to watch for, and specific measures to help avoid adverse effects).
- Monitor the effectiveness of comfort and safety measures and compliance with the regimen.

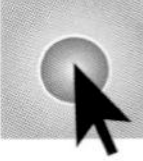

WEB LINKS

Health care providers and patients may want to consult the following Internet sources:

http://bnfc.org The BNF for Children provides UK health care professionals with authoritative and practical information on the selection and clinical use of medicines in children.

http://cks.library.nhs.uk The National Health Service Clinical Knowledge Summaries provides evidence-based practical information on the common conditions observed in primary care.

http://www.bnf.org.uk The BNF provides UK health care professionals with authoritative and practical information on the selection and clinical use of medicines.

http://www.nhsdirect.nhs.uk The National Health Service Direct service provides patients with information and advice about health, illness and health services.

http://www.who.int/ith The World Health Organization provides information on the main health risks for travellers.

Points to Remember

- Helminths are worms that cause disease by invading the human body. Helminths that affect humans include nematodes (round-shaped worms) such as hookworms, threadworms, whipworms and roundworms.
- Threadworms (pinworms) are the most frequent cause of helminth infection in the United Kingdom, and roundworms called *Ascaris* are the most frequent cause of helminth infections throughout the world.
- Platyhelminths (flatworms) include tapeworms (cestodes) and flukes (trematodes).
- Some helminths invade body tissues and can seriously damage lymphatic tissue, lungs, CNS, heart, liver and so on. These include trichinosis-causing tapeworms, which are found in undercooked pork; filariae, which occur when worms block the lymphatic system; schistosomiasis-causing flukes, which can invade the liver, lungs, CNS and other tissues; and hydatid disease with the formation of cysts in various organs.
- Anthelmintic drugs affect metabolic processes that are either different in worms than in human hosts or are not found in humans. These agents all cause death of the worm by interfering with normal functioning of the worm.
- Prevention is a very important part of the treatment of helminths. Thorough hand washing; laundering of bed linens, pyjamas and underwear to destroy ova that are shed during the night; and daily disinfection of toilet facilities and of bathroom floors periodically help stop the spread of these diseases. In addition,

proper sanitation and hygiene in food preparation and storage is essential for reducing the incidence of these infestations.

- Patient teaching is important for decreasing the stress and anxiety that may occur when individuals are diagnosed with a worm infestation.

CRITICAL THINKING SCENARIO 12-1

Anthelmintics

The Situation

Veronica, a 33-year-old female, spent several years working for a voluntary organization in Africa. Before returning to the United Kingdom, she travelled overland through Africa. Since her return 1 week ago she has not being feeling well with symptoms including headache, fever, aching muscles, abdominal pain and a persistent cough. On examination, her general practitioner noted hepatomegaly (enlarged liver), splenomegaly (enlarged spleen), lymphadenopathy (swollen lymph nodes) and pneumonia. Further tests indicated that she had chronic schistosomiasis. She was treated with praziquantel.

Critical Thinking

- What are the important nursing implications for Veronica?
- Are the other patients or workers in the hospital exposed to any health risks? What sort of educational programme should be developed to teach them about this disease and to allay any fears or anxieties they may have?
- What special interventions are needed to explain the drug therapy and any adverse effects or warning signs that Veronica should be watching for?

Discussion

The nursing staff should contact the local health department to determine whether the local sewer system can properly handle contaminated wastes. In this case, the staff learned that the snail's intermediate host does not live in this country, so the hazards posed by this waste are small, and normal disposal of the wastes should be appropriate.

Although praziquantel is not as toxic as some drugs, it does have unpleasant side-effects. Veronica should be warned that the drug could cause including nausea, vomiting, abdominal pain, headache, diarrhoea, dizziness, drowsiness and malaise.

Nursing Care Guide for Veronica: Anthelmintic Agents

Assessment: History and Examination

- Allergies to this drug, renal or liver dysfunction
- CNS: orientation, affect
- Skin: colour, lesions, texture
- GI: abdominal and liver evaluation, including hepatic function tests
- Genitourinary: renal function tests

Nursing Diagnoses

- Nausea, abdominal pain and diarrhoea related to GI effects
- Headache and dizziness related to CNS effects
- Potential for seizures if cerebral schistosomiasis are present
- Unable to carry out daily living activities due to malaise
- Disturbed personal identity related to diagnosis and treatment
- Fear related to health issues
- Deficient knowledge regarding drug therapy

Implementation

- Identification of ova and parasites before beginning therapy
- Provide comfort and safety measures: small, frequent meals; safety precautions; hygiene measures; maintenance of nutrition
- Monitor nutritional status as needed
- Provide support and reassurance to deal with drug effects, discomfort and diagnosis
- Provide patient teaching regarding drug name, dosage regimen, adverse effects and precautions to report and hygiene measures to observe

(continued)

Anthelmintics *(continued)*

Evaluation

- Evaluate drug effects: resolution of helminth infection, microfilariae are no longer present in blood
- Monitor for adverse effects: GI alterations, CNS changes and dizziness and confusion
- Monitor for drug–drug interactions
- Evaluate effectiveness of patient teaching programme
- Evaluate effectiveness of comfort and safety measures

Patient Teaching for Veronica

☐ This drug is called an anthelmintic. It works to destroy certain helminths, or worms, that have invaded your body.

☐ It is important that you take the full course of the drug – three doses the first day; then retesting to repeat this course if needed to ensure that all of the worms, in all phases of their life cycle, have disappeared from your body.

☐ You may take this drug with meals or with a light snack to help decrease any stomach upset that you may experience. Swallow the tablets whole and avoid holding them in your mouth for any length of time because a very unpleasant taste may occur.

☐ Common effects of this drug include:

- *Nausea and vomiting:* take the drug with food, and eat small, frequent meals.
- *Dizziness and drowsiness:* if this occurs, avoid driving a car or operating dangerous machinery. Change positions slowly to avoid falling or injury.

☐ Report any of the following conditions to your health care provider: fever, chills, rash, headache, weakness, or tremors.

☐ Take the complete course of drug that has been prescribed. Never use this drug to self-treat any other infection or give it to any other person.

☐ Tell any doctor, nurse, or other health care provider that you are taking this drug.

☐ Keep this drug and all medications out of the reach of children.

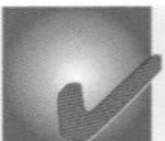

CHECK YOUR UNDERSTANDING

Answers to the questions in this chapter may be found in the answer key in the back of the book.

Multiple Choice

Select the most appropriate answer to the following.

1. To ensure effective treatment of threadworm infections, the nurse should teach the patient and family to
   a. keep nails long so cutting will not introduce more infection.
   b. launder underwear, bed linen and pyjamas every day.
   c. boil all drinking water.
   d. maintain a clear liquid diet for at least 7 to 10 days.

2. If a patient is suspected of having an *Ascaris* infection, assessment of that patient would reveal
   a. cough, fever and signs of pulmonary infestation.
   b. cardiac arrhythmias.
   c. seizures and disorientation.
   d. bloody diarrhoea.

3. Schistosomiasis is an infection caused by
   a. a protozoan carried by a mosquito.
   b. improperly cooked pork.
   c. a fluke which spends part of its life cycle in a snail.
   d. eating food contaminated by faecal material.

4. A patient has travelled to Egypt and come home with schistosomiasis. The family is very concerned about spreading the disease. Important teaching information that could help the family would include which of the following:
   a. Strict hand washing will stop the spread of the disease.
   b. Isolating the patient will be necessary to stop the spread of the disease.
   c. Carefully cooking all of the patient's food will help to stop the spread of the disease.

d. The snail that is needed for the life cycle of this worm does not live in this climate, and the disease cannot be spread without this species of snail.

5. Mebendazole is the most commonly used anthelmintic. It would be a drug of choice for treating
   a. threadworms, roundworms, whipworms and hookworms.
   b. trichinosis and flukes.
   c. pork tapeworm and threadworms.
   d. all stages of schistosomal infections.

6. Patient teaching regarding the use of anthelmintics should include counselling about
   a. the use of oral contraceptives.
   b. the importance of maintaining nutrition during therapy.
   c. the use of oral anticoagulants.
   d. cardiac drug effects.

7. Patients may experience anxiety about the diagnosis and treatment of helmintic infections. Teaching may help to alleviate this anxiety and should include
   a. what they may experience if the worms are passed from the body.
   b. focus on the cleanliness of the home.
   c. measures to isolate the organism in the home.
   d. criticism of their personal hygiene practices.

Extended Matching Questions

Select **all** that apply.

1. An adult client is being treated with mebendazole for a threadworm infection. Appropriate nursing diagnoses that might apply to this patient would include
   a. Disturbed personal identity related to treatment.
   b. Abdominal distension related to worm infestation.
   c. Itchy anal area.
   d. Risk for social isolation related to quarantine conditions.
   e. Impaired physical mobility related to muscle infestation.
   f. Deficient knowledge related to drug therapy.

Definitions

Define the following terms.

1. cestode ______________________________

2. trematode ______________________________

3. nematode ______________________________

4. threadworm ______________________________

5. roundworm ______________________________

6. schistosomiasis ______________________________

7. trichinosis ______________________________

8. whipworm ______________________________

Bibliography

British Medical Association and Royal Pharmaceutical Society of Great Britain (2008). *British National Formulary*. London: BMJ & RPS Publishing. *This publication is updated biannually: it is imperative that the most recent edition is consulted.*

British Medical Association and Royal Pharmaceutical Society of Great Britain. (2007). *British National Formulary for Children*. London: BMJ & RPS Publishing. *This publication is updated annually: it is imperative that the most recent edition is consulted.*

Brunton, L., Lazo, J. S., Parker, K., Goodman, L. S., & Gilman, A. G. (2005). *Goodman and Gilman's the pharmacological basis of therapeutics* (11th ed.). London: McGraw-Hill.

Howland, R. D., & Mycek, M. J. (2005). *Pharmacology* (3rd ed.). Philadelphia: Lippincott Williams & Wilkins.

Lee, G., & Bishop, P. (2006). *Microbiology and infection control for health professionals* (5th ed.). Australia: Pearson Education.

Murray, P. R., Rosenthal, K. S., & Pfaller, M. A. (2005). *Medical microbiology* (3rd ed.). Philadelphia: Elsevier Mosby.

Porth, C. M., & Matfin, G. (2008). *Pathophysiology: Concepts of altered health states* (8th ed.). Philadelphia: Lippincott Williams & Wilkins.

Rang, H. P., Dale, M. M., Ritter, J. M., & Flower, R. J. (2007). *Rang and Dale's pharmacology* (6th ed.). Philadelphia: Churchill Livingstone.

CHAPTER 13

Antineoplastic Agents

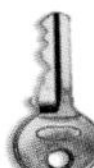

KEY TERMS

alopecia
anaplasia
angiogenesis
antineoplastic drug
apoptosis
autonomy
bone marrow suppression
carcinoma
metastasis
neoplasm
oncogenesis
sarcoma

LEARNING OBJECTIVES

Upon completion of this chapter, you will be able to:

1. Describe the nature of cancer and the changes the body undergoes when cancer occurs.
2. Describe the therapeutic actions, indications, pharmacokinetics, contraindications, most common adverse effects, and important drug–drug interactions associated with each class of antineoplastic drugs: alkylating drugs, platinum compounds, antimetabolites, cytotoxic antibacterials, mitotic inhibitors, hormones and hormone modulators, cancer cell-specific drugs and miscellaneous drugs.
3. Discuss the use of antineoplastic drugs across the lifespan.
4. Compare and contrast the key drugs for each class of antineoplastic drugs with other drugs in that class.
5. Consider the precautions health care professionals must take when handling antineoplastic drugs.
6. Outline the nursing considerations and teaching needs for patients receiving antineoplastic drugs.

ALKYLATING DRUGS

busulfan
carmustine
chlorambucil
cyclophosphamide
estramustine
ifosfamide
lomustine
melphalan
thiotepa
treosulfan

PLATINUM COMPOUNDS

carboplatin
cisplatin
oxaliplatin

ANTIMETABOLITES

capecitabine
cladribine
clofarabine
cytarabine
fludarabine
fluorouracil
gemcitabine
mercaptopurine
methotrexate
nelarabine
pemetrexed
raltitrexed
tegafur with uracil
tioguanine

CYTOTOXIC ANTIBACTERIALS

bleomycin
dactinomycin
daunorubicin
doxorubicin
epirubicin
idarubicin
mitomycin
mitoxantrone

MITOTIC INHIBITORS

docetaxel
etoposide
paclitaxel
vinblastine
vincristine

vindesine
vinorelbine

HORMONES AND HORMONE MODULATORS

anastrazole
bicalutamide
buserelin
cyproterone
exemestane
flutamide
fulvestrant
goserelin
letrozole
leuprorelin
medroxyprogesterone
megestrol
tamoxifen
toremifene
triptorelin

CANCER CELL-SPECIFIC DRUGS

alemtuzumab
bevacizumab
bortezomib
cetuximab
dasatinib
erlotinib
imatinib
porfimer sodium
rituximab
sorafenib
sunitinib
temoporfin
trastuzumab

MISCELLANEOUS ANTINEOPLASTIC DRUGS

aldesleukin
amsacrine
arsenic trioxide
bexarotene
crisantaspase
dacarbazine
hydroxycarbamide
irinotecan
mitotane
pentostatin
procarbazine
temozolomide
topotecan
tretinoin

ANTINEOPLASTIC ADJUNCTIVE THERAPY

dexrazoxane
calcium folinate
calcium levofolinate
disodium folinate
palifermin
mesna
rasburicase

One branch of chemotherapy involves drugs developed to act on and kill or alter human cells – the **antineoplastic drugs**, which are designed to fight **neoplasms** or cancers. When chemotherapy is mentioned, most people think of cancer treatment. Antineoplastic drugs alter human cells in a variety of ways and are intended to have a greater impact on the abnormal cells that make up the neoplasm or cancer than on normal cells. This area of pharmacology, which has grown in recent years, now includes many drugs that act on or are part of the immune system; these substances fight the cancerous cells using components of the immune system instead of destroying cells directly (see Chapter 14). This chapter discusses the classic antineoplastic approach and those drugs that are used in cancer chemotherapy.

Neoplasms

Cancer is one of the leading causes of death in the Western world. In the United Kingdom, more than one in four of all deaths are caused by cancer where nearly half of these deaths are accounted for by cancers of the lung, bowel, breast and prostate (Cancer Research UK, 2009). Cancer can affect a person at any age, but certain forms of cancer are more likely to affect particular age groups, for example children are more susceptible to cancers of the haematopoietic and nervous systems, whereas adults are more likely to develop lung, breast, testicular and colorectal cancer.

All cancers start with a single cell that is genetically different from the other cells in the surrounding tissue; that is there is a mutation in the genetic material or DNA. To understand how normal cells transform into a cancerous cell by the process of **oncogenesis**, it is important to first understand how cell growth and repair is normally controlled.

A number of different genes including tumour suppressor genes, proto-oncogenes and those involved in DNA repair and programmed cell death or **apoptosis**, are responsible for maintaining normal cell growth and replication. The genes responsible for repairing DNA are particularly important in (1) repairing any damage that may occur to the other genes and (2) ensuring that potentially malignant cells are prepared for elimination. Collectively, these genes ensure that cells replicate appropriately, and the potential for unregulated cell replication and thus tumour development is removed. However, a mutation to any one of these regulatory genes can lead to oncogenesis; for example damage to DNA repair genes prevents the normal repair mechanisms from occurring and can lead to mutations in other genes involved in the maintenance of normal cell growth and replication. In particular, mutations in the proto-oncogenes lead to the production of oncogenes and subsequent unregulated cell growth. Mutations in the tumour suppressor genes have the same effect.

As the mutated cell divides, the abnormalities are passed on to daughter cells, eventually producing a tumour or neoplasm that has characteristics quite different from the

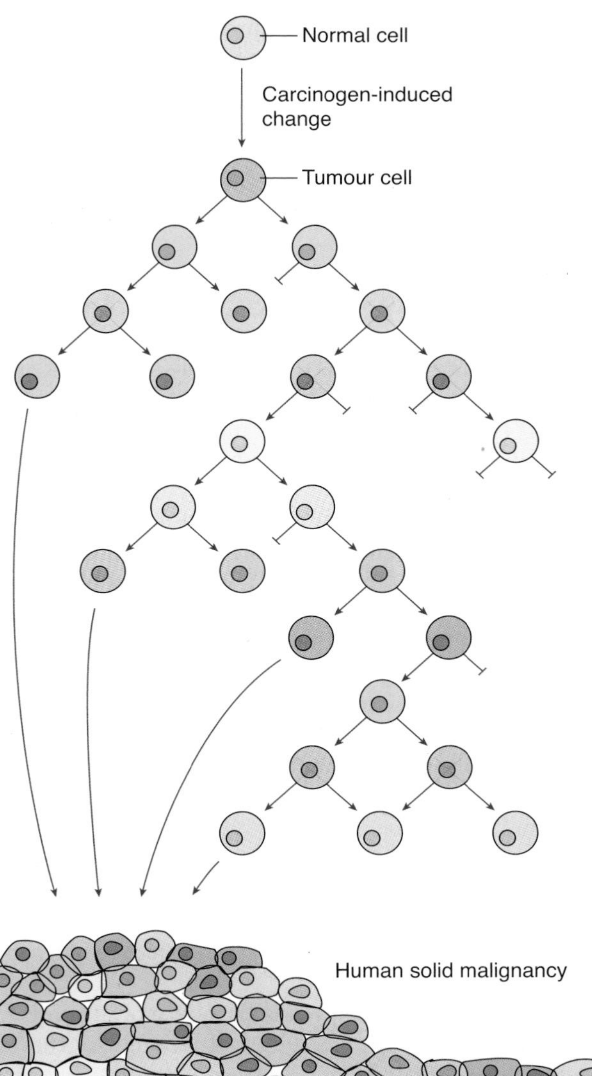

FIGURE 13.1 Tumour development from one cell, with somatic mutations occurring during cell division as the tumour grows.

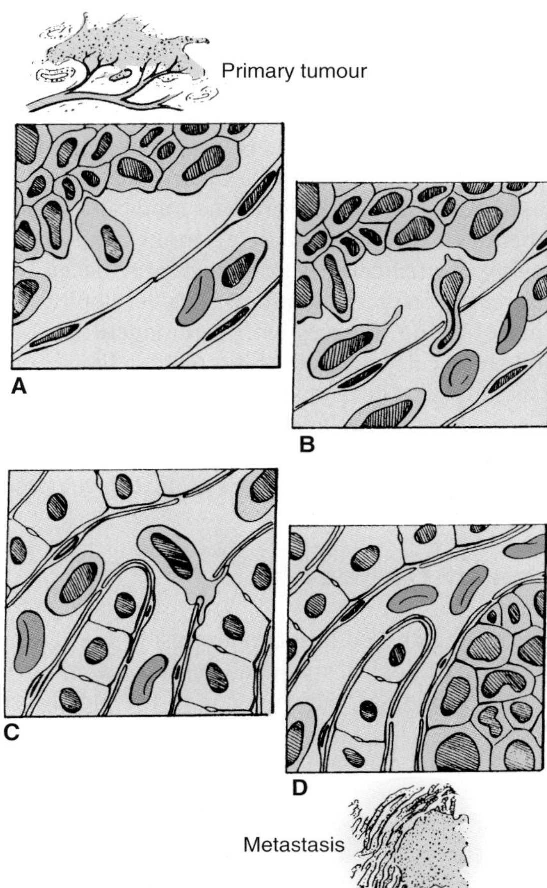

FIGURE 13.2 Metastasis of cancer cells. **(A)** Primary tumour grows and invades the surrounding tissues. **(B)** Tumour cells move into the endothelium and basement membrane of the surrounding capillary. **(C)** Tumour cells shed in lungs, brain or liver become trapped and penetrate the capillary wall to establish themselves in this new environment. **(D)** Cancer cells proliferate at the new site, which requires a conducive environment with blood supply and nutrition.

original tissue (Figure 13.1). The cancerous cells exhibit **anaplasia**, a loss of cellular differentiation and organization, which leads to a loss of their ability to function normally. They also exhibit **autonomy**, growing without the usual homeostatic restrictions that regulate cell growth and control, allowing the cells to form a tumour.

Over time, these neoplastic cells grow uncontrollably, invading and damaging healthy tissue in the area and even undergoing **metastasis**, or travelling from the place of origin in either blood or lymph to develop new tumours in other areas of the body where conditions are favourable for cell growth (Figure 13.2). The abnormal cells release enzymes that generate blood vessels (**angiogenesis**) in the area to supply both oxygen and nutrients to the cells, thus contributing to their growth. Overall, the cancerous cells rob the host cells of energy and nutrients and block normal lymph and vascular vessels as the result of pressure and intrusion on normal cells, leading to a loss of normal cellular function.

The body's immune system can damage or destroy some neoplastic cells: T cells, which recognize the abnormal cells and destroy them; antibodies, which form in response to parts of the abnormal cell protein; interferons and tumour necrosis factor all play a role in the body's attempt to eliminate the abnormal cells before they become uncontrollable and threaten the life of the host. Once the neoplasm has grown and enlarged, it may overwhelm the immune system, which is no longer able to manage the problem.

Causes of Cancer

What causes the cells to mutate and become genetically different is not always understood. In some cases, a genetic predisposition to such a mutation can be found. In some types of cancer, for example familial breast and ovarian cancer, there is a definite genetic link. In other cases, a viral infection, for example human papilloma virus and cervical cancer; hepatitis B virus and hepatocellular carcinoma, may be responsible. Cigarette smokers are at increased risk of developing oral and lung cancers because the chemicals in the cigarette smoke are constantly destroying normal cells, which must be replaced rapidly, increasing the chances of mutant cells developing. People working or living in areas with carcinogenic or cancer-causing chemicals in the air, water or even the ground are at increased risk of developing mutant cells as a reaction to these toxic chemicals. Cancer clusters are often identified in such high-risk areas. Most likely, a combination of both genetic and environmental factors leads to development of the neoplasm.

Types of Cancer

Cancers can be divided into two groups: (1) solid tumours and (2) haematological malignancies such as the leukaemias and lymphomas, which occur in the blood-forming organs.

Solid tumours may originate in any body organ and may be further divided into **carcinomas**, or tumours that originate in epithelial cells; and **sarcomas**, or tumours that originate in the mesenchyme and are made up of embryonic connective tissue cells. Examples of carcinomas include granular cell tumours of the breast, bronchogenic tumours arising in cells lining the bronchial tubes and squamous and basal tumours of the skin. Sarcomas include osteogenic tumours, which form in bone, and rhabdomyosarcomas, which occur in skeletal muscles.

Antineoplastic Drugs

Antineoplastic drugs can work by affecting cell survival or by boosting the immune system in its efforts to combat the abnormal cells. Chapter 16 discusses the immune drugs used to combat cancer. This chapter focuses on those drugs that affect cell survival. The antineoplastic drugs that are commonly used today include the alkylating drugs, antimetabolites, cyototoxic antibacterials, mitotic inhibitors, hormones and hormone modulators, a new group of drugs that specifically target cancer cells.

As discussed in Chapter 6, all cells progress through a cell cycle (see Figure 6.6 in Chapter 6). Different types of cells progress at different rates. Rapidly multiplying cells, or cells that replace themselves quickly, include those that line the gastrointestinal (GI) tract and those in hair follicles, skin and bone marrow. These cells complete the cell cycle every few days. Cells that proceed very slowly through the cell cycle include those in the breasts, testicles and ovaries.

Cancer cells tend to move through the cell cycle at about the same rate as their cells of origin; malignant cells that remain in a dormant phase for long periods are difficult to destroy. These cells can emerge long after cancer treatment has finished – after weeks, months or years – to begin their division and growth cycle all over again. For this reason, antineoplastic drugs are often given in sequence over periods, in the hope that the drugs will affect the cancer cells as they emerge from dormancy or move into a new phase of the cell cycle. Following successful treatment, there may be no detectable sign of cancerous cells. These patients are said to be in remission. Health care professionals will not use the term 'cured' because there is a small chance that the cancer may return; however, as more time passes the probability of the cancer returning is reduced.

Cancer treatment can be a long and debilitating experience. The adverse effects are often unpleasant and it is essential that patients understand the importance of returning every few weeks to go through the chemotherapy, with its adverse effects.

Cancer treatment is aimed at destroying cancer cells through several methods, including surgery to remove them, and either stimulation of the immune system, radiation therapy or drug therapy to destroy them during various phases of the cell cycle. To do this effectively, and without too much damage to the patient, combination therapy is often most successful. Surgery followed by radiation and/or chemotherapy, is very effective with some cancers. A collection of chemotherapeutic drugs that work at different phases of the cell cycle is frequently most effective in treating many cancers.

The goal of cancer therapy, much like that of anti-infective therapy, is to limit the offending cells enough so that the immune system can take care of them without causing too much toxicity to the host. However, this is a particularly difficult task when using antineoplastic drugs, because these drugs are not specific to mutant cells; they also affect normal cells. In most cases, antineoplastic drugs primarily affect rapidly multiplying cells, which have many cells in many phases of the cell cycle (e.g. those in the hair follicles, GI tract and bone marrow). Much research is being done to develop drugs that will affect the function of only the abnormal cells.

Some antineoplastic drugs influence fertility as a result of toxic effects on ova and sperm production. In addition, most antineoplastic drugs are usually selective for rapidly growing cells, so they are dangerous during pregnancy. The possible occurrence of serious foetal effects makes pregnancy a contraindication to the use of these drugs. Health care professionals handling these drugs are also at risk and should ensure they follow guidelines (Box 13.1).

Many antineoplastic drugs often jeopardize the immune system by causing **bone marrow suppression**, inhibiting the blood-forming components of the bone marrow and

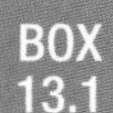

BOX 13.1 Safe Management of Antineoplastic Drugs

Antineoplastic drugs affect cell division in tumour cells and also normal cells. The effect on normal cells is responsible for many of the observed adverse effects in patients. Health care professionals responsible for the preparation and administration of antineoplastic drugs and the disposal of contaminated equipment and patient waste are also at risk of experiencing some of the harmful effects associated with these drugs (Health and Safety Executive, 2003). Staff who are either pregnant or breast-feeding are particularly vulnerable and are advised not to handle antineoplastic drugs.

The most common routes of exposure are contact with the skin or mucous membranes, inhalation and ingestion. The risk of exposure can be reduced by the wearing of suitable protective clothing including gowns, aprons, gloves, eye protection and face masks to reduce the likelihood of inhalation. Provision of a designated area for the reconstitution of antineoplastic drugs should also reduce the risks.

Only trained nurses are permitted to administer chemotherapy unsupervised. Qualified nurses must adhere to local guidelines for the safe handling, administration and disposal of antineoplastic drugs; the procedures for different routes of administration; be able to recognize and manage medical emergencies associated with administration including anaphylaxis and extravasation; and ensure that all appropriate drugs are prescribed to reduce the adverse effects associated with antineoplastic drugs. Nursing staff must also be clear of the procedure for the management of spillages.

interfering with the body's normal protective actions against abnormal cells. Other specific adverse effects may occur with particular drugs. The patient's haematological profile must always be assessed for toxic effects.

A cancerous mass may be so large that no therapy can arrest its growth without killing the patient. In such cases, cancer chemotherapeutic drugs are used as palliative therapy to shrink the size of the tumour and alleviate some of the signs and symptoms of the cancer, decreasing pain and increasing function. Here the goal of drug therapy is not to cure the disease but to try to improve the patient's quality of life in a situation in which there is no cure. The effect of the antineoplastic drugs on people of different ages is discussed in Box 13.2.

Other drugs are under development that target specific areas of the human genome. In the future, antineoplastic drugs may be able to target abnormal cells and not affect the healthy cells. This could relieve the suffering of many patients undergoing cancer chemotherapy. Some emerging antineoplastic drugs are discussed in Box 13.3.

Several drugs are used for their ability to block angiogenesis, for example bevacizumab. By blocking the development of new blood vessels to feed the tumour, the growing cells in the tumour will lack nutrition and oxygen and will not be able to survive.

BOX 13.2 DRUG THERAPY ACROSS THE LIFESPAN

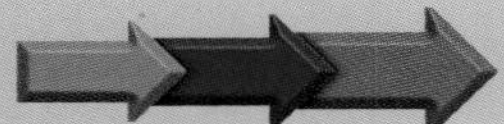

Antineoplastic Drugs

CHILDREN

Antineoplastic protocols have been developed for the treatment of most paediatric cancers. Combination therapy is stressed to eliminate as many of the mutant cells as possible. Dosage and timing of these combinations is crucial. Double checking of dosage, including recalculating desired dose and verifying the drug amount with another nurse, is essential practice when giving these toxic drugs to children.

Bone marrow activity should be monitored very carefully and the dosage adjusted accordingly. Children also need to be monitored closely for hydration and nutritional status. The nutritional needs of a child are greater than those of an adult, and this needs to be considered when formulating a care plan. Body image problems, lack of energy and the need to protect the child from exposure to infection can isolate a child receiving antineoplastic drugs. The total care plan of the child needs to include social, emotional and intellectual stimulation.

When administering any drug to children, always consult the most recent edition of the British National Formulary for Children.

ADULTS

The adult receiving antineoplastic drugs is confronted with many dilemmas that the nurse needs to address. Changes in body image are common with loss of hair, skin changes, GI complaints and weight loss. Fear of the diagnosis and the treatment is also common. Networking support systems and providing teaching, reassurance and comfort can have a tremendous impact on the success of the drug therapy.

Antineoplastic drugs are toxic to the developing cells of the foetus and pregnant women should not receive the therapy. This places these women in a difficult situation: the drug therapy can have serious adverse effects on the foetus, and not using the drug therapy can be detrimental to the mother. Education, support and referrals to appropriate specialists are important. Women of childbearing age are urged to use barrier contraceptives if either they or their partner are taking antineoplastic drugs. Nursing mothers should find another method of feeding the baby, to prevent the adverse effects to the foetus that occurs when these drugs cross into breast milk.

OLDER ADULTS

Older adults may be more susceptible to the central nervous system (CNS) and GI effects of some of these drugs. Older patients should be monitored for hydration and nutritional status regularly. Safety precautions should be introduced if CNS effects occur, including assistance with mobility and use of supports.

Many older patients have decreased renal and/or hepatic function. Many of these drugs depend on the liver and kidney for metabolism and excretion. Renal and liver function tests should be done before (baseline) and periodically during the use of these drugs and dosage should be adjusted accordingly.

Protecting these patients from exposure to infection and injury is a very important aspect of their nursing care. Older patients can be naturally immunosuppressed because of their age, and giving drugs that further depress the immune system can lead to infections that are serious and difficult to treat. Monitor blood counts carefully, and arrange for rest or reduced dosage as indicated.

BOX 13.3 FOCUS ON **EVIDENCE**

New Drugs for the Battle against Cancer

Arsenic trioxide, usually known as a poison in forensic medicine, has been approved for the induction and remission of promyelocytic leukaemia (PML) in patients whose disease is refractory to conventional therapy and whose leukaemia is characterized by t(15:17) translocation of *PML/RAR-α* gene expression. The patient needs to be screened carefully for toxic reactions, including prolonged QT interval and heart block, electrolyte disturbances, hyperglycaemia and thrombocytopenia.

A new generation of antineoplastic drugs known as PARP (poly (ADP-ribose) polymerase) inhibitors are currently in clinical trials to treat women carrying mutations in the *BRCA1* or *BRCA2* gene (*BR*east *CA*ncer genes 1 and 2 are involved in DNA repair). Women with mutations in either of these genes have a 50% to 80% chance of developing breast cancer and an increased risk of developing ovarian cancer (Cancer Research UK, 2009). The PARP enzyme plays a role in DNA repair: the enzyme binds to the break in the DNA and attracts repair proteins to the area. The new PARP inhibitors specifically target the PARP repair mechanism in cancer cells (Bryant *et al.*, 2005; Di Cosimo & Baselga, 2008). Clinical trials are investigating if PARP inhibitors can decrease tumour size.

FOCUS ON **PATIENT SAFETY**

Some adverse effects of therapy are so unpleasant that some patients may try alternative and herbal therapies. For the patient's safety in such situations, the nurse should be prepared to alert the patient to advantages and disadvantages of these therapies. If a patient has an unexpected reaction to a prescribed drug, ask whether they are using alternative therapies. Many of these drugs are untested, and interactions and adverse effects are not well documented.

Alkylating Drugs

This class of antineoplastic drugs are the most widely used in cancer chemotherapy. The oldest drugs in this class are the nitrogen mustards. Modifications of the structure of these drugs have led to the development of the nitrosoureas. Alkylating drugs produce their cytotoxic effects by adding an alkyl group to DNA nucleotides, usually guanine. The alkylated guanine nucleotides can bind to other guanine nucleotides in the same strand or crosslink with guanine nucleotides in other chains. This interlinking interferes with DNA replication (Figure 13.3). Alkylating drugs are regarded as *cell cycle-phase nonspecific* because they affect cells that are in the resting phase (G_0 phase) as well as dividing cells in the S phase

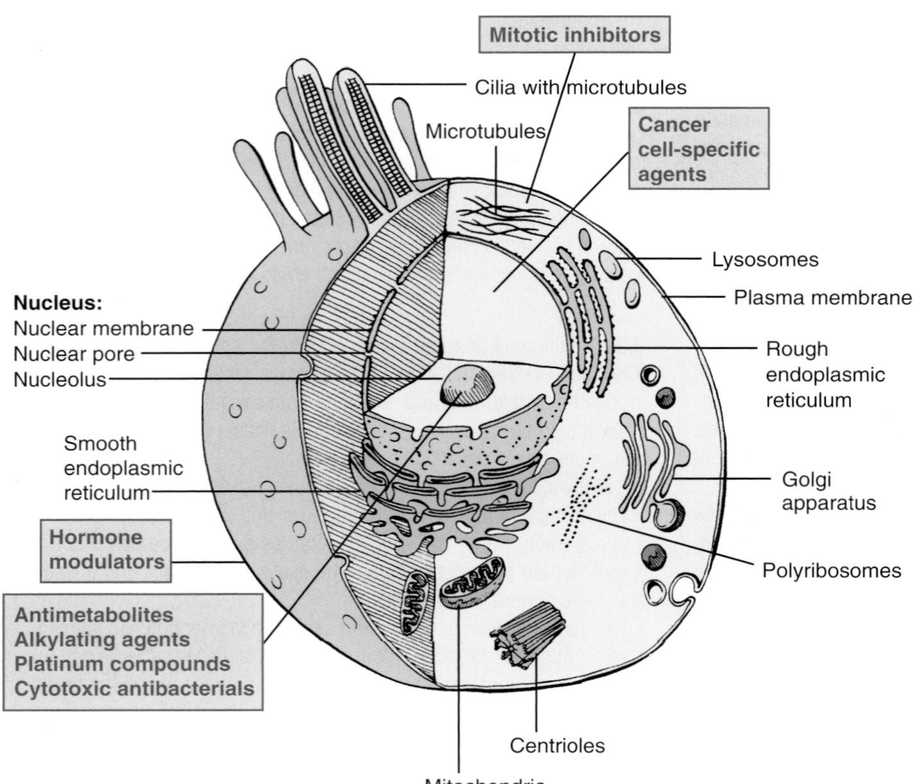

FIGURE 13.3 Sites of action of noncell cycle-specific antineoplastic agents.

Table 13.1 DRUGS IN FOCUS

Alkylating Drugs

Drug Name	Usual Indications
busulfan	Treatment of chronic myeloid leukaemia; also used as a conditioning treatment before haematopoietic stem-cell transplantation **Special considerations:** Dosing monitored by effects on bone marrow; can induce hepatoxicity; alopecia is common
carmustine	Treatment of brain tumours, non-Hodgkin's lymphomas and multiple myelomas; available in implantable form for treatment of glioblastoma **Special considerations:** Dosage determined by bone marrow toxicity
chlorambucil	Treatment of chronic lymphocytic leukaemia (CLL), non-Hodgkin's lymphoma and Hodgkin's disease **Special considerations:** Toxic to bone marrow; dosing based on bone marrow response
cyclophosphamide	Treatment of lymphoma, CLL, soft tissue and osteogenic sarcoma **Special considerations:** Haemorrhagic cystitis is a potentially fatal side-effect; alopecia is common
estramustine	Combined preparation of chlormethine and an oestrogen; used to treat prostate cancer **Special considerations:** can cause cardiovascular disorders
ifosfamide	Similar to cyclophosphamide **Special considerations:** Often given with mesna to reduce risk of urothelial damage
lomustine	Alternative therapy for Hodgkin's disease; used to treat malignant melanoma **Special considerations:** administered at 4- to 6-week intervals. Immune suppression and GI effects are common
melphalan	Nitrogen mustard; treatment for multiple myeloma, advanced ovarian and breast cancers **Special considerations:** Oral route is preferred; pulmonary fibrosis, bone marrow suppression and alopecia are common
thiotepa	Treatment of bladder or breast cancer **Special considerations:** Fatigue, infertility, and bone marrow suppression are the most common side-effects
treosulfan	Treatment of ovarian cancer **Special considerations:** Skin pigmentation is a common side-effect

(period of DNA and RNA synthesis); they are moderately more active against dividing cells than nondividing cells. They are most useful in the treatment of slow-growing cancers.

Therapeutic Actions and Indications

The alkylating drugs disrupt cellular mechanisms that affect DNA synthesis, causing apoptotic cell death. They are effective against various lymphomas; leukaemias; myelomas; some ovarian, testicular and breast cancers and bladder cancer. Table 13.1 lists the various alkylating drugs, their indications and specific information about each drug. These drugs are not used interchangeably.

Pharmacokinetics

The alkylating drugs vary in their degree of absorption, and little is known about their distribution in the tissues. They are metabolized and sometimes activated in the liver (e.g. ifosfamide and cyclophosphamide), with many of these drugs using the cytochrome P450 enzyme systems. They are also excreted in the urine, so caution must be used in patients with hepatic or renal dysfunction.

Contraindications and Cautions

These drugs are contraindicated during pregnancy and breast-feeding because of the potential harm to the foetus or neonate. Caution should be used when giving alkylating drugs to any individual with a known allergy to any of the alkylating drugs; with bone marrow suppression, *which is often the index for redosing and dosing levels;* or with suppressed renal or hepatic function, *which may interfere with metabolism or excretion of these drugs and often indicates a need to change the dosage.*

Adverse Effects

Adverse effects frequently encountered with the use of these alkylating drugs are listed here. Haemorrhagic cystitis is associated with alkylating drugs; especially ifosfamide and cyclophosphamide. The risk of developing haemorrhagic cystitis can be reduced by increasing fluid intake and taking mesna, a cytoprotective (cell-protecting) drug (Box 13.4).

Haematological effects include bone marrow suppression, with reduced number of either circulating white

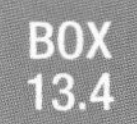

Alkylating Drugs and Haemorrhagic Cystitis

The sulphydryl compound mesna is a cytoprotective agent used to reduce the incidence of haemorrhagic cystitis caused by acrolein, an urotoxic metabolite of ifosfamide and cyclophosphamide. Mesna chemically reacts with the acrolein and is given at the time of the alkylating drug. An antiemetic may be useful in reducing the nausea and vomiting associated with mesna.

BOX 13.5 Antiemetics and Cancer Chemotherapy

Antineoplastic drugs can directly stimulate the chemoreceptor trigger zone (CTZ) in the medulla to induce nausea and vomiting. These drugs also cause cell death, which releases many toxins into the system and which in turn stimulate the CTZ. As patients expect nausea and vomiting with the administration of antineoplastic drugs, the higher cortical centres of the brain can stimulate the CTZ to induce vomiting just with the thought of chemotherapy.

A variety of antiemetic drugs has been used in the course of antineoplastic therapy. Sometimes a combination of drugs is most helpful. Drugs that are known to help in treating antineoplastic chemotherapy-induced nausea and vomiting include the following:

- Domperidone acts specifically at the CTZ and is used as a pretreatment for mild emetogenic cytotoxic drugs. This drug does not easily traverse the blood–brain barrier and therefore has fewer adverse effects on the CNS, for example sedation, than other antiemetics.
- Metoclopramide inhibits dopamine receptors at low concentrations and is especially effective if combined with either a corticosteroid or a centrally acting blocker such as lorazepam.
- Ondansetron blocks serotonin receptors in the GI tract and CTZ and is one of the most effective antiemetics for the treatment of patients at high risk of nausea and vomiting, especially when combined with a corticosteroid such as dexamethasone.
- Prochlorperazine, a phenothiazine, is an antagonist at dopamine D_2 receptors in the CTZ. This drug has strong antiemetic actions and can be administered either orally (oral or buccal) or as an intramuscular injection.
- Aprepitant blocks neurokinin 1 receptors in the CNS, blocking the nausea and vomiting caused by severely emetogenic antineoplastic drugs, particularly cisplatin. Patients at high risk of emesis are usually prescribed aprepitant in combination with ondansetron and dexamethasone.
- The benzodiazepine lorazepam is particularly effective in reducing the anticipatory symptoms (e.g. anxiolytic) associated with receiving chemotherapy.

Nausea and vomiting are unavoidable aspects of many chemotherapeutic regimens. However, treating the patient as the chemotherapy begins, using combination regimens, and providing supportive nursing care can help to alleviate some of the distress associated with these adverse effects.

blood cells (leukopenia), platelets (thrombocytopenia), red blood cells (anaemia) or all three (pancytopenia), as secondary effects of these drugs on the rapidly multiplying cells of the bone marrow. GI effects include nausea, vomiting, anorexia, diarrhoea and mucous membrane deterioration, all of which are related to the drugs' effects on the rapidly multiplying cells of the GI tract (Box 13.5). Hepatic toxicity and renal toxicity may occur, depending on the exact mechanism of action. **Alopecia**, or hair loss, related to effects on the hair follicles, may also occur. All drugs that cause cell death can also cause a potentially toxic increase in uric acid levels. Rasburicase can be used to manage uric acid levels in patients with haematological malignancy (Box 13.6).

BOX 13.6 Managing Rising Uric Acid Levels Associated With Tumour Lysis

Tumour lysis is the breakdown of a large amount of cells from the tumour leading to elevated serum uric acid levels. The uric acid can form crystals and block the renal tubule. Tumour lysis is most commonly associated with leukaemia, lymphoma and solid tumour malignancies. Rasburicase is indicated for the management of plasma uric acid levels in patients receiving antineoplastic therapy for a haematological malignancy and at high risk of tumour lysis. Rasburicase is administered either before or during chemotherapy for up to 7 days as a single daily intravenous (IV) infusion. Uric acid levels should be monitored frequently.

Clinically Important Drug–Drug Interactions

Alkylating drugs that are known to cause hepatic or renal toxicity should be used cautiously with any other drugs that have similar effects. In addition, drugs that are toxic to the liver may adversely affect drugs that are metabolized in the liver or that act in the liver (e.g. oral anticoagulants). Specific drug–drug interactions for each agent should be checked in a current copy of the British National Formulary.

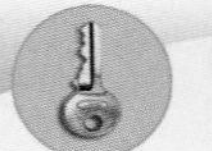

Key Drug Summary: *Cyclophosphamide*

Indications: Treatment of chronic lymphocytic leukaemia, malignant lymphomas, soft tissue and osteogenic sarcoma, cancers of the ovary, breast and bladder, rheumatoid arthritis

Actions: Activated in the liver to produce its cytotoxic actions. Alkylates cellular DNA, interfering with the replication of susceptible cells

Pharmacokinetics:

Route	Onset	Peak
Oral	Varies	1 h
IV	Varies	

$T_{1/2}$: 7 hours (for cyclophosphamide rather than active metabolites), metabolized in the liver and excreted in the urine

Adverse effects: Nausea, vomiting, alopecia, haemorrhagic cystitis, anorexia, hepatotoxicity, cardiotoxicity, bone marrow suppression, sterility, cancer

Platinum Compounds

The mechanism of action of platinum compounds is similar to that of the alkylating drugs. After diffusion into the cells, the platinum complexes bind to guanine nucleotides and form links both within and between DNA strands. This disrupts DNA replication. Of the platinum compounds, cisplatin is active against the widest range of cancers (Table 13.2).

Pharmacokinetics

Administered parenterally, the platinum compounds are bound to plasma proteins to varying extents. With the exception of oxaliplatin, these drugs are excreted largely unchanged in the urine. Caution must be used in patients with renal dysfunction. Oxaliplatin is metabolized to produce both active and inactive metabolites; these metabolites are subsequently excreted in the urine.

Contraindications and Cautions

These drugs are contraindicated during pregnancy and breast-feeding because of the potential harm to the foetus or neonate. Caution should be used when giving platinum compounds to any individual with a known allergy to any of the platinum compounds; or with suppressed renal function, *because of the potential for further damage to kidney function.*

Adverse Effects

In addition to the adverse effects associated with other cytotoxic drugs, that is nausea, vomiting and alopecia; the platinum compounds can also cause nephrotoxicity (particularly cisplatin), ototoxicity and peripheral neuropathies.

Clinically Important Drug–Drug Interactions

There is an increased risk of nephrotoxicity and ototoxicity when platinum compounds are administered with diuretics or antibiotics. There is also a risk of pulmonary toxicity if taken with other cytotoxic drugs, specifically bleomycin and methotrexate.

Always consult a current copy of the British National Formulary for further guidance.

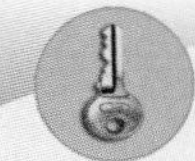

Key Drug Summary: *Cisplatin*

Indications: Single or combination therapy for testicular, lung, cervical, bladder, head and neck and ovarian cancers

Actions: Prevents DNA replication in susceptible cells. A cell cycle-phase nonspecific antineoplastic drug

Pharmacokinetics:

Route	Onset	Peak
IV	Varies	20–30 min

$T_{1/2}$: initially 25–50 minutes, and then 58–73 hours; excreted mainly in urine

Adverse effects: Nausea, vomiting, alopecia, nephrotoxicity, ototoxicity, peripheral neuropathy, bone marrow suppression, electrolyte imbalances (magnesium and calcium), sterility

Table 13.2 DRUGS IN FOCUS

Platinum Compounds

Drug Name	Usual Indications
carboplatin	Treatment of advanced ovarian cancer and small-cell lung cancer **Special considerations:** Dose calculated on renal function rather than body weight; adverse effects associated with cisplatin are reduced with carboplatin
cisplatin	Single or combination therapy for testicular, lung, cervical, bladder, head and neck and ovarian cancers **Special considerations:** Neurotoxic (ototoxicity), nephrotoxic (requires renal monitoring) and can cause serious hypersensitivity reactions. Premedicate with antiemetics and dexamethasone
oxaliplatin	Treatment of metastatic carcinoma of the colon or rectum when disease progresses after standard therapy. Combined with fluorouracil and folinic acid **Special considerations:** As for cisplatin

Antimetabolites

Antimetabolites are drugs that have chemical structures similar to those of various natural metabolites that are necessary for the growth and division of rapidly growing neoplastic cells and normal cells. Antimetabolites substitute for those needed metabolites but as they cannot be metabolized by the cancer cells, they prevent normal cellular function. The use of these drugs has been somewhat limited because of the ability of neoplastic cells to develop resistance to these drugs rather rapidly. For this reason, these drugs are usually administered as part of a combination therapy.

Therapeutic Actions and Indications

The antimetabolites inhibit DNA production in cells that depend on certain natural metabolites to produce their DNA. Many of these drugs inhibit thymidylate synthetase, DNA polymerase or dihydrofolate reductase, all of which are necessary for DNA synthesis. Methotrexate is a folic acid antagonist and inhibits dihydrofolate reductase. In turn, this prevents the synthesis of purine nucleotides required for DNA synthesis. Many of the remaining antimetabolites are analogues of the nucleotides purine or pyrimidine (Table 13.3). These analogues are similar in structure to

Table 13.3 DRUGS IN FOCUS

Antimetabolites

Drug Name	Usual Indications
capecitabine	Metabolized to fluorouracil, a pyrimidine analogue. Treatment of advanced colon cancer and metastatic colorectal cancer; as second-line treatment of metastatic breast cancer with or without docetaxel. Combination therapy of advanced gastric cancer **Special considerations:** Severe diarrhoea can occur – monitor hydration and nutrition; monitor for bone marrow suppression
cladribine	A purine analogue. Treatment of active hairy cell leukaemia; unresponsive CLL **Special considerations:** Severe bone marrow depression can occur – monitor patient closely and reduce dosage as needed; fever is common, especially early in treatment
clofarabine	Treatment of patients 1–21 years of age with acute lymphocytic leukaemia (ALL) after at least two relapses on other regimens **Special considerations:** GI toxicity, bone marrow suppression and infection are common
cytarabine	Inhibits pyrimidine synthesis. Remission induction of acute myeloblastic leukaemias and treatment of lymphomatous meningitis; used in combination with other agents **Special considerations:** GI effects and cytarabine syndrome (fever, myalgia, bone pain, chest pain, rash, conjunctivitis and malaise) are common – this syndrome sometimes responds to corticosteroids; alopecia may occur
fludarabine	A purine analogue. Treatment of advanced B cell CLL with no progress with at least one other treatment **Special considerations:** Bone marrow suppression and infection are common. Respiratory complications are common and patients are usually given co-trimoxazole to prevent pneumocystis infections
fluorouracil	Inhibits pyrimidine synthesis. Treatment of various GI cancers and breast cancer; topical treatment of malignant or premalignant skin lesions **Special considerations:** GI toxicity, bone marrow suppression, mouth ulcers and fatigue are common
gemcitabine	An analogue of cytarabine. Palliative treatment of advanced or metastatic nonsmall cell lung cancer and advanced bladder cancer with or without cisplatin; metastatic pancreatic cancer, and combined treatment with paclitaxel of relapsed metastatic breast cancer **Special considerations:** GI effects are relatively mild; skin rashes; respiratory complications and flulike symptoms
mercaptopurine	A purine analogue. Maintenance therapy of acute leukaemias; management of Crohn's disease and ulcerative colitis **Special considerations:** Bone marrow toxicity and GI toxicity are common; hyperuricaemia is a concern – ensure that the patient is well hydrated during therapy; hepatotoxicity – liver function should be monitored
methotrexate	A dihydrofolate reductase inhibitor. Treatment of leukaemias, choriocarcinomas, non-Hodgkin's lymphoma, psoriasis and rheumatoid arthritis **Special considerations:** Hypersensitivity reactions can be severe; liver and genitourinary toxicity and GI complications are common; mucositis; monitor for bone marrow suppression and increased susceptibility to infections
pemetrexed	A pyrimidine analogue. Combined with cisplatin to treat malignant pleural mesothelioma in patients whose disease is unresectable or who are not candidates for surgery; locally advanced or metastatic nonsmall cell lung cancer as a single agent after other chemotherapy **Special considerations:** Pretreat with folic acid and vitamin B_{12}; monitor for bone marrow suppression and GI effects
raltitrexed	A pyrimidine analogue. Palliative treatment of advanced colorectal cancer where fluorouracil and folinic acid are inappropriate **Special considerations:** Significant GI effects and myelosuppression
tegafur	Given in combination with uracil and calcium folinate to manage metastatic colorectal cancer **Special considerations:** fatigue, GI effects and bone marrow suppression are common
tioguanine	Inhibits purine synthesis. Treatment of acute and chronic myeloid leukaemias **Special considerations:** Bone marrow suppression, GI and liver toxicity; monitor bone marrow status to determine dosage and redosing; ensure that the patient is well hydrated during therapy to minimize hyperuricaemia – patient may respond to rasburicase

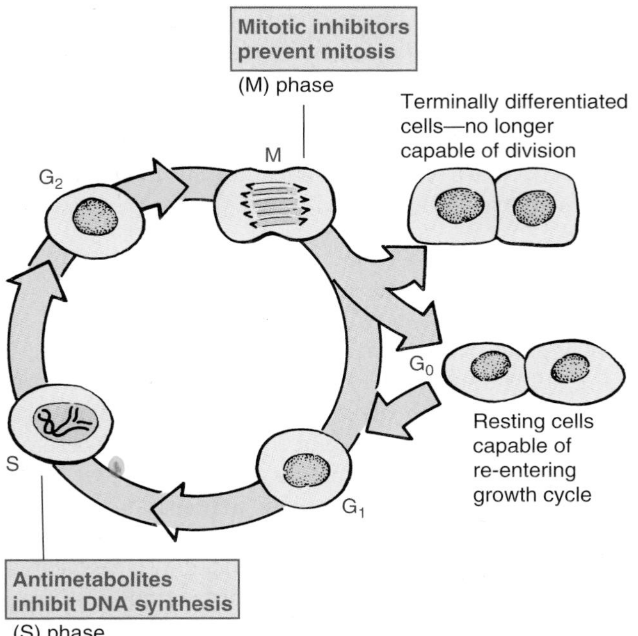

FIGURE 13.4 Sites of action of cell cycle–specific antineoplastic agents.

the natural precursors required for DNA synthesis and by substituting for the normal nucleotide they interfere with individual steps involved in DNA synthesis.

The antimetabolites are considered to be S phase-specific in the cell cycle: they are most effective in rapidly dividing cells, in which they prevent cell replication, leading to cell death (Figure 13.4). The antimetabolites are indicated for the treatment of various leukaemias, including some GI and basal cell cancers. Table 13.3 lists the antimetabolites, their indications and specific information about each drug.

Pharmacokinetics

Methotrexate is well absorbed from the GI tract and is mostly excreted unchanged in the urine. Patients with renal impairment may require reduced dosage and increased monitoring when taking methotrexate. Methotrexate readily crosses the blood–brain barrier. Cladribine, clofarabine, cytarabine, fluorouracil, gemcitabine, pemetrexed and raltitrexed are less well absorbed from the GI tract and are administered parenterally. These drugs are metabolized either in the liver or kidneys; many are excreted unchanged in the urine, making it important to monitor patients with hepatic or renal impairment who are receiving these drugs. Mercaptopurine and tioguanine are absorbed slowly from the GI tract and metabolized in the liver and excreted in the urine.

Contraindications and Cautions

All of these drugs are contraindicated during pregnancy and lactation because of the potential risk to the neonate. Caution should be used when administering antimetabolites to any individual with a known allergy to any of the antimetabolites; with bone marrow suppression, *which is often the index for redosing and dosing levels;* with renal or hepatic dysfunction, *which might interfere with the metabolism or excretion of these drugs and often indicates a need to change the dosage;* and with known GI ulcerations or ulcerative diseases *that might be exacerbated by the effects of these drugs.* Capecitabine and tegafur should be used with caution in patients with cardiovascular disease. Methotrexate should also be avoided in patients with significant pleural effusions or ascites, accumulation of fluid in the pleural cavity and peritoneal cavity, respectively.

Adverse Effects

Haematological effects include bone marrow suppression, with leukopenia, thrombocytopenia, anaemia and pancytopenia, secondary to the effects of the drugs on the rapidly multiplying cells of the bone marrow. Toxic GI effects include nausea, vomiting, anorexia, diarrhoea and mucous membrane deterioration, all of which are related to drug effects on the rapidly multiplying cells of the GI tract. CNS effects include headache, drowsiness, aphasia, fatigue, malaise and dizziness. Patients should be advised to take precautions if these conditions occur. As with alkylating drugs, effects of the antimetabolites may include possible hepatic toxicity or renal toxicity depending on the exact mechanism of action. Alopecia may also occur.

Methotrexate, when given in very high doses, can lead to nephrotoxicity and even death. Calcium folinate (and calcium levofolinate) is an active form of folinic acid that is used to 'rescue' normal cells from the adverse effects of methotrexate therapy, for example methotrexate-induced mucositis or myelosuppression, or overdose. Calcium folinate is given orally or intravenously at the time of methotrexate therapy.

Clinically Important Drug–Drug Interactions

Antimetabolites known to cause hepatic or renal toxicity should be used with care with any other drugs known to have the same effect. In addition, drugs that are toxic to the liver may adversely affect drugs that are metabolized in the liver or that act in the liver (e.g. oral anticoagulants). Specific drug–drug interactions for each agent should be checked in your nursing drug guide.

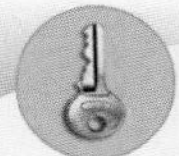

Key Drug Summary: *Methotrexate*

Indications: Treatment of choriocarcinoma, non-Hodgkin's lymphoma, meningeal cancer; maintenance therapy of childhood acute lymphoblastic leukaemia; symptomatic control of severe psoriasis, rheumatoid arthritis and Crohn's disease

Actions: Inhibits dihydrofolate reductase, leading to inhibition of DNA synthesis and inhibition of cellular replication; affects the most rapidly dividing cells

Pharmacokinetics:

Route	Onset	Peak
Oral	Varies	1–4 h
IV	Rapid	0.5–2 h

$T_{1/2}$: 2–4 hours, excreted unchanged in the urine

Adverse effects: Fatigue, nausea and vomiting, diarrhoea, ulcerative stomatitis, nephrotoxicity, temporary effect on liver function, severe bone marrow suppression, bruising, skin may darken, rashes, interstitial pneumonitis, chills, fever, anaphylaxis and alopecia (less frequently)

Cytotoxic Antibacterials

Cytotoxic antibacterials are not selective for bacterial cells; they are also toxic to human cells. Because these drugs tend to be more toxic to cells that are multiplying rapidly, they are useful in the treatment of certain cancers. These cell cycle phase nonspecific drugs interfere with cellular DNA transcription and causing cell death (see Figure 13.4). Some cytotoxic antibacterials break up DNA links, and others prevent DNA synthesis. Like other cytotoxic drugs, the main adverse effects are seen in cells that multiply rapidly: cells in the bone marrow, GI tract and skin.

Therapeutic Actions and Indications

The cytotoxic antibacterials interfere with DNA synthesis by inserting themselves between guanine–cytosine base pairs in the DNA chain. This intercalation process prevents the uncoiling of the DNA helix by the enzyme topoisomerase II. This enzyme normally breaks the bonds between the strands, allowing the DNA to unwind in preparation for DNA transcription by RNA polymerase. By preventing the strands from unwinding, the process of replication is prevented. Topoisomerase II is also responsible for ligating or 'sticking together' DNA strands, an important step in DNA replication and repair. These cytotoxic antibacterials also prevent broken DNA strands from resealing which leads to cell death.

Table 13.4 lists the cytotoxic antibacterials, their indications and specific information about each drug. These drugs

Table 13.4 DRUGS IN FOCUS

Cytotoxic Antibacterials

Drug Name	Usual Indications
bleomycin	Palliative treatment of metastatic germ cell cancer and non-Hodgkin's lymphoma **Special considerations:** Severe skin and hypersensitivity (fevers and chills) reactions may occur; pulmonary fibrosis can be a serious problem – baseline and periodic chest radiographs and pulmonary function tests are necessary. Does not cause bone marrow suppression
dactinomycin	Part of combination drug regimen in the treatment of a variety of paediatric cancers; potentiates the effects of radiation therapy **Special considerations:** Bone marrow suppression and GI toxicity, which may be severe, limit the dose; local extravasation can cause necrosis: infusion should be stopped and the area aspirated
daunorubicin	Treatment of acute leukaemias; available in a liposomal form for treatment of AIDS-associated Kaposi's sarcoma **Special considerations:** Complete alopecia is common, and GI toxicity and bone marrow suppression may also occur; severe necrosis may occur at sites of local extravasation
doxorubicin	Treatment of a number of acute leukaemias, Hodgkin's and non-Hodgkin's lymphomas, paediatric malignancies and bladder cancer **Special considerations:** Complete alopecia is common; GI toxicity and bone suppression may occur; severe necrosis may occur at sites of local extravasation; toxicity is dose related – an accurate record of each dose received is important in determining dosage. Cardiotoxicity can occur with higher doses and cardiac function should be monitored before and after treatment
epirubicin	Treatment of breast, ovarian, stomach and bowel cancer **Special considerations:** May cause cardiotoxicity and delayed cardiomyopathy; monitor for myelosuppression and hyperuricaemia; severe local cellulitis and tissue necrosis can occur with extravasation
idarubicin	Combination therapy for treatment of haematological malignancies and second-line treatment of breast cancer **Special considerations:** May cause severe bone marrow suppression, which dictates dosage; associated with cardiac toxicity, which can be severe; GI toxicity and local necrosis with extravasation are also common; it is essential to monitor heart and bone marrow function to protect the patient from potentially fatal adverse effects
mitomycin	Treatment of disseminated adenocarcinoma of the stomach and pancreas; breast and bladder cancers **Special considerations:** Severe pulmonary toxicity, alopecia, and injection site, renal and GI toxicity occur. Haematological indices should be monitored
mitoxantrone	Treatment of adult nonlymphocytic leukaemias, non-Hodgkin's lymphoma and metastatic breast cancer **Special considerations:** Severe bone marrow suppression may occur and limits dosage; alopecia, GI toxicity and congestive heart failure can occur; monitor bone marrow activity and cardiac activity to adjust dosage or discontinue drug as needed

should not be used in conjunction with radiotherapy because the cumulative toxic effects of both forms of treatment are significant. Their potentially serious adverse effects may limit their usefulness in patients with pre-existing diseases and in those who are debilitated and therefore more susceptible to these effects.

Pharmacokinetics

The cytotoxic antibacterials are not well absorbed from the GI tract and are given IV or injected into specific sites. They are metabolized in the liver (sometimes to produce active metabolites) and excreted in the urine at various rates. Many of them have very long half-lives (45 hours for idarubicin, more than 5 days for mitoxantrone). Daunorubicin and doxorubicin do not cross the blood–brain barrier, but they are widely distributed in the body and are taken up by the heart, lungs, kidneys and spleen.

Contraindications and Cautions

All of cytotoxic antibacterials are contraindicated for use during pregnancy and lactation because of the potential risk to the foetus and neonate. Caution should be used when giving cytotoxic antibacterials to an individual with a known allergy to the antibacterials or related antibacterials. Care should also be taken in patients with the following conditions: bone marrow suppression, *which is often the index for redosing and dosing levels;* suppressed renal or hepatic function, *which might interfere with the metabolism or excretion of these drugs and often indicates a need to change the dosage;* and pulmonary problems with bleomycin or mitomycin, or cardiac problems with doxorubicin, idarubicin or mitoxantrone, *which are specifically toxic to these systems.*

The cytotoxic antibacterials are particularly irritating and direct skin contact should be avoided. Health care professionals can minimize the personal risk by wearing protective clothing (including gloves and eye protection) and ensuring the drug vials and syringes are disposed of appropriately.

Adverse Effects

Adverse effects frequently encountered with the use of these antibacterials include bone marrow suppression, with leukopenia, thrombocytopenia, anaemia and pancytopenia, secondary to the effects of the drugs on the rapidly multiplying cells of the bone marrow. Toxic GI effects include nausea, vomiting, anorexia, diarrhoea and mucositis, all of which are related to drug effects on the rapidly multiplying cells of the GI tract. As with the alkylating drugs and antimetabolites, effects of cytotoxic antibacterials may include renal or hepatic toxicity, depending on the exact mechanism of action. Specific drugs are also toxic to the heart, for example doxorubicin, epirubicin; and lungs, for example bleomycin, mitomycin. Alopecia may also occur.

Cytotoxic antibacterials can cause severe tissue necrosis if extravasation occurs (Box 13.7). Dexrazoxane is a powerful intracellular chelating agent and can be used to treat extravasation associated with these drugs. In addition, dexrazoxane can also protect the cardiotoxicity associated with doxorubicin.

BOX 13.7 FOCUS ON **CLINICAL SKILLS**

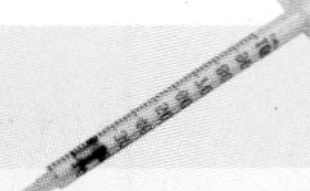

Preventing and Treating Extravasation

Many antineoplastic drugs are delivered parenterally, for example via an IV infusion. Extravasation occurs when the injected drug infiltrates into the tissues surrounding the vein. When an IV antineoplastic drug extravasates, serious tissue damage can occur. These drugs are toxic to cells, and the resulting tissue injury can result in severe pain, scarring, nerve and muscle damage, infection, and in very severe cases require amputation of the limb.

Prevention is the best way to deal with extravasation. Interventions that can help to prevent extravasation include the following: use a central line known as a Hickman catheter rather than a peripheral vein; avoid small veins on the wrist or digits; never use an existing line unless it is clearly open and running well; monitor for any sign of extravasation by checking the site frequently and asking the patient to report any discomfort in the area.

If extravasation does occur, local guidelines for the management of extravasation should be followed and specialist advice sought. In all cases, the infusion should be stopped and the cannula left in place so that as much of the drug can be aspirated as possible. There are specific antidotes available to use with some antineoplastic drugs which are usually administered through the same IV line to allow infiltration of the tissue. Corticosteroids can be used to reduce the inflammation as can cold compresses. Analgesics may also be required for pain relief.

Clinically Important Drug–Drug Interactions

Cytotoxic antibacterials that are known to cause hepatic or renal toxicity should be used with care with any other drugs known to have the same effect. Drugs that result in toxicity to the heart or lungs should be used with caution with any other drugs with the same toxicity.

Always consult a current copy of the British National Formulary for further guidance.

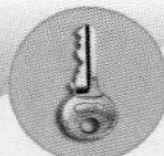

Key Drug Summary: *Doxorubicin*

Indications: To produce regression in acute leukaemias, Hodgkin's and non-Hodgkin's lymphomas, paediatric malignancies and bladder cancer

Actions: Binds to DNA and inhibits DNA synthesis in susceptible cells, causing cell death; also prevents the resealing of breaks in the DNA caused by the enzyme topoisomerase II

Pharmacokinetics:

Route	Onset	Peak
IV	Rapid	2 h

$T_{1/2}$: 12 minutes, then 3.3 hours, then 29.6 hours; metabolized in the liver to the active metabolite doxorubicinol; metabolites excreted in the bile, faeces and urine

Adverse effects: Cardiac toxicity (congestive heart failure, arrhythmias), complete but reversible alopecia, nausea, vomiting, mucositis, red-coloured urine, myelosuppression, fever, chills, rash (e.g. hand–foot syndrome)

Mitotic Inhibitors

Mitotic inhibitors are naturally occurring substances that kill cells as the process of mitosis begins (see Figure 13.4). The *vinca alkaloids* (vinblastine, vincristine and vindesine [vinorelbine is a semisynthetic alkaloid]) and *taxanes* (docetaxel and pacliataxel) have the same mechanism of action and inhibit DNA synthesis.

Therapeutic Actions and Indications

The mitotic inhibitors interfere with the ability of a cell to divide in different ways. The vinca alkaloids bind to the protein tubulin and prevent tubulin from polymerizing into microtubules. Inhibiting this step in the M phase of the cell cycle blocks DNA synthesis, causing cell death. The taxanes also act on microtubules, but promote microtubule formation and then prevent their breakdown. By suspending microtubules in this state, mitosis cannot take place. Etoposide prevents cell division in a similar way to doxorubicin by binding to topoisomerase II and causing breaks in the DNA strands. Table 13.5 lists the mitotic inhibitors, their indications, and specific information about each drug. These drugs are not interchangeable and each has a specific use.

Pharmacokinetics

Generally, these drugs are not well absorbed from the GI tract and are usually given intravenously. Oral formulations of

Table 13.5 DRUGS IN FOCUS

Mitotic Inhibitors

Drug Name	Usual Indications
docetaxel	Treatment of advanced metastatic breast cancer together with other antineoplastic agents, second-line treatment of nonsmall cell lung cancer, hormone-resistant prostate cancer, gastric adenocarcinoma and head and neck cancer **Special considerations:** Monitor patient closely for hypersensitivity reactions; severe fluid retention can occur – premedicate with dexamethasone and monitor for weight gain
etoposide	Treatment of testicular cancers refractory to other agents; nonsmall cell lung carcinomas and lymphomas **Special considerations:** Fatigue, GI toxicity, bone marrow depression and alopecia are common side-effects; avoid direct skin contact with the drug, use protective clothing and goggles; monitor bone marrow function to adjust dosage; rapid fall in blood pressure can occur during IV infusion – monitor patient carefully. Take steps to prevent extravasation
paclitaxel	Treatment of advanced ovarian cancer in combination with cisplatin and metastatic breast cancer where first-line treatment was unsuccessful; in combination with cisplatin to treat nonsmall cell lung cancer; and advanced AIDS-related Kaposi's sarcoma **Special considerations:** Anaphylaxis and severe hypersensitivity reactions have occurred – premedicate with a corticosteroid, antihistamine and an histamine H_2 antagonist; monitor very closely during administration; also monitor for bone marrow suppression; cardiotoxicity and neuropathies have occurred
vinblastine	Treatment of various leukaemias, lymphomas and sarcomas (including Kaposi's); breast, lung and bladder cancer **Special considerations:** For IV administration only. GI toxicity, CNS effects (e.g. paraesthesia), and total loss of hair are common; antiemetics may help; monitor injection sites for reactions. Avoid contact with the drug
vincristine	Treatment of acute leukaemia, various lymphomas and sarcomas (lung and breast) **Special considerations:** For IV administration only. Extensive CNS effects are common (including sensory loss, paraesthesia and constipation); GI toxicity, bronchospasm, local irritation at injection IV site, and hair loss commonly occur; can cause temporary bladder incontinence. Avoid contact with the drug
vindesine	Treatment of acute lymphoblastic leukaemia and lung cancer. Less frequently used for melanoma or breast cancer **Special considerations:** For IV administration only. GI toxicity, paralytic ileus, hair loss and bone marrow suppression are common. Bronchospasm and CNS toxicity can also occur. Cardiac function must be monitored regularly. Avoid contact with the drug
vinorelbine	Treatment of unresectable advanced nonsmall cell lung cancer; second-line treatment of advanced breast cancer where cytotoxic antibiotics have failed **Special considerations:** For IV administration only. GI and CNS toxicity are common; total loss of hair, local reaction at injection site, and bone marrow depression also occur. Antiemetics may be helpful if reaction is severe. Administered on a weekly basis: prepare a calendar with return dates. Avoid contact with the drug

etoposide and vinorelbine are available. They are metabolized in the liver and excreted primarily in the faeces, making them safer for use in patients with renal impairment than those antineoplastic drugs that are cleared through the kidney.

Contraindications and Cautions

Mitotic inhibitors should not be used during pregnancy or lactation because of the potential risk to the foetus or neonate. Caution should be used when giving these drugs to anyone with a known allergy to the drug or related drugs. Care should also be taken in patients with the following conditions: bone marrow suppression, *which is often the index for redosing and dosing levels*; hepatic or renal (etoposide only) dysfunction, *which could interfere with the metabolism or excretion of these drugs and may indicate a need to reduce the dosage*.

Adverse Effects

Adverse effects frequently encountered with the use of mitotic inhibitors include bone marrow suppression, with leukopenia, thrombocytopenia, anaemia and pancytopenia, secondary to the effects of the drugs on the rapidly multiplying cells of the bone marrow. GI effects include nausea, vomiting, anorexia, diarrhoea and mucositis. As with the other antineoplastic drugs, effects of the mitotic inhibitors may include possible hepatic toxicity, depending on the exact mechanism of action. Alopecia may also occur. These drugs also cause necrosis and cellulitis if extravasation occurs, so injection sites should be regularly monitored and appropriate action taken as needed. CNS effects including paraesthesia, motor weakness and sensory loss, are more common with the vinca alkaloids. With the exception of etoposide, the mitotic inhibitors should only be administered intravenously. Intrathecal injection can cause severe neurotoxic effects and death.

Clinically Important Drug–Drug Interactions

The more significant interactions occur between mitotic inhibitors and antibacterials, antifungals, anticoagulants, antiepileptics and antipsychotics. Mitotic inhibitors that are known to be toxic to the liver or the CNS should be used with care with any other drugs known to have the same adverse effect. A current copy of the British National Formulary should be consulted for further guidance on specific drug–drug interactions for each agent.

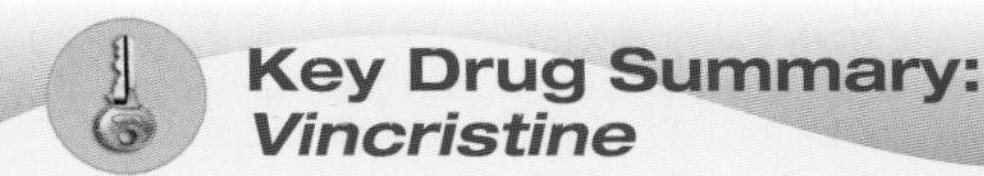

Key Drug Summary: *Vincristine*

Indications: Acute leukaemia, Hodgkin's disease, non-Hodgkin's lymphoma, breast and lung cancer

Actions: Arrests mitotic division at the stage of metaphase through the inhibition of microtubule formation

Pharmacokinetics:

Route	Onset	Peak
IV	Varies	15–30 min

$T_{1/2}$: 5 minutes, then 2.3 hours, then 85 hours; metabolized in the liver and excreted in the faeces and urine

Adverse effects: Abdominal cramps, constipation, peripheral neuropathy, fatigue, leukopenia and reduced resistance to fight infection, bruising, anaemia, possible alopecia

Hormones and Hormone Modulators

Some cancers, particularly those involving the breast tissue, ovaries, uterus, prostate and testes, are sensitive to hormones and may be dependent on the presence of a hormone. For example, oestrogen receptor sites on breast tumour cells can react with circulating oestrogen, stimulating the tumour cells to grow and divide. Several antineoplastic drugs are used to block or interfere with these receptor sites so as to prevent growth of the cancer and in some situations to actually cause cell death. Some hormones are used to block the release of gonadotrophic hormones in breast or prostate cancer if the tumours are responsive to gonadotrophic hormones.

Therapeutic Actions and Indications

The hormones and hormone modulators used as antineoplastics are receptor site-specific or hormone-specific to block the stimulation of growing cancer cells that are sensitive to the presence of that hormone (see Figure 13.3). Table 13.6 lists the hormones and hormone modulators, their uses and specific information about each drug. These drugs are mainly indicated for the treatment of breast cancer in postmenopausal women. In particular, tamoxifen is used to treat cancer cells which overexpress receptors for oestrogen.

Other drugs are indicated for the treatment of prostatic cancers that are dependent on the hormone testosterone, for example goserelin. Goserelin, a gonadotrophin-releasing hormone analogue, initially increases the release of luteinizing hormone from the pituitary gland and stimulates testosterone production. Long-term administration of goserelin leads to a decline in luteinizing hormone levels through a negative feedback system. Consequently, testosterone production is reduced and the stimulus for tumour growth is removed.

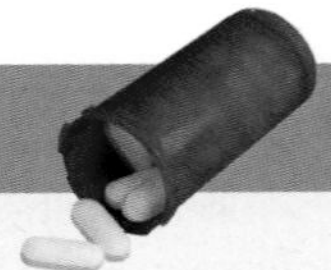

Table 13.6 DRUGS IN FOCUS

Hormones and Hormone Modulators

Drug Name	Usual Indications
anastrazole	Adjuvant treatment of breast cancer in postmenopausal women either alone or after tamoxifen therapy; treatment of postmenopausal women with advanced breast cancer. Tumours must be oestrogen-receptor positive **Actions:** Antioestrogen drug; an aromatase inhibitor which blocks oestrogen production without effects on adrenal hormones **Special considerations:** GI effects, signs and symptoms of menopause – hot flushes, mood swings, oedema, vaginal dryness and itching; bone pain and fractures, and back pain, treatable with analgesics, may also occur; monitor lipid concentrations in patients at risk for high cholesterol level
bicalutamide	In combination with a gonadorelin analogue or surgical castration for the treatment of advanced prostate cancer; sole or combined therapy for the treatment of locally advanced prostate cancer **Actions:** Antiandrogen drug that competitively binds androgen receptor sites **Special considerations:** Gynaecomastia and breast tenderness occur in 33% of patients; GI complaints are common; hot flushes, hirsutism, decreased libido and impotence are also common
buserelin	Treatment of advanced prostate cancer **Actions:** Analogue of gonadotrophin-releasing hormone (GnRH); causes a decrease in gonadotrophin release **Special considerations:** Causes hypertension and palpitations; glucose intolerance, alterations in lipid levels, thrombocytopenia, leucopenia and CNS effects (anxiety, changes in memory, fatigue). Pretreat with either cyproterone or flutamide for 3 days to reduce the initial surge in testosterone release caused by buserelin. Monitor patients for possible ureteral obstruction during the first 2 weeks, and prostate specific antigen and testosterone levels regularly
cyproterone	Treatment of prostate cancer. Also used to reduce the sudden increase in testosterone secretion observed with the initial use of GnRH analogues **Actions:** Antiandrogenic drug, inhibits androgen uptake and binding on target cells **Special considerations:** Can cause hepatotoxicity – patients should have their liver function evaluated prior, during and after treatment with cyproterone. Withdraw if hepatoxicity occurs.
diethylstilbestrol	Treatment of breast cancer in postmenopausal women and prostatic cancer **Actions:** A synthetic nonsteroidal oestrogen; inhibits the hypothalamic–pituitary–gonadal axis thereby reducing the synthesis of oestrogen (in the treatment of breast cancer) and testosterone (in the treatment of prostate cancer) **Special considerations:** Used less frequently because of significant adverse effects, including nausea, sodium retention and consequent oedema, and thromboembolism. Impotence and gynaecomastia occur in men and withdrawal bleeding; hypercalcaemia and bone pain can occur in women
ethinylestradiol	Palliative treatment of advanced prostatic cancer **Actions:** A synthetic nonsteroidal oestrogen; inhibits the enzyme 5-α reductase in the testis which reduces the release of testosterone and delays tumour progression **Special considerations:** Refer to diethylstilbestrol
exemestane	Adjuvant treatment of advanced breast cancer in postmenopausal women whose disease has progressed after tamoxifen therapy or where antioestrogen treatment has been unsuccessful **Actions:** Inactivates aromatase, lowering circulating oestrogen levels and preventing the conversion of androgens to oestrogen **Special considerations:** Avoid use in premenopausal women, or those with liver or renal dysfunction; hot flushes, headache, GI upset, anxiety and depression are common
flutamide	Treatment of metastatic prostate cancer unresponsive to GnRH analogues. Also used to reduce the sudden increase in testosterone secretion observed with the initial use of GnRH analogues **Actions:** Antiandrogenic drug, inhibits androgen uptake and binding on target cells **Special considerations:** May cause liver toxicity, so liver function should be monitored regularly; associated with impaired fertility and gynaecomastia; nausea, vomiting and diarrhoea are also common
fulvestrant	Treatment of hormone receptor-positive metastatic or locally advanced breast cancer in postmenopausal women with disease progression after antioestrogen therapy **Actions:** Competitively binds to oestrogen receptors, downregulating the oestrogen receptor protein in breast cancer cells **Special considerations:** Hot flushes, depression, headache and GI upset are common; mark calendar with monthly injection dates; injection site reactions may occur
goserelin	Treatment of prostatic cancer and early hormone-receptor positive and advanced breast cancers; management of endometriosis **Actions:** Synthetic GnRH analogue that inhibits pituitary release of luteinizing hormone and thus testosterone **Special considerations:** Causes hot flushes, sweating, sexual dysfunction and gynaecomastia. Pretreat with either cyproterone or flutamide for 3 days to reduce the initial surge in testosterone release caused by goserelin. Monitor male patients for possible ureteral obstruction during the first 2 weeks, and prostate specific antigen and testosterone levels regularly
letrozole	Adjuvant treatment of postmenopausal women with hormone-receptor positive early and advanced breast cancer **Actions:** Inactivates aromatase, lowering circulating oestrogen levels and preventing the conversion of androgens to oestrogen **Special considerations:** GI toxicity, osteoporosis, bone fractures, alopecia, hot flushes and CNS depression are common effects
leuprorelin	Treatment of advanced prostate cancer; also used to treat endometriosis **Actions:** Analogue of GnRH; causes a decrease in gonadotrophin release **Special considerations:** Monitor cancer patient's prostate-specific antigen levels periodically; monitor bone density and serum calcium levels; warn patient that there may be difficulties voiding in the first few weeks. Other adverse effects include bone pain, hot flushes and pain at injection site. Pretreat with either cyproterone or flutamide for 3 days to reduce the initial surge in testosterone release caused by leuprorelin. Monitor prostate specific antigen and testosterone levels regularly

Table 13.6 DRUGS IN FOCUS *(Continued)*

Hormones and Hormone Modulators	
medroxyprogesterone	Treatment of endometrial cancer; less frequently used to treat breast or renal cell cancer **Actions:** A synthetic derivative of progesterone that suppresses gonadotrophin production resulting in a decrease in ovarian oestrogen secretion and removal of the growth-stimulating effects of oestrogen on oestrogen-sensitive tumour cells **Special considerations:** Adverse effects are mild: may cause nausea, weight gain and fluid retention
megestrol	Treatment of endometrial cancer; less frequently used to treat breast or renal cell cancer **Actions:** Refer to medroxyprogesterone **Special considerations:** Refer to medroxyprogesterone
tamoxifen	In combination with surgery to treat breast cancer in women of all ages; treatment of anovulatory infertility. Can prevent cancer in women at high risk of breast cancer **Actions:** Oestrogen receptor antagonist; competes with oestrogen for receptor sites in target tissues **Special considerations:** Signs and symptoms of menopause are common effects; light-headedness, headache, nausea, oedema and visual disturbances can occur. There is an increased risk of thromboembolism in patients receiving tamoxifen following surgery or immobility
toremifene	Treatment of metastatic breast cancer in women with oestrogen receptor-positive disease **Actions:** Binds to oestrogen receptors and prevents growth of breast cancer cells **Special considerations:** Side-effects are similar to tamoxifen
triptorelin	Treatment of advanced prostate cancer. Also used to treat endometriosis and precocious puberty, and to reduce the size of uterine fibroids prior to surgery **Actions:** Analogue of GnRH, causes a decrease in gonadotrophin release, leading to a suppression of testosterone production **Special considerations:** Common side-effects in females are related to the signs and symptoms of the menopause; in men, side-effects include gynaecomastia. Male patients should be pretreated with either cyproterone or flutamide for 3 days to reduce the initial surge in testosterone release caused by triptorelin. Monitor prostate specific antigen and testosterone levels regularly

Pharmacokinetics

Most of these drugs are administered orally and where this is the case, they are readily absorbed from the GI tract, metabolized in the liver and excreted in the urine. Caution must be used with any patient who has hepatic or renal impairment. These drugs cross the placenta and enter into breast milk and are contraindicated during pregnancy where blocking of oestrogen effects or any gonadotropic effects can lead to foetal death and serious problems for the mother; and during lactation because of toxic effects on the neonate.

Contraindications and Cautions

In addition to pregnancy and lactation, some of these drugs are contraindicated in severe hepatic dysfunction and those patients with a history of thromboembolism. Caution should be used when giving hormones and hormone modulators to anyone with a known allergy to any of these drugs. Care should also be taken in patients with bone marrow suppression, *which is often the index for redosing and dosing levels*, and in those with renal or hepatic dysfunction, *which could interfere with the metabolism or excretion of these drugs and often indicates a need to change the dosage*. Endometrial hyperplasia is a contraindication to the use of toremifene, *which can cause endometrial changes*.

Adverse Effects

Adverse effects frequently encountered with the use of these drugs involve the effects that are seen when sex hormones are blocked or inhibited. In women, menopause-associated effects are common including hot flushes, vaginal spotting and dryness, mood swings and depression. Hypercalcaemia is also encountered as the calcium is extracted from bones in the absence of oestrogen activity to promote calcium deposition. In males, gynaecomastia and reduced fertility are common. Other effects include bone marrow suppression, GI toxicity and hepatic dysfunction. An initial tumour flare may be associated with the gonadotrophin-releasing hormone analogues where the initial increase in testosterone production causes tumour progression. Concomitant treatment with an antiandrogen such as bicalutamide or cyproterone can reduce the tumour flare.

Clinically Important Drug–Drug Interactions

If hormones and hormone modulators are taken with oral anticoagulants, there is often an increased risk of bleeding. Care should also be taken with any drugs that might increase serum lipid levels.

Always consult a current copy of the British National Formulary for further guidance.

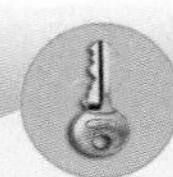

Key Drug Summary: *Tamoxifen*

Indications: Can be used to treat women of all ages with oestrogen-receptor positive tumours. Treatment of early breast cancer following surgery to reduce risk of metastases, advanced breast cancer; reduction in occurrence of contralateral breast cancer in patients receiving adjuvant tamoxifen therapy and reduction in incidence of breast cancer in some women at high risk for breast cancer; treatment of anovulatory infertility

Actions: A potent antioestrogenic agent; competes with oestrogen for oestrogen receptor sites in target tissues, such as the breast, to reduce tumour growth

Pharmacokinetics:

Route	Onset	Peak
Oral	Varies	4–7 h

$T_{1/2}$: 7–14 days; metabolized in the liver and excreted in the faeces

Adverse effects: Hot flushes, vaginal bleeding, menstrual irregularities, pelvic pain, headache, nausea, vomiting, oedema, cerebrovascular accident, pulmonary emboli, decreased platelet count, tumour flare

Cancer Cell-Specific Drugs

There are a number of different groups of drugs which fall into this category including tyrosine kinase inhibitors, proteasome inhibitors and monoclonal antibodies. Two drugs used in photodynamic treatment are porfimer sodium and temoporfin. These drugs accumulate in the cancerous tissues and become cytotoxic once activated by a laser light.

Drugs which specifically target cancer cells are associated with fewer of the more traditional adverse effects (e.g. alopecia, nausea and vomiting) associated with other antineoplastic drugs because they affect noncancerous cells to a lesser extent. Table 13.7 lists each of the drugs in this category and provides details on their uses, mechanism of action and specific information including adverse effects.

Tyrosine Kinase Inhibitors

The tyrosine kinase inhibitors include dasatinib, erlotinib, imatinib, sorafenib and sunitinib. Tyrosine kinases are involved in many signalling pathways that control the development of cancerous cells. For example, imatinib prevents activation of the tyrosine kinase receptor for platelet-derived growth factor, a protein involved in regulating cell growth and division and, in particular, the formation of new blood vessels (angiogenesis). Importantly, imatinib also selectively inhibits the Bcr/Abl tyrosine kinase which

Table 13.7 DRUGS IN FOCUS

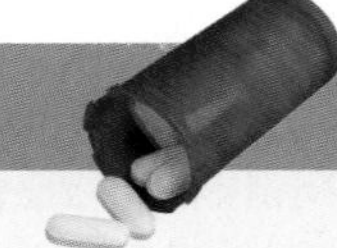

Cancer Cell-specific Agents

Drug Name	Usual Indications
Tyrosine Kinase Inhibitors	
dasatinib	Treatment of chronic myeloid and acute lymphoblastic leukaemias in patients who failed to respond to previous therapy **Actions:** Inhibits the growth-promoting activities of the typrosine kinase **Special considerations:** Many adverse effects including GI toxicity, arrhythmias, cardiac failure, haemorrhage, hypertension and oedema. Contraindicated in breast-feeding
erlotinib	Combined with gemcitabine for the treatment of metastatic pancreatic cancer; treatment of locally advanced or metastatic nonsmall cell lung cancer after failure of at least one other drug regimen **Actions:** Inhibits tyrosine kinase associated with epidermal growth factor (EGF), expressed on the surface of normal and cancer cells. Blocks the tumourigenic effects associated with EGF receptor activation **Special considerations:** Mainly GI effects, headache and rashes. Less common adverse effects are serious to fatal interstitial lung disease and hepatic failure – liver function should be monitored. Do not use during pregnancy
imatinib	Treatment of CML where transplantation is not suitable or for patients in chronic phase after interferon α therapy, or in blast crisis. Also used to treat patients with c-kit-positive unresectable or metastatic malignant GI stromal tumours (GIST); treatment of ALL: in combination for newly diagnosed ALL or monotherapy for relapsed cases **Actions:** Inhibits platelet-derived growth factor and the Bcr–Abl tyrosine kinase created by the Philadelphia chromosome abnormality in CML, inhibiting cell proliferation and inducing apoptosis. Tumour growth is inhibited **Special considerations:** GI upset is a problem – arrange for small, frequent meals; provide analgesics for headache and muscle pain; monitor full blood count, liver function and for oedema to arrange for dosage reduction if needed. Contraindicated in pregnancy and breast-feeding

Table 13.7 DRUGS IN FOCUS *(Continued)*

Cancer Cell-specific Agents	
sorafenib	Alternative treatment for advanced renal cell carcinoma **Actions:** Inhibits multiple kinases that are involved in growth signalling and proliferation. Also blocks tumour angiogenesis **Special considerations:** GI disturbances are common. Hypertension, haemorrhage, depression and peripheral neuropathies can also occur. Contraindicated in pregnancy and breast-feeding
sunitinib	Treatment of advanced or metastatic renal cell carcinoma. Also used to treat patients with unresectable or metastatic malignant GIST where imatinib has failed **Actions:** Inhibits multiple tyrosine kinase that are involved in cell proliferation and tumour angiogenesis **Special considerations:** Similar adverse effects to sorafenib. Contraindicated in breast-feeding
Proteasome Inhibitors	
bortezomib	Treatment of multiple myeloma in patients with disease progression after at least one other therapy **Actions:** A proteasome inhibitor; proteasomes are large protein complexes that maintain cell homeostasis and protein production. Without the proteasome a number of cell signalling pathways are disrupted leading to apoptosis and inhibition of tumour angiogenesis **Special considerations:** May cause peripheral neuropathies, postural hypotension and thrombocytopenia. Contraindicated in breast-feeding
Monoclonal Antibodies	
alemtuzumab	Treatment of unresponsive CLL **Actions:** Lyses B lymphocytes **Special considerations:** Associated with a cytokine release reaction characterized by fever, nausea, vomiting, dyspnoea and allergic reactions, occasionally fatal. Patients should be pretreated with an antihistamine and analgesic.
bevacizumab	First-line treatment of metastatic colorectal and breast cancer with other antineoplastic drugs **Actions:** this antibody is directed against vascular endothelial growth factor (VEGF). Bevacizumab binds to VEGF and inhibits binding to the VEGF receptor thereby preventing the growth of new blood vessels to maintain the tumour **Special considerations:** Use with caution in patients with intra-abdominal inflammation and cardiovascular disease including hypertension and thromboembolism. Can also cause haemorrhage
cetuximab	Combination therapy for metastatic colorectal cancer where other approaches have failed; also used with radiotherapy to treat advanced head and neck squamous cell cancer **Actions:** binds to the EGF receptor and prevents receptor activation, thereby reducing tumour growth and metastasis **Special considerations:** Can cause hypersensitivity reactions; patients should be pretreated with an antihistamine to prevent airway obstruction
panitumumab	Treatment of metastatic colorectal cancers expressing EGF receptors that are unresponsive to other therapies **Actions:** binds to the EGF receptor and inhibits EGF stimulation of tumour cells expressing EGF receptors, inhibiting tumour cell proliferation **Special considerations:** Can cause dermatological reactions. Patients should be monitored for hypomagnesaemia and hypocalcaemia
rituximab	Monotherapy or combined therapy of either untreated or refractory follicular lymphoma. Also used to treat CD-20 positive diffuse large-B-cell lymphoma **Actions:** Lyses B lymphocytes and also sensitizes resistant cells to other antineoplastic agents **Special considerations:** Refer to alemtuzumab. Rituximab should be used with caution by patients with a history of cardiovascular disease
trastuzumab	Treatment of early and metastatic breast cancer where tumours are positive for human EGF receptor-2 (HER-2). Trastuzumab is given in combination with other antineoplastic drugs in the treatment of metastatic breast cancer or as monotherapy when other approaches have failed **Actions:** this antibody is directed against the HER-2 receptor. Upon binding to the receptor, trastuzumab induces the patients immune response and the cell is destroyed **Special considerations:** Can only be used in tumours expressing HER-2. Side-effects include hypersensitivity reactions, GI disturbances, cardiotoxicity and CNS effects
Photodynamic Treatment	
porfimer sodium	Treatment of nonsmall cell lung cancer and oesophageal cancer **Actions:** After accumulating in malignant tissue, porfimer sodium is activated using a laser **Special considerations:** Patients should avoid exposure to sunlight for one month following treatment. Contraindicated in pregnancy, breast-feeding and porphyria
temoporfin	Treatment of advanced head and neck squamous cell carcinoma unresponsive to other therapies **Actions:** Refer to porfimer sodium **Special considerations:** Refer to porfimer sodium

is created by the Philadelphia chromosome abnormality in chronic myeloid leukaemia. This inhibits proliferation and induces apoptosis in Bcr/Abl positive cells thereby inhibiting tumour growth.

These drugs are administered orally and absorbed from the GI tract at different rates. The main site of metabolism is the liver, requiring caution in patients with hepatic impairment and when using drugs affected by the cytochrome P450 enzyme system, for example St. John's wort decreases the effectiveness of these drugs and should be avoided. Excretion occurs via the faeces and urine with half-lives ranging anything from 5 hours up to 60 hours for sunitinib. These drugs should not be used during pregnancy or in lactation.

The bone marrow suppression, alopecia and severe GI effects associated with more traditional antineoplastic therapy do not occur with these drugs. Nausea, vomiting and diarrhoea are still the most frequently observed adverse effects.

Proteasome Inhibitors

Proteasomes are large protein complexes residing in the nucleus and cytoplasm. Their role is to regulate the breakdown of cellular regulatory proteins involved in the cell cycle. Inhibition of the proteasomes by the drug bortezomib disrupts the replication of tumour cells and induces apoptosis, consequently slowing tumour growth. Administered intravenously, bortezomib is metabolized in the liver by enzymes belonging to the cytochrome P450 system. The metabolites are excreted in faeces and urine. Because bortezomib is metabolized by cytochrome P450 enzymes, there is potential for numerous drug interactions. The half-life varies with the disease being treated, ranging from 9 to 15 hours. Bortezomib can be used with caution during pregnancy but is contraindicated in breast-feeding. Renal and liver function should be monitored closely.

Monoclonal Antibodies

This class of drugs target cancer cells that express specific antigenic proteins on their cell surface. These antibodies are designed to recognize the membrane-bound proteins expressed on the cancer cells (Box 13.8). Once the antibody binds to the protein, the cancer cell is then attacked and lysed by the host's immune system. Panitumumab has a slightly different mechanism of action: this drug binds to epidermal growth factor (EGF) receptors expressed on colorectal cancer cells. By binding to this receptor, panitumumab inhibits cell activation and consequently cell death occurs.

These drugs are administered intravenously. There is limited information available on the pharmacokinetic properties of these drugs.

BOX 13.8 FOCUS ON **EVIDENCE**

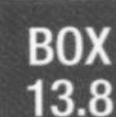

Trastuzumab (Herceptin) in the Treatment of Breast Cancer

Trastuzumab is currently the only monoclonal antibody available for the treatment of breast cancer. It is licensed for use by patients either in the early stages of breast cancer or once the tumour has metastasized. This treatment can only be used to treat breast cancer cells which overexpress receptors for human EGF, HER2. This receptor is a growth factor receptor and when activated signals the cells to grow. Trastuzumab binds to the receptor and prevents the growth factor from triggering cell growth. Between 15% and 25% of breast cancer patients are HER2 positive, that is the HER2 protein is present on the surface of their tumour cells. To qualify for trastuzumab treatment, patients must have already undergone surgery and chemotherapy (and possibly radiotherapy). Cardiac function must be monitored before and throughout treatment because trastuzumab can have cardiotoxic effects.

A number of large-scale studies are currently underway examining the long-term prognosis of patients with early stage breast cancer who are receiving trastuzumab in combination with other standard antineoplastic therapies. The HERA study (HERceptin Adjuvant study) is a worldwide study following patients to monitor the efficacy and the safety of the drug. Early results (the study is due for completion in 2011) have shown that women treated with trastuzumab and other antineoplastic drugs had improved disease-free survival rates improved by 33% to 52% (Jahanzeb, 2008). However, these are early results and the long-term prognosis of patients taking trastuzumab has yet to be finalized.

The most significant adverse effect associated with rituximab, trastuzumab and alemtuzumab is the risk of a cytokine release reaction during infusion of the drug. This occurs in response to the large amounts of cytokines released from the dying cancer cells. This reaction can cause death and current recommendations include premedication with an analgesic and an antihistamine. Corticosteroids may also be useful in reducing the risk.

Miscellaneous Antineoplastic Drugs

Many other drugs that do not fit into one of the previously discussed groups are used as antineoplastics to cause cell death. These drugs are used for treating a wide variety of cancers. Table 13.8 lists the unclassified antineoplastic drugs, their indications and anticipated adverse effects.

Table 13.8 DRUGS IN FOCUS

Miscellaneous Antineoplastics

Drug Name	Usual Indications
aldesleukin	Treatment of metastatic renal cell carcinoma **Actions:** An analogue of the cytokine interleukin-2. Thought to induce T lymphocyte mediated tumour regression **Special considerations:** Must be administered by subcutaneous injection. Can cause bone marrow suppression, hepatic, renal, CNS and thyroid toxicity
amsacrine	Treatment of acute myeloid leukaemia **Actions:** Mechanism of action not clearly defined but believed to prevent the resealing of breaks in the DNA caused by the enzyme topoisomerase II leading to cell death **Special considerations:** Causes bone marrow suppression and hypokalaemia – can lead to cardiac arrhythmias
arsenic trioxide	Induction and consolidation in patients with acute promyelocytic leukemia (APL) who are refractory to or relapsed from standard therapy **Actions:** Causes damage to fusion proteins and DNA failure leading to cell death **Special considerations:** Monitor for cardiac toxicity; do not use during pregnancy
bexarotene	Refractory treatment of cutaneous T-cell lymphoma **Actions:** A synthetic retinoic acid drug that binds to retinoid X receptors and leads to decreased cell proliferation and apoptosis of some types of cancer cells **Special considerations:** Can cause hyperlipidaemia and hypothyroidism
crisantaspase	Treatment of acute lymphoblastic leukaemia **Actions:** Catalyses the hydrolysis of asparagines, which is required by the leukaemic cells. The leukaemic cells are unable to synthesize proteins and undergo apoptosis **Special considerations:** Most common side-effects are nausea, vomiting, pancreatitis, neurotoxicity and depression, hepatic dysfunction and hyperglycaemia. Contraindicated in pregnancy and breast-feeding.
dacarbazine	Treatment of metastatic malignant melanoma and as second-line therapy in combination with other drugs for the treatment of Hodgkin's disease **Actions:** Disrupts DNA function and synthesis leading to cell cycle arrest and apoptosis **Special considerations:** Bone marrow depression leading to increased infection and anaemia; severe nausea and vomiting, and sensitivity to sunlight are the most common effects. Extravasation can cause tissue necrosis or cellulitis – use extreme care and monitor injection sites regularly
hydroxycarbamide	Treatment of chronic myeloid leukaemia; combined with radiotherapy in the treatment of cervical cancer **Actions:** Inhibits enzymes essential for the synthesis of DNA, causing cell death **Special considerations:** The most common side-effects include bone marrow depression, nausea and rashes. Renal function and haematological profiles should be monitored
irinotecan	Treatment of metastatic colorectal cancer after treatment with fluorouracil; can also be used together with fluorouracil **Actions:** Disrupts DNA strands during DNA synthesis via inhibition of topoisomerase I, causing cell death **Special considerations:** Can cause severe bone marrow depression, which regulates dose of the drug; causes diarrhoea, anorexia and alopecia
mitotane	Treatment of inoperable adrenocortical carcinoma **Actions:** Cytotoxic to corticosteroid-forming cells of the adrenal gland **Special considerations:** Can cause GI toxicity, CNS toxicity with vision and behavioural changes, adrenal insufficiency; monitor for adrenal insufficiency and arrange for replacement therapy as indicated
pentostatin	Treatment of hairy cell leukaemia **Actions:** A purine analogue which reduces DNA synthesis in rapidly dividing cells leading to cell death **Special considerations:** Can cause severe bone marrow suppression and immunosuppression
procarbazine	Used in combination therapy for treatment of Hodgkin's lymphoma **Actions:** Inhibits DNA, RNA and protein synthesis, leading to cell death **Special considerations:** Bone marrow toxicity; GI toxicity and hypersensitivity also limit use in some patients; severity of adverse effects regulates the dose of the drug
Temozolomide	Combined with radiotherapy to treat glioblastoma multiforme; treatment of refractory malignant glioma **Actions:** Related to dacarbazine in structure. An alkylating agent that prevents proliferation of tumour cells by inhibiting DNA synthesis **Special considerations:** Monitor bone marrow closely; especially toxic in women and older patients
topotecan	Treatment of patients with metastatic ovarian cancer after failure of other agents **Actions:** Disrupts DNA strands during DNA synthesis via inhibition of topoisomerase I, causing cell death **Special considerations:** Can cause severe bone marrow depression, which regulates the dose of the drug; total alopecia, GI toxicity, and CNS effects may also limit the use of the drug
tretinoin	Induction of remission in acute promyelotic leukaemia **Actions:** tretinoin is an endogenous metabolite of retinol and induces terminal differentiation in leukaemic cells **Special considerations:** Can cause retinoic acid syndrome, fatal if multiorgan failure occurs. Other side-effects include GI toxicity, CNS and cardiovascular effects. Patients should have liver function, serum calcium, plasma lipids and haematological screen monitored before and throughout treatment

General Nursing Considerations for Patients Receiving Antineoplastic Drugs

Assessment: History and Examination

Screen for the following, *which will alert you to specific cautions or contraindications to the use of the drug:*

- History of allergy to the recommended antineoplastic drug or adjunct therapy
- Establish if patient is currently taking other medications or herbal therapies which may potentially interact with the proposed drug treatment
- Bone marrow suppression
- Renal or hepatic dysfunction
- GI ulcers (when prescribing antimetabolites, mitotic inhibitors or antineoplastic antibiotic drugs)
- Hypercalcaemia and hypercholesterolaemia (when prescribing hormones and hormone modulators)
- Pregnancy or lactation

Physical assessment should be performed *to establish baseline data for determining the effectiveness of the drug and the occurrence of any adverse effects associated with drug therapy*. Include screening for orientation and reflexes *to evaluate any CNS effects*; respiratory rate and adventitious sounds *to monitor the disease* and *to evaluate for respiratory or hypersensitivity effects*; blood pressure and pulse *to monitor for systemic or cardiovascular effects*; and bowel sounds *to monitor for GI effects*. Evaluate the full blood count with differential, serum calcium levels (hormones and hormone modulators) and renal and liver function tests *to monitor for dosage adjustment as needed and to evaluate toxic drug effects*. Regular evaluation of injection sites should be performed *to check for signs of extravasation or inflammation*.

See Critical Thinking Scenario 13-1 for a full discussion of assessing and evaluating antineoplastic therapy with breast cancer.

Nursing Diagnoses

The patient receiving antineoplastic drugs may have the following nursing diagnoses related to drug therapy:

- Acute pain related to GI, CNS, local effects of drug
- Disturbed body image related to alopecia and effects on the skin, impaired fertility
- Fear, anxiety related to diagnosis and treatment
- Deficient knowledge regarding drug therapy

Implementation With Rationale

- Arrange for complete blood count and platelet count tests before, periodically during, and after therapy *to monitor bone marrow function*. Discontinue the drug or reduce the dose as needed.
- Avoid direct skin or eye contact with the drug. Wear protective clothing and goggles while preparing and administering the drug *to prevent toxic reaction to the drug*.
- Administer medication according to scheduled protocol and in combination with other drugs as indicated *to improve effectiveness*.
- Monitor injection sites *to arrange appropriate treatment for extravasation, local inflammation or cellulitis*.
- Ensure that the patient is well hydrated *to decrease risk of renal toxicity*.
- Protect the patient from exposure to infection because *bone marrow suppression will limit the patient's immune/inflammatory responses*.
- Provide small, frequent meals, frequent mouth care, and dietary consultation as appropriate *to maintain nutrition when GI effects are severe*. Antiemetics may be helpful in some cases (see Box 13.4).
- Arrange for proper head covering at extremes of temperature if alopecia occurs; a wig, scarf, or hat is important for *maintaining body temperature*. If alopecia is an anticipated effect of drug therapy, suggest the patient obtains a wig or head covering before hair loss occurs *to promote self-esteem and a positive body image*.
- Provide patient teaching *to enhance patient knowledge about drug therapy and to promote compliance regarding:*
    - The appropriate dosage regimen, including dates to return for further doses.
    - The importance of covering the head at extremes of temperature if alopecia is anticipated.
    - The need to try to maintain nutrition if GI effects are severe.
    - The need to avoid exposure to infection from others. Patients should also be taught how to recognize the signs of infection (fever, chills) and what action to take in the event of a suspected infection.
    - The need to plan appropriate rest periods, because fatigue and weakness are common effects of the drugs.
    - Possible dizziness, headache and drowsiness; if these occur the patient should avoid driving or using dangerous equipment.

- The possibility of impaired fertility.
- The importance of not taking the drugs during pregnancy and of using barrier contraceptives.

Evaluation

- Monitor patient response to the drug (alleviation of cancer being treated, palliation of signs and symptoms of cancer).
- Monitor for adverse effects (bone marrow suppression, GI toxicity, neurotoxicity, alopecia, renal or hepatic dysfunction, cardiac or respiratory dysfunction, local reactions at the injection site).
- Evaluate the effectiveness of the teaching plan (patient can recognize possible adverse effects, and specific measures to help avoid adverse effects).

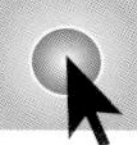

WEB LINKS

Health care providers and patients may want to consult the following Internet sources:

http://bnfc.org The BNF for Children provides UK health care professionals with authoritative and practical information on the selection and clinical use of medicines in children.

http://cks.library.nhs.uk The National Health Service Clinical Knowledge Summaries provide evidence-based practical information on the common conditions observed in primary care.

http://www.bnf.org.uk The BNF provides UK health care professionals with authoritative and practical information on the selection and clinical use of medicines.

http://www.cancerbackup.org.uk This site provides extensive information for patients and their families.

http://www.cancerresearchuk.org Cancer Research UK is a charity working to understand how to prevent, diagnose and treat different cancers. Patients can find information on symptoms, treatments and side-effects. There is also a database of current clinical trials.

http://www.christie.nhs.uk The Christie Hospital in Manchester is one of the leading cancer centres in Europe offering: high-quality diagnosis, treatment and care for cancer patients; world-class research and education in all aspects of cancer.

http://www.lymphoma.org.uk This site is run by the Lymphoma Association and provides information and support to patients with lymphatic cancer and their families.

http://www.lymphoma-net.org Information for patients with non-Hodgkin's lymphoma.

http://www.nhsdirect.nhs.uk The National Health Service Direct service provides patients with information and advice about health, illness and health services.

http://www.nice.org.uk The National Institute for Health and Clinical Excellence provides guidance on public health, new and existing treatments within the NHS and also information on the most appropriate care for patients.

http://www.teenagecancertrust.org This charitable trust provides teenagers and young adults with information.

Points to Remember

- Cancers arise from a single abnormal cell that multiplies and grows.
- Cancers can manifest as diseases of the blood and lymph tissue or as growth of tumours arising from epithelial cells (carcinomas) or from mesenchymal cells and connective tissue (sarcomas).
- Cancer cells lose their normal function (anaplasia), develop characteristics that allow them to grow in an uninhibited way (autonomy), have the ability to travel to other sites in the body that are conducive to their growth (metastasis) and can stimulate the production of blood vessels to bring nutrients to the growing tumour (angiogenesis).
- Antineoplastic drugs affect both normal cells and cancer cells by disrupting cell function and division at various points in the cell cycle; new drugs are being developed, such as kinase inhibitors, to target cancer cell-specific functions.
- Cancer drugs are usually most effective against cells that multiply rapidly (i.e. proceed through the cell cycle quickly). These cells include most neoplasms, bone marrow cells, cells in the GI tract and cells in the skin or hair follicles.
- The goal of cancer chemotherapy is to decrease the size of the neoplasm so that the human immune system can deal with it.
- Antineoplastic drugs are often given in combination so that they can affect cells in various stages of the cell cycle, including cells that are emerging from rest or moving to a phase of the cycle that is disrupted by these drugs.
- Adverse effects associated with antineoplastic therapy include effects caused by damage to the rapidly multiplying cells, such as bone marrow suppression, which may limit the drug use; GI toxicity, with nausea, vomiting, mouth sores and diarrhoea; and alopecia (hair loss).
- Chemotherapeutic drugs should not be used during pregnancy or lactation because they may result in potentially serious adverse effects on the rapidly multiplying cells of the neonate.

CRITICAL THINKING SCENARIO 13-1

Antineoplastic Therapy and Breast Cancer

The Situation

A 34-year-old woman, Barbara, is a teacher with two young daughters. She noticed a slightly painful lump under her arm when showering. About 2 weeks later, she found a mass in her right breast. Initial patient assessment found that she had no other underlying medical problems, no allergies and took no medications. Her family history was most indicative: many of the women in her family – her mother, maternal grandmother, aunt and an older sister – died of breast cancer before the age of 50. All data from the initial examination, including an evaluation of the lump in the upper outer quadrant of her breast and the presence of a fixed axillary node, were recorded as baseline data for further drug therapy and treatment. Barbara underwent a mastectomy and biopsy. The biopsy report indicated Stage 4 infiltrating ductal carcinoma (28 of 35 lymph nodes were positive for tumour), invasive breast cancer. The mastectomy was followed radiotherapy and a course of doxorubicin, cyclophosphamide and paclitaxel.

Critical Thinking

- What are the important nursing implications for Barbara? *Think about the outlook for Barbara, based on her biopsy results and her family history.*
- What impact will this disease have on Barbara's job and her family? *Think about the adverse drug effects that can be anticipated.*
- How can good patient teaching help Barbara to anticipate and cope with these many changes and unpleasant effects?
- What future concerns should be addressed or at least approached at this point in the treatment of Barbara's disease? What are the implications for her two daughters? How can the daughters be helped to cope with their mother's disease, as well as the prospects for their future?

Discussion

The extent of Barbara's disease, as evidenced by the biopsy results, does not signify a very hopeful prognosis. In this case, the overall nursing care plan should take into account not only the acute needs related to surgery and drug therapy, but also future needs related to potential debilitation and even the prospect of death. Immediate needs include comfort and teaching measures to help Barbara deal with the mastectomy and recovery from the surgery. She should be given an opportunity to discuss her feelings and thoughts with appropriate health care professionals.

The adverse effects associated with the antineoplastic drugs she will be given should be explained and possible ways to cope should be discussed. These effects include the following:

- *Alopecia* – Barbara should be reassured that her hair will grow back within 3 to 6 months of the end of treatment. Some patients are entitled to a free wig from the National Health Service. She should be reminded to cover her head in extremes of temperature.
- *Nausea and vomiting* – these effects will most often occur immediately after the drugs are given. Antiemetics can be given to relieve the adverse effects. Some antiemetics are more effective at preventing nausea and vomiting than stopping them once they have started, so it is sometimes recommended that the antiemetics are taken regardless of whether the patient feels sick directly after treatment.
- *Bone marrow suppression* – this will make Barbara more susceptible to disease, which could be a problem for a teacher and a mother with young children. Ways to avoid contact and infection, as well as warning signs to report immediately (e.g. elevated body temperature), should be discussed.
- *Mouth sores* – stomatitis and mucositis are common problems. Frequent, gentle teeth cleaning can help. The patient should be encouraged to maintain fluid intake and nutrition.
- Barbara's daughters are in a very high-risk group for this disease, so the importance of frequent examinations as they grow up needs to be stressed. Her daughters may be encouraged to have prophylactic mastectomies.

Nursing Care Guide for Barbara: Antineoplastic Drugs

Assessment: History and Examination

- Allergies to any of these drugs, renal or hepatic dysfunction, pregnancy or lactation, bone marrow suppression, or GI ulceration

Antineoplastic Therapy and Breast Cancer *(continued)*

- Concurrent use of: clozapine, pentastatin, phenytoin, itraconazole, digoxin, rosiglitazone, nelfinavir or ritonavir, which could interact with these drugs
- Local: evaluation of injection site
- Skin: colour (skin may darken), lesions, texture
- CNS: orientation, affect, reflexes
- GI: abdominal, liver evaluation
- Laboratory tests: baseline complete blood count and platelet count; renal and hepatic function tests

Nursing Diagnoses

- Acute pain related to GI, CNS and skin effects
- Imbalanced nutrition: less than body requirements related to GI effects
- Disturbed body image related to diagnosis, therapy, adverse effects
- Deficient knowledge regarding drug therapy

Implementation

- Ensure safe administration of the drug
- Provide comfort and safety measures: mouth and skin care, rest periods, safety precautions, antiemetics as needed, maintenance of nutrition and head covering
- Provide support and reassurance to deal with drug effects, discomfort and diagnosis
- Provide patient teaching regarding drug name, adverse effects, precautions to take, signs and symptoms to report and comfort measures to observe

Evaluation

- Evaluate drug effects: resolution of cancer
- Monitor for adverse effects: GI toxicity, bone marrow suppression, blood clots (associated with pain, redness and swelling in a leg or breathlessness), numbness or tingling in hands or feet, renal and hepatic damage, alopecia, extravasation of drug
- Monitor for drug–drug interactions as listed
- Evaluate effectiveness of patient teaching programme
- Evaluate effectiveness of comfort and safety measures

Patient Teaching for Barbara:

Antineoplastic drugs work to destroy cells at various phases of their life cycle. The drugs are given in combination to affect the cells at these various stages. These drugs are prescribed to kill cancer cells that are growing in the body. These drugs also affect normal cells and, therefore, sometimes cause many adverse effects. Your drug combination includes doxorubicin, cyclophosphamide and paclitaxel.

☐ These drugs are given in a 21-day cycle: the drugs are administered on the first day of treatment followed by a rest period of 3 weeks. This cycle of treatment is repeated between four and six times over the course of 3 to 4 months.

☐ Common adverse effects of these drugs include:

- *Nausea and vomiting* – antiemetic drugs may help. Your health care provider will be with you to help if these effects occur.
- *Loss of appetite* – it is very important to keep up your strength. Choose to eat food items that appeal to you. Some meals could be replaced with a nutritious drink. Try to eat when you feel hungry, regardless of the time of day.
- *Loss of hair* – your hair will grow back, although its colour or consistency may be different from what it was originally. You can choose to wear a wig, hat or scarf. It is very important to keep your head covered in extremes of temperature and to protect yourself from sun, heat and cold. Much of the body's heat can be lost through the head and not protecting yourself could cause serious problems.
- *Mouth sores* – frequent mouth care is very helpful. Try to avoid very hot or spicy foods.
- *Fatigue* – frequent rest periods and careful planning of your day's activities can be very helpful.
- *Bleeding* – you may bruise more easily than you normally do, and your gums may bleed while you are brushing your teeth. Special care should be taken when shaving or brushing your teeth. Avoid activities that might cause an injury, and avoid medications that contain aspirin.
- *Susceptibility to infection* – Avoid people with infections or colds. In some cases, the people who are caring for you may wear gowns and masks to protect you from their germs.
- *Colour of urine* – doxorubicin may turn the colour of your urine red shortly after administration.

☐ Report any of the following to your health care provider: bruising and bleeding, fever, chills, sore throat, difficulty breathing and swelling in your ankles or fingers. Pain to the chest, arm or neck may indicate cardiac complications.

(continued)

Antineoplastic Therapy and Breast Cancer *(continued)*

- ☐ It is very important to take the complete regimen that has been ordered for you. Cancer cells grow at different rates, and they go through rest periods during which they are not susceptible to the drugs. The disease must be attacked over time to eradicate the problem.
- ☐ Tell any doctor, nurse or other health care provider that you are taking this drug.
- ☐ Try to maintain a balanced diet while you are taking this drug. Drink 10 to 12 glasses of water each day during the drug therapy.
- ☐ Use a barrier contraceptive while you are taking this drug. These drugs can cause serious effects to a developing foetus and precautions must be taken to avoid pregnancy. If you think that you are pregnant, consult your health care provider immediately.
- ☐ You need to have periodic blood tests and examinations while you are taking this drug. These tests help guard against serious adverse effects and may be needed to determine the next dose of your drug.

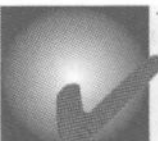

CHECK YOUR UNDERSTANDING

Answer to the questions in this chapter may be found in the answer key in the back of the book.

Multiple Choice

Select the most appropriate answer to the following.

1. Many properties of neoplastic cells are different from those of normal cells, with the exception of
   a. anaplasia.
   b. metastasis.
   c. mitosis.
   d. autonomy.

2. Carcinomas are tumours that originate in
   a. the mesenchyma and are made up of embryonic connective tissue cells.
   b. the bone marrow and affect the blood.
   c. the striated muscle.
   d. epithelial cells.

3. The goal of traditional antineoplastic drug therapy is to
   a. reduce the size of the mass of abnormal cells so that the immune system can take care of destroying them.
   b. eradicate all of the abnormal cells that have developed.
   c. destroy all cells of the originating type.
   d. stimulate the immune system to destroy the neoplastic cells.

4. Cancer can be a difficult disease to treat because
   a. cells no longer progress through the normal cell cycle.
   b. cells can develop resistance to drug therapy.
   c. cells can remain in the dormant state for long periods and emerge months to years later.
   d. the exact cause of cancer is not known.

5. Antineoplastic drugs destroy human cells. They are most likely to cause cell death among healthy cells that
   a. have poor cell membranes.
   b. are rapidly turning over and progress through their cell cycle rapidly.
   c. are in dormant tissues.
   d. are across the blood–brain barrier.

6. Cancer treatment usually occurs in several different treatment phases. In assessing appropriateness of another round of chemotherapy for a particular patient, the nurse would evaluate
   a. hair loss.
   b. bone marrow function.
   c. anorexia.
   d. hydration status.

7. It is important to explain to women that chemotherapeutic drugs should not be used during pregnancy because
   a. the tendency to cause nausea and vomiting will be increased.
   b. of potentially serious adverse effects on the rapidly multiplying cells of the foetus.
   c. bone marrow toxicity could alter hormone levels.
   d. patients may be weakened by the drug regimen.

8. Most cancer drugs are most effective against
   a. slowly growing cells.
   b. cells in the dormant phase of the cell cycle.
   c. cells that multiply rapidly and go through the cell cycle quickly.
   d. cells that have moved from their normal site in the body.

Matching

Match the word with the appropriate definition.

1. ____________________ anaplasia
2. ____________________ alopecia
3. ____________________ carcinoma
4. ____________________ metastasis
5. ____________________ neoplasm
6. ____________________ sarcoma
7. ____________________ autonomy
8. ____________________ antineoplastic

A. Tumours in the mesenchyma, composed of embryonic connective tissue cells
B. Drugs used to combat cancer
C. Tumours starting in epithelial cells
D. Loss of organization and structure
E. To travel throughout the body via lymph and circulation
F. New growth or cancer
G. Loss of hair
H. Loss of normal controls and reactions that limit cell growth and spreading

Bibliography and References

British Medical Association and Royal Pharmaceutical Society of Great Britain. (2008). *British National Formulary*. London: BMJ & RPS Publishing. *This publication is updated biannually: it is imperative that the most recent edition is consulted.*

British Medical Association and Royal Pharmaceutical Society of Great Britain. (2008). *British National Formulary for Children*. London: BMJ & RPS Publishing. *This publication is updated annually: it is imperative that the most recent edition is consulted.*

Brunton, L., Lazo, J. S., Parker, K., Goodman, L. S., & Gilman, A. G. (2005). *Goodman and Gilman's the pharmacological basis of therapeutics* (11th ed.). London: McGraw-Hill.

Bryant, H. E., Schultz, N., Thomas, H. D., Parker, K. M., Flower, D., Lopez, E., et al. (2005). Specific killing of BRCA-2 deficient tumours with inhibitors of poly(ADP-ribose) polymerase. *Nature, 434*, 913–917.

Di Cosimo, S., & Baselga, J. (2008). Targeted therapies in breast cancer: where are we now? *European Journal of Cancer, 44*, 2781–2790.

Health and Safety Executive. (2003). Safe handling of cytotoxic drugs. Available from www.hse.gov.uk *[The specific guidelines for individual Trusts should be consulted]*

Howland, R. D., & Mycek, M. J. (2005). *Pharmacology* (3rd ed.). Philadelphia: Lippincott Williams & Wilkins.

Jahanzeb, M. (2008). Adjuvant trastuzumab therapy for HER-2 positive breast cancer. *Clinical Breast Cancer, 8*(4), 324–333.

National Institute for Health and Clinical Excellence. (2006). *Familial breast cancer: The classification and care of women at risk of familial breast cancer in primary, secondary and tertiary care*. Available from www.nice.org.uk/CG041

Porth, C. M., & Matfin, G. (2008). *Pathophysiology: Concepts of altered health states* (8th ed.). Philadelphia: Lippincott Williams & Wilkins.

Rang, H. P., Dale, M. M., Ritter, J. M., & Flower, R. J. (2007). *Rang and Dale's pharmacology* (6th ed.). Philadelphia: Churchill Livingstone.

Simonsen, T., Aarbakke, J., Kay, I., Coleman, I., Sinnott, P., & Lysaa, R. (2006). *Illustrated pharmacology for nurses.* London: Hodder Arnold.

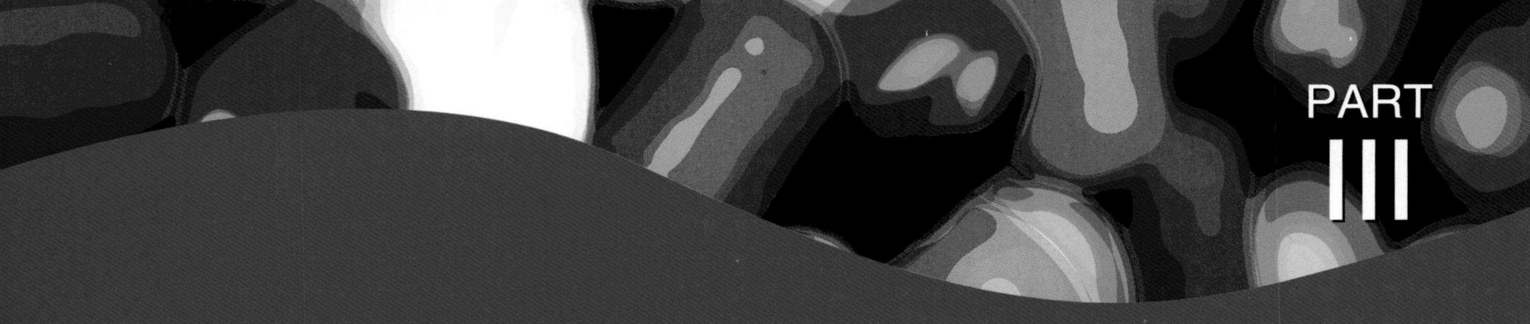

PART III

Drugs Acting on the Immune System

CHAPTER 14

Introduction to the Immune Response and Inflammation

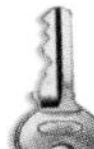

KEY TERMS

antibodies
antigen
arachidonic acid
autoimmune disease
B cells
bradykinin
chemotaxis
complement system
cytokines
dendritic
diapedesis
granulocytes
histamine
human leukocyte antigen
immune system
immunoglobulins (IgG, IgE, IgA, IgM)
interferons
interleukins
kinin system
leukocytes
lymphocytes
macrophages
major histocompatibility complex
mononuclear phagocytes
mononuclear phagocyte system (MPS)
myeloid cells
natural killer (NK) cells
phagocytes
phagocytosis
polymorphic
plasma cell
pyrogen
T cells

LEARNING OBJECTIVES

Upon completion of this chapter, you will be able to:

1. List four natural body defences against infection.
2. Outline the sequence of events in the inflammatory response.
3. Correlate the events in the inflammatory response with the clinical picture of inflammation.
4. Describe the cells associated with the body's fight against infection and their basic functions.
5. Outline the sequence of events in an antibody-related immune reaction and correlate these events with the clinical presentation of such a reaction.

The body has many defence systems in place to keep it intact and to protect it from external stressors. These stressors include bacteria, viruses and other pathogens, material foreign to the body such as insect stings and organ transplants and also trauma or exposure to extremes of environmental conditions. The same defence systems that protect the body also help to repair it after cellular trauma or damage. Understanding the basic mechanisms involved in these defence systems helps to explain the actions of the drugs that affect the immune system and inflammation.

Barrier Defences (innate immunity)

Anatomical barriers prevent the entry of foreign pathogens and serve as important lines of defence in protecting the body. These defences are collectively known as nonspecific responses.

Skin

The skin is the first line of defence. The skin acts as a watertight physical barrier to protect the internal tissues and organs of the body. Glands in the skin secrete chemicals that destroy or repel many pathogens. The skin sloughs off daily, making it difficult for any pathogen to colonize on the skin. Finally, nonharmful bacteria living on the skin can aid the destruction of disease-causing pathogens.

Mucous Membranes

Mucous membranes line the areas of the body that are directly exposed to the external environment but do not have the benefit of skin protection. These body areas include the respiratory tract, which is exposed to air; the gastrointestinal (GI) tract, which is exposed to anything ingested by mouth; and the genitourinary (GU) tract, which is exposed to many pathogens from the rectal area. Like the skin, the mucous membrane is a physical barrier to invasion. It also secretes sticky mucus, which traps invaders and inactivates them for later destruction and removal by the body. The mucus works much like flypaper trapping flies.

In the respiratory tract, the mucous membrane is lined with tiny, hair-like processes called *cilia*. The cilia sweep any captured pathogens or foreign materials upward toward the mouth, either to be swallowed or to cause irritation to the area and be removed by a cough or a sneeze.

In the GI tract, the mucous membrane serves as a protective coating, preventing erosion of GI cells by the acidic environment of the stomach, the digestive enzymes of the small intestine and the waste products that accumulate in the large intestine. The mucous membrane also secretes mucus that serves as a lubricant throughout the GI tract to facilitate movement of the food bolus and of waste products.

In the GU tract, the mucous membrane provides direct protection against injury and trauma and traps any pathogens in the area for destruction by the body.

Gastric Acid

The stomach secretes acid in response to many stimuli. The acidity of the stomach not only aids digestion, but also destroys many would-be pathogens that are either ingested or swallowed after removal from the respiratory tract.

Other nonspecific responses include: the production of tears, lysozymes in saliva and bladder flushing.

Cellular Defences

Any foreign pathogen that manages to get past the barrier defences will encounter the **mononuclear phagocyte system** (MPS) which produces an inflammatory response and the **immune system** which provides protection from subsequent infection.

Leukocytes

Stem cells in the bone marrow produce two types of white blood cells or **leukocytes**: lymphocytes and myeloid cells. The **lymphocytes** are the key components of the immune system and consist of T cells, B cells and natural killer (NK) cells (see later discussion of the immune response). The **myeloid cells** develop into a number of different cell types that are important in both the basic inflammatory response and the immune response. Myeloid cells can be further subdivided into two groups: the **granulocytes** (neutrophils, basophils, eosinophils and mast cells) and **mononuclear phagocytes** (monocytes, macrophages and dendritic cells; Figure 14.1).

Granulocytes

Neutrophils, basophils, eosinophils and mast cells are myeloid cells that have a bi- or multilobed nucleus (Figure 14.2). They are collectively known as granulocytes because their cytoplasm is full of granules containing a large number of chemicals that are important in removing infection by killing the infectious agents and by attracting more granulocytes and immune cells to the area.

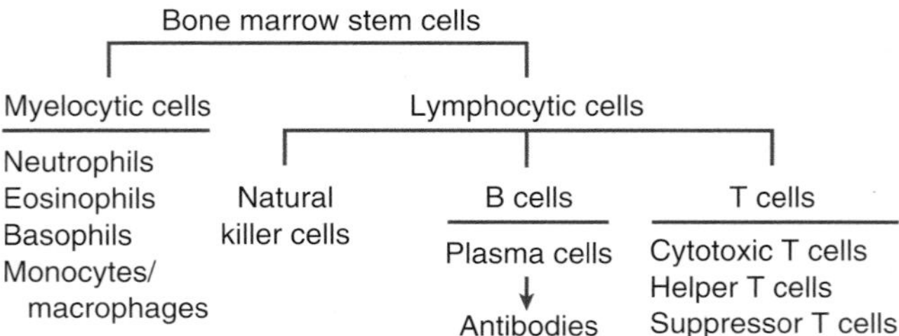

FIGURE 14.1 Types of white blood cells, or leukocytes, produced by the body.

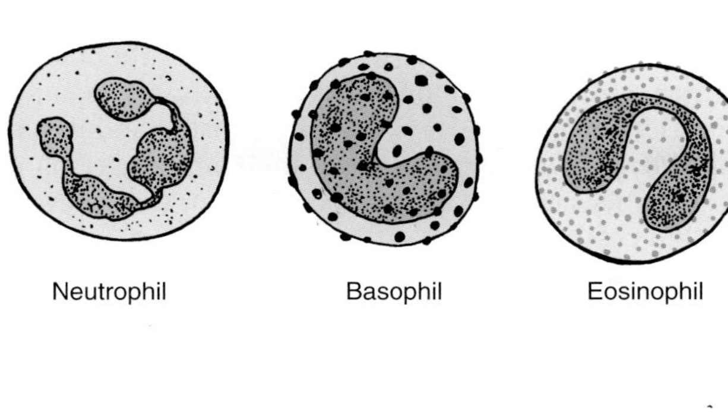

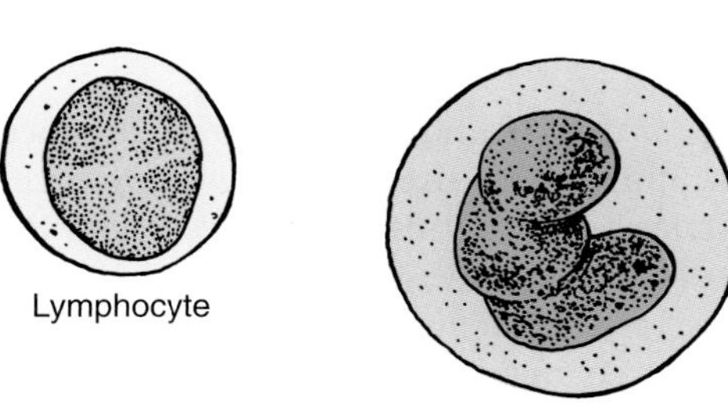

FIGURE 14.2 Appearance of various types of leukocytes.

Neutrophils

Neutrophils, also known as polymorphonuclear leukocytes, are the most abundant white cells in the blood. They are capable of **diapedesis** (moving from the bloodstream to the tissues) and of **phagocytosis** (engulfing and digesting foreign material). When the body is injured or invaded by a pathogen, neutrophils rapidly move to the site of the insult to attack the foreign substance. Because neutrophils are able to engulf and digest foreign material, they are also known as **phagocytes**.

Basophils

Basophils are circulating myeloid cells that are not capable of diapedesis or phagocytosis. When they encounter infection they release the chemical contents of their granules and help to initiate and maintain an inflammatory response. The granule contents include histamine, heparin and other chemicals used in the inflammatory response.

Eosinophils

Eosinophils are myeloid cells that, like neutrophils, are capable of diapedesis and phagocytosis. They play a role in protection against parasitic worms, but are often found at sites of allergic reactions, particularly in asthmatic lungs. It is thought that in these conditions they initiate and propagate inflammation by releasing the granule contents which include toxic proteins that help kill parasites and molecules that attract and activate immune and inflammatory cells.

Mast Cells

Mast cells are basophils that do not circulate; they are found in all tissues, and in higher numbers in the respiratory and GI tracts and in the skin. They release many of the chemical mediators of the inflammatory and allergic responses when they are stimulated by local irritation, including histamine, bradykinin, prostaglandins and leukotrienes.

Mononuclear Phagocytes

These are long-lived myeloid cells that, unlike granulocytes, do not contain large amounts of cytoplasmic granules. They have two important functions: they phagocytose, digest and destroy foreign material; and they activate cells of the immune system by presenting the digested contents on their cell surface (see T Cells and Major Histocompatibility Complex).

Monocytes

Monocytes are the mononuclear phagocytes of the blood. They continuously leave the blood to become **macrophages** and **dendritic** cells in the tissues, but they also help to protect the circulation from infection. In response to foreign material they supply the tissues with large numbers of macrophages.

Macrophages

Once monocytes leave the blood they can become long-lived macrophages that remain fixed in the tissue where they can phagocytose foreign material (**antigens**) which triggers their release of proinflammatory molecules. There are different types of macrophages in specific tissues, such as the Kupffer cells in the liver, the cells in the alveoli of the respiratory tract and the microglia in the central nervous system (CNS). Macrophages not only help remove foreign material, including pathogens, from the body but they also phagocytose debris from dead cells and necrotic tissue from injury sites, so that the body can heal. Macrophages respond to chemical mediators released by other immune and inflammatory cells to increase the intensity of a response and to facilitate the body's reaction.

Dendritic cells

Dendritic cells are found throughout the tissues, in higher numbers in mucosal and lymphoid tissue. They are very active phagocytic cells and their main function is to digest foreign proteins and present the fragments (peptides) to immune lymphocytes (T cells), causing their activation (see The Immune Response). Dendritic cells are essential for effective immune responses.

The Inflammatory Response

The inflammatory response is the local reaction of the body to invasion or injury. Any insult to the body that injures cells or tissues sets into action a series of events and chemical reactions.

Cell injury causes the activation of the **kinin system**, which is discussed here; the clotting cascade, which starts blood clotting; and the plasminogen system, which starts the dissolution of blood clots. The last two systems are discussed in Part VIII of this book, 'Drugs Acting on the Cardiovascular System'.

Bradykinin is a chemical mediator which causes local vasodilation to bring more blood to the injured area and to allow white blood cells to escape into the tissues. It also stimulates nerve endings to cause pain, which alerts the body to the injury. Bradykinin also causes the release of **arachidonic acid** from the cell membrane. Arachidonic acid is the precursor of other substances that act like local hormones – they are released from cells, cause an effect in the immediate area and are then broken down. These include:

- Prostaglandins, of which some augment the inflammatory reaction and others block it
- Leukotrienes, of which some cause vasodilation and increased capillary permeability and others can block the reactions
- Thromboxanes, which cause local vasoconstriction and facilitate platelet aggregation and blood coagulation

Aspirin blocks the enzymes that convert arachidonic acid into prostaglandins and thromboxanes, resulting instead in its conversion into epi-lipoxin, a potent anti-inflammatory molecule.

Another locally mediated response occurs at the same time as the above events. Injury to a cell membrane causes the local release of **histamine**. Histamine causes vasodilation, which brings more blood and blood components to the area; it changes capillary permeability, making it easier for neutrophils and blood chemicals to leave the bloodstream and enter the injured area; and it stimulates pain perception. These activities bring neutrophils to the area to phagocytose and get rid of the pathogen, or to remove the cell that has been injured.

Some leukotrienes have a property called **chemotaxis**, which is the ability to attract and stimulate neutrophils and other macrophages in the area. As the neutrophils become active and other chemicals are released into the area, they can injure or destroy local cells. The destruction of a cell results in the release of various lysosomal enzymes from it. These enzymes lyse or destroy the dead cell's membranes and cellular proteins. They are an important part of biological recycling and the breakdown of once-living tissues after death. In the case of an inflammatory reaction, they can cause local cellular breakdown and further inflammation, which can develop into a vicious cycle leading to cell death.

Many inflammatory diseases, such as rheumatoid arthritis and systemic lupus erythematosus, are examples of these uncontrolled cycles. The prostaglandins and leukotrienes are important to the inflammatory response because they act to moderate the reaction, thus preventing this destructive cycle from happening on a regular basis. Many of the drugs used to control the inflammatory and immune systems modify or interfere with these inflammatory reactions.

Clinical Presentation

Activation of the inflammatory response produces a characteristic clinical picture. *Heat, swelling, redness* and *pain* describe a typical inflammatory reaction. Heat occurs because of the increased blood flow to the area. Swelling occurs because of the fluid that leaks into the tissues as a result of the change in capillary permeability. Redness is related again to the increase in blood flow caused by the vasodilation. Pain comes from the activation of pain fibres by histamine and the kinin system. These signs and symptoms occur anytime a cell is injured (Figure 14.3).

Once the inflammatory response is under way and neutrophils become active, engulfing and digesting injured cells or the invader, they release a chemical called interleukin-1 (IL-1) that is a natural **pyrogen**, or fever-causing substance. This pyrogen resets specific neurons in the hypothalamus to maintain a higher body temperature, seen clinically as a fever. The higher temperature acts as a catalyst to many of the body's chemical reactions, making the inflammatory and immune responses more effective. Treating fevers remains a controversial subject because lowering a fever decreases the efficiency of the immune and inflammatory responses.

The leukotrienes (activated through the kinin system) cause myalgia and arthralgia (muscle and joint pain); common signs and symptoms of various inflammatory diseases, which also cause reduced activity and save energy. All of these chemical responses make up the total clinical picture of an inflammatory reaction.

The Immune Response

If a pathogen manages to get past the initial defences provided by the skin and gastric secretions, the granulocytes, monocytes and macrophages will initiate an inflammatory response with almost immediate effect and at the same time the dendritic cells will start the process leading to a specific immune response to the pathogen. The immune response is carried out by the lymphocytes and if this is the first time the person has encountered the pathogen it takes several days before the immune response becomes effective. On subsequent encounters with the same pathogen, the immune system remembers it and removes it before it can cause disease; this is the basis of vaccination.

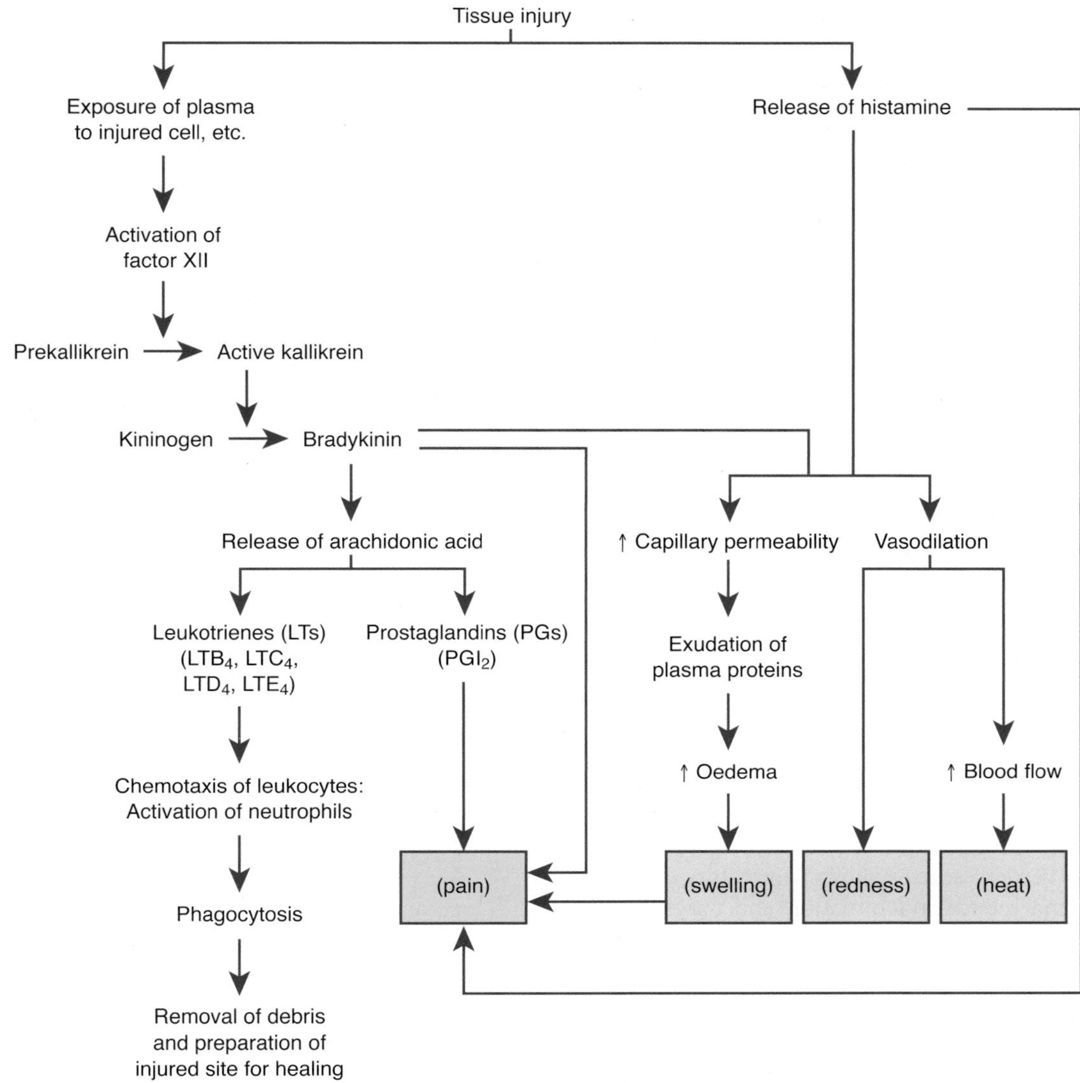

FIGURE 14.3 The inflammatory response in relation to the four cardinal signs of inflammation.

Lymphoid Tissues and Lymphocytes

Lymphoid tissues that play an essential part in the cellular defence system include the bone marrow, thymus (a bipolar gland located in the middle of the chest, which becomes smaller with age), spleen, lymph nodes and lymphoid tissue throughout mucosal surfaces of the respiratory and GI tracts.

There are three major types of lymphocyte: **B cells**, **T cells** and **natural killer (NK) cells**. Each B cell and T cell (but not NK cell) has receptors on its surface that recognize the foreign molecules (antigens) of the pathogen and on each B and T cell the specificity of the receptors for antigen is different. Together, the millions of different B and T cells circulating in the body provide comprehensive protection against foreign invaders.

All lymphocytes are generated from stem cells in the bone marrow, where NK cells and B cells reach maturity before entering the circulation, but the T cells have to go to the thymus for maturation (the name T cell means thymus-derived). Once mature, the lymphocytes recirculate through the blood and tissues, regularly entering the spleen, lymph nodes and mucosal lymphoid tissues to sample the resident dendritic cells that are presenting foreign antigens in order to start an immune response. If the lymphocytes recognize specific antigens here, they proliferate, become activated and then move back into the circulation to patrol the tissues for infection.

Natural Killer Cells

NK cells act as intermediaries between the innate and adaptive immune system; they patrol in the circulation and tissues, killing tumours and cells infected with viruses and at the same time secreting proinflammatory **cytokines** (locally acting hormone-like molecules).

T Cells

T cells are the most important cells in the adaptive immune response: they provide help to other immune cells; they directly kill cells that are infected and keep both the immune and the inflammatory responses under control.

T cells recognize foreign peptides (short amino acid sequences from digested proteins) on the surface of antigen-presenting cells: the dendritic cells, macrophages and B cells. The antigen-presenting cells attach the peptides to a self-protein called **major histocompatibility complex (MHC)** (see section below). Each T cell has membrane receptors that specifically bind to a particular peptide associated with self-MHC, thus activating the T cell.

There are three major types of T cell:

1. *Helper T cells* help B cells to produce antibodies and cytotoxic T cells to kill infected cells. They can also activate macrophages to kill intracellular bacteria and produce proinflammatory cytokines.
2. *Cytotoxic T cells* kill cells that are infected with intracellular pathogens such as viruses and some bacteria. They can also kill tumour cells that express tumour-specific antigens that appear to be foreign to the body and they secrete large amounts of proinflammatory cytokines to facilitate the removal of cells that have been killed.
3. *Regulatory T cells* control the helper and cytotoxic T cells, particularly to reduce their activity once infection has been cleared. They also secrete anti-inflammatory cytokines to control and reduce inflammation and prevent cellular destruction from a continued inflammatory reaction.

Major Histocompatibility Complex

All cells and tissues (except red blood cells) express self-proteins on their surface membranes that belong to a group known as the MHC. The MHC is used by T cells and NK cells to identify infected cells, tumours and transplanted cells. The genetic code for the MHC is carried on chromosome 6 and it is highly **polymorphic** (many different forms in different individuals); this means it is very unusual for two people to have exactly the same code (except for monozygotic twins). The MHC genes produce several proteins called histocompatibility antigens, or **human leukocyte antigens** (**HLA**, the name for human MHC). T cells identify foreign peptides attached to HLA and can also recognize foreign HLA on transplanted tissues leading to an immune response and rejection of the transplant. NK cells recognise a *lack* of self-HLA on cells; this can occur in infected cells and in tumours. NK cells attack a transplant with a different HLA from the patient because of the absence of self-HLA on the transplanted cells.

B Cells

B cells respond to foreign material by secreting **antibodies** that specifically bind to it and aid its removal. Antibodies are protein molecules collectively known as **immunoglobulins**. The antibody response is called *humoral immunity*, whereas the response by cytotoxic T cells and NK cells is called *cell-mediated immunity*. When an antigen binds to the receptors on the B cell membrane (these receptors are in fact antibody molecules embedded in the membrane), the B cell is activated to proliferate (to increase the number of antigen-specific B cells) and to differentiate into either a **plasma cell** that secretes antibodies or a long-lived memory B cell that patrols the body in case of reinfection.

Function of antibodies

By binding to pathogens, antibodies can aid their removal in a variety of ways: on the mucous membranes they can prevent pathogens from entering the body; in the blood and tissue fluid they make the pathogens easier to be phagocytosed by the neutrophils (which have receptors for bound antibodies) and they start an enzyme cascade reaction by the **complement system** that destroys the pathogen by punching holes in its membrane, activates platelets to form a clot and prevent the spread of infection, attracts more neutrophils by chemotaxis and activates local mast cells to release histamines causing vasodilation and increased vascular permeability.

During an infection, while some antigens remain embedded in the pathogen, others might be secreted (e.g. tetanus toxin) or get into the circulation as small soluble molecules when the pathogen dies. When antibodies bind to these soluble antigens they form insoluble antigen–antibody complexes that precipitate in small blood capillaries in the joints and skin and activate the complement system, resulting in local inflammation where the complexes are deposited.

When an antigen or pathogen is first encountered, a primary antibody response is started. This is characterized by circulating antibodies with weak antigen-binding but strong complement-activating properties, but after several days the amount and strength of antibody binding increases and the antibody is now more effective at removing the pathogen. This is dependent on antigen-specific T helper cells that communicate with the antigen-activated B cells in the lymphoid tissues.

Types of antibody

There are four main types of antibody which have different roles in antigen removal, but a single B cell can make only one type of antibody at any one time. The different types of antibody are known as immunoglobulin classes:

- **IgM** is the first antibody produced in the primary response without the need for T cell help. IgM antibodies have low binding affinity for antigen but are efficient at activating complement.
- **IgG** is the most abundant immunoglobulin in the blood. These antibodies have high binding affinity for antigen; their production is dependent on T cell help.

- **IgA** protects the mucous membranes; it is found in tears, saliva, mucus and bile. It is produced by plasma cells lying underneath the mucosal tissues and gets transported across the mucosal epithelium into the secretions. Its major role is to prevent infectious agents from entering the body through the mucous membranes.
- **IgE** is present in very small amounts in the blood but it is increased in parasitic infections. IgE binds to mast cells and is responsible for allergies such as hay fever.

Acquired Immunity

The process of antibody formation and the production of memory B and T cells is called acquired immunity and can be a lifelong reaction. For example, a person exposed to chickenpox will have a mild respiratory reaction when the virus (varicella) first enters cells in the respiratory tract. There will then be a 2- to 3-week incubation when the virus replicates in internal organs and some of the infected cells are killed by NK cells. During this time the body starts to produce IgM and IgG antibodies and cytotoxic T cells. The infected cells eventually rupture and eject more viruses into the system. These move to the skin causing a vesicular rash. More vesicles will form until the adaptive immune response is strong enough for circulating antibodies to prevent the virus from entering new cells and the cytotoxic T cells are able to kill the infected ones. Fever, myalgia and arthralgia are all part of the immune response to the virus. Not all of the invading chickenpox viruses get destroyed; some enter the CNS to safely hibernate away from the antibodies and cytotoxic T cells and the clinical signs and symptoms resolve. (Varicella can enter the CNS and stay dormant for many years. The antibodies and T cells are not able to cross into the CNS and the virus remains unaffected while it stays there. The adaptive T cells response is essential in preventing virus from re-emerging.) The plasma cells will continue to make a supply of IgG and IgA antibodies for use in any future exposure to the chickenpox virus and prevent the infection evolving into a clinical case because the viruses are inactivated immediately on entering the body so they are unable to multiply. Older patients with weakened immune systems that produce fewer antibodies and have fewer cytotoxic T cells, people who are immunosuppressed and individuals who have depleted their immune system fighting an infection are at risk for development of shingles if they had chickenpox earlier in their lives. The latent virus is able to leave the CNS along a nerve root because the adaptive T cell response is suppressed and slow to respond. Eventually the immune response usually responds to the varicella and the signs and symptoms of shingles resolve.

Other Mediators

Several other factors also play an important role in the immune reaction. **Interferons** are chemicals that are produced by cells that have been invaded by viruses and possibly by other stimuli. The interferons prevent viral replication and also suppress malignant cell replication and tumour growth.

Interleukins are cytokines secreted by active leukocytes and myeloid cells to influence other leukocytes. IL-1 activates T and B cells to initiate an immune response. IL-2 is released from active T cells to stimulate production of more T cells, particularly regulatory T cells and to increase the activity of B cells, cytotoxic cells and NK cells. Interleukins, especially IL-1, also cause fever, arthralgia, myalgia and slow-wave sleep induction—all things that help the body to conserve energy for use in fighting off the invader. Several other growth and chemotactic factors are released by lymphocytes and basophils that promote the growth of B cells, activate macrophages and platelets and attract neutrophils and eosinophils to the area.

Tumour necrosis factor (TNF) is a cytokine produced by macrophages and T cells that inhibits tumour growth and can actually cause tumour regression. It is also highly proinflammatory. Anti-TNF therapy is very successful in some patients with acute rheumatoid arthritis. This therapy either uses an antibody to TNF that blocks the action of the cytokine by preventing it from binding to its receptor on the cell membrane, or it uses a soluble form of the TNF receptor which removes all the TNF from the blood and tissue fluid.

All of these cytokines act as communication factors within the inflammatory and immune systems, allowing the coordination of both the inflammatory and the immune response.

Interrelationship of the Immune and Inflammatory Responses

The immune and inflammatory responses work together to protect the body and to maintain a level of homeostasis within the body. Helper T cells stimulate the activity of B cells and T cells. Regulatory T cells monitor the chemical activity in the body and act to suppress B-cell and T-cell activity when the foreign antigen is under control. Both B cells and T cells ultimately depend on an effective inflammatory reaction to achieve the end goal of destruction of the foreign protein or cell (Figure 14.4).

Pathophysiology Involving the Immune System

Several conditions can arise that cause problems involving the immune system. These conditions, many of which are treated by drugs that stimulate or suppress the immune system, include neoplasm, viral infection, allergy, autoimmune disease and transplant rejection.

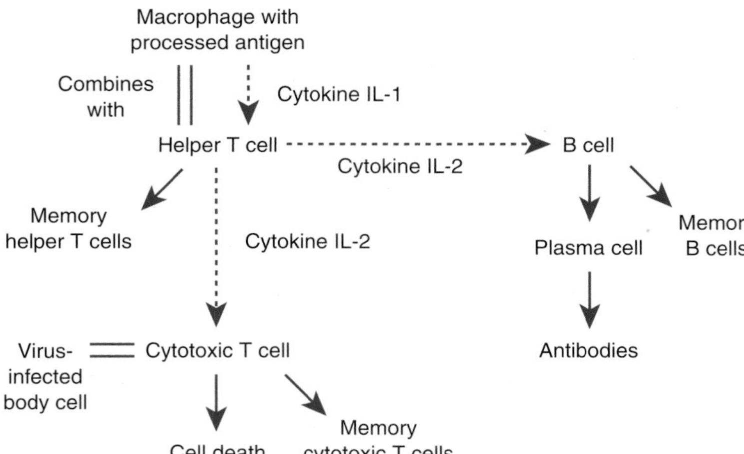

FIGURE 14.4 The cell-mediated immune response. Activation of a T cell by a non-self cell results in responses that destroy the foreign cell.

Viral Invasion of Cells

Viruses can survive only by invading a host cell that provides the nourishment necessary for viral replication. Once inside a cell, viruses can escape recognition by cytotoxic T cells by preventing the expression of MHC on the cell surface. These virally infected cells can be killed by NK cells but this is not a very effective way in removing the infection. In some cases the virus stimulates a T cell response to normal cellular components. This is one theory for the development of autoimmune disease.

Neoplasms

Neoplasms occur when mutant cells escape the normal surveillance of the immune system and begin to grow and multiply. This can happen in many ways. For example, ageing causes a decreased efficiency of the immune system, allowing some cells to escape. Location of the mutant cells can present a problem for getting lymphocytes to an area to respond. Mutant cells in breast tissue, for example, are not well perfused with blood and may escape detection until they are quite abundant. Sometimes cells are able to avoid detection by the T cells until the growing mass of cells is so large that the immune system cannot deal with it. A weakly antigenic tumour may develop; such a tumour elicits a mild response from the immune system and somehow tricks the T cells into allowing it to survive.

Allergy

It is not clear why some people are susceptible to developing allergies to commonly encountered environmental antigens such as pollen and house dust mite, but very often both IgE and eosinophils are involved. As these immune components are important in dealing with parasitic helminth worm infections it has been suggested that parasite infection prevents the development of allergies (Zaccone *et al.*, 2007).

Autoimmune Disease

Autoimmune disease occurs when the body responds to specific self-antigens to produce antibodies or cell-mediated immune responses against its own cells. The actual cause of autoimmune disease is not known, but theories speculate that (1) it could be a result of response to a cell that was invaded by a virus, leading to antibody production to similar cells; (2) production of autoantibodies is a normal process that goes on all the time, but in a state of immunosuppression the regulatory T cells do not control autoantibody production or autoreactive T cells; (3) there is a genetic predisposition to develop autoantibodies, or (4) it is a mixture of two or more of the above. Examples of autoimmune disease include rheumatoid arthritis, multiple sclerosis and myasthenia gravis.

Transplant Rejection

With the growing field of organ transplantation, more is being learned about the reaction to foreign cells that are introduced into the body. Effort is always made to match a donor's HLA molecules as closely as possible to those of the recipient for histocompatibility. The more closely the foreign cells can be matched, the less aggressive will be the immune reaction to the donated tissue. Self-transplantation, or autotransplantation, results in no immune response. All other transplants produce an immune reaction. Both the helper and cytotoxic T cells are activated by the presence of the foreign cells and release cytokines to stimulate an immune and inflammatory reaction, resulting in the destruction of the foreign tissue. Patients receiving organ transplants are now routinely given drugs such as ciclosporin and tacrolimus that prevent the activation of new T cells, prolonging the life of the graft.

Points to Remember

- The body has several defence mechanisms in place to protect it from injury or foreign invasion: the skin, mucous membranes, normal flora, gastric acid and the inflammatory and immune responses.
- The inflammatory response is an innate response to any cell injury.
- The clinical presentation of an inflammatory reaction is heat, redness, swelling and pain.
- Several types of T cells exist: cytotoxic T cells, helper T cells and regulatory T cells.
- Cytotoxic T cells destroy infected cells and tumour cells. Helper T cells stimulate the immune and inflammatory reactions. Regulatory T cells dampen the immune and inflammatory responses to conserve energy and prevent cellular damage.
- B cells recognise specific proteins or foreign antigens. Once in contact with that antigen, the B cell produces antibodies (immunoglobulins) that react with it directly.
- Reaction of an antibody with an antigen activates the complement cascade of proteins and lyses the pathogen or precipitates an aggressive inflammatory reaction around it.
- Cytokines are involved in communication among parts of the immune system and in local response to invasion. Any of these chemicals has the potential to alter the immune response.
- The T cells, B cells and inflammatory reaction work together to protect the body from invasion, limit the response to that invasion and return the body to a state of homeostasis.
- Patient problems that occur within the immune system include the development of neoplasms, viral invasions of cells that trigger immune responses, allergy, autoimmune diseases and rejection of transplanted organs.

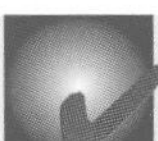

CHECK YOUR UNDERSTANDING

Answers to the questions in this chapter may be found in the answer key in the back of the book.

Multiple Choice

Select the most appropriate response to the following.

1. Antibodies are
   a. carbohydrates.
   b. secreted by activated T cells.
   c. not found in circulating γ-globulins.
   d. effective only against specific antigens.

2. B and T cells are similar in that they both
   a. secrete antibodies.
   b. play important roles in the immune response.
   c. are activated in the thymus.
   d. release cytotoxins to destroy cells.

3. Which of the following is not a cytokine?
   a. IL-2
   b. Antibody
   c. TNF
   d. Interferon

4. As part of the nonspecific defence against infection
   a. blood flow and vascular permeability to proteins increase throughout the circulatory system.
   b. particles in the respiratory tract are engulfed by phagocytes.
   c. B cells are released from the bone marrow.
   d. neutrophils release lysosomes, heparin and kininogen into the extracellular fluid.

5. B cells respond to an initial antigen challenge by
   a. reducing in size.
   b. immediately producing antigen-specific antibodies.
   c. producing a large number of cells that are unlike the original B cell.
   d. producing new cells that become plasma cells and memory cells.

6. Treating fevers remains a controversial subject because
   a. fevers make people feel ill.
   b. higher temperatures act as catalysts to many of the body's chemical reactions, so the inflammatory and immune responses are more effective.
   c. higher temperatures can suppress the body's normal metabolism.
   d. higher temperatures can alter the body's hormone levels, particularly progesterone.

7. T cells are programmed in the thymus and can become any of the following *except*:
   a. cytotoxic T cells.
   b. helper T cells.
   c. regulatory T cells.
   d. antibody-secreting T cells.

8. Interleukins are:
   a. chemicals released when a virus enters a cell.
   b. chemicals secreted by activated leukocytes to influence other leukocytes.
   c. part of the kinin system.
   d. activated by arachidonic acid.

Extended Matching Questions

Select **all** that apply.

1. Which of the following statements could be used to describe a neutrophil?
   a. They possess the property of phagocytosis.
   b. When activated, they release a pyrogen that causes fever.
   c. When the body is injured, they are produced rapidly and in large numbers.
   d. They are not capable of movement outside the circulatory system.
   e. They are most often seen in response to an allergic reaction.
   f. They float around in the blood and release chemicals in response to injury.

2. The inflammatory response is activated whenever cell injury occurs. An inflammatory response would involve which of the following activities?
   a. Activation of Factor XII
   b. Vasodilation in the area of the injury
   c. Generalized oedema and tumour development
   d. Changes in capillary permeability to allow proteins to leak out of the capillaries
   e. Activation of complement
   f. Production of interferon

True or False

Indicate whether the following statements are true (T) or false (F).

_____ 1. You are walking in a daisy field and get stung by what looks like a wasp. You should apply ice to the area to contain the venom.

_____ 2. You have a hard, reddened, warm area on your arm. You should apply ice to the affected area to keep the hardness, redness and warmth from spreading.

_____ 3. You have a hard, reddened, warm area on your arm. You should apply heat to the area to increase the blood flow to provide inflammatory and immune factors to the site.

_____ 4. Having your tonsils removed will prevent further upper respiratory infections.

_____ 5. Basophils are the first white blood cells at the site of an injury.

_____ 6. All white blood cells possess the property of phagocytosis.

_____ 7. Chemotaxis is the ability to move within the tissues.

_____ 8. Plasma cells are large and active B cells.

_____ 9. The thymus is responsible for the activation and programming of the B cells.

_____ 10. Applying ice to an injection site will decrease the pain of the injection but will also decrease the absorption of the injected substance.

Definitions

Define the following terms.

1. interleukin ____________________

2. pyrogen ____________________

3. antibody ____________________

4. chemotaxis ____________________

5. neutrophil ____________________

6. antigen ____________________

Bibliography and References

Brunton, L., Lazo, J. S., Parker, K., Goodman, L. S., & Gilman, A. G. (2005). *Goodman and Gilman's the pharmacological basis of therapeutics* (11th ed.). London: McGraw-Hill.

Ganong, W. (2003). *Review of medical physiology* (21st ed.). Norwalk: Appleton & Lange.

Marieb, E. N., & Hoehn, K. (2004). *Human anatomy & physiology* (7th ed.). San Francisco: Pearson Benjamin Cummings.

Peakman, M., & Vergani, D. (1997). *Basic and clinical immunology.* New York: Churchill-Livingstone.

Porth, C. M., & Matfin G. (2008). *Pathophysiology: Concepts of altered health states* (8th ed.). Philadelphia: Lippincott Williams & Wilkins.

Stites, D. P., Terr, A. I., & Parslow, T. G. (eds.). (1997). *Medical immunology* (9th ed.). Stamford: Appleton & Lange.

Wood, P. (2006). *Understanding immunology* (2nd ed.). London: Pearson Education.

Zaccone P., Burton, O. T., & Cooke, A. (2007). Interplay of parasite-driven immune responses and autoimmunity. *Trends in Parasitology, 24*(1), 35–42.

CHAPTER

15

Anti-inflammatory Agents

KEY TERMS

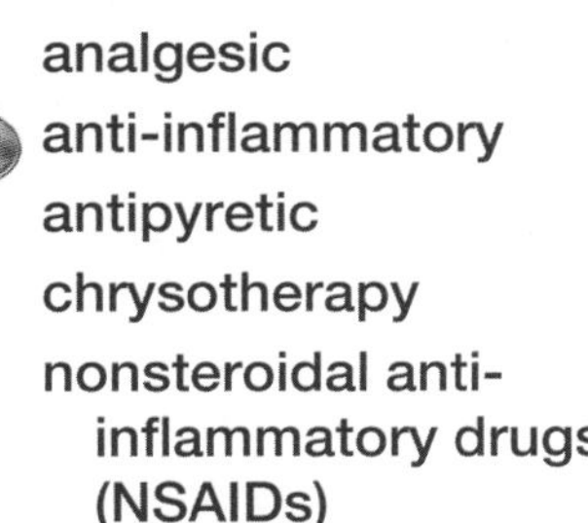

analgesic
anti-inflammatory
antipyretic
chrysotherapy
nonsteroidal anti-inflammatory drugs (NSAIDs)
salicylates

LEARNING OBJECTIVES

Upon completion of this chapter, you will be able to:

1. Describe the sites of action of the various anti-inflammatory agents.
2. Describe the therapeutic actions, indications and pharmacokinetics associated with each class of anti-inflammatory agent.
3. Describe the contraindications, most common adverse reactions and important drug–drug interactions associated with each class of anti-inflammatory agent.
4. Discuss the use of anti-inflammatory drugs across the lifespan.
5. Compare and contrast the key drugs for each class of anti-inflammatory drugs with the other drugs in that class.
6. Outline the nursing considerations and teaching needs for patients receiving each class of anti-inflammatory agents.

SALICYLATES

aspirin
balsalazide
choline salicylate
mesalazine
olsalazine
sulfasalazine

NONSTEROIDAL ANTI-INFLAMMATORY DRUGS

aceclofenac
acemetacin
azapropazone
celecoxib
dexibuprofen
dexketoprofen
diclofenac
etodolac
etoricoxib
fenbufen
fenoprofen
flurbiprofen
ibuprofen
indometacin
ketoprofen
ketorolac
mefenamic acid
meloxicam
nabumetone
naproxen
piroxicam
sulindac
tenoxicam
tiaprofenic acid
tolfenamic acid

ANTI-RHEUMATOID DRUGS

Disease-Modifying Anti-rheumatic Drugs (DMARDs)
gold salts (auranofin, sodium aurothiomalate) penicillamine
Cytokine Modulators
abatacept
adalimumab
anakinra
etanercept
infliximab
rituximab

RELATED DRUGS

paracetamol
hyaluronidase derivatives (hylan G-F 20, sodium hyaluronate)

The inflammatory response is designed to protect the body from injury and pathogens. It employs a variety of potent chemical mediators to produce the reaction that helps to destroy pathogens and promote healing. Inflammation is the first stage in tissue repair. As the body reacts to these chemicals, it produces some signs and symptoms of disease, such as swelling, pain, fever, aches and pains. Occasionally, the inflammatory response becomes a chronic condition and can actually result in body damage, leading to increased inflammatory reactions. **Anti-inflammatory** agents generally block or alter the chemical reactions associated with the inflammatory response to stop one or more of the signs and symptoms of inflammation.

Anti-inflammatory Agents

Several different types of drugs are used as anti-inflammatory agents. Corticosteroids (discussed in Chapter 35) are used systemically to block the inflammatory and immune systems. Blocking these important protective processes may produce many adverse effects, including decreased resistance to infection. Corticosteroids are also used topically to produce a local anti-inflammatory effect with fewer adverse effects. Antihistamines (discussed in Chapter 54) are used to block the actions of histamine in the initiation of the inflammatory response. In this chapter, discussion of anti-inflammatory agents focuses on salicylates, nonsteroidal anti-inflammatory drugs (NSAIDs) and other related drugs.

Salicylates are popular anti-inflammatory agents, not only because of their ability to block the inflammatory response, but also because of their **antipyretic** (fever-reducing) and **analgesic** (pain-inhibiting) properties. They are generally available without prescription and are relatively nontoxic when used as directed.

Nonsteroidal anti-inflammatory drugs (NSAIDs) are some of the most widely used drugs in the world. They provide strong anti-inflammatory and analgesic effects yet do not have the adverse effects associated with the corticosteroids.

Paracetamol is also a widely used agent. It has antipyretic and analgesic properties but does not have the anti-inflammatory effects of the salicylates or the NSAIDs.

Many anti-inflammatory drugs are available over-the-counter (OTC); therefore, there is potential for abuse and overdosing. In addition, patients may take these drugs and block the signs and symptoms of an underlying illness, thus potentially causing the misdiagnosis of a problem. Patients may also combine these drugs and unknowingly induce toxicity. All of these drugs have adverse effects that can be dangerous if toxic levels of drug accumulate in the body.

Salicylates

Salicylates are some of the oldest anti-inflammatory drugs used. They were originally extracted from willow bark, poplar trees and other plants to treat fever, pain and what we now

BOX 15.1 DRUG THERAPY ACROSS THE LIFESPAN

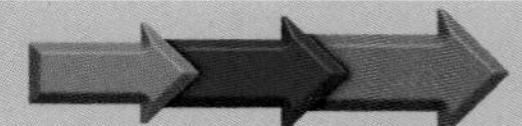

Anti-inflammatory Agents

CHILDREN

Children are more susceptible to the gastrointestinal (GI) and central nervous system (CNS) effects of these drugs. Care must be taken to make sure that the child receives the correct dose of any anti-inflammatory agent. This can be a problem because many of these drugs are available in OTC pain, cold, flu and combination products. Parents need to be taught to read the label to find out the ingredients and the dosage they are giving the child.

Paracetamol is probably the most used anti-inflammatory drug for children. Care must be taken to avoid overdosage which can cause severe hepatotoxicity.

Aspirin should not be used by children under the age of 16 years because of the potential risk of Reye's syndrome; a fatal disease associated with giving aspirin to children with viral illnesses, for example chicken pox.

Diclofenac, ibuprofen, mefenamic acid, naproxen and piroxicam are the NSAIDs approved for use in children.

Children with arthritis may receive treatment with the gold salt, sodium aurothiomalate, or etanercept. They must be monitored closely for toxic effects.

When administering any drug to children, always consult the most recent edition of the British National Formulary for Children.

ADULTS

Adults need to be cautioned about the presence of these drugs in many OTC products and taught to be aware of exactly what they are taking to avoid serious toxic effects. They should also be cautioned to report OTC drug use to their health care provider when they are receiving any other prescription drug, to avoid possible drug-drug interactions and the masking of signs and symptoms of disease.

Pregnant and nursing women should not use these drugs unless the benefit clearly outweighs the potential risk to the foetus or neonate. The salicylates, NSAIDs and gold products have potentially severe adverse effects on the neonate and possibly the mother. Paracetamol can be used cautiously if an analgesic or antipyretic is needed. Nondrug measures should be taken when possible to decrease the potential risk. These women also need to be urged to avoid OTC drugs unless they are suggested by their health care providers.

OLDER ADULTS

Older patients may be more susceptible to the GI and CNS effects of some of these drugs. However, dosage adjustment is not needed for many of these agents.

Increased toxicity has been associated with naproxen, ketorolac and ketoprofen when they are used by older patients. These NSAIDs should be avoided if possible.

call inflammation. Today they are produced synthetically and include:

- Aspirin, one of the most widely used drugs for treating inflammatory conditions, is available OTC.
- Balsalazide is a new drug that is delivered intact to the colon, where it delivers a local anti-inflammatory effect for patients with ulcerative colitis.
- Choline salicylate is used to treat oral ulceration.
- Mesalazine is a unique compound that releases aspirin in the large intestine for a direct anti-inflammatory effect in ulcerative colitis or other conditions involving inflammation of the large intestine.
- Olsalazine is converted to mesalazine in the colon and has the same direct anti-inflammatory effects.
- Sulfasalazine is used to treat Crohn's disease, ulcerative colitis and rheumatoid arthritis (RA).

Therapeutic Actions and Indications

Salicylates inhibit the synthesis of prostaglandins, important mediators of inflammatory reactions (Figure 15.1). The antipyretic effect of salicylates is related to the release of pyrogens, chemicals released by macrophages in response to toxins released by bacteria. Pyrogens stimulate the production of prostaglandins in the thermoregulatory centre of the hypothalamus, re-setting the 'thermostat'. Salicylates inhibit the production of prostaglandins and prevent re-setting of the thermostat. At low levels, aspirin also affects platelet aggregation by inhibiting the synthesis of thromboxane A_2, a potent vasoconstrictor that normally increases platelet aggregation and blood clot formation. At higher levels, aspirin inhibits the synthesis of prostacyclin, a vasodilator that inhibits platelet aggregation (see Chapter 15 for further actions of aspirin).

Salicylates are indicated for the treatment of mild to moderate pain, fever and numerous inflammatory conditions, including rheumatoid arthritis (RA) and osteoarthritis (see Box 15.1). Aspirin at low doses is indicated for the prevention of transient ischemic attack (TIA) and cerebrovascular accidents (CVA) in adults with a history of emboli. It is also indicated to reduce the risk of death and myocardial infarction (MI) in patients with a history of MI or unstable angina.

Pharmacokinetics

Salicylates are readily absorbed directly from the stomach, reaching peak levels within 5 to 30 minutes. They are

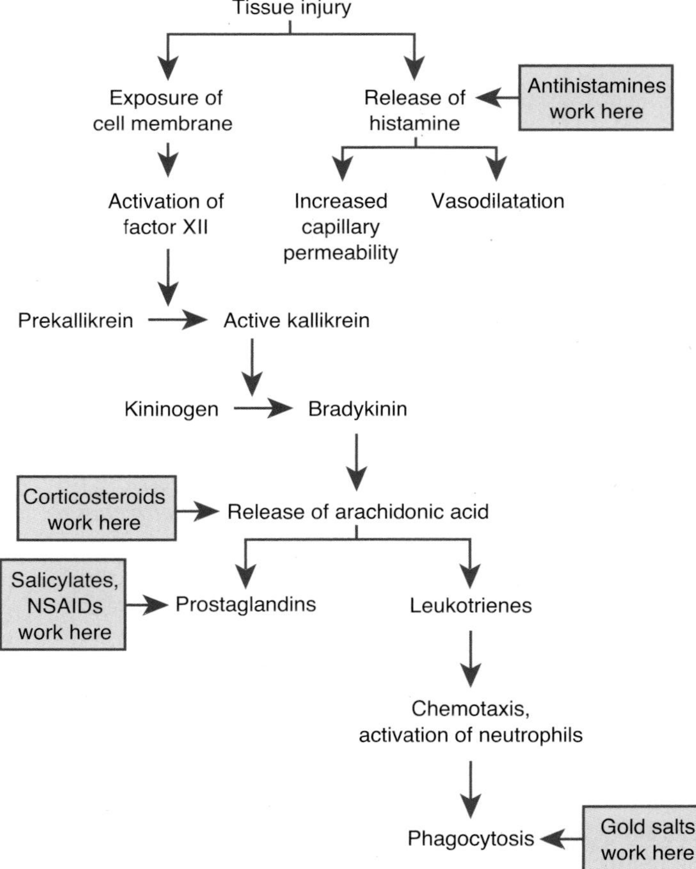

FIGURE 15.1 Sites of action of anti-inflammatory agents.

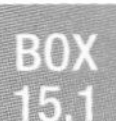

BOX 15.1 FOCUS ON **CLINICAL SKILLS**

Rheumatoid Arthritis (RA)

Pathophysiology

RA is a chronic, systemic disease that affects people of all ages. It is considered to be an autoimmune disease. Patients with RA usually have high levels of rheumatoid factor (RF), an antibody to immunoglobulin G (IgG). RF interacts with circulating IgG to form immune complexes, which deposit in the synovial fluid of joints as well as in the eye and small vessels. The formation of these immune complexes activates complement and precipitates an inflammatory reaction. During the immune reaction, lysosomal enzymes are released that destroy the tissues surrounding the joint. This destruction of normal tissue causes a further inflammatory reaction and a cycle of destruction and inflammation ensues. Over time, the joints become severely damaged and deformed and the synovial space fills with scar tissue.

Effects of Disease

The patient with RA is in chronic pain, related to the release of chemicals involved in the inflammatory process and the pressure of the swelling tissues in the joint capsule. At this time there is no cure for RA. Treatment is aimed at relieving the signs and symptoms of inflammation and delaying the progressive damage to the joints and maintaining mobility. Patients may progressively lose the use of the joint, which affects mobility as well as the ability to carry on the activities of daily living. Depression may also be a common side-effect. Patients with RA also have an increased risk of cardiovascular disease as the inflammation can have systemic effects.

Clinical Skills

Specific nursing interventions can help to alleviate some of the signs and symptoms of RA and help the patient to cope with the disease. These interventions include physical therapy; range-of-motion exercises; application of hot and cold packs to the joints; weight-bearing exercises; spacing activities throughout the day to make the most of energy and movement reserves; and assistance devices for normal daily activities (e.g. big handles on utensils and pans to help patients do things for themselves when they cannot grasp small handles). Thorough teaching about drug regimens can also help prevent adverse effects and increase concordance.

Patients may have to progress through a series of drugs as various agents lose their effectiveness. Aspirin, NSAIDs, gold salts or one of the cytokine modulators, for example infliximab and etanercept; that suppress the rheumatic disease process may all be used at one time or another. Patients with RA will benefit from a relationship with a consistent, reliable health care provider who listens, offers support and has knowledge of new drugs and treatments to improve the quality of life. Many community support and information groups are available as resources to patients and to health care providers who work with these patients. For a listing of available resources in your area, contact the Arthritis Care charity.

metabolized in the liver and excreted in the urine, with a half-life of 15 minutes to 12 hours, depending on the salicylate involved. Salicylates cross the placenta and enter breast milk; they are not indicated for use during pregnancy or lactation because of the potential adverse effects to the neonate and associated bleeding risks for the mother.

Contraindications and Cautions

Salicylates are contraindicated in the presence of known allergy to salicylates, other NSAIDs (more common with a history of nasal polyps, asthma because blocking prostaglandins in the airways results in bronchoconstriction, or chronic urticaria); bleeding abnormalities, *because of the changes in platelet aggregation associated with these drugs;* impaired renal function, *because the drug is excreted in the urine;* children under the age of 15 years, *because of the risk of Reye's syndrome;* surgery or other invasive procedures scheduled within 1 week, *because of the risk of increased bleeding;* and pregnancy or lactation, *because of the potential adverse effects on the neonate or mother.*

Adverse Effects

The adverse effects associated with salicylates may be the result of direct drug effects on the stomach (nausea, dyspepsia, heartburn, epigastric discomfort, ulceration with occult bleeding; occasionally major haemorrhage) and on clotting systems (blood loss, bleeding abnormalities). Aspirin inhibits prostaglandins in the stomach thereby increasing the release of gastric acid and the potential for gastric ulceration. It should be taken with food and enteric coated if taken continuously. Salicylism can occur with high levels of aspirin; dizziness, tinnitus (ringing in the ears), difficulty in hearing, nausea, vomiting, diarrhoea, mental confusion and lassitude can occur. Acute salicylate toxicity may occur at doses of 20 to 25 g in adults or 4 g in children. Signs of salicylate toxicity include hyperpnoea, tachypnoea, haemorrhage, excitement, confusion, pulmonary oedema, convulsions, tetany, metabolic acidosis, fever, coma and cardiovascular, renal and respiratory collapse.

Clinically Important Drug–Drug Interactions

The salicylates interact with many other drugs, primarily because of alterations in absorption, effects on the liver, or extension of the therapeutic effects of the salicylate or the interacting drug (or both). The list of interacting drugs in the British National Formulary should be consulted before adding or removing a salicylate from any drug regimen.

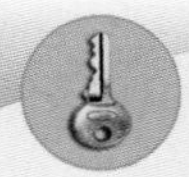

Key drug Summary: *Aspirin*

Indications: Treatment of mild to moderate pain, fever, inflammatory conditions; reduction of risk of TIA or stroke; reduction of risk of MI

Actions: Inhibits the synthesis of prostaglandins; blocks the effects of pyrogens in the hypothalamus; inhibits platelet aggregation by blocking thromboxane A_2

Pharmacokinetics:

Route	Onset	Peak	Duration
Oral	5–30 min	0.25–2 h	3–6 h
Rectal	1–2 h	4–5 h	6–8 h

$T_{1/2}$: 15 minutes to 12 hours; metabolized in the liver and excreted in the urine

Adverse effects: Nausea, vomiting, heartburn, epigastric discomfort, gastric ulceration (for nonenteric coated tablets) with occult bleeding, hypersensitivity reactions – angioedema, bronchospasm and rashes, dizziness and tinnitus.

Nursing Considerations for Patients Receiving Salicylates

Assessment: History and Examination

Screen for any of the following, *which could be contraindications or cautions for the use of the drug:* known allergies to any salicylates or NSAIDs; renal disease; bleeding disorders; child under the age of 16 years; influenza; and pregnancy or lactation, asthma, present or past gastric ulcers.

Include screening *for baseline status before beginning therapy and for any potential adverse effects:* the presence of any skin lesions; temperature; orientation, reflexes, pulse, blood pressure, perfusion; respirations and adventitious sounds; liver evaluation; bowel sounds; and full blood count, liver and renal function tests, urinalysis, stool occult blood and clotting times.

Establish if patient is currently taking other medications or herbal therapies which may potentially interact with salicylates.

Nursing Diagnoses

The patient receiving salicylates may have the following nursing diagnoses related to drug therapy:

- Ineffective breathing pattern if asthmatic and sensitive to NSAIDs
- Ineffective pain management due to inappropriate drug or dosage
- Potential for exacerbation of asthma due to drug sensitivity
- Potential for damage to cranial nerve VIII due to drug sensitivity
- Potential for gastric upsets due to drug actions
- Potential for gastric bleeding due to drug actions
- Lack of knowledge regarding dosage and actions and adverse effects

Implementation With Rationale

- Administer with food (if GI upset is severe; provide small, frequent meals *to alleviate GI effects*).
- Administer drug as indicated; monitor dosage *to avoid toxic levels.*
- Monitor for severe reactions *and provide emergency procedures* if they occur.
- Arrange for supportive care and comfort measures (rest, environmental control) *to decrease body temperature or to alleviate inflammation.*
- Provide thorough patient education, including measures to avoid adverse effects and warning signs of problems, as well as proper administration, *to increase knowledge about drug therapy and to increase compliance with drug regimen.*
- Offer support and encouragement *to deal with the drug regimen.*

Evaluation

- Monitor patient response to the drug (improvement in condition being treated, relief of signs and symptoms of inflammation).
- Monitor for adverse effects (GI upset, CNS changes, bleeding).
- Evaluate effectiveness of teaching plan (patient can name drug, dosage, adverse effects to watch for, specific measures to avoid adverse effects).
- Monitor effectiveness of comfort measures and compliance with the drug regimen.

Nonsteroidal Anti-inflammatory Drugs (NSAIDs)

The NSAIDs have become one of the most commonly used groups of drugs in the world. The choice of NSAID depends on personal experience and the patient's response to the drug. A patient may have little response to one NSAID and a huge response to another. It may take several trials to determine the drug of choice for any particular patient.

Therapeutic Actions and Indications

The anti-inflammatory, analgesic and antipyretic and adverse effects of the NSAIDs are largely related to inhibition of prostaglandin synthesis (see Figure 15.1). The NSAIDs block two enzymes, known as cyclo-oxygenase-1 (COX-1) and cyclo-oxygenase-2 (COX-2). COX-1 is present in all tissues and seems to be involved in many homeostatic functions, including blood clotting, protecting the stomach lining by inhibiting the release of gastric acid and maintaining sodium and water balance in the kidney. COX-1 converts arachidonic acid into a range of prostaglandins as needed. COX-2 is active at sites of trauma or injury when more prostaglandins are required, but it does not seem to be involved in the other tissue functions. By interfering with this part of the inflammatory reaction, NSAIDs block inflammation before all of the signs and symptoms can develop. Most NSAIDs are relatively nonselective and therefore block both COX-1 and COX-2. This explains why patients who take NSAIDs quite often experience G-I effects. The selective COX-2 inhibitors are thought to act only at sites of trauma and injury to more specifically block the inflammatory reaction.

The adverse effects associated with most NSAIDs are related to inhibition of both COX-1 and COX-2 enzymes and changes in the functions that they influence – GI integrity, blood clotting and sodium and water balance. The selective COX-2 inhibitors are designed to affect only the activity of COX-2, the enzyme that becomes active in response to trauma and injury. They do not interfere with COX-1, which is needed for normal functioning of these systems. Consequently, these drugs should not have the associated adverse effects seen when both COX-1 and COX-2 are inhibited. Recent studies suggest that they may block some protective responses in the body, such as vasodilation and inhibited platelet clumping, which could lead to cardiovascular problems (see Box 15.2).

The NSAIDs are indicated for relief of the signs and symptoms of RA and osteoarthritis, musculoskeletal disorders, for relief of mild-to-moderate pain, for treatment of primary dysmenorrhoea and acute gout and for fever reduction.

The NSAIDs are also an important group of drugs used with morphine in managing cancer pain including metastatic bone pain.

Pharmacokinetics

The NSAIDs are rapidly absorbed from the GI tract, reaching peak levels in 1 to 3 hours. They are metabolized in the liver and excreted in the urine. NSAIDs cross the placenta and cross into breast milk and are not recommended during pregnancy and lactation because of the potential adverse effects on the foetus or neonate.

BOX 15.2 Cyclo-Oxygenase (COX-2) Inhibitors

Originally, there were a number of COX-2 inhibitors in the market; however, several were withdrawn because of an increased risk of cardiovascular mortality compared with a placebo group. The Adenoma Prevention with Celecoxib study showed a two- to three-fold increase in cardiovascular (CV) events among patients using the drug compared with placebo over 33 months (Solomon *et al.*, 2005). There did seem to be a dose correlation, with more events in the group using a higher dose. A nearly identical study, the PreSAP trial (Prevention of Spontaneous Adenomatous Polyps), showed no increase in CV events in the group using celecoxib. In the meantime, the COX-2 inhibitors valdecoxib and rofecoxib have stayed off the market until appropriate guidelines and controls are in place for their return. Celecoxib and etoricoxib are still approved for use but packaging information includes warnings that there is potential risk for increased CV events as well as the risk of GI bleeding. Health care providers should use caution in recommending these drugs to anyone with an established CV risk and should only be prescribed to patients at high risk of developing gastric ulcers.

Celecoxib and etoricoxib are used for the acute and long-term treatment of rheumatoid and osteoarthritis, particularly in patients who cannot tolerate the GI effects of other NSAIDs (see Critical Thinking Scenario 15-1); for ankylosing spondylitis and acute gout. Celecoxib is also being studied for its potential ability to block angiogenesis in various cancers.

Contraindications and Cautions

The NSAIDs are contraindicated in the presence of allergy to any NSAID or aspirin; this includes those in whom attacks of asthma, angioedema, urticaria or rhinitis have been precipitated by aspirin or any other NSAID. Additional contraindications are cardiovascular dysfunction, *because of the varying effects of the prostaglandins*; peptic ulcer or known GI bleeding, *because of the potential to exacerbate the GI bleeding*; and pregnancy or lactation, *because of potential adverse effects on the neonate or mother*. Caution should be used with hepatic or renal dysfunction *which could alter the metabolism and excretion of these drugs* and patients with cardiac impairment and with any other known allergies, *which indicate increased sensitivity*; and with the elderly and those with asthma due to the potential for bronchoconstriction.

Adverse Effects

Patients receiving NSAIDs often experience nausea, dyspepsia, GI pain, constipation, diarrhoea or flatulence caused by direct GI effects of the drug. The potential for ulceration and/or GI bleeding is often a cause of discontinuation of the drug. Oral preparations containing misoprostol which has prostaglandin-like actions can limit the gastric effects of NSAIDs. Headache, dizziness, drowsiness and fatigue also occur frequently and could be related to prostaglandin activity in the CNS. Bleeding, platelet inhibition and even bone marrow depression have been reported with chronic use and are probably related to the blocking of prostaglandin activity. Rash and mouth sores may occur and severe hypersensitivity and cases of anaphylactic shock have been reported. Patients with asthma may experience a worsening of their asthma symptoms.

Clinically Important Drug–Drug Interactions

The most significant drug–drug interactions occur with other NSAIDs or aspirin; antibacterials; anticoagulants; antidepressants; hypoglycaemics; anticonvulsants; antipsychotics; antivirals; cyclosporine; cytotoxics; diuretics; and lithium. There is also potential for decreased antihypertensive effect of β-blockers if these drugs are combined; and there have been reports of lithium toxicity, especially when combined with ibuprofen. Patients who receive these combinations should be monitored closely and appropriate dosage adjustments should be made by the prescriber.

Always consult a current copy of the British National Formulary for further guidance.

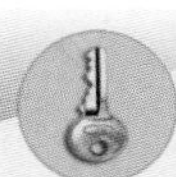

Key drug Summary: *Ibuprofen*

Indications: Relief of the signs and symptoms of RA and osteoarthritis; relief of mild-to-moderate pain; treatment of primary dysmenorrhoea, sore throat and dental pain; postoperative analgesia; fever reduction (including postimmunisation pyrexia). It can be used in the management of cancer pain in conjunction with opioids.

Actions: Inhibits prostaglandin synthesis by blocking cyclo-oxygenase-1 and -2 receptor sites, leading to anti-inflammatory, analgesia and antipyretic effects

Pharmacokinetics:

Route	Onset	Peak	Duration
Oral	30 min	1–2 h	4–6 h

$T_{1/2}$: 1.8–2.5 hours; metabolized in the liver and excreted in the urine

Adverse effects: GI disturbances (nausea, dyspepsia, ulceration and bleeding, constipation), headache, dizziness, somnolence, fatigue, rash and hypersensitivity reactions particularly bronchospasm.

Nursing Considerations for Patients Receiving NSAIDs

Assessment: History and Examination

Screen for any of the following, *which could be contraindications or cautions for the use of the drug:* known allergies to any salicylates or NSAIDs; hepatic or renal disease; cardiovascular dysfunction; and GI bleeding or peptic ulcer, asthma.

Include *screening for baseline status before beginning therapy and for any potential adverse effects:* temperature; orientation, reflexes, pulse, blood pressure and perfusion; bowel sounds; and full blood count, liver and renal function tests, urinalysis, stool occult, blood and serum electrolytes.

Nursing Diagnoses, Implementation and Evaluation

Refer to the Nursing Considerations section for the salicylates.

Paracetamol

Paracetamol is one of the most frequently used drugs to treat moderate-to-mild pain and fever. It is often used in place of the NSAIDs or salicylates. In contrast to the NSAIDs, paracetamol has weaker anti-inflammatory actions. Paracetamol is also available as a compound preparation with the opioid analgesic, codeine, to form co-codamol.

Therapeutic Actions and Indications

The exact mechanism of action of paracetamol is still unknown; however, it is known to reduce prostaglandin synthesis in the CNS. This may be via inhibition of another isoform of the cyclo-oxygenase enzyme, COX-3, but this remains to be determined.

Paracetamol possesses good analgesic and anti-pyretic properties and is indicated for the treatment of pain and fever associated with a variety of conditions, including influenza; for the prophylaxis of fever associated with children receiving immunisations; and for the relief of musculoskeletal pain associated with arthritis.

Pharmacokinetics

Paracetamol is rapidly absorbed from the GI tract, reaching peak levels in 0.5 to 1 hour. It is extensively metabolized in the liver and excreted in the urine, with a half-life of between 2 to 4 hours. Caution should be used in patients with hepatic or renal impairment, which could interfere with metabolism and excretion of the drug, leading to toxic

FOCUS ON **PATIENT SAFETY**

Paracetamol is found in numerous OTC products for treating pain, colds, flu and allergies. These products are available without a prescription. Many people are unaware of their potential hazards and they do not report the use of these products to their health care provider, even when specifically asked about drug use.

Patients, or parents, seeking relief from the signs and symptoms associated with the common cold or flu may take more than one of these products, hoping to relieve a stuffy nose, headache, or cough by combining products containing paracetamol. Many people do not read the product labels, relying instead on the advertised use. The consequence is many reports of people overdosing on paracetamol while following the dosage guidelines. In addition, patients who take liquid forms of these products may use an inaccurate measuring device (like a teaspoon from a cutlery set) and inadvertently overdose. Health care providers need to be alert for signs and symptoms of paracetamol toxicity – initially nausea, vomiting and GI upset. They need to ask patients specifically about whether they are using OTC products to reduce pain, control coughs, or help them sleep through the night. Overdose with paracetamol is particularly dangerous as it may cause hepatic damage, which is sometimes not apparent for 4 to 6 days.

The education of parents and patients about this potential hazard should not wait until a disaster occurs but should be incorporated into general health promotion opportunities.

Patients should be taught how to read labels, monitor dosage and measure liquid medications, what signs and symptoms of overdose to watch for and what to do if any occur.

levels. Therapeutic doses of paracetamol are safe for use during pregnancy or lactation.

Contraindications and Cautions

Paracetamol should be used cautiously in hepatic or renal dysfunction, or chronic alcoholism *because of associated toxic effects.* In patients the normal daily maximum dose may need to be decreased.

Adverse Effects

Adverse effects associated with paracetamol use are rare but can include thrombocytopaenia and leukopaenia and neutropaenia, skin rash and hypotension. Hepatotoxicity is a potentially fatal adverse effect usually associated with chronic use and overdose (10–15g) and is related to direct toxic effects on the liver.

Clinically Important Drug–Drug Interactions

There is an increased risk of bleeding with oral anticoagulants because of effects on the liver; of toxicity with chronic alcohol ingestion because of toxic effects on the liver. If these combinations cannot be avoided, appropriate dosage adjustment should be made and the patient should be monitored closely.

Always consult a current copy of the British National Formulary for further guidance.

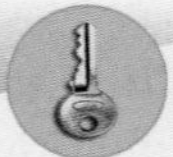

Key drug Summary: *Paracetamol*

Indications: Treatment of mild-to-moderate pain, fever, or signs and symptoms of the common cold or flu; musculoskeletal pain associated with arthritis and rheumatic disorders

Actions: Acts directly on the hypothalamus to cause sweating, which will reduce fever; mechanism of action as an analgesic is not fully understood

Pharmacokinetics:

Route	Onset	Peak	Duration
Oral	Varies	0.5–1 h	3–6 h

$T_{1/2}$: 2–4 hours; metabolized in the liver and excreted in the urine

Adverse effects: Rash, bone marrow suppression (causing blood disorders), hypotension with IV form

NOTE 10 to 15g of paracetamol taken within 24 hours can cause severe hepatocellular necrosis. Nausea and vomiting, the only early features of poisoning usually settle within 24 hours. Liver damage is maximal 3 to 4 days after ingestion and may lead to encephalopathy and haemorrhage and even death. Patients who have taken an overdose of paracetamol therefore need to be transferred to hospital urgently. Acetylcysteine helps to protect the liver if infused within 24 hours of ingesting paracetamol. (BNF, 2007).

Drugs Used to Suppress the Rheumatic Disease Process

The most commonly used drugs to treat RA are the NSAIDs and the *disease-modifying antirheumatic drugs (DMARDs).* Whereas the NSAIDs can only reduce the pain associated with RA, the DMARDs can slow the progress of the disease. These drugs are specifically used to block the inflammation and tissue damage associated with RA. Unlike NSAIDs these drugs do not produce an immediate therapeutic effect but require 4 to 6 months of treatment for a full response. Other DMARDs include sulfasalazine, methotrexate (Chapter 14), the antimalarial chloroquine (Chapter 12), penicillamine, azathioprine (Chapter 17) and gold compounds. Cytokine modulators have also proved highly effective in the treatment of RA.

In addition to the DMARDs, the immunosuppressant drug leflunomide directly inhibits an enzyme, inosine monophosphate dehydrogenase. This enzyme is active in the autoimmune process that leads to RA, preventing the signs and symptoms of inflammation and blocking the structural damage this inflammation can cause. Leflunomide is indicated for the treatment of active RA to relieve symptoms and to slow the progression of the disease. It has been associated with severe hepatic toxicity and the patient's liver function needs to be monitored closely.

The hyaluronidase derivatives, sodium hyaluronate and hylan G-F 20, are used to treat osteoarthritis of the knee. These drugs have elastic and viscous properties and are injected (weekly for 3–5 weeks) directly into the joints of patients with severe osteoarthritis of the knee. They seem to cushion and lubricate the joints and relieve the pain associated with degenerative arthritis.

Disease-Modifying Antirheumatic Drugs (DMARDs)

Some patients with rheumatic inflammatory conditions do not respond to the usual anti-inflammatory therapies and their conditions worsen despite weeks or months of standard pharmacological treatment. Some of these patients respond to treatment with gold salts, also known as **chrysotherapy**. Gold can be given orally as auranofin, or by intramuscular injection as sodium aurothiomalate.

Penicillamine, a metabolite of penicillin, is given orally to treat severe RA.

Therapeutic Actions and Indications

Gold salts are absorbed by macrophages, which results in inhibition of phagocytosis (see Figure 15.1). As phagocytosis is blocked, the release of lysosomal enzymes is inhibited and tissue destruction is decreased. This action allows gold salts to suppress and prevent some arthritis and synovitis. Gold salts are indicated to treat selected cases of rheumatoid and juvenile RA in patients whose disease has been unresponsive to standard therapy. These drugs do not repair damage; they prevent further damage and so are most effective if used early in the disease.

The exact mechanism of action of penicillamine is unclear but it is known to lower the immunoglobulin M (IgM) rheumatoid factor levels and levels of interleukin-1, relieving the signs and symptoms of inflammation. It may take 2 to 3 months of therapy before a response is noted. Penicillamine is also a metal-chelator and can be used to 'mop-up' heavy metals in heavy metal poisoning.

Pharmacokinetics

Gold salts are absorbed at different rates, depending on their route of administration. They are widely distributed throughout the body but seem to concentrate in the hypothalamic-pituitary-adrenocortical system, the adrenal and renal cortices, as well as the synovial joints. The gold salts are excreted in urine and faeces. These drugs cross the placenta and cross into breast milk. They have been shown to be teratogenic in animal studies and should not be used during pregnancy or lactation. Barrier contraceptives should be recommended to women of childbearing age and another method of feeding the baby should be used if gold therapy is needed in a lactating woman.

Only approximately half the dose of penicillamine is absorbed into the systemic circulation. The absorption of penicillamine is decreased if taken with iron salts or antacids; if these are given together, they should be separated by at least 2 hours. Penicillamine is excreted unchanged in the urine. This drug should not be used during pregnancy or lactation.

Contraindications and Cautions

Gold salts can be quite toxic and are contraindicated in the presence of any known allergy to gold, severe debilitation, renal or hepatic impairment, blood dyscrasias, systemic lupus erythematosus, recent radiation treatment, history of urticaria and eczema, or toxic levels of heavy metals and pregnancy or lactation.

Penicillamine is contraindicated in the presence of any known allergy to penicillamine or penicillin, renal dysfunction, lupus erythematosus or pregnancy.

Adverse Effects

A variety of adverse effects are common with the use of gold salts and are probably related to their deposition in the tissues and effects at that local level: stomatitis, colitis, diarrhoea and other GI inflammation; pulmonary fibrosis; bone marrow depression; nephrotic syndrome; dermatitis, pruritus and exfoliative dermatitis; and allergic reactions ranging from flushing, fainting and dizziness to anaphylactic shock.

Penicillamine is associated with a potentially fatal myasthenic syndrome, bone marrow depression and assorted hypersensitivity reactions.

Clinically Important Drug–Drug Interactions

Gold salts should not be combined with penicillamine, antimalarials, cytotoxic drugs, or immunosuppressive agents other than low-dose corticosteroids because of the potential for severe toxicity.

Penicillamine should not be administered with gold salts or other drugs known to be nephrotoxic because of the increased risk of toxicity. In addition, penicillamine should not be given with antipsychotics.

Always consult a current copy of the British National Formulary for further guidance.

Cytokine Modulators

Cytokine modulators are a relatively new approach to relieving the pain and suffering of patients with acute RA. National Institute for Health and Clinical Excellence (2007) guidance currently dictates that a cytokine modulator can only be prescribed if the patient has failed to respond to standard therapy; that is if the patient has already tried two DMARDs.

Therapeutic Actions and Indications

Cytokine modulators currently available for use are abatacept, adalimumab, anakinra, etanercept, infliximab and rituximab. They are used to treat moderate-to-severe RA. Most are used together with methotrexate.

- *Abatacept* inhibits the activation of cytotoxic T lymphocytes important in the inflammatory process. This drug is given via IV infusion.
- *Adalimumab* and *infliximab* are both monoclonal antibodies against the pro-inflammatory cytokine tumour necrosis factor (TNF). Infliximab has been associated with reduced resistance to severe infections and patients should be tested for tuberculosis before and throughout treatment.
- *Anakinra* is an interleukin-1 (IL-1) receptor antagonist. It blocks increased levels of IL-1, which is responsible for the degradation of cartilage in RA. This drug must be given each day by subcutaneous injection and is often used in combination with other drugs that suppress the rheumatic disease process.
- *Etanercept* contains genetically engineered TNF receptors derived from Chinese hamster ovary cells. These receptors react with free-floating TNF released by active leukocytes in autoimmune inflammatory disease to prevent the damage caused by TNF. Etanercept is indicated for subcutaneous use to treat severe, active and progressive RA; juvenile idiopathic arthritis; severe ankylosing spondylitis and psoriatic arthritis. The drug has been associated with the development of serious demyelinating disorders, including multiple sclerosis. It can also cause severe myelosuppression and increased risk of infections. Patients using this drug need to be monitored very closely.
- *Rituximab* is a monoclonal antibody that lyses the B lymphocytes involved in the inflammatory process. Although mainly used as a chemotherapeutic, rituximab can be used to treat severe RA. Some side-effects including nausea, vomiting and allergic reactions can occur during intravenous infusion. Patients will require close monitoring.

Contraindications and Cautions

These drugs are contraindicated in pregnancy or lactation, *because of the potential for adverse effects on the foetus or neonate;* and acute infection, *because of the blocking of normal inflammatory pathways.* The cytokine modulators should be used cautiously in patients with liver or renal impairment; a predisposition to infections, a history of heart failure or demyelinating disorders, *which could be exacerbated by these drugs.*

Adverse Effects

A variety of adverse effects are common with the use of these drugs, including local irritation at injection sites, increased risk of infection, nausea, abdominal pain, deterioration of heart conditions and blood disorders. Etanercept is associated with severe bone marrow suppression, as well as serious CNS disorders, including multiple sclerosis.

Clinically Important Drug–Drug Interactions

The cytokine modulators should not be used together because of an increased risk of side-effects, including serious infections. They should not be administered at the same time as a live vaccine.

Always consult a current copy of the British National Formulary for further guidance.

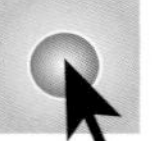

WEB LINKS

Health care providers and patients may want to consult the following Internet sources:

http://cks.library.nhs.uk The National Health Service Clinical Knowledge Summaries provides evidence-based practical information on the common conditions observed in primary care.

http://www.arthritiscare.org.uk Arthritis Care provides information and support to patients.

http://www.bnf.org.uk The BNF provides UK healthcare professionals with authoritative and practical information on the selection and clinical use of medicines.

http://www.bnfc.org.uk The same information as found on the BNF web site, but with regard to the clinical use of medicines for children.

http://www.nhsdirect.nhs.uk The National Health Service Direct service provides patients with information and advice about health, illness and health services.

http://www.nice.org.uk The National Institute for Health and Clinical Excellence (NICE) is an independent organization responsible for providing national guidance on promoting good health and preventing and treating ill health.

http://www.rheumatoid.org.uk The National Rheumatoid Arthritis Society site provides information and support for people with RA and juvenile idiopathic arthritis. It is a useful resource for families, friends and carers and also health professionals with an interest in RA.

Points to Remember

- The inflammatory response, which is important for protecting the body from injury and invasion, produces many of the signs and symptoms associated with disease, including fever, aches and pains and lethargy.
- Chronic or excessive activity by the inflammatory response can lead to the release of lysosomal enzymes and tissue destruction.
- Anti-inflammatory drugs block various chemicals associated with the inflammatory reaction. Anti-inflammatory drugs may also have antipyretic (fever-blocking) and analgesic (pain-blocking) activities.
- The salicylates and NSAIDs block the enzymes COX-1 and COX-2 involved in the synthesis of prostaglandins responsible for pain and inflammation. The exact mechanism of action of paracetamol is not clearly understood but it is known to inhibit prostaglandin synthesis in the CNS to lower fever and relieve pain possibly by inhibiting COX-3.
- The DMARDs include gold salts and penicillamine and are used to slow the development of the inflammatory process in RA.
- Cytokine modulators can suppress the rheumatic disease process in one of several ways: (i) inhibition of T lymphocyte activation; (ii) monoclonal antibodies against TNF, TNF receptors or B lymphocytes; and (iii) antagonist of interleukin-1 receptors. Each drug slows progression of the disease and the degradation of cartilage.
- Salicylates can cause acidosis and eighth cranial nerve damage. NSAIDs are most associated with GI irritation and bleeding. Paracetamol can cause serious liver toxicity.
- The gold salts cause many systemic inflammatory reactions. The cytokine modulators are associated with local injection site irritation and increased susceptibility to infection.
- Many anti-inflammatory drugs are available OTC and care must be taken to prevent abuse or overuse of these drugs.

CRITICAL THINKING SCENARIO 15-1

NSAID Use and Rheumatoid Arthritis

The Situation

Alfred is a 56-year-old man with a 14-year history of RA. He is seen in the clinic for review of his arthritis and he says that his medicines are not helping him. On examination, it is found that Alfred's range of motion, physical examination of joints and overall presentation has not changed since his last visit. Alfred states that he has been taking diclofenac, as prescribed, for his arthritis, but he found that he was feeling nauseous after taking it. He read the advice label and it stated this was a side-effect so he stopped taking the diclofenac regularly and only used it occasionally when his pain was worse.

Critical Thinking

- Think about the pathophysiology of RA and how the drugs prescribed act on the inflammatory process.
- How can the nurse best explain the disease and the drug regimen to this patient?
- What could be contributing to Alfred's perception that his condition has worsened?
- What alternative therapy could be prescribed to Alfred to manage his condition?
- What nursing interventions would be appropriate to help Alfred cope with his disease and his need for medication?

Discussion

Alfred should be offered encouragement and support to deal with his progressive disease and the drug regimen required. The fact that his physical status has not changed but he perceives that the condition is worse may reflect other underlying problems that are making it more difficult for him to cope with chronic pain and limitations. The nurse should explore his social situation, any changes in his living situation and support services. An examination should be done to determine whether other physical problems have emerged that could be adding to his sense that things are getting worse. The actions of diclofenac on the arthritic process should be reviewed in basic terms. Find out if he is taking the drug on an empty stomach. His medication should be taken with food.

If Alfred has been having GI complaints with the diclofenac, he can be encouraged to take the drug with food and to have small, frequent meals to keep stomach

(continued)

NSAID Use and Rheumatoid Arthritis *(continued)*

acid levels at a more steady state. Ibuprofen has the lowest risk of GI side-effects, therefore, Alfred may like to try ibuprofen instead, but he should be advised that this also needs to be taken with food. As a further alterative Alfred could be offered a suppository form of diclofenac.

Nursing Care Guide for Alfred: NSAIDs and Rheumatoid Arthritis

Assessment: History and Examination

Assess Alfred's health history for allergies to NSAIDs; cardiovascular dysfunction; renal or hepatic impairment; ulcerative GI disease, peptic ulcer; asthma and concurrent use of aspirin, antibacterials; anticoagulants; antidepressants; antidiabetics; anticonvulsants; antipsychotics; antivirals; cyclosporine; cytotoxics; diuretics; lithium and β-adrenergic blockers

Focus the physical examination on the following areas:

- Musculoskeletal system: joint assessment, range of movement
- Skin: colour, perfusion
- CV: pulse, cardiac auscultation, blood pressure
- GI: liver evaluation, epigastric symptoms
- Lab tests: full blood count, liver and renal function tests

Implementation

- Ensure proper administration of the drug.
- Administer with food
- Provide support and comfort measures to deal with adverse effects: small, frequent meals; safety measures if CNS effects occur
- Provide patient education regarding drug name, dosage, side-effects, precautions and warnings to report; supplementary measures to help decrease arthritis pain.
- Refer him to a physiotherapist/massage therapist

Evaluation

- Evaluate drug effects: decrease in signs and symptoms of inflammation.
- Monitor for adverse effects: rash, GI upset, GI bleeding
- Monitor for drug–drug interactions as listed.
- Evaluate effectiveness of patient education programme.
- Evaluate effectiveness of comfort/safety measures.

Patient Education for Alfred

- ☐ You have been prescribed diclofenac to help relieve the signs and symptoms of your RA. Diclofenac works as an analgesic and anti-inflammatory drug. It works in the body to decrease inflammation and to relieve the signs and symptoms of inflammation, such as pain, swelling, heat, tenderness and redness. It does not cure your arthritis, but will help you to live with it more comfortably.
- ☐ Take your diclofenac exactly as prescribed, every day.
- ☐ Some of the following adverse effects may occur:
  - *Nausea, abdominal discomfort: You should* take the drug with food and eating small, frequent meals may help. If these effects persist, consult with your health care provider.
  - *Drowsiness, dizziness:* Avoid driving or performing tasks that require alertness if you experience any of these problems.
  - *Headache:* If this becomes a problem, consult with your health care provider. Do not self-treat with more aspirin or other analgesics.
- ☐ Tell any health care provider who is taking care of you that you are taking this drug.
- ☐ Avoid using other over-the-counter preparations while you are taking this drug. If you feel that you need one of these drugs, consult with your health care provider for the most appropriate choice. Many of these drugs may also contain aspirin and could cause an overdose.
- ☐ Report any of the following to your health care provider: fever, rash, GI pain, nausea or itching.
- ☐ Keep this drug and all medications out of the reach of children.

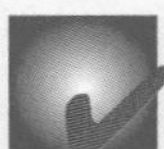

CHECK YOUR UNDERSTANDING

Answers to the questions in this chapter may be found in the answer key in the back of the book.

Multiple Choice

Select the most appropriate response to the following:

1. An analgesic is a drug that reduces
   a. fever.
   b. swelling.
   c. redness.
   d. pain.
2. An antipyretic is a drug that can block
   a. pain.
   b. swelling.
   c. fever.
   d. inflammation.
3. Salicylates are very popular anti-inflammatory agents for all of the following reasons, *except they*
   a. have antipyretic properties.
   b. have analgesic properties.
   c. are available without a prescription.
   d. must be given parenterally.
4. The NSAIDs affect the COX-1 and COX-2 enzymes. By blocking COX-2 enzymes, the NSAIDs block inflammation and the signs and symptoms of inflammation at the site of injury or trauma. By blocking COX-1 enzymes, these drugs block
   a. fever regulation.
   b. prostaglandins that protect the stomach lining.
   c. swelling in the periphery.
   d. liver function.
5. Your patient has been receiving ibuprofen for many years to relieve the pain of osteoarthritis. Assessment of the patient should include
   a. an electrocardiogram.
   b. full blood count with differential.
   c. respiratory auscultation.
   d. renal evaluation.
6. Patients taking NSAIDs should be taught to avoid the use of OTC medications without checking with their prescriber because
   a. many of the OTC preparations contain NSAIDs and inadvertent toxicity could occur.
   b. no one should take more than one type of pain reliever at a time.
   c. increased GI upset could occur.
   d. there is a risk of Reye's syndrome.
7. Chronic or excessive activity by the inflammatory response can lead to
   a. loss of white blood cells.
   b. coagulation problems.
   c. release of lysosomal enzymes and tissue destruction.
   d. adrenal suppression.

Extended Matching Questions

Select **all** that apply.

1. A patient is being treated for severe RA. The nurse could anticipate treatment with which of the following.
   a. Etanercept
   b. Gold therapy
   c. Hylan G-F 20
   d. Ketoprofen
   e. Interferon β-2a
   f. Methotrexate

Matching

Match the word with the appropriate definition.

1. ____________________ anti-inflammatory
2. ____________________ antipyretic
3. ____________________ analgesic
4. ____________________ salicylates
5. ____________________ NSAIDs
6. ____________________ pyrogens
7. ____________________ chrysotherapy

A. Treatment with gold salts
B. Nonsteroidal anti-inflammatory drugs
C. Blocking the prostaglandin system to prevent inflammation
D. Blocking the effects of the inflammatory response
E. Blocking pain sensation
F. Substances that elevate the body's temperature
G. Blocking fever

Bibliography and References

British Medical Association and Royal Pharmaceutical Society of Great Britain (2008). *British National Formulary*. London: BMJ & RPS Publishing. *This publication is updated biannually: it is imperative that the most recent edition is consulted.*

British Medical Association and Royal Pharmaceutical Society of Great Britain (2008). *British National Formulary for Children*. London: BMJ & RPS Publishing. *This publication is updated annually: it is imperative that the most recent edition is consulted.*

Ganong, W. (2005). *Review of medical physiology* (22nd ed.). New York: McGraw-Hill.

Howland, R. D. & Mycek, M. J. (2005). *Pharmacology* (3rd ed.). Philadelphia: Lippincott Williams & Wilkins.

National Institute for Health and Clinical Excellence. (2007). Adalimumab, Etanercept and Infliximab for the treatment of rheumatoid arthritis. Available from www.nice.org.uk

Porth, C. M. & Matfin G. (2008). *Pathophysiology: Concepts of altered Health States* (8th ed.). Philadelphia: Lippincott Williams & Wilkins.

Rang, H. P., Dale, M. M., Ritter, J. M. & Flower, R. J. (2007). *Rang and Dale's pharmacology.* (6th ed.). Philadelphia: Churchill Livingstone.

Simonsen, T., Aarbakke, J., Kay, I., Coleman, I., Sinnott, P. & Lysaa, R. (2006). *Illustrated pharmacology for Nurses.* London: Hodder Arnold.

Solomon, S., McMurray, J. J. V., Pfeffer, M. A. Wittes, J., Fowler, R., Finn, P., Anderson, W. F., Zauber, A., Hawk, E., Bertagnolli, M. (2005) *Cardiovascular Risk Associated with Celecoxib in a Clinical Trial for Colorectal Adenoma Prevention.* The New England Journal of Medicine 352:1071–1080.

CHAPTER 16

Immune Modulators

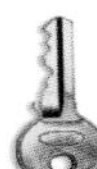

KEY TERMS

immune stimulant

immune suppressant

monoclonal antibodies

recombinant DNA technology

LEARNING OBJECTIVES

Upon completion of this chapter, you will be able to:

1. Describe the sites of actions of the various immune modulators.
2. Describe the therapeutic actions, indications, pharmacokinetics associated with each class of immune modulator.
3. Describe the contraindications, most common adverse reactions and important drug–drug interactions associated with each class of immune modulator.
4. Discuss the use of immune modulators across the lifespan.
5. Compare and contrast the key drugs for each class of immune modulator with the other drugs in that class and with drugs in other classes.
6. Outline the nursing considerations and teaching needs for patients receiving each class of immune modulator.

IMMUNE STIMULANTS

Interferons

interferon α-2a
interferon α-2b
interferon α-n3
interferon β-1a
interferon β-1b
interferon γ-1b
peginterferon α-2a
peginterferon α-2b

Interleukins

aldesleukin

T-and B-cell Modulators

levamisole

IMMUNE SUPPRESSANTS

T- and B-cell Suppressors

azathioprine
ciclosporin
glatiramer acetate
mycophenolate
pimecrolimus
sirolimus
tacrolimus

Interleukin Receptor Antagonist

anakinra

Monoclonal Antibodies

adalimumab
alemtuzumab
basiliximab
bevacizumab
cetuximab
daclizumab
efalizumab
erlotinib
infliximab
natalizumab
omalizumab
palivizumab
pegaptanib
rituximab
trastuzumab

As the name implies, immune modulators are used to modify the actions of the immune system. **Immune stimulants** are used to energize the immune system when it is exhausted from fighting prolonged invasion or needs help fighting a specific pathogen or cancer cell. **Immune suppressants** are used to block the normal effects of the immune system in cases of organ transplantation (in which nonself cells are transplanted into the body and destroyed by the immune reaction) and in autoimmune disorders (in which the body's defences recognize self-cells as foreign and work to destroy them).

The knowledge base about the actions and components of the immune system is constantly growing and changing. As new discoveries are made and interactions understood, new applications will be found for modulating the immune system in a variety of disorders. (Box 16.1 for their use in a variety of age groups. Box 16.2 discusses the use of immune modulators during pregnancy.)

BOX 16.2

Focus on Sex Considerations: Immune Modulators and Pregnancy

Generally, immune modulators are contraindicated for use during pregnancy and lactation, largely because these drugs have been associated with foetal abnormalities, increased maternal and foetal infections and suppressed immune responses in nursing babies. Female patients should be informed of the risk of using these drugs during pregnancy and receive counselling in the use of barrier contraceptives. The use of barrier contraceptives is advised because the effects of oral contraceptives may be altered by liver changes or by changes in the body's immune response, potentially resulting in unplanned pregnancy.

If a patient taking immune modulators becomes pregnant or decides that she wants to become pregnant, she should discuss this with her health care provider and review the risks associated with use of the drug or drugs being taken. The monoclonal antibodies should be used with caution during pregnancy and lactation.

Immune Stimulants

Immune stimulants include the interferons, which are naturally released from human cells in response to viral invasion; the interleukins, synthetic compounds much like the interleukins that communicate between lymphocytes, which stimulate cellular immunity and inhibit tumour growth; and a T- and B-cell modulator called levamisole, which restores immune function and also stimulates immune system activity (Figure 16.1).

Interferons

Interferons are naturally produced and released by human cells that have been invaded by viruses. They may also be released from cells in response to other stimuli. A number of interferons are available for use today. Several are produced by **recombinant DNA technology**, including interferon α-2a, interferon α-2b, peginterferon α-2a, peginterferon α-2b and interferon β-1b. Interferon β-1a is produced from Chinese hamster ovary cells. Interferon γ-1b is produced by *Escherichia coli* bacteria. The interferon of choice depends on the condition being treated.

BOX 16.1

DRUG THERAPY ACROSS THE LIFESPAN

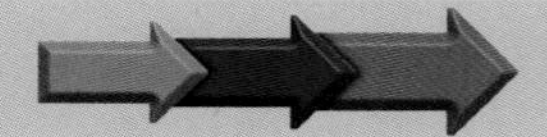

Immune Modulators

CHILDREN

Most of the drugs that affect the immune system are not recommended for use in children or have not been tested in children. The exceptions – interferon α-2b, azathioprine, ciclosporin, tacrolimus and palivizumab – should be used cautiously, monitoring the child frequently for infection, gastrointestinal (GI), renal, haematological or central nervous system (CNS) effects.

The immune suppressants (azathioprine, ciclosporin and tacrolimus) are usually needed in higher doses for children than for adults to achieve the same therapeutic effect.

Protecting the child from infection and injury is a very important part of the care of a child taking an immune modulator.

When administering any drug to children, always consult the most recent edition of the British National Formulary for Children.

ADULTS

Both the adult patient who is receiving a parenteral immune modulator and a significant other should learn the proper technique for injection, disposal of needles and special storage precautions for the drug. It is important to stress ways to avoid exposure to infection and injury to prevent further complications. The patient should be encouraged to seek regular follow-up and medical care.

Immune modulators are contraindicated during pregnancy and lactation because of the potential for adverse effects on the foetus or neonate and complications for the mother. Women of childbearing age should be advised to use barrier contraceptives while taking these drugs and, if breast-feeding, should be counselled to find another method of feeding the baby. Some of these drugs impair fertility and the patient should be advised of this fact before taking the drug.

OLDER ADULTS

Older patients may be more susceptible to the effects of the immune modulators, partly because the ageing immune system is less efficient and less responsive.

These patients need to be monitored closely for infection, GI, renal, hepatic and CNS effects. Baseline renal and liver function tests can help to determine whether a decreased dosage will be needed before beginning the therapy.

These patients are more susceptible to infection; therefore, they need to receive extensive teaching about ways to avoid infection and injury.

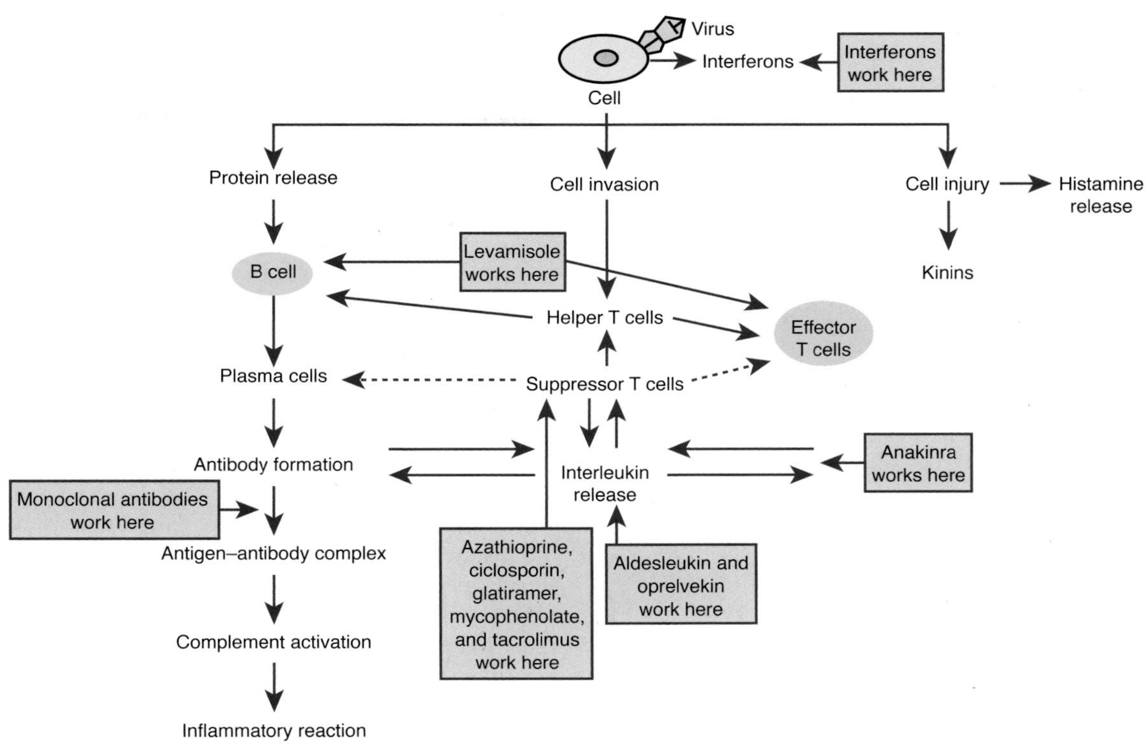

FIGURE 16.1 Sites of action of the immune modulators.

Therapeutic Actions and Indications

Interferons act to prevent virus particles from replicating inside other cells. They also stimulate interferon receptor sites on noninvaded cells to produce antiviral proteins, which prevent viruses from entering the cell. In addition, interferons have been found to inhibit tumour growth and replication. Interestingly, interferon γ-1b also acts like an interleukin, stimulating phagocytes to be more aggressive.

Interferons are indicated for treating selected leukaemias (α-2a, α-2b); multiple sclerosis (β-1a, β-1b; Box 16.3); chronic hepatitis B or chronic hepatitis C (α-2b); chronic hepatitis C; acquired immune deficiency syndrome (AIDS)-related Kaposi's sarcoma (α-2a, α-2b and unlabelled uses for several other interferons); and severe infections caused by chronic granulomatous disease (γ-1b). Most of the interferons are being tested for the treatment of various cancers and AIDS-related problems.

Pharmacokinetics

The interferons are generally well absorbed after subcutaneous or intramuscular injection. They are broken down in the tissues and seem to be excreted primarily through the kidneys. Many of them have been shown to be teratogenic in animals and therefore should not be used during human pregnancy. Use of barrier contraceptives is advised for women of childbearing age. It is not known whether these drugs cross into breast milk, but because of the potential adverse effects on the baby, it is advised that the drugs should not be used during lactation unless the benefits to the mother clearly outweigh any risks to the baby.

Contraindications and Cautions

The use of interferons is contraindicated during pregnancy and lactation *because of the potential risk to the foetus or neonate.* Caution should be used in the presence of known cardiac disease *because hypertension and arrhythmias have been reported with the use of these drugs;* with myelosuppression *because these drugs may further suppress the bone marrow;* and with CNS dysfunction of any kind *because of the potential for CNS depression and personality changes that have been reported.*

Always consult a current copy of the British National Formulary for further guidance.

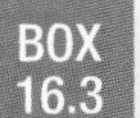

BOX 16.3 NICE Guidance on the Treatment of Multiple Sclerosis

Based on clinical and cost-effectiveness, the National Institute for Health and Clinical Excellence (NICE) decided in January 2002 that interferon-β and glatiramer acetate should no longer be recommended for the treatment of multiple sclerosis on the National Health Service in England and Wales. However those receiving these treatments may continue until they, in agreement with their consultant, decide to stop.

Adverse Effects

The adverse effects associated with the use of interferons are related to the immune or inflammatory reaction that is being stimulated (e.g. lethargy, myalgia, arthralgia, anorexia, nausea). Other commonly seen adverse effects include headache, dizziness, bone marrow depression, depression and suicidal ideation, photosensitivity and liver impairment.

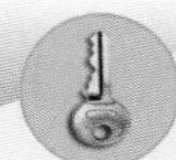

Key Drug Summary: Interferon α-2b

Indications: Hairy cell leukaemia, malignant melanoma, lymph or liver metastases, AIDS-related Kaposi's sarcoma, chronic hepatitis B and C (in combination with ribavirin).

Actions: Inhibits the growth of *tumour* cells in some lymphomas and solid tumours and enhances the immune response

Pharmacokinetics:

Route	Onset	Peak
IM, Sub-cut	Rapid	3–12 h
IV	Rapid	End of infusion

$T_{1/2}$: 2–3 hours; metabolized in the kidney, excretion is unknown

Adverse effects (usually dose dependant); hypersensitivity, thyroid abnormalities dizziness, confusion, rash, dry skin, anorexia, nausea, bone marrow suppression, hypoglycaemia alopecia, ocular side-effects and depression flu-like symptoms.

Interleukins

Interleukins are chemicals produced by leukocytes to communicate with other leukocytes. Interleukin-2 stimulates cellular immunity by increasing the activity of natural killer (NK) cells, platelets and cytokines. Two interleukin-2 preparations are available for use. Aldesleukin is a human interleukin-2 produced by recombinant DNA technology using *E. coli* bacteria. It is licensed for use in metastatic renal carcinoma.

Therapeutic Actions and Indications

Natural interleukin-2 is produced by helper T cells to activate cellular immunity and inhibit tumour growth by increasing lymphocyte numbers and their activity. When interleukins are administered, there are increases in the number of NK cells and lymphocytes, in cytokine activity and in the number of circulating platelets. Aldesleukin is indicated for the treatment of specific renal carcinomas and is also being investigated for use in the treatment of AIDS and AIDS-related disorders.

Pharmacokinetics

The interleukins are rapidly distributed after injection and are primarily cleared from the body by the kidneys. They were shown to be damaging to the embryo and teratogenic in animal studies and should not be used in human during pregnancy. Use of barrier contraceptives is recommended for women of childbearing age who require one of these drugs. It is not clear whether the drugs cross into breast milk, but it is recommended that they not be used during lactation; if they must be used, another method of feeding the baby should be chosen because of the potential for adverse effects in the baby.

Contraindications and Cautions

Interleukins are contraindicated in the presence of any allergy to an interleukin or *E. coli*-produced product and during pregnancy and lactation. Caution should be used with renal, liver, or cardiovascular impairment *because of the adverse effects of the drugs.*

Always consult a current copy of the British National Formulary for further guidance.

Adverse Effects

The adverse effects associated with the interleukins can be attributed to their effect on the body during inflammation (e.g. lethargy, myalgia, arthralgia, fatigue, fever). Respiratory difficulties, CNS changes and cardiac arrhythmias have also been reported and the patient should be monitored for these effects and the drug stopped if they do occur.

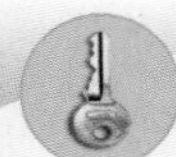

Key Drug Summary: Aldesleukin

Indications: Metastatic renal cell carcinoma in adults; treatment of metastatic melanomas produces, tumour shrinkage in a small number of patients.

Actions: Activates human cellular immunity and inhibits tumour growth through increases in lymphocytes, platelets and cytokines

Pharmacokinetics:

Route	Onset	Peak	Duration
Sub-Cut	5 min	13 min	3–4 h

$T_{1/2}$: 85 min; metabolized in the kidney and excreted in the urine

Adverse effects: Mental status changes, dizziness, hypotension, sinus tachycardia, arrhythmias, pruritus, nausea, vomiting, diarrhoea, anorexia, GI bleed, bone marrow suppression, respiratory difficulties, fever, chills, pain

T- and B-Cell Modulators

The drug levamisole is an immune stimulant that restores suppressed immune function in certain situations.

Therapeutic Actions and Indications

Levamisole stimulates B cells to produce antibodies, enhancing T cell activity and increase the activity of both monocytes and macrophages. Levamisole is indicated for the treatment of Dukes' stage C colon cancer after surgical resection and in conjunction with fluorouracil therapy. With further research, the indications may be expanded to include other carcinomas.

Pharmacokinetics

Levamisole is readily absorbed from the GI tract, reaching peak levels in 1.5 to 2 hours. It is extensively metabolized in the liver and excreted in the urine, with a half-life of 16 hours. Levamisole was embryotoxic in animal studies and should not be used during pregnancy. Women of childbearing age should be advised to use barrier contraceptives. It is not known whether levamisole crosses into breast milk, but because of the potentially severe adverse effects it could have on a neonate, it is recommended that the drug not be used during lactation.

Contraindications and Cautions

Levamisole is contraindicated in the presence of any known allergy to levamisole or its components and in pregnancy and lactation *because of possible adverse effects to the foetus or neonate.*

Adverse Effects

The most common adverse effects seen with levamisole are related to immune stimulation (flu-like effects: fatigue, lethargy, myalgia, arthralgia, fever). Other adverse effects that have been reported include GI upset, nausea, taste perversions and diarrhoea; dizziness, headache and depression; bone marrow depression; dermatitis; and hair loss.

Clinically Important Drug–Drug Interactions

There is a possibility of a disulphiram-type reaction if this drug is combined with alcohol. Patients should be cautioned to avoid this combination. There is also a possibility of increased phenytoin levels and toxicity if levamisole is combined with phenytoin. If such a combination cannot be avoided, phenytoin levels should be monitored and appropriate dosage reductions made.

Always consult a current copy of the British National Formulary for further guidance.

Nursing Considerations for Patients Receiving Immune Stimulants

Assessment: History and Examination

Screen for any of the following conditions, *which would contraindicate or require cautious use of the drug:* known allergies to any of these drugs or their components; pregnancy or lactation; hepatic, renal, or cardiac disease; bone marrow depression; and CNS disorders, including seizures.

Include screening *for baseline status before beginning therapy and for any potential adverse effects:* presence of any skin lesions; weight; temperature; orientation, reflexes; pulse, blood pressure, electrocardiogram (ECG), heart rhythm; liver evaluation; full blood count (FBC), liver and renal function tests; and assessment of condition being treated.

Establish if patient is currently taking other medications or herbal therapies, which may potentially interact with the immune stimulants.

Nursing Diagnoses

The patient receiving immune stimulants may have the following nursing diagnoses related to drug therapy:

- Acute pain related to CNS, GI and flu-like effects
- Imbalanced nutrition: less than body requirements related to flu-like symptoms
- Anxiety related to diagnosis and drug therapy
- Deficient knowledge regarding drug therapy

Implementation with Rationale

- Arrange for laboratory tests before and periodically during therapy, including FBC and differential, *to monitor for drug effects and adverse effects.*
- Administer drug as indicated; instruct the patient and a significant other if injections are required *to ensure that the drug will be given even if the patient is not able to administer it.*
- Monitor for severe reactions and *arrange to discontinue drug immediately if they occur.*
- Arrange for supportive care and comfort measures for flu-like symptoms (e.g. rest, environmental control, paracetamol) *to help the patient cope with the drug effects.* Ensure that the patient is well hydrated during therapy *to prevent severe adverse effects.*
- Instruct female patients in the use of barrier contraceptives *to avoid pregnancy during therapy because of the potential for adverse effects on the foetus.*
- Provide thorough patient education, including measures to avoid adverse effects, warning signs of

problems and proper administration, *to increase knowledge about drug therapy and to increase compliance with the drug regimen.*
- Offer support and encouragement *to deal with the diagnosis and the drug regimen.*

Evaluation

- Monitor patient response to the drug (improvement in condition being treated).
- Monitor for adverse effects (flu-like symptoms, GI upset, CNS changes, bone marrow depression).
- Evaluate the effectiveness of the teaching plan (patient can name drug, dosage, adverse effects to watch for, specific measures to avoid adverse effects).
- Monitor the effectiveness of comfort measures and compliance with the regimen.

Immune Suppressants

Immune suppressants are often used in conjunction with corticosteroids, which block the inflammatory reaction and decrease initial damage to cells. They are especially beneficial in cases of organ transplantation and in the treatment of autoimmune diseases. The immune suppressants include T- and B-cell suppressors, an interleukin receptor antagonist and **monoclonal antibodies**–antibodies produced by a single clone of identical B cells that react with specific antigens.

Patients receiving immune suppressants are at high risk of infection and cancers, therefore they need to be forewarned to avoid situations in which exposure to infection may be high (e.g. crowds, working in the soil, visiting hospitals or sick friends, interacting with children during flu and cold season). They should also avoid activities that may cause injury, which leads to infection. Protective strategies include wearing masks and heavy gloves, delaying vaccinations, knowing the signs and symptoms of infection that warrant medical care and obtaining regular physical examinations and screenings for diseases of developing neoplasms.

T- and B-Cell Suppressors

Several T- and B-cell immune suppressors are available for use. Only one, ciclosporin, is used to suppress rejection in a variety of transplantation scenarios. It is also the most commonly used immune suppressant. Ciclosporin is extensively metabolized in the liver by the cytochrome P450 system and is primarily excreted in the bile. Ciclosporin was embryotoxic in animal studies and crosses into breast milk. The drug should not be used during pregnancy or lactation and women of childbearing age should be advised to use barrier contraceptives.

- *Azathioprine* is used specifically to prevent rejection in renal transplants and to treat rheumatoid arthritis (an autoimmune disorder) in selected patients. It is rapidly absorbed from the GI tract, reaching peak levels in 1 to 2 hours. This drug is metabolized in the liver and red blood cells. It was highly teratogenic in animal studies and crosses into breast milk. Because of the potential effects on the foetus or neonate, the drug should not be used during pregnancy or lactation and women of childbearing age should be advised to use barrier contraceptives.
- *Glatiramer acetate* is used specifically to reduce the number of relapses in multiple sclerosis, a disease thought to be related to an autoimmune reaction. Little is known about the pharmacokinetics of this drug. Some of it is immediately hydrolyzed on injection, some enters the lymph system and some may actually reach the systemic circulation. It is not known whether this drug crosses the placenta or crosses into breast milk, therefore use during pregnancy and lactation should be reserved for those situations in which the benefit to the mother clearly outweighs the potential risk to the foetus or neonate.
- *Mycophenolate* is an oral drug used with ciclosporin and corticosteroids to prevent organ rejection after renal, hepatic or heart transplantation. It is readily absorbed and immediately metabolized to its active metabolite. Most of the metabolized drug is then excreted in the urine. Caution should be used if serious renal impairment exists and the dosage should be lowered. Mycophenolate was teratogenic in animal studies and women of childbearing age should be advised to use barrier contraceptives whenever this drug is used. It is not known whether mycophenolate crosses into human breast milk, but because of the potential for adverse effects in the baby, it should not be used during lactation.
- *Sirolimus* is used to prevent organ rejection in patients receiving renal transplants and should be used with ciclosporin and corticosteroids. It is being studied for use in the treatment of psoriasis. Sirolimus is rapidly absorbed from the GI tract, reaching peak levels in 1 hour. It is extensively metabolized in the liver, partly by the cytochrome P450 system. Reduced dosage may be needed if hepatic impairment is present. The drug is then excreted primarily in the faeces. Sirolimus was embryotoxic in animal studies and should not be used during pregnancy unless the benefit to the mother clearly outweighs the potential risks to the foetus. It is not known whether sirolimus crosses into breast milk, but because of the potential for serious adverse effects in the baby, the drug should not be used during lactation.
- *Tacrolimus* is used to prevent liver or renal transplant rejection and is being studied for use in multiple other transplant scenarios. This drug is rapidly absorbed from the GI tract, reaching peak levels in 1.5 to 3.5 hours. It is extensively metabolized in the liver by the cytochrome P450 system and excreted in the urine. Lower doses of the drug may be needed in the presence of hepatic or renal impairment, which would interfere with the metabolism and excretion

of the drug. Tacrolimus crosses the placenta and has been associated with foetal hyperkalaemia and renal dysfunction. Avoid use in pregnancy unless the benefit to the mother clearly outweighs the risk to the foetus. It crosses into breast milk and is contraindicated during lactation because of the potential for serious adverse effects on the baby.

Therapeutic Actions and Indications

The exact mechanism of action of the T- and B-cell suppressors is not wholly defined. It has been shown that they block antibody production by B cells, inhibit suppressor and helper T cells and modify the release of interleukins and IL-2 (see Figure 16.1). It is also thought that ciclosporin, tacrolimus and sirolimus inhibit IL-2 production by T cells. Azathioprine and mycophenolate are purine synthesis inhibitors. Glatiramer acetate is a polymer of four amino acids found in myelin basic protein and is thought to shift the T cell response to myelin basic protein in multiple sclerosis from pro-inflammatory to anti-inflammatory.

The T- and B-cell suppressors are indicated for the prevention and treatment of specific transplant rejections. Many of the T- and B-cell suppressors are used to treat a variety of autoimmune disorders and other transplant rejections as unlabeled uses for the drugs.

Contraindications and Cautions

The use of T- and B-cell suppressors is contraindicated in the presence of any known allergy to the drug or its components and during pregnancy and lactation *because of the potential adverse effects on the foetus or neonate.* Caution should be used with renal or hepatic impairment, *which could interfere with the metabolism or excretion of the drug* and in the presence of known neoplasms, *which potentially could spread with immune system suppression.*

Adverse Effects

Patients receiving these drugs are at increased risk for infection and for the development of neoplasms because of their blocking effect on the immune system. Other potentially dangerous adverse effects include hepatotoxicity, renal toxicity, renal dysfunction and pulmonary oedema. Patients may experience headache, tremors, and secondary infections such as acne, GI upset, diarrhoea and hypertension.

Clinically Important Drug–Drug Interactions

There is an increased risk of toxicity if these drugs are combined with other drugs that are hepatotoxic or nephrotoxic. Extreme care should be used if such combinations are necessary. Other reported drug–drug interactions are drug specific.

Always consult a current copy of the British National Formulary for further guidance.

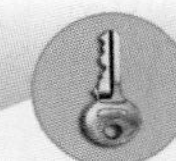

Key Drug Summary: Ciclosporin (cyclosporin)

Indications: Prophylaxis for organ rejection in kidney, liver and heart transplants (used with corticosteroids); treatment of chronic rejection in patients previously treated with other immunosuppressants; treatment of rheumatoid arthritis and recalcitrant psoriasis

Actions: Reversibly inhibits immunocompetent lymphocytes; inhibits T-helper cells and T-suppressor cells, lymphokine production and release of interleukin-2 and T-cell growth factor

Pharmacokinetics:

Route	Onset	Peak
Oral	Varies	3.5 h
IV	Rapid	1–2 h

$T_{1/2}$: 19–27 hours; metabolized in the liver and excreted in the bile and urine

Adverse effects: Tremor, hypertension, gum hyperplasia, renal dysfunction, diarrhoea, hirsutism, acne, bone marrow suppression, dose-dependant increase in creatinine and urea in the first few weeks.

Interleukin Receptor Antagonist

Anakinra specifically antagonizes human interleukin-1 receptors, blocking the activity of interleukin-1. Interleukin-1 levels are elevated in response to inflammation or immune reactions and are thought to be responsible for the degradation of cartilage that occurs in rheumatoid arthritis.

Therapeutic Actions and Indications

Anakinra is used to reduce the signs and symptoms of moderately to severely active rheumatoid arthritis in patients 18 years of age and older who have not responded to the traditional antirheumatic drugs.

Pharmacokinetics

Anakinra is absorbed slowly following subcutaneous injection, reaching peak effects in 3 to 7 hours. It is metabolized in the tissues with a 4 to 6 hour half-life and excreted in the urine. The drug may cross the placenta and may enter breast milk.

Contraindications and Cautions

Anakinra is contraindicated in pregnancy and lactation and in patients with renal impairment and a history of asthma or immunosuppression, or any active infection. There is an increased risk of infection whenever this drug is used and the patient needs to be protected from exposure to infections and monitored closely after any invasive procedures. Immunizations cannot be given while the patient is on this drug.

Adverse Effects

Headache, sinusitis, nausea, diarrhoea, upper respiratory tract infections and injection site reactions are among the most common adverse effects.

Clinically Important Drug–Drug Interactions

Patients who are also receiving etanercept must be monitored very closely because severe and even life-threatening infections have occurred.

Always consult a current copy of the British National Formulary for further guidance.

Monoclonal Antibodies

Antibodies that attach to specific receptor sites are being developed to respond to very specific situations. Every year, several new monoclonal antibodies are marketed, exemplifying the rapid pace with which these agents are being developed and approved for clinical use.

Therapeutic Actions and Indications

- *Adalimumab* is a monoclonal antibody specific for human tumour necrosis factor. It keeps the inflammatory reaction in check by reacting with and deactivating the free-floating tumour necrosis factor released by active leukocytes. It is used for reducing the signs and symptoms and preventing the structural damage associated with rheumatoid arthritis.
- *Alemtuzumab* is a monoclonal antibody specific for lymphocytes; it is used for the treatment of B-cell chronic lymphocytic leukaemia in patients who have been treated with alkylating agents and have failed fludarabine therapy.
- *Basiliximab* and *daclizumab* are monoclonal antibodies to interleukin-2 receptor sites on activated T lymphocytes; they react with those sites and block cellular response to allograft transplants. They are approved for use in preventing renal transplant rejection and are used in conjunction with ciclosporin and corticosteroids.
- *Bevacizumab* is a monoclonal antibody used with fluorouracil as an antineoplastic agent for the first-line treatment of patients with metastatic colon or rectal cancer.
- *Cetuximab* is a monoclonal antibody specific to epidermal growth factor receptor sites. It is used for the treatment of advanced epidermal growth factor–expressing colorectal cancer.
- *Efalizumab* is a monoclonal antibody specific for an antigen on human leukocytes. It prevents the adhesion of leukocytes to certain other cells. It is used for the treatment of adult patients with moderate-to-severe plaque psoriasis who are candidates for systemic therapy. This drug is associated with increased susceptibility to infections and reduced platelet counts and bleeding.
- *Erlotinib* is an oral agent for the treatment of locally advanced or metastatic nonsmall cell lung cancer. Its use is reserved for patients whose disease has progressed after other therapies.
- *Infliximab* is a monoclonal antibody to tumour necrosis factor. It is used to decrease the signs and symptoms of Crohn's disease in patients who do not respond to conventional therapy and for the treatment of fistulating Crohn's disease. It also is approved for use with methotrexate in the treatment of progressing moderate to severe rheumatoid arthritis.
- *Natalizumab* is a monoclonal antibody that was approved for decreasing the frequency of clinical exacerbations of multiple sclerosis. It is recommended as a possible treatment for people with rapidly evolving severe relapsing-remitting multiple sclerosis.
- *Omalizumab* is a monoclonal antibody to immunoglobulin E, an important factor in allergic reactions. It is used for the treatment of asthma with a strong allergic component and for patients with seasonal rhinitis that is not well controlled with traditional medications.
- *Palivizumab* is a monoclonal antibody to the antigenic site on respiratory syncytial virus (RSV); it inactivates the virus. It is used to prevent RSV disease in high-risk children.
- *Pegaptanib* is a monoclonal antibody injected into the vitreous fluid of the eye once every 6 weeks. It is specific for the treatment of neovascular (wet) age-related macular degeneration.
- *Rituximab* is a monoclonal antibody to specific sites on activated B lymphocytes; it is used in the treatment of CD 20-positive, follicular B-cell non-Hodgkin's lymphoma.
- *Tositumomab* combined with iodine^{131} is given to treat CD20-positive, follicular B-cell non-Hodgkin's lymphoma patients whose disease is refractory to rituximab and who have relapsed on therapy. There is a high risk of cytopenia with this drug.
- *Trastuzumab* is a monoclonal antibody that reacts with human epidermal growth factor receptor 2 (HER2), a genetic defect that is seen in certain metastatic breast cancers. It is used in the treatment of metastatic breast cancer in tumours that overexpress HER2.

Pharmacokinetics

Monoclonal antibodies must be injected. They are processed by the body like other antibodies. It is not known whether they cross the placenta or enter breast milk, but because of the potential for adverse effects, they should not be used during pregnancy or lactation unless the benefit clearly outweighs the potential risk to the foetus or neonate.

Contraindications and Cautions

Monoclonal antibodies are contraindicated in the presence of fluid overload. They should be used cautiously with fever (treat the fever before beginning therapy), previous administration of the monoclonal antibody *(serious hypersensitivity reactions can occur with repeat administration)* and pregnancy or lactation.

Adverse Effects

The most serious adverse effects associated with the use of monoclonal antibodies are acute pulmonary oedema (dyspnoea, chest pain, wheezing), which is associated with severe fluid retention and cytokine release syndrome (flu-like symptoms that can progress to third-spacing of fluids and shock). Other adverse effects that can be anticipated include fever, chills, malaise, myalgia, nausea, diarrhoea, vomiting and increased susceptibility to infection.

Clinically Important Drug–Drug Interactions

Use caution and arrange to reduce the dosage if a monoclonal antibody is combined with any other immunosuppressant drug because severe immune suppression with increased infections and neoplasms can occur.

Always consult a current copy of the British National Formulary for further guidance

Nursing Considerations for Patients Receiving Immune Suppressants

Assessment: History and Examination

Screen for the following, *which could be contraindications or cautions to use of the drug:* any known allergies to any of these drugs or their components; pregnancy or lactation; renal or hepatic impairment; and history of neoplasm.

Include screening *for baseline status before beginning therapy and for any potential adverse effects:* presence of any skin lesions; weight; temperature; orientation, reflexes; pulse, blood pressure, ECG; liver evaluation; FBC, liver and renal function tests; and assessment of condition being treated. Establish if patient is currently taking other medications or herbal therapies, which may potentially interact with the immune suppressants.

Nursing Diagnoses

The patient receiving immune suppressants may have the following nursing diagnoses related to drug therapy:

- Acute pain related to CNS, GI and flu-like effects
- Risk for infection related to immune suppression
- Imbalanced nutrition: less than body requirements, related to nausea and vomiting
- Deficient knowledge regarding drug therapy

Implementation With Rationale

- Arrange for laboratory tests before and periodically during therapy, including FBC, differential and liver and renal function tests, *to monitor for drug effects and adverse effects.*
- Administer the drug as indicated; instruct the patient and a significant other if injections are required *to ensure proper administration of the drug.*
- Protect the patient from exposure to infections and maintain strict aseptic technique for any invasive procedures *to prevent infections during immunosuppression.*
- Arrange for supportive care and comfort measures for flu-like symptoms (rest, environmental control, paracetamol or ibuprofen) *to decrease patient discomfort and increase therapeutic compliance.*
- Monitor nutritional status during therapy; provide small, frequent meals, mouth care and nutritional consultation as necessary *to ensure adequate nutrition.*
- Instruct female patients in the use of barrier contraceptives *to avoid pregnancy during therapy because of the risk of adverse effects to the foetus.*
- Provide thorough patient education, including measures to avoid adverse effects, warning signs of problems and proper administration, *to increase knowledge about drug therapy and to increase compliance with the drug regimen.*
- Offer support and encouragement *to help the patient deal with the diagnosis and the drug regimen.*

Evaluation

- Monitor patient response to the drug (prevention of transplant rejection; improvement in autoimmune disease or cancer; prevention of RSV disease; improvement in signs and symptoms of Crohn's disease or rheumatoid arthritis).
- Monitor for adverse effects (flu-like symptoms, GI upset, increased infections, neoplasms, fluid overload).
- Evaluate the effectiveness of the teaching plan (patient can name drug, dosage, adverse effects to watch for, specific measures to avoid adverse effects).
- Monitor the effectiveness of comfort measures and compliance to the regimen.

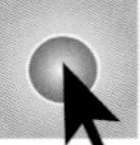

WEB LINKS

Health care providers and patients may want to consult the following Internet sources:

http://cks.library.nhs.uk/ The National Health Service Clinical Knowledge Summaries provides evidence-based practical information on the common conditions observed in primary care.

http://www.bnf.org.uk/ The BNF provides UK health care professionals with authoritative and practical information on the selection and clinical use of medicines.

http://www.mssociety.org.uk/ The Multiple Sclerosis Society supports patients with multiple sclerosis.

http://www.nhsdirect.nhs.uk The National Health Service Direct service provides patients with information and advice about health, illness and health services.

http://www.nice.org.uk National Institute for Health and Clinical Excellence (NICE) is an independent organisation responsible for providing national guidance on promoting good health and preventing and treating ill health.

Points to Remember

- Immune stimulants boost the immune system when it is exhausted from fighting off prolonged invasion or needs help fighting a specific pathogen or cancer cell.
- Immune suppressants are used to depress the immune system when needed to prevent transplant rejection or severe tissue damage associated with autoimmune disease.
- Interferons are naturally released from cells in response to viral invasion; they are used to treat various cancers and warts.
- Interleukins stimulate cellular immunity and inhibit tumour growth; they are used to treat very specific cancers.
- Adverse effects seen with immune stimulants are related to the immune response (flu-like symptoms, including fever, myalgia, lethargy, arthralgia and fatigue).
- Immune suppressants are used in a variety of specific transplantation situations. Research is ongoing to extend the use of various immune suppressants to other situations, including various autoimmune disorders.
- Increased susceptibility to infection and increased risk of neoplasm are potentially dangerous effects associated with the use of immune suppressants. Patients need to be protected from infection, injury and invasive procedures.

CRITICAL THINKING SCENARIO 16-1

Holistic Care for a Transplantation Patient

The Situation

After waiting on a transplant list for 4 years, Terry received a human heart transplant to replace his heart, which had been severely damaged by cardiomyopathy. Before getting the transplant, Terry was bedridden, on oxygen and near death. The transplant has given Terry a ‘new lease of life’, and he is determined to do everything possible to stay healthy and improve his activity and lifestyle. Currently, he is maintained on ciclosporin, mycophenolate and corticosteroids.

Critical Thinking

- What important teaching facts would help Terry to achieve his goal? *Think about the psychological impact of the heart transplant and the ‘new lease of life’.*
- What activity, dietary and supportive guidelines should be outlined for Terry?
- What impact will Terry’s drug regimen have on his plans?
- How can all of the aspects of his condition and medical care be coordinated to give Terry the best possible advantages for the future?

Discussion

Terry’s medical regimen will include a very complicated combination of rehabilitation, nutrition, drug therapy and prevention. Terry should know the risks of transplant rejection and the measures that will be used to prevent it. He also should know the names of his medications and when to take them, the signs and symptoms of rejection to watch for and what to do if they occur. Terry must understand the need to prevent exposure to infections and the precautions required, such as avoiding crowded areas and people with known diseases, avoiding injury and taking steps to maintain cleanliness and avoid infection if an injury occurs.

Holistic Care for a Transplantation Patient *(continued)*

The medications Terry is taking may cause him to experience flu-like symptoms, which can be quite unpleasant. A restful, quiet environment may help to decrease his stress. Paracetamol may be ordered to help alleviate the fever, aches and pains.

Terry may also experience GI upset, nausea and vomiting related to drug effects. A nutritional consultation may be requested to help Terry maintain a good nutritional state. Frequent mouth care and small, frequent meals may help. Proper nutrition will help Terry to recover, heal and maintain his health.

Terry's primary health care provider will need to work with the transplantation surgeon, rehabilitation team, nutritionist and cardiologist to coordinate a total programme that will help Terry to avoid problems and make the most of his transplanted heart.

Nursing Care Guide for Terry: Ciclosporin, Mycophenolate and Corticosteroids

Assessment: History and Examination

- Assess for history of allergies to any immune suppressant, renal or hepatic impairment, history of neoplasm, concurrent use of cholestyramine, theophylline, phenytoin, other nephrotoxic drugs, digoxin, lovastatin, diltiazem, metoclopramide, nicardipine, amiodarone, androgens, azole antifungals, macrolides; grapefruit juice.
- Review physical examination findings, including orientation, reflexes, affect (neurological); temperature and weight (general); pulse, cardiac auscultation, blood pressure, oedema, ECG (cardiovascular); liver evaluation (GI); and laboratory test results (FBC, liver and renal function tests, condition being treated).

Nursing Diagnoses

- Acute pain related to CNS, GI, flu-like symptoms
- Risk for infection related to immune suppression
- Imbalanced nutrition: less than body requirements related to GI effects
- Deficient knowledge regarding drug therapy

Implementation

- Arrange for laboratory tests before and periodically during therapy.
- Administer drug as indicated.
- Protect patient from exposure to infection.
- Provide supportive and comfort measures to deal with adverse effects.
- Monitor nutritional status and intervene as needed.
- Provide patient education regarding the drugs and their dosage, adverse effects, precautions and warning signs to report to care provider.

Evaluation

- Evaluate drug effects: prevention of transplant rejection, improvement of autoimmune disease.
- Monitor for adverse effects: infection, flu-like symptoms, GI upset, fluid overload, neoplasm.
- Monitor for drug–drug interactions and drug–food interactions.
- Evaluate effectiveness of patient education programme and of comfort and safety measures.

Patient Education for Terry: Ciclosporin, Mycophenolate and Corticosteroids

- ☐ You will need to take a combination of drugs to prevent your body from rejecting your new organ. These drugs include ciclosporin, mycophenolate and corticosteroids. They suppress the activity of your immune system and prevent your body from rejecting any transplanted tissue.
- ☐ You should never stop taking your drugs without consulting your health care provider. If your prescription is low or you are unable to take the medication *for any* reason, notify your health care provider.
- ☐ You should not take your ciclosporin with grapefruit juice.
- ☐ Some of the following adverse effects may occur:
  - *Nausea, vomiting:* Taking the drug with food and eating small frequent meals may help. It is very important that you maintain good nutrition. A consult with a nutritionist may be needed to help you if these GI problems are severe.
  - *Diarrhoea:* This may not decrease; ensure ready access to bathroom facilities.
  - *Flu-like symptoms:* Rest and a cool, peaceful environment may help; paracetamol may be ordered to help relieve discomfort.
  - *Rash, mouth sores:* Frequent skin and mouth care may ease these effects.
- ☐ You will be more susceptible to infection because your body's normal defences will be decreased. You should avoid crowded places, people with known infections and working in soil. If you notice any signs of illness or infection, notify your health care provider immediately.

(continued)

Holistic Care for a Transplantation Patient *(continued)*

- ☐ Tell any doctor, nurse, or other health care provider involved in your care that you are taking these drugs.
- ☐ You will need to schedule periodic blood tests and perhaps biopsies while you are being treated with these drugs.
- ☐ Report any of the following to your health care provider: unusual bleeding or bruising, fever, sore throat, mouth sores, fatigue and any other signs of infection or injury.
- ☐ Keep your medications safely out of the reach of children and pets and do not share medications with anyone else.

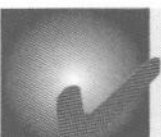

CHECK YOUR UNDERSTANDING

Answers to the questions in this chapter may be found in the answer key in the back of the book.

Multiple Choice

Select the most appropriate response to the following.

1. You would not expect to use an immune suppressant when working with treatment of
   a. transplant rejection.
   b. autoimmune disease.
   c. the number of relapses in multiple sclerosis.
   d. aggressive cancers.

2. Interferon α-n3 would be the drug of choice for
   a. treatment of leukaemias.
   b. treatment of multiple sclerosis.
   c. intralesional treatment of warts.
   d. treatment of Kaposi's sarcoma.

3. Patient education for a patient receiving an interferon would include
   a. proper use of oral contraceptives.
   b. use of aspirin to control adverse effects.
   c. importance of exercise and cardiovascular workouts.
   d. proper methods for drawing up and injecting the drug.

4. Patients receiving an immune stimulant may experience any of the clinical signs of immune response activity, including
   a. flu-like symptoms (arthralgia, myalgia, fatigue, anorexia).
   b. diarrhoea.
   c. constipation.
   d. headache.

5. Organ transplants are often rejected by the body because the T cells recognize the transplanted cells as foreign and try to destroy them. Treatment with an immune suppressant would
   a. activate antibody production.
   b. stimulate interleukin release.
   c. stimulate thymus secretions.
   d. block the inflammatory reaction and initial damage to the transplanted cells.

6. You might use a monoclonal antibody in treating
   a. warts.
   b. herpes zoster.
   c. metastatic breast cancers with tumours that overexpress HER2.
   d. Kaposi's sarcoma.

Extended Matching Questions

Select **all** that apply.

1. The nurse is assigned to care for a client who is receiving immune suppressants. The nurse would continually assess the client for which of the following anticipated adverse effects?
   a. Development of cancers
   b. Increased risk of infection
   c. Cardiac standstill
   d. Development of secondary infections
   e. Increased bleeding tendencies
   f. Hepatomegaly

2. Teaching points that the nurse would incorporate into the care of a client receiving ciclosporin would include which of the following?
   a. Use barrier contraceptives to avoid pregnancy.
   b. If mouth sores occur, try to restrict eating as much as possible.
   c. Dilute the solution with milk, chocolate milk, or orange juice and drink immediately.
   d. Avoid drinking grapefruit juice when on this drug.
   e. Stop taking the drug if GI upset or fever occurs.
   f. Refrigerate the oral solution.

Definitions

Define the following terms.

1. autoimmune______________________________

2. interferon______________________________

3. interleukin______________________________

4. monoclonal antibodies____________________

5. immune suppressant________________________

Fill in the Blanks

1. ________________ ________________are specific antibodies produced by a single clone of B cells to react with a specific antigen.

2. The following monoclonal antibodies are used in the prevention of renal transplant rejection: ________________, ________________ and ________________.

3. Infliximab is used to treat________________disease in patients who do not respond to other therapy.

4. Palivizumab was developed for the prevention of ________________in children who are at high-risk.

5. Treatment of metastatic breast cancer with tumours that overexpress HER2 is specifically the indication for________________ .

6. ________________is used for the treatment of relapsed follicular B-cell non-Hodgkin's lymphoma B lymphocytes.

7. The treatment of asthma with a strong allergic component is the main indication for________________ .

8. ________________is specifically used to treat B-cell chronic lymphocytic leukaemia.

Bibliography

British Medical Association and Royal Pharmaceutical Society of Great Britain (2008). *British National Formulary*. London: BMJ & RPS Publishing. *This publication is updated biannually: it is imperative that the most recent edition is consulted.*

British Medical Association and Royal Pharmaceutical Society of Great Britain (2008). *British National Formulary for Child*. London: BMJ & RPS Publishing. *This publication is updated annually: it is imperative that the most recent edition is consulted.*

Howland, R. D., & Mycek, M. J. (2005). *Pharmacology*. (3rd ed.). Philadelphia: Lippincott Williams & Wilkins.

Marieb, E. N., & Hoehn, K. (2004). *Human anatomy & physiology* (7th ed.). San Francisco: Pearson Benjamin Cummings.

National Institute for Health and Clinical Excellence (2003). Management of multiple sclerosis in primary and secondary care. Available from http://www.nice.org.uk

Porth, C. M., & Matfin G. (2008). *Pathophysiology: Concepts of altered health states* (8th ed.). Philadelphia: Lippincott Williams & Wilkins.

Rang, H.P., Dale, M.M., Ritter, J.M., & Flower, R.J. (2007). *Rang and Dale's pharmacology.* (6th ed.). Philadelphia: Churchill Livingstone.

Simonsen, T., Aarbakke, J., Kay, I., Coleman, I., Sinnott, P., & Lysaa, R. (2006). *Illustrated pharmacology for Nurses.* London: Hodder Arnold

CHAPTER 17

Vaccines and Sera

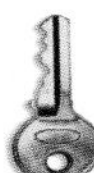

KEY TERMS

active immunity
antitoxins
immunoglobulin
immunization
passive immunity
vaccine

LEARNING OBJECTIVES

Upon completion of this chapter, you will be able to:

1. Define the terms active immunity and passive immunity.
2. Describe the therapeutic actions, indications, pharmacokinetics associated with each vaccine.
3. Describe the contraindications, most common adverse reactions and important drug–drug interactions associated with each vaccine.
4. Discuss the use of vaccines and sera across the lifespan, including recommended immunization schedules.
5. Compare and contrast the key drugs for each class of vaccine and immune serum with others in that class.
6. Outline the nursing considerations and teaching needs for patients receiving a vaccine or immune serum.

VACCINES

Bacterial Vaccines

haemophilus influenza B conjugate vaccine
haemophilus influenza B conjugate vaccine with hepatitis B vaccine
meningococcal group C conjugate vaccine
meningococcal polysaccharide A,C,W135
pneumococcal vaccine, polyvalent
pneumococcal 7-valent conjugate vaccine typhoid vaccine
tuberculosis (Bacillus Calmette-Guérin [BCG]; live)
typhoid vaccine (live)

Toxoids

diphtheria, tetanus, acellular pertussis combined and inactivated poliovirus vaccines absorbed
diphtheria (low dose), tetanus, acellular pertussis combined and inactivated poliovirus vaccines absorbed
diphtheria, tetanus and inactivated poliovirus vaccines absorbed

Viral Vaccines

hepatitis A vaccine, inactivated
hepatitis A vaccine, inactivated, with hepatitis B recombinant vaccine
hepatitis A vaccine, inactivated with typhoid vaccine
hepatitis B vaccine
influenza virus vaccine inactivated
intranasal Japanese encephalitis vaccine
measles virus vaccine, live attenuated
measles, mumps, rubella vaccine (MMR; live)
poliovirus vaccine, inactivated
rabies vaccine
rubella virus vaccine
yellow fever vaccine

IMMUNOGLOBULINS

normal immunoglobulin

Specific immunoglobulins

anti-D immunoglobulin
hepatitis B immunoglobulin
rabies immunoglobulin
tetanus immunoglobulin
varicella-zoster immunoglobulin

Immunization against infective disease has led to a remarkable fall in the incidence of these diseases. Prudent, prophylactic medical care requires the routine administration of certain vaccines to prevent diseases before they occur. Box 17.1 discusses the use of vaccines and immunological products among various age groups.

Immunization

Immunization is the process of artificially stimulating **active immunity** by exposing the body to weakened or less toxic proteins associated with specific disease-causing organisms. The goal is to cause an immune response without having the patient suffer the full course of a disease. Children are routinely immunized against many infections that were once quite devastating. For example, smallpox was one of the first diseases against which children were immunized. Today, smallpox is considered to be eradicated worldwide.

Immunity

Immunity is a state of relative resistance to a disease that develops after exposure to the specific disease-causing agent. People are not born with immunity to diseases, so they must acquire immunity by stimulating the production of antibodies and other components of the immune mechanism.

Active immunity occurs after vaccination when the body recognizes a foreign protein and begins producing antibodies and other components of the immune mechanism to react with that specific protein or antigen.

Vaccines can either be:

- *Live attenuated forms* of the bacteria (*Mycobacterium bovis;* BCG) or virus (measles, mumps and rubella; MMR). These vaccines have the ability to stimulate an immune response by mimicking natural exposure to the antigen and stimulating the production of antibodies. The result is usually long lasting. These vaccines should not be administered to pregnant women unless the risk to the mother outweighs the risk to the foetus.
- *Inactivated forms* of the bacteria (typhoid) or virus (hepatitis B). Immunity with these forms may require an initial series of doses to provoke adequate antibody response; and a booster is usually required. Duration of immunity may vary from months to years.
- *Detoxified forms* (toxoid; e.g. tetanus). These vaccines usually involve one dose of a toxin produced by a micro-organism rendered harmless.

After plasma cells are formed to produce antibodies, specific memory cells that produce the same antibodies are created. If the specific foreign protein is introduced into the body again, these memory cells react immediately to release antibodies. Active immunity can last for years and in some cases a lifetime. Active immunity can also exist in newborn babies as IgG antibodies cross the placenta; in this case immunity may only last for the first 6 months.

BOX 17.1 **DRUG THERAPY ACROSS THE LIFESPAN**

CHILDREN

Routine immunizations for children have become a standard of care in the United Kingdom (**for immunization schedules please see the latest edition of the BNF or check http://www.immunisation.nhs.uk**). Parents should receive written records of immunizations given to their children to ensure continuity of care. Parent education is a very important aspect of the immunization procedure. Parents may need reassurance and educational materials when concerns about the safety of immunizations arise (see Box 17.2).

Simple comfort measures of applying a cool compress at the injection site, paracetamol to reduce fever or aches and pains, comfort from parents or caregivers; will help the child deal with the immunization experience. The parent should report adverse reactions to any immunization. Sensitive children may receive divided doses of their immunizations to help prevent adverse reactions.

When administering any drug to children, always consult the most recent edition of the British National Formulary for Children.

ADULTS AND OLDER ADULTS

There are a number of reasons why adults should receive certain immunizations. For example, adults who are travelling to areas with high risk of particular diseases–and who may not have previously been exposed to those diseases–are advised to be immunized. Advice should be sought from their general practitioner (GP) or specialist travel clinics.

In addition, adults with chronic diseases (e.g. heart, liver, kidney, respiratory disease) or adults over the age of 65 years are advised to be immunized yearly with an influenza vaccine and once with a pneumococcal pneumonia vaccine. Vaccines provide some protection against diseases that can prove dangerous for people with chronic lung, cardiovascular (CV) or endocrine disorders. The influenza vaccine changes yearly, depending on predictions of which flu strain might be emergent in that year (recommended annually by the World Health Organisation). The pneumonia vaccine contains 23 different strains and is believed to offer lifetime protection.

Tetanus boosters are only recommended for adults with any injury that potentially could precipitate a tetanus infection.

Diphtheria, pertussis, tetanus, haemophilus B, polio, meningitis, tuberculosis (BCG) and MMR are all standard childhood immunizations today. The use of vaccines is not without controversy. Severe reactions, although rare, have occurred. The central reporting of adverse effects or suspected adverse effects via the Medicines and Healthcare products Regulatory Agency, Yellow Card scheme may help to clarify concerns about reactions to immunizations

Adults may also require immunizations in certain situations: exposure, travel to an area endemic in a disease they have not had and have not been immunized against and occupations that are considered high risk.

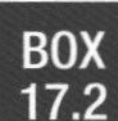

BOX 17.2 FOCUS ON THE **EVIDENCE**

Studies find no link between MMR Vaccine and Autism

Despite media attention and widespread speculation originally made in 1998, extensive reviews undertaken on behalf of the Medical Research Council and the Council for Safety in Medicines have failed to find any evidence to suggest link between autism, bowel disease and the MMR vaccine.

Source: www.immunisation.nhs.uk and www.mmrthefacts.nhs.uk

Passive immunity occurs when preformed antibodies are injected and react with a specific antigen. These antibodies can originate from animals that have been infected with the disease or from humans who have had the disease and have developed antibodies. The circulating antibodies act the same as those produced from plasma cells, recognizing the foreign protein and attaching to it, rendering it harmless. Unlike active immunity, passive immunity is limited. It lasts only as long as the circulating antibodies last because the body does not produce its own antibodies.

Contraindications and Cautions

The use of vaccines is contraindicated in an immunocompromised patient or the presence of immune deficiency *because the vaccine could cause disease and the body would not be able to respond as anticipated;* during pregnancy *because of potential effects on the foetus and on the success of the pregnancy–live vaccines because of risk to the foetus, unless the benefit to the mother is greater than the risk to the foetus or neonate;* with known allergies to any of the components of the vaccine (i.e. eggs; refer to each individual vaccine for specifics); or in patients who are receiving immunoglobulin or who have received blood or blood products within the last 3 months *because a serious immune reaction could occur*.

Caution should be used any time a vaccine is given to a child with a history of febrile convulsions or cerebral injury, or in any condition in which a potential fever would be dangerous. Caution also should be used in the presence of any acute infection. Anaphylaxis with an initial dose of a vaccine is contraindicated for further doses.

Adverse Effects

Adverse effects of vaccines vary, most are associated with the immune or inflammatory reaction that is being stimulated: moderate fever, rash, malaise, chills, drowsiness, anorexia, vomiting and irritability. Pain, redness, swelling and even nodule formation at the injection site are not uncommon; while others may produce a very mild form of the disease. In rare instances severe hypersensitivity reactions have been reported.

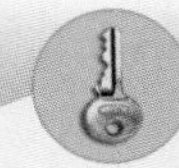

Key Drug Summary: Measles, Mumps and Rubella (MMR) Vaccine

Indications: Active immunization against MMR (and congenital rubella syndrome) in children older than 15 months and adults

Actions: Attenuated MMR viruses produce a modified infection and stimulate active immune reaction with the production of antibodies to these viruses. Each child should receive two doses of the MMR vaccine prior to starting nursery or primary school. The first dose should be when the child is 13 months old and a single booster dose before the child enters school.

Pharmacokinetics:

Route	Onset	Peak
IM	Rapid	3–12 h

$T_{1/2}$: Unknown; metabolism occurs in the tissues, excretion is unknown

Adverse effects: malaise, fever, rash, burning or stinging wheal or flare at site of injection (usually lasting 2–3 days), febrile convulsions and high fever are rare.

Nursing Considerations for Patients Receiving Vaccines

Assessment: History and Examination

Screen for any of the following, *which could be contraindications or cautions for use of the drug:* known allergies to any vaccines or to the components of the one being used; pregnancy; recent administration of immunoglobulin or blood products; immunodeficiency; and acute infection.

Include screening *for baseline status before beginning therapy and for any potential adverse effects:* presence of any skin lesions; temperature; pulse, blood pressure, perfusion.

Establish if patient is currently taking other medications or herbal therapies, which may potentially interact with vaccines.

Nursing Diagnoses

The patient receiving a vaccine may have the following nursing diagnoses related to drug therapy:

- Acute pain related to gastrointestinal (GI) and flu-like effects and localized reaction at injection site
- Ineffective tissue perfusion if severe reaction occurs
- Deficient knowledge regarding drug therapy

Implementation With Rationale

- Do not use to treat acute infection; *a vaccine is only used to prevent infection with future exposures.*
- Do not administer if the patient exhibits signs of acute infection or immune deficiency *because the vaccine can cause a mild infection and can exacerbate acute infections.*
- Do not administer if the patient has received blood, blood products, or immunoglobulin within the past 3 months *because a severe immune reaction could occur.*
- Arrange for proper preparation and administration of the vaccine; check on the timing and dosage of each injection *because dosage, preparation and timing vary with individual vaccines.*
- Maintain emergency equipment on standby, including adrenaline, *in case of severe hypersensitivity reaction.*
- Arrange for supportive care and comfort measures for flu-like symptoms (rest, environmental control, paracetamol) and for injection discomfort (paracetamol, resting arm) *to promote patient comfort.*
- Provide thorough patient education, including measures to avoid adverse effects, warning signs of problems and the need to keep a written record of immunizations, *to increase knowledge about drug therapy and to increase compliance with the drug regimen.*
- Provide a written record of the immunization, including the need to return for booster immunizations and timing of the boosters, if necessary, *to increase patient compliance with medical regimens.*

Evaluation

- Monitor patient response to the drug (prevention of disease, appropriate antibody levels).
- Monitor for adverse effects (flu-like symptoms; GI upset; local pain, swelling, nodule formation at injection site).
- Evaluate the effectiveness of the teaching plan (patient can name drug, dosage, adverse effects to watch for, has written record of immunizations).
- Monitor the effectiveness of comfort measures and adherence to the regimen.

Immunoglobulins and Anti-toxins

As explained earlier, passive immunity can be achieved by providing preformed antibodies to a specific antigen. These antibodies are found in immunoglobulins, which may contain antibodies to toxins, venins, bacteria, viruses, or even red blood cell antigenic factors. The term **immunoglobulin** is usually used to refer to sera that contain antibodies to specific bacteria or viruses. Immunoglobulins were originally obtained from animals, which led to many hypersensitivity reactions. Currently the majority of immunoglobulins are obtained from a pool of approximately 1000 donations of human plasma. The protection is immediate following injection and may last for several weeks. Examples of immunoglobulins include:

- Normal immunoglobulin is administered by intramuscular (IM) injection and is used to provide protection against hepatitis A and measles.
- Hepatitis B immunoglobulin is given to individuals who may have been exposed to the hepatitis B virus. It is also offered to provide protection in individuals who are at high risk of infection, including babies born to mothers with hepatitis B infection. It is administered by IM injection.
- Rabies immunoglobulin is given to individuals following an animal bite or exposure in a high-risk area. The wound should be cleaned and then the immunoglobulin filtered into the site of the wound. Any remaining immunoglobulin can be given by IM injection.
- Tetanus immunoglobulin should be administered by IM injection following a tetanus prone wound in an un-immunized individual. The administration may be accompanied by an antibiotic (e.g. metronidazole).
- Varicella-zoster immunoglobulin is only recommended for those individuals, at risk of developing severe chicken pox or the herpes zoster infection. *Consult the current edition of the British National Formulary (BNF) for detailed examples of those at increased risk.*
- Anti-D immunoglobulin is administered to rhesus-negative mothers to prevent the formation of antibodies to rhesus-negative foetal cells. This is given by deep IM injection within 72 hours of the sensitization period (this includes birth, miscarriage or termination). National Institute for Health and Clinical Excellence guidelines now recommend that Anti-D immunoglobulin is routinely given to all rhesus-negative mothers.

The terms **anti-toxin** and antivenom are used to refer to immunoglobulin that have antibodies to very specific toxins that might be released by invading pathogens or to venom that might be injected through spider or snake bites.

Therapeutic Actions and Indications

Immunoglobulins are used to provide passive immunity to a specific antigen or disease. They may also be used as prophylaxis against specific diseases after exposure in patients who are immunosuppressed. In addition, immunoglobulin may be used to lessen the severity of a disease after known or suspected exposure. See Figure 17.1 for sites of action of immunoglobulin and anti-toxins.

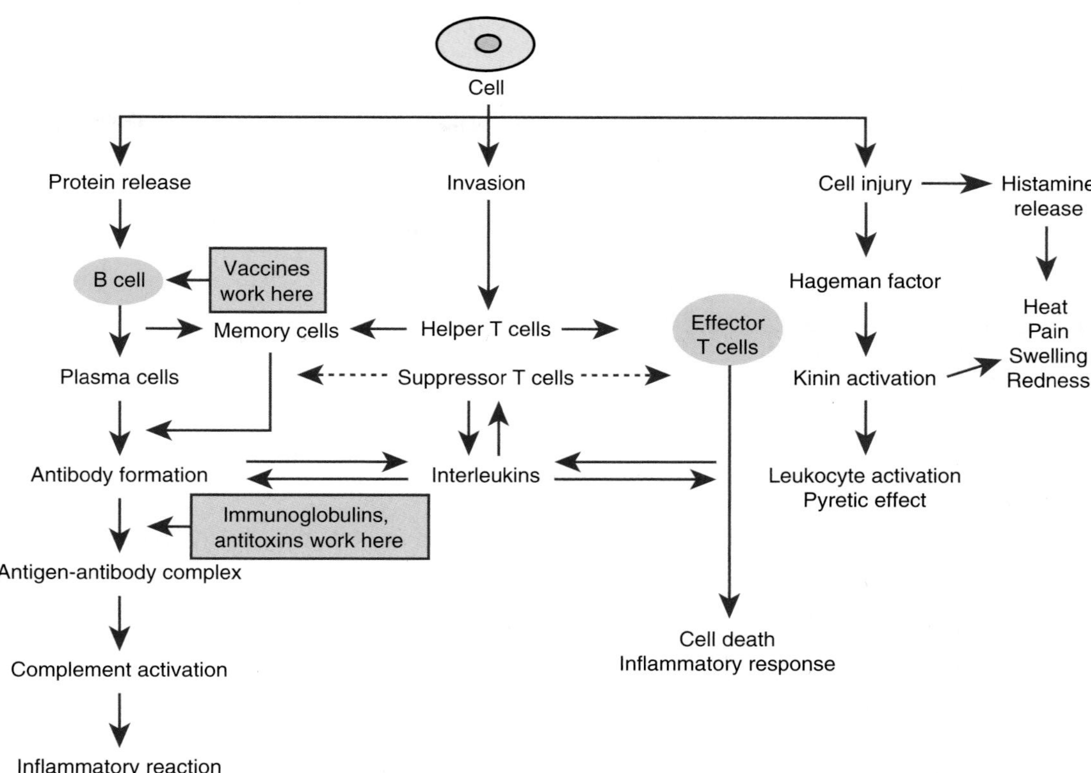

FIGURE 17.1 Sites of action of vaccines, immunoglobulins and antitoxins.

Contraindications and Cautions

Immunoglobulins are contraindicated in the presence of a history of severe reaction to any immunoglobulin or to products similar to the components of the sera. They should be used with caution during pregnancy because of potential risk to the foetus.

Adverse Effects

Adverse effects can be attributed to the effect of immunoglobulin on the immune system (rash, nausea, vomiting, chills and fever). Local reactions are very common: swelling, tenderness, pain, muscle stiffness at the injection site.

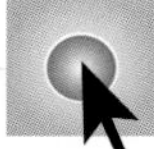

WEB LINKS

Health care providers and patients may want to consult the following Internet sources:

http://cks.library.nhs.uk/ The National Health Service Clinical Knowledge Summaries provides evidence-based practical information on the common conditions observed in primary care.

http://www.bnf.org.uk/ The BNF provides UK health care professionals with authoritative and practical information on the selection and clinical use of medicines.

http://www.fco.gov.uk The Foreign and Commonwealth Office provides health advice to overseas travellers

http://www.immunisation.nhs.uk A National Health Service site providing comprehensive and up-to-date information on vaccines, disease and immunization in the United Kingdom.

http://www/mmrthefacts.nhs.uk A National Health Service site providing evidence to support the safety of the triple vaccine, MMR.

http://www.nhsdirect.nhs.uk The National Health Service Direct service provides patients with information and advice about health, illness and health services.

http://www.nice.org.uk National Institute for Health and Clinical Excellence (NICE) is an independent organization responsible for providing national guidance on promoting good health and preventing and treating ill health.

Points to Remember

- Immunity (relative resistance to a disease) may be active or passive. Active immunity results from the body making antibodies against specific proteins for immediate release if the individual is re-exposed to the protein. Passive immunity results from the injection of preformed antibodies to a specific protein; this offers protection against the protein only for the life of the circulating antibodies.

- Vaccines are given to stimulate active immunity in a person who is at high risk of exposure to specific diseases. Immunizations are a standard part of preventive medicine.
- Vaccines contain live, inactivated or detoxified forms of the virus or bacteria containing specific antigens that stimulate the production of antibodies to that protein, thus providing active immunity.
- Immunoglobulins provide preformed antibodies to specific proteins for people who have been exposed to them or are at high risk for exposure.
- Patients should be advised to keep a written record (in addition to their medical notes) of all immunizations or immunoglobulin used. Booster doses may be needed to further stimulate antibody production.

CRITICAL THINKING SCENARIO 17-1

Educating a Parent about Vaccines

The Situation

Sue is a 25-year-old, first-time mother who has brought her 2-month-old daughter to the well-baby clinic for a routine check up. The baby is found to be healthy, growing well and within normal parameters for her age. At the end of the visit, the nurse prepares to give the baby the first of her routine immunizations. Sue becomes concerned and expresses fears about the risk of autism and infant deaths associated with immunizations.

Critical Thinking

- What information should Sue be given about immunizations?
- What nursing interventions would be appropriate at this time? *Think of ways to explain the importance of immunizations to Sue while supporting her concerns for the welfare of her baby.*
- How can this experience be incorporated into a teaching plan for Sue?

Discussion

Sue should be reassured before the baby is immunized. The nurse can tell her that in the past infant deaths were reported, but that efforts continue to make the vaccines pure. Careful monitoring of the child and the child's response to each immunization can help avoid such problems. Reassure Sue that the immunizations will prevent her daughter from contracting many, sometimes deadly, diseases.

The recommended schedule of immunizations should be given to Sue so that she is aware of what is planned and how the various vaccines are spaced and combined. She should be encouraged to monitor the baby after each injection for fever, chills and flu-like reactions. When she gets home, she can medicate the baby with paracetamol to avert many of these symptoms before they happen. Sue should also be told that the injection site might be sore, swollen and red, but that this will pass in a couple of days.

Sue should be encouraged to write down all of the immunizations that the baby has had and to keep this information handy for easy reference. She should also be encouraged to record any adverse effects that occur after each immunization. If reactions are uncomfortable, it is possible to split doses of future immunizations.

The nurse should give Sue a chance to express her concerns and fears. First-time parents may be more anxious than experienced ones when dealing with issues involving a new baby. To alleviate Sue's anxiety, the nurse should advise Sue on what to do and who to contact if a severe reaction occurs and if she wants to discuss any questions or concerns.

Nursing Care Guide for Sue's Baby: Vaccines

Assessment: History and Examination

- Allergies to the serum base, acute infection, immunosuppression
- General: temperature
- CV: pulse, cardiac auscultation, oedema, perfusion, central capillary refill
- Respiratory: respirations, adventitious sounds
- Skin: lesions
- Joints: normal movement for age

Nursing Diagnoses

- Acute pain related to infection and flu-like symptoms
- Ineffective tissue perfusion if severe reaction occurs
- Deficient knowledge by mother regarding drug therapy

Implementation

- Ensure proper preparation and administration of vaccine within appropriate time frame.

Educating a Parent about Vaccines *(continued)*

- Provide supportive and comfort measures to deal with adverse effects: anti-inflammatory/antipyretic, local heat application, rest and a quiet environment.
- Provide parent teaching regarding drug name, adverse effects and precautions and warning signs to report.
- Provide emergency life support if needed for acute reaction.

Evaluation

- Evaluate drug effects: serum titres reflecting immunization (if appropriate).
- Monitor for adverse effects: pain, flu-like symptoms and local discomfort.
- Evaluate effectiveness of parent teaching programme.
- Evaluate effectiveness of comfort and safety measures.
- Evaluate effectiveness of emergency measures if needed.

Patient Education for Sue

- ☐ This immunization will help your baby to develop antibodies to protect her against diphtheria, tetanus and pertussis. The baby will develop antibodies to these diseases and this will prevent the baby from contracting one of these potentially deadly diseases in the future.
- ☐ The injection site might be sore and painful. Heat applied to the area may help this discomfort.
- ☐ Adverse effects that the baby might experience include fever, muscle aches, joint aches, fatigue, malaise, crying and fretfulness. Paracetamol may help these discomforts; check with your health care provider for the correct dose to use for the baby. Rest and a quiet environment may also help the baby to feel better.
- ☐ The adverse effects should pass within 2 to 3 days. If they seem to be causing undue discomfort or persist longer than a few days, notify your health care provider.
- ☐ Booster immunizations are required for this immunization. Your GP's surgery will inform you of when the next immunization is required.
- ☐ Please contact your health care provider if you have any questions or concerns.

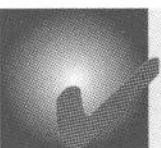

CHECK YOUR UNDERSTANDING

Answers to the questions in this chapter may be found in the answer key in the back of the book.

Multiple Choice

Select the most appropriate response to the following.

1. Vaccines are used to stimulate
   a. passive immunity to a foreign protein.
   b. active immunity to a foreign protein.
   c. serum sickness.
   d. a mild disease in healthy people.

2. Common adverse effects associated with routine immunizations would *not* include
   a. difficulty in breathing.
   b. fever and rash.
   c. drowsiness and fretfulness.
   d. pain, redness, swelling and nodule formation at the site of injection.

3. A 6-month-old child would *not* be a candidate for
   a. diphtheria, tetanus, pertussis vaccine.
   b. *H. influenza* B vaccine.
   c. poliovirus vaccine.
   d. Varicella-zoster vaccine.

4. Adults over the age of 65 and people who are at high risk for complications of influenza should receive a flu vaccine. This is repeated every year because
   a. the immunity wears off after a year.
   b. the strains of virus predicted to cause the flu change every year.
   c. a booster injection will activate the immune system.
   d. older people do not produce good antibodies.

5. You should check a patient's record to make sure that tetanus booster shots have been given
   a. only with exposure to anaerobic bacteria.
   b. every 2 years.

c. every 5 years.
d. every 10 years.

6. A nurse suffers a needle stick after injecting a patient with suspected hepatitis B. The nurse should
   a. have repeated titres to determine whether she was exposed to hepatitis B and, if she was, have hepatitis immunoglobulin.
   b. immediately receive hepatitis immunoglobulin and begin hepatitis B vaccines if she has not already received them.
   c. start antibiotic therapy immediately.
   d. go on sick leave until all screening tests are negative.

7. A patient is to receive immunoglobulin after exposure to hepatitis A. The patient has a previous history of allergies to various drugs. Before giving the immunoglobulin, the nurse should
   a. make sure that emergency equipment is readily available in case of a dramatic immune reaction.
   b. premedicate the patient with aspirin.
   c. make sure all of the patient's vaccinations are up to date.
   d. make sure the patient has a ride home.

Extended Matching Questions

Select **all** that apply.

1. A public education campaign to stress the importance of childhood immunizations should include which of the following points?
   a. Prevention of potentially devastating diseases outweighs the discomfort and risks of immunization.
   b. Routine immunization is standard practice in the United Kingdom.
   c. The practice of routine immunizations has virtually wiped out many previously deadly or debilitating diseases.
   d. The risk of severe adverse reactions is on the rise and is not being addressed.
   e. If you have a family history of autism or bowel disorder, you should not have your child immunized.
   f. The discomfort associated with the immunization can be treated with over-the-counter drugs and passes quickly.

2. A mother brings her child to his 18-month well-baby visit. The nurse would not give the child his routine immunizations in which of the following situations?
   a. He cried at his last immunization.
   b. He developed a fever or rash after his last immunization.
   c. He currently has a fever and symptoms of a cold.
   d. He is allergic to aspirin.
   e. He is currently taking oral corticosteroids.
   f. His siblings are all currently being treated for a viral infection.

3. When assessing the medical record of an older adult to evaluate the status of his immunizations, the nurse would be looking for evidence of which of the following?
   a. Yearly pneumococcal vaccination
   b. Yearly flu vaccination
   c. Tetanus booster every 10 years
   d. Tetanus booster every 5 years
   e. MMR vaccine if born after 1957

True or False

Indicate whether the following statements are true (T) or false (F).

_______ 1. Tetanus vaccines will provide active immunity against tetanus toxins.

_______ 2. Active immunity occurs when the host is stimulated to make antibodies to a specific antigen.

_______ 3. γ-globulin provides a good form of passive immunity to patients exposed to a specific antigen.

_______ 4. Vaccines are used to promote active immunity.

_______ 5. Vaccines are only used to prevent infection with future exposures.

_______ 6. Serious reactions have occurred to routine immunizations in the past.

_______ 7. Patients will not experience any discomfort after an immunization injection.

Bibliography

British Medical Association and Royal Pharmaceutical Society of Great Britain. (2008). *British National Formulary*. London: BMJ & RPS Publishing. *This publication is updated biannually: it is imperative that the most recent edition is consulted.*

British Medical Association and Royal Pharmaceutical Society of Great Britain. (2008). *British National Formulary for Children*. London: BMJ & RPS Publishing. *This publication is updated annually: it is imperative that the most recent edition is consulted.*

Brunton, L., Lazo, J. S., Parker, K., Goodman, L. S., & Gilman, A. G. (2005). *Goodman and Gilman's The Pharmacological Basis of Therapeutics* (11th ed.). London: McGraw-Hill.

Howland, R. D., & Mycek, M. J. (2005). *Pharmacology* (3rd ed.). Philadelphia: Lippincott Williams & Wilkins.

Marieb, E. N., & Hoehn, K. (2004). *Human anatomy & physiology* (7th ed.). San Francisco: Pearson Benjamin Cummings.

Rang, H. P., Dale, M. M., Ritter, J. M., & Flower, R. J. (2007). *Rang and Dale's pharmacology* (6th ed.). Philadelphia: Churchill Livingstone.

Simonsen, T., Aarbakke, J., Kay, I., Coleman, I., Sinnott, P., & Lysaa, R. (2006). *Illustrated pharmacology for nurses*. London: Hodder Arnold.

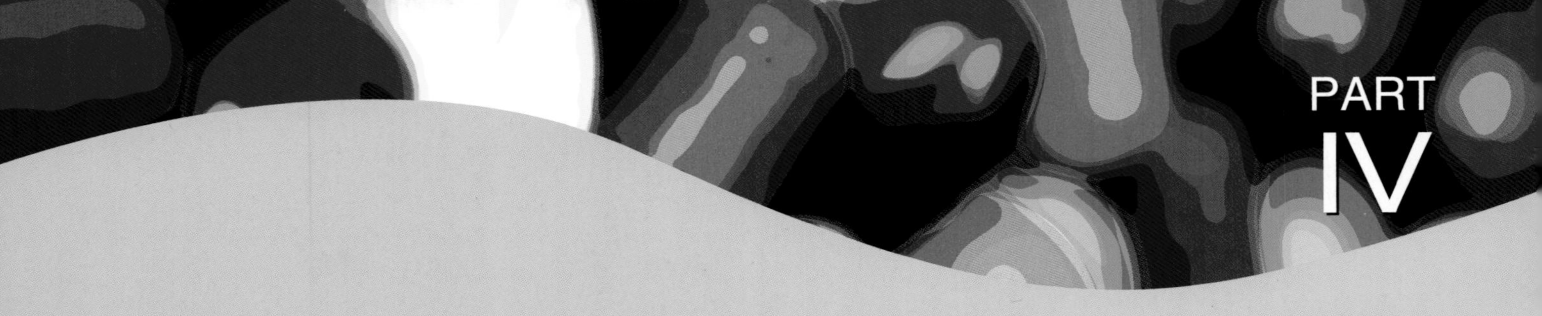

PART IV

Drugs Acting on the Central and Peripheral Nervous Systems

CHAPTER 18

Introduction to Nerves and the Nervous System

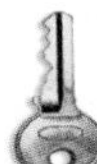

KEY TERMS

absolute refractory period
action potential
afferent
axon
brain stem
cerebellum
cerebral hemispheres
dendrite
depolarization
diencephalon
effector
efferent
exocytosis
limbic system
motor neuron
myelin sheath
nerve
neuron
neurotransmitter
repolarization
sensory neuron
soma
synapse

LEARNING OBJECTIVES

Upon completion of this chapter, you should be able to:

1. Label the parts of a neuron and describe the functions of each part.
2. Describe an action potential, including the roles of the various electrolytes involved.
3. Explain what a neurotransmitter is, where it comes from and its functions at the synapse.
4. Describe the function of the cerebral cortex, cerebellum, diencephalon, brain stem and spinal cord.

The nervous system is responsible for controlling the functions of the human body, analysing incoming stimuli and integrating internal and external responses. The nervous system is composed of the central nervous system (CNS; the brain and spinal cord) and the peripheral nervous system (PNS). The PNS is composed of **sensory neurons** that take information to the CNS and **motor neurons** that carry information away from the CNS to muscles and glands. The autonomic nervous system (ANS), which is discussed in Chapter 28, regulates automatic or unconscious responses to stimuli.

Physiology of the Nervous System

The nervous system operates through the use of electrical impulses and chemical messengers to transmit information throughout the body and to respond to internal and external stimuli. The structural unit of the nervous system is the nerve cell, or **neuron**. The billions of neurons that make up the nervous system are organized to allow movement; realization of various sensations; response to internal and external stimuli and learning, memory, thinking and emotion.

Neurons

The neuron is the structural unit of the nervous system. The human body contains about 14 billion neurons. About 10 billion of these are located in the brain and the remaining 4 billion are found in the spinal cord and PNS.

Neurons have several distinctive cellular features. Each neuron is made up of a cell body, or **soma**, which contains the nucleus, cytoplasm and various granules and other particles (Figure 18.1). A typical **motor neuron** has short, branch-like projections known as **dendrites** that cover most of the surface of the soma. These structures, which provide increased surface area, bring information in from other neurons. One end of the soma extends into a long process that does not branch out until the very end of the process. This elongated process is called the **axon**, and it emerges from the soma at the axon hillock (see Figure 18.1). The axon of a neuron can be extremely short, or can extend up to a metre or more. The axon carries information from a neuron to be transmitted to **effector** cells – cells in muscles, glands or other neurons. This transmission occurs at the end of the axon, where the axon branches out into the axon terminal.

The axons of many neurons are packed closely together into bundles of neurons. These bundles are then grouped together with connective tissue to form a **nerve**. Nerves are classified according to the direction in which they transmit information. **Afferent** or **sensory** nerves carry information from the periphery to the CNS. In contrast, **efferent** or **motor** nerves carry information from the CNS to the periphery to stimulate muscles or glands. Most nerves are mixed as they contain both sensory and motor fibres.

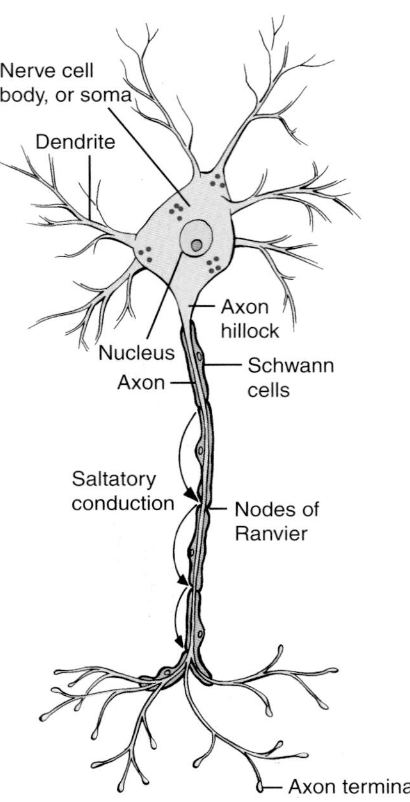

FIGURE 18.1 The neuron, functional unit of the nervous system.

Any damage to nervous tissue is serious because mature neurons do not usually divide to produce additional neurons to repair a damaged area, for example as a result of reduced oxygen supply to an area of the brain. However, depending upon the severity and also the location of the damage, some neurons in the PNS are able to repair themselves. A damaged neuron in the CNS, or a peripheral neuron damaged severely or close to the cell body is unlikely to recover. Not only is this neuron likely to die but also the neurons that the damaged neuron stimulates. However, if the cell body remains undamaged, the severed axon may be able to regenerate.

Action Potentials

Neurons transmit information by conducting electrical impulses called **action potentials**. Neuronal plasma membranes, which are capable of conducting action potentials along the entire surface, send messages to nearby neurons or to effector cells that may be located centimetres to metres away via this electrical communication system. Like all plasma membranes, neuronal plasma membranes have various channels or pores that control the movement of substances into and out of the cell. Some of these channels allow the movement of either sodium (Na^+), potassium (K^+) or calcium (Ca^{2+}) ions. When these channels open, ions diffuse across the membrane down their concentration gradients to create electrical currents – it is this movement of ions that creates the electrical impulses and enables neurons to conduct information.

As described in Chapter 6, there is a difference between the ionic makeup of the cytoplasm and that of the extracellular fluid; for example there is a higher concentration of Na^+ outside the cell compared to the cytoplasm, and a higher concentration of K^+ inside the cell compared to outside. There is also a difference in the permeability of the plasma membrane to the two ions: the plasma membrane is more permeable to K^+ than Na^+. When cells are at rest, K^+ leave the cell down their concentration gradient through 'leak' ion channels making the cell more negative inside. As the plasma membrane is less permeable to Na^+ at rest, fewer Na^+ enter the cell to balance the loss of positive charge. Also there are a larger number of negatively charged proteins on the inside of the cell. As a result, the cytoplasmic side of the plasma membrane becomes negatively charged compared to the outside. This difference in charge is called the resting membrane potential and is maintained by the Na^+/K^+-ATPase pump.

Stimulation of a neuron causes **depolarization**, which means that the Na^+ channels open in response to the stimulus, and Na^+ flows into the cell, down the established concentration gradient. The electrical charge on the inside of the plasma membrane changes from negative to positive. This sudden depolarization of membrane potential, called the **action potential** (Figure 18.2), lasts less than a microsecond. At the peak of the action potential the Na^+ channels start to close or inactivate, reducing the membrane permeability to Na^+. At the same time the K^+ channels open and K^+ flows out of the cell, down the concentration gradient. As a result, the membrane potential rapidly falls as the inside of the cell becomes more negative again, a process called **repolarization.** The action potential generated at one point along the plasma membrane stimulates the generation of an action potential in adjacent portions of the plasma membrane, and the stimulus travels the length of the plasma membrane.

Neurons can respond to stimuli several hundred times per second, but for a given stimulus to cause an action potential, it must have sufficient strength and must occur when the plasma membrane is able to respond – that is when it has repolarized and the Na^+ and K^+ have been returned to the correct sides of the membrane. A neuron cannot be stimulated again while in a depolarized state: this is known as the **absolute refractory period** and ensures that the electrical impulse is transmitted in one direction only. The balance of Na^+ and K^+ across the plasma membrane must be re-established before another action potential can be propagated. Following repolarization there is a brief period where too much K^+ leaves the cell. This is called hyperpolarization and ensures the action potential proceeds to the end of the axon.

Neurons require energy in the form of glucose, oxygen and the correct balance of the electrolytes Na^+ and K^+ for the action potential, and Ca^{2+} which is necessary for the release of chemical transmitter from the axon terminal. If an individual has anoxia or hypoglycaemia, the neurons might not be able to maintain the Na^+/K^+-ATPase pump leading to an imbalance in electrolyte levels. The individual may experience a range of symptoms or become unresponsive to stimuli.

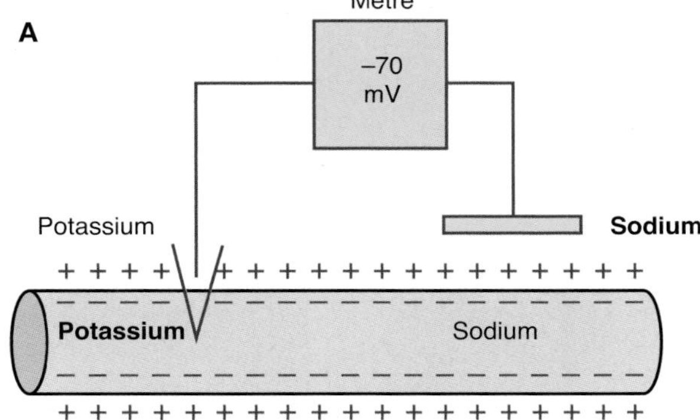

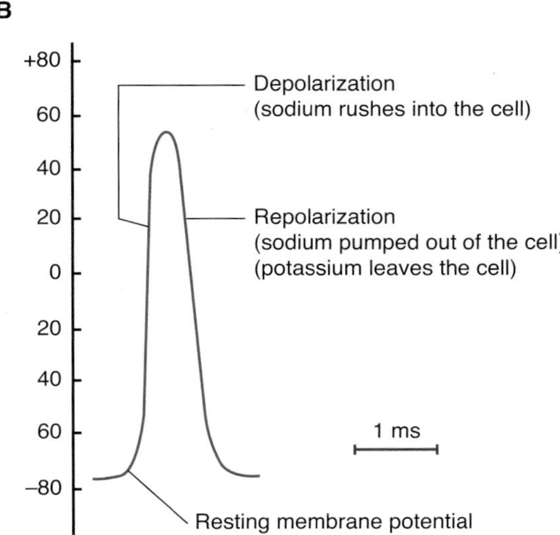

FIGURE 18.2 The action potential. **(A)** A segment of an axon showing that, at rest, the inside of the membrane is relatively negatively charged and the outside is positively charged. A pair of electrodes placed as shown would record a potential difference of about –70 mV; this is the resting membrane potential. **(B)** An action potential of about 1 ms that would be recorded if the axon shown in **A** were brought to threshold. At the peak of the action potential, the charge on the membrane reverses polarity.

Many axons, particularly those that are either large or long, are myelinated; that is they are covered by a fatty layer called a **myelin sheath**. The presence of a myelin sheath protects the axon and acts as an insulator to increase the speed of electrical conduction. In the CNS, the myelin sheath is formed by oligodendrocytes and those in the PNS are formed by Schwann cells. Both oligodendrocytes and Schwann cells are located at specific intervals along the axons (Figure 18.3) and wrap themselves around the axon many times. Between the oligodendrocytes and Schwann cells are areas of uncovered plasma membrane called the

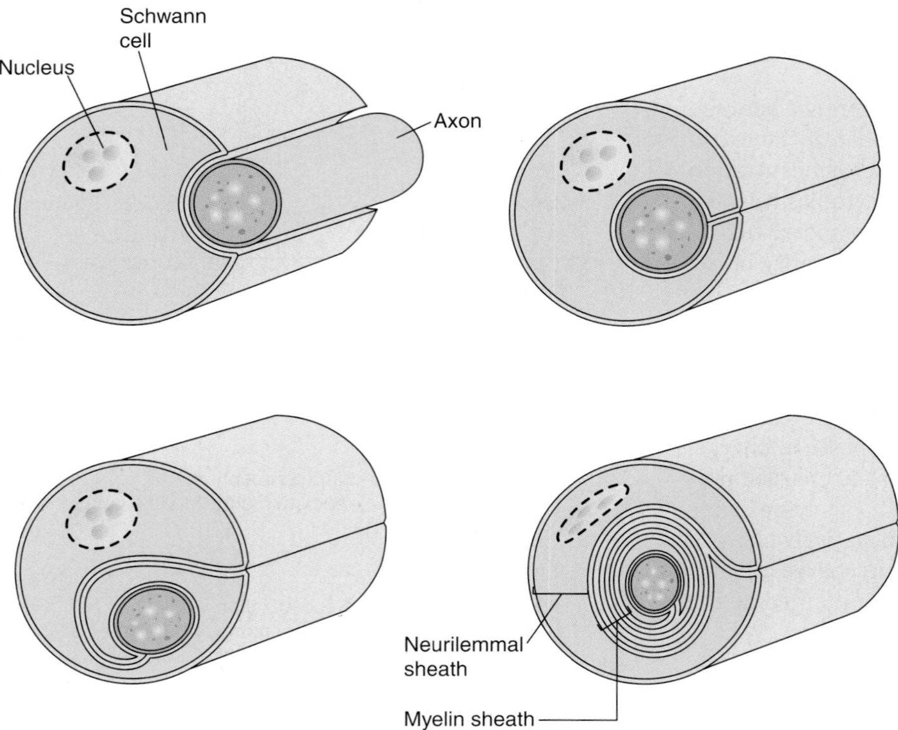

FIGURE 18.3 Formation of a myelin sheath in a peripheral axon. Successive wrappings of the Schwann cell membranes form the sheath, with most of the Schwann cell cytoplasm left outside the myelin. Therefore, the neurilemmal death of Schwann cells is outside the myelin sheath.

nodes of Ranvier. Both oligodendrocytes and Schwann cells insulate the axons, meaning that conduction of electrical impulses only occurs at the nodes of Ranvier. Therefore, the electrical impulses 'leap' between the nodes of Ranvier: an action potential excites one section of axon, and the electrical impulse then 'skips' from one node to the next, generating an action potential. As the membrane is forming fewer action potentials, the speed of conduction is much faster and the neuron is protected from using up energy to form multiple action potentials. This node-to-node mode of conduction is termed *saltatory conduction.*

If the myelin sheath becomes damaged in any way, conduction does not occur. A stimulus may simply be 'lost' along the nerve, as in the neurological disease, multiple sclerosis. Multiple sclerosis is primarily an autoimmune disorder that attacks and eventually destroys the myelin sheaths of axons in the CNS and PNS. The myelin is replaced by plaques and the axons degenerate and die. The disease is characterized by a progressive loss of nerve cells resulting in loss of muscle function.

Synapses

When the action potential reaches the end of an axon, the electrical impulse comes to a halt. At this point the stimulus no longer travels using an electrical mechanism. The transmission of information between two neurons or between a neuron and a gland or muscle cell is chemical. Neurons communicate with other neurons or effectors at the neuronal **synapse** (Figure 18.4). The synapse is made up of a presynaptic neuron, the synaptic cleft and the postsynaptic effector cell. When the electrical stimulus reaches the end of a neuron, Ca^{2+} channels open and an influx of Ca^{2+} causes the presynaptic neuron to release a chemical called a **neurotransmitter** into the synaptic cleft. The neurotransmitter diffuses across the synapse and binds to its receptors on the postsynaptic neuron to cause a reaction.

Neurotransmitters

Neurotransmitters stimulate postsynaptic cells either by exciting or by inhibiting them. The reaction that occurs when a neurotransmitter stimulates a receptor site will depend on the specific neurotransmitter released into the synapse and the receptors it activates. A neuron may produce only one type of neurotransmitter, using starting materials such as tyrosine or choline from the extracellular fluid. The neurotransmitter is then packaged into vesicles. During the action potential the Ca^{2+} channels in the plasma membrane open allowing Ca^{2+} entry. The vesicles move towards and fuse with the presynaptic membrane of the axon and deposit the neurotransmitter into the synaptic cleft. This process is called **exocytosis.** Once released into the synapse, the neurotransmitter binds to specific receptors to cause a reaction. When the cell repolarizes, Ca^{2+} leaves the cell, and exocytosis stops.

To return the effector cell to a resting state so that it can be stimulated again, if needed, neurotransmitters must be inactivated. Neurotransmitters may be either reabsorbed by the presynaptic neuron in a process called reuptake (a recycling effort to reuse the materials and save resources)

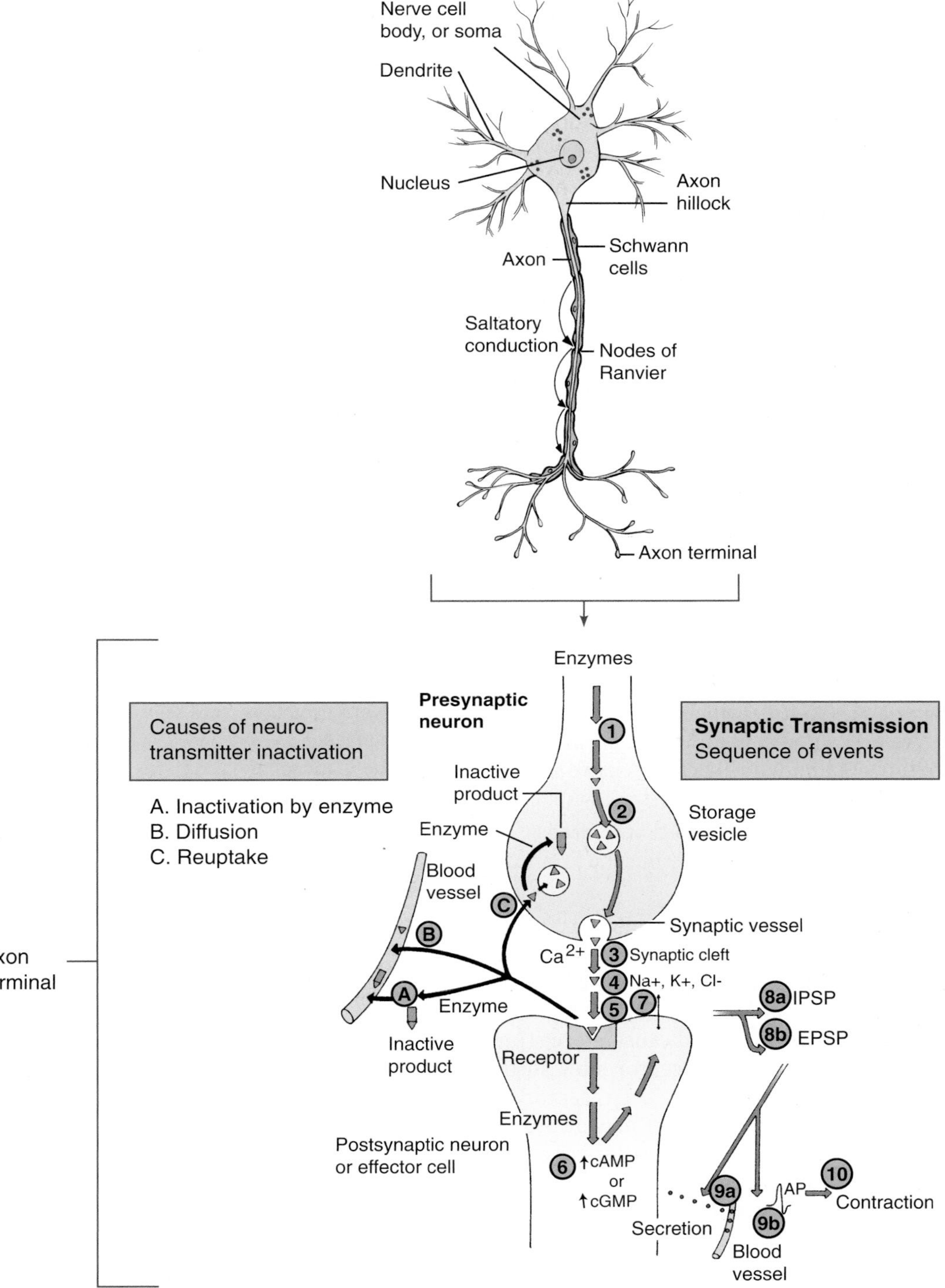

FIGURE 18.4 The sequence of events in synaptic transmission: **(1)** synthesis of the neurotransmitter; **(2)** uptake of the neurotransmitter into storage vesicles; **(3)** release of the neurotransmitter by an action potential in the presynaptic neuron; **(4)** diffusion of the neurotransmitter across the synaptic cleft; **(5)** binding of the neurotransmitter to the receptor; **(6)** either a sequence of events leading to activation of second messengers within the postsynaptic neuron or **(7)** a change in permeability of the postsynaptic membrane to one or more ions, causing either **(8a)** an inhibitory postsynaptic potential (IPSP) or **(8b)** an excitatory postsynaptic potential (EPSP). Characteristic responses of the postsynaptic cell are as follows: **(9a)** the gland secretes hormones; **(9b)** the muscle cells have an action potential; and **(10)** the muscle contracts. The action of the neurotransmitter is terminated by one or more of the following processes: **(A)** inactivation by an enzyme; **(B)** diffusion out of the synaptic cleft and removal by the vascular system and **(C)** reuptake into the presynaptic nerve followed by storage in a synaptic vesicle or deactivation by an enzyme.

or broken down by enzymes in the area (e.g. monoamine oxidase breaks down the neurotransmitter noradrenaline; the enzyme acetylcholinesterase breaks down the neurotransmitter acetylcholine). Several neurotransmitters have been identified. The following are examples of selected neurotransmitters:

- *Acetylcholine*, which communicates between nerves and muscles, is also important as the preganglionic neurotransmitter throughout the ANS and as the postganglionic neurotransmitter in the parasympathetic nervous system and in several pathways in the brain (see Chapter 28).
- *Noradrenaline* and *adrenaline* are catecholamines. Noradrenaline is released by most nerves (except those in the sweat glands) in the sympathetic division of the ANS (see Chapter 28). Both noradrenaline and adrenaline are classified as hormones when they are released into the bloodstream from the adrenal medulla when stimulated by sympathetic nerves. These neurotransmitters also occur in high levels in particular areas of the brain, such as the limbic system.
- *Dopamine*, which is found in high concentrations in certain areas of the brain, is involved in the co-ordination of impulses and responses, both motor and intellectual.
- *γ-aminobutyric acid (GABA)*, which is found in the brain, inhibits nerve activity and is important in preventing over excitability or stimulation such as seizure activity.
- *Serotonin* or *5-hydroxytryptamine (5-HT)*, which is also found in the limbic system, is important in arousal and sleep, as well as in preventing depression and promoting motivation.

Many of the drugs that affect the nervous system involve altering the activity at the synapse. These drugs can have several functions, including blocking the reuptake of neurotransmitters so that they are present in the synapse in greater quantities and cause more stimulation of receptor sites; blocking receptor sites so that the neurotransmitter cannot stimulate the receptor site; blocking the enzymes that break down neurotransmitters to cause an increase in neurotransmitter concentration in the synapse; stimulating specific receptor sites when the neurotransmitter is not available and causing the presynaptic neuron to release greater amounts of the neurotransmitter.

Central Nervous System

The CNS consists of the brain and the spinal cord. The bones of the vertebrae protect the spinal cord, and the bones of the skull protect the brain. In addition, the meninges, which are membranes that cover the nerves in the brain and spinal cord, and the fluid inside and around the brain and spinal cord called cerebrospinal fluid, provide further protection.

The blood–brain barrier, a functioning boundary, also plays a defensive role in keeping toxins and proteins out of the brain and preventing their contact with the sensitive and fragile neurons. The blood–brain barrier represents a therapeutic challenge to drug treatment of brain-related disorders because a large percentage of drugs are either not lipid-soluble or are carried bound to plasma proteins and are unable to cross into the brain.

Anatomy of the Brain

The brain can be divided into four regions: (1) cerebral hemispheres, (2) diencephalon, (3) brain stem (midbrain, pons and medulla) and (4) cerebellum (Figure 18.5). The cerebral hemispheres are the largest components of the brain and are made up of two hemispheres joined together by an area called the corpus callosum. The **cerebral hemispheres** contain an area called the cerebral cortex which is divided into lobes. It is the cerebral cortex that contains the sensory neurons, which receive nerve impulses, and the motor neurons which send signals to skeletal muscles. The different areas of the cerebral cortex responsible for receiving and sending information to specific areas of the body have been mapped, as have other functional areas (Figure 18.6). The cerebral cortex also contains areas that co-ordinate speech and communication and seem to be the area where learning takes place.

The **diencephalon** contains the thalamus, the hypothalamus and epithalamus. The thalamus transfers sensations such as cold, heat, pain, touch and muscle position to the cerebral cortex. The hypothalamus, which is poorly protected by the blood–brain barrier, acts as a major sensor for activities in the body. Areas of the hypothalamus are responsible for temperature control, water balance, appetite and fluid balance. In addition, the hypothalamus plays a central role in the endocrine system and in the ANS. The epithalamus assists the hypothalamus in regulating the sleep–wake cycle.

The **brain stem** contains the midbrain, pons and medulla oblongata. The midbrain is located between the diencephalon and the pons. Nerve fibre tracts pass through the brain stem on route from the spinal cord to the diencephalon and cerebrum. The substantia nigra is also located here, an area that, with the basal nuclei, contributes to motor function. Degeneration of neurons in the substantia nigra and basal nuclei leads to Parkinson's disease. The pons is situated between the midbrain and the medulla and acts as conduction pathway for nerves travelling between the cerebral cortex and lower brain areas, including the cerebellum. The pons also plays a role in controlling the rate and depth of respiration. The medulla oblongata is vitally important in maintaining body homeostasis and contains areas controlling basic, vital functions, such as the respiratory centres, which together with the pons controls breathing; the cardiovascular centres, which regulate blood pressure; and the swallowing centre, which co-ordinates the complex swallowing reflex.

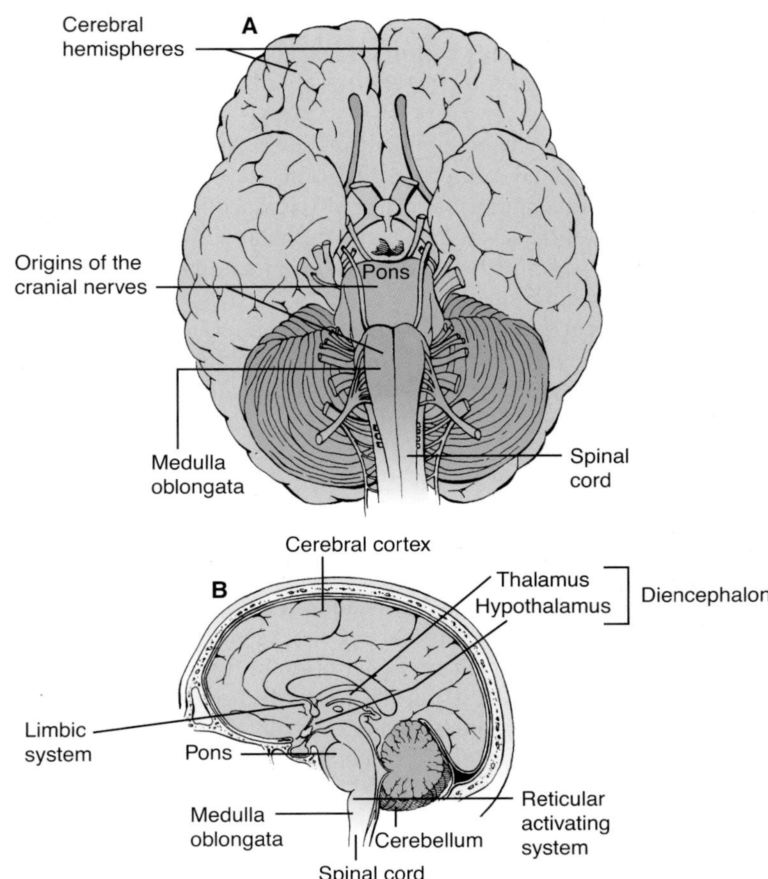

FIGURE 18.5 Anatomy of the brain. **(A)** A view of the underside of the brain. **(B)** The medial or midsagittal view of the brain.

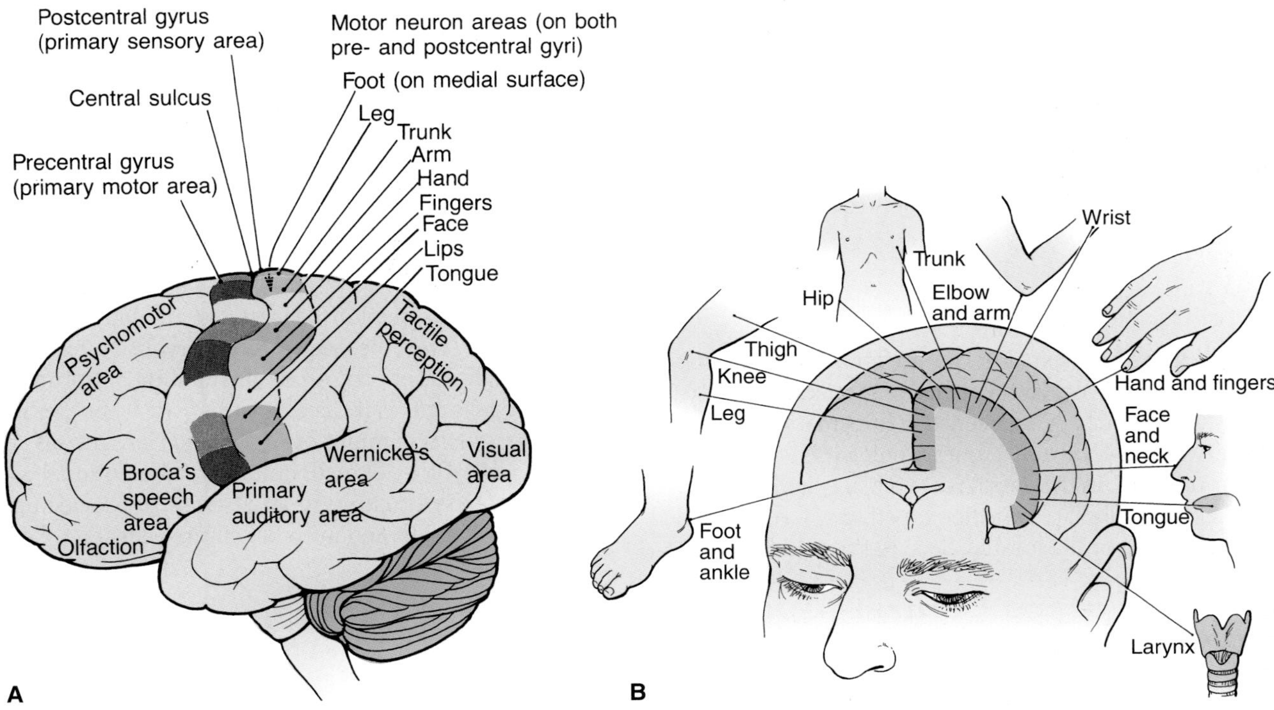

FIGURE 18.6 Functional areas of the brain. **(A)** Topographical organization of functions of control and interpretation in the cerebral cortex. **(B)** Areas of the brain that control specific areas of the body. Size indicates relative distribution of control.

The **cerebellum** is located behind the pons, and co-ordinates the motor function that regulates posture, balance and with the cerebral cortex participates in the control of voluntary muscle activity.

There are a number of networks of neurons in the brain that work together but may project to different areas of the brain and, therefore, cannot be localized to a specific area of the brain. One of these systems is the reticular activating system (RAS), which extends through the medulla oblongata, pons and midbrain and can project to the hypothalamus, thalamus, cerebellum and spinal cord. The RAS controls arousal and awareness of stimuli and contains the sleep centre. The RAS filters the billions of incoming messages, selecting only the most significant for response. Another example is the **limbic system** which includes many structures in the cerebral cortex and subcortex. The limbic system contains high levels of three neurotransmitters: adrenaline, noradrenaline and serotonin. Stimulation of neurons in the limbic system, which appears to be responsible for the expression of emotions, can lead to feelings of anger, pleasure and stress. This neuronal network seems to be largely responsible for the human aspect of brain function. Drug therapy aimed at alleviating emotional disorders such as depression and anxiety often involves attempting to alter the levels of adrenaline, noradrenaline and serotonin in these areas.

Cranial Nerves

There are 12 pairs of cranial nerves: two pairs of nerves emerge from the forebrain and the remaining 10 pairs originate in the brain stem (see Figure 18.5). The cranial nerves are involved in sensation (sight, smell, hearing, balance, taste, touch, pain and temperature) and some muscle activity of the head and neck (e.g. chewing, eye movement, facial expression). Cranial nerve X, the vagus nerves, are the only nerves to extend beyond the head and neck to the thorax and abdomen where nerve fibres supply the heart, lungs and abdominal organs.

Spinal Nerves

A total of 31 pairs of spinal nerves are attached to the spinal cord. Each spinal nerve has two components or roots: a sensory root which brings sensory information from the periphery to the CNS; and a motor root, which cause movement or reaction. In the dorsal roots of the spinal nerves, the neuronal cell bodies are collected together in a region called the **dorsal root ganglia** located close to the spinal cord.

Functions of the Central Nervous System

The brain is responsible for co-ordinating reactions to the constantly changing external and internal environment. In all animals, the function of this organ is essentially the same. The human component involving emotions, learning and conscious response takes the human nervous system beyond a simple reflex.

Sensory Functions

Millions of sensory impulses are constantly entering the CNS from peripheral receptors. Many of these impulses go directly to specific areas of the brain designated to deal with input from particular areas of the body or from the senses (see Figure 18.6). The responses that occur as a result of these stimuli can be altered by efferent neurons that respond to emotions through the limbic system, to learned responses stored in the cerebral cortex, or to autonomic input mediated through the hypothalamus.

Motor Functions

Many motor neurons travelling from the cerebrum to the spinal cord pass through the medulla oblongata at a region called the pyramids; the tracts passing through here are known as pyramidal tracts and are responsible for skilled and purposeful movements. Other motor neurons arise from other regions of the brain and do not pass through the pyramids; these are known as extrapyramidal tracts. The extrapyramidal motor system co-ordinates motor activity for unconscious activities such as posture and gait. Some drugs may interfere with the extrapyramidal system and cause parkinsonian-like symptoms of tremors, shuffling gait and lack of posture and position stability.

Clinical Significance of Drugs That Act on the Nervous System

The features of the human nervous system, including the complexities of the human brain, sometimes make it difficult to predict the exact reaction of a particular patient to a given drug. When a drug is used to affect the nervous system, the occurrence of many systemic effects is always a possibility because the nervous system affects the entire body. The chapters in this section address the individual classes of drugs used to treat disorders of the nervous system, including their adverse effects. An understanding of the actions of specific drugs makes it easier to anticipate what therapeutic and adverse effects might occur. In addition, nurses should consider all of the learned, cultural and emotional aspects of the patient's situation in an attempt to provide optimal therapeutic benefit and minimal adverse effects.

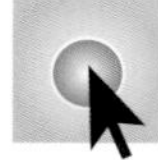

WEB LINK

http://www.innerbody.com To explore the virtual nervous system, visit this Internet site.

Points to Remember

- The nervous system, which consists of the CNS and the PNS, is responsible for control of the human body, analysis of stimuli coming into the system and integration of internal and external responses to stimuli.
- Although neurons do not reproduce, they can, in some cases, regenerate injured parts if the soma and axon hillock remain intact.
- Efferent nerves take information from the CNS to effector sites; afferent nerves are sensory nerves that take information towards the CNS.
- Nerves transmit information by way of electrical charges called action potentials. An action potential is a sudden change in membrane charge from negative to positive. It is caused when stimulation of a nerve opens Na^+ channels and allows Na^+ to flow into the cell.
- When the transmission of action potentials reaches the axon terminal, it causes entry of Ca^{2+} into the neuron and the release of chemicals called neurotransmitters, which cross the synaptic cleft to stimulate an effector cell, which can be another neuron, a muscle, or a gland.
- A neurotransmitter must be produced by a neuron (each neuron can produce only one kind); it must be released into the synapse when the neuron is stimulated; it must bind to a receptor site to cause a reaction and it must be immediately broken down or removed from the synapse so that the cell can be ready to be stimulated again.
- Much of the drug therapy in the nervous system involves receptors and the release or reuptake and breakdown of neurotransmitters.
- The CNS consists of the brain and spinal cord, which are protected by bone and meninges.
- The cerebral cortex consists of two hemispheres, which regulate the communication between sensory and motor neurons and are the sites of thinking and learning.
- The diencephalon contains the hypothalamus, thalamus and epithalamus. These areas co-ordinate internal and external responses and direct information into the cerebral cortex. They also play a role in regulating sleep patterns.
- The brainstem contains the midbrain, pons and medulla oblongata. These areas form part of nerve conduction pathways and also contain the centres that control basic, vital functions such as regulating the heart and respiration.
- The cerebellum regulates posture, balance and voluntary muscle activity.
- The mechanisms of learning and processing learned information are not fully understood. Emotion-related factors influence the human brain, which handles stimuli and responses in complex ways.
- Much remains to be learned about the human brain and how drugs influence it. The actions of many drugs that have known effects on human behaviour are not understood.

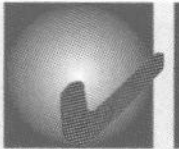

CHECK YOUR UNDERSTANDING

Answers to the questions in this chapter may be found in the answer key in the back of the book.

Multiple Choice

Select the best answer to the following.

1. The cerebellum
   a. initiates voluntary muscle movement.
   b. helps regulate the tone of skeletal muscles.
   c. if destroyed, would result in the loss of all voluntary skeletal activity.
   d. contains the centres responsible for the regulation of body temperature.

2. The neuron synapse
   a. is not resistant to electrical current.
   b. cannot become exhausted.
   c. has a synaptic cleft.
   d. transfers information at the speed of electricity.

3. Which of the following could result in the initiation of an action potential?
   a. Depolarizing the membrane
   b. Decreasing the extracellular K^+ concentration
   c. Increasing the activity of the Na^+/K^+-ATPase active transport system
   d. Stimulating the nerve with a threshold electrical stimulus during the absolute refractory period of the membrane

4. Neurotransmitters are
   a. produced in the muscle to communicate with nerves.
   b. the chemicals used to stimulate or suppress effectors at the synapse.
   c. usually found in the diet.
   d. nonspecific in their action on various nerves.

5. The limbic system is an area of the brain that
   a. is responsible for coordination of movement.
   b. is responsible for the special senses.

c. is responsible for the expression of emotions.
d. controls sleep.

6. The brainstem contains areas responsible for
   a. vomiting, swallowing, respiration, arousal and sleep.
   b. learning.
   c. motivation and memory.
   d. movement.

Extended Matching Questions

Select all that apply.

1. In explaining the importance of a constant blood supply to the brain, the nurse would tell the student which of the following?
   a. Energy is needed to maintain neuron membranes and cannot be produced without oxygen.
   b. Little glucose is stored in neurons, so a constant supply is needed.
   c. The brain needs a constant supply of insulin and thyroid hormone.
   d. The brain swells easily and needs the blood supply to reduce swelling.
   e. Circulating aldosterone levels maintain the fluid balance in the brain.

Matching

Match the word with the appropriate definition.

1. ____________________ action potential
2. ____________________ afferent
3. ____________________ axon
4. ____________________ dendrite
5. ____________________ depolarization
6. ____________________ effector
7. ____________________ efferent
8. ____________________ nerve
9. ____________________ cerebral hemispheres
10. ____________________ brainstem

A. Motor neurons
B. Long projection from a neuron that carries information from one nerve to another nerve or effector
C. Neurons or groups of neurons that bring information to the CNS
D. Location of the control centres for the heart and respiration
E. Interprets sensory inputs and controls skeletal muscle activity
F. A collection of neurons arranged longitudinally
G. The electrical signal by which neurons send information
H. Muscle, a gland, or another nerve stimulated by a nerve
I. Reversing the membrane charge from negative to positive
J. Short projection on a neuron that transmits information

Definitions

Define the following terms

1. neuron____________________
2. neurotransmitter____________________
3. limbic system____________________
4. Schwann cell____________________
5. myelination____________________
6. soma____________________
7. synapse____________________
8. repolarization____________________

Bibliography

Bear, M. F., Connors, B. W., & Paradiso, M. A. (2007). *Neuroscience: Exploring the brain* (3rd ed.). Philadelphia: Lippincott, Williams & Wilkins.

Ganong, W. (2005). *Review of medical physiology* (22nd ed.). New York: McGraw-Hill.

Guyton, A., & Hall, J. (2005). *Textbook of medical physiology* (11th ed.). Philadelphia: W. B. Saunders.

Howland, R. D., & Mycek, M. J. (2005). *Pharmacology* (3rd ed.). Philadelphia: Lippincott Williams & Wilkins.

Marieb, E. N., & Hoehn, K. (2009). *Human anatomy & histology* (8th ed.). San Francisco: Pearson.

Porth, C. M., & Matfin, G. (2008). *Pathophysiology: Concepts of altered health states* (8th ed.). Philadelphia: Lippincott Williams & Wilkins.

CHAPTER

19

Anxiolytic and Hypnotic Agents

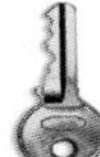

KEY TERMS

anxiety

anxiolytic

barbiturate

benzodiazepine

γ-aminobutyric acid (GABA)

hypnosis

hypnotic

ligand-gated ion channels

sedation

sedative

LEARNING OBJECTIVES

Upon completion of this chapter, you will be able to:

1. Define the states that are affected by anxiolytic or hypnotic agents.
2. Describe the therapeutic actions, indications, pharmacokinetics, contraindications, most common adverse reactions and important drug–drug interactions associated with each class of anxiolytic or hypnotic agent.
3. Discuss the use of anxiolytic or hypnotic agents across the lifespan.
4. Compare and contrast the key drugs for each class of anxiolytic or hypnotic drug with the other drugs in that class.
5. Outline the nursing considerations and teaching needs for patients receiving each class of anxiolytic or hypnotic agent.

BENZODIAZEPINES

alprazolam
chlordiazepoxide
diazepam
flurazepam
loprazolam
lormetazepam
lorazepam
nitrazepam
oxazepam
temazepam

BARBITURATES

amobarbital
butobarbital
secobarbital

OTHER ANXIOLYTIC AND HYPNOTIC DRUGS

buspirone
chloral hydrate
clomethiazole
promethazine
triclofos sodium
zaleplon
zolpidem
zopiclone

The drugs discussed in this chapter are used to alter an individual's responses to the environment. They have been called **anxiolytics**, because they can prevent feelings of tension or fear; **sedatives**, because they can calm patients and make them unaware of their environment and **hypnotics**, because they can cause sleep. In the past, a given drug would simply be used at different dosages to yield each of these effects. Further research into how the brain reacts to outside stimuli has resulted in the increased availability of specific drugs that produce particular goals and avoid unwanted adverse effects. Use of these drugs does vary across the lifespan (Box 19.1).

States Affected by Anxiolytic and Hypnotic Drugs

Anxiety

Anxiety is a feeling of tension, nervousness, apprehension or fear that usually involves unpleasant reactions to a stimulus, whether actual or unknown. Anxiety is often accompanied by signs and symptoms of the sympathetic stress reaction (see Chapter 28); including sweating, fast heart rate, rapid breathing and elevated blood pressure. Mild anxiety, a relatively common reaction, may serve as a stimulus or motivator in some situations. A person who feels anxious about being alone in a poorly lit alleyway at night may be motivated to take extra safety precautions. But when anxiety becomes overwhelming or severe, it can interfere with the activities of daily living and lead to medical problems related to chronic stimulation of the sympathetic nervous system. A severely anxious person may, for example, be afraid to leave the house or to interact with other people. In these cases, treatment is warranted. Anxiolytic drugs may be used to decrease the feeling of anxiety, possibly in conjunction with psychological approaches.

Sedation

The loss of awareness and reaction to environmental stimuli is termed **sedation**. This condition may be desirable in patients who are restless, nervous, irritable or overreacting to stimuli. Although sedation is also anxiolytic, it may frequently lead to drowsiness and this could be a concern for patients who need to be alert and responsive in their normal lives. Alternatively, this drowsiness may be desirable for patients who are about to undergo surgery or other procedures and who are receiving medical support. The choice of drug will depend on the situation in which it will be used and keeping the related adverse effects in mind.

Hypnosis

Extreme sedation results in further central nervous system (CNS) depression and sleep, or **hypnosis**. Hypnotics are used to help people fall asleep by causing sedation. Drugs that are effective hypnotics act on the reticular activating system

BOX 19.1 DRUG THERAPY ACROSS THE LIFESPAN

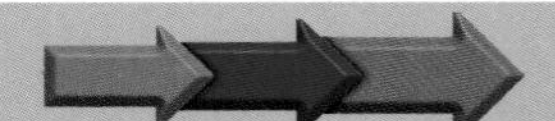

Anxiolytic and Hypnotic Agents

CHILDREN

There must be strong justification for the use of anxiolytic and hypnotic drugs with children. Anxiolytics should only be used to relieve acute anxiety caused by fear, for example, of surgery. The use of hypnotics should also be limited to occasional use, for example for night terrors and sleepwalking. Only diazepam, nitrazepam, chloral hydrate, triclofos sodium and promethazine are suitable for use by children and have established paediatric doses. The benzodiazepines midazolam and temazepan can be used as sedatives prior to surgery or other procedures.

When administering any drug to children, always consult the most recent edition of the British National Formulary for Children.

ADULTS

Adults using these drugs for the treatment of insomnia need to be cautioned that they are for short-term use only. The reason for the insomnia should be sought (e.g. medical, hormonal or anxiety problems). Other methods for helping to induce sleep – established routines, relaxing activities before bed, a warm bath, limiting alcohol and caffeine-containing substances – should be encouraged before drugs are prescribed.

The drowsiness associated with these drugs may affect driving or the operation of machinery. Liver function should be evaluated before and periodically during therapy, if necessary. These drugs are contraindicated during pregnancy and lactation because of the potential for adverse effects on the foetus and possible sedation of the baby. The antihistamines may be the safest to use, with caution, if an anxiolytic or hypnotic drug must be used at any time during pregnancy.

OLDER ADULTS

Nondrug measures to reduce anxiety and to help induce sleep are important with older patients. The patient should be screened for physical problems, neurological deterioration, or depression, all of which could contribute to the insomnia or anxiety.

Older patients are more susceptible to the adverse effects of these drugs, from unanticipated CNS effects to increased sedation, dizziness and confusion. Hypnotics should only be prescribed with caution to older adults. The anxiolytic dose should be reduced and the patient monitored very closely for toxic effects. Safety measures should be provided if CNS effects do occur. Baseline liver and renal function tests should be performed, and these values should be monitored periodically for any changes that would indicate a need to decrease dosage further or to stop taking the drug.

(RAS) and block the brain's response to incoming stimuli. Hypnosis, therefore, is the extreme state of sedation, in which the person no longer senses or reacts to incoming stimuli.

Benzodiazepines

Benzodiazepines are the most frequently used group used as anxiolytic and hypnotic drugs, although dependence and tolerance can occur even after a few weeks. These drugs should only be used in the short-term treatment of acute disorders. Withdrawal of benzodiazepines should be a gradual process to reduce the possibility of confusion or psychosis developing.

Therapeutic Actions and Indications

The benzodiazepines act in the limbic system and the RAS to enhance the effects of the inhibitory neurotransmitter, **γ-aminobutyric acid (GABA**; Figure 19.1). GABA is the main inhibitory neurotransmitter in the brain and modulates the activity of excitatory pathways. There are two subtypes of GABA receptors: $GABA_A$ and $GABA_B$. The $GABA_A$ receptors are located on the postsynaptic membrane and are the target for the benzodiazepines and barbiturates (see following sections). The $GABA_A$ receptors in the CNS are **ligand-gated ion channels** which allow the entry of chloride (Cl^-) ions into the neuron. Once GABA binds to the receptor, the ion channel opens allowing Cl^- to enter the neuron, making the inside of the cell more negative in relation to the outside, i.e. the cell becomes hyperpolarized which inhibits the neuronal activity in those areas of the brain associated with anxiety and sleep. The benzodiazepines do not cause a direct opening of the Cl^- channel; instead, these drugs enhance the effects of GABA by increasing the affinity of the receptors for GABA.

The benzodiazepines are indicated for the treatment of the following conditions: short-term anxiety disorders, alcohol withdrawal, insomnia, hyperexcitability and agitation, and preoperative relief of anxiety and tension to aid in balanced anaesthesia.

The benzodiazepines include the following:

- *Alprazolam* is indicated for the short-term treatment of anxiety. Patients may experience a 'hangover' effect the following day, for example drowsiness, lightheadedness, headache, confusion, vertigo.
- *Chlordiazepoxide* is also used for the short-term treatment of anxiety and as an adjunct in alcohol withdrawal. This drug has a long duration of action.
- *Diazepam*, in addition to its anxioloytic and hypnotic effects, is used as an anticonvulsant in status epilepticus and febrile convulsions. This drug has a long duration of action.

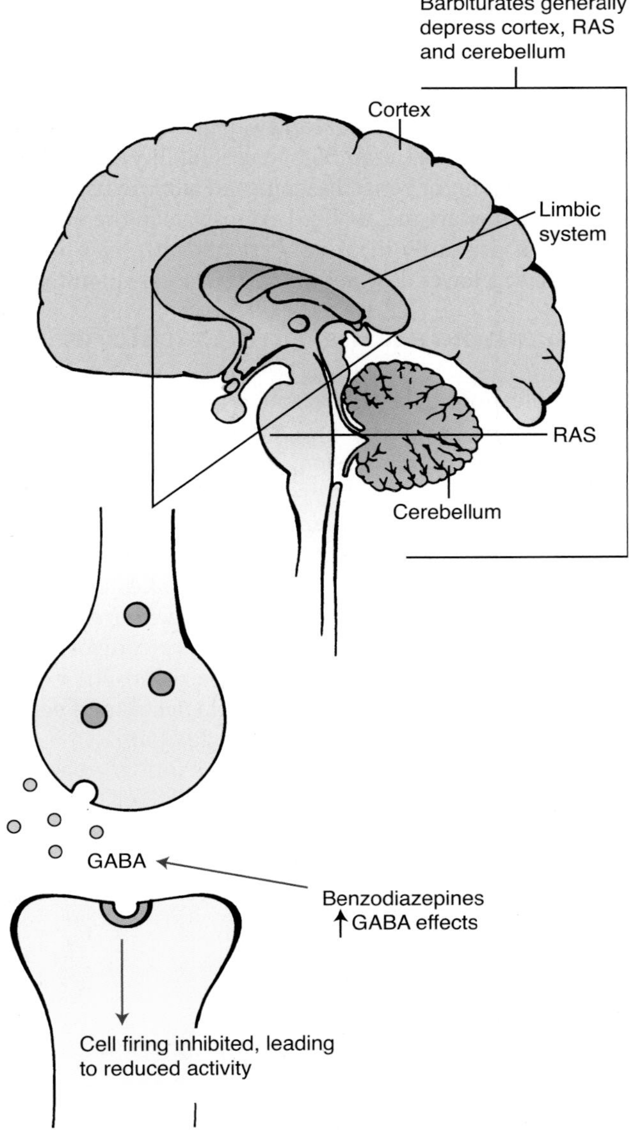

FIGURE 19.1 Sites of action of the benzodiazepines and barbiturates.

- *Flurazepam* and *nitrazepam* are used for the short-term treatment of insomnia. Their effects are prolonged and can cause drowsiness the following day. Flurazepam has a long duration of action.
- *Loprazolam, lormetazepam* and *temazepam* are all short-acting drugs used in the short-term treatment of insomnia. The drowsiness usually associated with hypnotics is reduced with these drugs; however, there can be withdrawal symptoms.
- *Lorazepam*, like diazepam, can also be used as an anticonvulsant. One of the short-acting benzodiazepines, lorazepam can also be used to treat panic disorders.
- *Oxazepam* is another short-acting benzodiazepine indicated for the short-term treatment of anxiety.

Pharmacokinetics

The benzodiazepines are well absorbed from the gastrointestinal (GI) tract, with peak levels achieved in 30 minutes to 2 hours. They are lipid-soluble and well distributed throughout the body; however, their high lipid solubility can result in the accumulation of benzodiazepines in adipose tissue. The benzodiazepines are metabolized extensively in the liver and excretion is primarily in urine. Patients with liver disease must receive a lower dose and should be closely monitored.

Contraindications and Cautions

Contraindications to benzodiazepines include allergy to any benzodiazepine; psychosis, *which could be exacerbated by sedation;* respiratory depression, sleep apnoea, depression or anxiety, *all of which could be exacerbated by the depressant effects of these drugs* and severe hepatic impairment *which could lead to toxic plasma benzodiazepine concentrations.*

In addition, benzodiazepines are contraindicated in pregnancy *because there is a risk of neonatal withdrawal syndrome* and should only be used for seizure control where the benefits to the mother outweigh the risk to the foetus. Breast-feeding is also a contraindication *because of potential adverse effects on the neonate (e.g. sedation).*

Caution should be used in patients with muscle weakness, myasthenia gravis or a history of drug or alcohol abuse. The metabolism and excretion of these drugs in elderly or debilitated patients or those with renal or hepatic dysfunction, *may be altered resulting in toxicity.* Dosage adjustments are usually needed for such patients.

Adverse Effects

The adverse effects of benzodiazepines are associated with the impact of these drugs on the central and peripheral nervous systems. Tolerance, when patients require an increased dose of the benzodiazepine to produce the desired response, can occur. As tolerance increases, the patient can also become physically dependent on the drug; although prescribed users tend not to become psychologically dependent (or addicted) to benzodiazepines (O'Brien, 2005). The drug dependence becomes evident when the patient stops the benzodiazepine treatment: abrupt cessation of these drugs may lead to a withdrawal syndrome characterized by anxiety, insomnia, anorexia, sweating and nightmares. ***Withdrawal of benzodiazepines should be a gradual process over a period of weeks to reduce the possibility of confusion or psychosis developing.***

Other nervous system effects include drowsiness, lightheadedness, amnesia, confusion (particularly in the elderly) and a paradoxical increase in aggressive behaviour may occur. The dose should be adjusted accordingly. Less frequent effects include blurred vision, headaches and vertigo.

Other adverse effects include dry mouth and GI disturbances. Cardiovascular problems may include hypotension; and there could be respiratory difficulties. Haematological conditions such as jaundice and anaemia may also occur. Genitourinary effects include urinary retention and hesitancy, loss of libido and changes in sexual functioning. Thrombophlebitis and local reactions may occur at local injection sites, and such sites should be monitored.

Refer to Box 19.2 for guidance on how to treat an overdose of benzodiazepines.

BOX 19.2 A Benzodiazepine Antidote

Flumazenil, a benzodiazepine antidote, acts by inhibiting the effects of the benzodiazepines at the GABA receptors. It is used to (1) treat benzodiazepine overdose, (2) reverse the sedation caused by benzodiazepines that are used as adjuncts for general anaesthesia and (3) reverse sedation produced for diagnostic tests or other medical procedures.

Flumazenil, which is available for intravenous (IV) use only, has a rapid onset of action that peaks 5 to 10 minutes after administration, with a duration of action of about 2 hours. Initially 200 μg is injected over the first 15 seconds followed by 100 μg at 60-second intervals if required. The maximum total dose is 1 or 2 mg if the patient is in intensive care. The cause of sedation must be questioned if the patient does not respond to the increased dose. If drowsiness returns after IV injection, an infusion of 100 to 400 μg flumazenil/hour can be set up. The dose should be adjusted according to the level of the patients' arousal (BNF, 2008).

If the patient has been taking a benzodiazepine for a long period, administration of flumazenil may precipitate a rapid withdrawal syndrome that requires supportive measures. Nausea, vomiting and flushing may be associated with use of flumazenil.

Clinically Important Drug–Drug Interactions

The risk of CNS depression increases if benzodiazepines are taken with alcohol or other CNS depressants, so such combinations should be avoided. In addition, the effects of benzodiazepines increase if they are taken with antibacterials, antifungals, cimetidine or disulfiram. If any of these drugs are used with benzodiazepines, patients should be monitored and the appropriate dosage adjustments made. There is also an increased risk of prolonged sedation with the concomitant use of antivirals.

Always consult a current copy of the British National Formulary for further guidance.

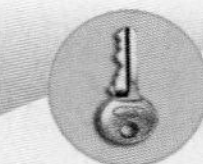

Key Drug Summary: *Diazepam*

Indications: Short-term management of anxiety disorders or insomnia, acute alcohol withdrawal, muscle relaxation, treatment of tetanus, status epilepticus, preoperative relief of anxiety and tension

Actions: Potentiate the inhibitory effects of the neurotransmitter GABA; may act in spinal cord and supraspinal sites to produce muscle relaxation

Pharmacokinetics:

Route	Onset	Peak	Duration
Oral	30–60 min	1–2 h	3 h
IM	15–30 min	30–45 min	3 h
IV	1–5 min	30 min	15–60 min
Rectal	Rapid	1.5 h	3 h

$T_{1/2}$: 20–40 hours (in older adults the $t_{1/2}$ may be extended to between 50 and 140 hours), metabolized in the liver, excreted in urine

Adverse effects: Drowsiness, confusion, ataxia, amnesia, muscle weakness, drug dependence. Occasionally headache, vertigo, hypotension, visual disturbances, dysarthria, tremor, GI disturbances, incontinence, urinary retention, changes in libido, blood disorders, jaundice and skin reactions

Nursing Considerations for Patients Receiving Benzodiazepines

Assessment: History and Examination

It may be necessary, depending on the patient, to screen for some or all of the following conditions, *which could be contraindications or cautions to the use of the drug:* any known allergies to benzodiazepines; impaired liver or kidney function, *which could alter the metabolism and excretion of a particular drug;* any condition *that might be exacerbated by the depressant effects of the drugs* (e.g. psychoses, respiratory disease, muscle weakness, acute alcohol intoxication); and pregnancy and lactation. Establish if patient is currently taking other medications or herbal therapies which may potentially interact with the benzodiazepine.

Include screening for baseline status before beginning therapy *to check for occurrence of any potential adverse effects.* Assess for the following: temperature and weight; affect, orientation and reflexes; pulse, blood pressure and perfusion; respiratory rate, adventitious sounds and presence of chronic pulmonary disease. Laboratory tests should include renal and liver function tests and full blood count. Refer to Critical Thinking Scenario 19-1 for a full discussion of nursing care for a patient dealing with anxiety.

Nursing Diagnoses

The patient receiving a benzodiazepine may have the following nursing diagnoses related to drug therapy:

- Disturbed thought processes and disturbed sensory perception (visual, kinaesthetic) related to CNS effects
- Risk for injury related to CNS effects
- Disturbed sleep pattern related to CNS effects
- Deficient knowledge regarding drug therapy

Implementation With Rationale

- Give parenteral forms only in emergency situations or if oral forms are not feasible or available, and switch to oral forms as soon as possible.
- Give IV drugs slowly *because these agents have been associated with hypotension, bradycardia and cardiac arrest.*
- Review the dosage of analgesics in patients receiving a benzodiazepine *to decrease potentiated effects and sedation.* Adjust the dose of both drugs accordingly to produce the most effective response for the patient, that is pain relief with minimal sedation.
- Advise patients taking these drugs to avoid operating heavy machinery and to take care with driving.
- Taper dosage gradually after long-term therapy in all patients. *Acute withdrawal could precipitate seizures in epileptic patients and psychosis in other patients or other symptoms of withdrawal.*
- Provide comfort measures *to help patients tolerate drug effects,* such as giving food with the drug if GI upset is severe, safety precautions, for example assistance with ambulation; and orientation.
- Provide thorough patient teaching, including drug name, prescribed dosage, measures for avoidance of adverse effects, and warning signs that may indicate possible problems. Instruct patients about the need for periodic monitoring and evaluation *to enhance patient knowledge about drug therapy and to promote concordance.*
- Suggest patients do not keep their medication beside their beds but in a cupboard in another room.
- Offer support and encouragement *to help the patient cope with the diagnosis and the drug regimen.*
- If necessary, use flumazenil (Box 19.2), the benzodiazepine antidote, *for treatment of overdose.*

Evaluation

- Monitor patient response to the drug (alleviation of signs and symptoms of anxiety, sleep, sedation).

- Monitor for adverse effects (sedation, hypotension, blood dyscrasias).
- Evaluate effectiveness of teaching plan (patient can give the drug name, dosage, possible adverse effects to watch for, specific measures to help avoid adverse effects, and the importance of continued follow-up).
- Monitor effectiveness of comfort measures and compliance with regimen (Critical Thinking Scenario 19-1).

Barbiturates

Barbiturates were once the anxiolytic/hypnotic drugs of choice. Not only is the likelihood of sedation and other adverse effects greater with these drugs than with newer anxiolytic/hypnotic drugs, but the risk of addiction and dependence is also greater. For these reasons, newer anxiolytic drugs have replaced the barbiturates in most instances. Three barbiturates, *amobarbital, butobarbital* and *secobarbital*, are indicated *only* for patients with severe intractable insomnia who are already taking barbiturates. Their use is generally avoided and specifically they should not be used by children, young adults, the elderly and debilitated patients.

Therapeutic Actions and Indications

The barbiturates are general CNS depressants that inhibit neuronal impulse conduction in the ascending RAS, depress the cerebral cortex, alter cerebellar function, and depress motor output (see Figure 19.1). Thus they can cause sedation, hypnosis, anaesthesia and, in extreme cases, coma and death. Their mechanism of action is similar to that of the benzodiazepines; however, they bind to a different site on the GABA receptor to increase the inhibitory actions of GABA.

Pharmacokinetics

The barbiturates are well absorbed, reaching peak levels in 20 to 60 minutes. They are metabolized in the liver to varying degrees, depending on the drug, and excreted in the urine. The longer-acting barbiturates tend to be metabolized more slowly and excreted to a greater degree unchanged in the urine. The barbiturates are known to induce liver enzymes, increasing the metabolism of the barbiturate broken down by that system, as well as that of any other drug that may be metabolized by the same enzyme system. Patients with hepatic or renal dysfunction require lower doses of the drug to avoid toxic effects and should be monitored closely. Barbiturates are lipid-soluble, readily crossing the placenta and entering breast milk.

Contraindications and Cautions

Contraindications to barbiturates include allergy to any barbiturate and a previous history of drug or alcohol abuse *because the barbiturates are more addictive than most other anxiolytics*. Other contraindications are latent or manifest porphyria (insufficient synthesis of haem for red blood cells), *which may be exacerbated*; marked hepatic impairment, *which may alter the metabolism*; and respiratory distress or severe respiratory dysfunction, *which could be exacerbated by the CNS depression caused by these drugs*. Pregnancy is a contraindication *because of potential adverse effects on the foetus*; congenital abnormalities have been reported with barbiturate use.

Caution should be used in patients with acute or chronic pain *because barbiturates can cause paradoxical excitement, masking other symptoms*; and with chronic hepatic, renal or respiratory diseases, *which could be exacerbated by the depressive effects of these drugs*. Care should be taken with lactating women *because of the potential for adverse effects on the infant*.

Adverse Effects

As previously stated, the adverse effects caused by barbiturates are more severe than those associated with other, newer sedatives/hypnotics. For this reason, barbiturates are no longer considered the mainstay for the treatment of anxiety. In addition, the development of physical tolerance and psychological dependence is more likely with the barbiturates than with other anxiolytics.

The most common adverse effects are related to general CNS depression. CNS effects may include drowsiness, a feeling of a 'hangover', dizziness, headaches, paradoxical excitement and ataxia (failure of muscular co-ordination). Hypersensitivity reactions and respiratory depression may also occur.

Clinically Important Drug–Drug Interactions

Increased CNS depression results if these agents are taken with other CNS depressants, including alcohol, antihistamines and other tranquilizers. If other CNS depressants are used, dosage adjustments are necessary.

In addition, because of an enzyme-induction effect of barbiturates in the liver, the following drugs may not be as effective as desired: oral anticoagulants, digoxin, tricyclic antidepressants, corticosteroids, oral contraceptives, oestrogens, metronidazole, chloramphenicol, doxycycline, β-blockers, calcium channel blockers, ciclosporin, sodium oxybate, thyroxine and antivirals. If these agents are given in combination with barbiturates, patients should be monitored closely; frequent dosage adjustments may be necessary to achieve the desired therapeutic effect.

Always consult a current copy of the British National Formulary for further guidance.

Nursing Considerations for Patients Receiving Barbiturates

Assessment: History and Examination

Screen for the following, *which could be contraindications or cautions for the use of the drug:* any known allergies to barbiturates or a history of addiction to sedative/hypnotic drugs, impaired hepatic or renal function *that could alter the metabolism and excretion of the drug,* respiratory dysfunction and pregnancy or lactation. Establish if patient is currently taking other medications or herbal therapies which may potentially interact with the barbiturate.

Include screening *for baseline status before beginning therapy and for the occurrence of any potential adverse effects.* Assess the following: temperature and weight; blood pressure and pulse, including perfusion; orientation and reflexes; respiratory rate and adventitious sounds.

Nursing Diagnoses

The patient receiving a barbiturate may have the following nursing diagnoses related to drug therapy:

- Disturbed thought processes and disturbed sensory perception (visual, auditory, kinaesthetic, tactile) related to CNS effects
- Risk of injury related to CNS effects
- Impaired gas exchange related to respiratory depression
- Risk of dependence
- Deficient knowledge regarding drug therapy

Implementation With Rationale

- Provide standby life-support facilities *in case of severe respiratory depression or hypersensitivity reactions.*
- Taper dosage gradually after long-term therapy, especially in patients with epilepsy. Acute withdrawal *may precipitate seizures in patients with epilepsy, cause psychosis in other patients or cause symptoms of withdrawal.*
- Provide comfort measures *to help patients tolerate drug effects,* including orientation as needed.
- Provide thorough patient teaching, including drug name, prescribed dosage, measures for avoidance of adverse effects, and warning signs that may indicate possible problems. Instruct patients about the need for periodic monitoring and evaluation *to enhance patient knowledge about drug therapy and to promote concordance.*
- Offer support and encouragement *to help the patient cope with the diagnosis and the drug regimen.*

Evaluation

- Monitor patient response to the drug (alleviation of signs and symptoms of anxiety, sleep, sedation).
- Monitor for adverse effects (sedation, hypoventilation, hepatic or renal dysfunction, hypersensitivity reactions, dependence).
- Evaluate effectiveness of teaching plan (patient can give the drug name, dosage, possible adverse effects to watch for, specific measures to help avoid adverse effects and the importance of continued follow-up).
- Monitor effectiveness of comfort measures and compliance with regimen.

Other Anxiolytic and Hypnotic Drugs

There are other drugs used to treat anxiety or to produce hypnosis that do not fall into either the benzodiazepine or the barbiturate group. These include the following:

- *Chloral hydrate* and *triclofos sodium* have been used to produce nocturnal sedation or preoperative sedation, but their use is now limited. They are rapidly absorbed from the GI tract and metabolized in the liver and kidney for excretion in the bile and urine. See Box 19.3 for an exercise in calculating the correct dosage for preparing a paediatric patient for a procedure.
- *Clomethiazole* is used as a hypnotic for elderly patients because the drowsiness experienced the following day with most of the other hypnotics is reduced.
- *Zaleplon, zolpidem* and *zopiclone* are hypnotics used for the short-term treatment of insomnia (up to 4 weeks). These drugs also act at the GABA receptor but do not have the same mechanism of action as the benzodiazepines. They are all metabolized in the liver and excreted in the urine. Caution should be used in patients with hepatic or renal impairment. Elderly patients are especially sensitive to these drugs; they should receive a lower dose and be monitored carefully.
- Antihistamines (*promethazine*) can be very sedating in some people and are available for night sedation and short-term occasional treatment of insomnia. Promethazine can also be used as a preoperative medication.
- *Buspirone,* a newer anxiolytic, is a serotonin (5-HT) receptor agonist. It reduces the signs and symptoms of anxiety without many of the CNS effects and severe

adverse effects associated with other anxiolytic drugs. It is rapidly absorbed from the GI tract, metabolized in the liver, and excreted in urine. Caution should be used in patients with hepatic or renal impairment.

BOX 19.3 **FOCUS ON CALCULATIONS**

Your 1-year-old patient, weighing 12 kg, is prescribed chloral hydrate as a hypnotic prior to a procedure. The order reads: 30 mg/kg. The drug comes in a syrup form as 200 mg/5 mL. How much syrup would you give?

First, calculate what the correct dose would be:

$$30 \text{ mg/kg} \times 12 \text{ kg} = 360 \text{ mg}$$

Set up the equation using available form = prescribed dose:

$$200 \text{ mg}/5 \text{ mL} = 360 \text{ mg/dose}$$

Then, cross-multiply:

$$\begin{aligned} 200 \text{ mg (dose)} &= 1800 \text{ mg (mL)} \\ \text{dose} &= 1800 \text{ mg (mL)} / 200 \text{ mg} \\ \text{dose} &= 9 \text{ mL} \end{aligned}$$

Always ask another nurse to double-check the accuracy of your calculations.

WEB LINKS

Health care providers and patients may want to consult the following Internet sources:

http://bnfc.org The BNF for Children provides UK health care professionals with authoritative and practical information on the selection and clinical use of medicines in children.

http://cks.library.nhs.uk The National Health Service Clinical Knowledge Summaries provides evidence-based practical information on the common conditions observed in primary care.

http://www.bnf.org.uk The BNF provides UK health care professionals with authoritative and practical information on the selection and clinical use of medicines.

http://www.nhsdirect.nhs.uk The National Health Service Direct service provides patients with information and advice about health, illness and health services.

Points to Remember

- Anxiety is a sense of tension, nervousness, apprehension or fear in response to an actual or an unknown stimulus. In the extreme, anxiety may produce physiological manifestations and may interfere with activities of daily life.
- Anxiolytics are drugs used to treat anxiety by depressing the CNS. They can also be used as muscle relaxants. When given at higher doses, these drugs may be sedatives or hypnotics.
- Sedatives block the awareness of and reaction to environmental stimuli, resulting in associated CNS depression that may cause drowsiness, lethargy and other effects. This action can be beneficial when a patient is very excited or afraid.
- Hypnotics further depress the CNS, particularly the RAS, to inhibit neuronal arousal and induce sleep.
- Benzodiazepines are a group of drugs used as anxiolytics and hypnotics. They bind to GABA receptor sites to enhance the inhibitory effects of GABA and depress the CNS. They can cause drowsiness, lethargy and other CNS effects.
- Barbiturates are an older class of drugs used as hypnotics. They are associated with potentially serious adverse effects and interact with many other drugs, and are therefore less desirable than the benzodiazepines or other anxiolytics.
- Buspirone, a newer anxiolytic drug, does not cause sedation or muscle relaxation. It is much preferred in certain circumstances (e.g. when a person must drive, go to work or maintain alertness) because of the absence of CNS effects.

CRITICAL THINKING SCENARIO 19-1

Benzodiazepines

The Situation

Penny, a 43-year-old mother of three teenage sons, visits her general practitioner's surgery for a routine physical examination. Results are unremarkable except for blood pressure of 145/90 mmHg, pulse rate of 98 bpm, and apparent tension. She is jittery, avoids eye contact, and sometimes appears teary-eyed. She says that she is having some problems dealing with 'life in general' and finds it very difficult to sleep at night. Her sons present many stresses and her husband, who is busy with his career, has little time to deal with issues at home. When he *is* home, he is very demanding. Overall, she feels lonely and has no outlet for her anger, tension or stress. She is reluctant to be prescribed an antidepressant and wants to seek alternative treatment approaches; however, she is keen to seek medical assistance for her insomnia so that she can face her current situation more effectively. A health care provider prescribes the benzodiazepine oxazepam to help Penny deal with her insomnia.

Critical Thinking

- What sort of crisis intervention would be most appropriate for Penny?
- What nursing interventions are helpful at this point?
- What nondrug interventions might be helpful?
- What other support systems could be used to help Penny deal with all that is going on in her life?
- Think about the overwhelming problems that Penny has to deal with on a daily basis and how oxazepam might change her approach to these problems. Could the problems actually get worse?
- Develop a care plan for the long-term care of Penny.

Discussion

Penny has been prescribed oxazepam to assist with her insomnia and not her anxiety or depression; an antidepressant is more appropriate for the latter. However, where insomnia is associated with stress arising during the day, oxazepam when taken at night may prove beneficial to her insomnia as well as her anxiety. The oxazepam prescribed for Penny may provide some immediate relief, enabling her to survive the 'crisis' period and plan changes in her life in general. However, the associated drowsiness and sedation may make coping with the problems in her life even more difficult. She should be taught the adverse effects of oxazepam, the warning signs of serious adverse effects, and the health problems to report.

A follow-up evaluation should be scheduled. Additional meetings with the same health care provider are important for the long-term solution to Penny's anxiety. Her need for drug therapy should be re-evaluated once she can discover other support systems and develop other ways of coping. Although oxazepam may be beneficial initially, it will not solve the problems that are causing anxiety, and in this case, the causes for the anxiety are specific. The oxazepam should only be considered as a short-term aid.

Unlike Penny, many patients in severe crisis do not consciously identify the many causes of stress, or stressors. However, Penny has identified a list of factors that makes her life stressful. This facilitates the development of coping strategies. She may find the following support systems helpful:

- Referral to a counsellor and involvement of the entire family in identifying problems and ways to deal with them.
- Support groups for women: having the opportunity to discuss problems and explore ways of dealing with them helps many people.

Nursing Care Guide for Penny: Oxazepam

Assessment: History and Examination

Allergies to oxazepam, psychoses, history of alcohol abuse, respiratory disease, impaired liver or kidney function, pregnancy, breast-feeding, concurrent use of alcohol, antibacterials, antivirals, phenytoin, valproate, sodium oxybate, omeprazole, cimetidine, disulfiram, theophylline

- Cardiovascular: blood pressure, pulse, perfusion
- CNS: orientation, affect, reflexes, vision
- GI: abdominal examination, bowel sounds

Nursing Diagnoses

- Potential for disturbed thought processes and disturbed sensory perception (visual, kinaesthetic) related to CNS effects
- Potential risk of injury related to CNS effects

(continued)

Benzodiazepines *(continued)*

- Potential for disturbed sleep patterns related to CNS effects
- Deficient knowledge regarding drug therapy

Implementation

- Provide comfort and safety measures, small meal, drug with food if GI upset occurs, bowel programme as needed; reduce dosage if other medications include narcotics; lower dose with renal or hepatic impairment.
- Limit prescription to preferably 1 week and no more than 3 weeks.
- Provide support and reassurance to deal with drug effects.
- Provide patient teaching regarding drug, dosage, adverse effects, safety precautions and unusual symptoms to report.

Evaluation

- Evaluate drug effects: relief of signs and symptoms of anxiety.
- Monitor for adverse effects, particularly sedation, drowsiness, insomnia, blood disorders and jaundice, GI upset, hepatic or renal dysfunction, cardiovascular effects.
- Monitor for drug–drug interactions.
- Evaluate effectiveness of patient teaching programme.
- Evaluate effectiveness of comfort and safety measures.

Patient Teaching for Penny

- ☐ The drug that has been prescribed for you is called oxazepam. It belongs to a class of drugs called benzodiazepines, which are used to relieve anxiety and the insomnia associated with anxiety. Common side-effects of this drug include:
  - *Drowsiness and light headedness:* avoid driving or performing hazardous tasks that require concentration if these effects occur.
  - *Constipation or diarrhoea:* these reactions usually pass with time. If they do not, consult with your health care provider for appropriate therapy.
  - *Vision changes, slurred speech, unsteadiness:* these effects also subside with time. Take extra care in your activities for the first few days. If these reactions do not go away after 3 or 4 days, consult your health care provider.
  - Report any of the following conditions to your health care provider: *rash, fever, confusion or depression.*
- ☐ Tell any doctor, nurse, or other health care provider involved in your care that you are taking this drug.
- ☐ Keep this drug and all medications safely away from children or pets.
- ☐ Avoid the use of over-the-counter medications or herbal therapies while you are taking this drug. If you think that you need one of these products, consult with your health care provider about the best choice because many of these products can interfere with your medication.
- ☐ Avoid alcohol while you are taking this drug. Combining alcohol and a benzodiazepine can cause oversedation.

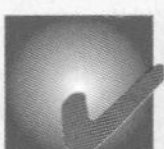

CHECK YOUR UNDERSTANDING

Answers to the questions in this chapter may be found in the answer key in the back of the book.

Multiple Choice

Select the most appropriate answer to the following.

1. Drugs that are used to alter a patient's response to the environment are called
   a. hypnotics.
   b. sedatives.
   c. antiepileptics.
   d. anxiolytics.

2. The benzodiazepines are the most frequently used anxiolytic drugs because they
   a. are anxiolytic at doses much lower than those needed for sedation or hypnosis.
   b. can also be stimulating.
   c. are more likely to cause physical dependence than older anxiolytic drugs.
   d. do not affect any neurotransmitters.

3. Barbiturates cause liver enzyme induction, which could lead to
   a. rapid metabolism and loss of effectiveness of other drugs metabolized by those enzymes.
   b. increased bile production.
   c. CNS depression.
   d. the need to periodically lower the barbiturate dose to avoid toxicity.

4. A person who could benefit from an anxiolytic drug for short-term treatment of insomnia would *not* be prescribed
   a. zolpidem.
   b. nitrazepam.
   c. buspirone.
   d. chloral hydrate.

5. Anxiolytic drugs block the awareness of and reaction to the environment. This effect would *not* be beneficial
   a. to relieve extreme fear.
   b. to moderate anxiety related to unknown causes.
   c. in treating a patient who must drive a vehicle for a living.
   d. in treating a patient who is experiencing a stress reaction.

6. Mr. Jones is the chief executive officer of a large company and has been experiencing acute anxiety attacks. His physical examination was normal, and he was diagnosed with anxiety. Considering his occupation and his need to be alert and present to large groups on a regular basis, the following anxiolytic would be a drug of choice for Mr. Jones:
   a. amobarbital.
   b. diazepam.
   c. promethazine.
   d. buspirone.

7. The benzodiazepines bind to
   a. GABA receptor sites in the RAS to cause inhibition of neuronal arousal.
   b. noradrenaline receptor sites in the sympathetic nervous system.
   c. acetylcholine receptor sites in the parasympathetic nervous system.
   d. monoamine oxidase to increase noradrenaline breakdown.

Extended Matching Questions

Select **all** that apply.

1. In assessing a patient who is experiencing anxiety, the nurse would expect to find which of the following?
   a. Rapid breathing
   b. Rapid heart rate
   c. Fear and apprehension
   d. Constricted pupils
   e. Decreased abdominal sounds
   f. Hypotension

2. Your client has a long history of anxiety and has always responded well to diazepam. She has just learned that she is pregnant and feels very anxious. She would like a prescription for diazepam to get her through her early anxiety. What rationale would the nurse use in explaining why this is not recommended?
   a. This drug should only be used in pregnancy if there is a clear indication for use, for example in seizure control.
   b. Babies born to mothers taking benzodiazepines may progress through a neonatal withdrawal syndrome.
   c. There is a risk of dependency with diazepam.
   d. This drug almost always causes miscarriage.
   e. The hormones the body produces during pregnancy will make you unresponsive to diazepam.
   f. This drug could have adverse effects on your baby; we should explore nondrug measures to help you deal with the anxiety.

Fill in the Blanks

1. ______________ is a feeling of tension, nervousness, apprehension or fear that usually involves unpleasant reactions to a stimulus, which is actual or unknown.

2. Mild anxiety may serve as a stimulus or ___________ in some situations.

3. _______________ are drugs that can calm patients and make them unaware of their environment.

4. Drugs that can cause sleep are called ____________.

5. Anxiolytics can prevent feelings of ______________ .

6. Patients who are restless, nervous, irritable or overreacting to stimuli could benefit from ____________.

7. Hypnosis or sleep can be caused by drugs that ______________the CNS.

8. ______________ are the most frequently used anxiolytic drugs.

Bibliography and References

British Medical Association and Royal Pharmaceutical Society of Great Britain. (2008). *British National Formulary*. London: BMJ & RPS Publishing. *This publication is updated biannually: it is imperative that the most recent edition is consulted.*

British Medical Association and Royal Pharmaceutical Society of Great Britain. (2007). *British National Formulary for Children*. London: BMJ & RPS Publishing. *This publication is updated annually: it is imperative that the most recent edition is consulted.*

Ganong, W. (2005). *Review of medical physiology* (22nd ed.). New York: McGraw-Hill.

Gilman, A., Hardman, J. G., & Limbird, L. E. (eds.). (2006). *Goodman and Gilman's the pharmacological basis of therapeutics* (11th ed.). New York: McGraw-Hill.

Howland, R. D., & Mycek, M. J. (2005). *Pharmacology* (3rd ed.). Philadelphia: Lippincott Williams & Wilkins.

O'Brien, C. P. (2005). Benzodiazepine use, abuse and dependence. *Journal of Clinical Psychiatry, 66*(S2), 28–33.

Porth, C. M., & Matfin, G. (2008). *Pathophysiology: Concepts of altered health states* (8th ed.). Philadelphia: Lippincott Williams & Wilkins.

Rang, H. P., Dale, M. M., Ritter, J. M., & Flower, R. J. (2007). *Rang and Dale's pharmacology* (6th ed.). Philadelphia: Churchill Livingstone.

Simonsen, T., Aarbakke, J., Kay, I., Coleman, I., Sinnott, P., & Lysaa, R. (2006). *Illustrated pharmacology for nurses*. London: Hodder Arnold.

CHAPTER 20

Antidepressant Agents

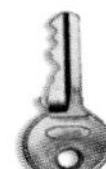

KEY TERMS

depression

MAO-A

MAO-B

monoamine oxidase (MAO)

monoamine oxidase inhibitor (MAOI)

selective serotonin reuptake inhibitor (SSRI)

tricyclic antidepressant (TCA)

tyramine

LEARNING OBJECTIVES

Upon completion of this chapter, you will be able to:

1. Describe the monoamine theory of depression.
2. Describe the therapeutic actions, indications, pharmacokinetics, contraindications, most common adverse reactions and important drug–drug interactions associated with each class of antidepressant.
3. Discuss the use of antidepressants across the lifespan.
4. Compare and contrast the key drugs for each class of antidepressant with the other drugs in that class and with drugs in the other classes of antidepressants.
5. Outline the nursing considerations and teaching needs for patients receiving each class of antidepressant.

TRICYCLIC ANTIDEPRESSANTS

clomipramine
doxepin
imipramine
lofepramine
nortriptyline
trimipramine

MONOAMINE OXIDASE INHIBITORS

isocarboxazid
moclobemide
phenelzine
tranylcypromine

SELECTIVE SEROTONIN REUPTAKE INHIBITORS

citalopram
escitalopram
fluoxetine
fluvoxamine
paroxetine
sertraline

OTHER ANTIDEPRESSANTS

duloxetine
flupentixol
mianserin
mirtazapine
reboxitine
trazodone
tryptophan
venlafaxine

Depression is an affective disorder (disorder of mood), which relates to people's feelings in response to their environment; whether positive and pleasant or negative and unpleasant. All people experience different affective states at various times in their lives depending upon the situations they find themselves in. These states of mind do not usually last very long and do not often involve extremes of happiness or sadness. If a person's mood goes far beyond the usual, normal 'ups and downs', he or she is said to have an affective disorder.

Depression and Antidepressants

Depression is the most common affective disorder in the world, affecting approximately 121 million people worldwide (WHO, 2009). In depression, feelings of sadness are much more severe and long-lasting than the suspected precipitating event and the mood of affected individuals is much more intense. The depression may not always be traceable to a specific event or stressor (i.e. having no external causes). Patients who are depressed may have little energy, sleep disturbances, a lack of appetite, decreased libido and inability to perform activities of daily living. They may describe overwhelming feelings of sadness, despair, hopelessness and inadequacy.

There are three main forms of depression:

1. *reactive* depression could be caused by a stressful event in an individuals life, such as bereavement; or as an adverse reaction to drug treatment.
2. *endogenous* depression for which there is no apparent precipitating cause.
3. *bipolar affective disorder* where a patient alternates between mania (characterized by feelings of elation) and depression.

The approach to treating depression is tailored to the severity and the frequency of the depressive episode(s) and the individuals personal needs (NICE, 2004). Patients with mild depression are recommended a self-help psychotherapy programme based on cognitive behavioural therapy, which aims to normalize the depressive thinking. Antidepressant therapy is not recommended at this stage because the risks to the patient outweigh the benefits. Patients are reassessed after a 2-week period and if found to be refractory to psychotherapy, antidepressant therapy should be considered. A patient with moderate-to-severe depression would be managed with a combination of antidepressant therapy, psychotherapy and social support.

Regardless of the severity of the depression, left untreated, that is without either psychotherapy or drug treatment; depression can interfere with a person's family life, job and social interactions and can produce multiple physical problems that can lead to further depression or, in extreme cases, suicide.

Monoamine Theory of Depression

Research on development of the drugs known to be effective in relieving depression led to formulation of the current hypothesis regarding the cause of depression. Depression is believed to result from a deficiency of the monoamine neurotransmitters, noradrenaline and serotonin (5-HT), in key areas of the brain. Both are released throughout the brain by neurons and bind to multiple receptors to regulate arousal, alertness, attention, mood, appetite and sensory processing. The neurotransmitter is then removed from the synaptic cleft by reuptake into the presynaptic neuron via an amine reuptake pump and re-packaged for release from the neuron. Any excess neurotransmitter is broken down by the enzyme **monoamine oxidase (MAO)** in the presynaptic neuron.

Deficiencies of noradrenaline and 5-HT may develop for three reasons. First, MAO may break them down and there will be less neurotransmitter available for release. Second, rapid firing of the neurons may lead to their depletion. Third, the number or sensitivity of post- and/or presynaptic receptors to noradrenaline or 5-HT may increase or decrease.

Depression may also occur as a result of other as yet unknown causes. This condition may be a syndrome that reflects either activity or lack of activity in a number of sites in the brain, including the reticular activating system, the limbic system and basal ganglia.

Drug Therapy

One way to manage depression is with the use of antidepressant drugs. The antidepressant drugs used today counteract the effects of neurotransmitter deficiencies by either inhibiting the enzymes that breakdown the monoamines or preventing the reuptake of monoamines into neurons. Both approaches lead to increased neurotransmitter levels in the synaptic cleft.

Antidepressants may be classified into three groups: (1) **tricyclic antidepressants (TCAs)**, (2) **MAO inhibitors (MAOIs)** and (3) **selective serotonin reuptake inhibitors (SSRIs)**. Other drugs that are used as antidepressants similarly increase the concentrations of these neurotransmitters in the synaptic cleft (Figure 20.1). For information on how antidepressants affect people of different ages, see Box 20.1.

Tricyclic Antidepressants

The TCAs all reduce the reuptake of the monoamine neurotransmitters 5-HT and noradrenaline into presynaptic neuron terminals (see Figure 20.1). There are a number of adverse effects associated with TCAs including sedation, hypotension, cardiovascular and antimuscarinic effects. These adverse effects are explained by the inhibitory action of TCAs on muscarinic, histamine and α-adrenergic receptors.

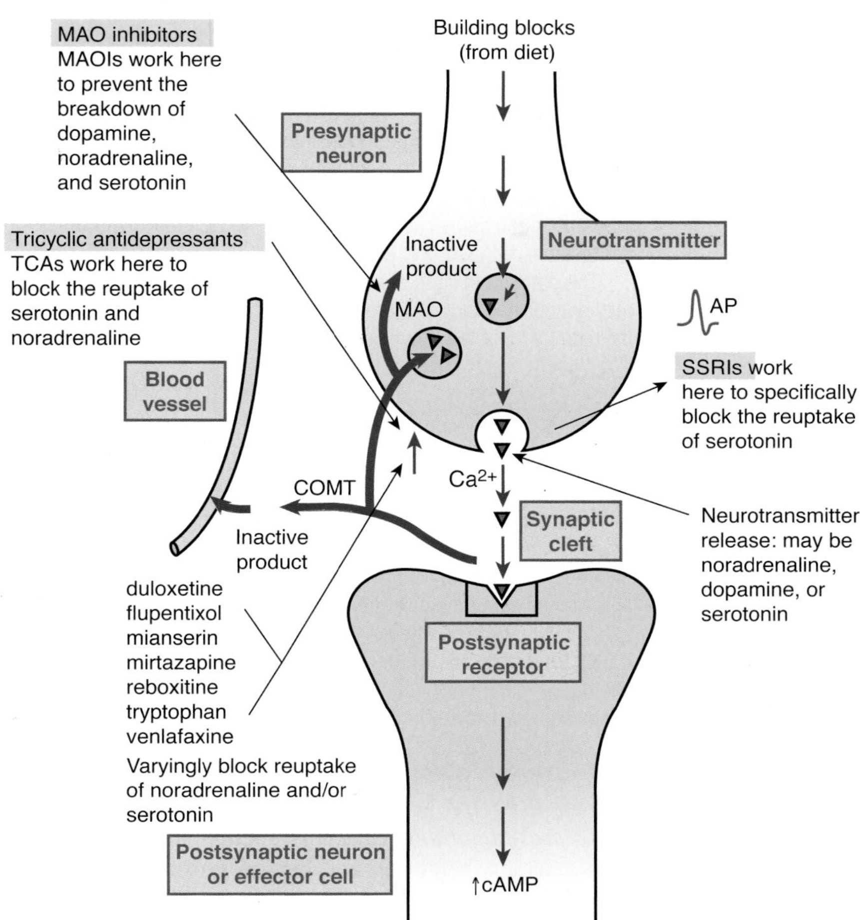

FIGURE 20.1 Sites of action for the antidepressants. cAMP, cyclic adenosine monophosphate; COMT, catecholamine-*O*-methyltransferase; MAOIs, monoamine oxidase inhibitors; TCAs, tricyclic antidepressants; SSRIs, selective serotonin reuptake inhibitors and other agents.

The TCAs have similar efficacies; therefore the choice of TCA will depend on individual response to the drug and tolerance of adverse effects. A patient who does not respond to one TCA may respond to another drug from this class. Table 20.1 lists the currently available TCAs, including the occurrence of sedation and other adverse effects. Amitriptyline and dosulepin are also effective TCAs; however, they are not recommended for the treatment of depression because there is a relatively high rate of fatality in overdosage (British National Formulary, 2008).

Therapeutic Actions and Indications

The inhibition of reuptake of the neurotransmitters, noradrenaline and 5-HT leads to an accumulation of these neurotransmitters in the synaptic cleft and increased stimulation of the postsynaptic receptors. The exact mechanism of action in decreasing depression is not known but is thought to be related to the accumulation of noradrenaline and 5-HT in certain areas of the brain.

TCAs are indicated for the relief of symptoms of depression and anxiety. The sedative effects of some of these drugs (dosulepin, doxepin, trimipramine) may make them more effective in patients whose depression is characterized by anxiety and sleep disturbances. Amitriptyline and nortriptyline are also used in the treatment of chronic, intractable pain, such as migraine. In addition, because TCAs are antimuscarinic, amitriptyline, imipramine and nortriptyline are effective in treating enuresis (bed-wetting) in children older than 7 years. Clomipramine is approved for use in the treatment of obsessive-compulsive disorders (OCDs).

Pharmacokinetics

The TCAs are well absorbed from the gastrointestinal (GI) tract, reaching peak levels in 2 to 4 hours. TCAs undergo significant first-pass metabolism so only 25% to 75% of the dose reaches the circulation. They are lipid-soluble allowing wide distribution in the tissues, including the brain. TCA metabolites from the liver are excreted in the urine: patients with hepatic impairment will require a lower dose of the drug to avoid toxic levels. The TCAs have relatively long half-lives, ranging from 8 to 46 hours. TCAs cross the placenta and enter breast milk and should not be used during pregnancy or lactation unless the benefit to

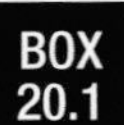

BOX 20.1 DRUG THERAPY ACROSS THE LIFESPAN

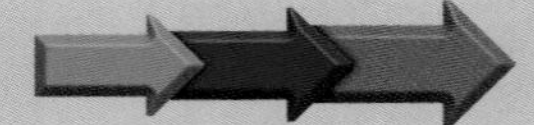

Antidepressant Agents

CHILDREN

Use of antidepressant drugs in children poses a challenge. The response of the child to the drug may be unpredictable and the long-term effects of many of these agents are not clearly understood. Underlying medical reasons for the depression should be ruled out before antidepressant therapy is considered.

The MAOIs should not be prescribed to children. The majority of TCAs are also not recommended for the treatment of depression in children. Doxepin can be used to treat depression in children over the age of 12 years. However, the TCAs can be used to treat nocturnal enuresis. Children should be monitored closely for adverse effects and dosage changes should be made as needed.

The SSRIs can cause serious adverse effects in children. Although there are established paediatric doses for some of these drugs, studies have shown an increase in harmful outcomes, such as suicidal behaviour and self-harm (Committee on Safety of Medicines, 2004). Where the clinical need is high and the benefits outweigh the risks, fluoxetine may be prescribed to children and adolescents, but these patients must be closely monitored, particularly for suicidal thoughts (see Box 20.2).

When administering any drug to children, always consult the most recent edition of the British National Formulary for Children.

ADULTS

Adults using these drugs should have medical causes for their depression ruled out before therapy commences. Thyroid disease, hormonal imbalance and cardiovascular disorders and certain types of medication can all lead to the signs and symptoms of depression.

The patient needs to understand that the effects of drug therapy may not be seen for 2 to 4 weeks and that it is important to continue the therapy for at least that long.

OLDER ADULTS

In older patients, the drug therapy should be continued for at least 6 weeks before evaluating the treatment outcome. Older patients may be more susceptible to the adverse effects of these drugs, from unanticipated central nervous system (CNS) effects to increased sedation, dizziness and even hallucinations. Dosages of all of these drugs need to be reduced and the patient monitored very closely for toxic effects. Safety measures should be provided if CNS effects do occur. Patients with hepatic or renal impairment should be monitored very closely while taking these drugs and doses adjusted accordingly.

the mother clearly outweighs the potential risk to foetus or neonate.

Contraindications and Cautions

Contraindications of TCAs include recent myocardial infarction *because TCAs can depress conduction pathways in the heart (characterized by a prolonged QT interval on an electrocardiogram [***ECG***]), which can predispose patients to fatal arrhythmias;* and the presence of hepatic or renal disease, *which could interfere with metabolism and excretion of these drugs and lead to toxic levels.*

Caution should be used with TCAs in patients with pre-existing cardiovascular disorders, particularly arrhythmias, *because of the cardiac stimulatory effects of the drug* and with *any condition that would be exacerbated by the antimuscarinic (parasympatholytic) effects,* such as angle-closure glaucoma, urinary retention and benign prostatic hypertrophy. Care should also be taken with patients with mental health problems, *who may exhibit a worsening of psychoses or paranoia* and with patients with bipolar disorder, *who may shift to a manic stage.* In addition, caution is necessary in patients with a history of seizures *because the seizure threshold may be decreased secondary to stimulation of the receptor sites.*

Adverse Effects

The adverse effects of TCAs are associated with the effects of the drugs on the CNS and on the peripheral nervous system. Sedation, confusion, disorientation, behavioural

Table 20.1 Tricyclic Antidepressants: Most Common Adverse Effects

	Common Adverse Effects			
Drug Name	*Sedation*	*Anticholinergic*	*Hypotension*	*Cardiovascular*
clomipramine	+++	+++	+++	+++
doxepin	+++	+++	++	++
imipramine	++	++	+++	++
lofepramine	++	++	++	++
nortriptyline	+	+	+	+
trimipramine	+++	++	++	++

++++ = marked effects; +++ = moderate effects; ++ = mild effects; + = negligible effects

disturbances, tremor, paraesthesia (tingling), blurred vision and tremors may occur.

Use of TCAs may lead to GI antimuscarinic effects, such as dry mouth, constipation, nausea, increased salivation, cramps and diarrhoea. Resultant genitourinary effects may include urinary retention and hesitancy, loss of libido and changes in sexual functioning. Cardiovascular effects such as postural hypotension, arrhythmias and tachycardia may also pose problems. Additional reported effects include weight gain or loss (occasionally), sweating, rashes, blurred vision and hypersensitivity reactions.

These adverse effects may be intolerable to some patients, who then stop taking the particular TCA. Abrupt cessation of all TCAs causes a withdrawal syndrome characterized by nausea, anorexia, headache, vertigo and sometimes hypomania and anxiety.

Clinically Important Drug–Drug Interactions

The key drug groups interacting with TCAs include: antiarrhythmics, β-blockers and antibacterials, where there is an increased risk of ventricular arrhythmias; antipsychotics, which may increase plasma TCA levels; and dopaminergics, where there is an increased risk of CNS toxicity. The sedation associated with some TCAs can be exacerbated by alcohol, antihistamines, anxiolytics and hypnotics.

Some drug groups such as antiseizure agents, may speed up the rate of TCA metabolism and therefore reduce plasma TCA levels; whereas cimetidine inhibits the metabolism of TCAs, increasing the plasma concentration of TCAs.

There is also an increased risk of hypertension when TCAs are combined with sympathomimetics and MAOIs. This combination should be avoided, especially in patients with underlying cardiovascular disease. Similarly, the plasma concentration of TCAs is increased by the SSRIs. *TCAs should not be prescribed until 2 weeks after stopping an MAOI (3 weeks if starting clomipramine or imipramine).*

TCAs may enhance or reduce the serum levels of anticoagulants leading to either an increased risk of bleeding or clotting, respectively. Blood tests should be performed frequently and appropriate dosage adjustments of the oral anticoagulant should be made.

Always consult a current copy of the British National Formulary for further guidance.

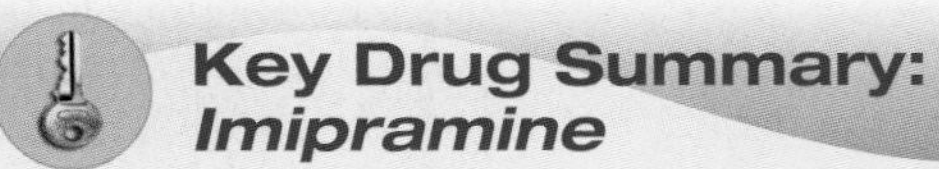

Key Drug Summary: *Imipramine*

Indications: Relief of symptoms of depression; nocturnal enuresis in children older than 7 years

Actions: Inhibits presynaptic reuptake of noradrenaline and 5-HT; antimuscarinic at CNS and peripheral receptors; sedating

Pharmacokinetics:

Route	Onset	Peak
Oral	Varies	2–4 h

$T_{1/2}$: 8–16 hours, metabolized in the liver, excretion in the urine

Adverse effects: sedation, antimuscarinic (parasympatholytic) effects, blurred vision, confusion, anxiety, headache, orthostatic hypotension, tachycardia, dry mouth, constipation, nausea, increased appetite and weight gain, urinary retention, sweating, tremor, rashes, interference with sexual function, endocrine side-effects (testicular enlargement, gynaecomastia), bone marrow depression

Nursing Considerations for Patients Receiving Tricyclic Antidepressants

Assessment: History and Examination

Screen for the following, *which could be contraindications or cautions for the use of the drug:* any known allergies to these drugs; impaired liver or kidney function, *which could alter metabolism and excretion of the drug*; glaucoma, benign prostatic hypertrophy, cardiac dysfunction or recent myocardial infarction, *all of which could be exacerbated by the effects of the drug*; and pregnancy or lactation. Determine whether the patient has a history of seizure disorders or a history of mental health problems. Establish if patient is currently taking other medications (e.g. MAOI) or herbal therapies, which may potentially interact with the TCA.

Include screening *for baseline status before beginning therapy and for any potential adverse effects.* Assess the following: affect, orientation and reflexes; vision; blood pressure, including orthostatic blood pressure; and pulse and perfusion. Obtain an ECG, as well as renal and liver function tests if the patient's history suggests potential problems.

Nursing Diagnoses

The patient receiving a TCA may have the following nursing diagnoses related to drug therapy:

- Acute pain related to antimuscarinic effects, headache, CNS effects
- Decreased cardiac output which could manifest as tiredness

- Disturbed thought processes and disturbed sensory perception (visual, kinaesthetic) related to CNS effects
- Risk of injury related to CNS effects
- Deficient knowledge regarding drug therapy

Implementation With Rationale

- Suicidal patients need to be under constant and close observation in a hospital setting or allowed to discuss their suicidal thoughts openly.
- Maintain initial dosage for 2 to 4 weeks *to evaluate the therapeutic effect.*
- Give the major portion of the dose at bedtime if drowsiness and antimuscarinic effects are severe *to decrease the risk of patient injury. Elderly and adolescent patients may not be able to tolerate larger doses.*
- If minor adverse effects occur, encourage the patient to persist with the treatment as tolerance to some of these effects does develop. Discontinue the drug slowly if major or potentially life-threatening adverse effects occur *to ensure patient safety.*
- Provide comfort measures *to help the patient tolerate drug effects.* These measures may include voiding before dosing, instituting a bowel programme as needed, taking food with the drug if GI upset is severe, drinking water for dry mouth and environmental control (temperature).
- Provide thorough patient teaching, including drug name, prescribed dosage, measures for avoidance of adverse effects and warning signs that may indicate possible problems. Instruct patients about the need for periodic monitoring and evaluation *to enhance patient knowledge about drug therapy and to promote concordance.*
- Offer support and encouragement *to help patients cope with the diagnosis and the drug regimen.*

Evaluation

- Monitor patient response to the drug (alleviation of signs and symptoms of depression).
- Monitor for adverse effects (sedation, antimuscarinic effects, hypotension, cardiac arrhythmias).
- Evaluate effectiveness of teaching plan (patient can give the drug name, dosage, possible adverse effects to watch for, specific measures to help avoid adverse effects and importance of continued follow-up).
- Monitor the effectiveness of comfort measures and concordance with the regimen.

Monoamine Oxidase Inhibitors

The MAOIs are used less frequently than TCAs and SSRIs and their related antidepressants because of the toxicity associated with interactions with other drugs and dietary components. Safer drugs that are usually just as effective have replaced them; however, they may still be of benefit to those patients who are unresponsive to other antidepressants. Agents still in use include: phenelzine, isocarboxazid, tranylcypromine and moclobemide. Phenelzine and isocarboxazid have reduced stimulant effects compared with tranylcypromine. The choice of a MAOI depends on the prescriber's experience and the individual's response. A patient who does not respond to one MAOI may respond to another.

Therapeutic Actions and Indications

The MAOIs irreversibly inhibit MAO, an enzyme found in some neurons and tissues (including the liver), that breaks down the amines noradrenaline, dopamine and 5-HT. There are two forms of the MAO enzyme: **MAO-A** and **MAO-B.** MAO-A prefers to break down 5-HT (but will also break down noradrenaline and dopamine) and is the main target for the MAOIs; and MAO-B will break down noradrenaline and dopamine. Inhibition of MAO will allow these amines to accumulate in the synaptic cleft and in neuronal vesicles, causing increased stimulation of the postsynaptic receptors and relief of depression. The MAOIs are generally indicated for treatment of the signs and symptoms of depression in patients who cannot tolerate or do not respond to other, safer antidepressants. The British National Formulary (2008) also states that MAOIs are more effective in phobic patients and depressed patients with atypical hypochondriacal features (e.g. worrying about health issues and aches and pains).

Pharmacokinetics

The MAOIs are well absorbed from the GI tract, reaching peak levels in 2 to 3 hours. They are metabolized in the liver by acetylation (an enzymatic process) and are excreted in the urine. Patients with liver or renal impairment and those known as 'slow acetylators' (i.e. MAOIs are metabolized at a slow rate) may require lowered doses to avoid exaggerated effects of the drugs. The MAOIs cross the placenta and enter breast milk. Use during pregnancy and lactation should be avoided unless the benefit to the mother clearly outweighs the potential risk to the foetus or neonate.

Contraindications and Cautions

Contraindications to the use of MAOIs include allergy to any of these antidepressants; phaeochromocytoma (tumour of the adrenal medulla releasing adrenaline and noradrenaline) *because an additional increase in noradrenaline levels with a MAOI could result in severe hypertension and cardiovascular emergencies;* and known abnormal CNS vessels or defects *because the potential increase in blood pressure and vasoconstriction associated with higher noradrenaline levels could precipitate a stroke.* Hepatic impairment *which could alter the metabolism of these drugs and lead to toxic levels* is also a contraindication.

In addition, caution should be used with patients with cardiovascular disease, including hypertension, coronary artery disease, angina and congestive heart failure, *which could be exacerbated by increased noradrenaline levels;* and in patients with epilepsy, *which could be exacerbated by the stimulation caused by these drugs;* or patients with diabetes mellitus *because these drugs may change the amount of oral hypoglycaemics or insulin the patient requires.* Care should also be taken with patients who are soon to undergo elective surgery *because of the potential for unexpected effects with noradrenaline accumulation during the stress reaction* and with female patients who are pregnant or breast-feeding *because of potential adverse effects to the foetus and neonate.*

Adverse Effects

The MAOIs are associated with more significant adverse effects than other classes of antidepressant drugs. These effects relate to the accumulation of noradrenaline in the synaptic cleft. Dizziness, excitement, nervousness, mania, hyperreflexia, tremors, confusion, insomnia, agitation and blurred vision may occur.

MAOIs can cause liver toxicity. Other GI effects can include constipation, anorexia, weight gain and dry mouth. Urinary retention and changes in sexual function may also occur. Cardiovascular effects can include postural hypotension, arrhythmias and the potentially fatal hypertensive crisis. This last condition is characterized by occipital headache, palpitations, neck stiffness, nausea, vomiting, sweating, dilated pupils, photophobia, tachycardia and chest pain. It may progress to intracranial bleeding and fatal stroke.

Clinically Important Drug–Drug Interactions

Drug interactions of MAOIs with other antidepressants include hypertensive crisis, coma and severe convulsions with TCAs and a potentially life-threatening 5-HT syndrome with SSRIs. *A period of 2 weeks should elapse after stopping a MAOI before beginning therapy with other antidepressants (3 weeks if starting clomipramine or imipramine). Conversely, a MAOI should not be started until 1 to 2 weeks after a tricyclic or other antidepressant therapy has finished (3 weeks in the case of clomipramine or imipramine).*

Note that MAOIs reduces the metabolism of 5-HT, noradrenaline and dopamine thereby increasing the levels of these transmitters in the synaptic cleft. Thus if MAOIs are given with other sympathomimetic drugs (e.g. methyldopa, pseudoephedrine), sympathomimetic effects increase and there is a risk of hypertensive crisis. Combinations with insulin or oral antidiabetic agents result in additive hypoglycaemic effects. Patients who receive these combinations must be monitored closely and appropriate dosage adjustments should be made. Concomitant use of the opioid analgesic pethidine and a MAOI can lead to hypotension, hyperpyrexia and coma. Pethidine should not be prescribed until 2 weeks after treatment with a MAOI has ceased.

Always consult a current copy of the British National Formulary for further guidance.

Clinically Important Drug–Food Interactions

Tyramine and other amines that are found in certain foods, beer and red wine are normally broken down by MAO enzymes in the wall of the GI tract and liver. Patients on MAOI therapy who ingest food or drink rich in tyramines will absorb larger quantities of tyramine into the systemic circulation resulting in increased blood pressure and the potential for hypertensive crisis. This reaction is also known as the ‘cheese’ reaction. In addition, tyramine causes the release of stored noradrenaline from nerve terminals, which further contributes to high blood pressure. Patients who take MAOIs should avoid the tyramine-containing foods listed in Table 20.2.

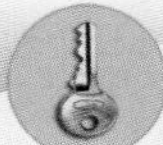

Key Drug Summary: *Phenelzine*

Indications: Treatment of patients with depression who are unresponsive to other antidepressive therapy or in whom other antidepressive therapy is contraindicated

Actions: Irreversibly inhibits MAO, allowing noradrenaline, 5-HT and dopamine to accumulate in the synaptic cleft; this accumulation is thought to be responsible for the clinical effects

Pharmacokinetics:

Route	Onset	Duration
Oral	Slow	48–96 h

$T_{1/2}$: 11 hours; metabolized in the liver, excreted in the urine

Adverse effects: Postural hypotension, dizziness. Less common effects include: vertigo, headache, over activity, hyperreflexia, tremors, agitation, nervousness, weakness, drowsiness, insomnia, fatigue, sweating, constipation, diarrhoea, urinary retention, dry mouth, oedema, potential for hypertensive crisis

Table 20.2 Tyramine-containing Foods

Foods High in Tyramine	Foods with Moderate Amounts of Tyramine	Foods with Low Amounts of Tyramine
Mature cheese	Meat extracts	Distilled alcohol: vodka, gin, Scotch, rye
Mature meats, fish or poultry: offal, game	Light beers and pale ale	Cheeses: mozzarella, cottage cheese, cream cheese
Yeast extracts (Bovril, Oxo, Marmite)	Avocados	Chocolate
Broad beans		Fruits: figs, raisins, grapes, pineapple, oranges, over-ripe bananas
Red wines: Chianti, burgundy, sherry, vermouth		Sour cream
Smoked or pickled meats, fish or poultry: pickled herrings, sausage, corned beef, salami, pepperoni		Soy sauce
		Yogurt

Nursing Considerations for Patients Receiving Monoamine Oxidase Inhibitors

Assessment: History and Examination

Screen for the following, *which could be contraindications or cautions for use of the drug*: any known allergies to these drugs; impaired liver function *that could alter the metabolism of the drug*; cardiac dysfunction; surgery; epilepsy; mental health conditions. Find out whether female patients are pregnant or breastfeeding. Establish if patient is currently taking other medications (e.g. SSRI) or herbal therapies, which may potentially interact with the MAOI.

Include screening *for baseline status before beginning therapy and for any potential adverse effects.* Assess the following: affect, orientation and reflexes; vision; blood pressure, including orthostatic blood pressure; and pulse and perfusion. Obtain an ECG and renal and liver function tests if the patient's history suggests potential problems.

Nursing Diagnoses

The patient receiving a MAOI may have the following nursing diagnoses related to drug therapy:

- Acute pain related to sympathomimetic effects, headache, CNS effects
- Potential for hypertensive crisis
- Decreased cardiac output which could manifest as tiredness
- Disturbed thought processes and disturbed sensory perception (visual, kinaesthetic) related to CNS effects
- Risk of injury related to CNS effects
- Deficient knowledge regarding drug therapy

Implementation With Rationale

- Suicidal patients need to be under constant and close observation in a hospital setting or allowed to discuss their suicidal thoughts openly.
- Monitor the patient for 2 to 4 weeks *to ascertain onset of full therapeutic effect.*
- Monitor blood pressure and orthostatic blood pressure carefully *to arrange for a slower increase in dosage as needed for patients who show a tendency towards postural hypotension.*
- Monitor liver function before and periodically during therapy and *arrange to decrease the drug dosage at the first sign of liver toxicity.*
- Decrease the drug dosage and monitor the patient carefully at any complaint of severe headache *to decrease the risk of severe hypertension and cerebrovascular effects.*
- Have phentolamine or another adrenergic blocker on standby *as treatment in case of hypertensive crisis.*
- Provide comfort measures *to help the patient tolerate drug effects.* These include voiding before dosing, instituting a bowel programme as needed, taking food with the drug if GI upset is severe, and environmental control (lighting, temperature, decreased stimulation).
- Provide a list of potential drug–food interactions that can cause severe toxicity *to decrease the risk of a serious drug–food interaction.* Encourage a diet that is low in tyramine-containing foods.
- Provide thorough patient teaching, including drug name, prescribed dosage, measures for avoidance of adverse effects and warning signs that may indicate possible problems. Instruct patients about the need for periodic monitoring and evaluation *to enhance patient knowledge about drug therapy and to promote concordance.*

- Offer support and encouragement *to help patients cope with the disease and the drug regimen.*

Evaluation

- Monitor patient response to the drug (alleviation of signs and symptoms of depression).
- Monitor for adverse effects (sympathomimetic effects, hypotension, cardiac arrhythmias, GI disturbances, hypertensive crisis).
- Evaluate the effectiveness of the teaching plan (patient can give the drug name, dosage, possible adverse effects to watch for, discuss specific measures to help avoid adverse effects, importance of continued follow-up and importance of avoiding foods high in tyramine).
- Monitor the effectiveness of comfort measures and concordance with the regimen.

Selective Serotonin Reuptake Inhibitors

SSRIs, the newest group of antidepressant drugs, do not have the many adverse effects associated with TCAs and MAOIs and are a better choice for many patients. SSRIs include the following agents:

- *Fluoxetine,* the first SSRI, has been successfully used to treat major depression, obsessive compulsive disorders (OCDs) and bulimia.
- *Fluvoxamine* is used to treat depression and OCDs.
- *Paroxetine* is indicated for the treatment of major depression, panic disorders, post-traumatic stress disorders, social anxiety disorders, general anxiety disorders and OCDs.
- *Sertraline* is used to treat depression, OCDs and post-traumatic stress disorders in women.
- *Citalopram* is indicated for the treatment of depression and panic disorder.
- *Escitalopram* is the active isomer of citalopram and is approved for the treatment of depressive illness, generalized anxiety disorders, panic disorders and social anxiety disorders.

With the SSRIs, a period of up to 4 weeks is necessary for realization of the full therapeutic effect. Patients may respond well to one SSRI and yet show little or no response to another one. The choice of drug will depend on the indications and individual response.

Therapeutic Actions and Indications

SSRIs specifically block the reuptake of 5-HT, with little to no known effect on noradrenaline. This action increases the levels of 5-HT in the synaptic cleft and may contribute to the antidepressant and other effects attributed to these drugs.

Pharmacokinetics

The SSRIs are well absorbed from the GI tract, metabolized in the liver and excreted in the urine and faeces. The half-life varies widely with the drug being used. The SSRIs have been associated with toxicity in animal studies and should be used during pregnancy only if the benefits to the mother clearly outweigh the potential risks to the foetus. There is also a risk of neonatal withdrawal. All SSRIs can enter breast milk but paroxetine and sertraline do so in very small quantities and are not thought to be harmful to the neonate. However, the other SSRI drugs should be either avoided or a different method of feeding the baby should be selected if a SSRI is required by the mother because of the adverse effects.

Contraindications and Cautions

The SSRIs are contraindicated in the presence of allergy to any of these drugs and during pregnancy and lactation *because of the potential for serious adverse effects on the neonate.* The SSRIs are also contraindicated in bipolar disorder. Caution should be used in patients with impaired renal or hepatic function *that could alter the metabolism and excretion of the drug, leading to toxic effects,* or with diabetes, epilepsy, cardiac disease and GI bleeding *which could be exacerbated by the stimulating effects of these drugs.* Recent studies have linked the incidence of suicidal ideation and suicide attempts to the use of these drugs in adolescent patients. Box 20.2 provides information of research into adverse effects of SSRIs in young people.

Adverse Effects

The adverse effects associated with SSRIs, which are related to the effects of increased 5-HT levels, include CNS effects such as headache, drowsiness, dizziness, insomnia, anxiety, tremor, agitation and seizures. GI effects such as nausea, vomiting, dyspepsia, diarrhoea, abdominal pain, dry mouth, anorexia, constipation and changes in taste often occur, as do genitourinary effects, including urinary retention, polyuria, menstrual irregularities and sexual dysfunction. Cardiovascular effects can include postural hypotension, tachycardia and palpitations. Other reported effects are sweating, hypersensitivity reactions, movement disorders and photosensitivity.

Clinically Important Drug–Drug Interactions

A combination of SSRIs and MAOIs should be avoided because of the risk of hypertensive crisis. *At least 2 to 4 weeks should be allowed between stopping one drug and*

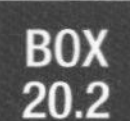

BOX 20.2 FOCUS ON THE **EVIDENCE**

Childhood Suicide and Antidepressants

In 1990 research revealed an increased risk of suicidal thoughts and behaviour in patients taking the SSRI, fluoxetine. The manufacturers of paroxetine subsequently demonstrated an increased risk of suicide-related adverse effects in children and adolescents taking paroxetine. The British Medicines and Healthcare Products Regulatory Agency and the U.S. Food and Drug Administration reviewed the SSRIs available for use by the paediatric population.

The data from these studies did not clearly establish a link between increased suicidal ideation and the use of these antidepressants, but the data also did not establish effectiveness in major depressive disorder in children for any of the drugs, except fluoxetine. The Committee on Safety of Medicines (2004) has advised that the balance between risks and benefits to children and adolescents is not favourable for any of the SSRIs except fluoxetine. Fluoxetine was the only SSRI effective in the treatment of depressive illness in paediatrics. However, if clinicians do decide to use one of the other SSRIs to treat children and adolescents, they must do so cautiously and monitor these patients for suicidal thoughts. Parents should be educated about the warning signs of suicide.

commencing another if switching between these groups of drugs. In addition, the use of SSRIs with TCAs results in increased therapeutic and toxic effects. If these combinations are used, patients should be monitored closely and appropriate dosage adjustments should be made.

Patients treated with SSRIs are at an increased risk of developing a severe reaction, including increased 5-HT effects, as well as increased photosensitivity if they are also taking St. John's wort. This herbal therapy is often used to self-treat depression; however, St. John's wort can induce liver metabolizing enzymes reducing the duration of action of other drugs metabolized by the same liver enzymes. It is important to warn any patient taking a SSRI not to combine it with herbal remedies without seeking advice from health care providers.

Always consult a current copy of the British National Formulary for further guidance.

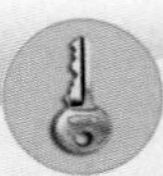

Key Drug Summary: *Fluoxetine*

Indications: Treatment of major depression, obsessive compulsive disorders and bulimia nervosa

Actions: Inhibits CNS neuronal reuptake of 5-HT with little effect on noradrenaline and little affinity for cholinergic sites

Pharmacokinetics:

Route	Onset	Peak
Oral	Slow	6–8 h

$T_{1/2}$: 2–4 weeks, metabolized in the liver, excreted in the urine and faeces

Adverse effects: Headache, nervousness, insomnia, drowsiness, impaired concentration, anxiety, tremor, postural hypotension, dizziness, sweating, rash, nausea, vomiting, diarrhoea, dry mouth, anorexia with weight loss, sexual dysfunction, upper respiratory infections, dyspnoea, alopecia, fever, urinary frequency

Nursing Considerations for Patients Receiving Selective Serotonin Reuptake Inhibitors

Assessment: History and Examination

Screen for the following conditions, *which could be contraindications or cautions for use of the drug*: any known allergies to SSRIs; history of mania; impaired liver or kidney function, *which could alter metabolism and excretion of the drug*; and diabetes mellitus. Find out whether female patients are pregnant or breast-feeding. Establish if patient is currently taking other medications (e.g. MAOI) or herbal therapies, which may potentially interact with the SSRI drug.

Include *screening for baseline status before beginning therapy and for any potential adverse effects.* Assess for the following: affect, orientation and reflexes; vision; blood pressure and pulse; respiratory rate and adventitious sounds; and bowel sounds on abdominal examination. Obtain renal and liver function tests if the patient's history suggests potential problems.

Nursing Diagnoses

The patient receiving an SSRI may have the following nursing diagnoses related to drug therapy:

- Acute pain related to GI, genitourinary CNS effects
- Disturbed thought processes and disturbed sensory perception (kinaesthetic, visual) related to CNS effects
- Imbalanced nutrition related to GI effects
- Potential for self-harm related to adverse effects of SSRIs
- Deficient knowledge regarding drug therapy

Implementation With Rationale

- Arrange for lower dosage in elderly patients and in those with renal or hepatic impairment *because of the potential for severe adverse effects.*
- Monitor patient for up to 4 weeks *to ascertain onset of full therapeutic effect before adjusting dosage.*
- Establish suicide precautions for severely depressed patients and limit the quantity of the drug dispensed *to decrease the risk of overdose.*
- Administer the drug once a day in the morning *to achieve optimal therapeutic effects.* If the dosage is increased or if the patient is having severe GI effects, the dosage can be divided.
- Suggest that patients use barrier contraceptives *to prevent pregnancy while taking this drug because serious foetal abnormalities can occur.*
- Provide comfort measures *to help patients tolerate drug effects.* These may include voiding before dosing, instituting a bowel programme as needed, taking food with the drug if GI upset is severe, or environmental control (lighting, temperature, stimuli).
- Provide thorough patient teaching, including the drug name, prescribed dosage, measures for avoidance of adverse effects and warning signs that may indicate possible problems. Instruct patients about the need for periodic monitoring and evaluation *to enhance patient knowledge about drug therapy and to promote concordance.*
- Offer support and encouragement *to help patients cope with the disease and the drug regimen.*

Evaluation

- Monitor patient response to the drug (alleviation of signs and symptoms of depression, OCD, bulimia, panic disorder).
- Monitor for adverse effects (sedation, dizziness, GI upset, respiratory dysfunction, genitourinary problems, skin rash).
- Evaluate effectiveness of the teaching plan (patient can give the drug name, dosage, possible adverse effects to watch for, specific measures to help avoid adverse effects, importance of continued follow-up and importance of avoiding pregnancy).
- Monitor the effectiveness of comfort measures and concordance with the regimen.

Other Antidepressants

Some other effective antidepressants do not fit into any of the three groups that have been discussed in this chapter. These drugs have varying effects on noradrenaline, 5-HT and histamine. Although it is not known how their actions are related to clinical efficacy, these agents may be most effective in treating depression in patients who do not respond to other antidepressants. Other antidepressants include the following:

- *Duloxetine* blocks both 5-HT and noradrenaline reuptake. It is indicated for the treatment of major depressive disorder, management of neuropathic pain associated with diabetic peripheral neuropathy and stress incontinence. Duloxetine has a half-life of 12 hours. Duloxetine should only be used in pregnancy if the potential benefit outweighs the risk and should be avoided if breast-feeding.
- *Mirtazapine* is an antagonist of α_2-adrenoceptors and 5-HT receptors and is used to treat major depression. It is rapidly absorbed from the GI tract, extensively metabolized in the liver and excreted in the urine. Mirtazapine has a half-life of 20 to 40 hours. This drug should be avoided in pregnancy and lactation.
- *Trazodone* is related to other TCAs and weakly blocks 5-HT reuptake; and is also an antagonist of 5-HT and histamine receptors. Effective in treating depression and anxiety, this drug is particularly useful where sedation is required during the treatment of the depression. It is readily absorbed from the GI tract, extensively metabolized in the liver and excreted in urine and faeces. Trazodone has a half-life of 3 to 6 hours. Trazodone should be avoided during pregnancy and lactation.
- *Venlafaxine* has fewer adverse CNS effects and is known to weakly block the reuptake of noradrenaline and 5-HT. It is very effective in treating some cases of depression and its popularity has increased with the introduction of an extended-release form that does away with the multiple daily doses that are required with the regular form. Venlafaxine is readily absorbed from the GI tract, extensively metabolized in the liver and excreted in urine. Venlafaxine has a half-life of 5 hours. Avoid during pregnancy and lactation unless the benefit to the mother clearly outweighs the potential risk to the neonate.
- *Flupentixol,* an antagonist of dopamine receptors, is used to treat depression and psychoses. Avoid during the final trimester of pregnancy and also during breast-feeding.
- *Mianserin* is related to other TCAs and is used to treat depression, especially where sedation is required. This drug inhibits α_2-adrenoceptors on the presynaptic membrane. Inhibition of these receptors increases the influx of calcium into the presynaptic neuron and increases

the exocytosis of neurotransmitter vesicles, including noradrenaline. This mechanism will increase the level of neurotransmitters circulating in the synaptic cleft. Mianserin should be avoided during pregnancy and while breast-feeding.

- *Reboxitine* is a selective noradrenaline reuptake inhibitor used to treat major depression. There are fewer adverse effects associated with this drug compared with other TCAs. Avoid during pregnancy and breast-feeding.
- *Tryptophan* can be used in combination with other antidepressants in patients resistant to standard antidepressant monotherapy. Tryptophan, an amino acid, is the precursor for the synthesis of 5-HT, therefore administering tryptophan will boost the synthesis and increase circulating levels of 5-HT. Caution should be applied if prescribing tryptophan during pregnancy and lactating.

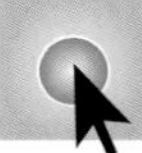

WEB LINKS

Health care providers and patients may want to consult the following Internet sources:

http://bnfc.org The BNF for Children provides UK health care professionals with authoritative and practical information on the selection and clinical use of medicines in children.

http://cks.library.nhs.uk The National Health Service Clinical Knowledge Summaries provides evidence-based practical information on the common conditions observed in primary care.

http://www.bnf.org.uk The BNF provides UK health care professionals with authoritative and practical information on the selection and clinical use of medicines.

http://www.nhsdirect.nhs.uk The National Health Service Direct service provides patients with information and advice about health, illness and health services.

http://www.mentalhealth.org.uk The Mental Health Foundation provides information, conducts research and campaigns to improve services for individuals affected by mental health problems.

http://www.mind.org.uk MIND, the National Association for Mental Health, is a charity offering support and guidance to patients with mental health illnesses and their families.

http://www.rcpsych.ac.uk The Royal College of Psychiatrists provides information and support to patients with a wide range of mental health illnesses.

Points to Remember

- Depression is an affective disorder characterized by overwhelming sadness, despair and hopelessness that is inappropriate with respect to the event or events that precipitated the depression. Depression is a very common problem; it is associated with many physical manifestations and is often misdiagnosed. It could be that depression is caused by a series of events that are not yet understood.
- The monoamine theory states that depression is caused by a deficiency of the amines – noradrenaline, 5-HT and dopamine – in certain key areas of the brain.
- Antidepressant drugs – TCAs, MAOIs and SSRIs – increase the concentrations of amines within the brain.
- Selection of an antidepressant depends on individual drug response and tolerance of associated adverse effects. The adverse effects of TCAs are sedating and antimuscarinic; those of MAOIs are CNS related and sympathomimetic. The adverse effects of SSRIs are fewer, but they do cause CNS changes.
- Other antidepressants are also effective in treating depression.

CRITICAL THINKING SCENARIO 20-1

Selective Serotonin Reuptake Inhibitors

The Situation

Debbie, a 46-year-old married woman, complains of weight gain, malaise, fatigue, sleeping during the day, loss of interest in daily activities and bouts of crying for no apparent reason. On examination, she weighs 6 kg more than the standard weight for her height; all other findings are within normal limits. In conversation with a nurse, Debbie says that in the past 10 months, she lost both of her parents and her only child left home to go to university. Debbie is prescribed fluoxetine and is given an appointment with a counsellor.

Critical Thinking

- What nursing interventions are appropriate at this time?
- What sort of crisis intervention would be most appropriate? *Balance the benefits of pointing out all of the*

Selective Serotonin Reuptake Inhibitors *(continued)*

losses and points of grief that you detect in Debbie's story with the risks of upsetting her strained coping mechanisms.

- What can Debbie expect to experience as a result of the SSRI therapy?
- How can you help Debbie cope during the lengthy period it takes to reach therapeutic effects?
- What other future interventions should be planned with Debbie?

Discussion

Many patients in severe crisis do not consciously identify the many things that are causing them stress. They have developed coping mechanisms to help them survive and cope with their day-to-day activities. However, Debbie seems to have reached her limit and she exhibits many of the signs and symptoms of depression. However, it is important to make sure that she does not have some underlying medical condition that could be contributing to her complaints. She may also be premenopausal, which could account for some of her problems.

It is hoped that the fluoxetine, a SSRI, will enable Debbie to regain her ability to cope and her normal mood. The drug should give her brain a chance to reach a new biochemical balance. Before she begins taking the fluoxetine, she should receive a written sheet listing the pertinent drug information, adverse effects to watch for, warning signs to report and a telephone number to call in case she has questions later or just needs to talk. The written information is especially important because she may not remember drug-related discussions or instructions clearly.

Once the SSRI reaches therapeutic levels, which can take as long as 4 weeks, Debbie may start to feel like her 'old self' and may be strong enough to begin dealing with her grief. She may recover from her need for the SSRI over time and use of the medication can then be gradually reduced and eventually discontinued.

Nursing Care Guide for Debbie: Fluoxetine

Assessment: History and Examination

- Allergies to fluoxetine or any other antidepressant SSRI; renal or hepatic dysfunction; pregnancy or lactation; diabetes
- Concurrent use of TCAs, cyproheptadine, lithium, MAO inhibitors, benzodiazepines, alcohol, other SSRIs, herbal remedies
- Cardiovascular: blood pressure, pulse
- CNS: orientation, reflexes, vision
- Respiratory: respiration, adventitious sounds
- GI: abdominal examination, bowel sounds
- Laboratory tests: hepatic and renal function tests if Debbie's history suggests potential problems

Nursing Diagnoses

- Acute pain related to GI, genitourinary, CNS effects
- Disturbed thought processes related to CNS effects
- Imbalanced nutrition related to GI effects
- Deficient knowledge regarding drug therapy

Implementation

- Administer drug in morning; divide doses if GI upset occurs.
- Provide comfort, safety measures; small meals; void before dosing; pain medication as needed; lower dose with renal or hepatic impairment.
- Provide support and reassurance to help Debbie deal with drug effects (4-week delay in full effectiveness).
- Provide patient teaching regarding drug dosage, adverse effect conditions to report and the need to use barrier contraceptives.

Evaluation

- Evaluate drug effects: relief of signs and symptoms of depression.
- Monitor for adverse effects: sedation, dizziness, insomnia; respiratory dysfunction; GI upset; genitourinary problems; rash.
- Monitor for drug–drug interactions.
- Evaluate effectiveness of patient teaching programme.
- Evaluate effectiveness of comfort and safety measures.

Patient Teaching for Debbie

- ☐ The drug that has been prescribed is called a selective serotonin reuptake inhibitor or SSRI. SSRIs change the concentration of serotonin in specific areas of the brain. An increase in serotonin level is believed to relieve depression.
- ☐ The drug should be taken once a day in the morning. If your dosage has been increased or if you are having stomach upset, the dose may be divided.

(continued)

Selective Serotonin Reuptake Inhibitors *(continued)*

- ☐ It may take as long as 4 weeks before you feel the full effects of this drug. Continue to take the drug every day during that time so that the concentration of the drug in your body eventually reaches effective levels.
- ☐ Common side-effects of SSRIs include the following:
  - *Dizziness, drowsiness, nervousnes and insomnia:* If these effects occur, avoid driving or performing hazardous or delicate tasks that require concentration.
  - *Nausea, vomiting and weight loss:* Small frequent meals may help. Monitor your weight loss; if it becomes excessive, consult your health care provider. Increased appetite and weight gain have also been reported and Debbie should be advised to maintain a balanced diet.
  - *Sexual dysfunction and flu-like symptoms:* These effects may be temporary. Consult with your health care provider if these conditions become bothersome.
- ☐ Report any of the following conditions to your health care provider: *rash, mania, seizures and severe weight loss.*
- ☐ Tell your doctors, nurses and other health care providers that you are taking this drug. Keep this drug and all medications out of the reach of children and pets. Do not take this drug during pregnancy because severe foetal abnormalities could occur. The use of barrier contraceptives is recommended while you are taking this drug. If you think that you are pregnant or would like to become pregnant, consult your health care provider.

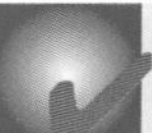

CHECK YOUR UNDERSTANDING

Answers to the questions in this chapter may be found in the answer key in the back of the book.

Multiple Choice

Select the best answer to the following.

1. The monoamine theory of depression states that depression is a result of
   a. an unpleasant childhood.
   b. GABA inhibition.
   c. deficiency of noradrenaline, dopamine or 5-HT in key areas of the brain.
   d. blockages within the limbic system, which controls emotions and affect.

2. When teaching a patient receiving TCAs, it is important to remember that they are associated with many antimuscarinic adverse effects. Teaching about these drugs should include anticipation of
   a. increased libido and increased appetite.
   b. polyuria and polydipsia.
   c. urinary retention, arrhythmias and constipation.
   d. hearing changes, cataracts and nightmares.

3. Adverse effects may limit the usefulness of TCAs with some patients. Nursing interventions that could alleviate some of the unpleasant aspects of these adverse effects include
   a. always administering the drug when the patient has an empty stomach.
   b. reminding the patient not to void before taking the drug.
   c. increasing the dosage to override the adverse effects.
   d. taking the major portion of the dose at bedtime to avoid experiencing drowsiness and the unpleasant antimuscarinic effects.

4. You might question an order for a MAOI as a first step in the treatment of depression, remembering that these drugs are reserved for use in cases in which there has been no response to other agents because MAOIs
   a. can cause hair loss.
   b. are associated with potentially serious drug–food interactions.
   c. are mostly recommended for use in surgical patients.
   d. are more expensive than other agents.

5. Your patient is being treated for depression and is started on fluoxetine. She calls you 10 days after the drug therapy has started to report that nothing has changed and she wants to try a different drug. You should
   a. try sertraline because some patients respond to one SSRI and not another.
   b. ask her to try a few days without the drug to see whether there is any difference.
   c. add an MAOI to her drug regimen to get an increased antidepressant effect.
   d. encourage her to keep taking the drug as prescribed because it usually takes up to 4 weeks to see the full antidepressant effect.

6. The drug of choice for a patient with a documented OCD who is also suffering from depression and occasional panic disorder would be
   a. phenelzine.
   b. paroxetine.
   c. tryptophan.
   d. imipramine.

7. Venlafaxine is a relatively new antidepressant that might be very effective for use in patients who
   a. have proven to be responsive to other antidepressants.
   b. can tolerate multiple side-effects.
   c. are reliable at taking multiple daily doses.
   d. have not responded to other antidepressants and would benefit from once-a-day dosing.

8. Depression is an affective disorder that is
   a. always precipitated by a specific event.
   b. most common in patients with head injuries.
   c. characterized by overwhelming sadness, despair and hopelessness.
   d. very evident and easy to diagnose in the clinical setting.

Extended Matching Questions

Select **all** that apply.

1. Depression is a very common affective disorder that strikes many people. In assessing a patient who might be suffering from depression, the nurse would expect to find which of the following?
   a. Lack of energy
   b. Hyperactivity
   c. Sleep disturbances
   d. Libido problems
   e. Confusion
   f. Decreased reflexes

2. A patient reports that he thinks he is taking an antidepressant, but he is not sure. In reviewing his medication history, which of the following drugs would be considered antidepressants?
   a. Tricyclics
   b. Cholinergics
   c. SSRIs
   d. MAOIs
   e. Angiotensin receptor antagonists
   f. Benzodiazepines

Fill in the Blanks

1. The amines linked to depression include ___________, ___________ and ___________.

2. The MAOIs block the___________of noradrenaline, leading to an accumulation of that neurotransmitter in the ___________.

3. The SSRIs block the___________of serotonin, leading to an increase in that neurotransmitter near the receptor sites.

4. The tricyclic antidepressants are believed to reduce the reuptake of___________and___________in all nerves that produce those neurotransmitters.

5. Patients taking MAOIs should avoid foods high in ___________ because of a risk of increased blood pressure.

6. Some of the drawbacks of tricyclic antidepressant therapy are the many_________________effects associated with the drugs, including dry mouth, urinary retention and constipation.

Bibliography and References

British Medical Association and Royal Pharmaceutical Society of Great Britain. (2008). *British National Formulary*. London: BMJ & RPS Publishing. *This publication is updated biannually: it is imperative that the most recent edition is consulted.*

British Medical Association and Royal Pharmaceutical Society of Great Britain. (2008). *British National Formulary for Children*. London: BMJ & RPS Publishing. *This publication is updated annually: it is imperative that the most recent edition is consulted.*

Brunton, L., Lazo, J. S., Parker, K., Goodman, L. S., & Gilman, A. G. (2005). *Goodman and Gilman's The Pharmacological Basis of Therapeutics* (11th ed.). London: McGraw-Hill.

Committee on Safety of Medicines. (2004). Report of the CSM Expert Working Group on the safety of selective serotonin reuptake inhibitor antidepressants. Available from http://www.mhra.gov.uk/Safetyinformation/

Gunnell, D., Spaeria, J., & Ashby, D. (2005). Selective serotonin reuptake inhibitors (SSRIs) and suicide in adults: meta-analysis of drug company data from placebo controlled, randomised controlled trials submitted to the MHRA's safety review. *British Medical Journal 330*: 385–390.

Howland, R. D., & Mycek, M. J. (2005). *Pharmacology* (3rd ed.). Philadelphia: Lippincott Williams & Wilkins.

National Institute for Health and Clinical Excellence. (2004). CG23 Depression: management of depression in primary and secondary care – NICE guidance (amended 2007). Available from http://www.nice.org.uk

National Institute for Health and Clinical Excellence. (2005). CG28 Depression in children and young people – NICE guidance. Available from http://www.nice.org.uk

Porth, C. M., & Matfin, G. (2008). *Pathophysiology: Concepts of altered health states* (8th ed.). Philadelphia: Lippincott Williams & Wilkins.

Rang, H. P., Dale, M. M., Ritter, J. M., & Flower, R. J. (2007). *Rang and Dale's Pharmacology*. (6th ed.). Philadelphia: Churchill Livingstone.

Simonsen, T., Aarbakke, J., Kay, I., Coleman, I., Sinnott, P., & Lysaa, R. (2006). *Illustrated Pharmacology for Nurses*. London: Hodder Arnold.

Timonen, M., & Liukkonen, T. (2008). Management of depression in adults. *British Medical Journal.* **336**: 435-439.

CHAPTER 21

Psychotherapeutic Agents

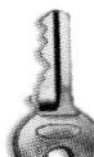

KEY TERMS

antipsychotic

attention-deficit hyperactivity disorder (ADHD)

bipolar affective disorder

narcolepsy

neuroleptic

schizophrenia

LEARNING OBJECTIVES

Upon completion of this chapter, you will be able to:

1. Describe the therapeutic actions, indications, pharmacokinetics, contraindications, most common adverse reactions and important drug–drug interactions associated with each class of psychotherapeutic agent.
2. Discuss the use of psychotherapeutic agents across the lifespan.
3. Compare and contrast the key drugs for each class of psychotherapeutic agent with other drugs in that class and with drugs in the other classes of psychotherapeutic agents.
4. Outline the nursing considerations and teaching needs for patients receiving each class of psychotherapeutic agent.

ANTIPSYCHOTIC (NEUROLEPTIC) DRUGS

Typical Antipsychotics

benperidol
chlorpromazine
flupentixol
fluphenazine
haloperidol
levomepromazine
pericyazine
perphenazine
pimozide
pipotiazine
prochlorperazine
sertindole
sulpiride
trifluoperazine
zuclopenthixol

Atypical Antipsychotics

amisulpride
aripiprazole
clozapine
olanzapine
quetiapine
risperidone
zotepine

ANTIMANIC DRUGS

carbamazepine
lithium
olanzapine
quetiapine
risperidone
valproic acid

CENTRAL NERVOUS SYSTEM STIMULANTS

atomoxetine
dexamfetamine
methylphenidate
modafinil

The drugs discussed in this chapter are used to treat behavioural disorders. These psychotherapeutic drugs are targeted at thought processes rather than affective states. Although these drugs do not cure any of these disorders, they do help patients function in a more acceptable manner and carry on activities of daily living. These drugs are used in both adults and children (Box 21.1).

Mental Health Disorders and Their Classification

Mental health disorders are now thought to be caused by some inherent dysfunction within the brain that leads to abnormal thought processes and responses. Most theories attribute these disorders to some sort of chemical imbalance in specific areas within the brain. Diagnosis of a mental health disorder is often based on distinguishing characteristics described in the *Diagnostic and Statistical Manual of Mental Disorders*, 4th edition *(DSM-IV)*, or *International Classification of Diseases (ICD-10)*. No diagnostic laboratory tests are available, therefore patient assessment and response must be carefully evaluated to determine the basis of a particular problem. Selected disorders are discussed here.

Patients with **bipolar affective disorder** (otherwise known as manic-depressive disorder) can experience periods of severe depression and also hyperactivity and excitement. Patients will often swing between these two states of mood. There is also a state of mania that combines both mania and depression called a mixed episode. In acute mania the person may lose touch with reality, such as experience psychosis. Bipolar affective disorder may reflect a biochemical imbalance followed by overcompensation on the part of neurons and their inability to re-establish stability.

Schizophrenia, the most common type of psychosis, can be very debilitating and prevents affected individuals from functioning in society. Characteristics of schizophrenia include positive and negative symptoms. The positive symptoms include hallucinations, paranoia, delusions, speech abnormalities and thought disorders; and the negative symptoms include withdrawal and apathy. Schizophrenia, which seems to have a very

BOX 21.1 DRUG THERAPY ACROSS THE LIFESPAN

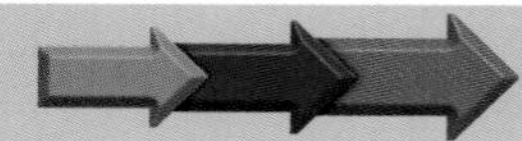

Psychotherapeutic Agents

CHILDREN

Some of these agents are indicated for childhood schizophrenia, Tourette syndrome, management of psychomotor agitation and violent behaviour (BNF, 2008). The long-term effects of many of these agents are not known, and parents should be informed of this fact. Of the antipsychotics, chlorpromazine, haloperidol, pimozide (over 12 years), quetiapine (over 12 years) and trifluoperazine are the only ones with established paediatric regimens. The child should be monitored carefully for adverse effects and developmental progress.

Children over the age of 12 years who present with a bipolar disorder, mania, recurrent depression or aggressive behaviour can be treated with lithium. The child should be monitored very closely for renal, central nervous system (CNS), cardiovascular (CV) and endocrine function.

Children with moderate attention-deficit hyperactivity disorders (ADHD) are generally referred to treatment programmes, such as cognitive behavioural therapy and social skills training (NICE, 2008). First-line treatment of more severe cases of attention-deficit hyperactivity disorders (ADHD) is with methylphenidate. Atomoxetine is used if the child is unresponsive or intolerant to methylphenidate (NICE, 2008).

When administering any drug to children, always consult the most recent edition of the British National Formulary for Children.

ADULTS

Antipsychotic Drugs

Antipsychotic drugs should be used very cautiously during pregnancy and lactation because of the potential for adverse effects on the foetus or neonate. A woman maintained on one of these drugs needs to be counselled about the risk to the foetus versus the risk of returning symptoms if the drug is stopped. Use should be reserved for situations in which the benefits to the mother far outweigh the potential risks to the neonate.

Antimanic Drugs

Adults using these drugs should be under regular care and should be monitored regularly (every 3 months) for adverse effects as lithium has a narrow therapeutic window. Patients should be monitored for blurred vision, ataxia, twitching and decreased level of consciousness as these are signs of overdose. Patients receiving lithium should be encouraged to maintain hydration and salt intake. They need to understand the importance of periodic monitoring of serum lithium levels. Renal and thyroid function should be assessed every 6 to 12 months. Women of childbearing age who need to take lithium should be advised to use barrier contraceptives while taking the drug because of the potential for serious congenital abnormalities. Lithium is contraindicated in breast-feeding.

OLDER ADULTS

Older patients may be more susceptible to the adverse effects associated with antipsychotic drugs, especially postural hypotension and hyper- or hypothermia in hot or cold weather (BNF, 2008). Safety measures should be provided if these effects occur.

Patients with renal impairment should be monitored very closely while taking lithium. Decreased dosages may be needed. They should be urged to maintain hydration and salt intake, which can be a challenge with some older patients. Patients should be aware of the initial signs of toxicity – sweating, increased urination, nausea and vomiting.

strong genetic association, may reflect a fundamental biochemical abnormality.

Attention-deficit hyperactivity disorders (ADHD) involve various conditions characterized by an inability to concentrate on one activity for longer than a few minutes and a state of hyperkinesis. These conditions are usually diagnosed in school-aged children and can continue into adulthood. ADHD is thought to affect between 3% and 9% of school-age children and young people in the United Kingdom (NICE, 2008).

Narcolepsy is characterized by daytime sleepiness and sudden periods of loss of wakefulness. This disorder may reflect problems with stimulation of the brain by the reticular activating system (RAS) or problems with response to that stimulation.

Antipsychotic Drugs

The **antipsychotic** drugs, which are essentially dopamine receptor blockers, are used to treat disorders that involve thought processes. These medications are also called **neuroleptic** agents because of their associated neurological adverse effects. At one time, these drugs were known as major tranquilizers. However, that name is no longer used because the primary action of these drugs is not sedation but a change in neuron stimulation and response (Figure 21.1).

Antipsychotics are classified as either (1) first-generation or *typical*, or (2) second-generation or *atypical*. The classic, typical antipsychotics are primarily dopamine D_2 receptor antagonists but also inhibit receptors for acetylcholine (muscarinic), histamine (H_1), noradrenaline and serotonin (5-HT). The lack of receptor specificity results in a number of adverse effects associated with multiple receptor blockade, including hypotension, antimuscarinic effects and extrapyramidal side-effects. The newer, atypical antipsychotics also block dopamine D_2 receptors and are associated with fewer of the side-effects on the motor system, such as tremor.

Table 21.1 lists the antipsychotics in use today and gives information about their relative potencies and associated adverse effects. Note that a patient who does not respond to one drug may react successfully to another agent. It is recommended that one of the atypical antipsychotic drugs is selected to treat patients with newly diagnosed schizophrenia and those finding it difficult to manage their condition (NICE, 2002). Those patients taking one of the older typical antipsychotics and who are still able to maintain control of their condition and tolerate the associated side-effects, should remain on the existing typical antipsychotic.

Therapeutic Actions and Indications

It is not understood which of the several actions of antipsychotics corrects the manifestations of schizophrenia. The typical antipsychotic drugs act by mainly antagonising

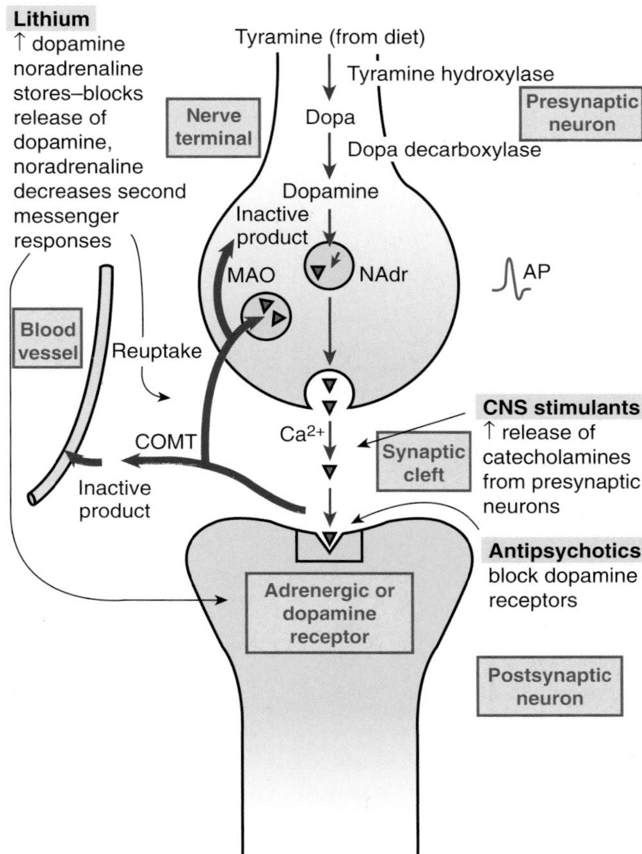

FIGURE 21.1 Sites of action of the drugs used to treat mental disorders: antipsychotics, central nervous system stimulants, lithium.

(blocking) dopamine receptors, preventing the stimulation of the postsynaptic neurons by dopamine. They also depress the RAS, limiting the stimuli coming into the brain, and they have antimuscarinic, antihistamine and α-adrenergic blocking effects, all related to the blocking of the dopamine receptor sites. Atypical antipsychotics also block dopamine receptors. The antipsychotics are indicated for schizophrenia and for manifestations of other psychotic disorders such as might occur with acute mania, especially those exhibiting aggression and agitation.

Pharmacokinetics

The antipsychotics are erratically absorbed from the gastrointestinal (GI) tract, depending on the drug and the preparation of the drug. Intramuscular doses provide four to five times the active dose as oral doses, requiring caution if switching between routes; however, the intramuscular injections are painful. Some of the antipsychotics (flupentixol, fluphenazine, haloperidol, pipotiazine, zuclopenthixol) are available as depot injections; whereby the drug is formulated in an oily solution for intramuscular injection. From the injection site the drug is slowly absorbed into the bloodstream. The injections are repeated

Table 21.1 Antipsychotics, Indicating Side-Effects Most Frequently Associated With Each Drug

Drug Name	Potency	Common Side-Effects			
		Sedation	*Anticholinergic*	*Hypotension*	*Extrapyramidal*
Typical Antipsychotics					
benperidol	High	+	+	+	+++
chlorpromazine	Low	+++	+++	+++	++
flupentixol	Low	–	–	+	++
fluphenazine	High	+	+	+	++++
haloperidol	High	+	+/–	+	++++
levomepromazine	Low	++++	++	+++	++
pericyazine	Medium	++	++++	++	+
perphenazine	High	+	+	+	++
pimozide	High	+	+	++	+++
pipotiazine	Medium	++	++++	++	+
prochlorperazine	Low	+	++	+	+++
sertindole	High	+	–	++	+
sulpiride	Low	+	–	–	+
trifluoperazine	High	+	+	+	+++
zuclopenthixol	High	++	+	+	+++
Atypical Antipsychotics					
amisulpride	Low	+	–	–	+
aripiprazole	Medium	+	–	–	–
clozapine	Low	++++	++	+++	+/–
olanzapine	High	++++	++	+++	+
quetiapine	Medium	++	+	++	+
risperidone	High	+	–	++	+
zotepine	Medium	+	+	–	–

at intervals of 1 to 4 weeks. This approach is most appropriate for patients who cannot comply with oral treatment.

The antipsychotics are widely distributed in the tissues and are often stored in the tissues, being released for up to 6 months after the drug is stopped. They undergo extensive metabolism in the liver and are excreted through the bile and urine. Children tend to metabolize these drugs faster than adults, and elderly patients tend to metabolize them more slowly. The antipsychotics cross the placenta and enter breast milk. They should not be used during pregnancy or lactation unless the benefit to the mother clearly outweighs the potential risk to the foetus or neonate.

Contraindications and Cautions

Antipsychotic drugs are contraindicated in the presence of underlying diseases *that could be exacerbated by the dopamine-blocking effects of these drugs*. They are also contraindicated in the following conditions, *which can be exacerbated by the drugs*: CNS depression, comatose states and phaechromocytoma (a tumour of the adrenal medulla that secretes adrenaline and noradrenaline). Prolongation of the QT interval is a contraindication to the use of pimozide, olanzapine, sertindole and zotepine, all of which can further prolong the QT interval, *leading to increased risk of serious cardiac arrhythmias.* Also contraindicated are hepatic impairment, Parkinson's disease, cardiovascular disease, history of circulatory collapse, bone marrow suppression and blood dyscrasias. It is best to avoid most antipsychotic drugs during pregnancy and breast-feeding *because of the potential of adverse effects on the foetus or neonate.* Some can be used with caution during pregnancy and breast-feeding.

Caution should be used in the presence of medical conditions *that could be exacerbated by the antimuscarinic effects of the drugs,* such as glaucoma, myasthenia gravis, peptic ulcer and urinary or intestinal obstruction. In addition, care should be taken in patients with seizure disorders *because the threshold for seizures could be lowered*; and in active alcoholism *because of potentiation of the CNS depression. The use of antipsychotics may result in bone marrow suppression, leading to blood dyscrasias*, so care should be taken with patients who are immunocompromised and those who have cancer.

Adverse Effects

The adverse effects associated with the antipsychotic drugs are related to their antidopamine, antimuscarinic, antihistamine and α-adrenergic activities. The most common CNS effects are sedation, weakness, tremor, drowsiness and extrapyramidal effects – pseudoparkinsonism, dystonia, akathisia, tardive dyskinesia (Figure 21.2) and potentially irreversible neuroleptic malignant syndrome. Antimuscarinic effects include dry mouth, nasal congestion, flushing, constipation, urinary retention, sexual impotence, glaucoma, blurred vision and photophobia. Cardiovascular effects, which are probably related to the dopamine-blocking effects, include hypotension, orthostatic hypotension, cardiac arrhythmias, congestive heart failure and pulmonary oedema. There is a risk of developing diabetes mellitus when atypical antipsychotic drugs are used, particularly clozapine and olanzapine. Consequently, when patients are maintained on any of the atypical antipsychotics, they should be monitored regularly for the signs and symptoms of diabetes mellitus. In addition, bone marrow suppression is a possibility with some antipsychotic agents.

Clinically Important Drug–Drug Interactions

Combining antipsychotics with β-blockers may lead to an increase in the effect of both drugs and should be avoided if possible. Antipsychotic-alcohol combinations result in an increased risk of CNS depression, and

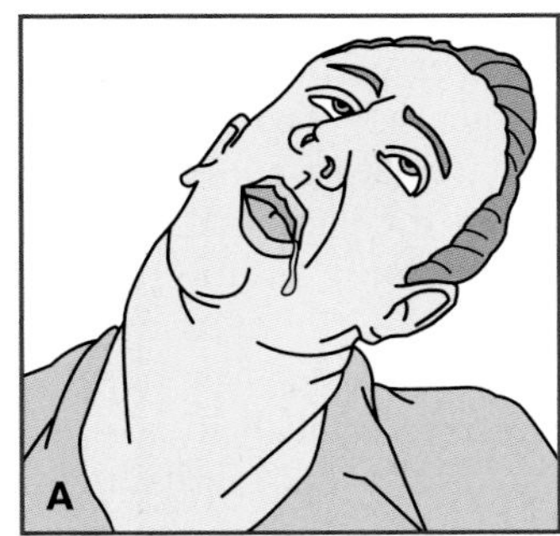

A. Dystonia—spasms of the tongue, neck, back and legs. Spasms may cause unnatural positioning of the neck, abnormal eye movements, excessive salivation.

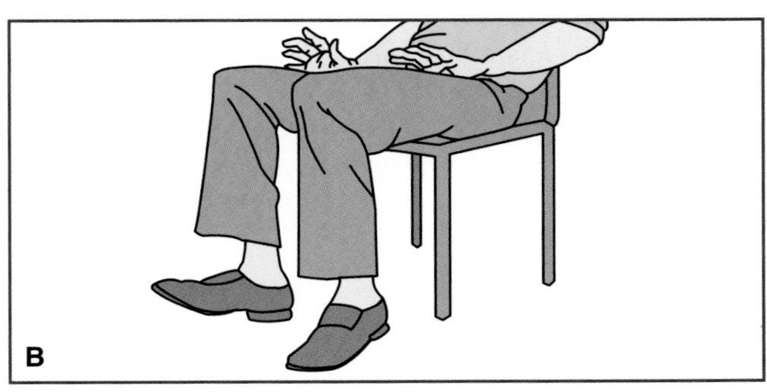

B. Akathisia—continuous restlessness, inability to sit still. Constant moving, foot tapping, hand movements may be seen.

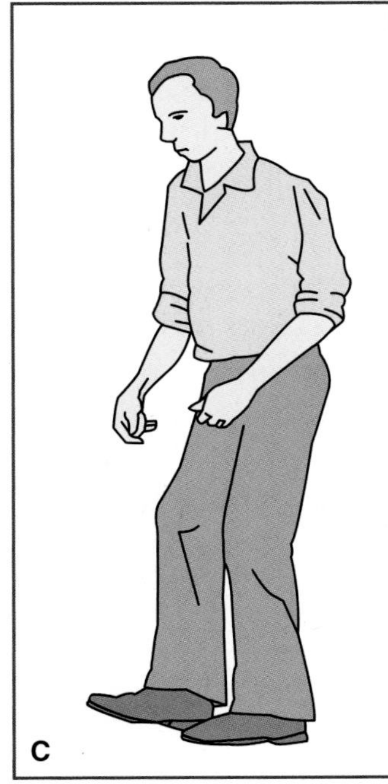

C. Pseudoparkinsonism—muscle tremors, cogwheel rigidity, drooling, shuffling gait, slow movements.

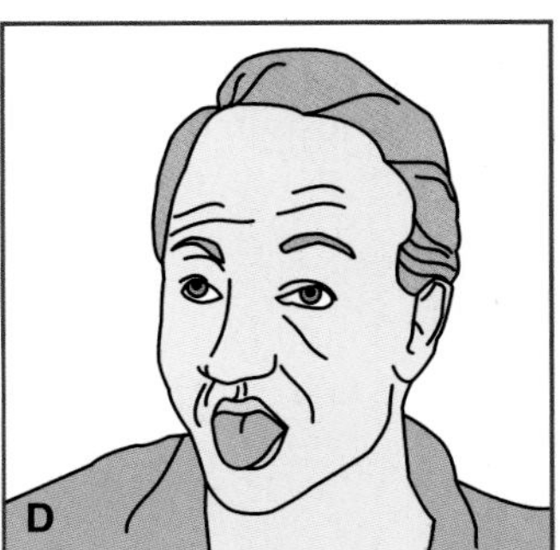

D. Tardive dyskinesia—abnormal muscle movements such as lip smacking, tongue darting, chewing movements, slow and aimless arm and leg movements.

FIGURE 21.2 Common neurological effects of antipsychotic drugs.

antipsychotic-antimuscarinic combinations lead to increased antimuscarinic effects, so dosage adjustments are necessary. Patients who take either of these combinations should be monitored closely for adverse effects, and supportive measures should be provided. Patients with schizophrenia should also be advised to avoid the use of evening primrose. This plant has been associated with increased symptoms and CNS hyperexcitability.

Always consult a current copy of the British National Formulary for further guidance.

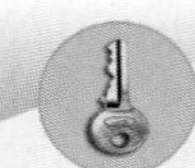

Key Drug Summary: *Chlorpromazine*

Indications: Management of manifestations of psychotic disorders; short-term management of severe anxiety, excitement and violent behaviour; intractable hiccups; antiemetic in palliative care

Actions: Blocks dopamine (D_1 and D_2), α-adrenergic, histamine H_1, muscarinic and serotonin (5-HT_2) receptors; depresses those parts of the brain involved in wakefulness and emesis

Pharmacokinetics:

Route	Onset	Peak	Duration
Oral	30–60 min	2–4 h	4–6 h
IM	10–15 min	15–20 min	4–6 h

$T_{1/2}$: 30 hours; extensive metabolism in the liver, excreted in the urine and faeces

Adverse effects: Marked drowsiness, extrapyramidal symptoms, hypotension, photophobia, blurred vision, dry mouth, nausea, vomiting, anorexia, urinary retention, photosensitivity

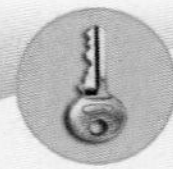

Key Drug Summary: *Clozapine*

Indications: Management of psychotic symptoms of schizophrenia (including psychosis in Parkinson's disease) who are unresponsive to standard antipsychotic drugs

Actions: Blocks dopamine (D_1 and D_2), α-adrenergic, histamine (H_1), muscarinic and serotonin (5-HT_2) receptors; depresses the RAS

Pharmacokinetics:

Route	Onset	Peak	Duration
Oral	Varies	1–6 h	Weeks

$T_{1/2}$: 8–16 hours; metabolized in the liver, excreted in the urine and faeces

Adverse effects: Drowsiness, fatigue, seizures, dizziness, syncope, headache, tachycardia, nausea, vomiting, anorexia, tremor, fever, neutropenia, agranulocytosis, myocarditis

Nursing Considerations for Patients Receiving Antipsychotic Drugs

Assessment: History and Examination

Screen for the following conditions, *which could be contraindications or cautions for the use of the drug*: any known allergies to these drugs, severe CNS depression, history of circulatory collapse, coronary disease including prolonged QT interval, respiratory depression, glaucoma, urinary or intestinal obstruction, thyrotoxicosis, epilepsy, bone marrow suppression, Parkinson's disease, phaeochromocytoma and pregnancy or lactation. Establish if patient is currently taking other medications or herbal therapies, which may potentially interact with the antipsychotic drug.

Include screening *for baseline status before beginning therapy and for any potential adverse effects.* Assess the following: temperature; skin colour and lesions; CNS orientation, affect, reflexes; bowel sounds and reported output; pulse, auscultation and blood pressure, including orthostatic blood pressure; respiration rate and adventitious sounds; and urinary output. Obtain liver and renal function tests, thyroid function tests, electrocardiogram (ECG) if appropriate, and full blood count.

Nursing Diagnoses

The patient receiving antipsychotics may have the following nursing diagnoses related to drug therapy:

- Impaired physical mobility related to extrapyramidal effects
- Risk of injury related to CNS effects and sedation
- Impaired elimination related to antimuscarinic effects
- Deficient knowledge regarding drug therapy
- Nonconcordance with drug therapy

Implementation With Rationale

- Do not allow the patient to crush or chew sustained-release capsules, *which will decrease their absorption and effectiveness.*

- If the patient receives parenteral forms, keep the patient supine for 30 minutes *to reduce the risk of orthostatic hypotension.*
- Consider warning the patient or the patient's guardians about the risk of development of tardive dyskinesias with continued use *so they are prepared for that neurological change.*
- Monitor full blood count *to arrange to discontinue the drug at signs of bone marrow suppression.*
- Arrange for gradual dose reduction after long-term use. *Abrupt withdrawal has been associated with gastritis, nausea, vomiting, dizziness, arrhythmias and insomnia.*
- Encourage frequent mouth care *to prevent dry mouth from becoming a problem.*
- Encourage the patient to empty bladder before taking a dose *if urinary hesitancy or retention is a problem.*
- Provide safety measures such as assistance with ambulation if CNS effects or orthostatic hypotension occurs *to prevent patient injury.*
- Provide for vision examinations *to determine ocular changes and arrange appropriate dosage change.*
- Provide thorough patient teaching, including drug name, prescribed dosage, measures for avoidance of adverse effects, warning signs that may indicate possible problems, and the need for monitoring and evaluation *to enhance patient knowledge about drug therapy and to promote concordance* (refer to Critical Thinking Scenario 21-1).
- Offer support and encouragement *to help patients cope with and maintain their drug regimen.*

Evaluation

- Monitor patient response to the drug (decrease in signs and symptoms of psychotic disorder).
- Monitor for adverse effects (sedation, antimuscarinic effects, hypotension, extrapyramidal effects, bone marrow suppression).
- Evaluate effectiveness of teaching plan (patient can give the drug name and dosage, possible adverse effects to watch for, specific measures to prevent adverse effects and warning signs to report).
- Monitor the effectiveness of comfort measures and concordance with the regime (see Critical Thinking Scenario 21-1).

Antimanic Drugs

Mania, the opposite of depression, is characterized by an elevated mood and excessive energy. Mania usually occurs in individuals with bipolar disorder, who experience a period of depression followed by a period of mania. There is increasing evidence to suggest that there is a genetic basis to this disease; however, the gene(s) responsible has yet to be identified (Owen *et al.*, 2007). The mainstay for treatment of mania is lithium (Table 21.2).

Lithium salts are taken orally for the management of manic episodes and prevention of future episodes. These very toxic drugs can cause severe CNS, renal and pulmonary problems that may lead to death. Lithium can also cause hypothyroidism. Despite the potential for serious adverse effects, lithium is used with caution because it is consistently effective in the treatment of mania. The therapeutically effective serum level is 0.5 to 1.0 mmol/l.

Also approved are the use of atypical antipsychotics, olanzapine and risperidone, for the short-term management

Table 21.2 DRUGS IN FOCUS

Antimanic Drugs

Drug Name	Usual Indications
carbamazepine	Prophylaxis of bipolar disorder in patients unresponsive to lithium
lithium	Treatment of mania, bipolar disorder and recurrent depression; maintenance therapy to prevent or diminish the frequency and intensity of future manic episodes; not recommended for children <12 years
olanzapine	Used to stabilize patient before lithium becomes effective; in combination with lithium or valproic acid
quetiapine	Adjunct or monotherapy for the treatment of manic episodes associated with bipolar disorder
risperidone	Used to stabilize patient before lithium becomes effective; in combination with lithium or valproic acid. Also available as a depot injection.
valproic acid	Treatment of manic episodes associated with bipolar disorder

of acute manic episodes of bipolar disorder in combination with lithium and valproic acid. Quetiapine, also an atypical antipsychotic, is also approved as an adjunct or as monotherapy for the treatment of manic episodes associated with bipolar disorder. Carbamazepine can be used for the prophylaxis of bipolar disorder in patients unresponsive to lithium.

Therapeutic Actions and Indications

Although the biochemical actions of lithium are known, the exact mechanisms responsible for decreasing the manifestations of mania are not understood. Lithium may alter sodium transport in nerve and muscle cells, thus affecting the excitability of these cells. Other proposed mechanisms include changes in gene expression, and a decrease in the level of second messengers inside neurons. These second messengers are important in the intracellular cascade of events occurring following receptor stimulation. This last mode of action may allow it to selectively modulate the responsiveness of hyperactive neurons that might contribute to the manic state.

Lithium is indicated for the treatment of manic episodes of bipolar or manic-depressive illness and for maintenance therapy to prevent or diminish the frequency and intensity of future manic episodes.

Pharmacokinetics

Lithium is readily absorbed from the GI tract, reaching peak levels in 2 to 4 hours. It follows the same distribution pattern in the body as water. It slowly crosses the blood–brain barrier. Lithium is excreted from the kidney, although about 80% is reabsorbed. During periods of sodium depletion or dehydration, the kidney reabsorbs more lithium into the serum, often leading to toxic levels. Therefore patients must be encouraged to maintain hydration while taking this drug. Lithium does cross the placenta and has been associated with congenital abnormalities. Women of childbearing age should be advised to use birth control while taking this drug. It also enters breast milk and can cause toxic effects in the baby. Breastfeeding should be discontinued while using lithium.

Contraindications and Cautions

Lithium is contraindicated in the presence of hypersensitivity to lithium. In addition, it is contraindicated in the following conditions: significant renal or cardiac disease *that could be exacerbated by the toxic effects of the drug*; a history of leukaemia; metabolic disorders, including sodium depletion, dehydration, and diuretic use *because lithium depletes sodium reabsorption and severe hyponatraemia may occur* (hyponatraemia leads to lithium retention and toxicity). Pregnancy and lactation are also contraindications *because of the potential for adverse effects on the foetus or neonate.* Caution should be used in any condition *that could alter sodium levels,* such as protracted diarrhoea or excessive sweating; with suicidal or impulsive patients; and in patients who have infection with fever, *which could be exacerbated by the toxic effects of the drug* or a history of hypothyroidism.

Adverse Effects

Serum lithium levels should be maintained between 0.5 to 1.0 mmol/l. The adverse effects associated with lithium are directly related to serum levels of the drug:

- Therapeutic level of 0.5 to 1.0 mmol/l: tremor, constipation, weight gain, oedema, polydipsia and cardiac arrhythmias.
- Between 1.5 and 2 mmol/l: diarrhoea, nausea and vomiting; blurred vision, muscle weakness, tremor, ataxia and dysarthria.
- Toxic lithium level above 2 mmol/l: hyperreflexia and hyperextension, seizures, hypotension, renal and circulatory failure, coma and even death is a significant possibility without appropriate treatment.

Clinically Important Drug–Drug Interactions

Some drug–drug combinations should be avoided. The following drugs will reduce the excretion of lithium, leading to increased plasma concentrations: angiotensin-converting enzyme inhibitors, nonsteroidal anti-inflammatory drugs, angiotensin-II receptor antagonists, loop diuretics, thiazides and potassium-sparing diuretics.

In contrast, the following drugs increase the excretion of lithium: antacids, acetazolamide and theophylline.

There is an increased risk of extrapyramidal symptoms and neurotoxicity when lithium is administered with other antipsychotics, particularly haloperidol and clozapine. There is also a risk of ventricular arrhythmias when lithium is combined with antiarrhythmics and the antipsychotic, sertindole.

Always consult a current copy of the British National Formulary for further guidance.

Nursing Considerations for Patients Receiving Lithium

Assessment: History and Examination

Screen for the following conditions, *which could be contraindications or cautions for the use of the drug*: any known allergies to lithium; renal or cardiovascular disease; dehydration; sodium depletion, use of diuretics, protracted sweating, or diarrhoea; suicidal or impulsive patients with severe depression; and pregnancy or lactation. Establish if patient is currently taking other medications or herbal therapies which may potentially interact with lithium.

Include screening *for baseline status before beginning therapy and for any potential adverse effects.* Assess the following: temperature; skin colour and lesions; CNS orientation, affect and reflexes; bowel sounds and reported output; pulse, auscultation and blood pressure, including orthostatic blood pressure; respiratory rate and adventitious sounds; and urinary output. Obtain liver and renal function tests, thyroid function tests, full blood count, and baseline ECG, and obtain serum lithium levels as appropriate.

Nursing Diagnoses

The patient receiving lithium may have the following nursing diagnoses related to drug therapy:

- Risk of injury related to CNS effects, including risk of self-harm
- Impaired urinary elimination related to renal toxic effects
- Disturbed thought processes related to CNS effects
- Disturbed sleep pattern
- Deficient knowledge regarding drug therapy
- Nonconcordance with drug regimen

Implementation With Rationale

- Monitor patient's emotional status: observe for mania and/or extreme depression.
- Measure serum lithium levels every 3 months *to monitor for toxic levels and to arrange for appropriate dosage adjustment.*
- Measure renal function and thyroid function every 6 to 12 months.
- Monitor electrolyte balance *to monitor for sodium imbalance.*
- Give the drug with food or milk *to alleviate GI irritation if GI upset is severe.*
- Ensure that the patient maintains adequate intake of salt and fluid *to decrease toxicity.*
- Monitor the patient's clinical status closely, especially during the initial stages of therapy, *to provide appropriate supportive management as needed.*
- Encourage frequent mouth care, *to increase secretions and decrease discomfort as needed.*
- Provide safety measures such as assistance with mobility if CNS effects occur *to prevent patient injury.*
- Provide thorough patient teaching, including drug name, prescribed dosage, measures for avoidance of adverse effects, warning signs that may indicate possible problems, and the need to avoid pregnancy while taking lithium *to enhance patient knowledge about drug therapy and to promote concordance.*
- Offer support and encouragement *to help the patient cope with and maintain their drug regimen.*

Evaluation

- Monitor patient response to the drug (decreased manifestations and frequency of manic episodes).
- Monitor for adverse effects (cardiovascular toxicity, renal toxicity, GI upset, respiratory complications, hypothyroidism).
- Evaluate the effectiveness of the teaching plan (patient can give the drug name and dosage and describe the possible adverse effects to watch for, specific measures to help avoid adverse effects, warning signs to report, and the need to avoid pregnancy).
- Monitor the effectiveness of comfort measures and concordance with the regimen.

Central Nervous System Stimulants

The CNS stimulants include the amphetamines and amphetamine-related drugs. They are used clinically to treat ADHD and narcolepsy. Paradoxically, these drugs calm hyperkinetic children and help them focus on one activity for a longer period. They also excite and redirect the arousal stimuli from the RAS (Figure 21.3). The CNS stimulants that are used to treat ADHD are methylphenidate and atomoxetine. Narcolepsy is treated with dexamfetamine and modafinil (Table 21.3).

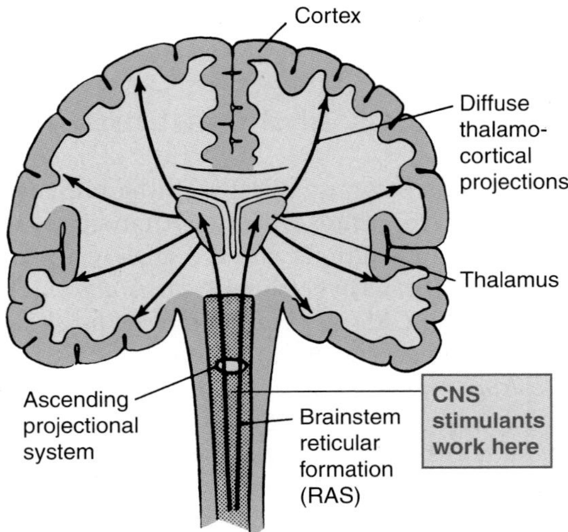

FIGURE 21.3 Site of action of the central nervous system (CNS) stimulants in the reticular activating system (RAS).

Table 21.3 DRUGS IN FOCUS

Central Nervous System Stimulants

Drug Name	Usual Indications
atomoxetine	Treatment of attention-deficit hyperactivity disorder in patients age ≥6 years
dexamfetamine	Treatment of narcolepsy and attention-deficit hyperactivity disorders
methylphenidate	Treatment of narcolepsy (unlicensed indication) and attention-deficit hyperactivity disorders
modafinil	Narcolepsy in adults, improving wakefulness in various sleep disorders and chronic shift work

Therapeutic Actions and Indications

The CNS stimulants act as cortical and RAS stimulants by increasing the release of catecholamines from presynaptic neurons, leading to an increase in stimulation of the postsynaptic neurons (Figure 21.1). The paradoxical effect of calming hyperexcitability through CNS stimulation seen in ADHD is believed to be related to increased stimulation of an immature RAS, which leads to the ability to be more selective in response to incoming stimuli.

The CNS stimulants are indicated for the treatment of attention deficit syndromes, including behavioural syndromes characterized by hyperactivity and distractibility, as well as narcolepsy and improvement of wakefulness in people with various sleep disorders.

Pharmacokinetics

These drugs are rapidly absorbed from the GI tract, reaching peak levels in 2 to 4 hours. They are metabolized in the liver and excreted in the urine, with half-lives ranging from 2 to 15 hours, depending on the drug. Dexamfetamine and modafinil should not be used during pregnancy or lactation. Atomoxetine and methylphenidate should be used only if the benefit to the mother clearly outweighs the potential risk to the foetus. Both drugs should be avoided whilst breast-feeding.

Contraindications and Cautions

The CNS stimulants are contraindicated in the presence of known allergy to the drug. Other contraindications include the following conditions: marked anxiety, agitation or hyperexcitability and hyperthyroidism, *which could be exacerbated by the CNS stimulation caused by these drugs*; history of drug dependence, including alcoholism, *because these drugs may result in physical and psychological dependence*; and pregnancy and lactation *because of the potential for adverse effects on the foetus or neonate.*

Caution should be used in patients with a history of seizures, *which could be potentiated by the CNS stimulation*; susceptibility to angle-closure glaucoma, *which could be exacerbated by the CNS stimulation caused by these drugs*; hepatic or renal impairment, *which could affect drug metabolism or excretion*; and with hypertension, *which could be exacerbated by the stimulatory effects of these drugs*. The height and weight of children should be monitored during long-term treatment.

Adverse Effects

The adverse effects associated with these drugs are related to the CNS stimulation they cause. CNS effects can include nervousness, insomnia, dizziness, headache and difficulty with accommodation resulting in blurred vision. Gastrointestinal effects such as anorexia, nausea and weight loss may occur. Cardiovascular effects can include hypertension, tachycardia, arrhythmias and angina. Skin rashes are a common reaction to some of these drugs. Physical and psychological dependence may also develop as can tolerance.

Clinically Important Drug–Drug Interactions

The combination of a CNS stimulant with a monoamine oxidase inhibitor (MAOI) leads to an increased risk of adverse effects and increased toxicity and should be avoided if possible. In addition, the combination of CNS stimulants with tricyclic antidepressants or phenytoin leads to a risk of increased drug levels. Patients who receive such a combination should be monitored for toxicity.

Always consult a current copy of the British National Formulary for further guidance.

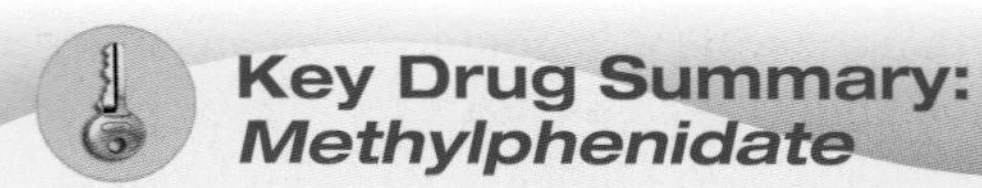

Indications: Attention deficit hyperactivity disorder and narcolepsy

Actions: Mild cortical stimulant with CNS actions similar to those of amphetamines

Pharmacokinetics:

Route	Onset	Peak	Duration
Oral	Varies	2 h	4–6 h

$T_{1/2}$: 2 hours; extensively metabolized in the liver; mainly excreted in the urine

Adverse effects: Nervousness, insomnia, changes in blood pressure, tachycardia, palpitations, arrhythmias, loss of appetite, nausea, vomiting, dyspepsia, dry mouth, anorexia, abdominal pain, depression, aggression, headache, drowsiness, dizziness, fever, rash, pruritis, alopecia

Nursing Considerations for Patients Receiving Central Nervous System Stimulants

Assessment: History and Examination

Screen for the following conditions, *which could be contraindications or cautions for the use of the drug*: any known allergies to the drug; glaucoma, anxiety or epilepsy; cardiac disease and hypertension; hyperthyroidism; pregnancy or lactation; a history of leukaemia; and history of drug dependency, including alcoholism. Establish if patient is currently taking other medications or herbal therapies, which may potentially interact with the stimulant.

Include screening *for baseline status before beginning therapy and for any potential adverse effects.* Assess the following: temperature; skin colour and lesions; CNS orientation and affect; ophthalmic examination; pulse, auscultation and blood pressure; respiratory rate and adventitious sounds; and urinary output. Obtain a full blood count.

Nursing Diagnoses

The patient receiving CNS stimulants may have the following nursing diagnoses related to drug therapy:

- Disturbed thought processes related to CNS effects of the drug
- Disturbed behaviour and sleep patterns
- Risk of injury related to CNS and visual effects of the drug
- Inadequate nutrition due to appetite suppression
- Potential for dependence
- Deficient knowledge regarding drug therapy

Implementation With Rationale

- Complete a full mental health and social assessment. Ensure proper diagnosis of behavioural syndromes and narcolepsy *because these drugs should not be used until underlying medical causes of the problem are ruled out.*
- Arrange to interrupt the drug periodically in children who are receiving the drug for behavioural syndromes *to determine whether symptoms recur and therapy should be continued.*
- Administer the drug before 6 PM *to reduce the incidence of insomnia.*
- Monitor vital signs *because stimulation of the CNS induces the release of catecholamines with a subsequent rise in heart rate and blood pressure.*
- Monitor weight (and height in children) and full blood count *to ensure early detection of adverse effects and proper interventions.* An ECG should be included if there is a history of cardiac disease either in the patient or family.
- Consult with the school nurse or counsellor *to ensure comprehensive care of school-aged children receiving CNS stimulants.*
- Provide safety measures such as assistance with ambulation if CNS effects occur *to prevent patient injury.*
- Monitor sleep-wake cycle *as CNS stimulation may disrupt normal sleep patterns.*
- Provide thorough patient teaching, including drug name, prescribed dosage, measures for avoidance of adverse effects, warning signs that may indicate possible problems, and the need for monitoring and evaluation *to enhance patient knowledge about drug therapy and to promote concordance.* Offer support and encouragement to help the patient cope with the drug regimen.

Evaluation

- Monitor patient response to the drug (decrease in manifestations of behavioural syndromes, decrease in daytime sleep and narcolepsy).
- Monitor for adverse effects (CNS stimulation, cardiovascular effects, rash, physical or psychological dependence, GI dysfunction).
- Evaluate the effectiveness of the teaching plan (patient can give the drug name and dosage, name possible adverse effects to watch for and specific measures to help avoid adverse effects, and describe the need for follow-up and evaluation).
- Monitor the effectiveness of comfort measures and concordance with the regimen.

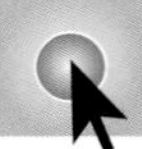

WEB LINKS

Health care providers and patients may want to consult the following Internet sources:

http://bnfc.org The BNF for Children provides UK health care professionals with authoritative and practical information on the selection and clinical use of medicines in children.

http://cks.library.nhs.uk The National Health Service Clinical Knowledge Summaries provides evidence-based practical information on the common conditions observed in primary care.

http://www.bnf.org.uk The BNF provides UK health care professionals with authoritative and practical information on the selection and clinical use of medicines.

http://www.nhsdirect.nhs.uk The National Health Service Direct service provides patients with information and advice about health, illness and health services.

http://www.mind.org.uk MIND is a mental health charity and can provide information to patients with a range of mental health problems.

http://www.rcpsych.ac.uk The Royal College of Psychiatrists provides information and support to patients with a wide range of mental health illnesses.

Points to Remember

- Mental health disorders are disorders of thought processes that may be caused by some inherent dysfunction within the brain. Psychoses are thought disorders.
- Schizophrenia, the most common psychosis, is characterized by delusions, hallucinations and inappropriate responses to stimuli.
- Mania is a state of hyperexcitability, one extreme of bipolar affective disorder.
- An ADHD is a behavioural syndrome characterized by hyperactivity and a short attention span.
- Narcolepsy is a disorder characterized by daytime sleepiness and sudden loss of wakefulness.
- Antipsychotics are dopamine-receptor blockers, but with antagonist action on other neurotransmitter receptors including 5-HT, muscarinic, α-adrenergic and histamine H_1. Side-effects include hypotension, antimuscarinic effects, sedation, and extrapyramidal effects, including parkinsonism, ataxia and tremors.
- Lithium is the treatment of choice for manic disorders. However, it is a very toxic salt and serum levels must be carefully monitored to prevent severe toxicity.
- CNS stimulants, which stimulate cortical levels and the RAS to increase RAS activity, are used to treat ADHD and narcolepsy. These drugs improve concentration and the ability to filter and focus incoming stimuli.

CRITICAL THINKING SCENARIO 21-1

Antipsychotic Drugs

The Situation

Beverley, a 36-year-old, single, professional woman, was diagnosed with chronic schizophrenia when she was a university student. Her condition has been well controlled with chlorpromazine, and she is able to maintain steady employment, live in her own home, and carry on a fairly active social life. At her last evaluation, she appeared to be developing bone marrow suppression, and her doctor decided to try to taper the drug dosage. As the dosage was being lowered, Beverley became withdrawn and listless, missed several days of work, and cancelled most of her social engagements. Afraid of interacting with people, she stayed in bed most of the time. She reported having thoughts of death and paranoid ideation about her neighbours that she was beginning to think might be true.

Critical Thinking

- What nursing interventions are appropriate at this time?
- What supportive measures might be useful to help Beverley cope with this crisis and allow her to function normally again?
- How does long-term therapy with phenothiazines affect dopamine receptors?
- What drug options should be tried?
- Are there any other options that might be useful?

Antipsychotic Drugs *(continued)*

Discussion

Beverley, an educated woman with a long history of taking antipsychotics, realizes the necessity of drug therapy to correct the chemical imbalance in her brain. She may need a different high-potency antipsychotic which does not affect bone marrow function to return her to the level of functioning she had reached before experiencing this setback. Her knowledge of her individual responses can be used to help select an appropriate drug and dosage. Her experiences may also facilitate her care planning and new drug regimen.

Beverley will need support to cope with problems at work—from her inability to go to work, to coping with feelings about not meeting her social obligations, to finding the motivation to get up and become active again. She may benefit from behaviour modification techniques that give her some control over her activities and allow her to use her knowledge and experience with her own situation to her advantage in forming a new medical regimen. She may need support in explaining her problem to her employer and her social contacts in ways that will help her avoid the prejudice associated with mental illness and will allow her every opportunity to return to her regular routine as soon as she can.

It may take several months to find the drug(s) that will bring Beverley back to a point of stabilization, therefore it is important to have a consistent, reliable health care team in place to support her through this stabilization period. She should have a reliable health worker to call when she has questions and when she needs support.

Nursing Care Guide for Beverley: Antipsychotic Drugs

Assessment: History and Examination

- Allergies to any of these drugs; CNS depression; cardiovascular disease; pregnancy or lactation; glaucoma; hypotension; seizures
- Concurrent use of antimuscarinics, barbiturate anaesthetics, alcohol, meperidine, β-blockers, adrenaline, noradrenaline, guanethidine
- Cardiovascular: blood pressure, pulse, orthostatic blood pressure
- CNS: orientation, affect, reflexes, vision
- Skin: colour, lesions, texture
- Respiratory: respiration, adventitious sounds
- GI: abdominal examination, bowel sounds
- Laboratory tests: thyroid, liver and renal function tests, full blood count

Nursing Diagnoses

- Impaired physical mobility related to extrapyramidal effects
- Risk of injury related to CNS effects
- Impaired urinary elimination related to antimuscarinic effects
- Potential for self-harm related to delusional thoughts
- Deficient knowledge regarding drug therapy

Implementation

- Give drug in evening; advise patient not to chew or crush sustained-release capsules.
- Provide comfort and safety measures: empty bladder before dosing; provide mouth care; institute safety measures if CNS effects occur; position patient to relieve dyskinesia discomfort; taper dosage after long-term therapy.
- Provide support and reassurance to help patient cope with drug effects and current worsening of symptoms.
- Teach patient about drug, dosage, adverse effects, conditions to report and precautions.

Evaluation

- Evaluate drug effects: relief of signs and symptoms of psychotic disorders.
- Monitor for adverse effects: sedation; antimuscarinic effects; extrapyramidal effects; cardiovascular effects; bone marrow suppression.
- Monitor for drug–drug interactions as listed.
- Evaluate effectiveness of patient teaching programme.
- Evaluate effectiveness of comfort and safety measures.

Patient Teaching for Beverley

- ☐ The drugs that are useful for treating schizophrenia are called antipsychotic or neuroleptic drugs. These drugs affect the activities of certain chemicals in your brain and are used to treat certain brain disorders.
- ☐ Drugs in this group should be taken exactly as prescribed. These drugs affect many body systems, therefore it is important that you have regular medical check-ups.
- ☐ Common effects of these drugs include:
  - *Dizziness, drowsiness and fainting:* Avoid driving or performing hazardous or delicate tasks that require concentration if these occur. Change position slowly. The dizziness usually passes after 1 to 2 weeks of drug use.

(continued)

Antipsychotic Drugs *(continued)*

- *Sensitivity to light:* Bright light might hurt your eyes and sunlight might burn your skin more easily. Avoid sun exposure: wear sunglasses and protective clothing when you must be out in the sun.
- *Constipation:* Consult with your health care provider if this becomes a problem.
- Report any of the following conditions to your health care provider: *sore throat, fever, rash, tremors, weakness and vision changes*

☐ Tell any doctor, nurse or other health care provider that you are taking this drug.

☐ Keep this drug and all medications out of the reach of children.

☐ Avoid the use of alcohol or other depressants while you are taking this drug. Try to limit your use of caffeine if you feel very tense or cannot sleep.

☐ Avoid the use of over-the-counter drugs while you are on this drug. Many of them contain ingredients that could interfere with the effectiveness of your drug. If you feel that you need one of these preparations, consult with your health care provider about the most appropriate choice.

☐ Take this drug exactly as prescribed. If you run out of medicine or find that you cannot take your drug for any reason, consult your health care provider. After this drug has been used for a period of time, additional adverse effects may occur if it is suddenly stopped. This drug should not be stopped suddenly.

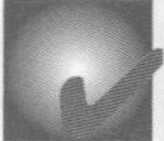

CHECK YOUR UNDERSTANDING

Answers to the questions in this chapter may be found in the answer key in the back of the book.

Multiple Choice

Select the most appropriate answer to the following.

1. The main mechanism of action of an antipsychotic agent is mainly as
   a. 5-HT reuptake inhibitors.
   b. noradrenaline blockers.
   c. inhibition of dopamine or reduction of dopamine in the brain.
   d. acetylcholine stimulators.
2. Antipsychotic drugs are also known as neuroleptic drugs because they
   a. cause numerous neurological effects.
   b. frequently cause epilepsy.
   c. are also minor tranquilizers.
   d. are the only drugs known to directly affect nerves.
3. Adverse effects associated with antipsychotic drugs are related to the drugs' effects on receptor sites and can include
   a. insomnia and hypertension.
   b. dry mouth, hypotension and glaucoma.
   c. diarrhoea and excessive urination.
   d. increased sexual drive and improved concentration.
4. Lithium toxicity can be dangerous. Patient assessment to evaluate for appropriate lithium levels would look for
   a. serum lithium levels greater than 2.0 mmol/l.
   b. serum lithium levels between 1.0 and 1.5 mmol/l.
   c. serum lithium levels less than 1.0 mmol/l.
   d. undetectable serum lithium levels.
5. ADHD (the inability to concentrate or focus on an activity) and narcolepsy (sudden episodes of sleep) are both most effectively treated with the use of
   a. neuroinhibitors.
   b. dopamine receptor blockers.
   c. antipsychotics.
   d. CNS stimulants.
6. Your patient, a 9-year-old boy, is starting a regime of methylphenidate to control an ADHD. Family teaching should include which of the following?
   a. This drug can be shared with other family members who might seem to need it.
   b. This drug may cause insomnia, weight loss and GI upset.
   c. Do not alert the school nurse to the fact that this drug is being taken because the child could have problems later on.
   d. This drug should not be stopped for any reason for several years.

7. Chlorpromazine is a potent antipsychotic that is associated with severe
   a. extrapyramidal effects.
   b. sedation.
   c. hypotension.
   d. antimuscarinic effects.

Extended Matching Questions

Select **all** that apply.

1. Before administering lithium to a client, the nurse should check for the concomitant use of which of the following drugs, which could cause serious adverse effects?
   a. Ibuprofen
   b. Haloperidol
   c. Thiazide diuretics
   d. Antacids
   e. Ketoconazole
   f. Theophylline

2. Dyskinesias are a common side-effect of antipsychotic drugs. Nursing interventions for the patient receiving antipsychotic drugs should include which of the following?
   a. Positioning to decrease discomfort of dyskinesias
   b. Implementing safety measures to prevent injury
   c. Encouraging the patient to chew tablets to prevent choking
   d. Careful teaching to alert the patient and family about this adverse effect
   e. Applying ice to the joints to prevent damage
   f. Pureeing all food to decrease the risk of aspiration

Matching

Match the following words with the appropriate definition.

1. ____________________schizophrenia
2. ____________________narcolepsy
3. ____________________ADHD
4. ____________________neuroleptic
5. ____________________mania
6. ____________________antipsychotic

A. A state of hyperexcitability
B. A behavioural syndrome characterized by an inability to concentrate
C. A mental disorder characterized by daytime sleepiness and sudden periods of loss of wakefulness
D. A drug used to treat a disorder of the thought processes; a dopamine receptor blocker
E. A psychotic disorder characterized by delusions, hallucinations, and thought and speech disturbances
F. An antipsychotic drug, so named because of the numerous neurological adverse effects caused by these drugs

Bibliography and References

Adams, M. P., Josephson, D. L., & Holland, L. N. (2005). *Pharmacology for nurses: A pathophysiologic approach.* New Jersey: Prentice Hall.

American Psychiatric Association. (2000). *Diagnostic and statistical manual of mental disorders*. (4th ed.) , Text Revision (DSM-IV-TR). Available from: http://www.psychiatryonline.com/

British Medical Association and Royal Pharmaceutical Society of Great Britain. (2008). *British National Formulary*. London: BMJ & RPS Publishing. *This publication is updated biannually: it is imperative that the most recent edition is consulted.*

British Medical Association and Royal Pharmaceutical Society of Great Britain. (2007). *British National Formulary for Children*. London: BMJ & RPS Publishing. *This publication is updated annually: it is imperative that the most recent edition is consulted.*

Gilman, A., Hardman, J. G., & Limbird, L. E. (Eds.). (2006). *Goodman and Gilman's the pharmacological basis of therapeutics* (11th ed.). New York: McGraw-Hill.

Howland, R. D., & Mycek, M. J. (2005). *Pharmacology* (3rd ed.). Philadelphia: Lippincott Williams & Wilkins.

Kumar, P., & Clark, M. (2005). *Clinical medicine.* (6th ed.). Edinburgh: Elsevier Saunders.

National Institute for Health and Clinical Excellence. (2002). Guidance on the use of newer (atypical) antipsychotic drugs for the treatment of schizophrenia. Available from http://www.nice.org.uk

National Institute for Health and Clinical Excellence. (2008). Attention deficit hyperactivity disorder. Diagnosis and management of ADHD in children, young people and adults. Available from http://www.nice.org.uk

National Institute for Health and Clinical Excellence. (2009). Schizophrenia. Core interventions in the treatment and management of schizophrenia in adults in primary and secondary care. Available from http://www.nice.org.uk

Owen, M. J., Carddock, N., & Jablensky, A. (2007). The genetic deconstruction of psychosis. *Schizophrenia Bulletin. 33*(4): 905–911.

Porth, C. M., & Matfin, G. (2008). *Pathophysiology: Concepts of altered health states* (8th ed.). Philadelphia: Lippincott Williams & Wilkins.

Rang, H. P., Dale, M. M., Ritter, J. M., & Flower, R. J. (2007). *Rang and Dale's pharmacology* (6th ed.). Philadelphia: Churchill Livingstone.

Simonsen, T., Aarbakke, J., Kay, I., Coleman, I., Sinnott, P., & Lysaa, R. (2006). *Illustrated pharmacology for nurses.* London: Hodder Arnold.

World Health Organisation. (2007). *International statistical classification of diseases and related health problems (10th Revision, ICD-10).* Available from: http://www.who.int/classifications/icd/

CHAPTER 22

Antiseizure Agents

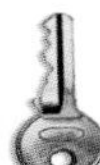

KEY TERMS

absence seizure
antiseizure agent
convulsion
epilepsy
focal seizure
generalized seizure
grand mal seizure
partial seizure
petit mal seizure
seizure
status epilepticus
tolerance
tonic–clonic seizure

LEARNING OBJECTIVES

Upon completion of this chapter, you will be able to:

1. Define the terms generalized seizure, tonic–clonic seizure, absence seizure, partial seizure and status epilepticus.
2. Describe the therapeutic actions, indications, pharmacokinetics, contraindications, most common adverse reactions and important drug–drug interactions associated with some of the major antiseizure drugs.
3. Discuss the use of antiseizure drugs across the lifespan.
4. Compare and contrast the key drugs with other antiseizure drugs.
5. Outline the nursing considerations and teaching needs for patients receiving antiseizure drugs.

DRUGS USED IN TREATING TONIC–CLONIC (GRAND MAL) SEIZURES

First line treatment

carbamazepine
lamotrigine
sodium valproate
topiramate

Second line treatment

clobazam
fosphenytoin
levetiracetam
oxcarbazepine
phenobarbital
phenytoin
primidone

DRUGS USED IN TREATING ABSENCE (PETIT MAL) SEIZURES

First line treatment

ethosuximide
lamotrigine
sodium valproate

Second line treatment

clobazam
clonazepam
phenobarbital sodium

DRUGS USED IN TREATING PARTIAL (FOCAL) SEIZURES

First line treatment

carbamazepine
lamotrigine
oxcarbazepine
sodium valproate
topiramate

Second line treatment

clobazam
fosphenytoin
gabapentin
levetiracetam
phenobarbital sodium

phenytoin
pregabalin
primidone
tiagabine
vigabatrin
zonisamide

DRUGS USED IN TREATING STATUS EPILEPTICUS

clonazepam
diazepam
fosphenytoin sodium
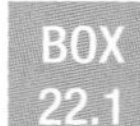 lorazepam
midazolam
paraldehyde
phenobarbital sodium
phenytoin sodium

Epilepsy is classified as a long-term condition. The most prevalent of the neurological disorders, epilepsy is not a single disease but a collection of different syndromes. All of these conditions are characterized by the same feature: sudden discharge of excessive electrical energy from nerve cells in the brain, which may be localized to one part of the brain or spread to both hemispheres, resulting in a **seizure**. There are different types of seizures. In some cases, motor nerves are stimulated, resulting in **convulsions**, with tonic–clonic muscle contractions that have the potential to cause injury; tics or spasms. Other discharges may stimulate autonomic or sensory nerves and cause very different effects, such as a barely perceptible, temporary lapse in consciousness or a sympathetic reaction. As epilepsy involves a loss of control, it can be very frightening to patients when they are first diagnosed (Box 22.1). Some people have auras, which give some prior warning of the onset of a seizure. Auras can take several forms, such as the person experiences an unusual taste or smell or visual disturbance.

The treatment of epilepsy varies widely, depending on the exact problem and its manifestations. The drugs used to manage epilepsy are called **antiseizures** (Box 22.2). The drug of choice for any given situation will depend on the type of epilepsy (Table 22.1) and patient **tolerance** for associated adverse effects.

Nature of Epilepsy

The form that a particular seizure takes depends on the location of the cells that initiate the electrical discharge and the neural pathways that are stimulated by the initial volley of electrical impulses. For the most part, epilepsy seems to be caused by abnormal neurons that are very sensitive to stimulation or over-respond for some reason. Seizures caused by these abnormal cells are called *primary seizures* because no underlying cause can be identified. In some cases, however, outside factors, such as head injury, drug overdose, environmental exposure; may precipitate seizures. Such seizures are often referred to as *secondary seizures*.

Classification of Seizures

Correct diagnosis of seizure type is very important for determining the correct medication to prevent future seizures while causing the fewest problems and adverse effects. Seizures may be grouped into two main types, and they are further classified within these two categories.

Generalized Seizures

Generalized seizures begin in one area of the brain and rapidly spread throughout both hemispheres of the brain.

BOX 22.1 FOCUS ON **CLINICAL SKILLS**

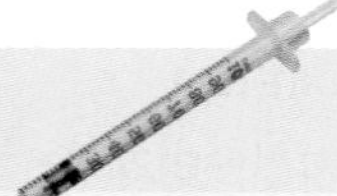

Educating and Counselling Patients with Epilepsy

Epilepsy is frightening to people who know little about the disease. A person who receives a diagnosis of epilepsy must deal with the stigma as well as the significance of the diagnosis. Individuals who are newly diagnosed with epilepsy must consider restrictions on their independence as well as the prospect of long-term chronic therapy for control of this problem.

Patients who are newly diagnosed with epilepsy have to cope not only with the stigma of epilepsy, but also with the loss of a driver's license (and potentially their means of employment). The Driver and Vehicle Licensing Agency allow patients to drive a car (but not a heavy goods vehicle or public transport) if they have remained seizure-free for a period of one year. Those patients who experience seizures only while asleep are allowed to drive if they have a 3-year period free from seizures during the day.

The nurse may be in the best position to help the patient adjust to these problems through patient teaching and referrals to community resources. Thorough patient teaching should include the following:

- Ways in which patients can educate family, friends and employers about the realities of the condition and its treatment.
- Actions to take if a seizure happens so that no injuries occur and no panic develops.
- The importance of encouraging patients with epilepsy to wear a MedicAlert identification, to alert any emergency caregivers to their condition and to what drugs they are taking if they are not able to speak for themselves.
- Contact information regarding other community support services.

There are many epilepsy support groups that can supply information on valuable resources. While patients are first adjusting to epilepsy and its implications, it may help to put them in contact with such organizations. The charity Epilepsy Action may be able to offer support groups, lists of resources and support.

BOX 22.2 DRUG THERAPY ACROSS THE LIFESPAN

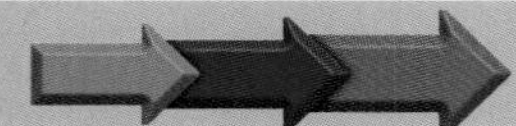

Antiseizure Agents

CHILDREN

Antiseizure drugs can have an impact on a child's learning and social development. Children may also be more sensitive to the sedating effects of some of these drugs. Children should be monitored very closely and often require a switch to a different agent or dosage adjustments based on their response.

Older children (usually up to 16 years of age) metabolize many of these drugs more quickly than adults and require a larger dosage per kilogram body weight to maintain therapeutic levels. Careful calculation of drug dosage using both weight and age are important in helping the child to receive the best therapeutic effect with the least toxicity. After the age of 16 years, many of these drugs can be given in the standard adult dose.

Parents of children receiving these drugs should receive consistent support and education about the seizure disorder and the medications being used to treat it. Many communities have local support groups that can offer lots of educational materials and support programmes. It is a very frightening experience to watch your child have a tonic–clonic seizure, and parents should be supported with this in mind.

When administering any drug to children, always consult the most recent edition of the British National Formulary for Children.

ADULTS

Adults using these drugs should be under regular care and monitored regularly for adverse effects. They should be encouraged to wear a MedicAlert identification to alert emergency personnel that antiseizure drugs are being taken. Adults also need education and support to deal with the stigma of having seizures as well as the lifestyle changes and drug effects that they may need to cope with.

Many of these drugs are associated with specific birth defects (e.g. neural tube defects); however, the risk of taking a woman with a seizure disorder off an antiseizure drug that has stabilized her condition may be greater than the risk of the drug to the foetus. Discontinuing the drug could result in status epilepticus, which has a high risk of hypoxia for both the mother and the foetus. In such cases, the mother should be informed of the potential risks. Folic acid supplements can be given to reduce the risk of neural tube defects. Although the plasma concentration of antiseizure drug can vary during pregnancy as a result of changes in blood volume, routine monitoring is only required if seizures increase or are likely to increase (NICE, 2004).

Women of child-bearing age should be urged to use barrier contraceptives while taking these drugs. If a pregnancy does occur, the woman should receive educational materials and counselling. Breast-feeding is safe when the drugs carbamazepine, lamotrigine and sodium valproate are given in *normal* doses.

OLDER ADULTS

Older patients may be more susceptible to the adverse effects of these drugs, especially depression of the central nervous system (CNS). Dosages of all of these drugs may need to be reduced, and the patient should be monitored very closely for toxic effects and to provide safety measures if CNS effects do occur.

Patients with renal or hepatic impairment should be monitored very closely. Baseline renal and liver function tests should be done and dosages adjusted as appropriate. Serum levels of the drug should be monitored closely in such cases to prevent serious adverse effects.

Patients who have a generalized seizure usually experience a loss of consciousness resulting from this massive electrical activity throughout the brain.

Generalized seizures are further classified into the following five types:

1. **Tonic–clonic seizures**, formerly known as **grand mal seizures**, are the most common type of seizure in all age groups. Tonic–clonic seizures generally last several minutes and involve dramatic tonic–clonic muscle contractions and a loss of consciousness. The recovery period is characterized by confusion, disorientation and exhaustion.
2. **Absence seizures**, formerly known as **petit mal seizures**, involve abrupt, brief (3- to 5-second) periods of self-limited loss of consciousness. During these seizures the individual stares into space and is temporarily unresponsive – this can be mistaken for daydreaming. There may be some muscle contraction, including rapid blinking of eyelids. Many people are not aware that a seizure is happening. This type of seizure frequently occurs in children, starting at about 3 years of age, and usually disappears by puberty. Some children may have multiple absence seizures per day.
3. **Myoclonic seizures** involve short, sporadic periods of muscle contractions that last for several minutes. They are relatively rare and are often secondary seizures.
4. **Febrile seizures** are related to very high fevers and usually involve convulsions. Febrile seizures most frequently happen in children between the ages of 6 months and 6 years and occur in approximately 3% of all children (Bellman & Peile, 2006). These seizures are usually self-limiting.
5. **Status epilepticus**, potentially the most dangerous of seizure conditions; is a state in which seizures rapidly recur again and again for up to 30 minutes with no rest in between. Status epilepticus is a medical emergency and if left untreated can lead to neurological damage and ultimately death. The prolonged muscle contractions increase the metabolic demands of the body and can lead to cerebral hypoxia. Patients should be administered oxygen and either diazepam or lorazepam.

Partial Seizures

Partial seizures, also called **focal seizures**, are so called because they involve only one area of the brain and usually originate from one site or focus. The presenting symptoms depend on exactly where in the brain the excessive electrical discharge is occurring. Partial seizures can be further classified as follows:

1. Simple partial seizures occur in a single area of the brain and may involve a single muscle movement or sensory alteration.

Table 22.1 Drugs Used to Treat Various Types of Seizures

Drug	Tonic–clonic	Absence	Myoclonic	Febrile	Status Epilepticus	Partial
Carbamazepine	1	—	—	—	—	1
Clobazam	2	2	—	—	—	2
Clonazepam	—	2	2	—	2	—
Diazepam	—	—	—	1	2	—
Ethosuximide	—	1	—	—	—	—
Fosphenytoin sodium	2	—	—	—	2	—
Gabapentin	—	—	—	—	—	2
Lamotrigine	1	2	2	—	—	1
Levetiracetam	2	—	2	—	—	2
Lorazepam	—	—	—	—	1	—
Midazolam	—	—	—	—	2	—
Oxcarbazepine	2	—	—	—	—	1
Paraldehyde	—	—	—	—	2	—
Phenobarbital	2	2	—	—	2	2
Phenytoin	2	—	2	—	2	2
Pregabalin	—	—	—	—	—	2
Primidone	2	—	—	—	—	2
Sodium valproate	1	1	1	—	—	1
Tiagabine	—	—	—	—	—	2
Topiramate	1	—	2	—	—	1
Vigabatrin	—	—	—	—	—	2
Zonisamide	—	—	—	—	—	2

2. Complex partial seizures involve complex sensory changes such as hallucinations, mental distortion, changes in personality, loss of consciousness and loss of social inhibitions. Motor changes may include involuntary urination, chewing motions and diarrhoea. The onset of complex partial seizures usually occurs by the late teens.

Partial seizures can spread to other areas of the cerebral hemispheres to become generalized; this type of seizure is known as a partial seizure with secondary generalization.

Antiseizure Drugs

The aim of antiseizure drugs is to reduce the excitability of the areas of the brain associated with hyperexcitability and seizure generation and therefore reduce the chance of sudden electrical outburst. Drugs used to treat seizures stabilize the nerve membranes in two ways – either directly, by altering sodium and calcium channels, or indirectly, by increasing the activity of γ-aminobutyric acid (GABA), an inhibitory neurotransmitter, and thereby decreasing excessive activity (see Figure 22.1). As they work generally on the CNS, sedation and other CNS effects often result. Associated adverse effects are often related to total brain stabilization (Figure 22.1).

It may be necessary to use combination therapy to manage seizures. Combining two or more drugs should only be considered when monotherapy with two first-line antiseizure drugs has failed to control seizures or if a patient has to take the maximum drug dose to remain free of seizures. There is a risk of increased toxicity and interactions when combining antiseizure drugs.

Inhibition of Voltage-Sensitive Sodium Channels

One of the most effective mechanisms of reducing neuronal excitability is to reduce the inflow of sodium ions through voltage-sensitive sodium channels. This will prevent the neuron from depolarizing and therefore the generation of action potentials. Some of the sodium channel inhibitors used to treat epilepsy demonstrate 'use-dependence', meaning that in areas of the brain where action potentials are firing repetitively, the drug is more effective at blocking the channels.

Phenytoin is the prototype drug belonging to the hydantoin group of compounds. The hydantoins are generally less

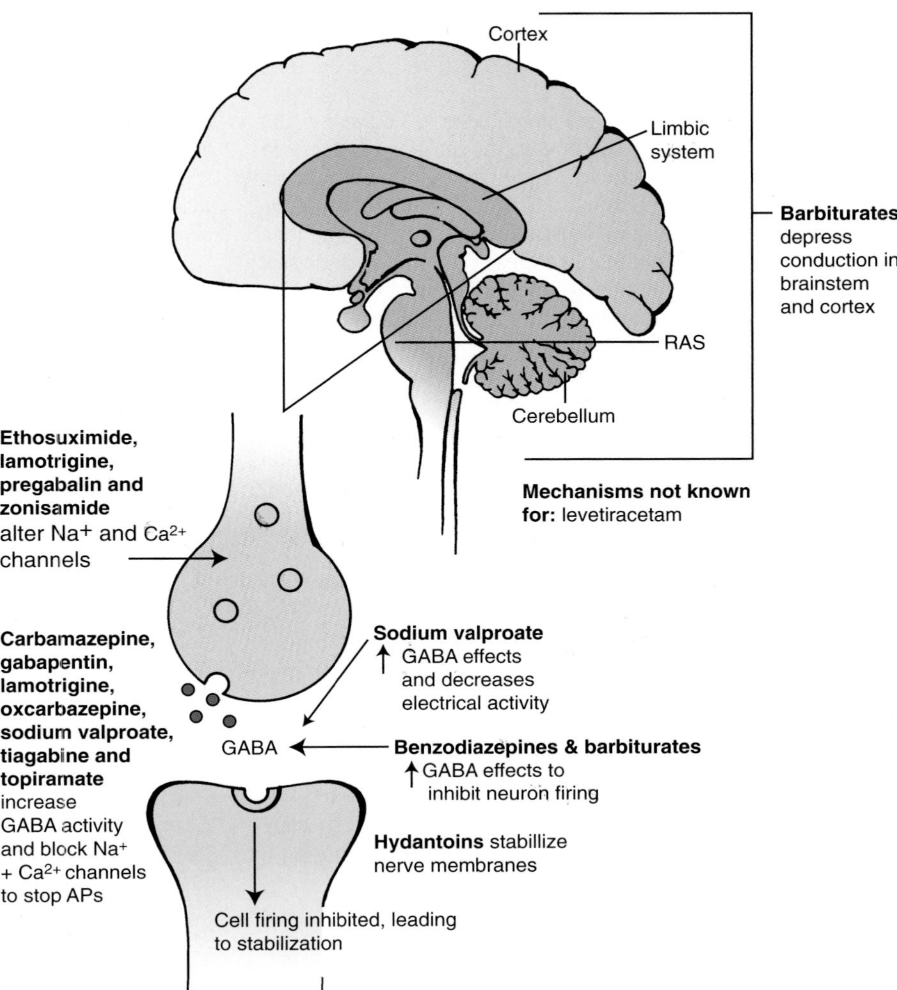

FIGURE 22.1 Sites of action of drugs used to treat various types of epilepsy. APs, action potentials; GABA, γ-aminobutyric acid; RAS, reticular activating system.

sedating than many other antiseizure drugs and may be the drugs of choice for patients who are not willing to tolerate sedation and drowsiness. Specific adverse effects with the hydantoins include bone marrow suppression, gingival hyperplasia (overgrowth of gum tissue), dermatological reactions (e.g. hirsutism, coarsening of facial skin) and liver toxicity. In many situations, less toxic drugs (e.g. the benzodiazepines) have replaced them.

Phenytoin is used in the treatment of many types of epilepsy, excluding absence seizures. It is available in oral and parenteral forms. The oral form is well absorbed from the gastrointestinal (GI) tract, metabolized in the liver and excreted in the urine. Phenytoin is a potent inducer of hepatic enzymes responsible for the metabolism of a range of drugs, including phenytoin (see Box 22.3). Induction of hepatic enzymes will speed up the metabolism of drugs that are metabolized by the same enzymes, such as anticoagulants. Phenytoin should not be given concurrently with cimetidine (used to treat gastric ulcers) as cimetidine causes phenytoin to reach toxic levels. Patients with hepatic impairment may be at risk of increased toxicity from phenytoin. Serum levels of phenytoin should be maintained between 10 and 20 mg/ml.

Fosphenytoin, a prodrug of phenytoin, is used for short-term control of status epilepticus and to prevent seizures after neurosurgery. It is given intramuscularly or intravenously. Fosphenytoin is metabolized in the liver to phenytoin and excreted in the urine. The therapeutic phenytoin serum levels peak about 10 to 20 minutes after the infusion, and the patient must be monitored closely for cardiovascular reactions during this period. Patients with hepatic and/or renal impairment are at increased risk of toxic effects because of alterations in metabolism and excretion of the drug. Such patients should be monitored routinely, and the dosage adjusted accordingly.

Carbamazepine, the most widely used antiseizure agent, is often the drug of choice for treatment of partial seizures with or without secondary generalization. Chemically related to the tricyclic antidepressants, it has also been used in the treatment of tonic–clonic seizures, trigeminal neuralgia and bipolar disorder. It has the ability to inhibit polysynaptic responses and to block sodium channels to

BOX 22.3 Metabolism of Antiseizure Agents

Most of the antiseizure agents are broken down in the liver by drug metabolizing enzymes. The hepatic drug metabolizing enzymes can be induced or inhibited by specific drugs, herbal therapies and certain foods and beverages. When a metabolizing enzyme is induced, this increases the rate of drug metabolism and removes the drug from the body more rapidly leading to a decrease in the pharmacological activity of the drug(s) metabolized by that enzyme. For example, phenytoin increases the metabolism of oestrogens leading to a reduced contraceptive effect.

In contrast, if an enzyme is inhibited, this slows the metabolism and can cause the drug to accumulate in the body leading to potential toxic levels. For example, the metabolism of carbamazepine is reduced when administered with some of the antidepressants. On frequent occasions patients are prescribed more than one drug and it is extremely important to determine if the drugs interact in any way to avoid either toxic plasma concentrations or reduced drug efficacy.

Always consult a current copy of the British National Formulary to ensure harmful drug–drug and drug-food interactions are avoided.

A number of the antiseizure drugs are known to induce hepatic enzymes including carbamazepine, oxcarbazepine, phenobarbital, phenytoin, primidone and topiramate. These drugs are usually substrates for the induced enzymes and therefore their own metabolism can also be increased. This can lead to tolerance where the patient observes diminished effects in response to the same drug concentration. Therefore treatment is usually commenced at a low dose, which is gradually increased over several weeks until the optimum plasma concentration is reached and seizures are prevented.

prevent the formation of repetitive action potentials in the abnormal focus. Carbamazepine is absorbed from the GI tract and metabolized in the liver by the cytochrome P450 system (see Chapter 2). It is excreted in the urine. Like phenytoin, carbamazepine is also a potent inducer of hepatic enzymes and should not be given with other antiseizure drugs (see Box 22.3).

Oxcarbazepine is approved for the treatment of partial seizures in adults and children over 6 years of age as monotherapy or in combination with other antiseizure drugs. Oxcarbazepine is a prodrug metabolized in the liver to a compound similar in action to carbamazepine. Completely absorbed from the GI tract, oxcarbazepine is extensively metabolized in the liver and excreted in the urine with a half-life of 2 and then 9 hours. The most common adverse effects include GI disturbances, depression of CNS activities and hyponatraemia – elderly patients and those taking diuretics should have regular monitoring of plasma sodium concentrations.

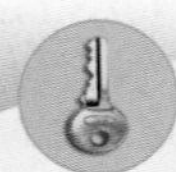

Key Drug Summary: *Carbamazepine*

Indications: Treatment of partial, tonic–clonic and mixed seizures; trigeminal neuralgia; prophylaxis of bipolar disorder

Actions: Stabilizes membrane potential through the inhibition of voltage-sensitive sodium ion channels.

Pharmacokinetics:

Route	Onset	Peak
Oral	Slow	4–5 h
SR oral	Slow	3–12 h

$T_{1/2}$: 25–65 hours, then 12–17 hours; metabolized in the liver, metabolites excreted in the urine and faeces

Adverse effects: Drowsiness, ataxia, dizziness, nausea, vomiting, arrhythmias, hepatitis, haematological disorders, Stevens–Johnson syndrome (a rare but severe condition characterized by inflammation of the oral mucosa, respiratory tract and genitalia), water retention and hyponatraemia. Treatment should start with a low dose due to the possibility of bone marrow suppression or hypersensitivity. Patients and carers must report symptoms such as fever, sore throat, rash, mouth ulcers, bruising or bleeding as soon as possible. This could indicate a blood, liver or skin disorder.

Sodium valproate reduces abnormal electrical activity in the brain via inhibition of sodium channels and may also increase GABA activity through the inhibition of two enzymes responsible for the inactivation of GABA. It is possible that sodium valproate may also enhance the postsynaptic action of GABA. Sodium valproate is indicated for all forms of epilepsy and is one of the drugs of choice for the treatment of tonic–clonic, absence and myoclonic seizures. Readily absorbed from the GI tract, sodium valproate is metabolized in the liver and excreted in the urine. It is sometimes associated with fatal hepatic toxicity, and liver function (serum levels of bilirubin and liver enzymes) should be regularly monitored.

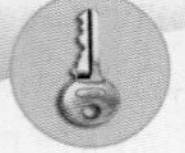

Key Drug Summary: *Sodium valproate*

Indications: Treatment of generalized tonic–clonic, absence and myoclonic seizures; may also be useful in treating atypical seizures; acute mania

Actions: Stabilization of neuronal membranes through inhibition of sodium channels; may also enhance GABA transmission

Pharmacokinetics:

Route	Onset
Oral	1–4 h
IV	5 min

$T_{1/2}$: 6–16 hours; metabolized in the liver, excreted in the urine

Adverse effects: GI disturbances including nausea, irritation and diarrhoea; weight gain, hair loss, liver dysfunction, pancreatitis, blood disorders. Patients and carers must report symptoms such as fever, sore throat, rash, mouth ulcers, bruising or bleeding as soon as possible. This could indicate a blood, liver or skin disorder.

Lamotrigine is one of the newer antiseizure drugs used as monotherapy or adjunctive therapy in the treatment of partial seizures, primary and secondarily generalized tonic–clonic seizures and in the treatment of seizures associated with Lennox–Gastaut syndrome (a form of absence seizure often associated with tonic or clonic seizures and mental deterioration) in adults and children 12 years of age and older. This drug inhibits voltage-sensitive sodium channels and also inhibits the calcium-dependent presynaptic release of excitatory neurotransmitters, such as glutamate. Lamotrigine is rapidly absorbed from the GI tract, metabolized in the liver, and primarily excreted in the urine. The half-life of lamotrigine is approximately 24 hours. It has been associated with very serious to life-threatening rashes, including Stevens–Johnson syndrome; and the drug should be discontinued at the first sign of any rash.

Topiramate is also a relatively new drug used as monotherapy and adjunctive therapy of tonic–clonic and partial seizures in adults and children 2 to 16 years of age. It is also approved for the prevention of migraine headaches, and as adjunct therapy in Lennox–Gastaut syndrome. The precise mechanism of action is not clear, but topiramate may inhibit sodium channels, increase GABA activity and prevent the binding of glutamate to excitatory amino acid receptors. Topiramate is rapidly absorbed from the GI tract, reaching peak levels in 2 hours. It is widely distributed and excreted unchanged in the urine. Patients with renal impairment should receive a reduced dosage of the drug. Acute myopia is an adverse effect of topiramate.

Inhibition of Voltage-Sensitive Calcium Channels

For the exocytosis of neurotransmitters to take place, calcium must enter the presynaptic neuron from the extracellular space through voltage-sensitive calcium channels. By preventing the entry of calcium into the neuron, exocytosis of excitatory neurotransmitters is inhibited, reducing the probability of action potentials occurring in postsynaptic neurons. In addition to lamotrigine mentioned above, ethosuximide, pregabalin and gabapentin all inhibit calcium channels.

Ethosuximide, a succinimide, is the drug of choice for treating absence seizures. This drug specifically inhibits calcium channels to suppress the abnormal electrical activity in the brain associated with absence seizures. Ethosuximide is readily absorbed from the GI tract following oral administration, reaching peak levels in about 3 hours. Twenty-five per cent of the drug is excreted in the urine unchanged; the rest is metabolized in the liver and the metabolites excreted in the urine. This drug should be avoided in patients with intermittent porphyria, which could be exacerbated by the adverse effects of these drugs.

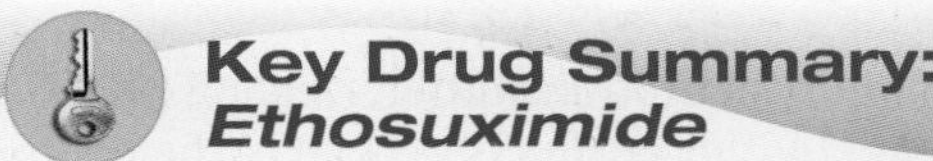

Key Drug Summary: *Ethosuximide*

Indications: Control of absence seizures

Actions: Inhibits calcium channels preventing calcium entry and neurotransmitter release. May act in inhibitory neuronal systems; suppresses the electroencephalogram (EEG) pattern associated with absence seizures; reduces frequency of attacks

Pharmacokinetics:

Route	Peak
Oral	3–7 h

$T_{1/2}$: 40–50 hours; mainly metabolized in the liver, excreted in the urine

Adverse effects: Drowsiness, ataxia, dizziness, irritability, nervousness, headache, blurred vision, pruritus (itching), Stevens–Johnson syndrome, nausea, vomiting, epigastric pain, anorexia, diarrhoea, bone marrow suppression, including potentially fatal pancytopenia (a reduction in the number of red and white blood cells). A full blood count should be taken. Patients and carers must report symptoms such as fever, sore throat, rash, mouth ulcers, bruising or bleeding as soon as possible.

Pregabalin has a high binding affinity for voltage-gated calcium channels. By modulating the calcium function in these neurons, this leads to a decreased release of neurotransmitters into the synaptic cleft and a decrease in neuronal activity. It is approved for the adjunctive treatment of adults with partial seizures and for the management of neuropathic pain and generalized anxiety disorder. Pregabalin is rapidly absorbed orally, reaching peak levels in 1.5 hours. Metabolism is negligible and approximately 98% is eliminated unchanged in the urine. The half-life is about 6.3 hours. The adverse effects most commonly seen with this drug are related to CNS depression – tremor, dizziness, somnolence and visual changes. Pregabalin can also cause feelings of well-being and euphoria and caution should be applied to patients who have a history of abuse of medications or alcohol.

Gabapentin is used as monotherapy or adjunctive therapy in the treatment of partial seizures and in the treatment of neuropathic pain. Gabapentin is an analogue of GABA. The precise mechanism of action of gabapentin is unclear but it is known to have a high affinity for voltage-gated calcium channels. Gabapentin is well absorbed from the GI tract and widely distributed in the body. It is excreted unchanged in the urine with a half-life of 5 to 7 hours.

Enhanced GABA Transmission

GABA is an inhibitory neurotransmitter. Binding of GABA to receptors, causes chloride channels to open in the neuronal plasma membrane. Chloride ions enter the neuron, causing hyperpolarisation, thus inhibiting neuronal transmission. This exerts a stabilizing influence and reduces the chances of an action potential occurring.

Antiseizure drugs can enhance GABA transmission in several ways, either by enhancing the opening of GABA receptors or by increasing the availability of GABA in the synaptic cleft, either through inhibition of the enzymes responsible for the breakdown of GABA or inhibition of reuptake mechanisms.

The benzodiazepines decrease excitability and conduction (see Figure 22.1) by selectively binding to a specific site on $GABA_A$ receptors and potentiating the binding of GABA to receptors. This results in an increased frequency of ion channel opening and an inhibitory response. They appear to act primarily in the limbic system and the reticular activating system (RAS), and also cause muscle relaxation and relieve anxiety without affecting cortical functioning substantially. In general, these drugs have limited toxicity and are well tolerated by most people. (See Chapter 19 for use of benzodiazepines as sedatives and anxiolytics) The benzodiazepines described here, diazepam, clonazepam, clobazam and lorazepam, are used as antiseizures; mainly in status epilepticus. Midazolam is also indicated (unlicensed) for the treatment of status epilepticus. [Midazolam has not received a licence to be used in the treatment of status epilepticus. This could be for several reasons: midazolam is either still under trial for treating this condition or awaiting licensing for a new purpose, i.e. midazolam is currently licensed for use as a premedication and the intention is this license will be extended for use as an antiseizure agent in status epilepticus.]

Diazepam, the prototype benzodiazepine, is useful in relieving tension, anxiety and muscle spasm. Available in oral, rectal and parenteral forms, it is used to treat status epilepticus, febrile convulsions, alcohol withdrawal, muscle spasm, short-term treatment of anxiety or insomnia, and is given to relieve preoperative anxiety. Diazepam is not used for long-term management of epilepsy. Diazepam is well absorbed from the GI tract, metabolized in the liver, and excreted in the urine. It has a long half-life of 20 to 50 hours.

Clonazepam is mainly used for the treatment of status epilepticus, and can also be used to treat myoclonic and atypical seizures. This drug is administered using either using IV injection or infusion, or oral preparations. Clonazepam may lose its effectiveness after 1 to 6 months (affected patients may respond to dosage adjustment). Clonazepam has a long half-life of 25 hours and is metabolized by the liver and excreted in the urine. *Clobazam* is related to clonazepam and is used orally as an adjunct therapy for tonic–clonic, absence and partial seizures.

Lorazepam is one of the first-line treatments for status epilepticus and its anxiolytic properties are exploited in the short-term treatment of anxiety and insomnia. With a half-life of approximately 14 hours, lorazepam is metabolized by the liver and excreted in the urine.

The barbiturates and barbiturate-like drugs also enhance the actions of GABA on $GABA_A$ receptors. They inhibit impulse conduction in the ascending RAS, depress the cerebral cortex, alter cerebellar function and depress motor nerve output. Because they depress nerve function, they can produce sedation, hypnosis, anaesthesia and deep coma. The degree of depression is dose related. These drugs block seizure activity at doses below those needed to cause hypnosis.

The antiseizure properties of the barbiturate, *phenobarbital,* were first recognized in 1912. In parenteral form, phenobarbital is used for the emergency control of status epilepticus. In addition, it is used orally for the long-term management of most forms of epilepsy, excluding absence seizures. Specifically, phenobarbital depresses conduction in the lower brainstem and the cerebral cortex and depresses motor conduction. This drug has very low lipid solubility, giving it a slow onset and a very long duration of activity. It is well absorbed from the GI tract and mainly metabolized in the liver and the metabolites excreted in the urine; the remaining drug is excreted unchanged in the urine. Phenobarbital is a powerful inducer of some liver enzymes and the concentration of other drugs in the plasma can be significantly reduced.

Primidone, which is structurally very similar to phenobarbital, is an alternative choice in the treatment of all seizures except absence seizures. It tends to have a longer half-life than phenobarbital and is available only in an oral form. A small starting dose should be prescribed; the dose can be increased gradually over weeks if necessary. Primidone may be combined with other agents to treat seizures that cannot be controlled by any other antiseizure agent. It is well absorbed from the GI tract, metabolized in the liver to phenobarbital metabolites, and excreted in the urine.

The most common adverse effects associated with the barbiturates and benzodiazepines, relate to CNS depression and its effects on body function: depression, confusion, drowsiness, lethargy, fatigue, constipation, dry mouth, anorexia, cardiac arrhythmias and changes in blood pressure, urinary retention and loss of libido. Barbiturates have a narrow therapeutic window particularly when combined with alcohol, which can lead to death from overdose.

In addition, benzodiazepines and phenobarbital may be associated with physical dependence and withdrawal syndrome. These drugs should only be withdrawn gradually (over 2–3 months or longer) under the supervision of a specialist. Abrupt withdrawal can lead to rebound seizures. Phenobarbital has also been linked to severe dermatological reactions and the development of drug tolerance related to changes in drug metabolism over time.

Tiagabine enhances GABA transmission by blocking the GABA reuptake into neurons and glial cells. Inhibition of this transporter increases the availability of GABA in the synaptic cleft; and because GABA is an inhibitory neurotransmitter, the result is a stabilizing of neuronal membranes and a decrease in excessive activity. Tiagibine is used as adjunct therapy in the treatment of partial seizures in adults and children 12 years and above. Tiagabine is rapidly absorbed from the GI tract, reaching peak levels in 45 minutes. It is metabolized in the liver by the cytochrome P450 enzyme system and excreted in the urine with a half-life of 4 to 7 hours. The main side-effects associated with tiagibine are diarrhoea, dizziness, drowsiness, tremor and impaired concentration.

Vigabatrin is structurally similar to GABA and inhibits the enzyme GABA transaminase, which is responsible for the metabolism of GABA. By inhibiting the breakdown of GABA, vigabatrin enhances inhibitory transmission mediated by GABA. Vigabatrin is administered orally in combination with other antiseizure drugs in the treatment of partial seizures. Significant side-effects associated with this drug include behavioural disturbances and defects in visual fields, thus this drug is limited to patients who are not adequately treated with other antiseizure drugs. Vigabatrin is well absorbed and largely excreted unchanged in the urine. The half-life is short at 6 hours.

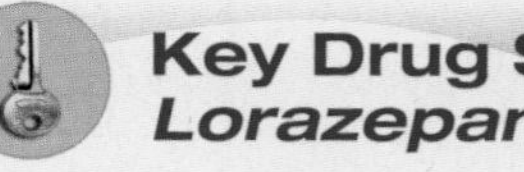

Key Drug Summary: Lorazepam

Indications: First choice drug in the treatment of status epilepticus and severe recurrent convulsive seizures; management of anxiety disorders; preoperative relief of anxiety and tension

Actions: Acts in the limbic system and reticular formation; potentiates the effects of GABA

Pharmacokinetics:

Route	Onset	Peak
IV	1–5 min	2 h

$T_{1/2}$: 14 hours; metabolized in the liver, excreted in the urine

Adverse effects: Drowsiness, sedation, depression, lethargy, apathy, fatigue, disorientation, paradoxical excitatory reactions, GI disturbances, incontinence, urinary retention; pain and thrombophlebitis on IV injection

Alternative Mechanisms of Action

Currently, two drugs fall into this category: *levetiracetam* and *zonisamide*.

Levetiracetam is a newer drug that is approved as a monotherapy or adjunct therapy in the treatment of partial seizures in adults and children. It can also be used as an adjunct therapy for myoclonic and tonic–clonic seizures. The mechanism of action of levetiracetam is not understood; its antiseizure action does not seem to be associated with any known mechanisms of inhibitory or excitatory neurotransmission. After rapid absorption from the GI tract, peak levels are reached in 1 hour. It undergoes some metabolism, but most of the drug is excreted unchanged in the urine with a half-life of 6 to 8 hours. Patients with renal dysfunction are more likely to experience toxic effects of the drug, and the dosage for these patients may need to be adjusted accordingly.

Zonisamide is a sulphonamide compound that inhibits voltage-sensitive sodium and calcium channels, thus stabilizing nerve cell membranes and inhibiting calcium-dependent presynaptic release of excitatory neurotransmitters. It is used as an adjunct to other drugs for the treatment of partial seizures. Zonisamide is well absorbed from the GI tract, reaching peak levels in 2 to 6 hours. It is primarily excreted unchanged in the urine, with a half-life of 63 hours. Patients who take this drug should maintain levels of hydration because there is a risk of developing renal calculi.

General Nursing Considerations for Patients Receiving Antiseizure Agents

See Chapter 19 for specific nursing considerations for patients receiving barbiturates or benzodiazepines.

Assessment: History and Examination

Screen for the following conditions, *which may be cautions or contraindications to the use of the drug*: any known allergies to these drugs; cardiac arrhythmias, hypotension, diabetes, coma, psychoses; porphyria; visual field defects; pregnancy and lactation; and renal or hepatic dysfunction. Obtain a description of seizures, including onset, aura, duration and recovery.

Include screening *for baseline status before beginning therapy and for any potential adverse effects.* Assess the following: skin colour and lesions; temperature; CNS orientation, affect, reflexes and bilateral grip strength; bowel sounds and reported output; pulse, auscultation and blood pressure; urinary output; and EEG if appropriate. Assess liver and renal function if the patient's history suggests potential problems.

Establish if patient is currently taking other medications or herbal therapies, which may potentially interact with the antiseizure agent. Patients are advised not to use the herb evening primrose or ginkgo because they can increase the risk of having seizures.

Nursing Diagnoses

Patients receiving antiseizures may have the following nursing diagnoses related to drug therapy:

- Acute pain related to GI, CNS and genitourinary effects
- Disturbed thought processes related to CNS effects
- Risk of injury related to CNS effects or effects of seizure
- Risk of infection related to bone marrow suppression
- Impaired skin integrity related to dermatological effects
- Deficient knowledge regarding drug therapy
- Loss of self-esteem related to the stigma of epilepsy or loss of self-control during a seizure.

Implementation With Rationale

- Ask the patient to report symptoms such as fever, sore throat, rash, mouth ulcers, bruising or bleeding as soon as possible *to limit reaction and prevent potentially serious reactions*. These symptoms could indicate a blood, liver or skin disorder. Specialist advice should also be sought if unusual depression or personality changes occur. Some antiseizure drugs have been associated with a small increased risk of suicidal thoughts and behaviour (Medicines and Healthcare products Regulatory Agency, 2008).
- With the exception of hypersensitivity or other adverse reactions, discontinue the drug slowly *because rapid withdrawal may precipitate absence seizures.*
- Take the medication exactly as prescribed, including the same manufacturer's product each time the prescription is refilled as *switching brands may result in alterations in seizure control.*
- Administer the drug with food *to alleviate GI irritation if GI upset is a problem.*
- Patients taking medication should be advised to avoid alcohol and caffeine, both of which can precipitate seizures.
- Monitor for adverse effects and provide appropriate supportive care as needed *to help the patient cope with these effects.*
- Monitor for drug–drug interactions *to arrange to adjust dosages appropriately if any drug is added or withdrawn from the drug regime.*
- Arrange for counselling for women of childbearing age who are taking these drugs. *These drugs have the potential to cause serious damage to the foetus,* and women should understand the risk of birth defects and use barrier contraceptives to avoid pregnancy (some of these drugs interact with oral contraceptives).
- Provide thorough patient teaching, including drug name and prescribed dosage, as well as measures for avoidance of adverse effects, warning signs that may indicate possible problems, and the need for monitoring and evaluation *to enhance patient knowledge about drug therapy and to promote compliance.* (See Critical Thinking Scenario 22-1.)
- Suggest the wearing of a MedicAlert bracelet *to alert emergency workers and health care providers about the use of an antiseizure drug.*
- Advise patients on general safety, such as avoid taking deep baths or swimming on your own, avoid using dangerous machinery.
- Avoid taking over-the-counter preparations and herbal remedies without prior consultation with the health care provider due to the potential for interaction between antiseizure medication and other drugs.

Evaluation

- Monitor patient response to the drug (decrease in incidence or absence of seizures).
- Monitor for adverse effects (CNS changes, GI disturbances, bone marrow suppression, severe dermatological reactions, liver toxicity, visual field defects, renal stones).
- Monitoring of plasma drug concentrations is required if toxicity or nonadherence to treatment is suspected, to adjust the dose of phenytoin,

to manage pharmacokinetic interactions or in specific clinical conditions such as status epilepticus.

- Evaluate effectiveness of teaching plan (patient can give the drug name and dosage and name possible adverse effects to watch for, and specific measures to prevent adverse effects; patient is aware of the risk of birth defects and the need to carry information about the diagnosis and use of this drug).
- A review should be held annually with a specialist to discuss drug effectiveness, tolerability, side-effects and adherence.

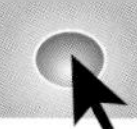

WEB LINKS

Health care providers and patients may want to consult the following Internet sources:

http://bnfc.org The BNF for Children provides UK health care professionals with authoritative and practical information on the selection and clinical use of medicines in children.

http://cks.library.nhs.uk The National Health Service Clinical Knowledge Summaries provides evidence-based practical information on the common conditions observed in primary care.

http://www.bnf.org.uk The BNF provides UK health care professionals with authoritative and practical information on the selection and clinical use of medicines.

http://www.dh.gov.uk The Department of Health provides information on the model for improving care for patients with long term conditions, including providing every patient with a personalized care plan.

http://www.direct.gov.uk The information on medical rules for all drivers can be found here (originally found under Driver and Vehicle Licensing Agency site).

http://www.epilepsy.org.uk Epilepsy Action is part of the British Epilepsy Association and provides information to patients and their families, including details of branches throughout the UK that can provide local support.

http://www.medicalert.org.uk MedicAlert is a registered charity providing a life-saving identification system for individuals with hidden medical conditions and allergies.

http://www.nhsdirect.nhs.uk The National Health Service Direct service provides patients with information and advice about health, illness and health services.

http://www.nice.org.uk The National Institute for Health and Clinical Excellence provides guidance on public health, new and existing treatments within the NHS and also information on the most appropriate care for patients.

Points to Remember

- Epilepsy is a collection of different syndromes, all of which have the same characteristic: a sudden discharge of excessive electrical energy from nerve cells located within the brain. This event is called a seizure.
- Seizures can be divided into two groups: generalized and partial (focal).
- Generalized seizures can be further classified as tonic–clonic (grand mal); absence (petit mal); myoclonic; febrile; and rapidly recurrent (status epilepticus).
- Partial (focal) seizures can be further classified as simple or complex.
- Drug treatment depends on the type of seizure that the patient has experienced and the toxicity associated with the available agents.
- Drug treatment is directed at stabilizing the overexcited nerve cell membranes and/or increasing the effectiveness of GABA, an inhibitory neurotransmitter.
- Adverse effects associated with antiseizures (e.g. insomnia, fatigue, confusion, suicidal thoughts, GI depression, bradycardia) reflect the CNS depression caused by the drugs.
- Other adverse effects include bone marrow depression, renal and hepatic impairment and hypersensitivity reactions.
- Many of the antiseizure drugs can have adverse effects on the foetus. However, uncontrolled epilepsy is a greater risk to the unborn child and mothers are advised to remain on the lowest dose possible.
- Patients treated with an antiseizure medication should be advised to wear a MedicAlert notification to alert emergency medical professionals to their epilepsy and their use of antiseizure drugs.

CRITICAL THINKING SCENARIO 22-1

Antiseizure Drugs

The Situation

Jonathan, an athletic, 18-year-old student, suffered his first seizure during a lesson. He seemed attentive and alert, and then he suddenly slumped to the floor and suffered a full tonic–clonic (grand mal) seizure. The other students were frightened and did not know what to do. Fortunately, the teacher was familiar with seizures and quickly reacted to protect Jonathan from hurting himself and to explain what was happening.

Jonathan was diagnosed with idiopathic (cause unknown) generalized epilepsy with tonic–clonic (grand mal) seizures. The carbamazepine he was prescribed was unable to control the seizures, and he suffered three more seizures in the next month – one at school and two at home. Jonathan is now undergoing re-evaluation for possible drug adjustment and counselling.

Critical Thinking

- What teaching implications should be considered when meeting with Jonathan? *Consider his age and the setting of his first seizure.*
- What problems might Jonathan encounter in school and in athletics related to the diagnosis and the prescribed medication? *Consider measures that may help him avoid some of the unpleasant side-effects related to this particular drug therapy.*
- What problems can be anticipated and confronted before they occur concerning laws that forbid individuals with newly diagnosed epilepsy from driving?
- Develop a teaching plan for Jonathan. How will you involve the entire family?

Discussion

On their first meeting, it is important for the nurse to establish a trusting relationship with Jonathan and his family. Jonathan requires a great deal of support and encouragement to cope with the diagnosis of epilepsy and the need for drug therapy. He may need to voice his concerns and discuss how he can return to school without worrying about having a seizure in class. The nurse should implement a thorough drug teaching plan, including a description of warning signs to watch for that should be reported to a health care professional. Jonathan should be encouraged to take the following preventive measures:

- Avoid driving, operating dangerous machinery or performing tasks that require alertness while drowsy and confused.
- Pace activities as much as possible to help deal with any fatigue and malaise.
- Take the drug with meals if GI upset is a problem.
- Avoid alcohol and caffeine, which may precipitate seizures.

This information should be given to both Jonathan and his family in written form for future reference, along with the name of a health care professional to contact with questions or comments. The importance of continuous medication to suppress the seizures should be stressed. The adverse effects of many of these drugs make it difficult for some patients to remain compliant with their drug regimen.

The nurse may be asked to meet with his family members, to provide support and encouragement to deal with his diagnosis and its implications. They need to know what seizures are, how the prescribed antiseizure drugs affect the seizures, what they can do when seizures occur, and complete information about the drugs he must take and their anticipated drug effects. In addition, it is important to work with family members to determine whether any particular stimulus that precipitated the seizures. In other words, was there any warning or aura? This may help with adjustment of drug dosages or avoidance of certain situations or stimuli that precipitate seizures. Family members should be encouraged to report and record any seizure activity that occurs.

Jonathan's condition is a chronic one that will require continual drug therapy and evaluation. He may be interested in referral to a support group for other young people with epilepsy, where he can share ideas, support and frustrations. He may need periodic re-teaching and should have the opportunity to ask additional questions. Jonathan should be encouraged to wear a MedicAlert tag so that emergency medical personnel are aware of his diagnosis and the medications he is taking.

Nursing Care Guide for Jonathan: Antiseizure Agents

Assessment: History and Examination

- Allergies to carbamazepine; history of cardiac arrhythmias, bone marrow suppression, porphyria, hepatic or renal dysfunction

Antiseizure Drugs *(continued)*

- Concurrent use of analgesics, antibacterials, anticoagulants, antidepressants, other antiseizures, antifungals, antimalarials, antipsychotics, antivirals, calcium channel blockers, ciclosporin, corticosteroids, diuretics, cimetidine
- Cardiovascular: blood pressure, pulse, peripheral perfusion
- CNS: orientation, reflexes, affect, strength, EEG
- Skin: colour, lesions, temperature
- Respiratory: respiratory rate and depth, adventitious sounds
- Laboratory tests: full blood count, liver and renal function tests

Nursing Diagnoses

- Acute pain related to GI, CNS and genitourinary effects
- Risk of injury related to CNS effects
- Disturbed thought processes related to CNS effects
- Deficient knowledge regarding drug therapy
- Impaired skin integrity related to dermatological effects
- Altered self-esteem due to stigma of having epilepsy or due to loss of control during a seizure
- Potential for depression due to having a long-term condition and/or restrictions on lifestyle

Implementation

- Specialist advice should be sought at first sign of blood or liver dysfunction or skin rash.
- Provide comfort and safety measures: give with meals.
- Provide support and reassurance to cope with diagnosis, restrictions and drug effects.
- Provide patient teaching regarding drug name, dosage, side-effects, symptoms to report, and the need to wear MedicAlert information; other drugs to avoid.

Evaluation

- Evaluate drug effects: decrease in incidence and frequency of seizures.
- Patient should report any adverse effects: GI effects (nausea, vomiting, anorexia, constipation or diarrhoea); CNS effects (dizziness, drowsiness, headache, confusion); abnormal heart beats. Immediate medical attention should be sought if the patient or carer recognizes the symptoms of fever, sore throat, rash, mouth ulcers, bruising or bleeding.
- Monitor for drug–drug interactions: increased depression with CNS depressants, alcohol; drugs as listed.
- Evaluate effectiveness of patient teaching programme.
- Evaluate effectiveness of comfort/safety measures.

Patient Teaching for Jonathan

- ☐ The drug that is being evaluated for you is called an antiseizure or antiepileptic drug. It is used to stabilize abnormal electrical activity in cells in the brain that are overactive and causing seizures.
- ☐ The timing of these doses is very important. To be effective, this drug must be taken regularly.
- ☐ Do not stop taking this drug suddenly. If for any reason you are unable to continue taking the drug, notify your health care provider at once. This drug must be slowly withdrawn (over 2 to 3 months or longer) under the guidance of the specialist when its use is discontinued.
- ☐ Common effects of these drugs include:
  - *Fatigue, weakness and drowsiness:* Try to space activities evenly throughout the day and allow rest periods to avoid these effects. Take safety precautions and avoid operating dangerous machinery if these conditions occur.
  - *Headaches:* These usually disappear as your body adjusts to the drug. If they persist and become too uncomfortable, consult with your health care provider.
  - *GI upset, loss of appetite and diarrhoea or constipation:* Taking the drug with food or eating small, frequent meals may help alleviate this problem.
  - Report any of the following conditions to your health care provider: *skin rash, fever, sore throat, mouth ulcers, and unusual bleeding or bruising.*
- ☐ It is advisable to wear a MedicAlert warning so that any person who takes care of you in an emergency will know that you are taking this drug.
- ☐ Tell any doctor, nurse or other health care provider involved in your care that you are taking this drug.
- ☐ Keep this drug and all medications out of the reach of children.
- ☐ Do not take any other drug, including over-the-counter medications and alcohol, without consulting with your health care provider. Many of these preparations interact with the drug and could cause adverse effects.

(continued)

Antiseizure Drugs *(continued)*

- ☐ Report and record any seizure activity that you have while you are taking this drug.
- ☐ Take this drug exactly as prescribed. Regular medical follow-up will be necessary to evaluate the effects of this drug on your body.
- ☐ Offer support and encouragement *to help the patient cope with the drug regimen.*

Evaluation

- Monitor patient response to the drug (decrease in incidence or absence of seizures; serum drug levels within the therapeutic range).
- Monitor for adverse effects (CNS changes, GI depression, arrhythmias, liver toxicity, blood disorders and severe dermatological reactions).
- Evaluate effectiveness of teaching plan (patient can give the drug name and dosage and name possible adverse effects to watch for, and specific measures to prevent adverse effects; patient is aware of the risk of birth defects and the need to carry information about the diagnosis and use of this drug).
- Monitor the effectiveness of comfort measures and compliance with the regimen.

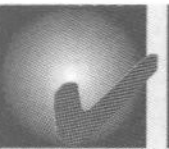

CHECK YOUR UNDERSTANDING

Answers to the questions in this chapter may be found in the answer key in the back of the book.

Multiple Choice

Select the best answer to the following.

1. Epilepsy is
   a. always characterized by grand mal seizures.
   b. only a genetic problem.
   c. the most prevalent neurological disorder.
   d. the name given to one brain disorder.

2. Generalized seizures could include all of the following except
   a. petit mal seizures.
   b. febrile seizures.
   c. grand mal seizures.
   d. partial seizures.

3. Patients who are maintained on an antiseizure drug should be encouraged to
   a. give up their driver's license.
   b. wear a MedicAlert notice.
   c. take antihistamines to help dry up secretions.
   d. keep the diagnosis a secret to avoid prejudice.

4. Drugs that are commonly used to treat grand mal seizures include
   a. barbiturates, benzodiazepines and hydantoins.
   b. barbiturates, antihistamines and local anaesthetics.
   c. hydantoins, phenobarbital and succinimides.
   d. benzodiazepines, succinimides and sodium valproate.

5. The drug of choice for the treatment of absence seizures is
   a. sodium valproate.
   b. diazepam.
   c. primidone.
   d. topiramate.

6. Focal or partial seizures
   a. start at one point and spread quickly throughout the brain.
   b. are best treated with benzodiazepines.
   c. involve only one area of the brain.
   d. are easily diagnosed and recognized.

7. Treatment of epilepsy is directed at
   a. blocking the transmission of nerve impulses into the brain.
   b. stabilizing overexcited nerve membranes and/or increasing the inhibitory neurotransmitter GABA.
   c. blocking peripheral nerve terminals.
   d. thickening the meninges to reduce brain electrical activity.

Extended Matching Questions

Select **all** that apply.

1. A patient has been stabilized on phenytoin for several years and has not experienced a grand mal seizure in more than 3 years. The patient decides to stop the drug because it no longer seems to be needed. In counselling the patient, the nurse should include which of the following points?
   a. He will always need this drug.
   b. This drug needs to be slowly tapered to avoid potentially serious adverse effects.
   c. He is probably correct and the drug is not needed.
   d. The drug should not be stopped until appropriate blood tests are done.
   e. Stopping the drug suddenly could precipitate seizures because the nerves will be more sensitive.

2. The most common adverse effects associated with antiseizure therapy reflect the depression of the CNS. In assessing a client on antiseizure therapy, the nurse would monitor the patient for which of the following?
   a. Hypertension
   b. Insomnia
   c. Confusion
   d. GI depression
   e. Tachycardia

Fill in the Blanks

1. ____________________, the most prevalent of the neurological disorders, is a collection of different syndromes, all characterized by a sudden discharge of excessive electrical energy from nerve cells located within the brain.

2. Sudden discharge of excessive electrical energy in the brain leads to a ________________ .

3. If motor nerves are stimulated by this sudden discharge of electrical energy, a_______________may occur with tonic–clonic muscle contractions.

4. Epilepsy is managed using a class of drugs called ____________________ .

5. Tonic–clonic seizures, formerly known as ____________________, involve dramatic tonic–clonic muscle contractions, loss of consciousness, and a recovery period that is characterized by confusion and exhaustion.

6. A petit mal seizure, now called a(n)_____________, involves abrupt, brief (3–5 seconds) periods of loss of consciousness.

7. Seizures that involve short, sporadic periods of muscle contractions that last for several minutes are called______________________ .

8. Seizures that are related to very high fevers and usually involve convulsions are called_________________ .

9. The most dangerous of seizure conditions is a state in which seizures rapidly recur again and again, which is referred to as ______________________ .

10. Partial or___________________seizures involve one area of the brain and do not spread throughout the entire brain.

Bibliography and References

Bellman, M., & Peile, E. (2006). *The normal child.* Philadelphia: Churchill Livingstone.

British Medical Association and Royal Pharmaceutical Society of Great Britain. (2008). *British National Formulary*. London: BMJ & RPS Publishing. *This publication is updated biannually: it is imperative that the most recent edition is consulted.*

British Medical Association and Royal Pharmaceutical Society of Great Britain. (2008). *British National Formulary for Children*. London: BMJ & RPS Publishing. *This publication is updated annually: it is imperative that the most recent edition is consulted.*

Brunton, L., Lazo, J. S., Parker, K., Goodman, L. S., & Gilman, A. G. (2005). *Goodman and Gilman's the pharmacological basis of therapeutics* (11th ed.). London: McGraw-Hill.

Galbraith, A., Bullock, S., Manias, E., Hunt, B., & Richards, A. (2007). *Fundamentals of Pharmacology. An Applied Approach for Nursing and Health.* (2nd ed.). Harlow: Pearson Education Ltd.

Howland, R. D., & Mycek, M. J. (2005). *Pharmacology* (3rd ed.). Philadelphia: Lippincott Williams & Wilkins.

Medicines and Healthcare products Regulatory Agency. (2008). Antiepileptics. Available from http://www.mhra.gov.uk

National Institute for Health and Clinical Excellence. (2004). *Clinical Guide 20: The epilepsies: the diagnosis and management of the epilepsies in adults and children in primary and secondary care.* Available from http://www.nice.org.uk

Porth, C. M., & Matfin, G. (2008). *Pathophysiology: Concepts of altered health states* (8th ed.). Philadelphia: Lippincott Williams & Wilkins.

Rang, H. P., Dale, M. M., Ritter, J. M., & Flower, R. J. (2007). *Rang and Dale's pharmacology* (6th ed.). Philadelphia: Churchill Livingstone.

Simonsen, T., Aarbakke, J., Kay, I., Coleman, I., Sinnott, P., & Lysaa, R. (2006). *Illustrated pharmacology for nurses.* London: Hodder Arnold.

CHAPTER 23

Antiparkinsonism Agents

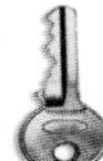

KEY TERMS

basal nuclei

bradykinesia

catechol-*O*-methyl transferase (COMT)

corpus striatum

dopaminergic

dopa-decarboxylase inhibitors

Parkinson's disease

substantia nigra

LEARNING OBJECTIVES

Upon completion of this chapter, you will be able to:

1. Describe the current theory of the cause of Parkinson's disease and correlate this with the clinical presentation of the disease.
2. Describe the therapeutic actions, indications, pharmacokinetics, contraindications, most common adverse reactions and important drug–drug interactions associated with therapies used to treat Parkinson's disease.
3. Discuss the use of antiparkinsonism drugs across the lifespan.
4. Compare and contrast the key drugs for each class of antiparkinsonism agents with the other drugs in that class and with drugs from the other classes used to treat the disease.
5. Outline the nursing considerations and teaching needs for patients receiving each class of antiparkinsonism agents.

DOPAMINERGICS

amantadine
apomorphine
bromocriptine
carbergoline
co-beneldopa
co-careldopa
entacapone
levodopa
pergolide
pramipexole
rasagiline
ropinirole
rotigotine
selegiline
tolcapone

ANTIMUSCARINICS

benzatropine
orphenadrine
procyclidine
trihexyphenidyl

Parkinsonism relates to a group of movement disorders. The most common cause of parkinsonism is **Parkinson's disease**, a progressive degenerative disorder of the central nervous system (CNS). Parkinson's disease could develop at any age (Box 23.1), but usually affects those in their 60s and 70s. Therapy is aimed at the management of signs and symptoms to provide optimal functioning for as long as possible.

Parkinsonism and Parkinson's Disease

Parkinsonism is characterized by tremor observed at rest, muscle rigidity, **bradykinesia** (extreme slowness or sluggishness of movement) and a lack of co-ordination. Rhythmic tremors develop, relatively inconspicuously at first. In some muscle groups, these tremors lead to rigidity and in others, weakness. Affected patients may have trouble maintaining position or posture and they may exhibit marked difficulties in performing intentional movements. As Parkinson's disease progresses, walking becomes a problem; a shuffling gait is a hallmark of the condition. In addition, patients may drool and their speech may become slow and slurred. As the cranial nerves are affected, patients develop a mask-like expression. The higher levels of the cerebral cortex are not affected, so a very alert and intelligent person may be trapped inside a progressively degenerating body.

Parkinson's disease is also known as *primary* or *idiopathic* parkinsonism, meaning the cause of the condition is unknown. However, a number of genetic mutations have now been identified therefore this categorization is not strictly accurate. *Secondary* parkinsonism refers to cases associated with drug toxicity, brain injuries or other medical conditions.

Causal Theories

Although the cause of Parkinson's disease is not known in every case, it is known that the signs and symptoms of the disease relate to damage to neurons in the **basal nuclei** of the brain. Theories about the cause of the degeneration range from generalized viral infection, blows to the head, brain infection, atherosclerosis and exposure to certain drugs and environmental factors, for example exposure to certain pesticides.

The mechanism that causes the signs and symptoms of Parkinson's disease is clearly understood. As described in Chapter 18, the motor cortex in the brain controls movement of voluntary muscles. The output of the motor cortex is modulated by impulses from other areas of the brain, including the basal nuclei and the thalamus. The basal nuclei are areas of grey matter lying deep within the cerebral hemispheres, which assist in co-ordinating motor activity for unconscious voluntary movements such as posture and gait. The basal nuclei includes the **substantia nigra** and **corpus**

BOX 23.1 DRUG THERAPY ACROSS THE LIFESPAN

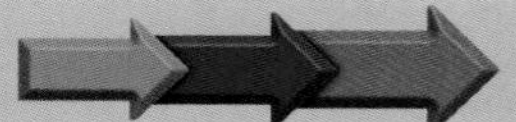

Antiparkinsonism Agents

CHILDREN

The safety and effectiveness of most of these drugs has not been established in children. There is no incidence of Parkinson's disease in children; however, children can experience parkinsonian symptoms as a result of drug effects, such as phenothiazines used to treat nausea and vomiting.

When administering any drug to children, always consult the most recent edition of the British National Formulary for Children.

ADULTS

The eventual dependence and lack of control that accompany Parkinson's disease are devastating to all patients and their families but may be particularly overwhelming to individuals in the prime of their life who value high degrees of autonomy, self-determination and independence. It is important for the nurse to assess all families with sensitivity to determine what convictions they hold and plan nursing care accordingly. Adults diagnosed with Parkinson's disease require extensive teaching, support and help in coping with the disease as well as with the effects of the drugs.

Women of childbearing age should be advised to use contraception when they are on these drugs. If pregnancy does occur, or is desired, they need counselling about the potential for adverse effects. Women who are nursing should be encouraged to find another method of feeding the baby because of the potential for adverse drug effects on the baby.

With the increasing interest in herbal and alternative therapies, it is important to stress the need to inform the health care provider about any other treatment being used. Vitamin B_6 can pose a serious problem for patients who are taking some of these drugs.

OLDER ADULTS

Although Parkinson's disease may affect individuals of any age, gender or nationality, the frequency of the disease increases with age. This debilitating condition, which affects more men than women, may be one of many chronic problems associated with ageing.

The drugs that are used to manage Parkinson's disease are associated with more adverse effects in older people with long-term problems. Both antimuscarinic and **dopaminergic** drugs aggravate glaucoma, benign prostatic hypertrophy, constipation, cardiac problems and chronic obstructive pulmonary diseases. Special precautions and frequent follow-up visits are necessary for older patients with Parkinson's disease and their drug dosages may need to be adjusted frequently to avoid serious problems. In many cases, other agents are given to counteract the effects of these drugs and patients then have complicated drug regimes with many associated adverse effects and problems. Consequently, it is essential for these patients to have extensive written protocols for their drugs.

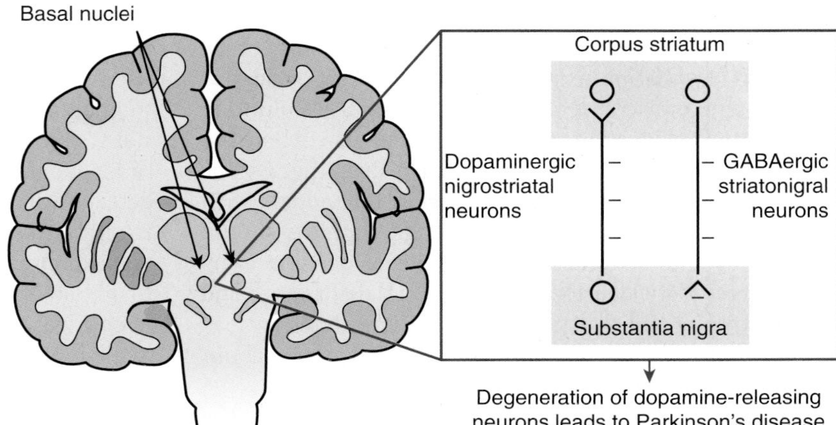

FIGURE 23.1 Schematic representation of the degeneration of neurons that leads to Parkinson's disease. Cells in the corpus striatum send impulses to the substantia nigra using GABA to inhibit activity. In turn, the substantia nigra sends impulses to the corpus striatum, using dopamine.

striatum (Figure 23.1) which together, regulate the activity of the motor cortex and assist in maintaining muscle tone.

Within the basal nuclei are groups of neurons, which release either dopamine, γ-aminobutyric acid (GABA) or acetylcholine (ACh). In Parkinson's disease there is a loss of dopaminergic neurons in the substantia nigra. The reduction in dopamine release from the dopaminergic neurons leads to reduced output from the motor cortex and the muscle rigidity and tremor observed in Parkinson's disease. As the number of dopaminergic neurons lost increases, the symptoms become progressively worse.

ACh also plays a role in the symptoms of Parkinson's disease. This excitatory neurotransmitter is released from neurons in the area of the corpus striatum to co-ordinate intentional movements of the body. The release of ACh is inhibited by dopamine. When there is a decrease in dopamine in the area as in Parkinson's disease, this leads to increased activity of the cholinergic neurons and the cholinergic neurons dominate. This neurotransmitter imbalance affects the functioning of the basal nuclei and of the cortical and cerebellar components of the extrapyramidal motor system. The extrapyramidal system is one that provides co-ordination for unconscious voluntary muscle movements, including those that control position, posture and movement. The result of this imbalance in the motor system is apparent as the manifestations of Parkinson's disease (see Figure 23.1).

Drug Therapy

Currently, there is no treatment that arrests the neuronal degeneration in Parkinson's disease and the eventual decline in patient function. Drug therapy remains the primary treatment and is aimed at restoring the balance between the declining levels of dopamine and the now-dominant cholinergic neurons (Figure 23.2). This may help to reduce the signs and symptoms of parkinsonism and restore normal

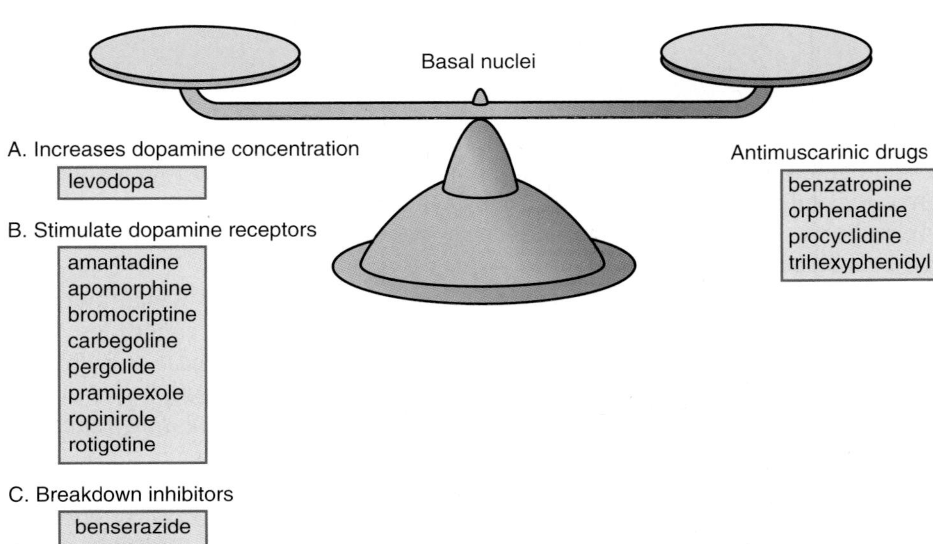

FIGURE 23.2 Drug therapy in treating Parkinson's disease is aimed at achieving a balance between the cholinergic effects and the effects of dopamine in the basal nuclei.

function for a time. Surgery (either surgical lesion in the thalamus, globus pallidus or subthalamic nucleus; or by deep brain stimulation using an implanted device) can also provide a temporary relief of tremor and abnormal voluntary movements (dyskinesia) and is considered in cases where the symptoms are not effectively controlled by drug therapy.

Total management of patient care in individuals with Parkinson's disease presents a challenge. Patients should be encouraged to be as active as possible, to perform exercises to prevent the development of skeletal deformities and muscle atrophy and to attend to their own care as long as they can. Both the patient and family need instruction about following drug protocols and monitoring adverse effects, as well as encouragement and support for coping with the progressive nature of the disease. The degenerative effects of this disease mean patients may become depressed and emotional and will require a great deal of psychological, as well as physical, support.

Dopaminergics

Dopaminergics, drugs that increase the effects of dopamine at receptor sites, are more effective than antimuscarinics in the treatment of parkinsonism. Dopamine itself cannot be used because it is rapidly broken down by enzymes in the wall of the GI tract, the liver and plasma. In addition, dopamine does not cross the blood–brain barrier. Drugs that are dopamine precursors, act like dopamine, or increase dopamine concentrations indirectly, must be used to increase dopamine levels in the brain. These drugs are effective as long as sufficient intact neurons remain in the substantia nigra to respond to increased levels of dopamine. After the neural degeneration has progressed beyond a certain point, patients no longer respond to these drugs.

Levodopa, a precursor of dopamine, crosses the blood–brain barrier where it is converted to dopamine. In this way, levodopa replenishes the depleted dopamine levels (see Critical Thinking Scenario 23-1). However, levodopa is rapidly metabolized to dopamine in the periphery and only a small amount reaches the brain. Levodopa is therefore given in combination with **dopa-decarboxylase inhibitors**, for example carbidopa (co-careldopa) or benserazide (co-beneldopa). In this combination form, carbidopa or benserazide inhibit the enzyme *dopa decarboxylase* in the periphery (carbidopa and benserazide are unable to cross the blood–brain barrier), diminishing the metabolism of levodopa in the gastrointestinal (GI) tract and in peripheral tissues and leading to higher levels crossing the blood–brain barrier. As these dopa-decarboxylase inhibitors decrease the amount of levodopa needed to reach a therapeutic level in the brain, the dosage of levodopa can be decreased, which reduces the incidence of adverse side-effects.

Entacapone and tolcapone are inhibitors of the enzyme **catechol-*O*-methyl transferase (COMT)**, which breaks down catecholamines, including dopamine. These drugs prevent the peripheral breakdown of levodopa and are used with levodopa and dopa-decarboxylase inhibitors to increase levels of levodopa reaching the brain (see Box 23.2). These drugs also increase the duration of action of levodopa and are useful for patients who experience a deterioration of symptoms between doses. Both drugs are readily absorbed from the GI tract, metabolized in the liver and excreted in urine and faeces. There is a risk of hepatotoxicity with tolcapone and is therefore contraindicated in liver disease. Both should be avoided during pregnancy and while breast-feeding.

Therapeutic Actions and Indications

The dopaminergic drugs are indicated for the relief of the signs and symptoms of Parkinson's disease. These drugs work by directly stimulating dopamine receptors in the substantia nigra. This action helps to restore the balance between the inhibitory and stimulating neurons. After degeneration has progressed to the extent that the nerves are damaged or gone, these drugs are no longer effective: these drugs control Parkinson's disease only as long as functioning dopamine receptors remain in the substantia nigra.

Pharmacokinetics

The dopaminergics are generally well absorbed from the GI tract and widely distributed in the body. Apomorphine must be given subcutaneously. The dopaminergics are metabolized in the liver and peripheral cells and excreted in the urine. These drugs can cross the placenta and most dopaminergics are not recommended for use during pregnancy. Pergolide, pramipexole, ropinirole and tolcapone can be used during pregnancy if the benefits to the mother clearly outweigh the potential risks to the foetus. Dopaminergics can also enter breast milk and should not be used during lactation because of the potential for adverse effects in the baby. Some may also suppress lactation.

Contraindications and Cautions

The dopaminergics are contraindicated in the following conditions: history of skin melanoma with levodopa *because this drug has been associated with the development of melanoma*; history of fibrotic disorders *because some dopaminergics can cause fibrotic reactions*; pregnancy *because these drugs cross the placenta and could adversely affect the foetus* and lactation *because of potential adverse effects on the baby or suppression of lactation.*

Caution should be *used with any condition that could be exacerbated by dopamine receptor stimulation*, such as cardiovascular disease, including myocardial infarction, arrhythmias, hypertension; pulmonary disease; fibrosis; history of peptic ulcers; angle-closure glaucoma; urinary tract obstruction; and psychiatric disorders. Care should also be taken in renal and hepatic disease, *which could interfere with the metabolism and excretion of these drugs. In particular, tolcapone can cause hepatotoxicity.*

Adverse Effects

The adverse effects associated with the dopaminergics usually result from stimulation of dopamine receptors. CNS effects may include anxiety, depression, nervousness, headache, malaise, fatigue, confusion, disturbed dreams, mental changes, blurred vision, muscle twitching and ataxia. Peripheral effects may include anorexia, nausea, vomiting, dysphagia, dyspepsia and constipation or diarrhoea; angina, cardiac arrhythmias, hypotension and palpitations; bizarre breathing patterns; urinary retention and urgency; and dry mouth, flushing, increased sweating and hot flushes. Bone marrow depression and hepatic dysfunction have also been reported. Patients on prolonged pergolide, bromocriptine or carbegoline therapy should be monitored for dyspnoea, persistent cough, chest or cardiac pain, cardiac failure and abdominal pain.

Clinically Important Drug–Drug Interactions

If the dopaminergic MAO-B and COMT inhibitors are combined with antidepressant treatments (other MAO inhibitors, tricyclics, selective serotonin reuptake inhibitors) or sympathomimetic drugs, therapeutic effects increase and a risk of hypertensive crisis exists. The antidepressant treatment should be stopped at least

BOX 23.2 Current Combination Therapy

A fixed-combination tablet is available for patients who are at a point in their Parkinson's disease where they require the addition of the adjunct drug entacapone. This fixed combination tablet contains levodopa, carbidopa and entacapone, reducing the number of tablets the patient needs to swallow each day. The tablet comes in three strengths:

- 50 mg levodopa, 12.5 mg carbidopa, 200 mg entacapone
- 100 mg levodopa, 25 mg carbidopa, 200 mg entacapone
- 150 mg levodopa, 37.5 mg carbidopa, 200 mg entacapone

Patients should be stabilized on each drug separately before switching to the correct preparation of the fixed-combination product. The usual dose is one tablet to a maximum of 10 tablets per day.

One of the major problems for patients who have taken levodopa for a long time is the 'on–off' effect, where the patient rapidly switches from dyskinesia (the 'on' phase) to hypokinesia and rigidity (the 'off' phase). This is extremely distressing for the patient. This effect is believed to relate to changes in the plasma concentration of levodopa.

This phenomenon is not seen with other treatments and therefore dopamine receptor agonists are often used as a first-line treatment. These drugs mimic the effects of dopamine and include the following:

- Apomorphine is approved for the intermittent treatment of hypomobility 'off' periods caused between doses and unpredictable on–off episodes seen in advanced Parkinson's disease. Often prescribed to those patients whose symptoms are not well controlled by co-careldopa, co-beneldopa or other dopaminergic agonists. Apomorphine is given subcutaneously with an antiemetic; there is a risk of hypotension with this drug and haemolytic anaemia if prescribed with levodopa, so the patient must be monitored closely.
- Bromocriptine, cabergoline, pergolide, pramipexole and ropinirole all bind to dopamine receptors in the CNS. They can be used either alone or as an adjunct to co-careldopa or co-beneldopa. Pramipexole and ropinirole are also approved for the treatment of restless legs syndrome. These drugs have the advantage of a longer duration of action meaning thereby that patients can reduce the frequency of dosing. When treating with pergolide, bromocriptine or carbegoline, patients should be monitored for fibrotic reactions in the lungs, heart and abdomen. The Committee for the Safety of Medicines (CSM) recommends that a chest X-ray should be obtained and serum creatinine (to assess renal function) and erythrocyte sedimentation rate (a nonspecific measure of inflammation) measured prior to treatment. Periodic spirometry tests can be used to assess lung function. Patients should also be monitored for dyspnoea (difficulty breathing), a persistent cough, chest pain, cardiac failure (oedema, hypertension) and abdominal pain or tenderness (CSM, 2008).
- Rotigotine is used as a monotherapy in the early stages of Parkinson's disease or as an adjunct to co-careldopa or co-beneldopa.

Other dopaminergic drugs either increase the amount of dopamine released or reduce dopamine metabolism. Amantadine, originally used as an antiviral agent, increases the amount of dopamine released from nerve terminals and is effective as long as there is a possibility of more dopamine release. This drug can help reduce the tremor and rigidity associated with Parkinson's disease.

Dopamine levels can also be boosted by reducing dopamine metabolism through inhibition of monoamine oxidase B (MAO-B), the enzyme that breaks down dopamine in the synaptic cleft. Selegiline and rasagiline are both irreversible inhibitors of MAO-B and can be used alone or as an adjunct to levodopa with dopa-decarboxylase inhibitors. Both drugs are well absorbed from the GI tract, extensively metabolized in the liver and excreted in urine. There is a potential interaction between selegiline and rasagiline and other MAO inhibitors (e.g. antidepressants) and sympathomimetics. The risk of MAO inhibitor-induced hypertensive effects (see Chapter 20) means patients should be urged to immediately report severe headaches and any other unusual symptoms that they have not experienced before. Both selegiline and rasagiline should be avoided during pregnancy and breast-feeding.

5 weeks before beginning therapy with either selegiline or rasagiline.

The combination of levodopa with vitamin B_6 or with phenytoin may lead to decreased efficacy of levodopa. In addition, patients who take dopaminergics should be cautioned to avoid over-the-counter vitamins; if such medications are used, the patient should be monitored closely because a decrease in effectiveness may result. Reduced effectiveness may also result if dopaminergics are combined with dopamine antagonists.

Always consult a current copy of the British National Formulary for further guidance.

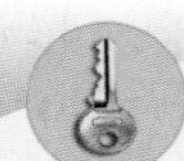

Key Drug Summary: Levodopa

Indications: Treatment of parkinsonism (but not drug-associated extrapyramidal symptoms)

Actions: A dopamine precursor which replaces the depleted dopamine associated with parkinsonism; crosses the blood–brain barrier, where it is converted to dopamine and acts as a replacement neurotransmitter

Pharmacokinetics:

Route	Onset	Peak	Duration
Oral	Varies	0.5–2 h	5 h

$T_{1/2}$: 1.5 hours; metabolized in the liver, excreted in the urine

Adverse effects: Abnormal involuntary movements (dyskinesia), increased hand tremor, anorexia, nausea, vomiting, insomnia, agitation, postural hypotension, dizziness, cardiac irregularities, hypomania and psychosis, depression, drowsiness, headache, flushing, sweating, GI bleeding.

Nursing Considerations for Receiving Dopaminergic Antiparkinsonism Drugs

Assessment: History and Examination

Screen for the following conditions, *which could be contraindications or cautions for the use of the drug*: any known allergies to these drugs or drug components; gastric ulceration; cardiac arrhythmias or underlying cardiac disease; postural hypotension; glaucoma; respiratory disease; pregnancy or lactation; and renal or hepatic dysfunction. With levodopa, check for skin lesions or history of melanoma. With apomorphine, check for prolonged QT interval using an electrocardiogram.

Include screening *to determine baseline status before beginning therapy and to monitor for any potential adverse effects.* Assess the following: temperature; skin colour and lesions; CNS orientation, affect, reflexes, bilateral grip strength and spasticity; vision; respiration and adventitious sounds; pulse, blood pressure and cardiac output (e.g. skin colour, peripheral temperature); and urinary output and bladder palpation. Check liver and renal function tests and full blood count.

Establish if patient is currently taking other medications or herbal therapies, which may potentially interact with the proposed drug.

Nursing Diagnoses

The patient taking a dopaminergic antiparkinsonism drug may have the following nursing diagnoses related to drug therapy:

- Acute pain related to GI, CNS and genitourinary (GU) effects
- Disturbed thought processes related to CNS effects
- Risk for injury related to CNS effects and incidence of postural hypotension
- Deficient knowledge regarding drug therapy

Implementation With Rationale

- Arrange to decrease dosage of the drug if therapy has been interrupted for any reason *to prevent acute peripheral dopaminergic effects.*
- Evaluate disease progress and signs and symptoms periodically and record *for reference of disease progress and drug response.*
- Give the drugs with meals *to alleviate GI irritation if GI upset is a problem.*
- Monitor bowel function and implement a bowel programme *if constipation is severe.*
- Ensure that the patient empties the bladder before taking the drugs *if urinary retention is a problem.*
- Establish safety precautions if CNS or vision changes occur *to prevent patient injury.*
- Monitor hepatic, renal and haematological tests periodically during therapy *to detect early signs of dysfunction and consider re-evaluation of drug therapy.*
- Provide support services and comfort measures as needed *to improve patient concordance.*
- Provide thorough patient teaching about topics such as the drug name and prescribed dosage, measures

to help avoid adverse effects, warning signs that may indicate problems and the need for periodic monitoring and evaluation *to enhance patient knowledge about drug therapy and to promote compliance.*

- Provide support *to help the patient cope with the disease and drug regimen.*

Evaluation

- Monitor patient response to the drug (improvement in signs and symptoms of parkinsonism).
- Monitor for adverse effects (CNS changes, urinary retention, GI depression, tachycardia, increased sweating, flushing). Fibrotic reactions (pulmonary, abdominal and pericardial) have been associated with bromocriptine, cabergoline and pergolide and patients taking these drugs should be monitored for dyspnoea, chest pain, cardiac failure and abdominal pain.
- Evaluate the effectiveness of the teaching plan (patient can give the drug name and dosage, name possible adverse effects to watch for and specific measures to prevent adverse effects and discuss the importance of continued follow-up).
- Monitor the effectiveness of comfort measures and concordance with the regimen.

Antimuscarinics

Antimuscarinics are drugs that oppose the effects of ACh at receptor sites in the substantia nigra and the corpus striatum, thus helping restore chemical balance in the area. The antimuscarinics used to treat parkinsonism are synthetic drugs that have been developed to have a greater affinity for cholinergic receptor sites in the CNS rather than those in the peripheral nervous system. However, they still block, to some extent, the cholinergic receptors of the parasympathetic nervous system's postganglionic effectors and are associated with the adverse effects resulting from this blockage (see Chapter 32), including slowed GI motility and secretions, with dry mouth and constipation, urinary retention, blurred vision and hallucinations.

Antimuscarinics used to treat Parkinson's disease include the following drugs:

- Benzatropine is available in intramuscular and intravenous forms.
- Orphenadrine is available in oral forms.
- Procyclidine is available in oral, intramuscular and intravenous forms.
- Trihexyphenidyl is available in oral forms.

Therapeutic Actions and Indications

The antimuscarinics block the action of ACh in the CNS to help normalize the ACh-dopamine imbalance. As a result, these drugs reduce the degree of rigidity and, to a lesser extent, the tremors associated with Parkinson's disease. The peripheral antimuscarinic effects that sometimes occur with the use of these drugs help alleviate some of the other adverse effects associated with Parkinson's disease, including drooling.

Although antimuscarinic drugs have been used in the past to treat parkinsonism, the dopaminergic drugs have replaced antimuscarinics as the first-line treatment. They are also ineffective in the treatment of tardive dyskinesia (repetitive, involuntary movements, e.g. lip smacking, tongue protrusion) observed in parkinsonism. However, these drugs are still used for the relief of symptoms of extrapyramidal disorders associated with the use of some drugs, including antipsychotic phenothiazines; and may be effective in controlling the excessive salivation that occurs with the use of neuroleptic medication. They may also be useful as adjunctive therapy and for patients who no longer respond to levodopa.

Pharmacokinetics

The antimuscarinic drugs are variably absorbed from the GI tract, reaching peak levels in 1 to 4 hours. They are metabolized in the liver and excreted by the kidneys. All of them cross the placenta and enter breast milk. They should be used during pregnancy and lactation only if the benefit to the mother clearly outweighs the potential risk to the foetus or neonate. The safety and efficacy for use in children have not been established.

Contraindications and Cautions

Antimuscarinics are contraindicated in the presence of allergy to any of these agents. They should be used with caution in cardiovascular disease, tachycardia and hypertension, *because of a loss of the suppressive effects of the parasympathetic division of the autonomic nervous system on the heart*; benign prostatic hyperplasia, GI obstruction and angle-closure glaucoma, *all of which could be exacerbated by the peripheral antimuscarinic effects of these drugs* and in myasthenia gravis, *which could be exacerbated by the blocking of ACh receptors at neuromuscular synapses.*

Caution should also be used in the following conditions: hepatic and renal dysfunction, *which could interfere with the metabolism and excretion of the drugs and lead to toxic levels*; pregnancy *because these drugs do cross the placenta* and lactation *because the drugs cross into breast milk and may cause adverse effects in infants.* In addition, these agents should be used with caution in individuals who work in hot environments *because reflex sweating may be blocked, placing patients at risk of heat stroke.*

Adverse Effects

The use of antimuscarinics for parkinsonism is associated with CNS effects, such as disorientation, confusion and impaired memory, related to the blocking of central ACh receptors. Agitation, restlessness, hallucinations and dizziness may also occur.

Anticipated peripheral antimuscarinic effects include dry mouth, nausea, vomiting and constipation related to decreased GI secretions and motility. In addition, tachycardia may occur, related to the inhibition of the suppressive cardiac effects of the parasympathetic nervous system; urinary retention and hesitancy related to an inhibition of bladder muscle activity and sphincter relaxation; blurred vision and photophobia related to pupil dilation and reduction in accommodation of the lens; and flushing and reduced sweating related to an inhibition of the sympathetic cholinergic sites that stimulate sweating.

Clinically Important Drug–Drug Interactions

When these antimuscarinic drugs are used with other drugs that have antimuscarinic properties, including the tricyclic antidepressants and the phenothiazines, there is a risk of potentially fatal paralytic ileus and an increased risk of toxic psychoses. If such combinations must be given, patients should be monitored closely. Dosage adjustments should be made and supportive measures should be taken.

Always consult a current copy of the British National Formulary for further guidance.

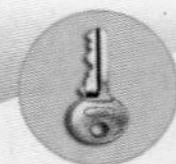

Key Drug Summary: *Orphenadrine*

Indications: Adjunct therapy for parkinsonism; relief of symptoms of extrapyramidal disorders that occur as adverse effects of phenothiazine therapy

Actions: Acts as an antimuscarinic, principally in the CNS, returning balance of neurotransmitters in the basal nuclei and reducing the severity of rigidity, akinesia and tremors; peripheral antimuscarinic effects help to reduce excessive salivation resulting in drooling and other secondary effects of parkinsonism

Pharmacokinetics:

Route	Onset	Peak	Duration
Oral	1 h	2–4 h	4–6 h

$T_{1/2}$: 13.2–20.1 hours (the $t_{1/2}$ increases with repeated dosing); metabolized in the liver and metabolites excreted by the kidneys

Adverse effects: Constipation, dry mouth, nausea, vomiting, tachycardia, euphoria, hallucinations, confusion, memory loss, anxiety, restlessness, dizziness, depression, blurred vision, mydriasis, urinary retention and rash

Nursing Considerations for Patients Receiving Antimuscarinic Antiparkinsonism Drugs

Assessment: History and Examination

Screen for the following conditions, *which could be contraindications or cautions to the use of the drug*: any known allergies to these drugs; GI obstruction; urinary dysfunction or obstruction; benign prostatic hypertrophy; cardiovascular disease; hypertension; angle-closure glaucoma; myasthenia gravis; pregnancy or lactation; hepatic dysfunction; and pyrexia.

Include screening *to determine baseline status before beginning therapy and to monitor for potential adverse effects.* Assess the following: temperature; skin colour and lesions; CNS orientation, affect, reflexes, bilateral grip strength and spasticity evaluation; respiration and adventitious sounds; pulse, blood pressure and cardiac output; bowel sounds and reported output; urinary output and bladder palpation; and liver and renal function tests if patients history suggests potential problems.

Establish if patient is currently taking other medications or herbal therapies, which may potentially interact with the proposed drug.

Nursing Diagnoses

The patient taking an antimuscarinic antiparkinsonism drug may have the following nursing diagnoses related to drug therapy:

- Acute pain related to GI, CNS and GU effects
- Disturbed thought processes related to CNS effects
- Risk for injury related to CNS effects
- Deficient knowledge regarding drug therapy

Implementation With Rationale

- Arrange to decrease dosage or discontinue the drug *if dry mouth becomes so severe that swallowing becomes difficult.* Provide frequent mouth care to help with this problem.
- Give the drug with caution and arrange for a decrease in dosage in hot weather or with exposure to hot environments *because patients are at increased risk for heat prostration because of decreased ability to sweat.*
- Give the drug with meals if GI upset is a problem, before meals if dry mouth is a problem and after meals if drooling occurs and the drug causes nausea. *These steps will facilitate compliance with drug therapy.*
- Monitor bowel function and institute a bowel programme *if constipation is a problem.*
- Ensure that the patient empties bladder before taking the drug *if urinary retention is a problem.*
- Establish safety precautions if CNS or vision changes occur *to prevent patient injury.*
- Provide thorough patient teaching about topics such as the drug name and prescribed dosage, measures to help avoid adverse effects, warning signs that may indicate problems and the need for periodic monitoring and evaluation *to enhance patient knowledge about drug therapy and to promote concordance.*
- Offer support and encouragement *to help the patient cope with the disease and drug regimen.*

Evaluation

- Monitor patient response to the drug (improvement in signs and symptoms of parkinsonism).
- Monitor for adverse effects (CNS changes, blurred vision, urinary retention, GI depression, tachycardia, heat intolerance, flushing).
- Evaluate the effectiveness of the teaching plan (patient can give the drug name and dosage, name possible adverse effects to watch for and specific measures to prevent adverse effects and discuss the importance of continued follow-up).
- Monitor the effectiveness of comfort measures and compliance with the regimen.

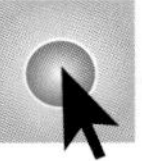

WEB LINKS

Health care providers and patients may want to consult the following Internet sources:

http://bnfc.org The BNF for Children provides UK health care professionals with authoritative and practical information on the selection and clinical use of medicines in children.

http://cks.library.nhs.uk The National Health Service Clinical Knowledge Summaries provides evidence-based practical information on the common conditions observed in primary care.

http://www.bnf.org.uk The BNF provides UK health care professionals with authoritative and practical information on the selection and clinical use of medicines.

http://www.nhsdirect.nhs.uk The National Health Service Direct service provides patients with information and advice about health, illness and health services.

http://www.parkinsons.org.uk The Parkinson's Disease Society is a registered charity and provides information and support to patients, their families and carers.

Points to Remember

- Parkinson's disease is a progressive, chronic neurological disorder for which there is no cure.
- Signs and symptoms of Parkinson's disease include tremor, changes in posture and gait, slow and deliberate movements (bradykinesia) and eventually drooling and changes in speech and loss of facial expression.
- Loss of dopamine-secreting neurons in the substantia nigra is characteristic of Parkinson's disease.
- Destruction of dopamine-secreting cells leads to an imbalance between excitatory cholinergic cells and inhibitory dopaminergic cells.
- Drug therapy for Parkinson's disease is aimed at restoring the dopamine-ACh balance. The signs and symptoms of the disease can be managed until the degeneration of neurons is so extensive that a therapeutic response no longer occurs.
- Dopaminergic drugs are used to increase dopamine levels or to directly stimulate dopamine receptors and antimuscarinic drugs are used to block the excitatory cholinergic receptors
- Many adverse effects are associated with the drugs used for treating Parkinson's disease, including CNS changes, antimuscarinic (atropine-like) effects and dopamine stimulation in the peripheral nervous system.

CRITICAL THINKING SCENARIO 23-1

Effects of Vitamin B_6 Intake on Levodopa Levels

The Situation

Colin, a 68-year-old man with well-controlled Parkinson's disease presents with severe nausea, anorexia, fainting spells and heart palpitations. He has been maintained on levodopa for the Parkinsonism symptoms and he claims to have followed his drug regimen religiously. According to Colin the only change in his lifestyle has been the addition of several health foods and vitamins. His daughter has introduced him to a new health regime, including natural foods and plenty of supplemental vitamins.

Critical Thinking

- Based on Colin's signs and symptoms, what has probably occurred?
- In Parkinson's disease, is it possible to differentiate between a deterioration of illness and a toxic reaction to a drug?
- What nursing implications should be considered when teaching Colin and his family about the effects of vitamin B_6 on levodopa levels?
- In what ways can the daughter cope with her role in this crisis?
- Develop a new care plan for Colin that involves all family members and that includes drug teaching.

Discussion

The presenting symptoms reflect an increase in Parkinson symptoms, as well as an increase in peripheral dopamine reactions (e.g. palpitations, fainting, anorexia, nausea). It is necessary to determine whether the problem involves a further degeneration in the neurons in the substantia nigra or the particular medication that Colin has been taking. In many patients, responsiveness to levodopa is lost as neural degeneration continues.

The explanation of the new lifestyle – full of grains, natural foods and vitamins – alerted a nurse to the possibility of excessive vitamin B_6 intake. In reviewing the vitamin bottles and some of the food packages supplied by Colin, it seemed that too much vitamin B_6, which speeds the conversion of levodopa to dopamine before it can cross the blood–brain barrier, might be the reason as to why his Parkinson's symptoms have recurred. It was decided to reduce the dose of levodopa temporarily until the excess vitamin B_6 was cleared.

The status of Colin's Parkinson's disease and his levodopa dose regimen should be re-evaluated. It would be wise to consider combining the drug with carbidopa to prevent some of the side-effects associated with levodopa monotherapy. To begin with the smallest dose possible should be used, with slow increases following to achieve the maximum benefit with the fewest side-effects.

In addition, the need to avoid excessive intake of vitamin B_6 should be emphasized. The entire family should be involved in an explanation of what happened and how this situation can be avoided in the future. This situation can serve as a good teaching example for staff, as well as presenting them with an opportunity to review drug therapy in Parkinson's disease and the risks and benefits of more extreme diets or vitamin supplementation.

Nursing Care Guide for Colin: Levodopa

Assessment: History and Examination

Assess history of chronic obstructive pulmonary disease, cardiovascular disease, hypotension, hepatic or renal dysfunction; psychosis; peptic ulcer, diabetes mellitus, osteomalacia, history of melanoma or glaucoma and/or concurrent use of MAOIs, phenytoin or pyridoxine.

Focus physical examination on:

- Cardiovascular: blood pressure, pulse rate, peripheral perfusion, electrocardiogram results
- CNS: orientation, affect, reflexes, grip strength
- GI: abdominal examination, bowel sounds
- Respiratory: respiration, adventitious sounds
- Laboratory tests: renal and liver function tests, full blood count

Nursing Diagnoses

- Risk of injury if patient becomes dizzy or faints
- Potential for dehydration and inadequate nutrition due to nausea
- Deficient knowledge regarding drug interactions

Implementation

- Provide comfort and safety: slow positioning changes; assess orientation; give drug with food; administer with carbidopa; have patient empty bladder before each dose.

Effects of Vitamin B_6 Intake on Levodopa Levels *(continued)*

- Provide support and reassurance to deal with disease and drug effects.
- Instruct the patient regarding drug dosage, effects and adverse symptoms to report and interactions.

Evaluation

- Evaluate drug effects: relief of signs and symptoms of Parkinson's disease
- Monitor for adverse effects: CNS effects; renal changes, urinary retention; GI effects (constipation); increased sweating or flushing.
- Monitor for drug–drug interactions: decreased effects with vitamin B_6.
- Evaluate effectiveness of patient teaching education.
- Evaluate effectiveness of comfort and safety measures.

Patient Education for Colin

- ☐ The drug that has been prescribed is called levodopa. It increases the levels of dopamine in the central areas of the brain and helps to reduce the signs and symptoms of Parkinson's disease.
- ☐ Often this drug is combined with carbidopa, which allows the correct levels of levodopa to reach the brain.
- ☐ People who take this drug must have their individual dosage needs adjusted over time.
- ☐ Common effects of this drug include:
  - *Fatigue, weakness and drowsiness:* Try to space activities evenly through the day; allow rest periods to avoid these side-effects. Take safety precautions and avoid driving or operating dangerous machinery if these conditions occur.
  - *Dizziness, fainting:* Change position slowly to avoid dizzy spells.
  - *Increased sweating, darkened urine:* This is a normal reaction. Avoid very hot environments.
  - *Headaches, difficulty sleeping:* These usually pass as the body adjusts to the drug. If they become too uncomfortable and persist, consult with your health care provider.
- ☐ Report any of the following to your health care provider: *uncontrolled movements of any body part, chest pain or palpitations, depression or mood changes, difficulty in emptying bladder and/or bowel, persistent nausea and vomiting.*
- ☐ Be aware that vitamin B_6 interferes with the effects of levodopa. If you feel that you need a vitamin product, consult with your health care provider about using an agent that does not contain vitamin B_6.
- ☐ Avoid eating large quantities of health foods that contain vitamin B_6, such as grains and bran. If you are taking co-careldopa, these precautions are not as important. Eat a normal well-balanced diet.
- ☐ Tell any doctor, nurse, or other health care provider involved in your care that you are taking this drug.
- ☐ Keep this drug and all medications out of the reach of children.
- ☐ Do not overexert yourself when you begin to feel better. Gradually increase your level of exercise to what you normally do.
- ☐ Take this drug exactly as directed and schedule regular medical checkups to evaluate the effects of this drug.

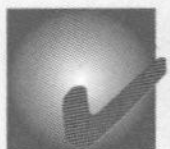

CHECK YOUR UNDERSTANDING

Answers to the questions in this chapter may be found in the answer key in the back of the book.

Multiple Choice

Select the most appropriate response to the following.

1. Parkinson's disease is a progressive, chronic neurological disorder that is usually
   a. associated with severe head injury.
   b. associated with chronic diseases.
   c. associated with ageing.
   d. affects people of all ages with equal frequency.

2. Parkinson's disease reflects an imbalance between inhibitory and stimulating activity of neurons in the
   a. reticular activating system.
   b. cerebellum.
   c. basal nuclei.
   d. limbic system.

3. The main underlying problem with Parkinson's disease seems to be a decrease in the neurotransmitter
   a. ACh.
   b. noradrenaline.
   c. dopamine.
   d. serotonin.

4. Antimuscarinic drugs act to
   a. block the stimulating effects of ACh in the brain to bring activity back into balance.
   b. block the signs and symptoms of the disease, making it more bearable.
   c. inhibit dopamine effects in the brain.
   d. increase the effectiveness of GABA.

5. Replacing dopamine in the brain would seem to be the best treatment for Parkinson's disease. This is difficult because dopamine
   a. is broken down in gastric acid.
   b. is not available in drug form.
   c. cannot cross the blood–brain barrier.
   d. cannot be absorbed across the GI tract.

6. A patient taking levodopa and over-the-counter vitamins might experience
   a. cure from Parkinson's disease.
   b. return of parkinsonian symptoms and increased blood pressure, pulse, respirations, sweating and feeling of tension.
   c. improved health and well-being.
   d. increased resistance to viral infections.

Extended Matched Questions

Select **all** that apply.

1. A patient asks the nurse to explain Parkinson's disease to him. Which of the following possible causes of Parkinson's disease might be included in the explanation?
   a. Adverse effect of drug therapy
   b. Head injury
   c. Viral infection
   d. Dementia
   e. Bacterial infection
   f. Birth defect

2. There is no therapy currently available that will stop the loss of neurons and the eventual decline of function in clients with Parkinson's disease. As a result, nursing care may involve which of the following interventions?
   a. Regular exercises to slow loss of function
   b. Support and education as drugs fail and new therapy is needed
   c. Community and family support networking
   d. Discontinuation of drug therapy to test for a cure
   e. Special vitamin therapy to slow the loss of the neurons
   f. Stereotactic neurosurgery to provide temporary improvement in symptoms

Bibliography and References

British Medical Association and Royal Pharmaceutical Society of Great Britain. (2008). *British National Formulary*. London: BMJ & RPS Publishing. *This publication is updated biannually: it is imperative that the most recent edition is consulted.*

British Medical Association and Royal Pharmaceutical Society of Great Britain. (2008). *British National Formulary for Children*. London: BMJ & RPS Publishing. *This publication is updated annually: it is imperative that the most recent edition is consulted.*

Brunton, L., Lazo, J. S., Parker, K., Goodman, L. S., & Gilman, A. G. (2005). *Goodman and Gilman's the pharmacological basis of therapeutics* (11th ed.). London: McGraw-Hill.

Committee for the Safety of Medicines. (2008). Fibrotic reactions, including cardiovalvulopathy, associated with chronic use. Available from http://www/mhra.gov.uk/Safetyinformation/

Ganong, W. (2005). *Review of medical physiology* (22nd ed.). New York: McGraw-Hill.

Howland, R. D., & Mycek, M. J. (2005). *Pharmacology* (3rd ed.). Philadelphia: Lippincott Williams & Wilkins.

National Institute for Health and Clinical Excellence. (2006). CG35 Parkinson's disease: diagnosis and management in primary and secondary care. Available from http://www.nice.org.uk

Porth, C. M., & Matfin, G. (2008). *Pathophysiology: Concepts of altered health states* (8th ed.). Philadelphia: Lippincott Williams & Wilkins.

Rang, H. P., Dale, M. M., Ritter, J. M., & Flower, R. J. (2007). *Rang and Dale's Pharmacology.* (6th ed.). Philadelphia: Churchill Livingstone.

Saltzman, E. W. (1996). Living with Parkinson's disease. *New England Journal of Medicine, 334*, 114–116

Simonsen, T., Aarbakke, J., Kay, I., Coleman, I., Sinnott, P., & Lysaa, R. (2006). *Illustrated pharmacology for nurses.* London: Hodder Arnold.

CHAPTER 24

Neuromuscular Junction Blocking Agents

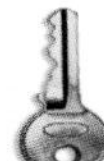

KEY TERMS

acetylcholine receptor site acetylcholinesterase

depolarizing

malignant hyperthermia

nondepolarizing

paralysis

sarcomere

sliding filament theory Troponin

LEARNING OBJECTIVES

Upon completion of this chapter you will be able to:

1. Draw and label a neuromuscular junction.
2. Describe the therapeutic actions, indications, pharmacokinetics associated with the depolarizing and nondepolarizing neuromuscular junction blockers.
3. Describe the contraindications, most common adverse reactions and important drug–drug interactions associated with the depolarizing and nondepolarizing neuromuscular junction blockers.
4. Discuss the use of neuromuscular junction blockers across the lifespan.
5. Outline the nursing considerations, including important teaching points, for patients receiving a neuromuscular junction blocker.

NONDEPOLARIZING NEUROMUSCULAR BLOCKERS

atracurium
cisatracurium
mivacurium
pancuronium
rocuronium
vecuronium

DEPOLARIZING NEUROMUSCULAR BLOCKER

suxamethonium

ANTICHOLINESTERASES USED IN ANAESTHESIA

edrophonium
neostigmine

During surgery drugs that affect the neuromuscular junction (NMJ), the NMJ blockers, are routinely used in combination with anaesthesia. They can be divided into two groups. One group, the **nondepolarizing** blockers (competitive muscle relaxants), includes those agents that act as antagonists to acetylcholine (ACh) at the NMJ and prevent depolarization of muscle cells. The actions of these drugs can be reversed by anticholinesterases. The other group, the **depolarizing** blockers that is suxamethonium act as an ACh agonist (mimicking ACh) at the NMJ, causing stimulation of the muscle cell and then preventing it from repolarizing. Both of these types of drugs are used to cause **paralysis**, or loss of muscular function, for performance of surgical procedures or facilitation of mechanical ventilation.

The Neuromuscular Junction

The NMJ blockers affect the normal functioning of muscles by interfering with the transmission of the action potential at the junction of the motor nerve and muscle fibre. The functional unit of a muscle, called a **sarcomere**, is made up of thin and thick filaments formed by actin and myosin molecules arranged in orderly stacks that give the sarcomere a striated or striped appearance (Figure 24.1). Normal muscle function involves the arrival of a nerve impulse at the motor nerve terminal, followed by the release of ACh into the synaptic cleft. The ACh interacts with the **acetylcholine receptor site** (nicotinic cholinergic receptors) on the effector side of the synapse, causing depolarization of the muscle membrane. This depolarization allows calcium ions, stored in T tubules to be released into the cell. The calcium binds to **troponin**, a chemical found throughout the sarcomere and the binding of troponin causes the exposure of myosin binding sites on the actin, allowing them to react with each other and cross bridges are formed. ACh is broken down by the enzyme **acetylcholinesterase**, freeing the receptor for further stimulation.

The actin and myosin molecules react with each other again and again, sliding along the filament and making it shorter. This is a contraction of the muscle fibre according to the **sliding filament theory**. As the calcium is removed from the cell during repolarization of the muscle membrane, the troponin is freed and once again prevents the actin and myosin from reacting with each other. The muscle filament then relaxes or slides back to the resting position. Muscle tone results from a dynamic balance between excitatory and inhibitory impulses to the muscle. Muscle paralysis or weakness may occur when ACh cannot react with the cholinergic muscle receptor or when the muscle cells cannot repolarize to allow new stimulation and muscle contraction.

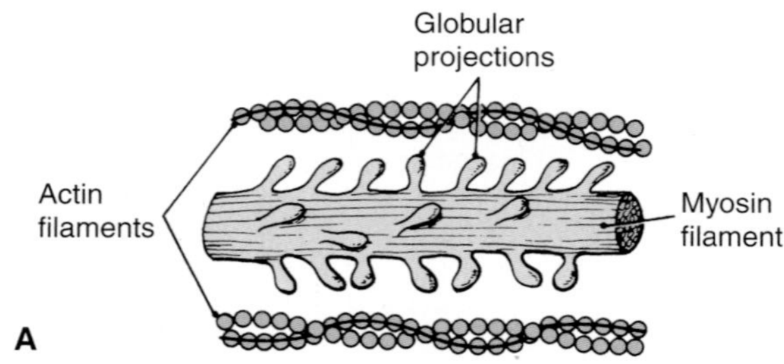

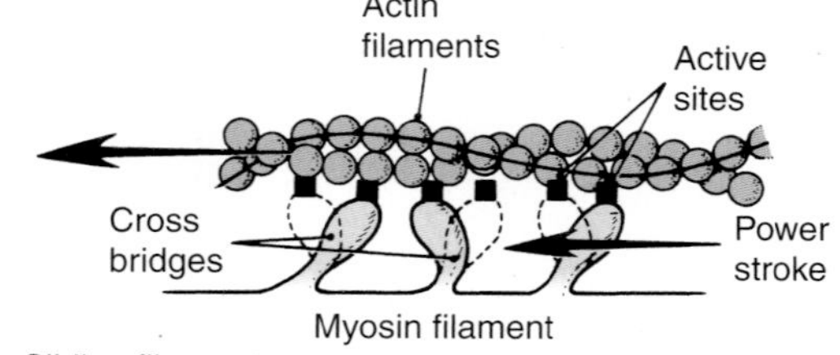

FIGURE 24.1 Sliding filament theory of muscle contraction.

Nondepolarizing Neuromuscular Junction (NMJ) Blockers (competitive muscle relaxants)

All nondepolarizing NMJ blockers are similar in structure to ACh and occupy the neuromuscular cholinergic receptor site, preventing ACh from reacting with the receptor. These agents do not cause activation of muscle cells and consequently muscle contraction does not occur. As they are not broken down by acetylcholinesterase, their effect is more long-lasting than that of ACh. NMJ blockers are used when clinical situations require muscle paralysis such as during the insertion of an endotracheal tube during assisted ventilation. Nondepolarizing blockers can be further classified by their duration of action as for example short acting (mivacurium), intermediate acting (atracurium) and long-acting (pancuronium). The action of nondepolarizing muscle relaxants may be reversed with anticholinesterases such as neostigmine.

Nursing Considerations for Patients Receiving Nondepolarizing Neuromuscular Junction Blockers

Assessment: History and Examination

Screen for the following conditions, *which could be cautions or contraindications to use of the drug*: any known allergies to these drugs; impaired liver or kidney function; myasthenia gravis; pregnancy or lactation; impaired cardiac or respiratory function; personal or family history of malignant hyperthermia; and fractures, closed angle glaucoma, or paraplegia, severe sepsis as risk of hyperkalaemia

Include screening *for baseline status before beginning therapy and for any potential adverse effects.* Assess the following: body temperature; skin, reflexes, pupil size and reactivity, muscle tone, pulse, blood pressure, electrocardiogram (ECG); respiration and adventitious sounds; abdominal examination; renal and liver function tests and serum electrolytes.

Establish if patient is currently taking other medications or herbal therapies which may potentially interact with the nondepolarizing NMJ blockers.

Nursing Diagnoses

The patient receiving an NMJ blocker may have the following nursing diagnoses related to drug therapy:

- Impaired gas exchange related to depressed respirations
- Impaired skin integrity related to immobility
- Impaired verbal communication
- Fear related to paralysis
- Deficient knowledge regarding drug therapy

Implementation With Rationale

- Administration of the drug should be performed by trained personnel (usually an anaesthetist) *because of the potential for serious adverse effects and the need for immediate ventilatory support.*
- Supplies and equipment should be on standby *to maintain airway and provide mechanical ventilation.*
- Do not mix the drug with any alkaline solutions such as barbiturates *because a precipitate may form, making it inappropriate for use.*
- Test patient response and recovery periodically if the drug is being given over a long period to maintain mechanical ventilation. *Discontinue the drug if response does not occur or is greatly delayed.*
- Monitor patient temperature *for prompt detection and treatment of malignant hyperthermia.*
- Keep dantrolene on standby *for treatment of malignant hyperthermia if it should occur.*
- Arrange for a small dose of a nondepolarizing NMJ blocker before the use of suxamethonium *to reduce the adverse effects associated with muscle contraction.*
- Maintain a cholinesterase inhibitor on standby *to overcome excessive neuromuscular blockade caused by nondepolarizing NMJ blockers.*
- Provide a peripheral nerve stimulator on standby *to assess the degree of neuromuscular blockade, if appropriate.*
- Provide comfort measures *to help the patient tolerate drug effects,* such as pain relief as appropriate; reassurance, support and orientation *for conscious patients unable to move or communicate*; skin care and turning *to prevent skin breakdown*; and supportive care *for emergencies such as hypotension and bronchospasm.*
- Monitor patient response closely (blood pressure, temperature, pulse, respiration, reflexes) *and adjust dosage accordingly to ensure the greatest therapeutic effect with minimal risk of toxicity.*
- Incorporate information on this drug into a thorough preoperative patient education plan *because most patients who receive the drug will be receiving teaching about a particular procedure and will be unconscious when the drug is given.* (See Critical Thinking Scenario 24-1.)
- Offer support and encouragement *to help the patient cope with drug effects.*

Depolarizing Neuromuscular Junction Blocker: Suxamethonium

Suxamethonium, a depolarizing NMJ blocker (muscular blocker) attaches to the ACh receptor site on the muscle cell and depolarizes the muscle cell membrane. This depolarization causes stimulation of the muscle and muscle contraction. Unlike ACh, suxamethonium is not broken down instantly and the result is a prolonged depolarization (contraction) of the muscle, which cannot be re-stimulated. Eventually a gradual repolarization occurs as continually stimulated channels in the cell membrane close. Certain ethnic groups can have a genetic predisposition for lengthened paralysis. Unlike nondepolarizing blockers its action cannot be reversed by anticholinesterases (these drugs will potentiate the effect). Recovery with suxamethonium is spontaneous. Bradycardia and excessive salivation can often occur with this drug therefore premedication with atropine is often associated with suxamethonium use.

Therapeutic Actions and Indications

All of the NMJ blockers are structurally similar to ACh and compete with ACh for muscle ACh receptor sites. They are hydrophilic, instead of lipophilic, so they do not readily cross the blood–brain barrier. The nondepolarizing NMJ blockers act by blocking the ACh receptor so that it cannot be stimulated. Depolarizing NMJ blockers prevent muscle movement by prohibiting the depolarization of the muscle membrane. The depolarizing NMJ blocker suxamethonium works by reacting with the ACh receptor and causing a prolonged depolarization, which causes first muscle contraction and then flaccid paralysis. Both effects cause muscles to stop responding to stimuli and paralysis occurs. Clinically, muscle twitching occurs when the drug is first given and is followed by flaccid paralysis. Suxamethonium has a rapid onset and a brief duration of action because it is broken down by cholinesterase in the plasma (Figure 24.2).

These drugs are indicated for any situation in which muscle paralysis is desired. The therapeutic uses of NMJ blocking are as follows:

- To serve as an adjunct to general anaesthetics during surgery, when reflex muscle movement could interfere with the surgical procedure or the delivery of gas anaesthesia.
- To facilitate mechanical intubation by preventing resistance to passing of the endotracheal tube and in situations in which patients 'fight' or resist the ventilator.
- To facilitate electroconvulsive therapy when intense skeletal muscle contractions as a result of electric shock could cause the patient broken bones or other injury.

Several NMJ blockers are available, with different times of onset and durations of activity. The drug of choice in any given situation is determined by the procedure being

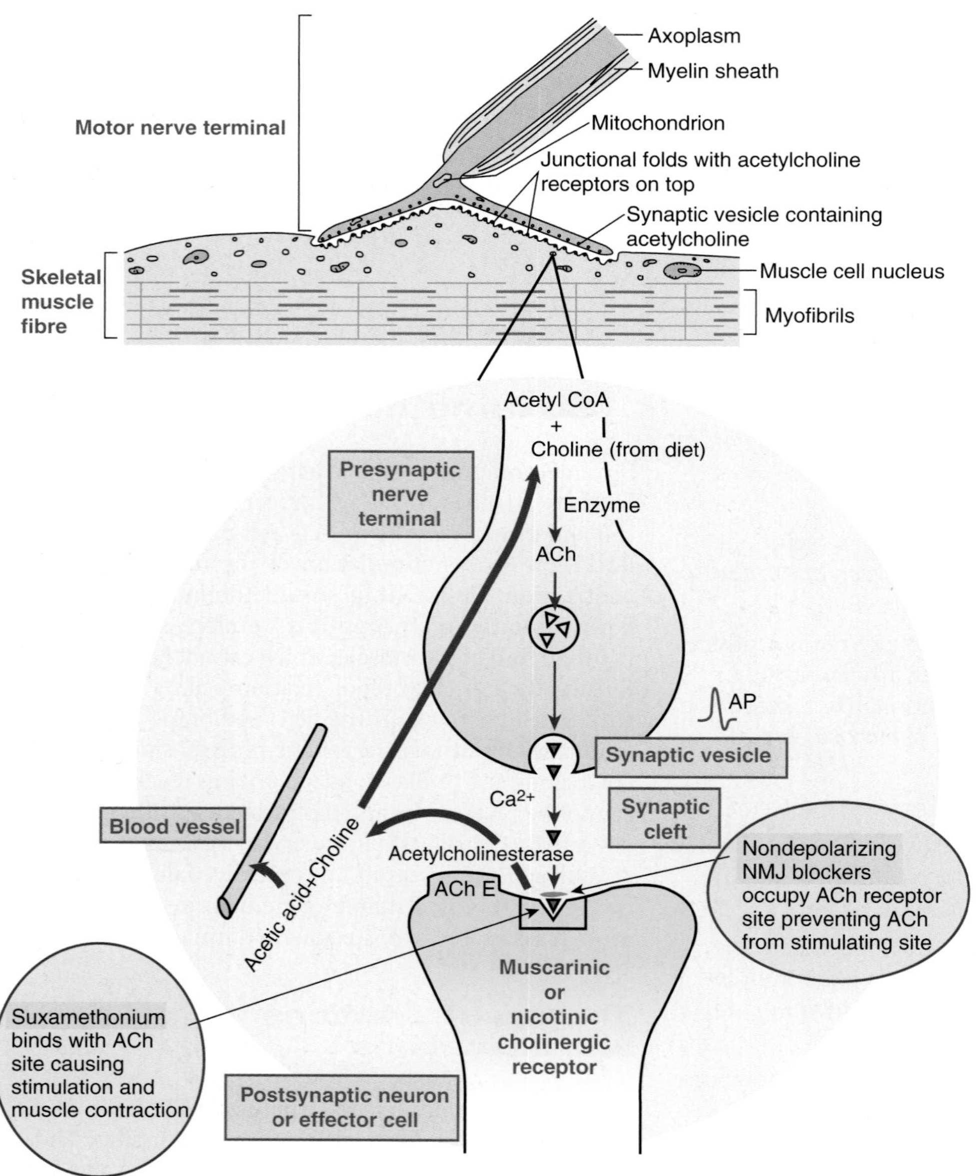

FIGURE 24.2 Sites of action of the neuromuscular junction (NMJ) blockers.

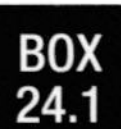

BOX 24.1 DRUG THERAPY ACROSS THE LIFESPAN

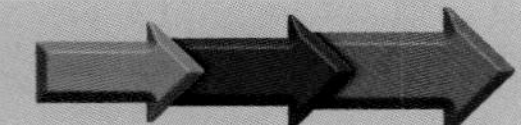

NMJ Blocking Agents

CHILDREN

Children require very careful monitoring and support after the use of NMJ blockers. These agents are used by anaesthetists who are skilled in their use and with full support services available.

The nondepolarizing NMJs are preferable because of the lack of muscle contraction with its resultant discomfort on recovery. Suxamethonium, a depolarizing agent; is usually preferred when a very short-acting, rapid-onset blocker is needed (e.g. for intubation).

When administering any drug to children, always consult the most recent edition of the British National Formulary for Children.

ADULTS

Adults need to be monitored closely for full return of muscle function. If suxamethonium is used, they need to be told that they will experience muscle pain and discomfort when the procedure is over.

The NMJ blockers are used during pregnancy and lactation only if the benefit to the mother outweighs the potential risk to the foetus or neonate.

OLDER ADULTS

Older patients often also have renal or hepatic impairment; therefore they are more likely to have toxic levels of the drug related to changes in metabolism and excretion. The older patient should receive special efforts to provide skin care to prevent skin breakdown, which is more likely with older skin. The older patient may require longer monitoring and regular orienting and reassuring.

performed, including the estimated time involved. For use of these drugs across the life span see Box 24.1.

Pharmacokinetics

In general, the NMJ blockers are metabolized in the serum, although metabolism is dependent on the liver to produce the needed plasma cholinesterases. Patients with hepatic impairment may experience prolonged effects of the drugs. Most of the metabolites are excreted in the urine. Patients with renal impairment may be at risk for increased toxicity from the drugs.

Contraindications and Cautions

The NMJ blockers are contraindicated in the following conditions: known allergy to any of these drugs; myasthenia gravis *because blocking of the ACh cholinergic receptors aggravates the neuromuscular disease* (which results from destruction of the ACh receptor sites) *and increases the muscular effects* (see Chapter 31); renal or hepatic disease, *which could interfere with the metabolism or excretion of these drugs, leading to toxic effects*; and pregnancy (some of these drugs are used in caesarean sections, but the dose needs to be decreased to protect the foetus).

Caution should be used in patients with any family or personal history of **malignant hyperthermia**, a serious adverse effect associated with these drugs that is characterized by extreme muscle rigidity, severe hyperpyrexia, acidosis and death in some cases, *because malignant hyperthermia can occur with the use of these drugs*. Caution should also be used in the following circumstances: pulmonary or cardiovascular dysfunction, *which could be made worse by the paralysis of the respiratory muscles and resulting changes in perfusion and respiratory function*; altered fluid and electrolyte imbalance, *which could affect membrane stability and muscular function*; some respiratory conditions *that could be made worse by the histamine release associated with some of these agents*; and lactation *because of the potential for adverse effects on the baby*.

In addition, suxamethonium should be used with caution in patients with closed-angle glaucoma or penetrating eye injuries *because intraocular pressure increases*; and in those with paraplegia or spinal cord injuries, *which could cause loss of potassium from the overstimulated cells and hyperkalaemia*. Extreme caution should be taken in the presence of genetic or disease-related conditions causing low plasma cholinesterase levels, such as cirrhosis, metabolic disorders, carcinoma, burns, dehydration, malnutrition, hyperpyrexia, thyroid toxicosis, collagen diseases and exposure to neurotoxic insecticides. *Low plasma cholinesterase levels may result in a very prolonged paralysis because suxamethonium is not broken down in the plasma and continues to stimulate the receptor site, leading to a need for prolonged support after use of the drug is discontinued.*

Adverse Effects

The adverse effects related to the use of NMJ blockers are associated with the paralysis of muscles. Profound and prolonged muscle paralysis is always possible and patients must be supported until they are able to resume voluntary and involuntary muscle movement. When the respiratory muscles are paralyzed, depressed respiration, bronchospasm and apnoea are anticipated adverse effects. NMJ blockers are never used without the presence of an anaesthetist who can provide artificial ventilation and deliver oxygen under positive pressure. Intubation is an anticipated procedure with these drugs.

The histamine release associated with many of the NMJ blockers can cause respiratory obstruction with wheezing and bronchospasm. Prolonged drug use may also result in gastrointestinal (GI) dysfunction related to paralysis of the muscles in the GI tract; constipation, vomiting, regurgitation and aspiration may occur. Decubitus ulcers may develop because the patient loses reflex muscle movement that protects the body from pressure sores. Hyperkalaemia may occur as a result of muscle membrane alterations.

In addition, suxamethonium is associated with muscle pain, related to the contraction of the muscles as a first reaction. A nondepolarizing NMJ blocker may be given first to prevent some of these contractions and the associated discomfort. Aspirin also alleviates much of this pain after the procedure. Malignant hyperthermia, which may occur in susceptible patients, is a very serious condition characterized by massive muscle contraction, sharply elevated body temperature, severe acidosis and if uncontrolled, death. This reaction is most likely with suxamethonium and treatment involves dantrolene (see Chapter 24) to inhibit the muscle effects of the NMJ blocker.

Always consult a current copy of the British National Formulary for further guidance.

Clinically Important Drug–Drug Interactions

Many drugs are known to react with the NMJ blockers. Some drug combinations result in an increased neuromuscular effect. A combination of NMJ blockers and aminoglycoside antibiotics (e.g. gentamicin) also leads to increased neuromuscular blockage. Patients who receive this drug combination require a lower dose of NMJ blocker and prolonged support and monitoring after the procedure.

Calcium channel blockers may also greatly increase the paralysis caused by NMJ blockers because of their effects on the calcium channels in the muscle. If the combination of NMJ blockers and calcium channel blockers cannot be avoided, the dose of the NMJ agent should be lowered and the patient should be monitored closely until complete recovery occurs.

If NMJ blockers are combined with cholinesterase inhibitors, the effectiveness of the NMJ blockers is decreased because of an accumulation of ACh in the synaptic cleft.

Combination with xanthines (e.g. theophylline, aminophylline) could result in reversal of the neuromuscular blockage. Patients receiving this combination of drugs should be monitored very closely during the procedure for the potential of early arousal and return of muscle function.

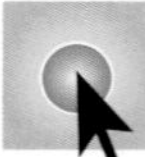

WEB LINKS

Health care providers and patients may want to consult the following Internet sources:

http://cks.library.nhs.uk The National Health Service Clinical Knowledge Summaries provides evidence-based practical information on the common conditions observed in primary care.

http://www.bnf.org.uk The BNF provides UK health care professionals with authoritative and practical information on the selection and clinical use of medicines.

http://www.nhsdirect.nhs.uk The National Health Service Direct service provides patients with information and advice about health, illness and health services.

http://www.rcoa.ac.uk The Royal College of Anaesthetists – a patient's guide to anaesthesia.

http://www.nice.org.uk National Institute for Health and Clinical Excellence (NICE) is an independent organization responsible for providing national guidance on promoting good health and preventing and treating ill health.

Points to Remember

- The nerves communicate with muscles at a point called the NMJ, using ACh as the neurotransmitter.
- NMJ blockers prevent skeletal muscle function.
- Nondepolarizing NMJ blockers prevent ACh from exciting the muscle and paralysis ensues because the muscle is unable to respond.
- Depolarizing NMJ blockers cause muscle paralysis by acting like ACh and exciting the muscle (depolarization), preventing repolarization and further stimulation of that muscle cell.
- NMJ blockers are primarily used as adjuncts to general anaesthesia, to facilitate endotracheal intubation, to facilitate mechanical ventilation and to prevent injury during electroconvulsive therapy.
- Adverse effects of NMJ blockers, such as prolonged paralysis, inability to breathe, weakness, muscle pain and soreness and effects of immobility, are related to muscle function blocking.
- Care of patients receiving NMJ blockers must include support and reassurance because communication is decreased with paralysis; vigilant maintenance of airways and respiration; prevention of skin breakdown; and monitoring for return of function.

CRITICAL THINKING SCENARIO 24-1

Using Suxamethonium in an Elderly Patient

The Situation

Kitty an 82-year-old woman in very good health has been admitted to the hospital for an exploratory laparoscopy to evaluate a probable abdominal mass. On admission, we learn that she had a history of mild hypertension that was well regulated by diuretic therapy. She received a baseline physical examination and preoperative instruction. On the morning of the surgery, it was noted that the anaesthetist planned to give her a general anaesthetic and suxamethonium to ensure muscle paralysis.

Critical Thinking

What nursing care plans should be made for Kitty? *Consider the patient's age and associated chronic problems that often occur with ageing. Also consider the support that she has available and potential physical and emotional support that she might need before and after this procedure. Use of a NMJ blocker in the elderly presents some nursing challenges that may not be seen with younger patients.*

What particular nursing care activities should be considered with Kitty?

What, if any, complications could arise if Kitty has electrolyte disturbances before surgery?

As Kitty has been maintained on long-term diuretic therapy, she is at special risk for electrolyte imbalance.

Discussion

Before surgery, the preoperative teaching should be reviewed with the patient. Kitty should be advised that she may experience back, neck and throat pain after the procedure. Reassure her that this is normal and that pain relief will be made available to alleviate the discomfort. Review deep breathing and coughing; she may need encouragement to clear secretions from her lungs and ensure full inflation. This is usually easier to do if it is a familiar activity. Kitty's serum electrolytes should be evaluated before surgery because potassium imbalance can cause unexpected effects with suxamethonium. Renal and hepatic function tests should also be performed to ensure that the dosage of the NMJ blocker is not excessive.

During the procedure, Kitty's cardiac and respiratory status should be monitored carefully for any potential problems; such effects are more common in people with underlying physical problems. Considering Kitty's age and potential circulatory problems, she should receive meticulous skin care and turning as soon as the procedure allows this kind of movement. Nursing staff must be near the patient until she has regained muscle control and the ability to communicate. She should be monitored for the need for pain relief and position adjustments.

Kitty will require additional teaching about her diagnosis and potential treatment. This should wait until she has regained full ability to communicate and is able to respond and participate in any discussion that may be held. At that time, she may require emotional support and encouragement. It may be necessary to contact available family or social service agencies regarding her physical and medical needs.

Nursing Care Guide for Kitty: Suxamethonium

Assessment: History and Examination

Assess for history of chronic obstructive pulmonary disease , cardiac disorders, myasthenia gravis, hepatic or renal dysfunction, fractures, glaucoma, and concurrent use of aminoglycosides or calcium channel blockers.

Focus the physical examination on the following;

- Cardiovascular (CV): Blood pressure, pulse rate, peripheral perfusion and ECG
- Central nervous system (CNS): orientation, affect and reflexes
- Skin: colour, texture and sweating
- Genitourinary: urinary output, bladder tone
- GI: abdominal examination
- Respiratory: respirations, adventitious sounds

Nursing Diagnoses

- Impaired gas exchange related to depressed respirations
- Impaired skin integrity related to immobility
- Deficient knowledge regarding drug therapy

(continued)

Using Suxamethonium in an Elderly Patient *(continued)*

- Impaired verbal communication, fear related to paralysis and inability to communicate

Implementation

- Provide comfort and safety measures: positioning, skin care, temperature control, pain medication as needed, maintain airway, ventilate patient.
- Provide support and reassurance to deal with paralysis and inability to communicate.
- Provide patient education about procedure being performed and what to expect.
- Assist with life support as needed.
- May need to premedicate with atropine to reduce risk of bradycardia and excessive salivation

Evaluation

- Evaluate drug effects: muscle paralysis.
- Monitor for adverse effects: CV effects (tachycardia with single use and bradycardia with repeated use) hypotension, respiratory distress, increased respiratory secretions), GI effects (constipation, nausea), skin breakdown, anxiety.
- Monitor for drug–drug interactions as indicated.
- Evaluate effectiveness of patient education programme and comfort and safety measures.
- Constantly monitor vital signs and watch for return of normal muscular function.

Patient Education for Kitty

☐ Before the surgery is performed, you will be given a drug to paralyze your muscles called a neuromuscular blocking agent. It is important that your muscles do not move at this time because it could interfere with the procedure.

☐ Common effects of these drugs include complete paralysis:

- You will not be able to move or to speak while you are receiving this drug.
- You will not be able to breathe on your own and you will receive assistance in breathing.
- This drug may not affect your level of consciousness and it can be very frightening to be unable to communicate with anyone around you. Someone will be with you, will try to anticipate your needs and will explain what is going on at all times.
- This drug may have no effect on your pain perception. Every effort will be made to make sure that you do not experience pain.
- You will be receiving suxamethonium; with this drug, you may experience back and throat pain related to muscle contractions that occur. You will be able to take aspirin to relieve this discomfort.
- Recovery of your muscle function may take 2 to 3 hours and someone will be nearby at all times until you have recovered from the paralysis.

Evaluation

- Monitor patient response to the drug (adequate muscle paralysis).
- Monitor for adverse effects (respiratory depression, hypotension, bronchospasm, GI slowdown, skin breakdown, fear related to helplessness and inability to communicate).
- Evaluate the effectiveness of the teaching plan (patient can relate anticipated effects of the drug and the recovery process).
- Monitor the effectiveness of comfort measures and compliance with the regimen.

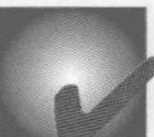

CHECK YOUR UNDERSTANDING

Answers to the questions in this chapter may be found in the answer key in the back of the book.

Multiple Choice

Select the most appropriate response to the following:

1. Nondepolarizing NMJ blockers
   a. antagonize ACh to prevent depolarization of muscle cells.
   b. act as agonists of ACh and cause depolarization of muscle cells.
   c. prevent the repolarization of muscle cells.
   d. are associated with painful muscle contractions on administration.

2. Suxamethonium has a rapid onset of action and a short duration of activity because it
   a. does not bind well to receptor sites.
   b. rapidly crosses the blood–brain barrier and is lost.
   c. is broken down by acetylcholinesterase that is found in the plasma.
   d. is very unstable.

3. Whenever NMJ blockers are used, the patient
   a. must be unconscious.
   b. must be intubated to ensure continuation of ventilation.
   c. will have no memory of any events.
   d. will have no adverse effects after the drug is stopped.

4. Malignant hyperthermia can occur with any NMJ blocker, but it most often occurs with suxamethonium. This disorder is treated with
   a. barbiturates.
   b. ice packs.
   c. dantrolene.
   d. diazepam.

5. Patient recovery from an NMJ blocker
   a. is predictable, based on the drug given.
   b. can be affected by genetic enzyme deficiency.
   c. can always be ensured because of the drug half-life.
   d. can be shortened by administration of oxygen.

6. When preparing NMJ blockers for administration, it is important that they are not
   a. mixed in with any alkaline solutions because a precipitate may form.
   b. exposed to light.
   c. mixed with any other drug.
   d. mixed with heparin.

Extended Matching Questions

Select **all** that apply.

1. An NMJ blocker would be a drug of choice to:
   a. facilitate endotracheal intubation
   b. facilitate mechanical ventilation
   c. prevent injury during electroconvulsive therapy
   d. relieve pain during labour and delivery
   e. treat myasthenia gravis
   f. treat a patient with a history of malignant hyperthermia

Bibliography

British Medical Association and Royal Pharmaceutical Society of Great Britain. (2008). *British National Formulary*. London: BMJ & RPS Publishing. *This publication is updated biannually: it is imperative that the most recent edition is consulted.*

British Medical Association and Royal Pharmaceutical Society of Great Britain. (2008). *British National Formulary for Children*. London: BMJ & RPS Publishing. *This publication is updated annually: it is imperative that the most recent edition is consulted.*

Ganong, W. (2005). *Review of medical physiology* (22nd ed.). New York: McGraw-Hill.

Howland, R. D., & Mycek, M. J. (2005). *Pharmacology* (3rd ed.). Philadelphia: Lippincott Williams & Wilkins.

Marieb, E. N., & Hoehn, K. (2004). *Human anatomy & physiology* (7th ed.). San Francisco: Pearson Benjamin Cummings.

Porth, C. M., & Matfin G. (2008). *Pathophysiology: Concepts of altered health states* (8th ed.). Philadelphia: Lippincott Williams & Wilkins.

Simonsen, T., Aarbakke, J., Kay, I., Coleman, I., Sinnott, P., & Lysaa, R. (2006). *Illustrated pharmacology for nurses.* London: Hodder Arnold.

CHAPTER

25

Muscle Relaxants

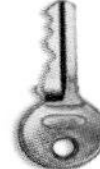

KEY TERMS

actin
basal ganglia
cerebellum
extrapyramidal tract
hypertonia
interneuron
myosin
pyramidal tract
reflex arc
spasticity

LEARNING OBJECTIVES

Upon completion of this chapter, you will be able to:

1. Describe a spinal reflex and discuss the pathophysiology of muscle spasm and muscle spasticity.
2. Describe the therapeutic actions, indications, pharmacokinetics associated with the centrally acting and the direct-acting skeletal muscle relaxants
3. Describe the contraindications, most common adverse reactions and important drug–drug interactions associated with the centrally acting and the direct-acting skeletal muscle relaxants.
4. Discuss the use of muscle relaxants across the lifespan.
5. Compare and contrast the key drugs baclofen and dantrolene with other muscle relaxants in their classes.
6. Outline the nursing considerations, including important teaching points, for patients receiving an anaesthetic.

CENTRALLY ACTING SKELETAL MUSCLE RELAXANTS

baclofen
carisoprodol
methocarbamol
orphenadrine
tizanidine
diazepam

DIRECT-ACTING SKELETAL MUSCLE RELAXANTS

botulinum toxin type A
botulinum toxin type B
dantrolene

Many injuries and accidents result in local damage to muscles, to the tendons, which attach muscles to other muscles or ligaments which attach muscles to bone. These injuries may lead to muscle spasm and pain, which may be of long duration and may interfere with normal functioning. Damage to neurons in the central nervous system (CNS) may cause a permanent state of muscle **spasticity** as a result of loss of the nerves that help maintain balance and control muscle activity.

Neuron damage, whether temporary or permanent, may be treated with skeletal muscle relaxants. Most skeletal muscle relaxants work in the brain and spinal cord, where they interfere with the control of muscle at the level of the motor neuron or the neuromuscular junction (NMJ). Others like the botulinum toxins and dantrolene enter muscle fibres directly (see Box 25.1).

Nerves and Movement

Posture, balance and movement are the result of a constantly fluctuating sequence of muscle contraction and relaxation. The neurones that regulate these actions are the spinal motor neurons. These neurons are influenced by higher-level brain activity in the **cerebellum** and **basal ganglia**, which provide coordination of contractions and in the cerebral cortex, which allows conscious thought to regulate movement.

Spinal Reflexes

The spinal reflexes are the simplest nerve pathways that monitor movement and posture (Figure 25.1). Spinal reflexes can be simple, involving an incoming sensory (afferent) neuron and an outgoing (efferent) motor neuron, or more complex, involving **interneurons** that communicate with the related centres in the brain. Simple **reflex arcs** involve sensory receptors in the periphery and spinal motor nerves. These reflexes are responsible for maintaining muscle tone and keeping an upright position against the pull of gravity. Other spinal reflexes may involve synapses with interneurons within the spinal cord, which adjust movement and response based on information from higher brain centres and coordinate movement and position.

Brain Control

Many areas within the brain influence the spinal motor nerves. Areas of the brainstem, the basal ganglia and the cerebellum modulate spinal motor nerve activity and help

BOX 25.1 DRUG THERAPY ACROSS THE LIFESPAN

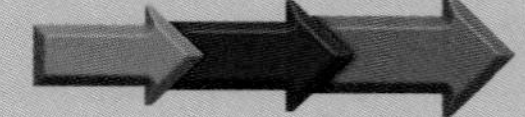

Skeletal Muscle Relaxants

CHILDREN

The safety and effectiveness of most of these drugs have not been established in children. Agents have been used but with adjustments to the adult dosage based on the child's age and weight.

Baclofen is often used to relieve the muscle spasticity associated with cerebral palsy. The child's carer needs detailed education about the use of the intrathecal infusion pump and how to monitor the child for therapeutic or adverse effects.

Methocarbamol is the drug of choice if a child needs to be treated for tetanus.

Dantrolene is used to treat upper motor neuron spasticity in children. The dosage is based on body weight and increases over time. The child should be screened regularly for CNS and gastrointestinal (GI) (including hepatic) toxicity.

When administering any drug to children, always consult the most recent edition of the British National Formulary for Children.

ADULTS

Adults being treated for acute musculoskeletal pain should be cautioned to avoid driving and to take safety precautions against injury because of the related CNS effects (dizziness and drowsiness).

Adults complaining of muscle spasm pain that may be related to anxiety often respond very effectively to diazepam, which is a muscle relaxant and anxiolytic (sedative).

Women of childbearing age should be advised to use contraception when they are taking these drugs. If a pregnancy does occur, or is desired, they should be offered counselling to discuss the potential for adverse effects. Women who are breast-feeding should be encouraged to find another method of feeding the baby because of the potential for adverse drug effects on the baby.

Premenopausal women are also at increased risk for the hepatotoxicity associated with dantrolene and should be monitored very closely for any change in hepatic function. They should be given written information about the prodrome syndrome that often occurs with the hepatic toxicity.

OLDER ADULTS

Older patients are more likely to experience the adverse effects associated with these drugs—CNS, GI and cardiovascular. Also older patients often have renal or hepatic impairment, they are more likely to have toxic levels of the drug related to changes in metabolism and excretion.

Carisoprodol is the centrally acting skeletal muscle relaxant of choice for older patients and for those with hepatic or renal impairment, although half the adult dose is recommended for elderly patients (as per British National Formulary [BNF] recommendations).

If dantrolene is required for an older patient, lower doses and more frequent monitoring are needed to assess for potential cardiac, respiratory and liver toxicity.

Older women who are receiving hormone replacement therapy are at the same risk for development of hepatotoxicity as premenopausal women and should be monitored accordingly.

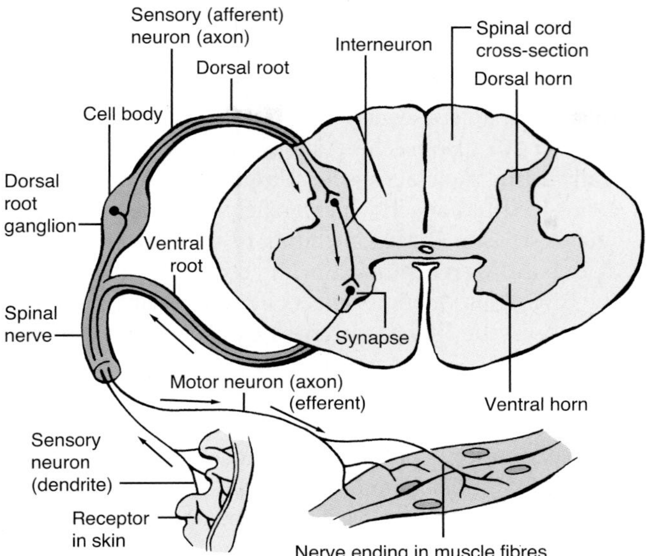

FIGURE 25.1 Reflex arc showing the pathway of impulses.

coordinate activity among various muscle groups; nerve areas within the cerebral cortex allow conscious, or intentional, movement. Nerves within the cortex send signals down the spinal cord, where they cross to the opposite side of the spinal cord before sending out nerve impulses to cause muscle contraction. In this way, each side of the cortex controls muscle movement on the opposite side of the body.

The motor pathways (or descending tracts) involve upper motor neurons (UMN) which originate in the motor cortex and track down to the spinal cord and lower motor neurons (LMN) which synapse the spinal cord and connect with the muscle fibres. The only exceptions are the cranial nerves as their UMN synapses with the LMN in the brainstem.

Different fibres control different types of movements. These fibres that control precise, intentional movement make up the **pyramidal tract** within the CNS. The **extrapyramidal tract** is composed of cells from the cerebral cortex as well as from several subcortical areas, including the basal ganglia and the cerebellum. This tract modulates or coordinates unconsciously controlled muscle activity and it allows the body to make automatic adjustments in posture or position and balance. The extrapyramidal tract controls lower-level, or crude, movements.

Neuromuscular Abnormalities

All of the areas mentioned work together to allow for a free flow of impulses into and out of the CNS to coordinate posture, balance and movement. When injuries, diseases and toxins affect the normal flow of information into and out of the CNS motor pathways, many clinical signs and symptoms may develop, ranging from simple muscle spasms to spasticity, or sustained muscle spasm and paralysis.

Muscle Spasm

Muscle spasms often result from injury to the musculoskeletal system – for example, overstretching a muscle, twisting a joint, or tearing a tendon or ligament. Other causes of muscle spasms include overmedication with antipsychotic drugs, epilepsy, hypocalcaemia, pain and debilitating neurologic disorders (Adams *et al.* 2005). These injuries can cause violent and painful involuntary muscle contractions. Patients with muscle spasms may experience inflammation, oedema, pain at the affected muscle, loss of co-ordination and reduced mobility. It is thought that these spasms are caused by the flood of sensory impulses coming to the spinal cord from the injured area. These impulses can be passed through interneurons to spinal motor nerves, which stimulate an intense muscle contraction. The contraction can reduce blood flow to the muscle fibres in the injured area, causing lactic acid to accumulate, resulting in pain. The new flood of sensory impulses caused by the pain may lead to further muscle contraction and a vicious cycle may develop (Box 25.2).

BOX 25.2 Summary of Muscle Contraction and Relaxation

Stimulus from nerve axon to NMJ (increase in sodium permeability along the motor neuron)

↓

Acetylcholine release into synaptic cleft by calcium dependant exocytosis

↓

Increased permeability of muscle cell membrane to sodium

↓

Rise in membrane potential (action potential generation)

↓

Transmission of action potential through T tubules

↓

Release of calcium from sarcoplasmic reticulum

↓

Binding of calcium to troponin—tropomyosin

↓

Sliding of **actin** on **myosin** with shortening of sarcomere unit

↓

Contraction of the muscle fibre

↓

Calcium pump moves calcium back to sarcoplasmic reticulum

↓

Unbinding of troponin—tropomyosin

↓

Release of actin and myosin binding

↓

Lengthening of sarcomere unit

↓

Relaxation of muscle fibre

Muscle Spasms

Muscle spasms are a very common, troublesome problem for many people. Over 12 million people worldwide have muscle spasms (Adams *et al.* 2005). Muscle spasms severe enough for drug therapy are often found in patients who have had other debilitating disorders such as stroke, injury, neurodegenerative disorders and cerebral palsy.

Muscle spasms may result from an increase in excitatory influences or a decrease in inhibitory influences within the CNS. The interruption in the balance among all of these higher influences within the CNS may lead to excessive stimulation of muscles, or **hypertonia**, in opposing muscle groups at the same time, a condition that may cause permanent structural changes. This control imbalance also results in a loss of coordinated muscle activity.

For example, the signs and symptoms of cerebral palsy and paraplegia are related to the disruption in the nervous control of the muscles. The exact presentation of any chronic neurological disorder depends on the specific nerve fibres, brain centres and tracts that are damaged.

Centrally Acting Skeletal Muscle Relaxants

The centrally acting skeletal muscle relaxants work in the CNS to interfere with the reflexes that are causing the muscle spasm. These drugs are often referred to as spasmolytics because they lyse or destroy spasm (see Box 25.1). These drugs include:

- Baclofen, which is used for the treatment of muscle spasticity associated with neuromuscular diseases such as multiple sclerosis, muscle rigidity and spinal cord injuries. This agent, which is available in oral and intrathecal forms, can be administered via a delivery pump for the treatment of central spasticity. Baclofen is often a drug of first choice due to its wide safety margin.
- Carisoprodol, which is indicated for the relief of discomfort associated with musculoskeletal pain. It may be safer than the other spasmolytics in older patients and in those with renal or hepatic dysfunction.
- Methocarbamol, which is recommended for the short-term relief of discomfort associated with painful, acute musculoskeletal conditions and also to alleviate signs and symptoms of tetanus. It is available in oral forms.
- Orphenadrine, another parenteral drug, which is available for the relief of acute, painful musculoskeletal conditions and in parkinsonism. This agent is also being tried for the relief of quinidine-resistant leg cramps.
- Tizanidine, which is approved for the acute and intermittent management of increased muscle tone spasticity associated with multiple sclerosis and spinal cord injury. It has been associated with liver toxicity and should be used with caution if a patient has hepatic dysfunction. It is also associated with hypotension in some patients. *Note*: As these drugs work in the upper levels of the CNS, there is a risk of depression with their use.
- Diazepam, a drug widely used as an anxiety agent (see Chapter 20), also has been shown to be an effective centrally acting skeletal muscle relaxant. It may be advantageous in situations in which anxiety may precipitate the muscle spasm. Diazepam binds to the γ-aminobutyric acid (GABA) receptor-chloride channels throughout the CNS. It produces its effects by suppressing neuronal activity in the limbic system and subsequent impulses that might be transmitted to the reticular activating system. Effects of this drug are suppression of abnormal neuronal foci that may cause seizures, calming without strong sedation, and skeletal muscle relaxation (Adams *et al.* 2005). It is commonly used for example for nurses suffering from severe back pain and spasms associated with back pain. The current recommendation is rest, and diazepam; 5 mg three times daily to relieve their pain.

In addition to these drugs other measures should be used to alleviate muscle spasm and pain. These include: resting the affected muscle; heat applications to increase blood flow to the area and to remove the pain-causing chemicals; physical therapy to return the muscle to normal tone and activity and anti-inflammatory agents (including nonsteroidal anti-inflammatory drugs [NSAIDs]) if the underlying problem is related to injury or inflammation may help.

Therapeutic Actions and Indications

Although the exact mechanism of action of these skeletal muscle relaxants is unknown, it is thought to involve action in the upper or spinal interneurons. Tizanidine is a centrally acting α_2-adrenergic agonist and is thought to increase inhibition of presynaptic motor neurons in the CNS. The primary indication for the use of centrally acting skeletal muscle agents is the relief of discomfort associated with acute, painful musculoskeletal conditions as an adjunct to rest, physical therapy and other measures.

Pharmacokinetics

Most of these agents are rapidly absorbed and metabolized in the liver. Baclofen is not metabolized, but like the other skeletal muscle relaxants, it is excreted in the urine. No conclusive studies exist regarding the effects of these agents during pregnancy and lactation; therefore, use should be limited to those situations in which the benefit to the mother clearly outweighs any potential risk to the foetus or neonate.

Contraindications and Cautions

Centrally acting skeletal muscle relaxants are contraindicated in the presence of any known allergy to any of these drugs and with skeletal muscle spasms resulting from rheumatic disorders. In addition, baclofen should not be used to treat any spasticity that contributes to locomotion, upright position, or increased function. *Blocking this spasticity results in loss of these functions.*

All centrally acting skeletal muscle relaxants should be used cautiously in the following circumstances: with a history of epilepsy *because the CNS depression and imbalance caused by these drugs may exacerbate the seizure disorder*; with cardiac dysfunction *because muscle function may be depressed*; with any condition marked by muscle weakness *that the drugs could make much worse*; and with hepatic or renal dysfunction, *which could interfere with the metabolism and excretion of the drugs, leading to toxic levels*. These agents should be used with caution in pregnancy or lactation *because of adverse effects to the foetus or neonate*.

Adverse Effects

The most frequently seen adverse effects associated with these drugs relate to the associated CNS depression: drowsiness, fatigue, weakness, confusion, headache and insomnia. GI disturbances, which may be linked to CNS depression of the parasympathetic reflexes, include nausea, dry mouth, anorexia and constipation. In addition, hypotension and arrhythmias may occur, again as a result of depression of normal reflex arcs. Urinary frequency, enuresis and feelings of urinary urgency reportedly may occur.

Clinically Important Drug–Drug Interactions

If any of the centrally acting skeletal muscle relaxants are taken with other CNS depressants or alcohol, CNS depression may increase. Patients should be cautioned to avoid alcohol while taking these muscle relaxants; if this combination cannot be avoided, they should take extreme precautions.

Always check the most up to date copy of the BNF for further details.

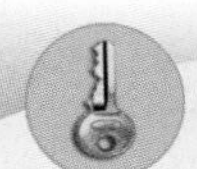

Key Drug Summary: *Baclofen*

Indications: Alleviation of signs and symptoms of spasticity; may be of use in spinal cord injuries or spinal cord diseases and for spasticity associated with multiple sclerosis

Actions: GABA analogue; exact mechanism of action is not understood; inhibits transmission at the spinal level and generally suppresses the CNS.

Pharmacokinetics:

Route	Onset	Peak	Duration
Oral	1 h	2 h	4–8 h
Intrathecal	30–60 min	4 h	4–8 h

$T_{1/2}$: 3–4 hours; not metabolized; excreted in the urine

Note: the dose should be increased slowly to avoid sedation and hypotonia

Adverse effects: Transient drowsiness, dizziness, weakness, fatigue, constipation, headache, insomnia, hypotension, nausea, urinary frequency

Nursing Considerations for Patients Receiving Centrally Acting Skeletal Muscle Relaxants

Assessment: History and Examination

Screen for the following conditions, *which could be cautions or contraindications for the use of the drug*: any known allergies to these drugs; cardiac depression, epilepsy, muscle weakness, rheumatic disorder; pregnancy or lactation; and renal or hepatic dysfunction.

Include screening *for baseline status before beginning therapy and for any potential adverse effects*. Assess the following: temperature; skin colour and texture; CNS orientation, affect, reflexes, bilateral grip strength and spasticity evaluation; bowel sounds and reported output; and liver and renal function tests.

Assess pain levels and monitor; determine location, duration and precipitating factors of the patient's pain.

Establish if patient is currently taking other medications or herbal therapies, which may potentially interact with the centrally acting skeletal muscle relaxants.

Nursing Diagnoses

The patient who is receiving a centrally acting skeletal muscle relaxant may have the following nursing diagnoses related to drug therapy:

- Acute pain related to GI and CNS effects
- Disturbed thought processes related to CNS effects

- Risk for injury related to CNS effects
- Deficient knowledge regarding drug therapy

Implementation With Rationale

- Provide additional measures to relieve discomfort – heat, rest for the muscle, NSAIDs, positioning – *to increase the effects of the drug at relieving the musculoskeletal discomfort.*
- Discontinue the drug at any sign of hypersensitivity reaction or liver dysfunction *to prevent severe toxicity.*
- If using baclofen, decrease the drug slowly over 1 to 2 weeks *to prevent the development of psychoses and hallucinations. Monitor for withdrawal reactions. Abrupt withdrawal of Baclofen may cause visual hallucinations, paranoid ideation and seizures.*
- Use baclofen cautiously in patients whose spasticity contributes to mobility, posture, or balance *to prevent loss of this function.*
- If the patient is receiving baclofen through a delivery pump, the patient should understand the pump, the reason for frequent monitoring and how to adjust the dose *to enhance patient knowledge and promote compliance.*
- Monitor respiratory status *to evaluate adverse effects and arrange for appropriate dosage adjustment or discontinuation of the drug.*
- Provide patient education, including drug name, prescribed dosage, methods to avoid adverse effects, warning signs that may indicate possible problems and the need for monitoring and evaluation *to enhance patient knowledge about drug therapy and to promote compliance.*
- Offer support and encouragement *to help the patient cope with the drug regimen.*

Evaluation

- Monitor patient response to the drug (improvement in muscle spasm and relief of pain; improvement in muscle spasticity).
- Monitor for adverse effects (CNS changes, GI depression, and urinary urgency).
- Evaluate the effectiveness of the teaching plan (patient can give the drug name and dosage, possible adverse effects and specific measures to prevent adverse effects and describe, if necessary, proper intrathecal administration.
- Monitor the effectiveness of comfort measures and compliance with the regimen.

Direct-acting Skeletal Muscle Relaxants

One drug is currently available for use in treating (general) spasticity that directly affects peripheral muscle contraction. This drug, dantrolene, has become important in the management of spasticity associated with neuromuscular diseases such as cerebral palsy (see Critical Thinking Scenario 25-1), multiple sclerosis, muscular dystrophy, polio, tetanus, quadriplegia and amyotrophic lateral sclerosis. This agent is not used for the treatment of muscle spasms associated with musculoskeletal injury or rheumatic disorders.

The botulinum toxins A and B bind directly to the receptor sites of motor nerve terminals and inhibit the release of acetylcholine, leading to local muscle paralysis. These two drugs are injected locally and used for specific muscle groups.

Therapeutic Actions and Indications

Dantrolene acts within skeletal muscle fibres, interfering with the release of calcium from the muscle tubules (Figure 25.2). This action prevents the fibres from contracting. Dantrolene does not interfere with neuromuscular transmissions and it does not affect the surface membrane of skeletal muscle. It is the drug of choice as it has few central adverse effects.

Dantrolene is indicated for the control of spasticity resulting from upper motor neuron disorders, including

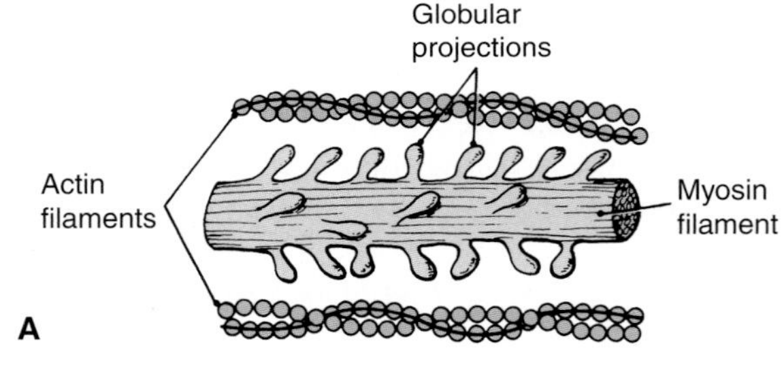

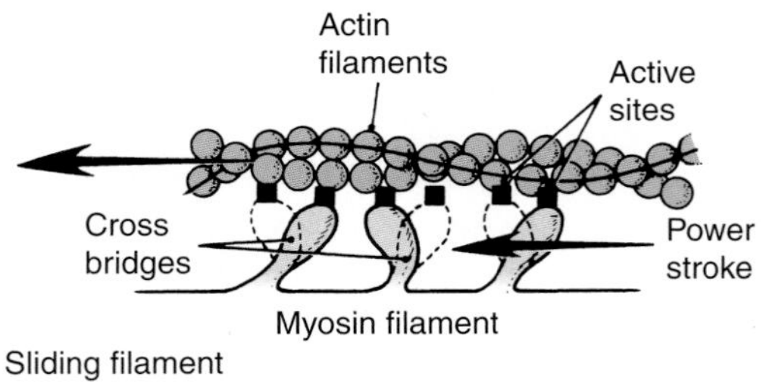

FIGURE 25.2 Sliding filament mechanism of muscle contraction. **(A)** The relationship between the myosin filament and the actin filament projections. **(B)** The bridges formed by the myosin filament along successive sites on the actin filaments, as outlined in Box 25.2.

spinal cord injury, myasthenia gravis, muscular dystrophy and cerebral palsy (oral form). It can also be used for spasms of the head and neck. It is especially useful for muscle spasms when they occur after spinal cord injury or stroke and in cases of cerebral palsy, multiple sclerosis and occasionally for the treatment of muscle pain after heavy exercise. Also used for the treatment of malignant hyperthermia. Continued long-term use is justified as long as the drug reduces painful and disabling spasticity. Long-term use results in a decrease in the amount and intensity of required nursing care.

Dantrolene is also indicated for the prevention of malignant hyperthermia, a state of intense muscle contraction and resulting hyperpyrexia. Malignant hyperthermia may occur as an adverse reaction to certain NMJ blockers that are used to induce paralysis during surgery. Dantrolene is used orally as preoperative prophylaxis in susceptible patients who must undergo anaesthesia and after acute episodes to prevent recurrence.

The agent is also used parenterally to treat malignant hyperthermia crisis.

Botulinum toxin type B is a direct-acting skeletal muscle relaxant that is approved for the reduction of the severity of abnormal head position and neck pain associated with cervical dystonia. Injections of 5000 to 10,000 units is given intramuscularly (IM) into the affected muscles, causing muscle relaxation and relieving the tight spasm that can distort head position and cause pain – please note ***this toxin is not interchangeable with other botulinum toxin preparations***.

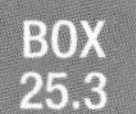

Sex Considerations: Understanding the Risks of Liver Damage with Dantrolene

Dantrolene is associated with potentially fatal hepatocellular injury. When liver damage begins to occur, patients often experience a warning syndrome, which includes anorexia, nausea and fatigue. The incidence of such hepatic injury is greater in women and in patients 35 years of age or above.

In women, a combination of dantrolene and oestrogen seems to affect the liver, thus posing a greater risk. Women of all ages may be at increased risk, because those entering menopause may be taking hormone replacement therapy. Patients older than 35 years of age are at increasing risk of liver injury because of the changing integrity of the liver cells that comes with age and exposure to toxins over time.

If a particular woman needs dantrolene for relief of spasticity, she should not be taking any estrogens (e.g. birth control pills, hormone replacement therapy) and she should be monitored closely for any sign of liver dysfunction. For safer relief of spasticity in these patients, baclofen may be helpful.

Pharmacokinetics

Dantrolene is slowly absorbed from the GI tract. It is metabolized in the liver with a half-life of 4 to 8 hours. Excretion is through the urine. Dantrolene crosses the placenta and was found to have toxic effects on the embryo in animal studies. Use should be reserved for those situations in which the benefit to the mother clearly outweighs the risk to the foetus. Dantrolene enters breast milk and is contraindicated for use during lactation. Safety for use in children younger than 5 years of age has not been established; because the long-term effects are not known, careful consideration should be given to use of the drug in children. The botulinum toxins are not generally absorbed systemically.

Contraindications and Cautions

Dantrolene is contraindicated in the following conditions: spasticity that contributes to locomotion, upright position, or increased function, *which would be lost if that spasticity were blocked*; active hepatic disease, *which might interfere with metabolism of the drug and because of known liver toxicity*; and lactation *because the drug may cross into breast milk and cause adverse effects in the infant*. The botulinum toxins are contraindicated in the presence of allergy to any component of the drug or with active infection at the site of the injection *because injecting the drug could aggravate the infection*.

Caution should be used with dantrolene in the following circumstances: in women and in all patients older than 35 years *because of increased risk of potentially fatal hepatocellular disease* (see Box 25.3) in patients with a history of liver disease or previous dysfunction, *which could make the liver more susceptible to cellular toxicity*; in those with respiratory depression, *which could be exacerbated by muscular weakness*; in those with cardiac disease *because cardiac muscle depression may be a risk*; and during pregnancy *because of the potential for adverse effects on the foetus*. Caution should be used with the botulinum toxins with any peripheral neuropathic disease; with neuromuscular disorders, *which could be exacerbated by the effects of the drug*; with pregnancy and lactation; and with any known cardiovascular disease.

Always consult the latest edition of the BNF for up to date information.

Adverse Effects

The most frequently seen adverse effects associated with dantrolene relate to drug-caused CNS depression: drowsiness, fatigue, weakness, confusion, headache and insomnia and visual disturbances. GI disturbances may be linked to direct irritation or to alterations in smooth muscle function caused by the drug-induced calcium effects. Such adverse GI effects may include GI irritation, diarrhoea, constipation and abdominal cramps. Dantrolene may also cause direct hepatocellular damage and hepatitis that can be fatal. Urinary frequency, enuresis and feelings of urinary urgency reportedly occur and crystalline urine with pain or burning on urination may result. In addition, several unusual adverse effects may occur, including acne, abnormal hair growth, rashes, photosensitivity, abnormal sweating, chills and myalgia.

The botulinum toxins have been associated with anaphylactic reactions; with headache, dizziness, muscle pain and paralysis; and with redness and oedema at the injection site.

Clinically Important Drug–Drug Interactions

If dantrolene is combined with oestrogens, the incidence of hepatocellular toxicity is apparently increased. If possible, this combination should be avoided. Dantrolene also interacts with OTC cough preparations and antihistamines, alcohol or other CNS depressants. Verapamil and other calcium channel blockers taken with dantrolene increase the risk of ventricular fibrillation and cardiovascular collapse. Patients with impaired cardiac or pulmonary function or hepatic disease should not take this drug. If the botulinum toxins are used with other drugs that interfere with neuromuscular transmission; NMJ blockers, quinidine, magnesium sulphate, anticholinesterases, or polymyxin – or with aminoglycosides, there is a risk of enhanced blocking effects. If any of these must be given in combination, extreme caution should be used.

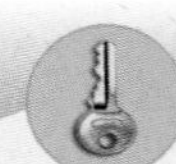

Key Drug Summary: *Dantrolene*

Indications: Control of clinical spasticity resulting from upper motor neuron disorders; preoperatively to prevent or attenuate the development of malignant hyperthermia in susceptible patients; intravenous (IV) for management of fulminant malignant hyperthermia

Actions: Interferes with the release of calcium from the sarcoplasmic reticulum within skeletal muscles, preventing muscle contraction; does not interfere with neuromuscular transmission

Pharmacokinetics:

Route	Onset	Peak	Duration
Oral	Slow	4–6 h	8–10 h
IV	Rapid	5 h	6–8 h

$T_{1/2}$: 9 hours (oral), 4–8 hours (IV); excreted in the urine

Adverse effects: Drowsiness, dizziness, weakness, fatigue, diarrhoea, hepatitis, myalgia, tachycardia, transient blood pressure changes, rash, urinary frequency

Nursing Considerations for Patients Receiving a Direct-acting Skeletal Muscle Relaxant

Assessment: History and Examination

Screen for the following conditions, *which could be cautions or contraindications for the use of the drug*: any known allergies to these drugs; cardiac depression; epilepsy; muscle weakness; respiratory depression; pregnancy and lactation; and renal or hepatic dysfunction.

Include screening *for baseline status before beginning therapy and for any potential adverse effects.* Assess the following: temperature; skin colour and lesions; CNS orientation, affect, reflexes, bilateral grip strength and spasticity; respiration and adventitious sounds; pulse, electrocardiogram (ECG) and cardiac output; bowel sounds and reported output; and liver and renal function tests.

Establish if patient is currently taking other medications or herbal therapies, which may potentially interact with the direct-acting skeletal muscle relaxants.

Nursing Diagnoses

The patient taking a direct-acting skeletal muscle relaxant may have the following nursing diagnoses related to drug therapy:

- Acute pain related to GI and CNS effects
- Disturbed thought processes related to CNS effects
- Risk for injury related to CNS effects
- Deficient knowledge regarding drug therapy

Implementation With Rationale

- Discontinue the drug at any sign of liver dysfunction. *Early diagnosis of liver damage may prevent permanent dysfunction. Arrange for the drug to be discontinued if signs of liver damage appear.* A prodrome, with nausea, anorexia and fatigue, is present in 60% of patients with evidence of hepatic injury.
- Monitor intravenous access sites for potential extravasation *because the drug is alkaline and very irritating to tissues.*
- Institute other supportive measures (e.g. ventilation, anticonvulsants as needed) for the treatment of malignant hyperthermia *to support the patient through the reaction.*
- *To monitor therapeutic effectiveness* periodically discontinue the drug for 2 to 4 days. A clinical impression of exacerbation of spasticity indicates a positive therapeutic effect and justifies continued use of the drug.

- Establish a therapeutic goal before beginning oral therapy (e.g. to gain or enhance the ability to engage in a therapeutic exercise programme; to use braces; to accomplish transfer manoeuvres) *to promote patient compliance and a sense of success with therapy.*
- If diarrhoea becomes severe discontinue the drug *to prevent dehydration and electrolyte imbalance.* The drug may be restarted at a lower dose.
- Provide thorough patient education, including drug name, prescribed dosage, measures to avoid adverse effects, warning signs that may indicate possible problems and the need for monitoring and evaluation *to enhance patient knowledge about drug therapy and to promote compliance.*
- Offer support and encouragement to help the patient cope with the drug regimen.

Evaluation

- Monitor patient response to the drug (improvement in spasticity, improvement in movement and activities).
- Monitor for adverse effects (CNS changes, diarrhoea, liver toxicity, urinary urgency).
- Evaluate the effectiveness of the teaching plan (patient can give the drug name and dosage, possible adverse effects to watch for and specific measures to prevent adverse effects and therapeutic goals).
- Monitor the effectiveness of comfort measures and compliance with the regimen.

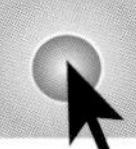

WEB LINKS

Health care providers and patients may want to consult the following Internet sources:

http://cks.library.nhs.uk The National Health Service Clinical Knowledge Summaries provides evidence-based practical information on the common conditions observed in primary care.

http://www.bnf.org.uk The BNF provides UK health care professionals with authoritative and practical information on the selection and clinical use of medicines.

http://www.nhsdirect.nhs.uk The National Health Service Direct service provides patients with information and advice about health.

http://www.nice.org.uk National Institute for Health and Clinical Excellence (NICE) is an independent organization responsible for providing national guidance on promoting good health and preventing and treating ill health.

http://www.ucp.org Information for patients and health care professionals about cerebral palsy research and treatment.

http://www.spinalcord.org Patient information regarding cerebral palsy

Points to Remember

- Movement and control of muscles is regulated by spinal reflexes and influences from higher-level CNS areas, including the basal ganglia, cerebellum and cerebral cortex.
- Higher-level controls of muscle activity include the pyramidal tract in the cerebellum, which regulates coordination of intentional muscle movement and the extrapyramidal tract in the cerebellum and basal ganglia, which coordinates crude movements related to unconscious muscle activity.
- Damage to a muscle or anchoring skeletal structure may result in the arrival of a flood of impulses to the spinal cord. Such overstimulation may lead to a muscle spasm or a state of increased contraction.
- Damage to motor neurons can cause muscle spasticity, with a lack of coordination between muscle groups and loss of coordinated activity, including the ability to perform intentional tasks and maintain posture, position and locomotion.
- Centrally acting skeletal muscle relaxants are used to relieve the effects of muscle spasm. Dantrolene, a direct-acting skeletal muscle relaxant, is used to control spasticity and prevent malignant hyperthermia.
- The botulinum toxin type B is used to reduce the severity of abnormal head position and neck pain associated with cervical dystonia. Botulinum toxin type A is used to improve the appearance of moderate to severe glabellar lines and to treat cervical dystonia, severe primary axillary hyperhidrosis and strabismus also blepharospasm associated with dystonia.

CRITICAL THINKING SCENARIO 25-1

Skeletal Muscle Relaxants for Cerebral Palsy

The Situation

Lee is 19 years old. He was diagnosed with cerebral palsy shortly after birth. He lives at home with his parents, they are his main carers. In the past few months, Lee's spasticity has progressed severely, making it impossible for him to carry out his daily activities without extensive assistance.

His parents attend the general practitioner (GP) surgery with Lee for advice and after clinical examination his GP suggests trying a course of dantrolene therapy. After learning about the risks of dantrolene-related hepatic dysfunction, Lee decides that the benefits of dantrolene therapy are more important to him than the risks of hepatotoxicity.

Therapy begins and the GP arranges a home visit by the district nurses in 4 days time to re-access Lee's condition.

Critical Thinking

What basic principles must be included in the nursing care plan for Lee for the district nurses? *Think about the importance of including any teaching or evaluation programmes for Lee's parents. Consider specific problems that could develop that Lee would be unable to handle on his own.*

What therapeutic goals might the nurse set with Lee and his parents? How might these be evaluated?

What additional drug-related information should be given to Lee and his parents?

Discussion

On the first visit to Lee's home the nurse should all realize that drug therapy and other measures, is needed to help Lee attain his full potential and make use of his existing assets. Step-by-step therapeutic goals should be established and written down for future reference. Small reachable goals, such as partially dressing himself, walking to the table for meals and managing parts of his daily hygiene routine are best at the beginning. Written goals provide a good basis for future evaluation when drug therapy is stopped briefly to determine its therapeutic effectiveness. It also helps Lee to remain positive and motivated by seeing his progress and improvement.

In addition, the nurse should perform a complete examination to obtain baseline observations. His pain and mobility should be assessed. Lee should be asked about any noticeable changes or problems since starting the drug. If improvement appears to have occurred, the dosage may be slowly increased until the optimal level of functioning has been achieved. The nurse is in a position to evaluate this.

While in the home, the nurse can also evaluate resources and environmental limitations and suggest improvements, (e.g. use of leg braces). The nurse could also provide additional pain relief measures, such as positional support, gentle massage, and moist heat or ice packs (drugs alone may not be sufficient to provide pain relief.)

Lee should also receive information, which includes a telephone number to call with questions or concerns; warning signs of liver disease; and a list of findings to report. The nurse should discuss follow-up appointments for liver function tests. Lee's parents should work closely with him to maximize his involvement in his care and to minimize unnecessary problems and confusion. The treatment involves a long-term commitment. A good working relationship among all members of the health care team is important to ensure continuity of care and optimal results.

Nursing Care Guide for Lee's: Muscle Relaxants

Assessment: History and Examination

Concentrate the health history on allergies to any skeletal muscle relaxants, respiratory depression, muscle weakness, hepatic or renal dysfunction and concurrent use of verapamil or alcohol.

Focus the physical examination on the following:

- Cardiovascular: blood pressure pulse rate, peripheral perfusion, ECG
- CNS: orientation, reflexes, grip strength
- Skin: colour, lesions, texture, temperature
- GI: abdominal examination, bowel sounds
- Respiratory: respiration, adventitious sounds
- Laboratory tests: renal and hepatic function

Nursing Diagnoses

- Acute pain related to GI, genitourinary and CNS effects (pain associated with muscle spasms).
- Risk for injury related to CNS effects and side-effects of drug

Skeletal Muscle Relaxants for Cerebral Palsy *(continued)*

- Disturbed thought processes related to CNS effects
- Deficient knowledge regarding drug therapy
- Impaired physical mobility, related to acute/chronic pain

Implementation

- Discontinue drug at first sign of liver dysfunction.
- Report signs of urinary retention, such as a feeling of urinary bladder fullness, distended abdomen and discomfort
- Provide comfort and safety measures: positioning, pain management as needed.
- Provide support and reassurance to help Lee deal with spasticity and drug effects.
- Teach Lee about drug, dosage, drug effects and symptoms of reportable serious adverse effects.

Evaluation

- Evaluate drug effects: relief of spasticity, improved daily function.
- Monitor for adverse effects: multiple CNS effects, respiratory depression, rash, skin changes, GI problems (diarrhoea, hepatotoxicity), urinary urgency or weakness.
- Monitor for drug–drug interactions: myocardial suppression with verapamil or alcohol.
- Evaluate effectiveness of patient education programme.

Patient Education for Lee

The drug prescribed for you is a direct-acting skeletal muscle relaxant called dantrolene. This drug makes spastic muscles relax. This drug may cause liver damage, so it is important that you have regular medical check-ups. Common side-effects of skeletal muscle relaxants, such as dantrolene, include:

- *Fatigue, weakness and drowsiness:* Try to pace activities evenly throughout the day and allow rest periods to avoid discouraging side-effects. If they become too severe, consult your doctor.
- *Dizziness and fainting:* Change position slowly to avoid dizzy spells. If these effects should occur, avoid activities that require coordination and concentration.
- *Diarrhoea:* Be sure to be near bathroom facilities if this occurs. This effect usually subsides after a few weeks.
- Report any of the following to your health care provider: *fever, chills, rash, itching, changes in the colour of your urine or stool, or a yellowish tint to the eyes or skin*
- Do not overexert yourself when you begin to feel better. Pace yourself.
- Take this drug exactly as directed and schedule regular medical checkups to evaluate the effects of this drug on your body.

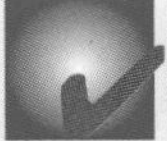

CHECK YOUR UNDERSTANDING

Answers to the questions in this chapter may be found in the answer key in the back of the book.

Multiple Choice

Select the most appropriate response to the following.

1. A muscle spasm often results from
   a. damage to the basal ganglia.
   b. CNS damage.
   c. injury to the musculoskeletal system.
   d. chemical imbalance within the CNS.

2. Muscle spasticity is the result of
   a. direct damage to a muscle cell.
   b. overstretching of a muscle.
   c. tearing of a ligament.
   d. damage to neurons within the CNS.

3. Signs and symptoms of tetanus, which includes severe muscle spasm, are best treated with
   a. baclofen.
   b. diazepam.
   c. carisoprodol.
   d. methocarbamol.

4. The drug of choice for a patient experiencing severe muscle spasms and pain precipitated by anxiety would be
   a. methocarbamol.
   b. baclofen.
   c. diazepam.
   d. carisoprodol.

5. Dantrolene differs from the other skeletal muscle relaxants because it
   a. acts in the highest levels of the CNS.
   b. is used to treat muscle spasms as well as muscle spasticity.
   c. can not be used to treat neuromuscular disorders.
   d. acts directly within the skeletal muscle fibre and not within the CNS.

6. The use of NMJ blockers may sometimes cause a condition known as malignant hyperthermia. The drug of choice for prevention or treatment of this condition is
   a. baclofen.
   b. diazepam.
   c. dantrolene.
   d. methocarbamol.

7. Dantrolene is associated with potentially fatal cellular damage. If your patient's condition is being managed with dantrolene, the patient should
   a. have repeated hearing tests during therapy.
   b. have renal function tests done monthly.
   c. be monitored for signs of liver damage and have liver function tests done regularly.
   d. have a thorough eye examination before and periodically during therapy.

Extended Matching Questions

Select all that apply.

1. Spasmolytics or centrally acting muscle relaxants block the reflexes in the CNS that lead to spasm. While a patient is taking one of these drugs, which of the following interventions should be implemented?
   a. Rest for the affected muscle
   b. Heat to the affected area
   c. Ice packs to the affected area
   d. Use of anti-inflammatory agents
   e. Body temperature check every 2 hours to watch for malignant hyperthermia
   f. Positioning to decrease pain and spasm

2. Muscle relaxants would be used to:
   a. treat spasticity related to spinal cord injury
   b. treat spasticity that contributes to locomotion, upright position, or increase in function
   c. treat spasticity that is related to toxins, such as tetanus
   d. treat spasticity that is a result of neuromuscular degeneration
   e. reduce the severity of head position associated with cervical dystonia
   f. reduce the appearance of frown lines (glabellar lines)

Matching

Match the following words with the appropriate definitions.

1. ____________________spasticity
2. ____________________hypertonia
3. ____________________hypotonia
4. ____________________basal ganglia
5. ____________________interneurons
6. ____________________pyramidal tract
7. ____________________extrapyramidal tract
8. ____________________cerebellum

A. Neurons that communicate between other neurons
B. Fibres within the CNS that control precise, intentional movement
C. Sustained contractions of muscles
D. Lower portion of the brain associated with coordination of muscle movements and voluntary muscle movement
E. State of excessive muscle response and activity
F. Lower area of the brain associated with coordination of unconscious muscle movements
G. Cells that coordinate unconsciously controlled muscle activity
H. State of limited or absent muscle response and activity

True or False

Indicate whether the following statements are true (T) or false (F).

_____ 1. The nerves that affect movement, position and posture are the spinal sensory neurons.

_____ 2. The basal ganglia and the cerebellum modulate spinal motor nerve activity and help coordinate activity between various muscle groups.

_____ 3. Fibres that control precise, intentional movement make up the extrapyramidal tract.

_____ 4. The pyramidal tract modulates or coordinates unconsciously controlled muscle activity and allows the body to make automatic adjustments in posture, position and balance.

_____ 5. Muscle spasticity is the result of damage to neurons within the CNS, rather than injury to peripheral structures.

_____ 6. Excessive stimulation of muscles is referred to as hypotonia.

_____ 7. Centrally acting skeletal muscle relaxants work in the CNS to interfere with the reflexes that are causing the muscle spasm.

_____ 8. Dantrolene acts within skeletal muscle fibres, interfering with the release of potassium from the muscle tubules, to prevent the fibres from contracting.

_____ 9. The primary indication for the use of centrally acting skeletal muscle agents is the relief of discomfort associated with acute, painful musculoskeletal conditions.

_____10. Centrally acting muscle relaxants should be used as an adjunct to rest, physical therapy and other measures.

Bibliography and References

Adams, M. P., Josephson, D. L., & Holland, L. N. (2005) *Pharmacology for nurses: A pathophysiologic approach*. New Jersey: Pearson Prentice Hall.

Britis Medical Association and Royal Pharmaceutical Society of Great Britain. (2008). *British National Formulary*. London: BMJ & RPS Publishing. *This publication is updated biannually: it is imperative that the most recent edition is consulted.*

Britis Medical Association and Royal Pharmaceutical Society of Great Britain. (2008). *British National Formulary for Children*. London: BMJ & RPS Publishing. *This publication is updated annually: it is imperative that the most recent edition is consulted.*

Ganong, W. (2005). *Review of medical physiology* (22nd ed.). New York: McGraw-Hill.

Howland, R. D., & Mycek, M. J. (2005). *Pharmacology* (3rd ed.). Philadelphia: Lippincott Williams & Wilkins.

Marieb, E. N., & Hoehn, K. (2004). *Human anatomy & physiology* (7th ed.). San Francisco: Pearson Benjamin Cummings.

Porth, C. M., & Matfin G. (2008). *Pathophysiology: Concepts of altered health states* (8th ed.). Philadelphia: Lippincott Williams & Wilkins.

Simonsen, T., Aarbakke, J., Kay, I., Coleman, I., Sinnott, P., & Lysaa, R. (2006). *Illustrated pharmacology for nurses*. London: Hodder Arnold.

CHAPTER 26

Opioids and Antimigraine Agents

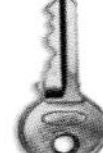

KEY TERMS

A fibres
A-δ and C fibres
endorphins
enkephalins
gate control theory
migraine headache
opioids
opioid agonists
opioid agonists–antagonists
opioid antagonists
opioid receptors
spinothalamic tracts
triptans ($5HT_1$ agonists)

LEARNING OBJECTIVES

Upon completion of this chapter, you will be able to:

1. Outline the gate theory of pain and explain therapeutic ways to block pain using the gate theory.
2. Describe the therapeutic actions, indications, pharmacokinetics associated with opioids and antimigraine drugs.
3. Describe the contraindications, most common adverse reactions and important drug–drug interactions associated with opioids and antimigraine drugs.
4. Discuss the use of opioids and antimigraine drugs across the lifespan.
5. Compare and contrast the key drugs morphine, pentazocine, naloxone, ergotamine and sumatriptan with other drugs in their respective classes.
6. Outline the nursing considerations, including important teaching points, for patients receiving an opioid or an antimigraine drug.

OPIOIDS

Opioid Agonists

codeine
fentanyl
hydromorphone
methadone
morphine
oxycodone
remifentanil

Opioid Agonists–Antagonists

buprenorphine
pentazocine

Opioid Antagonists

naloxone
naltrexone

ANTIMIGRAINE DRUGS

Triptans

almotriptan
eletriptan
frovatriptan
naratriptan
rizatriptan
sumatriptan
zolmitriptan

Pain, by definition, is a sensory and emotional experience associated with actual or potential tissue damage. The perception of pain is part of the clinical presentation in many disorders and is one of the hardest sensations for patients to cope with during the course of a disease or dysfunction. The drugs involved in the management of severe pain, whether acute or chronic, are discussed in this chapter. These agents all work in the central nervous system (CNS) – the brain and the spinal cord – to alter the way pain impulses arriving from peripheral nerves are processed. These agents can change the perception and tolerance of pain. Two major types of drugs are considered here: the **opioids**, the opium derivatives that are used to treat many types of pain and the **antimigraine** drugs, which are reserved for the treatment of **migraine headaches**, a type of severe headache. These drugs are used with patients of all ages (Box 26.1).

Pain Perception

Pain occurs whenever tissues are damaged. The injury to cells releases many chemicals, including kinins and prostaglandins, which stimulate specific sensory nerves (Figure 26.1). Two small-diameter sensory nerves, called the **A-δ (myelinated) and C (unmyelinated) fibres**, respond to stimulation by generating nerve impulses that produce pain sensations. Pain impulses from the skin, subcutaneous (Subcut) tissues, muscles and deep visceral structures are conducted to the dorsal, or posterior, horn of the spinal cord on these fibres via axons of 1st order neurons. In the spinal cord, these nerve fibres synapse with spinal cord nerve fibres (2nd order neurons) that then send impulses to the brain (via 3rd order neurons, forming the ascending tracts).

In addition, large-diameter sensory nerve fibres enter the dorsal horn of the spinal cord. These **A-β fibres** do not transmit pain impulses; instead, they transmit sensations associated with touch and temperature. The A-β fibres, which are larger and conduct impulses more rapidly than the smaller fibres, can actually block the ability of the smaller fibres to transmit their signals to the secondary neurons in the spinal cord. The dorsal horn, therefore, can be both excitatory and inhibitory with pain impulses that are transmitted from the periphery. The impulses reaching the dorsal horn are transmitted upward toward the brain by a number of specific ascending nerve pathways. These pathways run from the spinal cord into the thalamus, where they form synapses with various nerve cells that transmit the information to the cerebral cortex. These pathways are known as the **spinothalamic tracts**.

According to the **gate control theory**, the transmission of these impulses can be modulated all along these tracts (Figure 26.2). All along the spinal cord, the interneurons can act as 'gates' by blocking the ascending transmission of

BOX 26.1 DRUG THERAPY ACROSS THE LIFESPAN

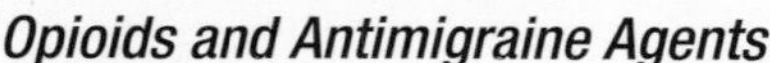

Opioids and Antimigraine Agents

CHILDREN

The safety and effectiveness of many of these drugs have not been established in children. If an opioid is used, the dosage should be calculated very carefully and the child should be monitored closely for the adverse effects associated with opioid use.

Opioids that have an established paediatric dose include codeine, fentanyl (but not transdermal fentanyl) and morphine.

Methadone is not recommended as an analgesic. If a child older than 13 years of age requires an opioid agonist–antagonist, buprenorphine is the drug of choice. Naloxone is the drug of choice for reversal of opioid effects and opioid overdose in children. None of the drugs used to treat migraines are recommended for use in children

When administering any drug to children, always consult the most recent edition of the British National Formulary for Children.

ADULTS

Adults being treated for acute pain should be reassured that the risk of addiction to an opioid during treatment is remote. They should be encouraged to ask for pain medication before the pain is acute, to get better coverage for their pain. Many institutions allow patients to self-regulate IV drips to control their own pain postoperatively. Adults requesting treatment for migraine headaches should be carefully evaluated before one of the antimigraine drugs is used to ensure that the headache being treated is of the type that can benefit from these drugs.

The opioids are contraindicated or should only be used with caution during pregnancy because of the potential for adverse effects on the foetus. These drugs enter breast milk and can cause opioid effects in the baby, so caution should be used during lactation. Morphine and meperidine are often used for analgesia during labour. The mother should be monitored closely for adverse reactions and, if the drug is used over a prolonged labour, the newborn infant should be monitored for opioid effects.

The ergots and the statins are contraindicated during pregnancy because of the potential for adverse effects in the mother and foetus. Women of childbearing age should be advised to use contraception while they are taking these drugs. Women who are nursing should be encouraged to find another method of feeding the baby because of the potential for adverse drug effects on the baby.

OLDER ADULTS

Older patients are more likely to experience the adverse effects associated with these drugs, including CNS, GI and CV effects. They often have renal or hepatic impairment; they are also more likely to have toxic levels of the drug related to changes in metabolism and excretion. The older patient should always be provided with safety measures (i.e. hand rails) when receiving one of these drugs in the hospital setting.

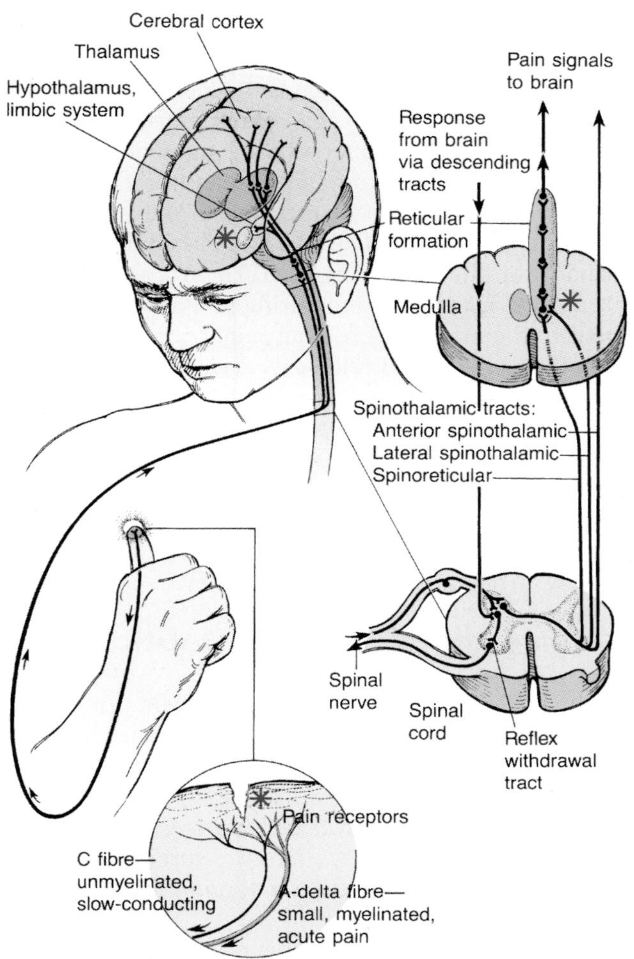

FIGURE 26.1 Neural pathways of pain.

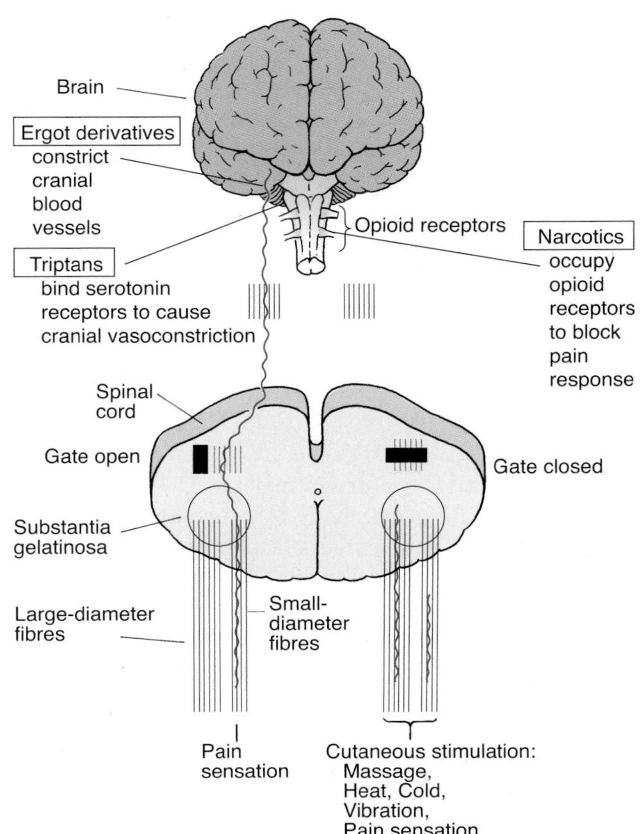

FIGURE 26.2 Gate control theory of pain. Narcotics occupy opioid receptors to block pain response. Ergot derivatives constrict cranial blood vessels, and triptans bind serotonin receptors to cause cranial vasoconstriction.

pain impulses. It is thought that the gates can be closed by stimulation of the larger A-β fibres (when the input from the A-β fibres is greater than that of the A-δ and the C fibres) and by descending impulses coming down the spinal cord from higher levels in such areas as the cerebral cortex, the limbic system and the reticular activating system.

The inhibitory influence of the higher brain centres on the transmission of pain impulses helps explain much of the mystery associated with pain. Several factors, including learned experiences, cultural expectations, individual tolerance and the placebo effect, can activate the descending inhibitory nerves from the upper CNS. Pain management usually involves the use of drugs, but it may also incorporate these other factors. The placebo effect, stress reduction, acupuncture and back rubs (which stimulate the A-β fibres) all can play an important role in the effective management of pain.

Opioids

The **opioids**, or narcotics were first derived from the opium plant. Although most opioids are now synthetically prepared, their chemical structure resembles that of the original plant alkaloids. All drugs in this class are similar in that they occupy specific **opioid receptors** in the CNS.

Opioid Receptors

Opioid receptors respond to naturally occurring peptides, the **endorphins** and the **enkephalins**. These receptors are found in the CNS, on nerves in the periphery and on cells in the gastrointestinal (GI) tract. In the brainstem, opioid receptors help to control blood pressure, pupil diameter, GI secretions and the chemoreceptor trigger zone (CTZ) that regulates nausea and vomiting, cough and respiration. In the spinal cord and thalamus, these receptors help to integrate and relate incoming information about pain. In the hypothalamus, they may interrelate the endocrine and neural response to pain. In the limbic system, the receptors incorporate emotional aspects of pain and response to pain. At peripheral nerve sites, the opioids may block the release of neurotransmitters that are related to pain and inflammation.

The opioid drugs that are used vary with the type of opioid receptors with which they react. This accounts for a change in pain relief, as well as a variation in the side-effects that can be anticipated. Four types of opioid receptors have been identified: **mu (μ), kappa (κ), beta (β) and sigma (σ).**

The μ-receptors are primarily pain-blocking receptors. Besides analgesia, μ-receptors also account for respiratory depression, a feeling of euphoria, decreased GI activity, pupil constriction and the development of physical dependence. The **κ**-receptors are associated with some analgesia and with pupillary constriction, sedation and dysphoria. Enkephalins react with **β**-receptors in the periphery to modulate pain transmission. The **σ**-receptors cause pupillary dilation and may be responsible for the hallucinations, dysphoria and psychoses that can occur with opioid use.

Opioid Agonists

The **opioid agonists** are drugs that react with the opioid receptors throughout the body to cause analgesia, sedation, or euphoria. Anticipated effects other than analgesia are mediated by the types of opioid receptors affected by each drug. The opioid agonists are classified as controlled substances because of the potential for the development of physical dependence while taking these drugs. The degree of control is determined by the relative ability of each drug to cause physical dependence.

Therapeutic Actions and Indications

The opioid agonists act at specific opioid receptor sites in the CNS to produce analgesia, sedation and a sense of well-being. They are used as antitussives and as adjuncts to general anaesthesia to produce rapid analgesia, sedation and respiratory depression. Indications for opioid agonists include relief of severe acute or chronic pain, preoperative medication, analgesia during anaesthesia and specific individual indications depending on their receptor affinity. (Box 26.2 describes how to calculate dosage for one opioid agonist).

In deciding which opioid to use in any particular situation, it is important to consider all of these aspects and to select the drug that will be most effective in each situation with the least adverse effects for the patient.

BOX 26.2 Sex Considerations: Headache Distribution

Headaches are distributed in the general population in a definite sex-related pattern. For example:

- Migraine headaches are three times more likely to occur in women than men.
- Cluster headaches are more likely to occur in men than in women.
- Tension headaches are more likely to occur in women than in men.

Pharmacokinetics

Intravenous (IV) administration is the most reliable way to achieve therapeutic levels of opioids. Intramuscular (IM) and Subcut administration offer varying rates of absorption and absorption is slower in female than in male patients. These drugs undergo hepatic metabolism and are generally excreted in the urine and bile. Half-life periods vary widely depending on the drug being used. These agents cross the placenta and should be used during pregnancy only if the benefit to the mother clearly outweighs the potential risk to the foetus. Extended release oxycodone has been associated with abuse because when the tablet is cut, crushed, or chewed, the entire dose of the drug is released at once. Pregnant women must be cautioned not to cut, crush, or chew these tablets. The opioids are known to enter breast milk, but there are no documented adverse effects on the baby. Many sources recommend waiting 4 to 6 hours after receiving an opioid to breast-feed the baby.

Contraindications and Cautions

The opioid agonists are contraindicated in the following conditions: pregnancy, labour, or lactation *because of potential adverse effects on the foetus or neonate, including respiratory depression*; diarrhoea caused by poisons *because depression of GI activity could lead to increased absorption and toxicity*; and after biliary surgery or surgical anastomoses *because of the adverse effects associated with GI depression and opioids.*

Caution should be used in patients with respiratory dysfunction, *which could be exacerbated by the respiratory depression caused by these drugs*; recent GI or genitourinary (GU) surgery; acute abdomen or ulcerative colitis, *which could become worse with the depressive effects of the opioids*; head injuries, alcoholism, delirium tremens, or cerebral vascular disease, *which could be exacerbated by the CNS effects of the drugs*; and liver or renal dysfunction, *which could alter the metabolism and excretion of the drugs.*

Adverse Effects

The most frequently seen adverse effects associated with opioid agonists relate to their effects on various opioid receptors. Respiratory depression with apnoea, cardiac arrest and shock may result from opioid-caused CNS respiratory depression. Orthostatic hypotension is commonly seen with some opioids. Such GI effects as nausea, vomiting, constipation and biliary spasm may occur as a result of CTZ stimulation and negative effects on GI motility. Neurological effects such as light-headedness, dizziness, psychoses, anxiety, fear, hallucinations, pupil constriction and impaired mental processes may occur as a result of the stimulation of CNS opioid receptors in the cerebrum, limbic system and hypothalamus. GU effects, including urethral spasm, urinary retention, hesitancy and loss of libido, may be related to direct receptor stimulation or to CNS activation of sympathetic pathways. In addition, sweating and dependence (both physical and psychological) are possible, more so with some agents than with others.

Clinically Important Drug–Drug Interactions

When opioid agonists are given with the barbiturate general anaesthetics, or with some phenothiazines and monoamine oxidase inhibitors (MAOIs), the likelihood of respiratory depression, hypotension and sedation or coma is increased. If these drug combinations cannot be avoided, patients should be monitored closely and appropriate supportive measures taken.

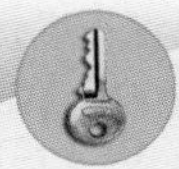

Key Drug Summary: *Morphine*

Indications: Relief of moderate-to-severe acute or chronic pain; preoperative medication; intraspinal to reduce intractable pain

Actions: Acts as an agonist at specific opioid receptors in the CNS to produce analgesia, euphoria and sedation

Pharmacokinetics:

Route	Onset	Peak	Duration
Oral	Varies	60 min	5–7 h
Subcut	Rapid	50–90 min	5–7 h
IM	Rapid	30–60 min	5–6 h
IV	Immediate	20 min	5–6 h

$T_{1/2}$: 1.5–2 hours; metabolized in the liver, excreted in the urine and bile

Adverse effects: Light-headedness, dizziness, sedation, nausea, vomiting, dry mouth, constipation, urethral spasm, respiratory depression, apnoea, circulatory depression, respiratory arrest, shock, cardiac arrest

Nursing Considerations for Patients Receiving Opioid Agonists

Assessment: History and Examination

Screen for the following conditions, *which could be cautions or contraindications for the use of the drug*; pregnancy; respiratory dysfunction; GI or biliary surgery; psychosis; convulsive disorders; diarrhoea caused by toxins; alcoholism or delirium tremens; and renal or hepatic dysfunction.

Include screening *for baseline status before beginning therapy and for any potential adverse effects.* Assess the following: CNS orientation, reflexes, pupil size; respiration and adventitious sounds; pulse, blood pressure and cardiac output; bowel sounds and bladder palpation.

Check liver and renal function tests, as well as electroencephalogram and electrocardiogram (ECG) as appropriate.

Establish if patient is currently taking other medications or herbal therapies, which may potentially interact with the opioid agonists.

Nursing Diagnoses

The patient receiving an opioid agonist may have the following nursing diagnoses related to drug therapy:

- Acute pain related to GI, CNS and GU effects
- Disturbed sensory perception (visual, auditory and kinaesthetic) related to CNS effects
- Impaired gas exchange related to respiratory depression
- Constipation related to GI effects
- Deficient knowledge regarding drug therapy

Implementation With Rationale

- Provide an opioid antagonist and equipment for assisted ventilation on standby during IV administration *to support the patient in case severe reaction occurs.*
- Monitor injection sites for irritation and extravasation *to provide appropriate supportive care if needed.*
- Monitor timing of analgesic doses. *Prompt administration may provide a more acceptable level of analgesia and lead to quicker resolution of the pain.*
- Use extreme caution when injecting an opioid into any body area that is chilled or has poor perfusion or shock *because absorption may be delayed. After repeated doses, an excessive amount is absorbed all at once.*
- Use additional measures for relief of pain, such as stress reduction *to increase the effectiveness of the opioid and reduce pain.*
- Reassure patients that the risk of addiction is minimal. *Most patients who receive opioids for medical reasons do not develop dependency syndromes.*
- Provide thorough patient teaching, including drug name and prescribed dosage, measures for avoidance of adverse effects, warning signs that may indicate

possible problems and the need for monitoring and evaluation, *to enhance patient knowledge about drug therapy and to promote compliance.* (See Critical Thinking Scenario 26-1.)

- Offer support and encouragement *to help the patient cope with the drug regimen.*

Evaluation

- Monitor patient response to the drug (relief of pain, cough suppression, sedation).
- Monitor for adverse effects (CNS changes, GI depression, respiratory depression, constipation).
- Evaluate the effectiveness of the teaching plan (patient can give the drug name and dosage and describe possible adverse effects to watch for, specific measures to prevent adverse effects and warning signs to report).
- Monitor the effectiveness of comfort measures and compliance with the regimen.

Opioid Agonists–Antagonists

The **opioid agonists–antagonists** stimulate certain opioid receptors but block other such receptors. These drugs, which have less abuse potential than the pure opioid agonists, all have about the same analgesic effect as morphine. Like morphine, they may cause sedation, respiratory depression and constipation. They have also been associated with more psychotic-like reactions and they may even induce a withdrawal syndrome in patients who have been taking opioids for a long period.

Available opioid agonists–antagonists include the following:

- Buprenorphine is recommended for treatment of mild-to-moderate pain; it is available for use in IM and IV forms.
- Pentazocine is available in an oral form, making it the preferred drug for patients who will be switched from parenteral to oral forms after surgery or labour.

Therapeutic Actions and Indications

The opioid agonists–antagonists act at specific opioid receptor sites in the CNS to produce analgesia, sedation, euphoria and hallucinations. In addition, they block opioid receptors that may be stimulated by other opioids. These drugs have three functions:

1 relief of moderate-to-severe pain,

2 adjuncts to general anaesthesia and

3 relief of pain during labour and delivery.

Pharmacokinetics

These drugs are readily absorbed after IM administration and reach rapid peak levels when given intravenously. They are metabolized in the liver and are excreted in urine or faeces. They are known to cross the placenta, but no adequate studies are available regarding their effects during pregnancy. They should be used during pregnancy only if the benefit to the mother clearly outweighs the risk to the foetus. They are used to relieve pain during labour, which provides a short-term exposure to the foetus. They are known to enter breast milk and should be used with caution during lactation because of the potential for adverse effects on the baby.

Contraindications and Cautions

Opioid agonists–antagonists are contraindicated in the presence of any known allergy to any opioid agonist–antagonist and during pregnancy and lactation *because of potential adverse effects on the neonate, including respiratory depression.* (However, these drugs may be used to relieve pain during labour and delivery.)

Caution should be used in cases of physical dependence on an opioid *because a withdrawal syndrome may be precipitated*; the opioid antagonistic properties can block the analgesic effect and intensify the pain. Opioid agonists–antagonists may be desirable for relieving chronic pain in patients who are susceptible to opioid dependence, but extreme care must be used if patients are switched directly from an opioid agonist to one of these drugs.

Caution should also be exercised in the following conditions: chronic obstructive pulmonary disease or other respiratory dysfunction, *which could be exacerbated by respiratory depression*; acute myocardial infarction (MI), documented coronary artery disease (CAD), or *hypertension that could be exacerbated by cardiac stimulatory effects of these drugs*; and renal or hepatic dysfunction *that could interfere with the metabolism and excretion of the drug.*

Pentazocine also may cause cardiac stimulation including arrhythmias, hypertension and increased myocardial oxygen consumption, which could lead to angina, MI, or congestive heart failure; *therefore, care must be taken in patients with known heart disease.*

Adverse Effects

The most frequently seen adverse effects associated with opioid agonists–antagonists relate to their effects on various opioid receptors. Respiratory depression with apnoea and suppression of the cough reflex is associated with the respiratory depression caused by the opioids. Nausea, vomiting, constipation and biliary spasm may occur as a result of CTZ stimulation and the negative effects on GI motility.

Light-headedness, dizziness, psychoses, anxiety, fear, hallucinations and impaired mental processes may occur as a result of the stimulation of CNS opioid receptors in the cerebrum, limbic system and hypothalamus. GU effects, including ureteral spasm, urinary retention, hesitancy and loss of libido, may be related to direct receptor stimulation or to CNS activation of sympathetic pathways. Although sweating and dependence, both physical and psychological, are possible, their occurrence is considered less likely than with opioid agonists.

Clinically Important Drug–Drug Interactions

When opioid agonists–antagonists, like opioid agonists, are given with barbiturate general anaesthetics, the likelihood of respiratory depression, hypotension and sedation or coma increases. If this combination cannot be avoided, patients should be monitored closely and appropriate supportive measures taken.

Use of opioid agonists–antagonists in patients who have previously received opioids puts these patients at risk. When such a sequence of drugs is used, patients require support and monitoring.

Always consult a current copy of the British National Formulary for further guidance.

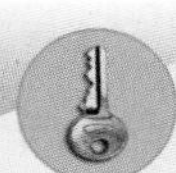

Key Drug Summary: *Pentazocine*

Indications: Relief of moderate-to-severe pain; preanaesthetic medication and a supplement to surgical anaesthesia

Actions: An agonist at specific opioid receptors in the CNS, producing analgesia and sedation; an agonist at σ-opioid receptors, causing dysphoria and hallucinations; acts at μ-receptors to antagonize the analgesia and euphoria

Pharmacokinetics:

Route	Onset	Peak	Duration
Oral, IM, Subcut	15–30 min	1–3 h	3 h
IV	2–3 min	15 min	3 h

$T_{1/2}$: 2–3 hours; metabolized in the liver, excreted in the urine and bile

Adverse effects: Light-headedness, dizziness, sedation, euphoria, nausea, vomiting, constipation, tachycardia, palpitations, sweating, urethral spasm, physical dependence

Nursing Considerations for Patients Receiving Opioid Agonists–Antagonists

Assessment: History and Examination

Screen for the following conditions, *which could be cautions or contraindications for the use of the drug*: any known allergies to these drugs or to sulphites; pregnancy or lactation; respiratory dysfunction; MI or CAD; and renal or hepatic dysfunction.

Include screening *for baseline status before beginning therapy and for any potential adverse effects.* Assess the following: CNS orientation and pupil size; respiration and adventitious sounds; pulse, blood pressure and cardiac output; bowel sounds and liver and renal function tests, as well as ECG.

Establish if patient is currently taking other medications or herbal therapies, which may potentially interact with the opioid agonists–antagonists.

Nursing Diagnoses

The patient receiving an opioid agonist–antagonist may have the following nursing diagnoses related to drug therapy:

- Acute pain related to GI and CNS effects
- Disturbed sensory perception (visual, auditory, kinaesthetic) related to CNS effects
- Impaired gas exchange related to respiratory depression
- Deficient knowledge regarding drug therapy

Implementation With Rationale

- Provide an opioid antagonist and equipment for assisted ventilation on standby during IV administration *to provide patient support in case of severe reaction.*
- Monitor injection sites for irritation and extravasation *to provide appropriate supportive care if needed.*
- Monitor timing of analgesic doses. *Prompt administration may provide a more acceptable level of analgesia and lead to quicker resolution of the pain.*
- Use extreme caution when injecting these drugs into any body area that is chilled or has poor perfusion or shock *because absorption may be delayed* and *after repeated doses an excessive amount is absorbed all at once.*
- Use additional measures to relieve pain *to increase the effectiveness of the opioid being given and reduce pain.*

- Institute comfort and safety measures, such as side rails *to ensure patient safety*; bowel programme as needed *to treat constipation*; environmental controls *to decrease stimulation*; and small meals *to relieve GI distress if GI upset is severe.*
- Reassure patients that the risk of addiction is minimal. *Most patients who receive these drugs for medical reasons do not develop dependency syndromes.*
- Provide thorough patient teaching, including drug name and prescribed dosage, as well as measures for avoidance of adverse effects, warning signs that may indicate possible problems and the need for monitoring and evaluation *to enhance patient knowledge about drug therapy and to promote compliance.* (See Critical Thinking Scenario 26-1.)
- Offer support and encouragement *to help the patient cope with the drug regimen.*

Evaluation

- Monitor patient response to the drug (relief of pain, sedation).
- Monitor for adverse effects (CNS changes, GI depression, respiratory depression, arrhythmias and hypertension).
- Evaluate the effectiveness of the teaching plan (patient can give the drug name and dosage and describe possible adverse effects to watch for, specific measures to prevent adverse effects and warning signs to report).
- Monitor the effectiveness of comfort measures and compliance with the regimen.

Opioid Antagonists

The **opioid antagonists** are drugs that bind strongly to opioid receptors, but they do not activate the receptors. These agents are useful in blocking unwanted adverse effects associated with opioids, such as respiratory depression and they play a role in the treatment of opioid overdose. These drugs do not have an appreciable effect in most people, but individuals who are addicted to opioids experience the signs and symptoms of withdrawal when rapidly receiving these drugs. The opioid antagonists in use today include the following:

- Naloxone is used IV, IM, or Subcut to reverse adverse effects of opioids and to diagnose suspected acute opioid overdose.
- Naltrexone is used orally in the management of alcohol or opioid dependence as part of a comprehensive treatment programme.

Therapeutic Actions and Indications

The opioid antagonists block opioid receptors and reverse the effects of opioids, including respiratory depression, sedation, psychomimetic effects and hypotension. Their effects are seen in people who have been using opioids or are dependent on opioids.

These agents are indicated for reversal of the adverse effects of opioid use, including respiratory depression and sedation and for treatment of opioid overdose. Naloxone is used to diagnose opioid overdose (the naloxone challenge).

Pharmacokinetics

These agents are well absorbed after injection and are widely distributed in the body. They undergo hepatic metabolism and are excreted primarily in the urine. There are no well-controlled studies during pregnancy, so they should be used during pregnancy only if the benefit to the mother clearly outweighs any potential risk to the foetus. They enter breast milk and should be used with caution during lactation because of the potential adverse effects on the baby.

Contraindications and Cautions

Opioid antagonists are contraindicated in the presence of any known allergy to any opioid antagonist. Caution should be used in the following circumstances: during pregnancy and lactation *because of potential adverse effects on the foetus and neonate*; with opioid addiction *because of the precipitation of a withdrawal syndrome*; and with cardiovascular (CV) disease *which could be exacerbated by the reversal of the depressive effects of opioids.*

Adverse Effects

The most frequently seen adverse effects associated with these drugs relate to the blocking effects of the opioid receptors. The most common effect is an acute opioid abstinence syndrome that is characterized by nausea, vomiting, sweating, tachycardia, hypertension and feelings of anxiety. CNS excitement and reversal of analgesia are especially common after surgery. CV effects related to the reversal of the opioid depression can include tachycardia, blood pressure changes, dysrhythmias and pulmonary oedema.

Always consult a current copy of the British National Formulary for further guidance.

Drug–Drug Interactions

To reverse the effects of buprenorphine, or pentazocine, larger doses of opioid antagonists may be needed.

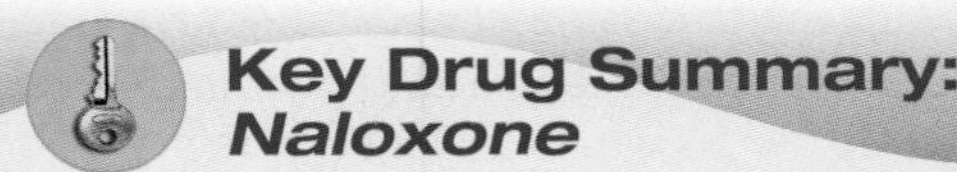

Key Drug Summary: Naloxone

Indications: Complete or partial reversal of opioid depression; diagnosis of suspected opioid overdose

Actions: Pure opioid antagonist; reverses the effects of the opioids, including respiratory depression, sedation and hypotension

Pharmacokinetics:

Route	Onset	Peak	Duration
IV	Unknown	2 min	4–6 h
IM, Subcut	Unknown	3–5 min	4–6 h

$T_{1/2}$: 30–81 min; metabolized in the liver, excreted in the urine

Adverse effects: Acute opioid abstinence syndrome (nausea, vomiting, sweating, tachycardia, a fall in blood pressure), hypotension, hypertension, pulmonary oedema

Migraine Headaches

The term *migraine headache* is used to describe several different syndromes, all of which include severe, throbbing headaches on one side of the head. This pain can be so severe that it can cause widespread disturbance, affecting GI and CNS function, including mood and personality changes.

Migraine headaches should be distinguished from cluster headaches and tension headaches. Cluster headaches usually begin during sleep and involve sharp, steady eye pain that lasts 15 to 90 minutes with sweating, flushing, tearing and nasal congestion. Tension headaches, which usually occur at times of stress, feel like a dull band of pain around the entire head and last from 30 minutes to 1 week. They are accompanied by anorexia, fatigue and a mild intolerance to light or sound.

There are at least two types of migraine headaches:

- Common migraines, which occur without an aura, cause severe, unilateral, pulsating pain that is frequently accompanied by nausea, vomiting and sensitivity to light and sound. Such migraine headaches are often aggravated by physical activity.
- Classic migraines are usually preceded by an aura, or a sensation involving sensory or motor disturbances, that usually occurs about half an hour before the pain begins. The pain and adverse effects are the same as those of the common migraine.

It is believed that the underlying cause of migraine headaches is arterial dilation. Headaches accompanied by an aura are associated with a hypoperfusion of the brain during the aura stage, followed by reflex arterial dilation and a hyper-perfusion. The underlying cause and continued state of arterial dilation are not clearly understood, but they may be related to the release of bradykinins, serotonin, or a response to other hormones and chemicals.

For many years, the one standard treatment for migraine headaches was acute analgesia, often involving an opioid, together with control of lighting and sound and the use of ergot derivatives. In the late 1990s, a new class of drugs, the triptans, was found to be extremely effective in treating migraine headaches without the adverse effects associated with ergot derivative use because of this ergot alkaloids are rarely used now.

There is some speculation that the female predisposition to migraine headaches may be related to the vascular sensitivity to hormones. Some women can directly plot migraine occurrence to periods of fluctuations in their menstrual cycle. The introduction of the triptan class of antimigraine drugs has been beneficial for many of these women.

Triptans

The **triptans** are a new class of drugs that cause cranial vascular constriction and relief of migraine headache pain in many patients. These **$5HT_1$ agonists** act on 5HT (serotonin) receptors (1B/1D). They are the preferred drug choice for migraine treatment in patients that do not respond to other analgesic treatment. These drugs are not associated with all of the vascular and GI effects of the ergot derivatives. The triptan of choice for a particular patient depends on personal experience and other pre-existing medical conditions. A patient may have a poor response to one triptan and respond well to another.

Available triptans include the following:

- Sumatriptan is used for the treatment of acute migraine attacks. It can be given orally, subcutaneously, or by nasal spray; when given by the Subcut route, it has proved very effective against cluster headaches. It is not recommended for use in elderly patients because they are more susceptible to the adverse effects of the drug, including decreased hepatic function, increased risk of hypertension and increased risk of CAD.
- Naratriptan is used orally only for the treatment of acute migraines. It has been associated with severe birth defects and is not recommended for patients with severe renal or hepatic dysfunction.
- Rizatriptan is used orally for the treatment of acute migraine attacks with or without aura. This drug is also available as an oral fast-dissolving tablet. This agent seems to have more angina-related effects, therefore it is not recommended for patients with a history of CAD. It has also been shown to cause foetal abnormalities in animal studies and should not be used during human pregnancy.

- Zolmitriptan is used orally for the treatment of acute migraine; it is also available in an orally disintegrating tablet, making it useful if swallowing is difficult.
- Amotriptan is approved for the treatment of acute migraine with or without aura in adults. This drug is reported to have fewer side-effects than the other triptans, but the effects of long-term use are not known
- Frovatriptan has the advantage of a long half-life. It is used orally as a treatment for acute migraines with or without aura. Although long-term studies are not available, it is thought that the longer half-life of this drug will prevent the rebound headaches that may be seen with other triptans.
- Eletriptan is only available as an oral agent and is used for the treatment of acute migraine with or without aura.

Therapeutic Actions and Indications

The triptans bind to selective serotonin receptor sites to cause vasoconstriction of cranial vessels, relieving the signs and symptoms of migraine headache. They are indicated for the treatment of acute migraine and are not used for prevention of migraines. Sumatriptan injection is also indicated for the treatment of cluster headaches.

Pharmacokinetics

The triptans are rapidly absorbed from many sites; they are metabolized in the liver (sumatriptan by monoamine oxidase [MAO]) and are primarily excreted in the urine. They cross the placenta and have been shown to be toxic to the foetus in animal studies. They should be used in pregnancy only if the benefit to the mother clearly outweighs any potential risks to the foetus. They have also been shown to enter breast milk and should be used with caution during lactation. The safety and efficacy of use in children have not been established.

Contraindications and Cautions

Triptans are contraindicated with any of the following conditions: allergy to any triptan; pregnancy *because of the possibility of severe adverse effects on the foetus*; and active CAD, *which could be exacerbated by the vessel-constricting effects of these drugs.* These drugs should be used with caution in elderly patients *because of the possibility of underlying vascular disease*; in patients with risk factors for CAD; in lactating women *because of the possibility of adverse effects on the infant*; and in patients with renal or hepatic dysfunction, *which could alter the metabolism and excretion of the drug.*

Adverse Effects

The adverse effects associated with the triptans are related to the vasoconstrictive effects of the drugs. CNS effects may include numbness, tingling, burning sensation, feelings of coldness or strangeness, dizziness, weakness, myalgia and vertigo. GI effects such as dysphagia and abdominal discomfort may occur. CV effects can be severe and include blood pressure alterations and tightness or pressure in the chest.

Always consult a current copy of the British National Formulary for further guidance.

Clinically Important Drug–Drug Interactions

Combining triptans with ergot-containing drugs results in a risk of prolonged vasoactive reactions.

There is a risk of severe adverse effects if these drugs are used within 2 weeks after discontinuation of an MAO inhibitor (MAOI) *because of the increased vasoconstrictive effects that occur.* If triptans are to be given, it should be clear that the patient has not received an MAOI within 2 weeks.

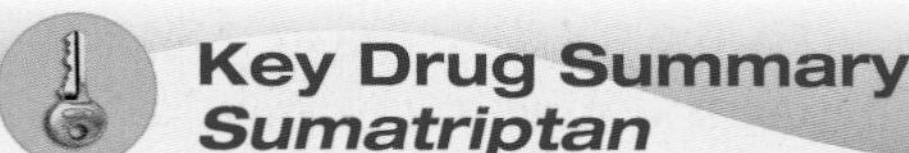

Key Drug Summary: *Sumatriptan*

Indications: Treatment of acute migraine; treatment of cluster headaches (Subcut route)

Actions: Binds to serotonin (5HT) receptors to cause vasoconstrictive effects on cranial blood vessels

Pharmacokinetics:

Route	Onset	Peak	Duration
Nasal spray	Varies	5–20 min	Unknown
Oral	1–1.5 h	2–4 h	Up to 24 h
Subcut	Rapid	1–5 h	Up to 24 h

$T_{1/2}$: 115 min; metabolized in the liver, excreted in the urine

Adverse effects: Dizziness, vertigo, weakness, myalgia, blood pressure alterations, tightness or pressure in the chest, injection site discomfort, tingling, burning sensations, numbness

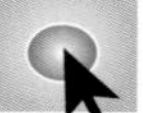

WEB LINKS

Health care providers and patients may want to consult the following Internet sources:

http://cks.library.nhs.uk The National Health Service Clinical Knowledge Summaries provides evidence-based practical information on the common conditions observed in primary care.

http://hcd2.bupa.co.uk/factsheets/html/migraine.html Information on migraines – support groups, treatment and research.

http://www.bnf.org.uk The BNF provides UK health care professionals with authoritative and practical information on the selection and clinical use of medicines.

http://www.nhsdirect.nhs.uk The National Health Service Direct service provides patients with information and advice about health, illness and health services.

http://www.britishpainsociety.org Information on pain, physiology and management of pain.

http://www.nice.org.uk National Institute for Health and Clinical Excellence (NICE) is an independent organization responsible for providing national guidance on promoting good health and preventing and treating ill health.

Points to Remember

- Pain occurs any time when tissue is injured and various chemicals are released. The pain impulses are carried to the spinal cord by small-diameter A-δ and C fibres, which form synapses with interneurons in the dorsal horn of the spinal cord.
- Opioid receptors, which are found throughout various tissues in the body, react with endogenous endorphins and enkephalins to modulate the transmission of pain impulses.
- Opioids, derived from the opium plant, react with opioid receptors to relieve pain. In addition, they lead to constipation, respiratory depression, sedation and suppression of the cough reflex and they stimulate feelings of well-being or euphoria.
- Opioids are controlled substances because they are associated with the development of physical dependence.
- The effectiveness and adverse effects associated with specific opioids are associated with their particular affinity for various types of opioid receptors.
- Opioid agonists react with opioid receptor sites to stimulate their activity.
- Opioid agonists–antagonists react with some opioid receptor sites to stimulate activity and block other opioid receptor sites. These drugs are not as addictive as pure opioid agonists.
- Opioid antagonists, which work to reverse the effects of opioids, are used to treat opioid overdose or to reverse unacceptable adverse effects.
- Migraine headaches are severe, throbbing headaches on one side of the head that may be associated with an aura or warning syndrome. These headaches are thought to be caused by arterial dilation and hyperperfusion of the brain vessels.
- Treatment of migraines may involve the use of triptans, a new class of selective serotonin receptor blockers, these cause CNS vasoconstriction but are not associated with many adverse systemic effects.

CRITICAL THINKING SCENARIO 26-1

Using Morphine to Relieve Pain

The Situation

David a 26-year-old, was involved in a car crash and suffered a fractured pelvis, a fractured left tibia, a fractured right humerus and multiple contusions and abrasions. The first 2 days after surgery, David was heavily sedated. The days following this he was given IV injections of morphine every 4 hours as needed for pain, although, David requested medication every 2 to 3 hours and became very agitated by the end of the prescribed 4 hours. David's physician decided to change the analgesia regimen to dihydrocodiene IM 4 to 6 hourly with regular nonsteroidal anti-inflammatory drugs (NSAIDs) for break-through pain, in order to wean David off the opioids. This regimen is slowly reduced as David's pain reduces.

Critical Thinking

What basic principles must be included in the nursing care plan for this patient? *Think about the difficult position the nurse is in when David begins demanding pain relief.*

What implications will David's agitation have on the way the staff responds to him and on other patients in the area?

What other nursing measures could be used to help relieve pain and make the opioid more effective?

What methods could be used to make David more in control of his situation and increase the chances that the pain relief being effective?

Discussion

In assessing David's response to drug therapy, you suspect that the morphine was not providing the desired therapeutic effect. Numerous research studies have shown that, in general, the dosage of opioids prescribed for acute pain relief provides inadequate analgesic coverage. It could be that the dose of morphine prescribed for David was just not sufficient to relieve his pain. This patient has

(continued)

Using Morphine to Relieve Pain *(continued)*

many causes of acute pain and will heal more quickly if the pain is managed better. He has requested more drugs because the dosage is too small or the intervals between doses are too long to effectively relieve his pain.

David may be very anxious about his injuries and the opportunity to express his feelings and concerns may relieve some of the tension associated with pain. He may fear that if he does not request the medication early, he will not get it by the prescribed time. The nursing staff can work on this concern and devise a way to reassure him that the medication will be delivered on time.

Cortical impulses can close gates as effectively as descending inhibitory pathways and stimulation of the cortical pathways through patient education and active involvement should be considered an important aspect of pain relief. As David's injuries are extensive, a long-term approach should be taken to his care. The sooner David can be involved, the better the situation will be for everyone involved.

Nursing Care Guide for David: Opioids

Assessment: History and Examination

- Assess history of allergies to any opioid drug, respiratory depression, GI or biliary surgery, hepatic or renal dysfunction, alcoholism, convulsive disorders.
- Focus the physical examination on the following:
- CV: blood pressure, pulse rate, peripheral perfusion, ECG
- CNS: orientation, reflexes,
- Skin: colour, temperature
- GI: abdominal examination, bowel sounds
- Respiratory: respiration, adventitious sounds
- Laboratory tests: renal and liver function tests

Nursing Diagnoses

- Acute pain related to GI, CNS, GU effects
- Disturbed sensory perceptions (visual, auditory, kinaesthetic) related to CNS effects
- Impaired gas exchange related to respiratory depression
- Deficient knowledge regarding drug therapy
- Constipation

Implementation

- Provide an opioid antagonist, facilities for assisted ventilation during IV administration.
- Provide comfort and safety measures: orientation, accurate timing of doses, monitoring for extravasation and additional measures for pain relief to increase effects.
- Provide patient teaching about the drug, dosage, drug effects and symptoms of serious reactions to report.

Evaluation

- Evaluate drug effects: relief of pain, sedation.
- Monitor for adverse effects: CNS effects (multiple), respiratory depression, rash, skin changes, GI depression, constipation.
- Monitor drug–drug interactions: increased respiratory depression, sedation, coma with barbiturate anaesthetics, MAOIs, phenothiazines.
- Evaluate effectiveness of patient teaching programme.
- Evaluate effectiveness of comfort and safety measures.

Patient Teaching for David

- ☐ An opioid is used to relieve pain. Do not hesitate to take this drug if you feel any discomfort. Remember that it is important to use the drug before the pain becomes severe and thus more difficult to treat.
- ☐ Common effects of these drugs include:
  - *Constipation:* Your health care provider will suggest appropriate measures to alleviate this common problem.
  - *Dizziness, drowsiness* and *visual changes:* If any of these occur, avoid driving, operating complex machinery, or performing delicate tasks. If these effects occur in the hospital, the side rails on the bed may be raised for your own protection.
  - *Nausea and loss of appetite:* Taking the drug with food may help. Lying quietly until these sensations pass may also help alleviate this problem.
  - Report any of the following to your health care provider: *severe nausea or vomiting, skin rash, or shortness of breath or difficulty breathing.*
  - Avoid the use of alcohol, antihistamines and other over-the-counter drugs while taking this drug. Many of these drugs could interact with this opioid.
  - Tell any doctor, nurse, dentist, or other health care provider involved in your care that you are taking this drug.
  - Take this drug exactly as prescribed. Regular medical follow-up is necessary to evaluate the effects of this drug on your body.

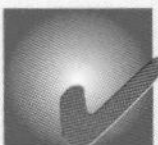

CHECK YOUR UNDERSTANDING

Answers to the questions in this chapter may be found in the answer key in the back of the book.

Multiple Choice

Select the most appropriate response

1. According to the gate control theory, pain
   a. is caused by gates in the CNS.
   b. can be blocked or intensified by the opening or closing of gates in the CNS.
   c. is caused by gates in peripheral nerve sensors.
   d. cannot be affected by learned experiences.

2. Opioid receptors are found throughout the body
   a. only in people who have become addicted to opiates.
   b. in increasing numbers with chronic pain conditions.
   c. and incorporate pain perception and blocking.
   d. and cause endorphin release.

3. Most opioids are controlled substances because they
   a. are very expensive.
   b. can cause respiratory depression.
   c. can be addictive.
   d. can be used only in a hospital setting.

4. Injecting an opioid into an area of the body that is chilled can be dangerous because
   a. an abscess will form.
   b. the injection will be very painful.
   c. absorption may be delayed and an excessive amount absorbed all at once.
   d. opioids are inactivated in cold temperatures.

5. Proper administration of an ordered opioid
   a. can lead to addiction.
   b. should be done promptly to prevent increased pain and the need for larger doses.
   c. would include holding the drug as long as possible until the patient really needs it.
   d. should rely on the patient's request for medication.

6. Migraine headaches
   a. occur during sleep and involve sweating and eye pain.
   b. occur with stress and feel like a dull band around the entire head.
   c. often occur when drinking coffee.
   d. are throbbing headaches on one side of the head.

7. The triptans are a class of drugs that bind to selective serotonin receptor sites and cause
   a. cranial vascular dilation.
   b. cranial vascular constriction.
   c. depression.
   d. nausea and vomiting.

8. The only triptan that has been approved for use in treating cluster headaches as well as migraines is
   a. naratriptan.
   b. rizatriptan.
   c. sumatriptan.
   d. zolmitriptan.

Extended Matching Questions

Select all that apply.

1. Opioids are drugs that react with opioid receptors throughout the body. The use of these drugs is associated with which of the following?
   a. Hypnosis
   b. Sedation
   c. Analgesia
   d. Euphoria
   e. Orthostatic hypotension
   f. Increased salivation

2. An opioid would be the analgesic of choice for a:
   a. patient with severe postoperative pain
   b. patient with severe, chronic obstructive pulmonary disease and difficulty in breathing
   c. patient with severe, chronic pain
   d. patient with ulcerative colitis
   e. patient with recent biliary surgery
   f. cancer patient with severe bone pain

Definitions

Define the following terms.

1. A-β fibres ______________________________

   ____

2. A-δ and C fibres ______________________________

   ____

3. gate control theory ______________________________

   ____

4. migraine headache ______________________________

   ____

5. opioids ______________________________

   ____

6. opioid agonists____________________________________

____

7. opioid agonists–antagonists ________________________

____

8. opioid antagonists__________________________________

____

9. opioid receptors___________________________________

____

10. triptan____

____

Bibliography and References

British Medical Association and Royal Pharmaceutical Society of Great Britain. (2008). *British National Formulary*. London: BMJ & RPS Publishing. *This publication is updated biannually: it is imperative that the most recent edition is consulted.*

British Medical Association and Royal Pharmaceutical Society of Great Britain. (2008). *British National Formulary for Children*. London: BMJ & RPS Publishing. *This publication is updated annually: it is imperative that the most recent edition is consulted.*

Ganong, W. (2005). *Review of medical physiology* (22nd ed.). New York: McGraw-Hill.

Howland, R. D., & Mycek, M. J. (2005). *Pharmacology* (3rd ed.). Philadelphia: Lippincott Williams & Wilkins.

Marieb, E. N., & Hoehn, K. (2004). *Human anatomy & physiology* (7th ed.). San Francisco: Pearson Benjamin Cummings.

Porth, C. M., & Matfin G. (2008). *Pathophysiology: Concepts of altered health states* (8th ed.). Philadelphia: Lippincott Williams & Wilkins.

Simonsen, T., Aarbakke, J., Kay, I., Coleman, I., Sinnott, P., & Lysaa, R. (2006). *Illustrated pharmacology for nurses.* London: Hodder Arnold

CHAPTER 27

General and Local Anaesthetic Agents

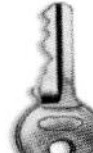

KEY TERMS

amnesia
analgesia
balanced anaesthesia
general anaesthetic
induction
local anaesthetic
plasma esterase
unconsciousness
volatile drugs (inhalation)

LEARNING OBJECTIVES

Upon completion of this chapter, you will be able to:

1. Describe the concept of balanced anaesthesia.
2. Describe the therapeutic actions, indications, pharmacokinetics and contraindications associated with general and local anaesthetics.
3. Describe the most common adverse reactions and important drug–drug interactions associated with general, regional and local anaesthetics.
4. Outline the preoperative and postoperative needs of a patient undergoing anaesthesia.
5. Compare and contrast the key drugs thiopental, midazolam, nitrous oxide, halothane, benzocaine and lidocaine with other drugs in their respective classes.
6. Outline the nursing considerations, including important teaching points, for patients receiving anaesthetics.

GENERAL ANAESTHETICS

Barbiturates

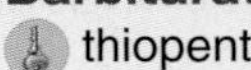
thiopental

Nonbarbiturate General Anaesthetics

etomidate
propofol

Benzodiazepines (sedation with amnesia)

diazepam
lorazepam
midazolam

Anaesthetic Gases

nitrous oxide (N_2O)

Volatile Liquids

desflurane
isoflurane
sevoflurane

LOCAL ANAESTHETICS

Esters

benzocaine
tetracaine

Amides

bupivacaine
levobupivacaine
lidocaine (lignocaine)
prilocaine
ropivacaine

Anaesthetics are drugs that are used to cause complete or partial **loss of sensation**. The anaesthetics can be subdivided into general and **local anaesthetics** depending on their site of action. **General anaesthetics** are central nervous system (CNS) depressants used to produce loss of pain sensation and consciousness. **Local anaesthetics** are drugs used to cause loss of pain sensation and feeling in a designated area of the body without the systemic effects associated with severe CNS depression. This chapter discusses various general and local anaesthetics.

General Anaesthetics

General anaesthesia is induced either by **inhalation** of a **volatile drug** or by the intravenous (IV) administration of a drug. Anaesthesia is maintained by either of these methods. When administering general anaesthetics, several different drugs are combined to achieve the following goals:

- **analgesia**, or loss of pain perception;
- **unconsciousness**, or loss of awareness of one's surroundings;
- **amnesia**, or inability to recall what took place.

General anaesthetics also block the body's reflexes. Blockage of autonomic reflexes prevents involuntary responses to injury that may compromise a patient's cardiac, respiratory, gastrointestinal (GI) and immune status. Blockage of muscle reflexes prevents jerking movements that might interfere with the success of the surgical procedure.

With the wide variety of drugs available, the anaesthetist has the opportunity to try to balance the therapeutic effects needed with the potential for adverse effects by utilising a variety of anaesthetic drugs. **Balanced anaesthesia** is the use of a combination of drugs, each with a specific effect, to achieve analgesia, muscle relaxation, unconsciousness and amnesia, rather than the use of a single drug. Balanced anaesthesia commonly involves the following agents:

- *Preoperative medications,* which may include the use of anticholinergics that decrease secretions to facilitate intubation and prevent bradycardia associated with neural depression.
- *Sedative-hypnotics,* which may include benzodiazepines to relax the patient, facilitate amnesia and decrease sympathetic stimulation.
- *Antiemetics* to decrease the nausea and vomiting associated with GI depression.

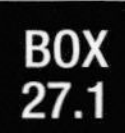

BOX 27.1 DRUG THERAPY ACROSS THE LIFESPAN

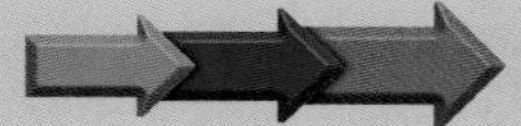

Anaesthetic Agents

CHILDREN

Children require very careful monitoring and support when being administered anaesthetic drugs and the anaesthetist needs to be very skilled at calculating dosage and balance during the procedure. They are at greater risk for complications after anaesthesia – laryngospasm, bronchospasm, aspiration and even death. Propofol is widely used for diagnostic tests and short procedures in children older than 3 years of age because of its rapid onset and metabolism and generally smooth recovery. Sevoflurane has a minimal impact on intracranial pressure and allows a very rapid induction and recovery with minimal sympathetic reaction. The dosage of anaesthetics may need to be higher in children and that factor will be considered by the anaesthetist.

Nursing care after general anaesthesia should include close monitoring, support and reassurance; assessment of the child for any skin breakdown related to immobility and safety precautions until full recovery has occurred.

Local anaesthetics are used in children in much the same way that they are used in adults. When topically applying a local anaesthetic, it is important to remember that there is greater risk of systemic absorption and toxicity with infants. Tight nappies can act like occlusive dressings and increase systemic absorption.

Bupivacaine, levobupivacaine and tetracaine do not have established doses for children younger than 12 years of age. Benzocaine should not be used in children younger than 1 year of age.

When administering any drug to children, always consult the most recent edition of the BNF for Children.

ADULTS

Adults require a considerable amount of teaching and support when receiving anaesthetics, including what will happen, what they will feel, how it will feel when they recover and the approximate time to recovery.

Adults should be monitored closely until fully recovered from general anaesthetics and should be cautioned to prevent injury when receiving local anaesthetics. It is important to remember to reassure and talk to adults who may be aware of their surroundings yet unable to speak due to short-term effects of the drugs.

Most of the general anaesthetics are not recommended for use during pregnancy because of the potential risk to the foetus. Short onset and local anaesthetics are frequently used at delivery. Use of a regional or other local anaesthetic is usually preferred if surgery is needed during pregnancy. During lactation, it is recommended that the mother wait 4 to 6 hours to feed the baby after the anaesthetic is used.

OLDER ADULTS

Older patients are more likely to experience the adverse effects associated with these drugs, including CNS, CV and dermatological effects. Thinner skin and the possibility of decreased perfusion to the skin makes them especially susceptible to skin breakdown during immobility. As older patients often also have renal or hepatic impairment, they are also more likely to have toxic levels of the drug related to changes in metabolism and excretion. The older patient should have safety measures in effect, special efforts to provide skin care to prevent skin breakdown are especially important with older skin. The older patient may require longer monitoring and greater reassurance. After general anaesthesia, it is very important to promote vigorous pulmonary drainage to decrease the risk of pneumonia.

- *Antihistamines* to decrease the chance of allergic reaction and to help dry up secretions.
- *Narcotics* to aid analgesia and sedation.

Many of these drugs are given before the anaesthetic to facilitate the process and some are maintained during surgery to aid the anaesthetic, allowing therapeutic effects at lower doses. For example, patients may receive a neuromuscular junction (NMJ) blocker and a rapid-acting IV anaesthetic to induce anaesthesia and then a gas anaesthetic to balance it during the procedure and allow easier recovery. Careful selection of appropriate anaesthetic agents, along with monitoring and support of the patient, helps to alleviate many problems. For the use of anaesthesia across the lifespan see Box 27.1.

Administration of General Anaesthetics

Anaesthesia is delivered by a physician (anaesthetist) trained in the delivery of these potent drugs with competence in using equipment for intubation, mechanical ventilation and full life support. During the delivery of anaesthesia, the patient can go though predictable stages, referred to as the depth of anaesthesia. These stages are as follows:

Stage 1: the analgesia stage refers to the loss of pain sensation, with the patient still conscious and able to communicate.

Stage 2: the excitement stage is a period of excitement and often combative behaviour, with many signs of sympathetic stimulation (e.g. tachycardia, increased respirations and blood pressure [BP] changes).

Stage 3: surgical anaesthesia, involves relaxation of skeletal muscles, return of regular respirations and progressive loss of eye reflexes and pupil dilation. Surgery can be safely performed in stage 3.

Stage 4: medullary paralysis is very deep CNS depression with loss of respiratory and vasomotor centre stimuli, in which death can occur rapidly.

Induction

Induction is the period from the beginning of anaesthesia until stage 3, or surgical anaesthesia is reached. The danger period for many patients during induction is stage 2 because of the systemic stimulation that occurs. Many times a rapid-acting anaesthetic is used to move quickly though this phase and into stage 3. NMJ blockers may be used during induction to facilitate intubation, which is necessary to support the patient with mechanical ventilation during anaesthesia.

Maintenance

Maintenance is the period from stage 3 until the surgical procedure is complete. A slower, more predictable anaesthetic, such as a gas anaesthetic, may be used to maintain the anaesthesia once the patient is in stage 3.

Recovery

Recovery is the period from discontinuation of the anaesthetic until the patient has regained consciousness, movement and the ability to communicate. During recovery, the patient must be continuously monitored to provide life support as needed and to monitor for any adverse effects of the drugs being used.

Nursing Considerations for Patients Receiving General Anaesthetics

Assessment: History and Examination

Screen for the following conditions, *which could be contraindications or cautions for the use of the drug*: any known allergies to general anaesthetics; impaired liver or kidney function; myasthenia gravis; personal or family history of malignant hyperthermia; and cardiac or respiratory disease.

Include screening *for baseline status before beginning therapy and for any potential adverse effects.*

Assess the following: temperature and weight; skin, reflexes, pupil size and reaction, pulse, BP and electrocardiogram (ECG); respiration and adventitious sound and renal and liver function tests.

Establish if the patient is currently taking other medications or herbal therapies, which may potentially interact with the general anaesthetic.

Nursing Diagnoses

The patient receiving a general anaesthetic may have the following nursing diagnoses related to drug therapy:

- Impaired gas exchange related to respiratory depression
- Impaired skin integrity related to immobility
- Disturbed thought processes and disturbed sensory perception related to CNS depression
- Deficient knowledge regarding drug therapy

Implementation With Rationale

- The drug must be administered by trained personnel (usually an anaesthetist) *because of the potential risks associated with its use.*
- Have equipment on standby to maintain airway and provide mechanical ventilation *when patient is not able to maintain respiration because of CNS depression.*
- Monitor temperature *for prompt detection and treatment of malignant hyperthermia.*

- Monitor pulse, respiration, BP, ECG and cardiac output continually during administration. In addition, monitor temperature and reflexes. *Dosage adjustment may be needed to alleviate potential problems and to maximise overall benefit with the least toxicity.*
- Monitor the patient until the recovery phase is complete and the patient is conscious and able to move and communicate *to ensure patient safety.*
- Provide comfort measures *to help the patient tolerate drug effects.* Provide pain relief as appropriate, along with reassurance and support *to deal with the effects of anaesthesia and loss of control*; skin care and turning *to prevent skin breakdown*; and supportive care *for conditions such as hypotension and bronchospasm.*
- Provide thorough patient education preoperatively, *realizing that most patients who receive the drug will be unconscious or will be receiving teaching about a particular procedure.*
- Information about the anaesthetic (e.g. what to expect, rate of onset, time to recovery) should be incorporated into the teaching plan *to prepare the patient to deal with the drug effects.*
- Offer support and encouragement *to help the patient cope with the procedure and the drugs being used.*

Evaluation

- Monitor patient response to the drug (analgesia, loss of consciousness).
- Monitor for adverse effects (respiratory depression, hypotension, bronchospasm, GI slowdown, skin breakdown, malignant hyperthermia).
- Evaluate the effectiveness of the teaching plan (patient can relate anticipated effects of the drug and the recovery process).
- Monitor the effectiveness of comfort measures and compliance with the regimen.

Types of General Anaesthetics

Several different types of drugs are used as general anaesthetics. These include barbiturate and nonbarbiturate anaesthetics, volatile liquids and gas anaesthetics.

Barbiturate Anaesthetics

The barbiturate anaesthetics are IV drugs used to induce rapid anaesthesia, which is then maintained with an inhaled drug. **Thiopental** is probably the most widely used of the IV anaesthetics. This agent has a very rapid onset of action and rapid recovery period. The patient may need additional analgesics after surgery because it has no analgesic properties,

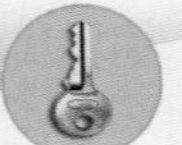

Key Drug Summary: *Thiopental*

Indications: Induction of anaesthesia, maintenance of anaesthesia; induction of a hypnotic state

Actions: Depresses the CNS to produce hypnosis and anaesthesia without analgesia

Pharmacokinetics:

Route	Onset	Duration
IV	1 min	20–30 min

$T_{1/2}$: 3–8 hours; metabolized in the liver, excreted in the urine

Adverse effects: Emergence delirium, cardiovascular (CV) depression, hypotension, respiratory depression sneezing salivation, hiccups, skin rashes, hypersensitivity.

Always check the latest addition of the British National Formulary (BNF) for up to date details.

Nonbarbiturate Anaesthetics

The other drugs used for IV administration in anaesthesia are nonbarbiturates with a wide variety of effects. Such anaesthetics include the following:

- Midazolam is the key drug nonbarbiturate anaesthetic. This agent has a rapid onset but does not reach peak effectiveness for 30 to 60 minutes. It is more likely to cause nausea and vomiting than are some of the other anaesthetics. It is a very potent amnesiac.
- Propofol is widely used as a very short-acting anaesthetic with a rapid onset of action, therefore it is often used for short procedures. It does not give the hangover effect on withdrawal. It often causes local burning on injection. It can cause bradycardia, hypotension and in extreme cases pulmonary oedema. The use of propofol has been associated with convulsions and anaphylaxis.
- Etomidate has very rapid onset and a rapid recovery period. It does not give the hangover effect often seen with thiopental. This agent is sometimes used for sedation of patients on ventilators. During the recover

phase, many patients experience myoclonic and tonic movements as well as nausea and vomiting. Etomidate can suppress adrenocortical function during continuous use therefore it should not be used for maintenance of anaesthesia.

Benzodiazepines

Benzodiazepines such as **diazepam, lorazepam and midazolam** are the most commonly used drug type for **premedication** before surgery. They have the effects of sedation, reducing anxiety and amnesia. These drugs can be given orally but may be given by IV injection. As they have no analgesic properties they will need to be administered with an analgesic, for example an opioid.

- Diazepam causes mild sedation with amnesia – it often has delayed the effect of drowsiness, which may occur several hours later. IV injection of diazepam has been associated with venous thombosis so other methods of administration are preferred.
- Lorazepam produces sedation for more than 90 minutes therefore it can be used as a premedication several hours before surgery. It has marked amnesic effects.

Key Drug Summary: Midazolam

Indications: Sedation, anxiety and amnesia before diagnostic, therapeutic, or endoscopic procedures; induction of anaesthesia; continuous sedation of intubated patients

Actions: Acts mainly at the limbic system and the reticular activating system (RAS); potentiates the effects of γ-aminobutyric acid; has little effect on cortical function; exact mechanism of action is not understood. Its recovery is much faster that diazepam.

Pharmacokinetics:

Route	Onset	Peak	Duration
Oral	30–60 min	12 h	2–6 h
IM	15 min	30 min	2–6 h
IV	3–5 min	30 min	2–6 h

$T_{1/2}$:1.8–6.8 hours; metabolized in the liver, excreted in the urine

Adverse effects: Transient drowsiness, sedation, drowsiness, lethargy, apathy, fatigue, disorientation, restlessness, constipation, diarrhoea, incontinence, urinary retention, bradycardia, tachycardia, phlebitis at IV injection site

Anaesthetic Gases

Like all inhaled anaesthetics, anaesthetic gases enter the bronchi, bronchioles and alveoli. They rapidly pass into the capillary system (as gases flow from areas of higher concentration to areas of lower concentration), where they are transported to the heart to be pumped throughout the body. These gases have a very high affinity for fatty tissue, including the lipid membrane of the nerves in the CNS. The gases pass quickly into the brain and cause severe CNS depression. Once the patient is in stage 3 of anaesthesia, the anaesthetist regulates the amount of gas that is delivered to ensure that it is sufficient to keep the patient unconscious but not enough to cause severe CNS depression. This is done by decreasing the concentration of the gas that is flowing into the respiratory system, creating a concentration gradient that results in the movement of gas in the opposite direction – out of the tissues and back to expired air.

- **Nitrous oxide** is **the key drug anaesthetic gas**. Although this agent is a very potent analgesic, it is the weakest of the gas anaesthetics and the least toxic. It moves so quickly in and out of the body that it can actually increase the volume of closed body compartments such as sinuses. Nitrous oxide is such a potent analgesic with rapid onset and recovery; it is often used for dental surgery. Nitrous oxide is usually combined with other agents for anaesthetic use (which allows for a reduction in the dose of other anaesthetic agents). Nitrous oxide is always given in combination with oxygen. Susceptible patients should be monitored for signs of hypoxia, chest pain and stroke.

Volatile Liquids

Inhaled anaesthetics are either gases or **volatile liquids** that are unstable at room temperature and release gases. These gases are then inhaled by the patient, so that these volatile liquids act like gas anaesthetics.

Most of the volatile liquids in use today are halogenated hydrocarbons such as the following:

- Desflurane has a rapid onset and rapid recovery. This agent is associated with a collection of respiratory reactions, including cough, increased secretions and laryngospasm. Therefore, it should be avoided in patients with respiratory problems and in those with increased sensitivity. In addition, its use is not recommended for induction in paediatric patients.
- Isoflurane has a rapid onset and recovery. It can cause muscle relaxation. Isoflurane is associated with hypotension, hypercapnia, muscle soreness and a bad taste in the mouth, but it does not cause cardiac arrhythmias or respiratory irritation as do some other volatile liquids.
- Sevoflurane is the newest of the volatile liquids. This agent has a very rapid onset of action and very rapid clearance therefore adverse effects are thought to be minimal.

Overview of General Anaesthetics

Therapeutic Actions and Indications

The mechanism of action of the general anaesthetics is not fully understood (Figure 27.1). It is known, however, that depression of the RAS and the cerebral cortex occurs. General anaesthetics are indicated for producing sedation, hypnosis, anaesthesia, amnesia and unconsciousness to allow performance of painful surgical procedures.

Pharmacokinetics

General anaesthetics tend to be lipid soluble and therefore are distributed widely throughout the body, including the CNS. They are generally metabolized in the liver; therefore they should be used with caution with patients who have hepatic dysfunction. They should only be used during pregnancy if they are clearly needed and the benefit to the mother outweighs any potential risk to the foetus as they can cross the placenta. Breastfeeding mothers should wait 4 to 6 hours after recovery from the anaesthetic before feeding the baby.

Contraindications and Cautions

These agents are contraindicated when there is an absence of suitable veins for IV administration, *which could be dangerous if life support measures became necessary and* IV *delivery of life-saving drugs is essential.*

Caution should be used in cases of severe CV disease, hypotension, or shock; conditions in which hypnotic effects may be prolonged or potentiated with increased intracranial pressure; and myasthenia gravis – *all of which could be exacerbated by the depressive effects of these drugs and may necessitate extra support and prolonged monitoring during surgery.*

Adverse Effects

The adverse effects associated with general anaesthetics are often associated with the depressive effects of these drugs and may include the following conditions: circulatory depression; hypotension; shock; decreased cardiac output; arrhythmias; respiratory depression, including apnoea, laryngospasm, bronchospasm, hiccups and coughing; headache; nausea and vomiting; prolonged somnolence; and in some cases delirium. The halogenated hydrocarbons may cause malignant hyperthermia, with extreme muscle rigidity, severe hyper-pyrexia, acidosis and in some cases death. If this condition occurs, it is treated with dantrolene. In addition, there is also always a risk of skin breakdown secondary to immobility when patients receive general anaesthetics.

Clinically Important Drug–Drug Interactions

Combinations of barbiturate anaesthetics and narcotics may produce apnoea more commonly than with other analgesics. The nonbarbiturate anaesthetic midazolam is associated with increased toxicity and length of recovery when used in combination with inhaled anaesthetics, other CNS depressants, narcotics, propofol, or thiopental. If any of these agents are used in combination, careful balancing of drug doses is necessary.

Always check the latest addition of the BNF for up to date details.

Risk Factors Associated with General Anaesthetics

Use of general anaesthetics involves widespread CNS depression, which is not without risks. Several factors must be taken into consideration before the use of general anaesthesia (which usually involves a series of drugs) aimed at achieving the best effect with the fewest side-effects. As general anaesthetics have wide systemic effects, individual patients should be evaluated for potential risks. When anaesthetic drugs are selected, the following factors are kept in mind so that the potential risk to each particular patient is minimized:

- *CNS factors:* Underlying neurological disease (e.g. epilepsy, stroke, myasthenia gravis) that presents a risk

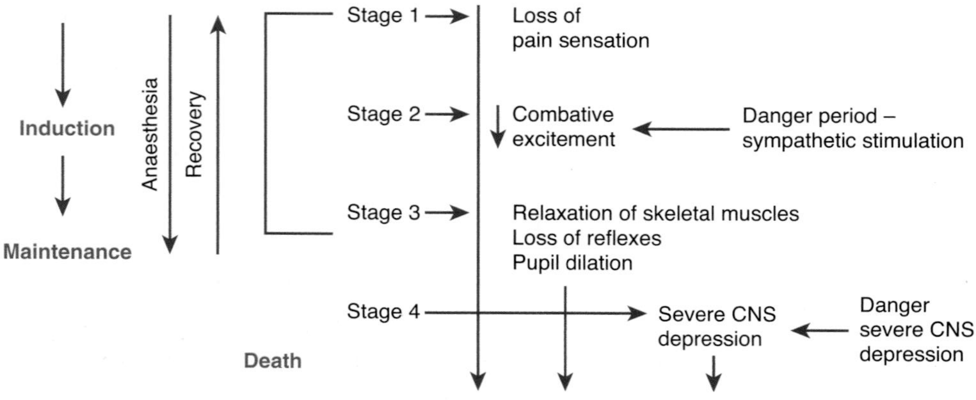

FIGURE 27.1 Stages of general anaesthesia.

for abnormal reaction to the CNS-depressing and muscle-relaxing effects of these drugs.

- *CV factors:* Underlying vascular disease, coronary artery disease, or hypotension, which put patients at risk for severe reactions to anaesthesia, such as hypotension and shock, dysrhythmias and ischemia.
- *Respiratory factors:* Obstructive pulmonary disease (e.g. asthma, chronic obstructive pulmonary disease, bronchitis), which can complicate the delivery of gas anaesthetics as well as the intubation and mechanical ventilation that must be used in most cases of general anaesthesia.
- *Renal and hepatic function:* Conditions that interfere with the metabolism and excretion of anaesthetics (e.g. acute renal failure, hepatitis) and could result in prolonged anaesthesia and the need for continued support during recovery. Toxic reactions to the accumulation of abnormally high levels of anaesthetic agents may even occur.

Local Anaesthetics

Local anaesthetics are drugs that cause a loss of sensation in limited areas of the body. They are used primarily to prevent the patient from feeling pain for varying periods of time after they have been administered in the peripheral nervous system. In increasing concentrations, local anaesthetics can also cause loss of the following sensations (in this sequence): temperature, touch, proprioception (position sense) and skeletal muscle tone. If these other aspects of nerve function are progressively lost, recovery occurs in the reverse order of the loss.

The local anaesthetics are very powerful reversible nerve blockers. Local anaesthetics work by causing a temporary interruption in the production and conduction of nerve impulses. They act by **blocking the sodium channels**, which normally infuse into the cell in response to stimulation and are involved in the propagation of the action potential. By preventing the sodium ions from entering the nerve, they stop the nerve from depolarizing. A particular section of the nerve cannot be stimulated and nerve impulses directed toward that section are lost when they reach that area.

It is very important that their effects be limited to a particular area of the body. They should not be absorbed systemically as systemic absorption could produce toxic effects on the nervous system and the heart (e.g. severe CNS depression, cardiac arrhythmias).

Modes of Administration

The way in which a local anaesthetic is administered helps increase its effectiveness by delivering it directly to the area where pain is felt. Local administration also decreases systemic absorption and related toxic effects (Figure 27.2).

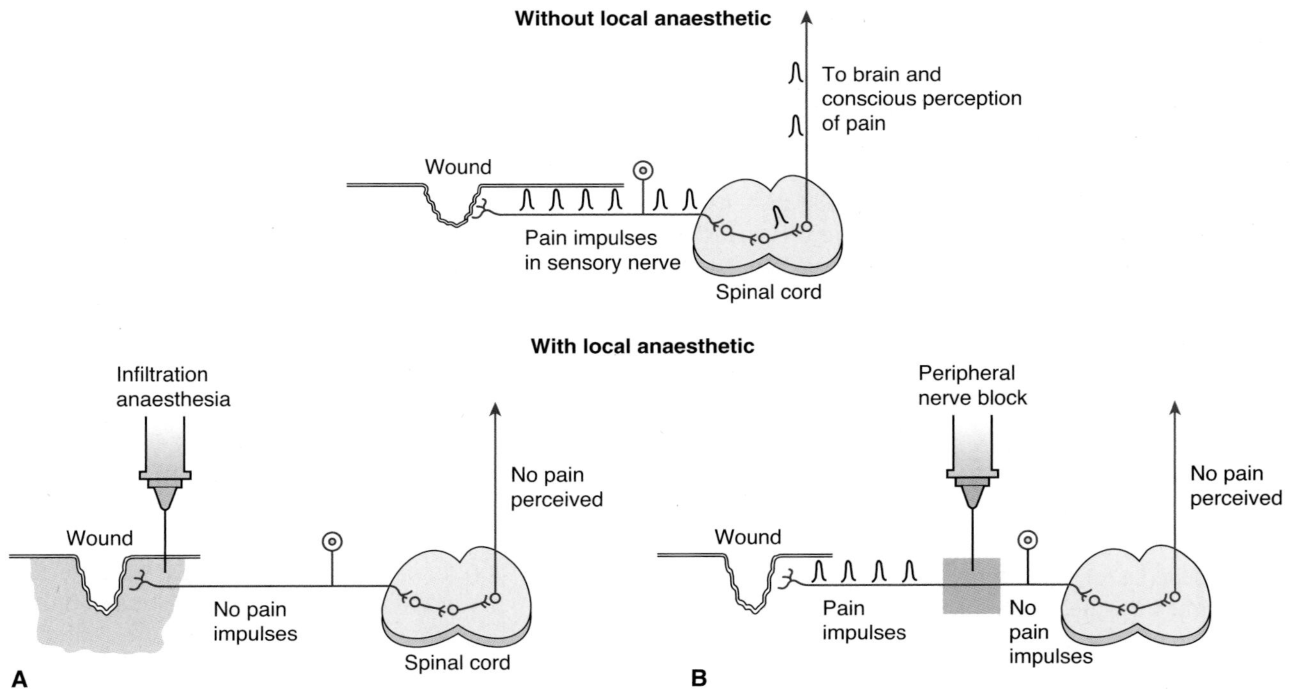

FIGURE 27.2 Mechanism of action of local anaesthetics. *Top*: An injury produces pain impulses (action potentials) that are conducted and transmitted in an area of the brain in which pain is perceived. **(A)** Conduction of the pain impulse has been blocked by infiltration anaesthetics at the site of the injury. **(B)** A nerve block at some distance from the injury. Local anaesthetics block the movement of sodium into the nerve and prevent nerve depolarization, stopping the transmission of the pain impulse.

There are five types of local anaesthetic administration: topical, infiltration, field block, nerve block.

Topical Administration

Topical anaesthesia involves applying a cream, lotion, ointment, or drop of a local anaesthetic to traumatized skin to relieve pain. It can also involve applying these to the mucous membranes in the eye, nose, throat, mouth, urethra, anus, or rectum to relieve pain or to anaesthetize the area to facilitate a medical procedure. Although systemic absorption is rare with topical application, it can occur if there is damage or breakdown of the tissues in the area.

Infiltration

Infiltration anaesthesia involves injecting the anaesthetic directly into the subcutaneous layer of tissue being treated (e.g. sutured, cut). This injection brings the anaesthetic into contact with the nerve endings in the area and prevents them from transmitting nerve impulses to the brain.

Field Block

Field block anaesthesia involves injecting the anaesthetic all around the area that will be affected by the operation. This is more intense than infiltration anaesthesia because the anaesthetic agent comes in contact with all of the nerve endings surrounding the area. This type of block is often used for tooth extractions.

Nerve Block

Nerve block anaesthesia involves injecting the anaesthetic at some point along the nerve or nerves that run to and from the region in which the loss of pain sensation or muscle paralysis is desired. These blocks are performed not in the surgical field, but at some distance from the field; they involve a greater area with potential for more adverse effects. Several types of nerve blocks are possible. A peripheral nerve block blocks the sensory and motor aspects of a particular nerve for relief of pain or for diagnostic purposes (e.g. digital block of the fingers or toes). With a central nerve block, the anaesthetic is injected into the roots of the nerves in the spinal cord. In epidural anaesthesia (often used during childbirth), the drug is injected into the space where the spinal nerves emerge from the spinal cord.

Characteristics of Local Anaesthetics

Several drugs may be used as local anaesthetics. The agent of choice depends on the method of administration, the length of time for which the area is to be anaesthetized and consideration of potential adverse effects.

Pharmacokinetics

The ester local anaesthetics, such as benzocaine; are broken down immediately in the plasma by enzymes known as **plasma esterases**. The amide local anaesthetics, such as lidocaine; are metabolized more slowly in the liver and serum levels of these drugs can increase and lead to toxicity. They should be used during pregnancy and lactation only if the benefit outweighs any potential risk to the foetus or neonate that could occur if the drug is inadvertently absorbed systemically.

Contraindications and Cautions

The local anaesthetics are contraindicated with any of the following conditions: heart block, *which could be greatly exacerbated with systemic absorption*; shock, *which could alter the local delivery and absorption of these drugs*; and decreased plasma esterases, *which could result in toxic levels of the ester-type local anaesthetics.*

Adverse Effects

The adverse effects of these drugs may be related to their local blocking of sensation (e.g. skin breakdown, self-injury, when the mouth area has been anaesthetized). Other problematic effects are associated with the route of administration and the amount of drug that is absorbed systemically. These effects are related to the blockade of nerve depolarization throughout the system. Effects that may occur include CNS effects such as headache, restlessness, anxiety, dizziness, tremors, blurred vision and backache; GI effects such as nausea and vomiting; CV effects such as peripheral vasodilation, myocardial depression, arrhythmias and BP changes, all of which may lead to fatal cardiac arrest; and respiratory arrest.

Clinically Important Drug–Drug Interactions

It is improtant that the anaesthetist is aware of all the drugs a patient is or has been taking.

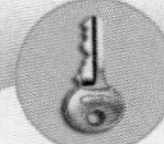

Key Drug Summary: *Lidocaine (lignocaine)*

Indications: Infiltration anaesthesia, peripheral and sympathetic nerve blocks, central nerve blocks, spinal and caudal anaesthesia, topical anaesthetic for skin or mucous membrane disorders

Actions: Blocks the generation and conduction of action potentials in sensory nerves by reducing sodium permeability, reducing the height and rate of rise of the action potential, increasing the excitation threshold and slowing conduction velocity

Pharmacokinetics:

Route	Onset	Peak	Duration
IM	5–10 min	5–15 min	2 h

Topical. Not generally absorbed systemically

$T_{1/2}$:10 min, then 1.5–3 hours; metabolized in the liver, excreted in the urine

Adverse effects: confusion, respiratory depression, hypotension, convulsions; rarely hypersensitivity reactions

Please refer to the latest edition of the BNF for up to date details.

Nursing Considerations for Patients Receiving Local Anaesthetics

Assessment: History and Examination

Screen for the following conditions, *which could be cautions or contraindications to the use of the drug*: any known allergies to these drugs; impaired liver function; low plasma esterases; heart block; shock; and pregnancy or lactation.

Include screening *for baseline status before beginning therapy and for any potential adverse effects.* Assess the following: weight, skin, pulse, BP, respiration; liver function tests and plasma esterases (if appropriate).

Establish if patient is currently taking other medications or herbal therapies, which may potentially interact with the local anaesthetic drug.

Nursing Diagnoses

The patient receiving a local anaesthetic may have the following nursing diagnoses related to drug therapy:

- Disturbed sensory perception (kinaesthetic, tactile) related to anaesthetic effect
- Impaired skin integrity related to immobility
- Risk for injury related to loss of sensation and mobility
- Deficient knowledge regarding drug therapy

Implementation With Rationale

- Have equipment on standby *to maintain airway and provide mechanical ventilation if needed.*
- Ensure that drugs for managing hypotension, cardiac arrest and CNS alterations are on standby *in case of severe reaction and toxicity.*
- Ensure that patients receiving spinal anaesthesia are well hydrated and remain lying down for up to 12 hours after the anaesthesia *to minimize headache.*
- Establish safety precautions *to prevent skin breakdown and injury during the time that the patient has a loss of sensation and/or mobility.*
- Provide comfort measures *to help the patient tolerate drug effects.* Provide pain relief as appropriate; reassurance and support *to deal with the effects of anaesthesia and loss of control*; skin care and turning *to prevent skin breakdown*; and supportive care for hypotension *to prevent shock or serious hypoxia.*
- Provide thorough patient education *to explain what to expect, safety precautions that will be needed and when to expect return of function.*
- Offer support and encouragement *to help the patient cope with the procedure and drugs being used.*

Evaluation

- Monitor patient response to the drug (loss of feeling in designated area).
- Monitor for adverse effects (respiratory depression, BP changes, arrhythmias, GI upset, skin breakdown, injury, CNS alterations).
- Evaluate the effectiveness of the teaching plan (patient can relate the anticipated effects of the drug and the re-covery process) (see Critical Thinking Scenario 27-1).

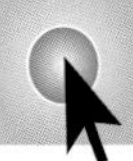

WEB LINKS

Health care providers and patients may want to consult the following Internet sources:

http://cks.library.nhs.uk The National Health Service Clinical Knowledge Summaries provides evidence-based practical information on the common conditions observed in primary care.

http://www.anaesthesia-analgesia.org Information on anaesthesia – physiology and research.

http://www.anaesthesiologyonline.com Information for patients about types of anaesthesia, research and teaching protocols.

http://www.bnf.org.uk The BNF provides UK health care professionals with authoritative and practical information on the selection and clinical use of medicines.

http://www.nhsdirect.nhs.uk The National Health Service Direct service provides patients with information and advice about health, illness and health services.

http://www.nice.org.uk National Institute for Health and Clinical Excellence is an independent organization responsible for providing national guidance on promoting good health and preventing and treating ill health.

http://www.pain.com Information on regional anaesthesia.

Points to Remember

- General anaesthetics are drugs used to produce pain relief, analgesia, amnesia, unconsciousness and to block muscle reflexes that could interfere with a surgical procedure or put the patient at risk of harm.
- The use of general anaesthetics involves a widespread CNS depression that could be harmful, especially in patients with underlying CNS, CV or respiratory diseases.
- Anaesthesia proceeds though predictable stages from loss of sensation to total CNS depression and death.
- Induction of anaesthesia is the period of time from the beginning of anaesthesia administration until the patient reaches surgical anaesthesia (stage 3).
- Balanced anaesthesia involves giving a variety of drugs, including anticholinergics, rapid IV anaesthetics, inhaled anaesthetics, NMJ blockers and narcotics.
- Patients receiving general anaesthetics should be monitored for any adverse effects and to provide reassurance and safety precautions until the recovery of sensation, mobility and ability to communicate.
- Local anaesthetics block the depolarization (sodium channels) of nerve membranes, preventing the transmission of pain sensations and motor stimuli.
- Local anaesthetics are administered to deliver the drug directly to the desired area and to prevent systemic absorption, which could lead to serious interruption of nerve impulses and response.
- Ester-type local anaesthetics are immediately destroyed by plasma esterases. Amide local anaesthetics are destroyed in the liver and have a greater risk of accumulation and systemic toxicity.
- Nursing care of patients receiving anaesthetics should include safety precautions to prevent injury and skin breakdown; support and reassurance to deal with the loss of sensation and mobility; and patient education regarding what to expect to decrease stress and anxiety.

CRITICAL THINKING SCENARIO 27-1

Local Anaesthesia

The Situation

Adam, a 32-year-old male athlete with a history of asthma (which could indicate pulmonary dysfunction) was admitted to the hospital for an inguinal hernia repair. At the patient's request, the surgeon elected to use a local anaesthetic employing spinal anaesthesia. As the extent of the repair was unknown, levobupivacaine, a long-acting anaesthetic, was selected. Adam remained alert (BP 120/64, P 62, R 14) and remained stable throughout the procedure. Two hours after the procedure, Adam appeared agitated (BP 154/68, P 88, R 18). Although he did not complain of discomfort, he did state that he was feeling anxious because he still had no feeling to the lower half of his body.

Critical Thinking

What safety precautions need to be taken?

What nursing interventions should be done at this point?

How could the patient be reassured? *Think about the anxiety level of the patient – an athlete who elected to have local anaesthesia may have a problem with control and feel somewhat vulnerable. Consider the anxiety that loss of mobility and sensation in the legs may cause in a person who makes his living as an athlete.*

In addition, consider the expected duration of action of levobupivacaine and the rate of return of function.

Discussion

Levobupivacaine is a long-acting anaesthetic with effects that may persist for several hours. The timing of the drug's effects should be explained to Adam and he should be monitored for a period of time to determine whether his agitated state and slightly elevated vital signs are a result of anxiety or an unanticipated reaction to the surgery or the drug. Life-support equipment should be on standby in case his condition is a toxic drug reaction or some unanticipated problem occurring after surgery.

The nurse is in the best position to perform the following interventions: explaining the effects of the drug and the anticipated recovery, keeping the patient as flat as possible to decrease the headache usually associated

Local Anaesthesia *(continued)*

with spinal anaesthesia; encouraging the patient to turn from side to side periodically to allow skin care to be performed and to alleviate the risk of pressure sore development; and staying with the patient as much as possible to reassure him and answer any questions he has.

An elevated systolic pressure with a normal diastolic pressure often is an indication of a sympathetic stress response. If the agitated state is caused by a stress reaction, the patient should return to normal. Teaching and comfort measures may be all that is needed to relieve the anxiety and ensure a good recovery.

Nursing Care Guide for Adam Local Anaesthesia

Assessment: History and Examination

Assess for allergies to local anaesthetics, cardiac disorders, vascular problems and hepatic dysfunction.

Focus physical examination on the following:

- CV: BP, pulse, peripheral perfusion,
- CNS: orientation, reflexes,
- Skin: colour, texture, sweating
- Respiratory: respiration, adventitious sounds
- Laboratory tests: liver function tests, plasma esterases (if appropriate)

Nursing Diagnoses

- Disturbed sensory perception (kinaesthetic, tactile) related to anaesthesia
- Impaired skin integrity related to immobility
- Risk for injury related to loss of sensation and mobility
- Deficient knowledge regarding drug therapy

Implementation

- Administer drug under strict supervision.
- Provide comfort and safety measures: positioning, skin care, handrails (if appropriate), pain management, antidotes on standby.
- Provide support and reassurance to deal with loss of sensation and mobility.
- Provide patient education about procedure being performed and what to expect.
- Provide life support as needed.

Evaluation

- Evaluate drug effects: loss of sensation, loss of movement.
- Monitor for adverse effects: CV effects (BP changes, arrhythmias), respiratory depression, GI upset, CNS alterations, skin breakdown and anxiety.
- Monitor for drug–drug interactions as indicated for each drug.
- Evaluate effectiveness of patient education programme and comfort and safety measures.
- Constantly monitor vital signs and muscular function and sensation as it returns.

Patient Education for Adam

Teaching about local anaesthetics is usually incorporated into the overall teaching plan about the procedure that the patient will undergo. Things to highlight with the patient would include:

☐ Discussion of the overall procedure:
  - What it will feel like? (any numbness, tingling, inability to move, pressure, pain)
  - Any anticipated discomfort
  - How long it will last?
  - Concerns during the procedure: report any discomfort and ask any questions as they arise

☐ Discussion of the recovery:
  - How long it will take?
  - Feelings to expect: tingling, numbness, pressure, itching
  - Sensation/pain that may be felt as the anaesthesia wears off
  - Measures to reduce pain in the area
  - Signs and symptoms to report (e.g. pain along a nerve route, palpitations, feeling faint, disorientation)

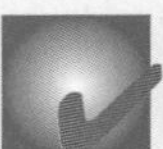

CHECK YOUR UNDERSTANDING

Answers to the questions in this chapter may be found in the answer key in the back of the book.

Multiple Choice

Select the most appropriate response to the following:

1. The most dangerous period for many patients undergoing general anaesthesia is during
   a. stage 1, when communication becomes difficult.
   b. stage 2, when systemic stimulation occurs.
   c. stage 3, when skeletal muscles relax.
   d. there is no real danger during general anaesthesia.

2. Recovery after a general anaesthetic refers to the period of time
   a. from the beginning of the anaesthesia until the patient is ready for surgery.
   b. during the surgery when anaesthesia is maintained at a certain level.
   c. from the discontinuation of the anaesthetic until the patient has regained consciousness, movement and the ability to communicate.
   d. when the patient is in the most danger of CNS depression.

3. While a patient is receiving a general anaesthetic, he or she must be continually monitored because
   a. the patient has no pain sensation.
   b. generalized CNS depression affects all body functions and could cause problems for patients with CNS, CV, or respiratory disorders.
   c. the patient cannot move.
   d. the patient cannot communicate.

4. Local anaesthetics are used to block feeling in specific body areas. If given in increasing concentrations, local anaesthetics can cause loss, in order, of the following:
   a. temperature sensation, touch sensation, proprioception and skeletal muscle tone.
   b. touch sensation, skeletal muscle tone, temperature sensation and proprioception.
   c. proprioception, skeletal muscle tone, touch sensation and temperature sensation.
   d. skeletal muscle tone, touch sensation, temperature sensation and proprioception.

Extended Matching Questions:

Select **all** that apply.

1. Comfort measures that are important for a patient receiving a local anaesthetic would include which of the following?
   a. Skin care and turning
   b. Reassurance over loss of control and sensation
   c. Use of antihypertensive agents
   d. Use of analgesics as needed
   e. Ice applied to the area involved
   f. Safety precautions to prevent injury

2. A nurse would anticipate the use of general anaesthetics to
   a. produce analgesia
   b. produce amnesia
   c. activate the RAS
   d. block muscle reflexes
   e. cause unconsciousness
   f. prevent nausea

3. Balanced anaesthesia combines different classes of drugs to achieve the best effects with the fewest adverse effects. Balanced anaesthesia usually involves the use of which of the following?
   a. Anticholinergics
   b. Narcotics
   c. Sedative/hypnotics
   d. Adrenergic β-blockers
   e. Calcium channel blockers
   f. Neuromuscular blocking agents

Fill in the Blanks

1. General anaesthetics are drugs used to produce ______________ and to block muscle reflexes that could interfere with a surgical procedure or put the patient at risk for harm.

2. Anaesthesia proceeds though predictable stages from __________ to total CNS depression and __________.

3. ________________ is the time from the beginning of anaesthesia administration until the patient reaches surgical anaesthesia.

4. __________________involves giving a variety of drugs, including anticholinergics, rapid IV anaesthetics, inhaled anaesthetics, NMJ blockers and narcotics.

5. Local anaesthetics block the_____________, preventing the transmission of pain sensations and motor stimuli.

6. The use of general anaesthetics involves a widespread __________________that could be harmful, especially in patients with underlying CNS, CV or respiratory diseases.

7. Patients receiving general anaesthetics should be monitored for any adverse effects, offered reassurance and provided with safety precautions until the recovery of ___________.

8. The adverse effects of local anaesthetics may be related to their local blocking of sensation; such effects may ___________.

Bibliography and References

British Medical Association and Royal Pharmaceutical Society of Great Britain. (2008). *British National Formulary*. London: BMJ & RPS Publishing. *This publication is updated biannually: it is imperative that the most recent edition is consulted.*

British Medical Association and Royal Pharmaceutical Society of Great Britain. (2008). *British National Formulary for Children*. London: BMJ & RPS Publishing. *This publication is updated annually: it is imperative that the most recent edition is consulted.*

Ganong, W. (2005). *Review of medical physiology* (22nd ed.). New York: McGraw-Hill.

Howland, R. D., & Mycek, M. J. (2005). *Pharmacology*. (3rd ed.). Philadelphia: Lippincott Williams & Wilkins.

Marieb, E. N., & Hoehn, K. (2004). *Human anatomy & physiology* (7th ed.). San Francisco: Pearson Benjamin Cummings.

Porth, C. M., & Matfin G. (2008). *Pathophysiology: Concepts of altered health states* (8th ed). Philadelphia: Lippincott Williams & Wilkins.

Simonsen, T., Aarbakke, J., Kay, I., Coleman, I., Sinnott, P., & Lysaa, R. (2006). *Illustrated pharmacology for nurses*. London: Hodder Arnold.

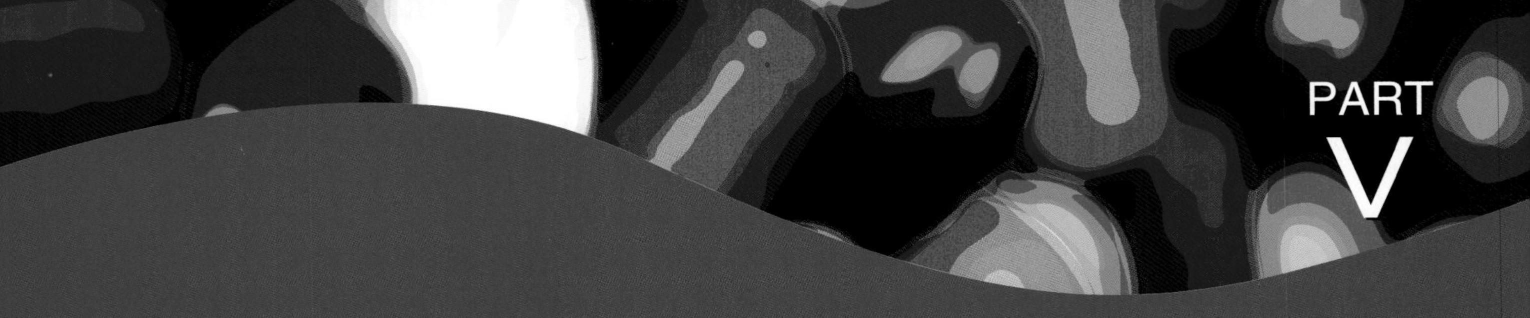

PART V

Drugs Acting on the Autonomic Nervous System

CHAPTER

28

Introduction to the Autonomic Nervous System

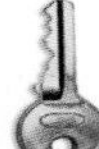

KEY TERMS

α-receptor
β-receptor
acetylcholinesterase
adrenergic receptors
afferent
autonomic nervous system
cholinergic neuron
cholinergic receptor
efferent
ganglia
monoamine oxidase (MAO)
muscarinic receptor
nicotinic receptor
parasympathetic division
sympathetic division

LEARNING OBJECTIVES

Upon completion of this chapter, you will be able to:

1. Describe how the autonomic nervous system differs anatomically from the rest of the nervous system.
2. Outline a sympathetic response and the clinical manifestation of this response.
3. Describe the α- and β-receptors found within the sympathetic division of the autonomic nervous system by sites and actions that follow the stimulation of each kind of receptor.
4. Outline the events that occur with stimulation of the parasympathetic division of the autonomic nervous system.
5. Define the terms muscarinic receptor and nicotinic receptor, giving an example of each.

The **autonomic nervous system** (ANS) is sometimes called the involuntary or visceral nervous system because it mostly operates with little conscious awareness of its activity. Working closely with the endocrine system, the ANS helps to regulate and integrate the body's internal functions. The ANS integrates parts of the central nervous system (CNS) and peripheral nervous system to automatically react to changes in the internal and external environment and therefore to maintain homeostasis.

General Functions

The main control centres for the ANS are located in the hypothalamus, the medulla and the spinal cord. Nerve impulses arising in peripheral structures are carried to these centres by **afferent** nerve fibres. Integrating centres in the CNS respond by sending out **efferent** impulses along the autonomic nerve pathways. These impulses adjust the functioning of various internal organs to keep the body's internal environment constant.

The ANS works to regulate, for example, blood pressure, heart rate, respiration, body temperature, water balance, urinary excretion and digestive functions. The fine control exerted by this system results from an interrelationship between opposing divisions of the autonomic system: the **sympathetic** and **parasympathetic divisions** (Figures 28.1 and 28.2).

In most peripheral nervous system activities, the CNS nerve body sends an impulse directly to an effector organ or muscle. The ANS does not send impulses directly to the periphery; instead nerve impulses are carried from the CNS to the outlying organs by way of a two-neuron system. Axons from neurons in the brain stem and spinal cord end in a collection of neuronal cell bodies that are packed together (known as **ganglia**) and located outside the CNS. These ganglia receive information from the *preganglionic neuron* that originated in either the brain stem or spinal cord and relay that information along *postganglionic neurons*. The postganglionic neurons transmit impulses to the neuroeffector cells – muscles, glands and organs.

Divisions of the Autonomic Nervous System

The ANS is divided into two branches (sympathetic and parasympathetic) that differ in three basic ways: (i) the location of the cells originating in the CNS, (ii) the location of the nerve ganglia, and (iii) the preganglionic and postganglionic neurons (Table 28.1).

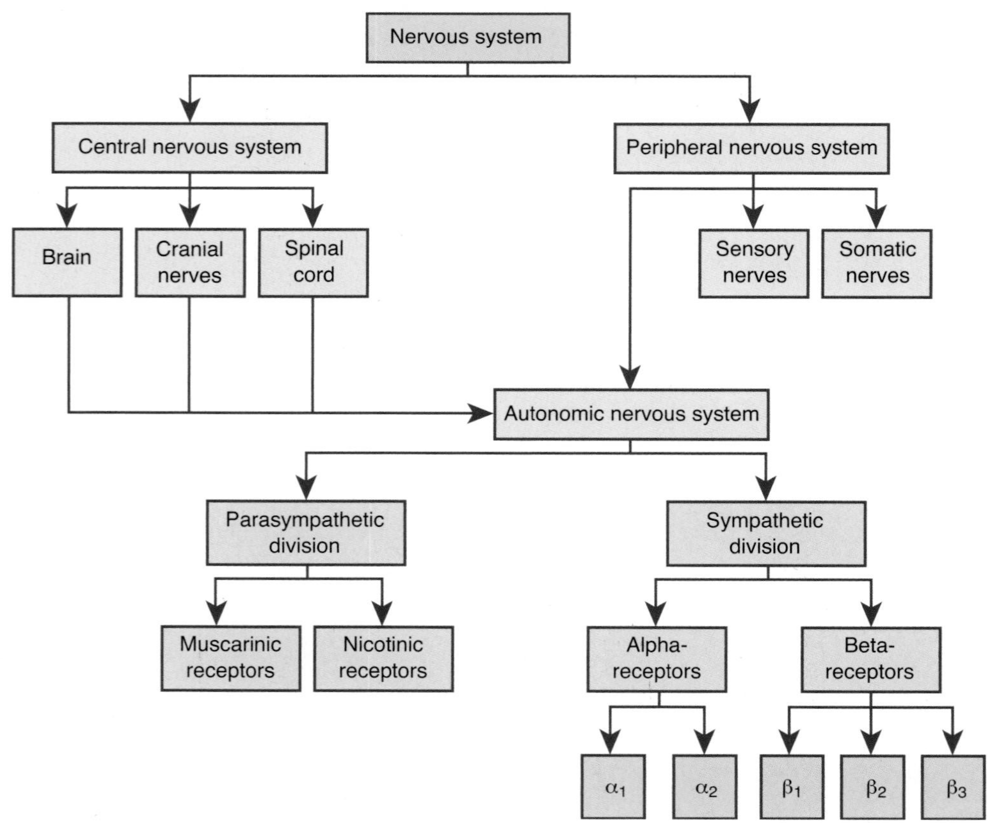

FIGURE 28.1 Organization of the nervous system.

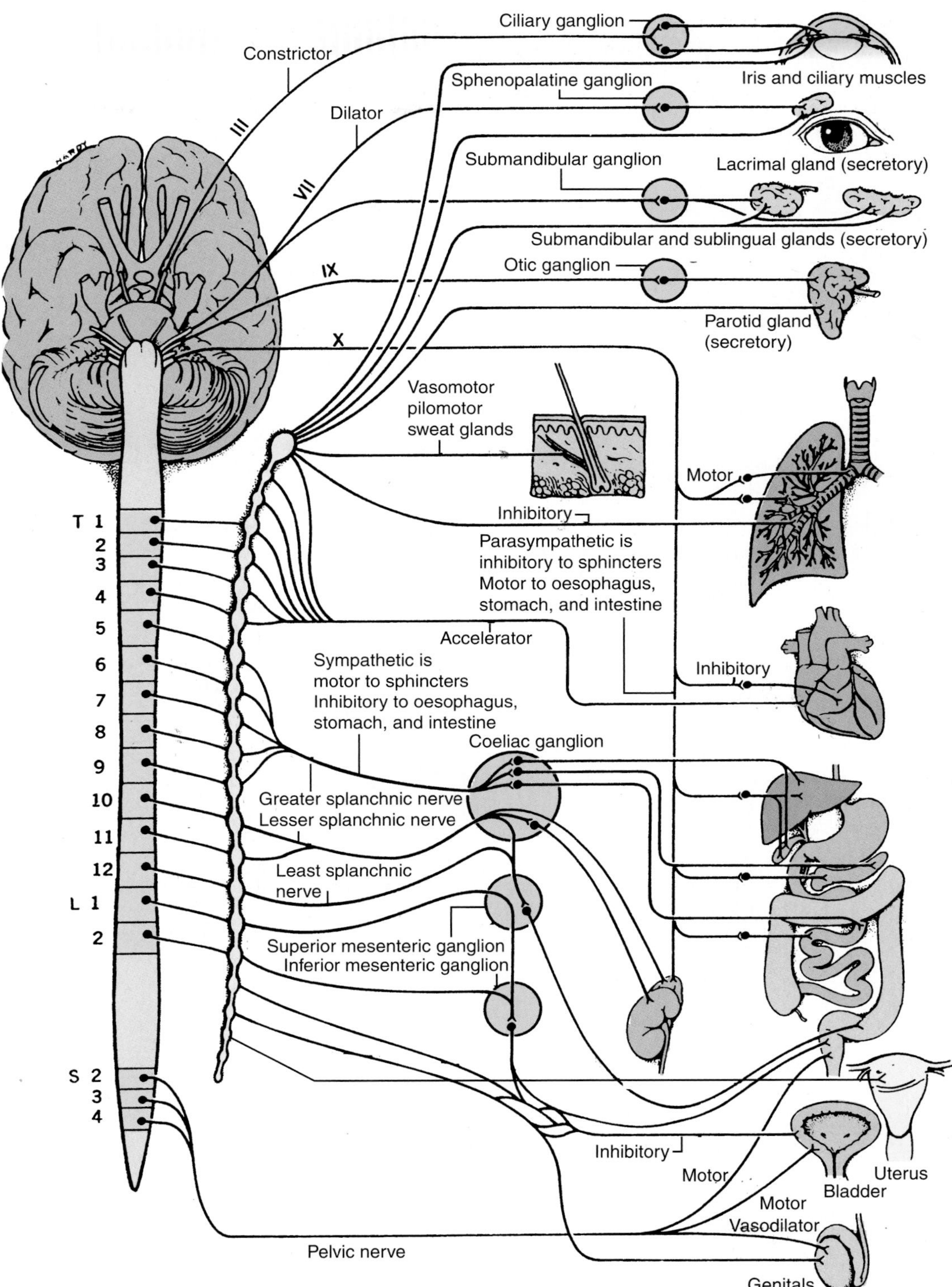

FIGURE 28.2 The autonomic nervous system. The parasympathetic, or craniosacral, division sends long preganglionic fibres that synapse with a second neuron in ganglia located close to or within the organs that are then innervated by short postganglionic fibres. The sympathetic, or thoracolumbar, division sends relatively short preganglionic fibres to the chains of paravertebral ganglia and to certain outlying ganglia. The second neuron shown sends relatively long postganglionic fibres to the organs it innervates.

Table 28.1 Comparison of the Sympathetic and Parasympathetic Divisions of the Autonomic Nervous System

Characteristic	Sympathetic Division	Parasympathetic Division
General response	Fight-or-flight	Rest-and-digest
Central Nervous System (CNS) nerve origin	Thoracic, lumbar spinal cord	Cranium, sacral spinal cord
Preganglionic neuron	Short axon	Long axon
Preganglionic neurotransmitter	Acetylcholine	Acetylcholine
Ganglia location	Next to spinal cord	Within or near effector organs
Postganglionic neuron	Long axon	Short axon
Postganglionic neurotransmitter	Noradrenaline	Acetylcholine
Neurotransmitter terminator	Monoamine oxidase (MAO), catechol-*O*-methyltransferase (COMT)	Acetylcholinesterase

The Sympathetic Division of the Nervous System

The **sympathetic division** of the nervous system (SNS) is responsible for preparing the body to respond to stress. Stress can be either internal, such as cell injury or death, or external, a perceived or learned reaction to various external situations or stimuli. The SNS is sometimes referred to as the 'fight-or-flight' system.

Anatomy

The SNS is also called the thoracolumbar system because the preganglionic neurons arise from the spinal nerves in the thoracic and lumbar sections of the spinal cord. After the spinal nerve exits the spinal cord, short preganglionic fibres leave the spinal nerve and synapse or communicate with one of the ganglia. Many of these ganglia are located in chains running down both sides of the spinal cord; the remaining ganglia lie in front of the spinal cord. The neurotransmitter released by these preganglionic neurons is acetylcholine (ACh). In turn, the ganglia sends out long postganglionic fibres that synapse with neuroeffectors, using noradrenaline as the main neurotransmitter. The exception to this two-neuron system is the adrenal medulla where the preganglionic fibres pass, without synapsing, from the spinal cord to the two adrenal medullae. The preganglionic fibres synapse directly with the adrenal medulla, which then secretes adrenaline and noradrenaline into the bloodstream.

Functions

Sympathetic system stimulation results in the following actions to prepare the body to fight-or-flight more effectively (Figure 28.3):

- Increased heart rate, blood pressure and blood flow to the skeletal muscles.

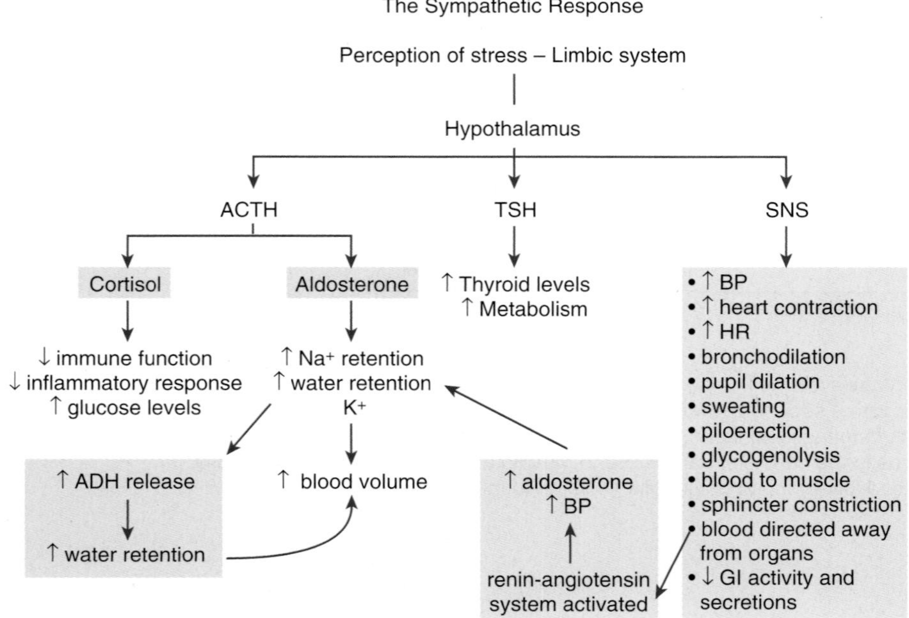

FIGURE 28.3 The 'fight-or-flight' response: the sympathetic stress reaction. ACTH, adrenocorticotrophic hormone; ADH, antidiuretic hormone; BP, blood pressure; GI, gastrointestinal; HR, heart rate; SNS, sympathetic nervous system; TSH, thyroid stimulating hormone.

- Increased respiratory efficiency: bronchi dilate to allow more air to enter with each breath, and the respiratory rate increases.
- Reduced motility and secretions in the gastrointestinal (GI) tract since there is no real need to digest food during a fight-or-flight situation. Digestion slows dramatically; sphincters constrict and defaecation does not occur.
- Diversion of blood from other internal organs, including the kidneys. This results in activation of the renin-angiotensin system (Chapter 41) and an increase in blood pressure and blood volume as water is retained by the kidneys. Sphincters in the urinary bladder are also constricted, preventing urination.
- Pupillary dilation, allowing more light to enter the eye, to improve vision in darkened areas.
- Sweating is increased to dissipate heat generated by the increased metabolic activity.
- Piloerection (hair standing on end) occurs to generate heat when the core body temperature is too low.
- Glucose is formed by glycogenolysis, to increase blood glucose levels and provide energy.
- Immune and inflammatory reactions are suppressed, to preserve energy that might otherwise be used by these activities.
- Corticosteroid hormones are released to regulate glucose activity and balance electrolytes.

Adrenergic Transmission

Sympathetic postganglionic neurons that synthesize, store and release noradrenaline are referred to as adrenergic neurons. Adrenergic neurons are also found within the CNS. The chromaffin cells of the adrenal medulla are also adrenergic because they synthesize, store and release noradrenaline and adrenaline. When the SNS is stimulated, the chromaffin cells secrete adrenaline and noradrenaline directly into the bloodstream to act on **adrenergic receptors** distributed around the body.

Noradrenaline Synthesis and Storage

Noradrenaline belongs to a group of structurally related chemicals called catecholamines that also include dopamine and adrenaline. Noradrenaline is made by the neurons using tyrosine obtained from the diet. Tyrosine is converted to dihydroxyphenylalanine (dopa) by tyrosine hydroxylase. The enzyme dopa decarboxylase, then converts dopa to dopamine, which in turn is converted to noradrenaline in adrenergic neurons. The noradrenaline is then stored in granules or vesicles within the neurons (Figure 28.4).

Noradrenaline Release

When the neuron is stimulated, the action potential travels down the axon and arrives at the axon terminal (see

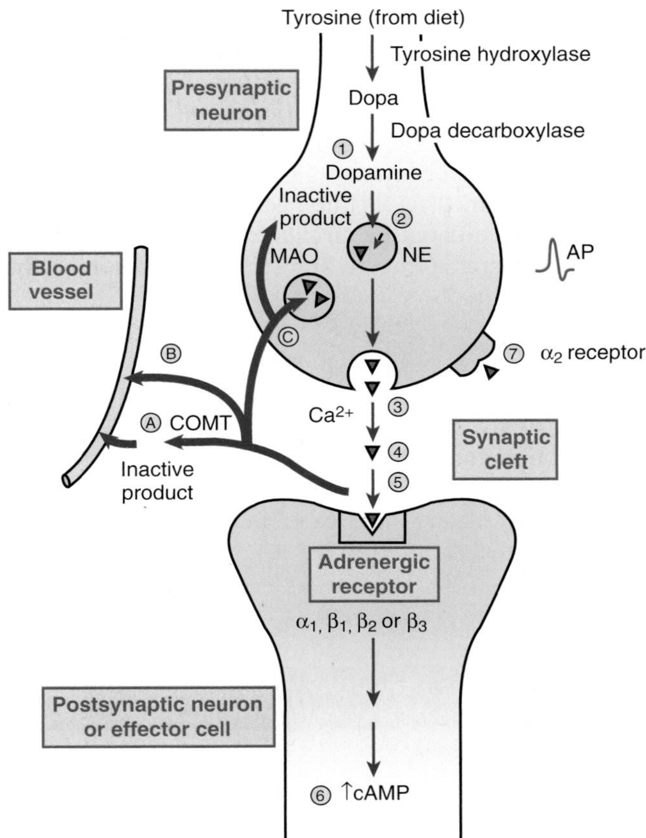

FIGURE 28.4 Sequence of events at an adrenergic synapse. *1.* Dopamine, a precursor of noradrenaline (NAdr), is synthesized from tyrosine in several steps. *2.* Dopamine is taken into the storage vesicle and converted to NAdr. *3.* Release of neurotransmitter by action potential (AP) in presynaptic neuron. *4.* Diffusion of neurotransmitter across synaptic cleft. *5.* Binding of neurotransmitter with receptor. The events resulting from NAdr's occupying of receptor sites depend on the nature of the postsynaptic cell. *6.* Interaction of NAdr with many β-receptors leads to increased synthesis of cyclic adenosine monophosphate (cAMP). *7.* Feedback control at α_2-receptors leads to decreased NAdr release from the presynaptic neuron. An enzyme, catechol-*O*-methyl transferase (COMT), inactivates the NAdr (A), but the most important way in which the action of NAdr is terminated is by reuptake into the presynaptic neuron (C), where it may be reused or inactivated by another enzyme, monoamine oxidase (MAO). The neurotransmitter may also diffuse away from the synaptic cleft (B).

Chapter 18). The action potential then depolarizes the axon membrane. This action causes calcium to enter the neuron, causing the storage vesicles to fuse with the cell membrane, and then release their load of noradrenaline into the synaptic cleft via exocytosis. The noradrenaline travels to specific adrenergic receptor sites on the effector cell on the other side of the synaptic cleft.

Adrenergic Receptors

The receptor sites that interact with neurotransmitters at adrenergic sites have been classified as **α-receptors** and **β-receptors**; which can be further subdivided into α_1-, α_2-, β_1-, β_2- and β_3-receptors (Table 28.2). It is known that these receptors respond to different concentrations of noradrenaline or different ratios of noradrenaline and adrenaline, that is they have different sensitivities. In addition to stimulation by neurotransmitter released from the axon in the immediate vicinity, **adrenergic receptors** can be further stimulated by circulating noradrenaline and adrenaline secreted directly into the bloodstream by the adrenal medulla.

α-Receptors

α_1-receptors are found in blood vessels, in the iris and in the urinary bladder. In blood vessels, they cause vasoconstriction and increase peripheral resistance, thus raising blood pressure. In the iris, they cause pupil dilation. In the urinary bladder, they cause increased closure of the internal sphincter.

α_2-receptors are located on nerve membranes and act as modulators of noradrenaline release. When noradrenaline is released from a nerve ending, it crosses the synaptic cleft to bind with its specific receptor site. Some of it also binds to α_2-receptor on the presynaptic membrane, reducing noradrenaline release through a negative feedback mechanism. In this way, the α_2-receptor helps to prevent over-stimulation of effector sites. These receptors are also found on the β cells in the pancreas, where they help to moderate the insulin release stimulated by SNS activation.

β-Receptors

β_1-receptors are found in the heart, where they stimulate increased myocardial activity and increased heart rate. **β_2-receptors** are found in the smooth muscle of blood vessels where stimulation leads to vasodilation. In the bronchi, β_2-receptors cause dilation; and in the periphery, they cause

Table 28.2 Physiological Effects of Specific Receptor Sites in the Autonomic Nervous System

Sympathetic Division	Parasympathetic Division
α_1-Receptors	**Muscarinic receptors**
Vasoconstriction	Pupil constriction
Increased peripheral resistance with increased blood pressure	Accommodation of the lens
Contracted piloerection muscles	Decreased heart rate
Pupil dilation	Increased gastrointestinal (GI) motility
Thickened salivary secretions	Increased GI secretions
Closure of urinary bladder sphincter	Increased urinary bladder contraction
Ejaculation	Penile erection
α_2-Receptors	Sweating
Negative feedback control of noradrenaline release from presynaptic neuron	**Nicotinic receptors**
Moderation of insulin release from the pancreas	Muscle contractions
β_1-Receptors	Release of noradrenaline and adrenaline from the adrenal medulla
Increased heart rate	Autonomic ganglia stimulation
Increased conduction through the atrioventricular node	
Increased myocardial contraction	
β_2-Receptors	
Vasodilation	
Bronchial dilation	
Increased breakdown of muscle and liver glycogen	
Release of glucagon from the pancreas	
Relaxation of uterine smooth muscle	
Decreased gastrointestinal (GI) muscle tone and activity	
Decreased GI secretions	
Relaxation of urinary bladder detrusor muscle	
β_3-Receptors	
Stimulation of lipolysis in adipose tissue	
Thermogenesis in adipose tissue and skeletal muscle	

increased muscle and liver breakdown of glycogen and increased release of glucagon from the α cells of the pancreas. Stimulation of β_2-receptors in the uterus results in relaxed uterine smooth muscle.

β_3-receptors are responsible for increased lipolysis or breakdown of fat for energy in peripheral tissues.

Termination of Transmission

Once noradrenaline has been released into the synaptic cleft, stimulation of the receptor site is terminated only once the noradrenaline has been inactivated. Most of the free unbound noradrenaline molecules are recycled and taken back up into the nerve terminal that released them in a process called reuptake. The neurotransmitter is then either repackaged into vesicles to be released later with nerve stimulation or broken down by **monoamine oxidase (MAO)**. Any noradrenaline that is absorbed into the circulation can be metabolized by catechol-*O*-methyl transferase (COMT).

The Parasympathetic Division of the Nervous System

In many areas, the **parasympathetic division** of the nervous system works in opposition to the SNS. This allows the autonomic system to maintain a fine control over internal homeostasis. For instance, the SNS increases heart rate and the parasympathetic system decreases it. Therefore, the ANS can influence heart rate by increasing or decreasing sympathetic activity or by increasing or decreasing parasympathetic activity. Whereas the SNS is associated with the stress reaction and expenditure of energy, the parasympathetic system is associated with activities that help the body to store or conserve energy, a 'rest-and-digest' response (Table 28.3).

Anatomy

The parasympathetic system is sometimes called the craniosacral division because the CNS neurons that originate

Table 28.3 Effects of Autonomic Stimulation

Effector Site	Sympathetic Reaction	Parasympathetic Reaction
Eye		
Iris radial muscle	Contraction (pupil dilates)	—
Iris sphincter muscle	—	Contraction (pupil constricts)
Ciliary muscle	—	Contraction (lens accommodates for near vision)
Lacrimal glands	—	↑ Secretions
Heart	↑ Rate, contractility	↓ Rate
	↑ Atrioventricular conduction	↓ Atrioventricular conduction
Blood vessels		
Skin, mucous membranes	Constriction	—
Skeletal muscle	Dilation	—
Bronchial muscle	Relaxation (dilation)	Constriction
Gastrointestinal tract		
Muscle motility and tone	↓ Activity	↑ Activity
Sphincters	Contraction	Relaxation
Secretions	↓ Secretions	↑ Activity
Salivary glands	Thick secretions	Copious, watery secretions
Gallbladder	Relaxation	Contraction
Liver	Glyconeogenesis	—
Urinary bladder		
Detrusor muscle	Relaxation	Contraction
Trigone muscle and sphincter	Contraction	Relaxation
Reproductive tracts		
Male	Ejaculation	Erection (vascular dilation)
Female	Uterine relaxation	—
Skin structures		
Sweat glands	↑ Sweating	—
Piloerector muscles	Contracted ('goose bumps')	—

parasympathetic impulses are found in the cranium (one of the most important being the vagus or tenth cranial nerve) and in the sacral area of the spinal cord (see Figure 28.1). The long preganglionic axons extend from the CNS to the ganglia located close to or within the organ that will be innervated. The postganglionic axons emerging from the ganglia are very short, going directly to the effector cell. The neurotransmitter used by both the preganglionic and postganglionic neurons is ACh.

Functions

Parasympathetic system stimulation results in the following actions:

- Increased motility and secretions in the GI tract to promote digestion and absorption of nutrients.
- Decreased heart rate and contractility to conserve energy and provide rest for the heart.
- Constriction of the bronchi, with increased secretions.
- Relaxation of the GI and urinary bladder sphincters, allowing removal of waste products.
- Pupillary constriction, decreasing the light entering the eye and decreasing stimulation of the retina.

These activities are aimed at increasing digestion, absorption of nutrients, and building of essential proteins, as well as a general conservation of energy.

Cholinergic Transmission

Neurons that use ACh as their neurotransmitter are called **cholinergic neurons**. There are four basic kinds of cholinergic neurons:

1. All preganglionic neurons in the ANS, both sympathetic and parasympathetic
2. Postganglionic neurons of the parasympathetic system and a few SNS neurons, such as those that re-enter the spinal cord and cause general body reactions such as sweating
3. Motor neurons on skeletal muscles
4. Cholinergic neurons within the CNS

Acetylcholine Synthesis and Storage

Under the action of the enzyme choline acetyltransferase, ACh is produced from choline obtained from the diet, and acetyl CoA. Like noradrenaline, the ACh is produced in the neuron and travels to the end of the axons, where it is packaged into vesicles.

Acetylcholine Release

The vesicles full of ACh migrate to the neuron membrane. When an action potential reaches the neuron terminal, calcium entering the cell causes the secretion of neurotransmitter into the synaptic cleft. The ACh travels across the synaptic cleft and binds to **cholinergic receptor** sites on the effector cells of organs and muscles (Figure 28.5).

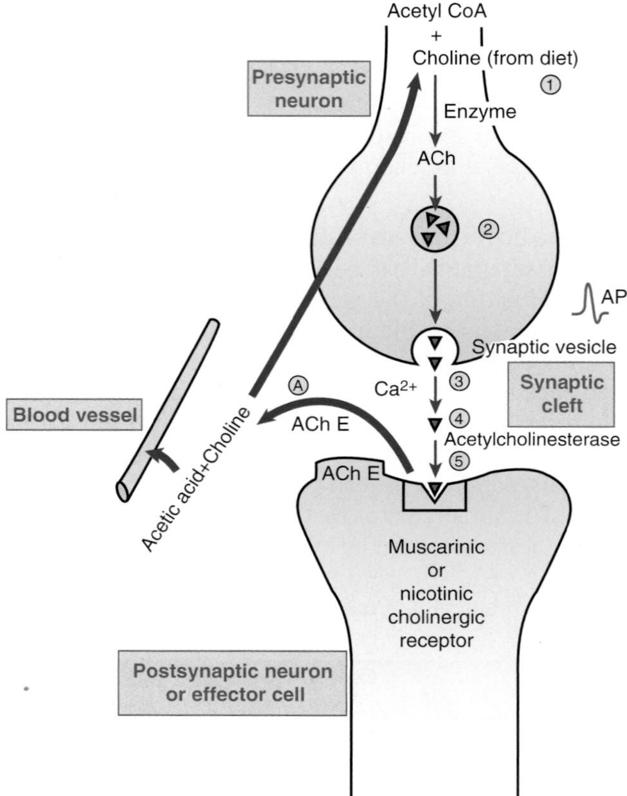

FIGURE 28.5 Sequence of events at a cholinergic synapse. *1.* Synthesis of acetylcholine (ACh) from choline and a cofactor (the enzyme is choline acetyltransferase, CoA). *2.* Uptake of neurotransmitter into storage (synaptic) vesicle. *3.* Release of neurotransmitter by action potential (AP) in presynaptic neuron. *4.* Diffusion of neurotransmitter across synaptic cleft. *5.* Binding of neurotransmitter with receptor. The events resulting from ACh's occupying of receptor sites depend on the nature of the postsynaptic cell. ACh excites some cells and inhibits others. An enzyme, acetylcholinesterase (AChE), found in the tissues and on the postsynaptic neuron, inactivates ACh (A). Some of the products diffuse into the circulation, but most of the choline formed is taken up and reused by the cholinergic neuron.

ACh receptors are classified as either **muscarinic** or **nicotinic receptors**.

Muscarinic Receptors

Muscarinic receptors can be found in visceral effector organs, in sweat glands and in some vascular smooth muscle. Stimulation of muscarinic receptors causes pupil constriction, increased GI motility and secretions (including saliva), increased urinary bladder contraction and a slowing of the heart rate.

Nicotinic Receptors

Nicotinic receptors are located in the CNS, the adrenal medulla, the autonomic ganglia and the neuromuscular junction. Stimulation of nicotinic receptors causes muscle contraction, autonomic responses, and release of noradrenaline and adrenaline from the adrenal medulla.

Termination of Transmission

Once the postsynaptic neuron has been stimulated by ACh, it is important to stop the stimulation and remove the ACh. The destruction of ACh is carried out by the enzyme **acetylcholinesterase** to form the chemically inactive compounds, acetic acid and choline. The choline is then recycled to produce additional ACh molecules.

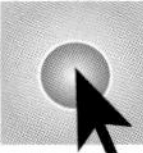

WEB LINK

To explore the virtual ANS, consult the following Internet source: http://www.InnerBody.com

Points to Remember

- The ANS works with the endocrine system to regulate internal functioning and maintain homeostasis.
- The ANS is divided into two branches, the sympathetic and the parasympathetic divisions.
- The two branches of the ANS work in opposition to maintain constant regulation of the internal environment and to allow rapid response to stress situations.
- The sympathetic nervous system, when stimulated, is responsible for the fight-or-flight response. It prepares the body for immediate reaction to stressors by increasing metabolism, diverting blood to large muscles, and increasing cardiac and respiratory function.
- The parasympathetic division, when stimulated, acts as a rest-and-digest response. It increases the digestion, absorption and metabolism of nutrients and slows metabolism and function to save energy.
- The sympathetic nervous system is composed of CNS cells arising in the thoracic or lumbar area of the spinal cord, short preganglionic axons, ganglia located near the spinal cord, and long postganglionic axons that react with effector cells. The neurotransmitter used by the preganglionic cells is ACh; the neurotransmitter used by the postganglionic cells is noradrenaline.
- The parasympathetic nervous system comprises CNS cells that arise in the cranium and sacral region of the spinal cord, long preganglionic axons that secrete ACh, ganglia located very close to or within the effector tissue, and short postganglionic axons that also secrete ACh.
- Noradrenaline is made by adrenergic neurons using tyrosine from the diet. It is packaged in storage vesicles that align on the axon membrane and is secreted into the synaptic cleft when the neuron is stimulated. Noradrenaline binds to specific receptor sites and is then broken down by MAO or COMT. The breakdown products are used to synthesize more noradrenaline.
- ACh is made by choline from the diet and packaged into storage vesicles to be released by the cholinergic neuron into the synaptic cleft. ACh is broken down to an inactive form almost immediately by acetylcholinesterase.
- Sympathetic nervous system adrenergic receptors are classified as α_1-, α_2-, β_1-, β_2- or β_3-receptors.
- Parasympathetic nervous system receptors are classified as muscarinic or nicotinic.

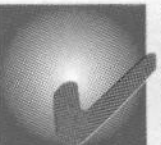

CHECK YOUR UNDERSTANDING

Answers to the questions in this chapter may be found in the answer key in the back of the book.

Multiple Choice

Select the best answer to the following.

1. The ANS functions to
   a. maintain balance and posture.
   b. maintain the special senses.
   c. regulate and integrate internal functions of the body.
   d. coordinate peripheral and central nerve pathways.

2. The ANS differs from other systems in the CNS in that it
   a. uses only peripheral pathways.
   b. affects organs and muscles by way of a two-neuron system.
   c. uses a unique one-neuron system.
   d. bypasses the CNS in all of its actions.

3. If you suspect that a person is very stressed and is experiencing a sympathetic stress reaction, you would expect to find
   a. increased bowel sounds and urinary output.
   b. constricted pupils and warm, flushed skin.
   c. slow heart rate and decreased systolic blood pressure.
   d. dilated pupils and elevated systolic blood pressure.

4. Stimulating only the β_2-receptors in the SNS would result in
   a. increased heart rate.
   b. increased myocardial contraction.
   c. vasodilation and bronchial dilation.
   d. uterine contraction.

5. Once a postganglionic receptor site has been stimulated, the neurotransmitter must be broken down immediately. The sympathetic nervous system breaks down postganglionic neurotransmitters using
   a. liver enzymes and acetylcholinesterase.
   b. acetylcholinesterase and MAO.
   c. COMT and liver enzymes.
   d. MAO and COMT.

6. The parasympathetic nervous system, in most situations, opposes the actions of the sympathetic division, allowing the ANS to
   a. generally have no effect.
   b. maintain a fine control over internal homeostasis.
   c. promote digestion.
   d. respond to stress most effectively.

7. Cholinergic neurons, i.e. those using ACh as their neurotransmitter, would *not* be found in
   a. motor neurons on skeletal muscles.
   b. preganglionic neurons in the sympathetic and parasympathetic nervous systems.
   c. postganglionic neurons in the parasympathetic nervous system.
   d. the adrenal medulla.

8. Stimulation of the parasympathetic nervous system would cause
   a. slower heart rate and increased GI secretions.
   b. faster heart rate and urinary retention.
   c. bronchial dilation.
   d. pupil dilation and muscle paralysis.

Extended Matching Questions

Select **all** that apply.

1. The sympathetic nervous system
   a. is also called the thoracolumbar system.
   b. is also called the fight-or-flight system.
   c. is also called the craniosacral system.
   d. uses ACh as its sole neurotransmitter.
   e. uses adrenaline as its sole neurotransmitter.
   f. is active during a stress reaction.

2. The parasympathetic nervous system
   a. is also called the craniosacral system.
   b. increases heart rate and blood pressure.
   c. has ganglia located close to the spinal cord.
   d. will dilate pupils.
   e. uses ACh as its sole neurotransmitter.
   f. increases gastric motility.

Matching

Match the following words with the appropriate definition.

1.____________________autonomic nervous system
2.____________________sympathetic nervous system
3.____________________parasympathetic nervous system
4.____________________ganglia
5.____________________adrenergic receptors
6.____________________cholinergic receptors
7.____________________β-receptors
8.____________________muscarinic receptors
9.____________________nicotinic receptors
10.____________________acetylcholinesterase
11.____________________monoamine oxidase

A. Closely packed group of nerve cell bodies
B. Fight-or-flight response mediator
C. Enzyme that breaks down noradrenaline
D. Cholinergic receptors that mediate muscle contraction
E. Rest-and-digest response mediator
F. Receptor sites on effectors that respond to ACh
G. Adrenergic receptors found in the heart, lungs and vascular smooth muscle
H. Receptor sites on effectors that respond to noradrenaline
I. Cholinergic receptors that increase secretion from the GI tract
J. Portion of the central and peripheral nervous systems that, with the endocrine system, functions to maintain internal homeostasis
K. Enzyme that deactivates ACh released from the neuron axon

Bibliography

Ganong, W. (2005). *Review of medical physiology* (22nd ed.). New York: McGraw-Hill.
Guyton, A., & Hall, J. (2005). *Textbook of medical physiology* (11th ed.). Philadelphia: W. B. Saunders.
Howland, R. D., & Mycek, M. J. (2005). *Pharmacology* (3rd ed.). Philadelphia: Lippincott Williams & Wilkins.
Marieb, E. N., & Hoehn, K. (2009). *Human anatomy & histology* (8th ed.). San Francisco: Pearson.

CHAPTER 29

Adrenergic Agents

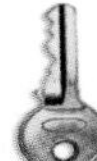

KEY TERMS

adrenergic agonist
α-agonist
β-agonist
glycogenolysis
sympathomimetic

LEARNING OBJECTIVES

Upon completion of this chapter, you will be able to:

1. Describe ways that sympathomimetic drugs act to produce effects on adrenergic receptors.
2. Describe the therapeutic actions, indications, pharmacokinetics, associated with adrenergic agents.
3. Describe the contraindications, most common adverse reactions and important drug–drug interactions associated with adrenergic agents.
4. Discuss the use of adrenergic agents across the lifespan.
5. Compare and contrast the key drugs dopamine and phenylephrine with other adrenergic agents.
6. Outline the nursing considerations, including important teaching points, for patients receiving an adrenergic agent.

α- AND β-ADRENERGIC AGONISTS

adrenaline
dobutamine
dopamine
ephedrine
metaraminol
noradrenaline

α-SPECIFIC ADRENERGIC AGONISTS

clonidine (α_1-specific)
phenylephrine

β-SPECIFIC ADRENERGIC AGONISTS

salbutamol
salmeterol
terbutaline

(ALSO SEE β-ADRENERGIC AGONISTS IN CHAPTER 54.)

Adrenergic agonists are also called **sympathomimetic** drugs because they mimic the effects of the sympathetic nervous system (SNS). The use of adrenergic agonists varies from ophthalmic preparations for dilating pupils (Box 29.1), inhalants to dilate the airways (Chapter 54) and systemic preparations used to support people who are in shock. They can be used in patients of all ages (Box 29.2).

Adrenergic Agonists

The therapeutic and adverse effects associated with these drugs are related to their stimulation of adrenergic receptor sites (Figure 29.1). That stimulation can be either direct, by occupation of the adrenergic receptor, or indirect, by modulation of the release of neurotransmitters from the axon. Some drugs act in both ways.

BOX 29.1 FOCUS ON **CLINICAL SKILLS**

Administering Ophthalmic Medications

Some of the adrenergic agonists are applied to the eye; it is important to review the administration technique. First, wash hands thoroughly. Do not touch the dropper to the eye or to any other surface. Have the patient tilt his or her head back or lie down and stare upward. Gently grasp the lower eyelid and pull the eyelid away from the eyeball. Instil the prescribed number of drops into the pouch formed by the eyelid and then release the lid slowly. Have the patient close the eye and look downward. Apply gentle pressure to the inside corner of the eye (the punctum) for 3 to 5 minutes to prevent drainage. Do not rub the eyeball and do not rinse the dropper. If more than one type of eye drop is being used, wait 5 minutes before administering the next one.

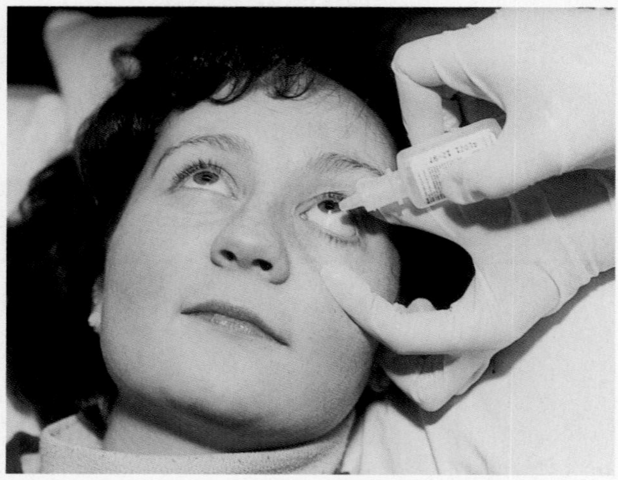

After gently exposing the lower conjunctival sac, the nurse administers an eyedrop (with permission from Taylor, C, Lillis, C, & LeMone, P. (2004). *Lippincott's photo atlas of medication administration.* Philadelphia: Lippincott Williams & Wilkins).

α- and β-Adrenergic Agonists

Drugs that are generally sympathomimetic – that is, they stimulate the adrenergic receptors (adrenoceptors). They are referred to as **α-** and **β-agonists** depending on the type of adrenoceptor they stimulate. The receptor subtypes include α_1, α_2, β_1, β_2, β_3. Some of these drugs are preparations of catecholamines.

Adrenaline (epinephrine) is a naturally occurring catecholamine that interacts with both α- and β-adrenergic receptors. It is used therapeutically in the treatment of shock, when increased blood pressure and heart contractility are essential; as one of the primary treatments for bronchospasm, by direct dilation of the bronchioles; as an ophthalmic agent; and to produce a local vasoconstriction that prolongs the effects of local anaesthetics.

Noradrenaline (Norepinephrine), another naturally occurring catecholamine, is not used as frequently as adrenaline. It is given intravenously to treat shock or during cardiac arrest to get sympathetic activity, but in recent years it has been replaced by dopamine.

Dopamine is the sympathomimetic of choice for the treatment of shock. It stimulates the heart and blood pressure but also causes a renal and splanchnic arteriole dilation that increases blood flow to the kidney, thus preventing the diminished renal blood supply and possible renal shutdown that can occur with adrenaline or noradrenaline.

Dobutamine is a synthetic catecholamine that has a slight preference for β_1-receptor sites. It is used in the treatment of congestive heart failure because it can increase myocardial contractility without much change in rate and does not increase the oxygen demand of the cardiac muscle, an advantage over all of the other sympathomimetic drugs.

Therapeutic Actions and Indications

The effects of the sympathomimetic drugs are mediated by the adrenergic receptors in target organs: heart rate increases with increased myocardial contractility, bronchioles dilate and respirations increase in rate and depth, vasoconstriction occurs with increase in blood pressure, intraocular pressure decreases, **glycogenolysis** (breakdown of glucose stores so that the glucose can be used as energy) occurs throughout the body, pupils dilate and sweating can increase (see Figure 29.1). These drugs are indicated for the treatment of hypotensive states or shock, bronchospasm and some types of asthma. As noted earlier, dopamine has become the drug of choice for the treatment of shock and hypotensive states because it causes an increase in renal blood flow and does not cause the renal shutdown that has been associated with other agents. Ephedrine is also widely used as a local nasal drug for the treatment of seasonal rhinitis.

BOX 29.2 **DRUG THERAPY ACROSS THE LIFESPAN**

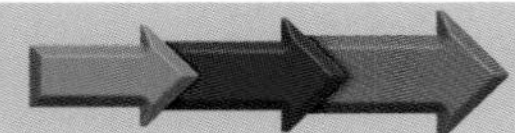

Adrenergic Agents

CHILDREN

Children are at greater risk for complications associated with the use of adrenergic agents, including tachycardia, hypertension, tachypnoea and GI complications. The dosage for these agents needs to be calculated from the child's body weight and age. It is good practice to have a second person check the dosage calculation before administering the drug to avoid potential toxic effects. Children should be carefully monitored and supported during the use of these drugs.

Phenylephrine is often found in over-the-counter (OTC) allergy and cold preparations and parents need to be instructed to be very careful with the use of these drugs – they should check the labels for ingredients monitor the recommended dosage and avoid combining drugs that contain similar ingredients.

ADULTS

Adults being treated with adrenergic agents for shock or a shock-like condition require constant monitoring and dosage adjustments based on their response. Patients who may be at increased risk for cardiac complications should be monitored very closely and started on a lower dose.

Adults using these agents for glaucoma or for seasonal rhinitis need to be cautioned about the use of OTC drugs and alternative therapies that might increase the drug effects and cause serious adverse effects.

Many of these drugs are used in emergency situations and may be used during pregnancy and lactation. In general, there are no adequate studies about their effects during pregnancy and lactation and in those situations they should be used only if the benefit to the mother is greater than the risk to the foetus or neonate.

OLDER ADULTS

Older patients are more likely to experience the adverse effects associated with these drugs, effecting their CNS, CV, GI and respiratory systems. Older patients often have renal or hepatic impairment, so they are also more likely to have toxic levels of the drug related to changes in metabolism and excretion. Older patients should be started on lower doses of the drugs and should be monitored very closely for potentially serious arrhythmias or blood pressure changes.

They should also be cautioned about the use of OTC drugs and complementary therapies that could potentially increase drug effects and cause serious adverse reactions.

Ephedrine is a synthetically produced plant alkaloid that stimulates the release of noradrenaline from nerve endings and directly acts on adrenergic receptor sites. Although it was once used for everything from the treatment of shock to chronic management of asthma and allergic rhinitis, its use in many areas is declining because of the availability of less toxic drugs with more predictable onset and action. It is used as a nasal decongestant in a topical, nasal form.

Metaraminol is a synthetic agent that is very similar to noradrenaline. It is given as a single parenteral injection to prevent hypotension by increasing myocardial contractility and causing peripheral vasoconstriction. Its use is limited to situations in which dopamine or noradrenaline cannot be used.

Always refer to the latest edition of the Children's British National Formulary when administering drugs to children.

Pharmacokinetics

These drugs are generally absorbed rapidly after injection or passage through mucous membranes. They are metabolized in the liver and excreted in the urine. The sympathomimetic drugs stimulate the SNS, therefore, they should be used during pregnancy and lactation only if the benefits to the mother clearly outweigh any potential risks to the foetus or neonate.

Contraindications and Cautions

The **α- and β-agonists** are contraindicated in patients with phaeochromocytoma *because the systemic overload of catecholamines could be fatal;* with tachyarrhythmias or ventricular fibrillation *because the increased heart rate and oxygen consumption usually caused by these drugs could exacerbate these conditions*; with hypovolaemia, *for which fluid replacement would be the treatment for the associated hypotension*; and with halogenated hydrocarbon general anaesthetics, (e.g. halothane), *which sensitize the myocardium to catecholamines and could cause serious cardiac effects.* Caution should be used with any kind of peripheral vascular disease (e.g. atherosclerosis, Raynaud's disease, diabetic endarteritis), *which could be exacerbated by systemic vasoconstriction.*

Adverse Effects

The adverse effects associated with the use of α- and β-adrenergic agonists may be associated with the drugs' effects on the SNS: arrhythmias, hypertension, palpitations, angina and dyspnoea related to the effects on the heart and cardiovascular (CV) system; nausea and vomiting, related to the depressant effects on the gastrointestinal (GI) tract; and headache, sweating and piloerection, related to the sympathetic stimulation.

Clinically Important Drug–Drug Interactions

Increased effects of tricyclic antidepressants (TCAs) and monoamine oxidase inhibitors (MAOIs) can occur because of the increased noradrenaline levels or increased receptor stimulation that occurs with both these drugs. There is an increased risk of hypertension if α- and β-adrenergic agonists are given with any other drugs that cause hypertension.

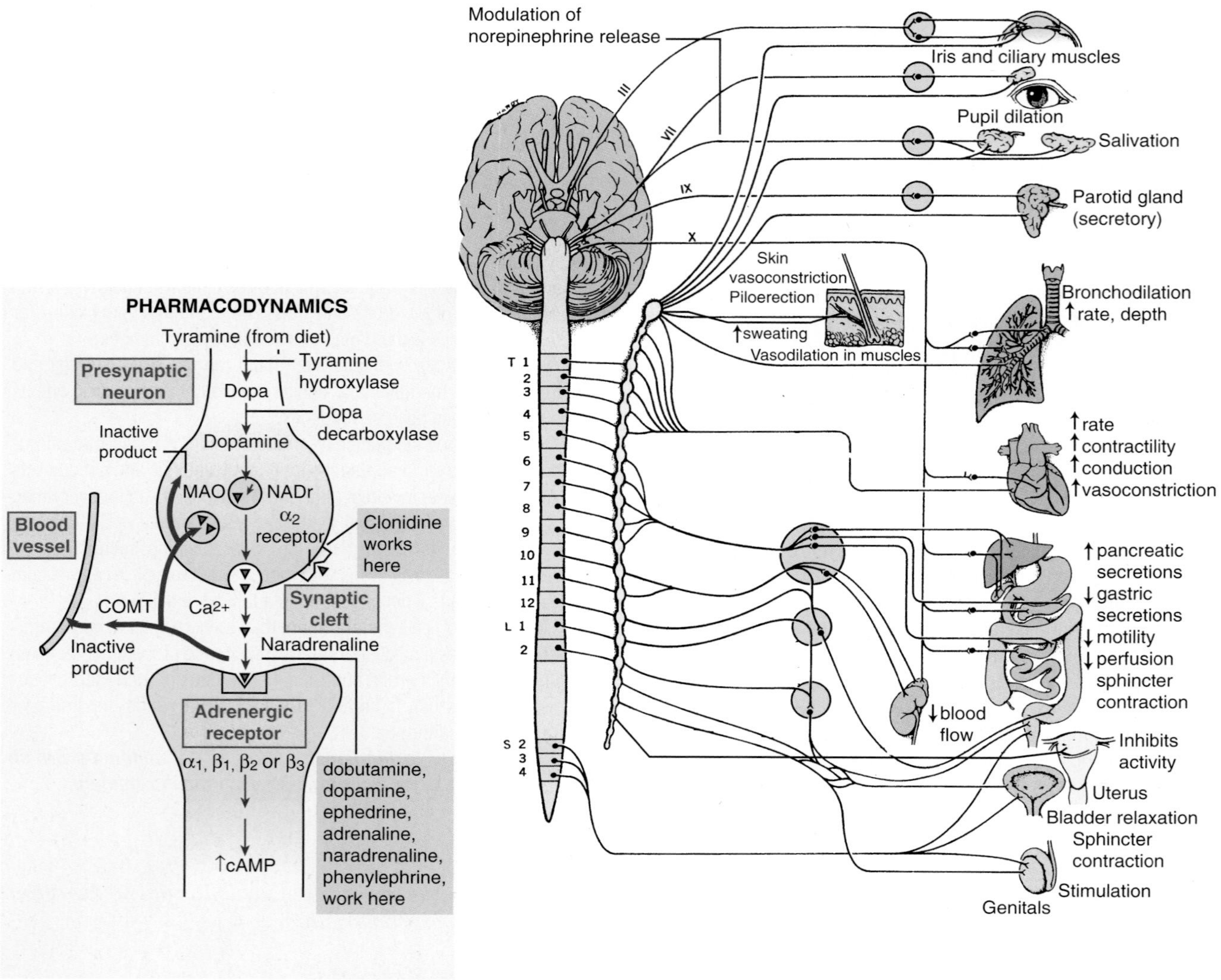

FIGURE 29.1 Pharmacodynamics of adrenergic agonists and associated physiologic reactions.

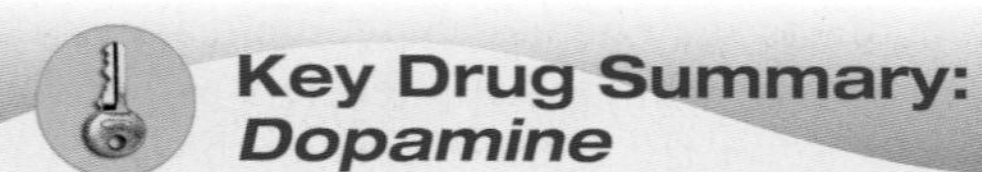

Key Drug Summary: *Dopamine*

Indications: Correction of haemodynamic imbalances present in shock

Actions: Acts directly and by the release of noradrenaline from sympathetic nerve terminals; mediates dilation of vessels in the renal and splanchnic beds to maintain renal perfusion while stimulating the sympathetic response

Pharmacokinetics:

Route	Onset	Peak	Duration
IV	1–2 min	10 min	Length of infusion

$T_{1/2}$: 2 min; metabolized in the liver, excreted in the urine

Adverse effects: Tachycardia, ectopic beats, anginal pain, hypotension, dyspnoea, nausea, vomiting, headache

Nursing Considerations for Patients receiving α- and β-Adrenergic Agonists

Assessment: History and Examination

Screen for the following conditions, *which could be cautions or contraindications to use of the drug*: any known allergies to these drugs; phaeochromocytoma, tachyarrhythmias or ventricular fibrillation, or hypovolaemia; general anaesthesia with halogenated hydrocarbon anaesthetics; and the presence of vascular disease, *which would require cautious use of the drug.*

Include screening *for baseline status before beginning therapy and for any potential adverse effects*: skin colour and temperature; pulse, blood pressure and ECG; respiration, adventitious sounds; urine output and electrolytes.

Establish if the patient is currently taking other medications or herbal therapies which may potentially interact with the α- and β-adrenergic agonists.

Nursing Diagnoses

The patient receiving an α- and β-agonist may have the following nursing diagnoses related to drug therapy:

- Acute pain related to CV and systemic effects
- Decreased cardiac output related to CV effects
- Ineffective tissue perfusion related to CV effects
- Reduced urinary output
- Deficient knowledge regarding drug therapy

Implementation With Rationale

- Use extreme caution in calculating and preparing doses of these drugs *because even small errors could have serious effects.* Always dilute drug before use, if it is not prediluted *to prevent tissue irritation on injection.*
- Monitor patient response closely (blood pressure, ECG, urine output, cardiac output) and adjust dosage accordingly *to ensure the most benefit with the least amount of toxicity.*
- Maintain phentolamine on standby *in case extravasation occurs*; infiltration of the site with 10 ml saline containing 5 to 10 mg phentolamine is usually effective in saving the area.
- Provide thorough patient education, including measures to avoid adverse effects, warning signs of problems and the need for monitoring and evaluation, *to enhance patient knowledge about drug therapy and to promote compliance.*
- Offer support and encouragement *to deal with the drug regimen.* (See Critical Thinking Scenario 29-1.)

Evaluation

- Monitor patient response to the drug (improvement in blood pressure, ocular pressure, and bronchial airflow).
- Monitor for adverse effects (CV changes, decreased urine output, headache, GI upset).
- Evaluate the effectiveness of the teaching plan (patient can name the drug, dosage, adverse effects to watch for, specific measures to avoid adverse effects).
- Monitor the effectiveness of comfort measures and compliance with regimen.

α-Specific Adrenergic Agonists

α-specific adrenergic agonists, or α-agonists, are drugs that bind primarily to α-receptors, rather than to β-receptors. Currently, two drugs are in this class phenylephrine and clonidine.

Phenylephrine, a potent vasoconstrictor with little or no effect on the heart or bronchioles, is used in many combination cold- and-allergy products. Topically it is used to treat allergic rhinitis and to relieve the symptoms of otitis media. Ophthalmically it is used to dilate the pupils for eye examination, before surgery, or to relieve elevated eye pressure associated with glaucoma.

Clonidine specifically stimulates central nervous system (CNS) α_2-receptors. This leads to decreased sympathetic outflow from the CNS because the α_2-receptors moderate the release of noradrenaline from the nerve axon. Clonidine is used to treat essential hypertension as a secondary, to treat chronic pain in cancer patients in combination with opiates and other drugs and to ease withdrawal from opiates. Given that it has centrally acting effects, clonidine is associated with many more CNS effects (bad dreams, sedation, drowsiness, fatigue and headache) than other sympathomimetics. It can also cause extreme hypotension, congestive heart failure and bradycardia owing to its centrally mediated effects; therefore it should be used carefully with any patient who is susceptible to such conditions. It is available in an oral and transdermal form and in injection form for epidural infusion to control pain.

Therapeutic Actions and Indications

The therapeutic effects of the α-specific adrenergic agonists come from the stimulation of α-receptors within the SNS (see Figure 29.1). The uses are varied, depending on the route of the drug and the drug being used. Clonidine is frequently used to treat essential hypertension. Phenylephrine is found in many cold and allergy products because it is so effective in constricting topical vessels and decreasing the swelling, signs and symptoms of rhinitis.

Pharmacokinetics

These drugs are generally well absorbed and reach peak levels in a short period – 20 to 45 minutes. They are widely distributed in the body, metabolized in the liver and primarily excreted in the urine. There are no adequate studies about use during pregnancy and lactation, so use should be reserved for situations in which the benefit to the mother outweighs any potential risk to the foetus or neonate.

Contraindications and Cautions

The α-specific adrenergic agonists are contraindicated in severe hypertension or tachycardia *because of possible additive effects*; narrow-angle glaucoma, *which could be exacerbated by arterial constriction*; or pregnancy *because of potential adverse effects on the foetus.*

Adverse Effects

Patients receiving these drugs often experience adverse effects that are extensions of the therapeutic effects or other sympathetic stimulatory reactions. CNS effects include feelings of anxiety, restlessness, depression, fatigue, strange dreams, blurred vision and personality changes. CV effects can include arrhythmias, electrocardiogram (ECG) changes, blood pressure changes and peripheral vascular problems. Nausea, vomiting and anorexia can occur, related to the GI-depressing effects of the sympathetic system. Genitourinary effects can include decreased urinary output, difficulty urinating, dysuria and changes in sexual function related to the sympathetic stimulation of these systems.

Clinically Important Drug–Drug Interactions

Phenylephrine combined with MAOIs can cause severe hypertension, headache and hyperpyrexia; this combination should be avoided. Increased sympathomimetic effects occur when phenylephrine is combined with TCAs; if this combination must be used, the patient should be monitored very closely.

Clonidine has a decreased antihypertensive effect if taken with TCAs and a paradoxical hypertension occurs if it is combined with propranolol. If these combinations are used, the patient response should be monitored closely and dosage adjustment made as needed.

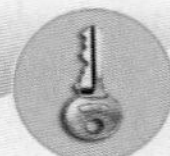

Key Drug Summary: *Phenylephrine*

Indications: Treatment of vascular failure in shock or drug-induced hypotension; to overcome paroxysmal supraventricular tachycardia; to prolong spinal anaesthesia; as a vasoconstrictor in regional anaesthesia; to maintain blood pressure during anaesthesia; topically for symptomatic relief of nasal congestion and as adjunctive therapy in middle ear infections; ophthalmically to dilate pupils and as a decongestant to provide temporary relief of eye irritation.

Actions: Powerful postsynaptic α-adrenergic receptor stimulant causing vasoconstriction and raising systolic and diastolic blood pressure with little effect on the β-receptors in the heart.

Pharmacokinetics:

Route	Onset	Duration
IV	Immediate	15–20 min
IM, Subcut	10–15 min	30–120 min
Topically	Very little systemic absorption occurs	

$T_{1/2}$: 47–100 hours; metabolized in the tissues and liver; excreted in urine and bile

Adverse effects: Fear, anxiety, restlessness, headache, nausea, decreased urine formation, pallor

Nursing Considerations for Patients Receiving α-Specific Adrenergic Agonists

Assessment: History and Examination

Screen for the following conditions, *which could be cautions or contraindications to use of the drug*: any known allergies to the drug; presence of any CV diseases, thyrotoxicosis, or diabetes, *which would require cautious use*; pregnancy or lactation; and chronic renal failure, *which could be exacerbated by drug use.*

Include screening *for baseline status before beginning therapy and for any potential adverse effects*: orientation, reflexes and vision *to monitor for CNS changes related to drug therapy*; blood pressure, pulse, ECG, peripheral perfusion and cardiac output *to establish a baseline and to monitor drug effects and adverse CV effects*; and urinary output and renal function tests *to monitor drug effects on the renal system.*

Nursing Diagnoses

The patient receiving an **α-agonist** may have the following nursing diagnoses related to drug therapy:

- Disturbed sensory perception (visual, kinaesthetic, tactile) related to CNS effects
- Risk for injury related to CNS or CV effects of drug
- Decreased cardiac output related to blood pressure changes, arrhythmias, or vasoconstriction
- Deficient knowledge regarding drug therapy

Implementation With Rationale

- Do not discontinue drug abruptly *because sudden withdrawal can result in rebound hypertension, arrhythmias, flushing and even hypertensive encephalopathy and death*; reduce drug dosage over 2 to 4 days.
- Do not discontinue drug before surgery; mark the patient's chart and monitor blood pressure carefully during surgery. *Sympathetic stimulation may alter the normal response to anaesthesia, as well as recovery from anaesthesia.*
- Monitor blood pressure, pulse, rhythm and cardiac output regularly, even with ophthalmic preparations *in order to adjust dosage or discontinue the drug if CV effects are severe.*
- When giving phenylephrine intravenously, maintain an α-blocking agent on standby *in case severe reaction occurs*; infiltrate any area of extravasation with phentolamine within 12 hours after extravasation *to preserve tissue.*
- Arrange for supportive care and comfort measures, including rest and environmental control *to decrease CNS irritation*; headache medication *to relieve discomfort*; safety measures if CNS effects occur *to protect the patient from injury;* and protective measures *if CNS effects are severe.*
- Provide thorough patient education, including dosage, potential adverse effects, safety measures, warning signs of problems and proper administration for each route used, *to enhance patient knowledge about drug therapy and to promote compliance.*
- Offer support and encouragement *to help the patient deal with the drug regimen.*

Evaluation

- Monitor patient response to the drug (improvement in condition being treated).
- Monitor for adverse effects (GI upset, CNS and CV changes).
- Evaluate the effectiveness of the teaching plan (patient can name drug, dosage, adverse effects to watch for and specific measures to avoid adverse effects).
- Monitor the effectiveness of comfort measures and compliance with the regimen.

β-Specific Adrenergic Agonists

Most of the drugs that belong to the class of β-specific adrenergic agonists, or β-agonists, are β_2-specific agonists, which are used to manage and treat bronchial spasm, asthma and other obstructive pulmonary conditions. These drugs, including salbutamol, salmeterol and terbutaline, are discussed in Chapter 53, which deals with drugs used to treat obstructive pulmonary diseases.

Nursing Considerations for Patients receiving β-Specific Adrenergic Agonists

Assessment: History and Examination

Screen for the following conditions, *which could be cautions or contraindications to the use of the drug*: any known allergies to any drug or any components of the drug; pulmonary hypertension; anaesthesia with halogenated hydrocarbons, *which sensitize the myocardium to catecholamines and could cause severe reaction*; eclampsia, uterine haemorrhage and intrauterine death, *which could be complicated by uterine relaxation or increased blood pressure*; pregnancy and lactation *because of potential effects on the foetus or neonate*; diabetes, thyroid disease, vasomotor problems, degenerative heart disease, or history of stroke, *all of which could be exacerbated by the sympathomimetic effects of the drugs.*

Physical assessment should include screening *for baseline status before beginning therapy and for any potential adverse effects*: skin colour and temperature; pulse, blood pressure and ECG; respiration; adventitious sounds; and urine output and electrolytes.

Establish if patient is currently taking other medications or herbal therapies, which may potentially interact with the β-specific adrenergic agonists.

Nursing Diagnoses

The patient receiving β-agonists may have the following nursing diagnoses related to drug therapy:

- Acute pain related to CV and systemic effects
- Decreased cardiac output related to CV effects
- Ineffective tissue perfusion related to CV effects
- Deficient knowledge regarding drug therapy

Implementation With Rationale

- Monitor patient pulse and blood pressure carefully during administration *in order to arrange to discontinue the drug at any sign of pulmonary oedema.*
- Arrange for supportive care and comfort measures, including rest and environmental control, *to relieve CNS effects*; provide headache medication and safety measures if CNS effects occur *to provide comfort and prevent injury*; avoid over-hydration *to prevent pulmonary oedema.*

- Provide thorough patient education, including the name of the drug, dosage, anticipated adverse effects, measures to avoid drug-related problems, warning signs of problems and proper administration techniques, *to enhance patient knowledge about drug therapy and to promote compliance.*
- Offer support and encouragement *to help the patient deal with the drug regimen.*

Evaluation

- Monitor patient response to the drug (improvement in condition being treated, stabilization of blood pressure, and prevention of preterm labour, cardiac stimulation).
- Monitor for adverse effects (GI upset, CNS changes, and respiratory problems).
- Evaluate the effectiveness of the teaching plan (patient can name drug, dosage, adverse effects to watch for, specific measures to avoid adverse effects).
- Monitor the effectiveness of comfort measures and compliance to the regimen.

WEB LINKS

Health care providers and patients may want to consult the following Internet sources:

http://cks.library.nhs.uk The National Health Service Clinical Knowledge Summaries provides evidence-based practical information on the common conditions observed in primary care.

http://www.bnf.org.uk The BNF provides UK health care professionals with authoritative and practical information on the selection and clinical use of medicines.

http://www.nice.org.uk The National Institute for Health and Clinical Excellence is an independent organization responsible for providing national guidance on promoting good health and preventing and treating ill health.

http://www.nhsdirect.nhs.uk The National Health Service Direct service provides patients with information and advice about health, illness and health services.

Points to Remember

- Adrenergic agonists are drugs used to stimulate the adrenergic receptors within the SNS. They are also called sympathomimetic drugs because they mimic the effects of the SNS.
- Sympathomimetic drugs are used when sympathetic stimulation is needed. The adverse effects associated with these drugs are usually also a result of sympathetic stimulation.
- α- and β-adrenergic agonists stimulate all of the adrenergic receptors in the SNS. They are used to induce a fight-or-flight response and are frequently used to treat shock.
- α-specific adrenergic agonists stimulate only the α-receptors within the SNS. Clonidine stimulates α_2-receptors and is used to treat hypertension because its action blocks release of noradrenaline from nerve axons. Phenylephrine is used in many cold and allergy remedies because it is a powerful local vasoconstrictor.
- Many of the β_2-specific adrenergic agonists are used to manage and treat asthma, bronchospasm and other obstructive pulmonary diseases.

CRITICAL THINKING SCENARIO 29-1

Adrenergic Agonist Toxicity

The Situation

Mark is a 26-year-old man who has recently moved to the northwest of England from Devon. He has been suffering from sinusitis, runny nose and cold-like symptoms for 2 weeks. He appears at an outpatient clinic with complaints of headache, 'jitters', inability to sleep, loss of appetite and a feeling of impending doom. He states that he feels 'on edge' and has not been productive in his job as a watch repairman and jewellery maker. According to his history, Mark has been treated with several different drugs for nocturnal enuresis, a persisting childhood problem. Only ephedrine, which he has been taking for 2 years, has been successful. He has no other significant health problems. He denies any side-effects from the use of ephedrine but does admit to self-medicating his nagging cold with OTC preparations – a nasal spray used four times a day and a combination

Adrenergic Agonist Toxicity *(continued)*

decongestant-pain reliever. A physical examination reveals a pulse of 104, blood pressure 154/86, respiratory rate of 16. The patient appears flushed and slightly diaphoretic.

Critical Thinking

What are the important nursing implications for Mark? *Think about the problems that confront a patient in a new area seeking health care for the first time.*

What could be causing the problems that Mark presents with? *The diagnosis of ephedrine overdose was eventually made based on the patient history of OTC drug use and the presenting signs and symptoms.*

Keeping in mind that this diagnosis means Mark has an over stimulated sympathetic stress reaction; what other physical problems can be anticipated? *Overwhelming feelings of anxiety and stress are influencing Mark's response to work and health care.*

What treatment should be planned and what teaching points should be covered for Mark?

Discussion

The first step in caring for Mark is establishing a trusting relationship to help alleviate some of the anxiety he is feeling. Seeking treatment in a new setting can be very stressful for patients under normal circumstances. In Mark's case, the sympathomimetic effects of the drugs that he has been taking make him feel even more anxious and jittery.

A careful patient history will help determine whether there are any underlying medical problems that could be exacerbated by these drug effects. A review of Mark's nocturnal enuresis and the treatments that have been tried will enhance understanding of his former health care and suggest possible implications for further study.

A careful review of the OTC drugs that Mark has been using will be informative for the patient; as well as for the health care providers. Who may not have the OTC drugs may not have been checked for those specific ingredients, but combining them to ease signs and symptoms often results in toxic levels and symptoms of overdose. Mark will need a full teaching programme about the effects of his adrenaline and which OTC drugs to avoid. The treatment for his current problems involves withdrawal of the OTC drugs; when these drug levels fall, the signs and symptoms will disappear. Mark may also wish to avoid nicotine and caffeine, because these stimulants could increase his 'jitters'.

Nursing Care Guide for Mark: Adrenergic Agonist Toxicity

Assessment: History and Examination

Assess the patient's history of drug allergies, CV dysfunction, phaeochromocytoma, narrow-angle glaucoma, prostatic hypertrophy, thyroid disease, or diabetes, as well as concurrent use of MAOIs, TCAs, ephedrine, or substances that alkalinize the urine.

Focus the physical examination on the following:

CV: Blood pressure, pulse rate, peripheral perfusion and ECG

CNS: orientation, reflexes peripheral sensation and vision

Skin: colour, temperature

GI: abdominal examination

Genitourinary: urine output, bladder percussion, prostate palpation

Respiratory: respiratory rate, adventitious sounds

Nursing Diagnoses

Decreased cardiac output related to CV effects

Acute pain related to CV and systemic effects

Impaired tissue perfusion related to CV effects

Deficient knowledge regarding drug therapy

Implementation

Ensure safe and appropriate administration of the drug.

Provide comfort and safety measures.

Monitor blood pressure, pulse rate and respiratory status throughout drug therapy.

Provide support and reassurance to deal with drug therapy and drug effects.

Provide patient education about drug name, dosage, side-effects, precautions and warning signs to report.

Evaluation

Evaluate drug effects: relief of enuresis.

Monitor for adverse effects: CV effects, dizziness, confusion, headache, rash, sweating, flushing and pupillary dilation.

Monitor for drug–drug interactions as indicated.

Evaluate effectiveness of patient education programme.

(continued)

Adrenergic Agonist Toxicity *(continued)*

Patient Education for Mark

☐ The drug that you have been taking is ephedrine. It is called an adrenergic agonist (or a sympathomimetic drug). Ephedrine acts by mimicking the effects of the SNS, which is the part of your nervous system that is responsible for your response to fear or danger (this is called the 'fight-or-flight' response). This drug triggers many effects in the body, so you may experience some undesired adverse effects. It is crucial to discuss the effect of the drug with your health care provider and to try to make the effect as tolerable as possible.

☐ Some of the following adverse effects may occur:

- *Restlessness or shaking:* If these occur, avoid driving, operating machinery, or performing delicate tasks.
- *Flushing or sweating:* Avoid warm temperatures and heavy clothing; frequent washing with cool water may help.
- *Heart palpitations:* If you feel your heart is beating too fast, or skipping beats, sit down for a while and rest. If the feeling becomes too uncomfortable, notify your health care provider.
- *Sensitivity to light:* Avoid glaring lights or wear sunglasses if in bright light. Be careful when moving between extremes of light because your vision may not adjust quickly.
- Report any of the following to your health care provider: *chest pain, difficulty in breathing, dizziness, headache, or changes in vision.*
- Do not stop taking this drug suddenly; make sure you have enough of your prescription. This drug dosage should be reduced gradually over 2 to 4 days when you are instructed to discontinue it by your health care provider.
- Avoid OTC medications, including cold and allergy remedies. If you feel that you need one of these, check with your health care provider first.

They should be used with caution in the presence of CV disease or vasomotor spasm *because these conditions could be aggravated by the vascular effects of the drug*; thyrotoxicosis or diabetes *because of the thyroid-stimulating and glucose-elevating effects of sympathetic stimulation*; lactation *because the drug may be passed to the infant and cause α-specific adrenergic stimulation*; or renal or hepatic impairment *which could interfere with metabolism and excretion of the drug.*

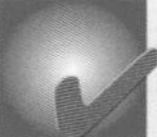

CHECK YOUR UNDERSTANDING

Answers to the questions in this chapter may be found in the answer key in the back of the book.

Multiple Choice

Select the most appropriate response to the following statements:

1. Adrenergic drugs, because of their action in the body, are also called
   a. sympatholytic agents.
   b. cholinergic agents.
   c. sympathomimetic agents.
   d. anticholinergic agents.

2. The adrenergic agent of choice for treating the signs and symptoms of seasonal rhinitis would be
   a. noradrenaline.
   b. phenylephrine
   c. dobutamine.
   d. dopamine.

3. An adrenergic agent that is being used to treat shock is being given intravenously and it infiltrates. The nurse should
   a. watch the area for any signs of necrosis.
   b. notify the physician and decrease the rate of infusion.
   c. remove the intravenous and have phentolamine ready to infuse into the area.
   d. apply ice and elevate the arm.

4. Phenylephrine, an α-agonist, is found in many cold and allergy preparations. Adverse effects that should be watched for would include
   a. urinary retention and pupil constriction.
   b. hypotension and slow heart rate.
   c. cardiac arrhythmias and increased appetite.
   d. cardiac arrhythmias and anxiety and restlessness.

5. Adverse effects associated with adrenergic agents are related to the generalized stimulation of the SNS and could include
   a. slowed heart rate.
   b. constriction of the pupils.
   c. hypertension.
   d. increased GI secretions.

6. A patient has elected to take an OTC cold preparation that contains phenylephrine. The patient should be advised not to take that drug if the patient has
   a. had thyroid or CV disease.
   b. a cough and runny nose.
   c. chronic obstructive pulmonary disease.
   d. has hypotension.

Extended Matching Questions

Select all that apply.

1. A nurse would question the prescription for an adrenergic agonist for a patient who is also receiving which of the following?
   a. anticholinergic drugs
   b. inhalational anaesthetics
   c. β-blockers
   d. benzodiazepines
   e. dopaminergic drugs
   f. TCAs

Definitions

Define the following terms.

1. adrenergic agonist____________________

2. α-agonist____________________

3. β-agonist____________________

4. glycogenolysis____________________

5. sympathomimetic____________________

Bibliography and References

British Medical Association and Royal Pharmaceutical Society of Great Britain (2008). *British National Formulary*. London: BMJ & RPS Publishing. *This publication is updated biannually: it is imperative that the most recent edition is consulted.*

British Medical Association and Royal Pharmaceutical Society of Great Britain (2008). *British National Formulary for Children*. London: BMJ & RPS Publishing. *This publication is updated annually: it is imperative that the most recent edition is consulted.*

Ganong, W. (2005). *Review of Medical Physiology* (22nd ed.). New York: McGraw-Hill.

Howland, R. D., & Mycek, M.J. (2005). *Pharmacology*. (3rd ed.). Philadelphia: Lippincott Williams & Wilkins.

Marieb, E. N., & Hoehn, K. (2004). *Human Anatomy & Physiology* (7th ed.). San Francisco: Pearson Benjamin Cummings.

Porth, C. M., & Matfin G. (2008). *Pathophysiology: Concepts of Altered Health States* (8th ed.). Philadelphia: Lippincott Williams & Wilkins.

Simonsen, T., Aarbakke, J., Kay, I., Coleman, I., Sinnott, P., & Lysaa, R. (2006). *Illustrated Pharmacology for Nurses*. London: Hodder Arnold.

CHAPTER

30

Adrenergic Blocking Agents

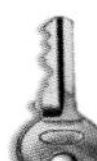

KEY TERMS

adrenergic blocking agents

α_1-selective adrenergic blocking agents

β-adrenergic blocking agents

β_1-selective

bronchodilating effect

specific adrenergic receptor sites

sympatholytic

phaeochromocytoma

LEARNING OBJECTIVES

Upon completion of this chapter, you will be able to:

1. Describe the effects of activating adrenergic receptors and correlate this with the clinical effects of blocking adrenergic receptors.
2. Describe the therapeutic actions, indications, pharmacokinetics and contraindications associated with adrenergic blocking agents.
3. Describe the most common adverse reactions and important drug–drug interactions associated with adrenergic blocking agents.
4. Discuss the use of adrenergic blocking agents across the lifespan.
5. Compare and contrast the key drugs labetalol, phentolamine, doxazosin, propranolol and atenolol with other adrenergic blocking agents.
6. Outline the nursing considerations, including important teaching points, for patients receiving an adrenergic blocking agent.

α- AND β-ADRENERGIC BLOCKING AGENTS

amiodarone
carvedilol
guanethidine
labetalol

α-ADRENERGIC BLOCKING AGENTS

phentolamine
phenoxybenzamine

α_1-SELECTIVE ADRENERGIC BLOCKING AGENTS

alfuzosin
doxazosin
prazosin
tamsulosin
terazosin

β-ADRENERGIC BLOCKING AGENTS

carteolol
nadolol
pindolol
propranolol
sotalol
timolol

β_1-SELECTIVE ADRENERGIC BLOCKING AGENTS

acebutolol
atenolol
betaxolol
bisoprolol
esmolol
metoprolol

Adrenergic blocking agents are also called **sympatholytic** drugs because they inhibit or block the effects of the sympathetic nervous system (SNS). The therapeutic and adverse effects associated with these drugs are related to their ability to react with **specific adrenergic receptor sites** without activating them. By occupying the adrenergic receptor site, they prevent noradrenaline (released from the nerve terminal or from the adrenal medulla) or circulating adrenaline; from activating the receptor, thus blocking the SNS effects.

Adrenergic Blockers

The therapeutic and the adverse effects associated with adrenergic blocking drugs are related to their ability to prevent the signs and symptoms associated with SNS activation.

The adrenergic blockers have varying degrees of specificity for the adrenergic receptor sites. For example, some can interact with all of the adrenergic sites (both α- and β-receptors denoted as α and β, respectively). Some are specific to α-receptors or even to just α_1-receptors. Some adrenergic blockers are specific to both β_1- and β_2-receptors, whereas others interact with just one type of β-receptor, either β_1- or β_2-receptors. This specificity allows the clinician to select a drug that will have the desired therapeutic effects without the undesired side-effects that occur when the entire SNS is blocked. In general, however, the specificity of these drugs depends on the concentration of drug in the body. Most specificity is lost with higher serum drug levels (Figure 30.1).

The effects of the adrenergic blocking agents vary with the age of the patient. (See Box 30.1 for more information.)

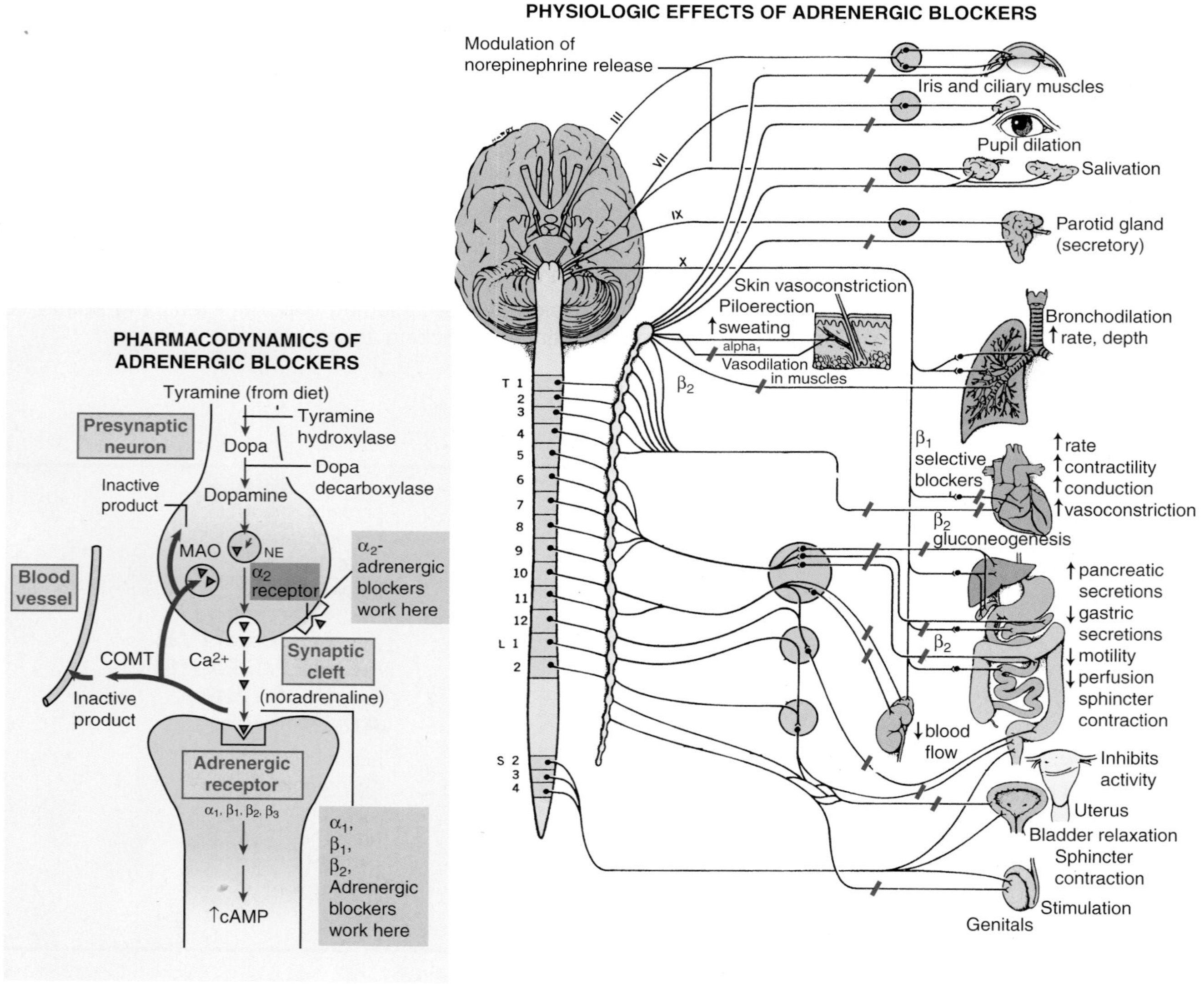

FIGURE 30.1 Site of action of adrenergic blockers and resultant physiologic responses. A bar indicates blocking of the effects indicated by those receptors.

BOX 30.1 DRUG THERAPY ACROSS THE LIFESPAN

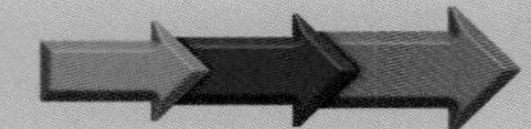

Adrenergic Blocking Agents

CHILDREN

Children are at greater risk of complications associated with the use of adrenergic blocking agents, including bradycardia, difficulty in breathing and changes in glucose metabolism. The safety and efficacy for use of these drugs has not been established for children younger than 18 years of age. If one of these drugs is used, the dosage for these agents needs to be calculated from the child's body weight and age. Two adrenergic blocking agents have established paediatric dosages and they might be the drugs to consider when one is needed: prazosin is used to treat hypertension and phentolamine is used but only for treatment of **phaeochromocytoma**. Children should be carefully monitored and supported during the use of these drugs.

When administering any drug to children, always consult the most recent edition of the British National Formulary (BNF) for Children.

ADULTS

Adults being treated with adrenergic blocking agents should be cautioned about the many adverse effects associated with the drugs. It needs to be emphasized to patients suffering from diabetes mellitus the importance of monitoring their plasma glucose levels because the sympathetic reaction usually alerts patients if they are going hypo or hyperglycaemic. Patients with severe thyroid disease are also at high risk when taking these drugs, as the symptoms of the condition can be masked, the patient should be monitored very closely. Propranolol and metoprolol are associated with more central nervous system (CNS) adverse effects than other adrenergic blockers, for example bronchoconstriction, so these drugs should not be given to patients who have a history of asthma or breathing difficulties.

OLDER ADULTS

Older patients often also have renal or hepatic impairment; therefore, they are more likely to have toxic levels of the drug related to changes in metabolism and excretion. The older patient should be started on lower doses of the drugs and should be monitored very closely for potentially serious arrhythmias or blood pressure changes. Bisoprolol is often a drug of choice for older patients who require an adrenergic blocker for hypertension because it is not associated with as many problems in the elderly and regular dosing profiles can be used.

α- and β-Adrenergic Blocking Agents

Drugs that block all adrenergic receptors are primarily used to treat cardiac-related conditions. **Amiodarone** blocks both α- and β-adrenergic receptors. It is used primarily in the treatment of arrhythmias (see Chapter 45). **Carvedilol** is used as part of combination therapy in the treatment of hypertension and congestive heart failure (CHF). A newer drug, **labetalol** is used intravenously and orally to treat hypertension and can be used with diuretics. Labetalol has also been used to treat hypertension associated with phaeochromocytoma and clonidine withdrawal. It may also be used to treat hypertension during pregnancy.

Therapeutic Actions and Indications

Adrenergic blocking agents competitively block the effects of noradrenaline at α- and β-receptors throughout the SNS. This action prevents the signs and symptoms associated with a sympathetic stress reaction and results in lower blood pressure, slower pulse rate and increased renal perfusion with decreased renin levels. These drugs are indicated to treat essential hypertension and may be used alone or with diuretics.

Pharmacokinetics

These drugs are well absorbed and distributed throughout the body. They are metabolized in the liver and excreted in faeces and urine. The half-life varies with the particular drug and preparation. The adrenergic blockers are not recommended for those under 18 years. There are no well-defined studies on the use of these drugs during pregnancy and lactation, so use should be reserved for those situations in which the benefit to the mother outweighs the potential risk to the neonate.

Contraindications and Cautions

The **α- and β-adrenergic blocking agents** should be used with caution in patients with diabetes because the usual signs and symptoms of hypoglycaemia and hyperglycaemia are lost when the SNS cannot respond. Caution also should be used with patients with a history of asthma or breathing difficulties as use of these drugs could lead to respiratory distress when the bronchodilating actions of noradrenaline actions are blocked (β_2).

These drugs are contraindicated in patients with bradycardia or heart block, which could be worsened by the slowed heart rate and conduction; asthma; shock or CHF and pregnancy or lactation because of the potential adverse effects on the foetus or neonate. There is a potential adrenoceptor blocking effect of some herbal or alternative therapies (see Box 30.2). Patients should be warned of this interaction.

Adverse Effects

The adverse effects associated with the use of α- and β-adrenergic blocking agents are usually associated with the drug's effects on the SNS. These effects can include dizziness, paresthesia, insomnia, depression, fatigue and vertigo, *which are related to the blocked effects of noradrenaline in the*

BOX 30.2 HERBAL AND ALTERNATIVE THERAPIES

Patients who use alternative therapies as part of their daily regimen should be cautioned about potential increased adrenergic blocking effects if the following alternative therapies are combined with adrenergic blocking agents:

- *Ginseng, sage* – increased antihypertensive effects (risk of hypotension and increased CNS effects)
- *Celery, coriander* – lower blood glucose (increased risk of severe hypoglycaemia)
- *Saw palmetto* – increased urinary tract complications

Further information on herbal medicines and complementary medicines can be found at: www.mhra.gov.uk

CNS. Nausea, vomiting, diarrhoea, anorexia and flatulence are *associated with the loss of the balancing sympathetic effect on the gastrointestinal (GI) tract and increased parasympathetic dominance.* Cardiac arrhythmias, hypotension, CHF, pulmonary oedema and cerebrovascular accident, or stroke, are *related to the lack of stimulatory effects and loss of vascular tone in the cardiovascular (CV) system.* Bronchospasm, cough, rhinitis and bronchial obstruction are *related to loss of the* ***bronchodilating effects*** *on the respiratory tract and vasodilation of the mucous membrane vessels.* Other effects reported include decreased exercise tolerance, hypoglycaemia and rash.

Clinically Important Drug–Drug Interactions

There is increased risk of excessive hypotension if any of these drugs are combined with the anaesthetic isoflurane. The effectiveness of diabetic agents is increased, leading to hypoglycaemia when such agents are used with these drugs; patients should be monitored closely and dosage adjustments made as needed. In addition, **carvedilol** has been associated with potentially dangerous conduction system disturbances when combined with **verapamil** or **diltiazem**; if this combination is used, the patient should be monitored continuously.

Always consult a current copy of the BNF for further guidance.

Nursing Considerations for Patients Receiving α- and β-Adrenergic Blocking Agents

Assessment: History and Examination

Screen for the following conditions, *which could be contraindications to use of the drug:* any known allergies to these drugs.

Presence of an underlying condition that could worsen following the administration of β-adrenergic blocking agents:

Bradycardia or heart blocks

Asthma, *by the loss of the bronchodilating effect of noradrenaline*

Shock or CHF, *due to loss of the sympathetic reaction*

Pregnancy or lactation *because of the potential adverse effects on the foetus or neonate*

Diabetes, *by the blocking of the sympathetic response and because the usual signs and symptoms of hypoglycaemia and hyperglycaemia are lost when the SNS cannot respond*

Bronchospasm, *which could progress to respiratory distress and the loss of the bronchodilating actions of noradrenaline.*

Include screening *for baseline status and any potential adverse effects*: skin colour, temperature; pulse, blood pressure, cardiac output, electrocardiogram (ECG); respiration and blood glucose levels and electrolytes.

Establish if the patient is currently taking other medications or herbal therapies which may potentially interact with the α- and β-adrenergic blocking agents.

Nursing Diagnoses

The patient receiving an α- or β-adrenergic blocker may have the following nursing diagnoses related to drug therapy:

- Acute pain related to CV and systemic effects
- Decreased cardiac output related to CV effects
- Ineffective airway clearance related to lack of bronchodilating effects
- Deficient knowledge regarding drug therapy

Implementation With Rationale

- Do not discontinue abruptly after chronic therapy *because hypersensitivity to catecholamines may develop and the patient could have a severe reaction*; reduce drug dose slowly over 2 weeks and monitor patient.
- Consult with the doctor about withdrawing the drug before surgery *because withdrawal is controversial; effects on the sympathetic system after surgery can cause problems.*
- Encourage the patient to adopt lifestyle changes, including diet, exercise, smoking cessation and decreasing stress *to aid in lowering blood pressure.*

- Monitor for postural hypotension and provide safety precautions, if this occurs *to prevent injury to the patient.*
- Monitor for any sign of liver failure *in order to arrange to discontinue the drug if this occurs.* (This effect is more likely to happen with carvedilol).
- Provide thorough patient teaching, including measures to avoid adverse effects, warning signs of problems and the need for monitoring and evaluation *to enhance patient knowledge about drug therapy and to promote compliance.*
- Offer support and encouragement *to help the patient deal with the drug regimen.*

Evaluation

- Monitor patient response to the drug (improvement in blood pressure and CHF).
- Monitor for adverse effects (CV changes, headache, GI upset, bronchospasm, liver failure).
- Evaluate the effectiveness of the teaching plan (patient can name drug, dosage, adverse effects to watch for, specific measures to avoid adverse effects).
- Monitor the effectiveness of comfort measures and compliance with the regimen.

α-Adrenergic Blocking Agents

Phaeochromocytoma is a tumour of the chromaffin cells of the adrenal medulla that periodically releases large amounts of noradrenaline and adrenaline into the circulatory system, resulting in severe hypertension and tachycardia. **Phenoxybenzamine** and **phentolamine** are used to treat **phaeochromocytoma.** Phenoxybenzamine is a powerful α-blocker that is used to manage phaeochromocytoma; unfortunately it has many side-effects. Phentolamine can be used to diagnose phaeochromocytoma and to prevent severe hypertension reactions caused by manipulation of the phaeochromocytoma before and during surgery.

Therapeutic Actions and Indications

Phentolamine and phenoxybenzamine block the postsynaptic α_1-adrenergic receptors, decreasing sympathetic tone in the vasculature and causing vasodilation, which leads to lowering of blood pressure. These drugs also block presynaptic α_2-receptors, preventing the feedback control of noradrenaline release. The result is an increase in the reflex tachycardia that occurs when blood pressure is lowered. This drug is used to diagnose and manage episodes of phaeochromocytoma. This drug is also used to rescue cells injured by noradrenaline or dopamine extravasation; it causes vasodilation and a return of blood flow to the area.

Pharmacokinetics

Phentolamine is rapidly absorbed after injection and is excreted in the urine. There are few data on its metabolism and distribution. Use of phentolamine and phenoxybenzamine during pregnancy or lactation should be reserved for those situations in which the benefit to the mother outweighs any potential risk to the foetus or neonate.

Contraindications and Cautions

The α-adrenergic blocking agents are contraindicated in the presence of coronary artery disease or myocardial infarction (MI) *because of the potential exacerbation of these conditions.*

Adverse Effects

Patients receiving phenoxybenzamine or phentolamine often experience postural hypotension, angina, MI, cerebrovascular accident, flushing, tachycardia and arrhythmia – *all of which are related to vasodilation and decreased blood pressure.* Weakness and dizziness often occur *as a reaction to the hypotension.* Nausea, vomiting and diarrhoea may also occur. Phenoxybenzamine use is associated with nasal congestion, decreased sweating, an inability to ejaculate and idiosyncratic profound hypotension within minutes of an intravenous infusion.

Clinically Important Drug–Drug Interactions

Ephedrine and adrenaline may have decreased hypertensive and vasoconstrictive effects if they are taken alongside phentolamine, because these agents work in opposing ways in the body. Increased hypotension may occur if this drug is combined with alcohol, which is also a vasodilator.

α_1-Selective Adrenergic Blocking Agents

α_1-selective adrenergic blocking agents are drugs that have a specific affinity for α_1-receptors. **Doxazosin** is used to treat hypertension and is also effective in the treatment of benign prostatic hyperplasia (BPH) (see Chapter 52). **Prazosin** alone is used to treat hypertension, or it may be used in combination with other drugs. **Terazosin** is used to treat hypertension as well as BPH (see Chapter 52). **Tamsulosin** and **alfuzosin** *are* used only in the treatment of BPH and are discussed later in the book (see Chapter 52).

Therapeutic Actions and Indications

The therapeutic effects of the α_1-selective adrenergic blocking agents come from their ability to block the postsynaptic α_1-receptor sites. This causes a decrease in vascular tone and vasodilation, which leads to a fall in blood pressure. These drugs do not block the presynaptic α_2-receptor sites; therefore the reflex tachycardia that accompanies a fall in blood pressure does not occur. These drugs can be used to treat BPH or hypertension, alone or as part of a combination therapy.

Pharmacokinetics

The α_1-selective adrenergic blocking agents are well absorbed and undergo extensive hepatic metabolism. *They therefore must be used with caution in patients with hepatic impairment.* They are excreted in the urine.

Contraindications and Cautions

The α_1-selective adrenergic blocking agents are contraindicated with lactation *because the drugs cross into breast milk and could have adverse effects on the neonate.* They should be used cautiously in the presence of CHF or renal failure *because their blood pressure-lowering effects could exacerbate these conditions and* with hepatic impairment, *which may alter the metabolism of these drugs.* Caution also should be used during pregnancy *because of the potential for adverse effects on the foetus.*

Adverse Effects

The adverse effects associated with the use of these drugs *are usually related to their effects of blocking the SNS.* CNS effects include dizziness, weakness, fatigue, drowsiness and depression. Nausea, vomiting, abdominal pain and diarrhoea may occur *as a result of direct effects on the GI tract and sympathetic blocking.* Anticipated CV effects include arrhythmias, hypotension, oedema, CHF and angina. *The vasodilation caused by these drugs can also cause flushing, rhinitis, reddened eyes and nasal congestion.*

Clinically Important Drug–Drug Interactions

Increased hypotensive effects may occur if these drugs are combined with any other vasodilating or antihypertensive drugs.

Always consult the most recent edition of the BNF for more details

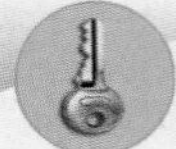

Key Drug Summary: *Doxazosin*

Indications: Treatment of mild-to-moderate hypertension or in combination with other antihypertensives; treatment of BPH.

Actions: Reduces total peripheral resistance through α-receptor blockade; does not affect heart rate or cardiac output; increases high-density lipoproteins while lowering total cholesterol levels.

Pharmacokinetics:

Route	Onset	Peak	Duration
Oral	Varies	2–3 h	Not known

$T_{1/2}$:22 hours, with hepatic metabolism and excretion in the bile, faeces and urine

Adverse effects: Postural hypotension, headache, fatigue, dizziness, vertigo, oedema, nausea, dyspepsia, sleep disturbances, diarrhoea, rhinitis and less frequently; tremor, rash, haematuria, thrombocytopaenia, leucopaenia hepatic jaundice, impotence and urinary incontinence

Nursing Considerations for Patients Receiving α_1-Selective Adrenergic Blocking Agents

Assessment: History and Examination

Screen for the following conditions, *which could be cautions or contraindications to the use of the drug*: presence of any CV diseases, *which may be contraindications to the use of these drugs*; and pregnancy or lactation, *which require caution for drug use.* Include screening *for baseline status and for any potential adverse effects*: assess orientation and reflexes to monitor for CNS changes related to drug therapy; blood pressure, pulse, ECG, peripheral perfusion and cardiac output; and urine output.

Establish if patient is currently taking other medications or herbal therapies which may potentially interact with the α_1-selective adrenergic blocking agents.

Nursing Diagnoses

The patient receiving an α-adrenergic blocking agent may also have the following nursing diagnoses related to drug therapy:

- Risk for injury related to CNS, CV effects of drug

- Decreased cardiac output related to blood pressure changes, arrhythmias, vasodilation
- Deficient knowledge regarding drug therapy

Implementation With Rationale

- Monitor heart rate and blood pressure very carefully *in order to arrange to discontinue the drug if adverse reactions are severe*; provide supportive management if needed.
- Inject phentolamine directly into the area of extravasation of adrenaline or dopamine *to prevent local cell death.*
- Arrange for supportive care and comfort measures, such as rest, environmental control and other measures, *to decrease CNS irritation*; provide headache medication *to alleviate patient discomfort*; arrange safety measures if CNS effects or orthostatic hypotension occur *to prevent patient injury.*
- Provide thorough patient teaching, including dosage, potential adverse effects, measures to avoid adverse effects and warning signs of problems, *to enhance patient knowledge about drug therapy and to promote compliance.*
- Offer support and encouragement *to help the patient deal with the drug regimen.*

Evaluation

- Monitor patient response to the drug (improvement in signs and symptoms of phaeochromocytoma, improvement in tissue condition after extravasation).
- Monitor for adverse effects (orthostatic hypotension, arrhythmias, CNS effects).
- Evaluate the effectiveness of the teaching plan (patient can name drug, dosage, adverse effects to watch for, specific measures to avoid adverse effects).
- Monitor the effectiveness of comfort measures and compliance to the regimen.

β-Adrenergic Blocking Agents

The **β-adrenergic blocking agents** are used to treat CV problems (hypertension, angina, migraine headaches) and to prevent reinfarction after an MI.

Propranolol has been approved for multiple uses, including treatment of hypertension, angina, idiopathic hypertrophic subaortic stenosis (IHSS)-induced palpitations, angina and syncope and certain cardiac arrhythmias induced by catecholamines or digoxin; prevention of reinfarction after MI; treatment of phaeochromocytoma; prophylaxis for migraine headache (which may be caused by vasodilation and is relieved by vasoconstriction); prevention of stage fright (which is a sympathetic stress reaction to a particular situation); and treatment of essential tremors. It is very effective in blocking all of the β-receptors in the SNS and was one of the first drugs of the class.

Since the introduction of propranolol, newer and more selective drugs have become available which are not associated with some of the adverse effects seen with total blockade of the SNS β-receptors. Pindolol is also used for the treatment of hypertension. The drug of choice would depend mostly on personal experience. Nadolol is used to treat hypertension and also for the chronic management of angina. It would be a drug of choice in an angina patient who is also hypertensive. **Sotalol** is reserved for use in the treatment of potentially life-threatening arrhythmias and is not recommended for any other use.

Therapeutic Actions and Indications

The therapeutic effects of these drugs are related to their competitive blocking of the β-adrenergic receptors in the SNS. The blockade of the β-receptors in the heart and in the juxtaglomerular apparatus in the nephron, accounts for most of the therapeutic benefits of these drugs. Decreased heart rate, contractility and excitability, as well as a membrane-stabilizing effect, lead to a decrease in arrhythmias, a decreased cardiac workload and decreased oxygen consumption. The juxtaglomerular cells are not stimulated to release renin, which further decreases the blood pressure. These effects are useful in treating hypertension and chronic angina and can help to prevent reinfarction after an MI by decreasing cardiac workload and oxygen consumption.

- **Propranolol** may be used to prevent 'stage fright', to alleviate situational anxiety by decreasing pulse and blood pressure and decreasing sweating and flushing. The mechanism of action in treating migraines is not clearly understood.
- **Timolol** is used topically to reduce intraocular pressure through its relaxing effects on the eye muscles. It is applied topically therefore it is not usually absorbed systemically from this route.

Pharmacokinetics

These drugs are absorbed from the GI tract and undergo hepatic metabolism. Food has been found to increase the bioavailability of propranolol, although this effect was not found with other β-adrenergic blocking agents (although absorption of **sotalol** is decreased by the presence of food). **Propranolol** also crosses the blood–brain barrier, but

carteolol, nadolol and **sotalol** do not, making them a better choice of drug if CNS effects occur with propranolol. These drugs are excreted in the urine. The use of any β-adrenergic blocker during pregnancy should be reserved for situations in which the benefit to the mother outweighs the risk to the foetus. In general, they should not be used during lactation *because of the potential for adverse effects on the baby.* The safety and efficacy for use of these drugs in children have not been established.

Contraindications and Cautions

β-adrenergic blocking agents are contraindicated with bradycardia or heart blocks, shock, or CHF, *which could be exacerbated by the cardiac-suppressing effects of these drugs*; with bronchospasm, chronic obstructive pulmonary disease (COPD), or acute asthma, *which could be made worse by the blocking of the sympathetic bronchodilation*; with pregnancy *because neonatal apnoea, bradycardia and hypoglycaemia could occur*; and with lactation *because of the potential effects on the neonate, which could include slowed heart rate, hypotension and hypoglycaemia.* These drugs should be used cautiously in patients with diabetes and hypoglycaemia *because of the blocking of the normal signs and symptoms of hypoglycaemia and hyperglycaemia*; with thyrotoxicosis *because of the adrenergic blocking effects on the thyroid gland*; or with hepatic dysfunction, *which could interfere with the metabolism of these drugs.* With propranolol avoid abrupt withdrawal especially in patients with bradycardia or heart block, shock, or CHF.

Adverse Effects

Patients receiving these drugs often experience the following adverse effects: CNS effects include fatigue, dizziness, depression, paresthesia, sleep disturbances, memory loss and disorientation. CV effects can include bradycardia, heart block, CHF, hypotension and peripheral vascular insufficiency. Pulmonary effects can range from difficulty breathing, coughing and bronchospasm to severe pulmonary oedema and bronchial obstruction. GI upset, nausea, vomiting, diarrhoea, gastric pain and even colitis can occur *as a result of unchecked parasympathetic activity and the blocking of the sympathetic receptors.* Genitourinary (GU) effects can include decreased libido, impotence and dysuria. Other effects that can occur include decreased exercise tolerance hypoglycaemia or hyperglycaemia (see Critical Thinking Scenario 30-1).

Clinically Important Drug–Drug Interactions

A paradoxical hypertension occurs when β-blockers are given with clonidine and an increased rebound hypertension with clonidine withdrawal may also occur. It is best to avoid this combination.

A decreased antihypertensive effect occurs when β-blockers are given with nonsteroidal anti-inflammatory drugs (NSAIDs); if this combination is used, the patient should be monitored closely and dosage adjustment should be made to achieve the desired control of blood pressure.

An initial hypertensive episode followed by bradycardia may occur if these drugs are given with adrenaline. Another interaction is the possibility of peripheral ischaemia if the β-blockers are taken in combination with ergot alkaloids.

When these drugs are given with insulin or antidiabetic agents, there is a potential for change in blood glucose levels. The patient also will not display the usual signs and symptoms of hypoglycaemia or hyperglycaemia. If this combination is used, the patient should monitor blood glucose levels frequently throughout the day and should be alert to new warnings about glucose imbalance.

For more interactions always refer to the current edition of the BNF

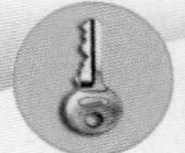

Key Drug Summary: Propranolol

Indications: Treatment of hypertension, angina pectoris, IHSS, supraventricular tachycardia, tremor; prevention of reinfarction after MI; adjunctive therapy in phaeochromocytoma; prophylaxis of migraine headache; management of situational anxiety

Actions: Competitively blocks β-adrenergic receptors in the heart and juxtaglomerular apparatus; reduces vascular tone in the CNS

Pharmacokinetics:

Route	Onset	Peak	Duration
Oral	20–30 min	60–90 min	6–12 h
IV	Immediate	1 min	4–6 h

$T_{1/2}$:3–5 hours with hepatic metabolism and excretion in the urine

Adverse effects: Allergic reaction, bradycardia, CHF, cardiac arrhythmias, cerebrovascular accident, pulmonary oedema, gastric pain, flatulence, impotence, decreased exercise tolerance, bronchospasm

For more interactions always refer to the current edition of the BNF

β_1-Selective Adrenergic Blocking Agents

The therapeutic effects of these drugs are related to their ability to selectively block β_1-receptors in the SNS. This selectivity occurs at therapeutic doses, but the selectivity is lost with doses higher than the recommended range.

Acebutolol is used for treating hypertension and premature ventricular contractions. **Atenolol**, which is more widely used, is prescribed to treat MI (but only within 12 hours of onset of symptoms), chronic angina and hypertension. **Betaxolol** is used to treat hypertension; it is also available as an ophthalmic agent to treat ocular hypertension and open-angle glaucoma. **Bisoprolol** is reserved for use in treating hypertension. **Esmolol** is available as an intravenous agent for the short-term treatment of supraventricular tachycardias, (e.g. atrial flutter, atrial fibrillation) and noncompensatory tachycardia when the heart rate must be slowed. **Metoprolol** is used to treat hypertension and has a modified-release form that only needs to be taken once a day. It is also used to treat angina, to treat stable and symptomatic CHF and to prevent reinfarction after MI. The **β_1-selective** blocker of choice depends on the condition or combination of conditions being treated and personal experience with the drugs.

Therapeutic Actions and Indications

The blockade of the β_1-receptors in the heart and in the juxtaglomerular apparatus accounts for most of the therapeutic benefit of these drugs. Decreased heart rate, contractility, excitability, as well as a membrane-stabilizing effect, lead to a decrease in arrhythmias, decreased cardiac workload and decreased oxygen consumption. The juxtaglomerular cells are not stimulated to release renin, which further decreases blood pressure. These effects are useful in treating hypertension and chronic angina and can help to prevent reinfarction after an MI by decreasing cardiac workload and oxygen consumption. These drugs are used to treat cardiac arrhythmias, hypertension and angina; to prevent reinfarction after MI (again only within first 12 hours after acute MI); and in ophthalmic form, to decrease intraocular pressure and to treat open-angle glaucoma. Metoprolol is also approved in the extended-release form for the treatment of stable, symptomatic CHF.

β-blockers including the cardioselective drugs should NOT be given to any patient with a history of asthma or breathing difficulties. If there is no other alternative then these drugs should be given with extreme care under supervision.

Pharmacokinetics

The β_1-selective adrenergic blockers are absorbed from the GI tract. The bioavailability of metoprolol is increased if it is taken in the presence of food. Like the other β-blockers, these drugs are metabolized in the liver and excreted in the urine. Metoprolol readily crosses the blood–brain barrier and may cause more CNS effects than acebutolol and atenolol, which do not cross. These drugs should not be used during pregnancy and lactation unless the benefit to the mother outweighs the potential risk to the foetus or neonate.

Contraindications and Cautions

The β_1-selective adrenergic blockers are contraindicated with sinus bradycardia, heart block, cardiogenic shock, CHF, or hypotension, *all of which could be exacerbated by the cardiac-depressing and blood pressure-lowering effects of these drugs*; and with lactation *because of the potential adverse effects on the neonate*. They should be used with caution in patients with diabetes, thyroid disease, or COPD *because of the potential for adverse effects on these diseases with sympathetic blockade*; and in pregnancy *because of the potential for adverse effects on the foetus.*

Adverse Effects

Patients receiving these drugs often experience adverse effects related to the blocking of β_1-receptors in the SNS. CNS effects include fatigue, dizziness, depression, paresthesia, sleep disturbances, memory loss and disorientation. CV effects can include bradycardia, heart block, CHF, hypotension and peripheral vascular insufficiency. Pulmonary effects ranging from rhinitis to bronchospasm and dyspnoea can occur; these effects are less likely to occur with these drugs when compared with the nonselective β-blockers. GI upset, nausea, vomiting, diarrhoea, gastric pain and even colitis can occur as a result of excessive parasympathetic activity and the blocking of the sympathetic receptors. GU effects can include decreased libido, impotence and dysuria. Other effects that can occur include decreased exercise tolerance, hypoglycaemia or hyperglycaemia and liver changes that are reflected in increased concentrations of liver enzymes.

Clinically Important Drug–Drug Interactions

A decreased hypertensive effect occurs if these drugs are given with clonidine, NSAIDs, rifampin, or barbiturates. If such a combination is used, the patient should be monitored closely and dosage adjustment made.

There is an initial hypertensive episode followed by bradycardia if these drugs are given with adrenaline. An increased risk for postural hypotension occurs if these drugs are taken with prazosin. If this combination is used, the patient must be monitored closely and safety precautions taken.

The selective β_1-blockers have increased hypotensive effects if they are taken with verapamil, cimetidine, or propylthiouracil. The patient should be monitored closely and appropriate dosage adjustment made.

Always consult a current copy of the BNF for further guidance.

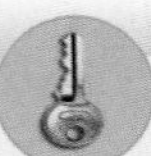

Key Drug Summary: *Atenolol*

Indications: Treatment of angina pectoris, hypertension, MI; unlabelled uses – prevention of migraine headaches, alcohol withdrawal syndrome, supraventricular tachycardias

Actions: Blocks β_1-adrenergic receptors, decreasing the excitability of the heart, cardiac output and oxygen consumption; decreases renin release, which lowers blood pressure

Pharmacokinetics:

Route	Onset	Peak	Duration
Oral	Varies	2–4 h	24 h
IV	Immediate	5 min	24 h

$T_{1/2}$: 6–7 hours, with excretion in the bile, faeces and urine

Adverse effects: Allergic reaction, dizziness, bradycardia, CHF, arrhythmias, gastric pain, flatulence, impotence, bronchospasm, decreased exercise tolerance, fatigue and coldness of the extremities

For more interactions always refer to the current edition of the BNF

Nursing Considerations for Patients receiving β_1-Selective Adrenergic Blocking Agents

Assessment: History and Examination

Screen for the following conditions, *which could be cautions or contraindications to the use of the drug*: bradycardia or heart blocks, shock, or CHF, *which could be exacerbated by the cardiac-suppressing effects of these drugs*; bronchospasm or COPD; pregnancy or lactation *because of the potential effects on the foetus or neonate*; diabetes or hypoglycaemia; and thyrotoxicosis.

Include screening *for baseline status and for any potential adverse effects*: skin colour, temperature; pulse, blood pressure, ECG; respiration, adventitious sounds; abdominal examination, urine output and electrolytes. Establish if patient is currently taking other medications or herbal therapies, which may potentially interact with the β_1-selective adrenergic blocking agents.

Nursing Diagnoses

The patient receiving β_1-adrenergic blockers may have the following nursing diagnoses related to drug therapy:

- Acute pain related to CNS, GI and systemic effects
- Decreased cardiac output related to CV effects
- Ineffective tissue perfusion related to CV effects
- Deficient knowledge regarding drug therapy

Implementation With Rationale

- Do not stop these drugs abruptly after chronic therapy but taper gradually over 2 weeks *to prevent the possibility of severe reactions.* Long-term use of these drugs can sensitize the myocardium to catecholamines and *severe reactions could occur.*
- Consult with the physician about discontinuing these drugs before surgery *because withdrawal of the drug before surgery when the patient has been maintained on the drug is controversial.*
- Give oral forms of the drug with food *to facilitate absorption.*
- Continuously monitor any patient receiving an intravenous form of these drugs *to detect severe reactions to sympathetic blockade and to ensure rapid response if these reactions occur.*
- Arrange for supportive care and comfort measures, including rest, environmental control and other measures, *to relieve CNS effects*; safety measures if CNS effects occur *to protect the patient from injury*; and small, frequent meals and mouth care *to relieve the discomfort of GI effects.*
- Provide thorough patient teaching, including the name of the drug, dosage, anticipated adverse effects, measures to avoid drug-related problems and warning signs of problems, as well as proper administration, as needed *to enhance patient knowledge about drug therapy and to promote compliance.*
- Offer support and encouragement *to help the patient deal with the drug regimen.*

Evaluation

- Monitor patient response to the drug (lowered blood pressure, fewer episodes of angina, lowered intraocular pressure).
- Monitor for adverse effects (GI upset, CNS changes, CV effects, loss of libido and impotence, potential respiratory effects).
- Evaluate the effectiveness of the teaching plan (patient can name drug, dosage, adverse effects to watch for, specific measures to avoid adverse effects).
- Monitor the effectiveness of comfort measures and compliance with the regimen.

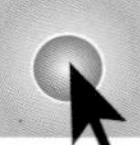

WEB LINKS

Health care providers and patients may want to consult the following Internet sources:

http://cks.library.nhs.uk The National Health Service Clinical Knowledge Summaries provides evidence-based practical information on the common conditions observed in primary care.

www.mhra.gov.uk The MHRA regulates a wide range of materials from medicines and medical devices to blood and therapeutic products/services that are derived from tissue engineering.

http://www.bnf.org.uk The BNF provides UK health care professionals with authoritative and practical information on the selection and clinical use of medicines.

http://www.bhf.org Patient information, support groups, diet, exercise and research information on hypertension and other CV diseases.

http://www.nhsdirect.nhs.uk The National Health Service Direct service provides patients with information and advice about health, illness and health services.

http://pmj.bmj.com/cgi/content/abstract Use of diuretics in CV diseases: (1) heart failure

http://www.nice.org.uk National Institute for Health and Clinical Excellence is an independent organization responsible for providing national guidance on promoting good health and preventing and treating ill health.

Points to Remember

- Adrenergic blocking agents or sympatholytic drugs block the effects of the SNS.
- Both the therapeutic and the adverse effects associated with these drugs are related to their blocking of the normal responses of the SNS.
- The α- and β-adrenergic blocking agents block all of the receptor sites within the SNS, which results in lower blood pressure, slower pulse and increased renal perfusion with decreased renin levels. These drugs are indicated for the treatment of essential hypertension. They are associated with many adverse effects, including lack of bronchodilation, cardiac suppression and diabetic reactions.
- Selective adrenergic blocking agents have been developed that, at therapeutic levels, have specific affinity for α- or β-receptors or for specific α_1-, β_1-, or β_2-receptor sites. This specificity is lost at levels higher than the therapeutic range.
- α-adrenergic drugs specifically block α-receptors of the SNS. At therapeutic levels, they do not block β-receptors.
- Nonselective α-adrenergic blocking agents are used to treat phaeochromocytoma, a tumour of the adrenal medulla.
- α_1-selective adrenergic blocking agents block the postsynaptic α_1-receptor sites, causing a decrease in vascular tone and a vasodilation that leads to a fall in blood pressure without the reflex tachycardia that occurs when the presynaptic α_2-receptor sites are also blocked.
- β-blockers are drugs used to block the β-receptors within the SNS. These drugs are used for a wide range of problems, including hypertension, situational anxiety, migraines, angina and essential tremors.
- Blockade of all β-receptors results in a loss of the reflex bronchodilation that occurs with sympathetic stimulation. This limits the use of these drugs in patients who smoke or have allergic or seasonal rhinitis, asthma or COPD.
- β_1-selective adrenergic blocking agents do not block the β_1-receptors that are responsible for bronchodilation and therefore are preferred in patients with respiratory problems.

CRITICAL THINKING SCENARIO 30-1

Nonselective β-Blockers (Propranolol)

The Situation

Ben a 59-year-old man had a MI last August. He recovered well and returned to his job as a salesman within 8 weeks. Shortly after he resumed working, he began to suffer vague, pressure-type chest pains. His cardiologist prescribed propranolol 10 mg QDS. Ben had no further problems until the following June, when he developed acute respiratory distress whilst resting at home. On the way to A&E he suffered an apparent respiratory arrest. He was admitted to the hospital and observed in the high dependency unit. It was found that Ben had a history of hayfever and allergic rhinitis during the pollen season but that he had never experienced such a severe reaction.

Critical Thinking

Why did Ben have such a severe reaction? What appropriate measures should be taken to ensure that Ben recovers fully and this episode does not reoccur?

What sort of support will Ben need after going through such a frightening experience?

Ben *has been taking propranolol for several months and needs to be weaned from it because the drug is somewhat responsible for the reaction that he experienced.*

What kind of teaching programme will need to be developed to help Ben deal with his medication, their effects and his underlying cardiac problem?

Discussion

Propranolol, a nonselective β-blocker, was prescribed for Ben to decrease the workload and oxygen consumption of the heart and to prevent another MI. He did well on the drug until the pollen season arrived. That is because propranolol, a nonselective β-blocker, prevented the compensatory bronchodilation that occurs when the SNS is stimulated. When the pollen reacted with Ben's airways, causing them to swell and become narrower, his swollen bronchial tubes were unable to allow air to flow through them. The result was bronchial constriction and respiratory distress that, in Ben's case, progressed to a respiratory arrest. Before he began taking propranolol, Ben had probably been effectively compensating for the swelling of the bronchi/bronchioles through bronchodilation and had never experienced such a reaction. Ben needs to be weaned of propranolol over a period of time. He should then be started on a specific β-adrenergic blocker, which should decrease cardiac workload without interfering with reflex bronchodilation.

A full teaching programme, including information on Ben's heart disease and details about his new specific β-adrenergic blocker, should be undertaken. Ben should receive written information about the drug, including warning signs to watch for and adverse effects that may occur.

Nursing Care Guide for Ben: Propranolol

Assessment: History and Examination

Review the patient's history for allergy to propranolol, CHF, shock, bradycardia, heart block, hypotension, COPD, thyroid disease, diabetes, respiratory impairment, concurrent use of: barbiturates, NSAIDs, piroxicam, lignocaine, cimetidine, phenothiazines, clonidine, theophylline and rifampin.

Focus the physical examination on the following:

CV: blood pressure, pulse, peripheral perfusion, ECG

CNS: orientation, reflexes, vision

Skin: colour, lesions, texture

GU: urinary output, sexual function

GI: abdominal, liver evaluation

Respiratory: respirations, adventitious sounds

Nursing Diagnoses

Decreased cardiac output related to CV effects

Acute pain related to CNS, GI, systematic effects

Impaired tissue perfusion, related to CV effects

Deficient knowledge regarding drug therapy

Implementation

Ensure safe and appropriate administration of drug.

Provide comfort and safety measures: temperature control; rest periods; small, frequent meals.

Monitor blood pressure, pulse and respiratory status throughout drug therapy.

Provide support and reassurance to deal with drug effects and discomfort, sexual dysfunction and fatigue.

Provide patient teaching regarding drug name, dosage, side-effects, precautions and warning signs to report.

Evaluation

Evaluate drug effects: blood pressure within normal limit, decrease in episodes of angina, stabilized cardiac rhythm.

Nonselective β-Blockers (Propranolol) *(continued)*

Monitor for adverse effects: CV effects: CHF; dizziness, confusion; sexual dysfunction; GI effects; hypoglycaemia; respiratory problems.

Monitor for drug–drug interactions as indicated.

Evaluate effectiveness of patient education programme

Evaluate effectiveness of comfort and safety measures.

Patient Education for Ben

- The drug that has been prescribed for you, propranolol, is a β-adrenergic blocking agent. A β-adrenergic blocking agent works to prevent certain stimulating activities that normally occur in the body in response to such factors as stress, injury, or excitement. You should learn to take your own pulse and monitor it daily. Your current pulse rate is 82 bpm.
- Never suddenly stop taking this medication. If you find that your prescription is running low, notify your general practitioner at once. This drug needs to be reduced over time to prevent severe reactions when its use is discontinued. Some of the following adverse effects may occur: *tiredness, weakness*: Try to stagger your activities throughout the day to allow rest periods. *Dizziness, drowsiness*: If these should occur, take care to avoid driving, operating dangerous machinery, or doing delicate tasks. Change position slowly to avoid dizzy spells.
- *Change in sexual function*: Be assured that this is a drug effect and discuss it with your health care provider.
- *Nausea, diarrhoea*: These GI discomforts often diminish with time. If they become too uncomfortable or do not improve, talk to your health care provider.
- Report any of the following to your health care provider: very slow pulse, difficulty breathing, swelling in the ankles or fingers, sudden weight gain, mental confusion or personality change, fever or rash.
- Avoid over-the-counter medications, including cold and allergy remedies. Many of these preparations contain drugs that could interfere with this medication. If you feel that you need one of these, check with your health care provider first.
- Tell any doctor, nurse, or other health care provider that you are taking these drugs, keep all medications out of the reach of children and do not share these drugs with other people.

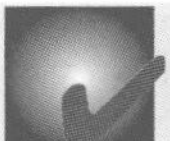

CHECK YOUR UNDERSTANDING

Answers to the questions in this chapter may be found in the answer key in the back of the book.

Multiple Choice

Select the most appropriate response to the following.

1. Adrenergic blocking drugs, because of their clinical effects, are also known as
   a. anticholinergics.
   b. sympathomimetic.
   c. parasympatholytics.
   d. sympatholytics.

2. You might give drugs that generally block all adrenergic receptor sites to treat
   a. signs and symptoms of allergic rhinitis.
   b. COPD.
   c. cardiac-related conditions.
   d. premature labour.

3. Phentolamine an α-adrenergic blocker, is most frequently used
   a. to prevent cell death after extravasation of intravenous dopamine or noradrenaline.
   b. to treat COPD.
   c. to treat hypertension.
   d. to block bronchoconstriction during acute asthma attacks.

4. You might administer an α_1-selective adrenergic blocking agent in the treatment of
   a. COPD.
   b. hypertension and BPH.
   c. erectile dysfunction.
   d. shock states and bronchospasm.

5. The β-blocker of choice for a patient who is hypertensive and has angina would be
   a. nadolol.
   b. pindolol.
   c. timolol.
   d. carteolol.

6. You would question an order for β_1-selective adrenergic blockers in the treatment of
   a. cardiac arrhythmias.
   b. hypertension.
   c. cardiogenic shock.
   d. open-angle glaucoma.

7. A smoker who is being treated for hypertension with a β-blocker should be treated with a
   a. nonselective β-blocker.
   b. β_2-specific β-blocker.
   c. β- and α-blockers.
   d. β_1-specific blocker.

8. You would caution a patient who is taking an adrenergic blocker
   a. to avoid exposure to infection.
   b. to stop the drug if he/she experiences flu-like symptoms.
   c. never to stop the drug abruptly because it needs to be tapered slowly.
   d. to avoid exposure to the sun.

Multiple Response

Select all that apply.

1. A nurse would question an order for a β-adrenergic blocker if the patient was also receiving what other drugs?
   a. Clonidine
   b. Salbutamol
   c. Aspirin
   d. NSAIDs
   e. Triptans
   f. Adrenaline

2. The β-adrenergic blocker propranolol is approved for a wide variety of uses. Which of the following would be approved indications?
   a. Migraine headaches
   b. Stage fright or situational anxiety
   c. Bronchospasm
   d. Reinfarction after an MI
   e. Erectile dysfunction
   f. Hypertension

True or False

Indicate whether the following statements are true (T) or false (F).

_____1. Adrenergic blocking agents are also called sympathomimetic drugs.

_____2. Drugs that block all adrenergic receptors are primarily used to treat cardiac-related conditions.

_____3. Adrenergic blocking agents competitively block the effects of noradrenaline at both α- and β-receptors throughout the SNS, causing the signs and symptoms associated with a sympathetic stress reaction.

_____4. The adverse effects associated with adrenergic blocking agents of cardiac arrhythmias, hypotension, CHF, pulmonary oedema, cerebral vascular accident, or stroke are related to the lack of stimulatory effects and loss of vascular tone in the CV system.

_____5. The therapeutic effects of α_1-selective adrenergic blocking agents come from their ability to block the postsynaptic α_1-receptor sites. This causes a decrease in vascular tone and vasodilation, which leads to a fall in blood pressure.

_____6. The β-adrenergic blocking agents are used to treat asthma and obstructive pulmonary diseases.

_____7. Propranolol is a widely prescribed drug that has been used to treat migraine headaches and stage fright (situational anxiety).

_____8. β-adrenergic blocking agents should not be stopped abruptly after chronic therapy but should be tapered gradually over 2 weeks.

Bibliography

British Medical Association and Royal Pharmaceutical Society of Great Britain. (2008). *British National Formulary*. London: BMJ & RPS Publishing. *This publication is updated biannually: it is imperative that the most recent edition is consulted.*

British Medical Association and Royal Pharmaceutical Society of Great Britain. (2008). *British National Formulary for Children*. London: BMJ & RPS Publishing. *This publication is updated annually: it is imperative that the most recent edition is consulted.*

Ganong, W. (2005). *Review of medical physiology* (22nd ed.). New York: McGraw-Hill.

Howland, R. D., & Mycek, M. J. (2005). *Pharmacology* (3rd ed.). Philadelphia: Lippincott Williams & Wilkins.

Marieb, E. N., & Hoehn, K. (2004). *Human anatomy & physiology* (7th ed.). San Francisco: Pearson Benjamin Cummings.

Porth, C. M., & Matfin G. (2008). *Pathophysiology: Concepts of altered health states* (8th ed.). Philadelphia: Lippincott Williams & Wilkins.

Simonsen, T., Aarbakke, J., Kay, I., Coleman, I., Sinnott, P., & Lysaa, R. (2006). *Illustrated pharmacology for nurses*. London: Hodder Arnold

CHAPTER 31

Cholinergic Agents

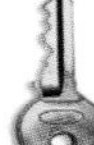

KEY TERMS

acetylcholinesterase
Alzheimer's disease
cholinergic
miosis
myasthenia gravis
nerve gas
parasympathomimetic

LEARNING OBJECTIVES

Upon completion of this chapter, you will be able to:

1. Describe the effects of cholinergic receptors and correlate these with the clinical effects of cholinergic drugs.
2. Describe the therapeutic actions, indications, pharmacokinetics associated with the direct- and indirect-acting cholinergic drugs.
3. Describe the contraindications, most common adverse reactions and important drug–drug interactions associated with the direct- and indirect-acting cholinergic drugs.
4. Discuss the use of cholinergic agents across the lifespan.
5. Compare and contrast the key drugs pilocarpine, rivastigmine and pyridostigmine with other cholinergic agents.
6. Outline the nursing considerations, including important education points, for patients receiving a cholinergic agent.

DIRECT-ACTING CHOLINERGIC DRUGS

bethanechol
pilocarpine

INDIRECT-ACTING CHOLINERGIC DRUGS

donepezil
distigmine
edrophonium
galantamine
neostigmine
pyridostigmine
rivastigmine

REVERSING AGENT

pralidoxime

Cholinergic drugs are chemicals that act at the same site as the neurotransmitter acetylcholine (ACh). These sites are found extensively throughout the parasympathetic nervous system, and therefore, stimulation of these sites produces a response similar to what is seen when the parasympathetic nervous system is activated. As a result, these drugs are often called **parasympathomimetic** drugs. The action of these drugs cannot be limited to a specific site: their effects can be widespread throughout the body and are usually associated with undesirable systemic effects.

Cholinergic Drugs

Cholinergic drugs increase the activity of ACh receptor sites throughout the body either directly or indirectly. Direct-acting cholinergic drugs occupy ACh receptor sites on effector cells of the postganglionic cholinergic nerves, causing increased stimulation of the ACh receptor. In contrast, indirect-acting cholinergic drugs inhibit the enzyme **acetylcholinesterase** to prevent the breakdown of ACh released from the nerve. These drugs produce their effects indirectly by increasing the level of ACh in the synaptic cleft, leading to increased stimulation of the cholinergic receptor site (Figure 31.1). The effects of these drugs differ across the lifespan, as discussed in Box 31.1.

Direct-acting Cholinergic Drugs

The direct-acting cholinergic drugs are similar to ACh and bind directly with receptor sites to cause the same reaction as ACh. These drugs tend to cause stimulation of the muscarinic receptors within the parasympathetic nervous system. This class of drugs is used systemically to increase bladder tone, urinary excretion and gastrointestinal (GI) secretions and topically as ophthalmic agents. However, the widespread parasympathetic activity of these drugs now means that their use today is infrequent; the more specific and less toxic drugs now available are preferred.

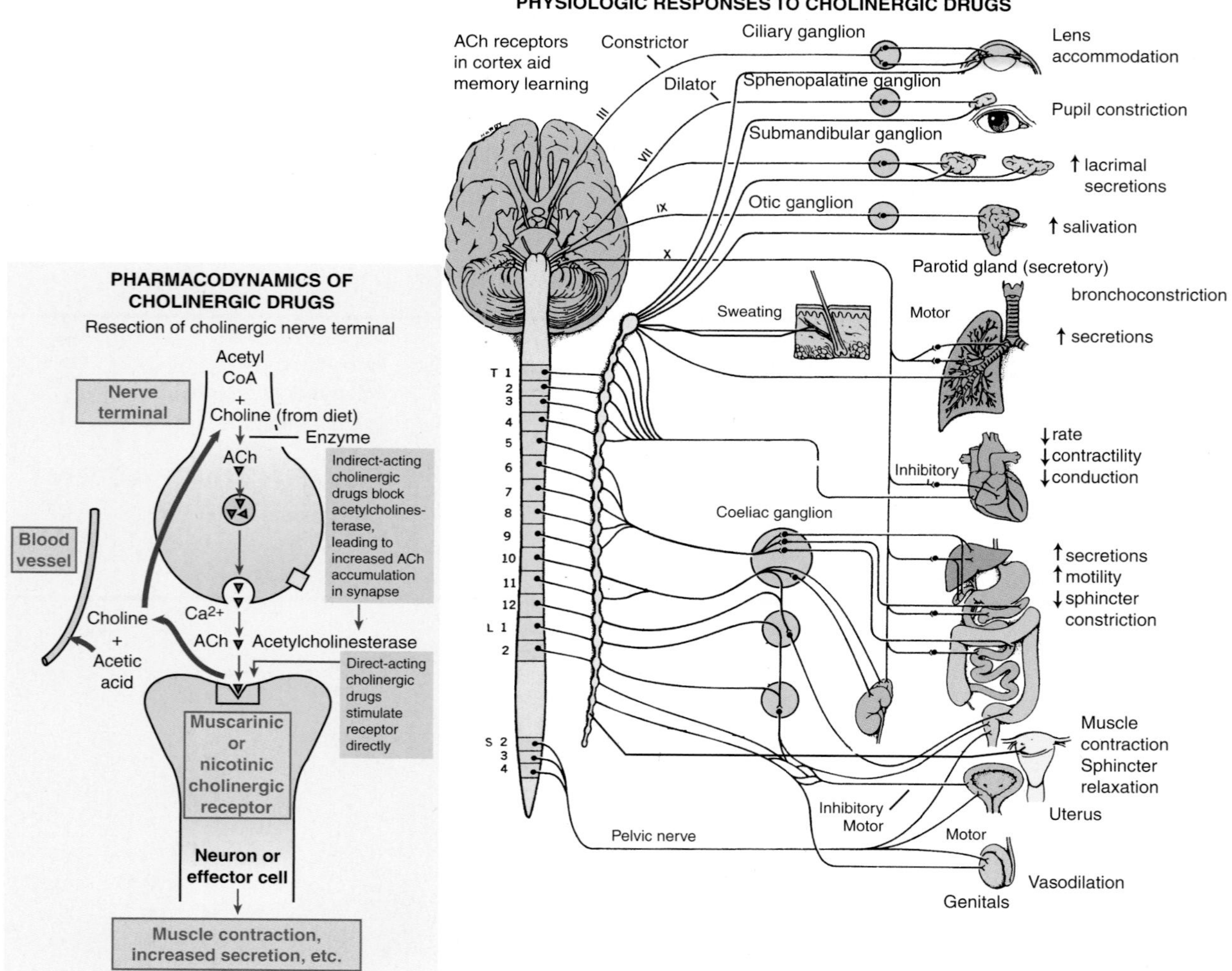

FIGURE 31.1 Pharmacodynamics of cholinergic drugs and associated physiologic responses.

BOX 31.1 **DRUG THERAPY ACROSS THE LIFESPAN**

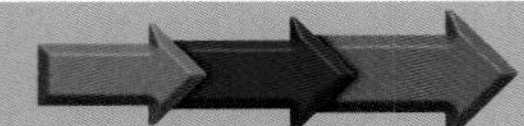

Cholinergic Agents

CHILDREN

Children may be more susceptible to the adverse effects associated with cholinergic drugs, including GI upset and diarrhoea, or increased salivation, which could lead to loss of bowel and bladder control and choking respectively, a problem that could cause stress in the child. Children should be monitored closely if these agents are used and should receive appropriate supportive care.

In children, the preferred approach to treating urinary retention is through catheterization. The systemic use of pilocarpine is not recommended in children. Distigmine, neostigmine and pyridostigmine are used in the control of myasthenia gravis, and neostigmine can also be used to reverse the effects of muscle relaxants used during surgery. Care should be taken in determining the appropriate dose based on weight. Edrophonium is used for the diagnosis of myasthenia gravis only.

When administering any drug to children, always consult the most recent edition of the British National Formulary for Children.

ADULTS

Adults should be cautioned about the many adverse effects that can be anticipated when using a cholinergic agent. Flushing, increased sweating, increased salivation, GI upset and urinary urgency occur frequently. The patient also needs to be aware that dizziness, drowsiness and blurred vision may occur and that driving and operating dangerous machinery should be avoided.

In general, there are no adequate studies about the effects of these drugs during pregnancy and lactation. Therefore, the cholinergic agents should be used only in those situations in which the benefit to the mother is greater than the risk to the foetus or neonate. Nursing mothers who require one of these drugs may be advised to find another way to feed the baby.

OLDER ADULTS

Older patients are more likely to experience the adverse effects associated with these drugs: central nervous system (CNS), cardiovascular, GI, respiratory and urinary. As many older patients often have renal or hepatic impairment, they are also more likely to reach toxic levels of the drug related to changes in drug metabolism and excretion.

The older patient should be started on lower doses of the drugs and should be monitored very closely for potentially serious arrhythmias or hypotension. Safety precautions should be established if the drug causes dizziness or drowsiness. Special efforts may also be needed to help the patient maintain fluid intake and nutrition if the GI effects become uncomfortable. Taking the drug with food and offering the patient several small meals throughout the day may alleviate some of these problems.

Therapeutic Actions and Indications

The direct-acting cholinergic drugs act at cholinergic receptors in the peripheral nervous system to mimic the effects of ACh and parasympathetic stimulation. These parasympathetic effects include slowed heart rate and decreased myocardial contractility, vasodilation, bronchoconstriction and increased secretions from bronchial mucous membranes, increased GI activity and secretions, increase in bladder tone, relaxation of GI and bladder sphincters and pupil constriction (see Figure 31.1).

Bethanechol has an affinity for the cholinergic receptors in the urinary bladder and increases the tone of the detrusor muscle of the bladder and relaxes the bladder sphincter to improve bladder emptying. Available for use orally, bethanechol can be used to treat nonobstructive postoperative and postpartum urinary retention by directly increasing muscle tone and relaxing the sphincters. However, the current preferred treatment is bladder catheterization. As bethanechol is not destroyed by acetylcholinesterase, the effects of this drug on the receptor site are of longer duration than that with stimulation by ACh.

Pilocarpine is available for topical use as an ophthalmic agent to induce **miosis**, or pupil constriction, to relieve the increased intraocular pressure of glaucoma and to allow surgeons to perform certain surgical procedures. When used topically, pilocarpine is not generally absorbed systemically and therefore not associated with severe adverse effects. Pilocarpine can also be used systemically to treat the dry mouth (xerostomia) associated with irradiation treatment of head and neck cancer and also the xerostomia and dry eyes (xerophthalmia) associated with Sjögren's syndrome.

Pharmacokinetics

The direct-acting cholinergic drugs are generally well absorbed and have relatively short half-lives, ranging from 1 to 6 hours. The metabolism and excretion of these drugs are not known but are believed to occur at the synaptic level and possibly in plasma (pilocarpine).

Contraindications and Cautions

These drugs are used sparingly *because of the potential undesirable systemic effects of parasympathetic stimulation.* They are contraindicated in the presence of any condition that would be exacerbated by parasympathetic effects, for example bradycardia, hypotension, vasomotor instability and cardiovascular disease *could be made worse by the cardiac- and cardiovascular-suppressing effects of the parasympathetic system.* Asthma and chronic obstructive pulmonary disorder *could be exacerbated by the increased parasympathetic effect, overriding the protective sympathetic bronchodilation.* Peptic ulcer, intestinal obstruction or recent GI surgery *could be negatively affected by the GI-stimulating effects of the peripheral nervous system.* Bladder obstruction or healing sites from recent bladder surgery *could be aggravated by the stimulatory effects on the bladder*. Epilepsy and parkinsonism symptoms could be affected by stimulation of ACh receptors in the brain. There is potential for serious adverse effects to the foetus and neonate with both bethanechol and pilocarpine, and therefore both drugs should be avoided during pregnancy and lactation.

Always consult a current copy of the British National Formulary for further guidance.

Adverse Effects

Patients should be cautioned about the potential adverse effects of these drugs. Even if the drug is being given as a topical ophthalmic agent, there is always a possibility that it will have systemic effects. The adverse effects associated with these drugs are related to increased parasympathetic activation. GI effects can include nausea, vomiting, cramps, diarrhoea, increased salivation and involuntary defaecation related to the increase in GI secretions and activity. Cardiovascular effects can include bradycardia, palpitations and hypotension related to the cardiac-suppressing effects of the PNS. Urinary tract effects can include a sense of urgency related to the stimulation of the bladder muscles and sphincter relaxation. Other effects may include flushing and increased sweating secondary to stimulation of the cholinergic receptors in the sympathetic nervous system. It is important that patients are monitored for dehydration, bradycardia and discomfort associated with increased GI activity.

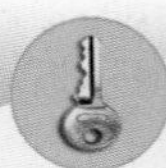

Key Drug Summary: *Pilocarpine*

Indications: Management of raised intraocular pressure; xerostomia (dry mouth) following irradiation therapy and xerostomia and xerophthalmia (dry eyes) associated with Sjögren's syndrome

Actions: Acts directly on cholinergic receptors to mimic the effects of ACh, constricts pupil and stimulates saliva production and lacrimation

Pharmacokinetics:

Route	Onset	Peak	Duration
Topical	5–10 min	20–30 min	6–8 h
Oral	30–90 min	60–90 min	1–6 h

$T_{1/2}$: Metabolism and excretion unknown; thought to be synaptic

Adverse effects: When used systemically, dyspepsia, diarrhoea, abdominal pain, nausea, vomiting, constipation, flushing, hypertension, palpitations, headache, dizziness, sweating and increased urinary frequency

Nursing Considerations for Patients Receiving Direct-acting Cholinergic Drugs

Assessment: History and Examination

Screen for the following conditions, *which could be cautions or contraindications to use of the drug: known allergies to these drugs*; bradycardia, vasomotor instability, peptic ulcer, obstructive urinary or GI diseases; recent GI or genitourinary surgery; asthma; parkinsonism or epilepsy and pregnancy or lactation, *all of which could be exacerbated or complicated by parasympathetic stimulation.* Establish if patient is currently taking other medications or herbal therapies which may potentially interact with the cholinergic drug.

Include screening *for baseline status before beginning therapy and for any potential adverse effects*: skin colour, lesions, temperature; pulse, blood pressure, electrocardiogram (ECG); respiration, adventitious sounds; and urine output and bladder tone (e.g. any patient observed changes in bladder activity – frequency of urination; colour, smell or amount of urine).

Nursing Diagnoses

The patient receiving a direct-acting cholinergic agonist may have the following nursing diagnoses related to drug therapy:

- Acute pain related to GI effects
- Decreased cardiac output related to cardiovascular effects related to blood pressure changes, arrhythmias, vasodilation
- Impaired urinary elimination related to effects on the bladder
- Deficient knowledge regarding drug therapy

Implementation With Rationale

- Ensure proper administration of ophthalmic preparations *to increase effectiveness of drug therapy.*
- Administer oral drug on an empty stomach *to decrease nausea and vomiting.*
- Monitor patient response closely, including blood pressure, ECG, urine output and cardiac output, and *arrange to adjust dosage accordingly to ensure the most benefit with the least amount of toxicity.* Maintain atropine on standby *to reverse overdose or counteract severe reactions.*
- Provide safety precautions if the patient reports poor visual acuity in dim light *to prevent injury.*
- Provide thorough patient education, including measures to avoid adverse effects and warning signs of problems as well as the need for monitoring and

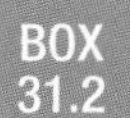

evaluation *to enhance patient knowledge about drug therapy and to promote concordance.*

- Offer support and encouragement *to help the patient deal with the drug regimen.*

Evaluation

- Monitor patient response to the drug (improvement in bladder function, miosis).
- Monitor for adverse effects (cardiovascular changes, GI stimulation, urinary urgency, respiratory distress).
- Evaluate the effectiveness of the education plan (patient can name drug, dosage, adverse effects to watch for, specific measures to avoid adverse effects, proper administration of ophthalmic drugs).
- Monitor the effectiveness of comfort and safety measures and compliance with the regimen.

Indirect-acting Cholinergic Drugs

The indirect-acting cholinergic drugs react chemically with acetylcholinesterase (the enzyme responsible for the breakdown of ACh) in the synaptic cleft to prevent the enzyme from breaking down ACh. As a result, the ACh that is released from the presynaptic neuron remains in the area and accumulates, stimulating the ACh receptors. These drugs work on all ACh receptors throughout the nervous system and at the neuromuscular junction (NMJ). Most of these drugs bind reversibly to acetylcholinesterase, so their effects will pass with time. However, certain cholinergic drugs are irreversible acetylcholinesterase-inhibiting agents and require special considerations (see Boxes 31.2 and 31.3). The indirect-acting cholinergic agents fall into two main categories: (1) agents used to treat myasthenia gravis and (2) newer agents used to treat Alzheimer's disease.

Myasthenia Gravis Drugs

Myasthenia gravis is a chronic muscular disease caused by a defect in neuromuscular transmission. It is an autoimmune disease in which antibodies are produced to the nicotinic ACh receptors at the NMJ. These antibodies cause gradual destruction of the nicotinic ACh receptors, causing the patient to have fewer and fewer receptor sites available for stimulation. The disease is marked by progressive weakness and lack of muscle control with periodic acute episodes. The disease can progress to paralysis of the diaphragm, preventing the patient from breathing and would prove fatal without intervention.

Drugs used to help patients with this progressive disease are acetylcholinesterase inhibitors. These drugs cause an accumulation of ACh in the synaptic cleft, providing a longer time period for ACh to stimulate available receptors.

Neostigmine is a synthetic drug that does not cross the blood–brain barrier but has a strong influence at the NMJ. With a duration of action of 2 to 4 hours, neostigmine must be administered every few hours, based on patient response, to maintain a therapeutic level. Pyridostigmine, although absorbed more efficiently than neostigmine, is less powerful and slower in action. In some cases, pyridostigmine is preferred to neostigmine in the management of myasthenia gravis because pyridostigmine has a longer duration of action (3 to 6 hours) and therefore does not need to be taken as frequently. Distigmine has the longest action compared with neostigmine and pyridostigmine; however, there is a danger of cholinergic crisis (see Box 31.4) if accumulation of

BOX 31.2 Organophosphates: Irreversible Acetylcholinesterase Inhibitors

Organophosphates, used as pesticides and also as **nerve gases** in conflict, are irreversible acetylcholinesterase inhibitors. These drugs are rapidly absorbed across mucous membranes and distributed throughout the body, permanently binding to acetylcholinesterase and causing an accumulation of ACh at nerve endings and a massive cholinergic response. Bradycardia, pupil constriction, nausea, diarrhoea, hypersalivation and breathing difficulties are all signs of poisoning. Muscle weakness and paralysis can lead to severe breathing difficulties and death.

If exposure to nerve gases is expected, individuals are given intramuscular injections of atropine (to temporarily block cholinergic activity and to activate ACh sites in the CNS) and pralidoxime (to reactivate the acetylcholinesterase to start breaking down ACh). An autoinjection is provided to military personnel who may be at risk. The injections are repeated until the skin becomes flushed and dry, the pupils dilated and tachycardia is recorded.

BOX 31.3 Pralidoxime: Antidote for Irreversible Acetylcholinesterase-Inhibiting Drugs

Pralidoxime, the antidote for irreversible acetylcholinesterase-inhibiting drugs, is given intravenously to reactivate the acetylcholinesterase blocked by these drugs. Acting within minutes after injection, this drug releases the enzyme allowing breakdown of the accumulated ACh.

Pralidoxime does not readily cross the blood–brain barrier and is therefore most useful for treating peripheral effects. Pralidoxime is also used with atropine (which does cross the blood–brain barrier and will block the effects of accumulated ACh at CNS sites) to treat organophosphate pesticide poisoning and nerve gas exposure (see Box 31.2), both of which cause inactivation of acetylcholinesterase.

Adverse effects associated with pralidoxime include dizziness, blurred vision, headache, drowsiness, hyperventilation and nausea. These effects are also seen with exposure to nerve gases and organophosphate pesticides, so it can be difficult to differentiate drug effects from those of poisoning.

BOX 31.4 FOCUS ON **PATIENT SAFETY**

Myasthenic Crisis Versus Cholinergic Crisis

Myasthenia gravis can run an unpredictable course throughout the patient's life. Some patients have a very mild presentation, for example drooping eyelids, and go into remission with no further signs or symptoms for several years. Others have a more severe course, with progressive muscle weakness and possible confinement to a wheelchair. Many times, the disease goes through an intense phase called a myasthenic crisis, marked by extreme muscle weakness and respiratory difficulty.

The variability of the disease and the tendency to have crises and periods of remission mean management of the drug dosage for a patient with myasthenia gravis is a genuine nursing challenge. If a patient goes into remission, a smaller dose will be needed. If a patient has a crisis, an increased dose will be needed. To further complicate the clinical picture, the presentation of a cholinergic overdose or cholinergic crisis is similar to the presentation of a myasthenic crisis. The patient with a cholinergic crisis presents with progressive muscle weakness and respiratory difficulty as the accumulation of ACh at the cholinergic receptor leads to reduced impulse transmission and muscle weakness. This is a crisis when the respiratory muscles are involved.

In a myasthenic crisis, the correct treatment is increased cholinergic drug. However, treatment of a cholinergic crisis requires withdrawal of the drug. The patient's respiratory difficulties usually necessitate acute medical attention. At this point, the drug edrophonium can be used as a diagnostic agent to distinguish between the two conditions. If the patient improves immediately after the edrophonium injection, the problem is a myasthenic crisis, which is improved by administration of the cholinergic drug. If the patient deteriorates, the problem is probably a cholinergic crisis and withdrawal of the patient's cholinergic drug along with intense medical support is indicated. Atropine helps to alleviate some of the parasympathetic reactions to the cholinergic drug. However, because atropine is not effective at the NMJ, only time will reverse the drug toxicity.

The patient will need support, education and encouragement to deal with the careful regulation of the cholinergic medication throughout the course of the disease. Nurses in the acute care setting need to be mindful of the difficulty in distinguishing drug toxicity from the need for more drug and be prepared to respond appropriately.

the drug occurs and so this drug is rarely used in the treatment of myasthenia gravis.

Edrophonium, with a very short duration of action (10 to 20 minutes), is primarily used as a diagnostic agent for myasthenia gravis (see Box 31.4). If a patient has a temporary reversal of symptoms after injection with edrophonium, this indicates a problem with the nicotinic ACh receptors at the NMJ.

Cholinergic Drugs Used to Treat Alzheimer's Disease

Alzheimer's disease, the most common form of dementia, is a progressive disorder involving neural degeneration, mainly in the brain cortex, leading to a marked loss of memory and an inability to carry on activities of daily living (also see Critical Thinking Scenario 31.1). The presence of deposits or 'plaques' of amyloid protein outside the neurons and neurofibrillary tangles (aggregation of a protein called tau) within the neurons leads to a progressive loss of ACh-producing neurons and their target neurons (Welsh-Bohmer & White III, 2009). In the past, many people with Alzheimer's disease would have been diagnosed with senile dementia or dementia. The cause of the disease is not yet known.

Three cholinergic drugs are currently available to slow the progression of this disease: donepezil, galantamine and rivastigmine are all recommended for use with mild to moderate Alzheimer's dementia. Patients diagnosed with the early to moderate stages of the disease before 2007 have been able to use donepezil, galantamine, rivastigmine and memantine (an *N*-methyl-D-aspartate receptor antagonist used to treat moderate to severe dementia in Alzheimer's disease). Changes in the National Institute for Health and Clinical Excellence (NICE) guidelines have stated that patients diagnosed after this date can use these drugs only if they are in the mild to moderate stages of the disease. Patients diagnosed before 2007 can continue to use these drugs. However, the Clinical Care guidelines recognize that there must be a degree of flexibility in what constitutes moderate disease (NICE, 2007).

The least expensive of the three drugs is prescribed first. However, if it is not suitable for the patient, another drug could be chosen. Donezepil requires administration on a once-a-day basis; this offers a distinct advantage in a disease that affects memory and the patient's ability to remember to take pills throughout the day.

Existing therapeutic strategies only reduce the progression of the disease and provide only modest improvements in symptoms. The aim is to now generate drugs which target the underlying disease processes that are involved in the pathogenesis of Alzheimer's disease, for example preventing the formation of plaques of amyloid protein and neurofibrillary tangles (Rafii & Aisen, 2009).

Therapeutic Actions and Indications

All of the indirect-acting cholinergic drugs work by blocking acetylcholinesterase at the synaptic cleft. This blocking allows the accumulation of ACh released from the nerve endings and leads to increased and prolonged stimulation of ACh receptor sites at all of the postsynaptic cholinergic sites.

These drugs can relieve the signs and symptoms of myasthenia gravis and increase muscle strength by accumulating ACh in the synaptic cleft at NMJs. The drugs preferred for use with myasthenia gravis are those that do not cross the blood–brain barrier. Drugs that do cross the blood–brain barrier and seem to affect mostly the cells in the cortex to increase ACh concentration are used in the treatment of Alzheimer's disease. Neostigmine and edrophonium, because of their rapid onset of action, are also used to reverse toxicity from muscle relaxants used to paralyse muscles during surgery (see Chapter 25).

Pharmacokinetics

These drugs are well absorbed and distributed throughout the body. The drugs used to treat myasthenia gravis do not cross the blood–brain barrier and are metabolized in the liver. The drugs used for Alzheimer's disease are metabolized in the liver mostly by the cytochrome P450 system, so caution must be used with hepatic impairment and with many interacting drugs.

Contraindications and Cautions

These drugs are contraindicated in patients with bradycardia or intestinal or urinary tract obstruction, *which could be exacerbated by the stimulation of cholinergic receptors.* With the exception of distigmine which should not be used during pregnancy, the other drugs can be used provided the potential benefits outweigh the risk to the foetus. Edrophonium, neostigmine and pyridostigmine can be used during lactation, but the other drugs should be avoided.

Caution should be used with any condition that could be exacerbated by cholinergic stimulation. Although the effects of these drugs are generally more localized to the cortex and the NMJ, the possibility of parasympathetic effects should be considered carefully in patients with asthma, coronary disease, peptic ulcer, arrhythmias, epilepsy or parkinsonism.

Always consult a current copy of the British National Formulary for further guidance.

Adverse Effects

The adverse effects associated with these drugs are related to the stimulation of the parasympathetic nervous system. GI effects can include nausea, vomiting, cramps, diarrhoea, increased salivation and involuntary defaecation related to the increase in GI secretions and activity caused by parasympathetic nervous system stimulation. Cardiovascular effects can include bradycardia, heart block, hypotension and cardiac arrest related to the cardiac-suppressing effects of the parasympathetic nervous system. Urinary tract effects can include a sense of urgency related to stimulation of the bladder muscles and sphincter relaxation. Miosis and blurred vision, headaches, dizziness and drowsiness can occur related to CNS cholinergic effects. Other effects may include flushing and increased sweating secondary to stimulation of the cholinergic receptors in the sympathetic nervous system.

Clinically Important Drug–Drug Interactions

There may be an increased risk of GI bleeding if these drugs are used with nonsteroidal anti-inflammatory drugs (NSAIDs) because of the combination of increased GI secretions and the GI mucosal erosion associated with the use of NSAIDs. If this combination is used, the patient should be monitored closely for any sign of GI bleeding. The effect of anticholinesterase drugs is decreased if they are taken in combination with any cholinergic drugs because these work in opposition to each other.

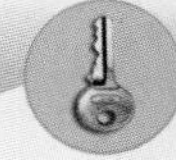

Key Drug Summary for Alzheimer's Disease: *Rivastigmine*

Indications: Treatment of mild-to-moderate dementia in Alzheimer's disease or Parkinson's disease

Actions: Reversible cholinesterase inhibitor that elevates ACh levels in the cortex, slowing the neuronal degradation of Alzheimer's disease

Pharmacokinetics:

Route	Onset	Peak	Duration
Oral	Varies	1h	8h
Transdermal patch	Varies	10–16 h (first patch)	8 h (second patch)

$T_{1/2}$: 1 hour (oral dose), 3 hours (after patch removal); metabolism is in the liver and excretion is mainly in the urine

Adverse effects: Nausea, vomiting, diarrhoea, dyspepsia, anorexia, abdominal pain; dizziness, headache, tremor, asthenia (loss of strength), agitation, confusion, sweating, weight loss

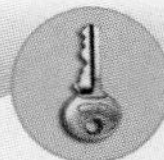

Key Drug Summary for Myasthenia Gravis: *Pyridostigmine*

Indications: Treatment of myasthenia gravis

Actions: Reversible cholinesterase inhibitor that increases the levels of ACh, facilitating transmission at the NMJ

Pharmacokinetics:

Route	Onset	Duration
Oral	35–45 min	3–6 h

$T_{1/2}$:1.9–3.7 hours; metabolism is in the liver and tissue and excretion is in the urine

Adverse effects: Nausea, vomiting, salivation, diarrhoea, bradycardia, cardiac arrest, lacrimation, miosis, dysphagia, increased bronchial secretions, urinary frequency and incontinence

Nursing Considerations for Patients Receiving Indirect-acting Cholinergic Drugs

Assessment: History and Examination

Screen for the following conditions, *which could be contraindications or cautions to use of the drug*: known allergies to any of these drugs; arrhythmias, coronary artery disease, hypotension, urogenital or GI obstruction, peptic ulcer, pregnancy, lactation or recent GI or genitourinary surgery, *which could limit use of the drugs*, and regular use of NSAIDs, cholinergic drugs or theophylline, *which could cause a drug–drug interaction.* Establish if patient is currently taking other medications or herbal therapies which may potentially interact with the cholinergic drug.

Include screening *for baseline status before beginning therapy and for any potential adverse effects*: assess orientation, affect, reflexes, ability to carry on activities of daily living (Alzheimer's drugs) and vision *to monitor for CNS changes related to drug therapy*; blood pressure, pulse, ECG, peripheral perfusion and cardiac output; urinary output and renal and liver function tests if the patient's history suggests potential problems *to monitor drug effects on the renal system and liver, which could change the metabolism and excretion of the drugs.*

Nursing Diagnoses

The patient receiving an indirect-acting cholinergic agonist may also have the following nursing diagnoses related to drug therapy:

- Disturbed thought processes related to CNS effects
- Acute pain related to GI effects
- Decreased cardiac output related to blood pressure changes, arrhythmias, vasodilation
- Deficient knowledge regarding drug therapy

Implementation With Rationale

- If the drug is given intravenously, administer it slowly, *to avoid severe cholinergic effects.*
- Maintain atropine on standby *as an antidote in case of overdose or severe cholinergic reaction.*
- Discontinue the drug if excessive salivation, diarrhoea, emesis or frequent urination becomes a problem *to decrease the risk of severe adverse reactions.*
- Administer the oral drug with meals *to decrease GI upset if it is a problem.*
- Mark the patient's chart and notify the surgeon if the patient is to undergo surgery *because prolonged muscle relaxation may occur if succinylcholine-type anaesthetics are used.* The patient will require prolonged support and monitoring.
- Monitor the patient being treated for Alzheimer's disease for any progress, *because the drug is not a cure and only slows progression*; refer families to supportive services.
- The patient who is being treated for myasthenia gravis and a significant other should receive instruction in drug administration, warning signs of drug overdose and signs and symptoms to report immediately *to enhance patient knowledge about drug therapy and to promote compliance.*
- Arrange for supportive care and comfort measures, including rest, environmental control and other measures, *to decrease CNS irritation*; headache medication *to relieve pain*; safety measures if CNS effects occur *to prevent injury*; protective measures if CNS effects are severe *to prevent patient injury*; and small, frequent meals if GI upset is severe *to decrease discomfort and maintain nutrition.*
- Provide thorough patient education, including dosage and adverse effects to anticipate, measures to avoid adverse effects and warning signs of problems, as well as proper administration for each route used *to enhance patient knowledge about drug therapy and to promote compliance.*
- Offer support and encouragement *to help the patient deal with the drug regimen.*

Evaluation

- Monitor patient response to the drug (improvement in condition being treated).
- Monitor for adverse effects (GI upset, CNS changes, cardiovascular changes, genitourinary changes).
- Evaluate the effectiveness of the education plan (patient can name drug, dosage, adverse effects to watch for, specific measures to avoid adverse effects, proper administration).
- Monitor the effectiveness of comfort measures and compliance to the regimen.

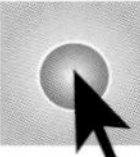

WEB LINKS

Health care providers and patients may want to consult the following Internet sources:

http://bnfc.org The BNF for Children provides UK health care professionals with authoritative and practical information on the selection and clinical use of medicines in children.

http://cks.library.nhs.uk The National Health Service Clinical Knowledge Summaries provides evidence-based practical information on the common conditions observed in primary care.

http://www.alzheimers.org.uk The Alzheimer's Society works to improve the quality of life of people affected by dementia in England, Wales and Northern Ireland.

http://www.bnf.org.uk The BNF provides UK health care professionals with authoritative and practical information on the selection and clinical use of medicines.

http://www.medicalert.org.uk MedicAlert is a registered charity providing a life-saving identification system for individuals with hidden medical conditions and allergies.

http://www.mgauk.org This association provides support and guidance to myasthenia gravis patients and their families.

http://www.nhsdirect.nhs.uk The National Health Service Direct service provides patients with information and advice about health, illness and health services.

Points to Remember

- Cholinergic drugs are chemicals that act at the same site as the neurotransmitter ACh, stimulating the parasympathetic nerves, some nerves in the brain and the NMJ.
- Direct-acting cholinergic drugs bind to ACh receptor sites to cause cholinergic stimulation.
- Use of direct-acting cholinergic drugs is limited by the systemic effects of the drug. They are used to cause miosis and to treat glaucoma; one agent is available to treat neurogenic bladder and bladder atony postoperative or postpartum, and another agent is available to increase GI secretions and relieve the dry mouth of Sjögren's syndrome.
- Indirect-acting cholinergic drugs are acetylcholinesterase inhibitors. They block acetylcholinesterase to prevent it from breaking down ACh in the synaptic cleft.
- Cholinergic stimulation by acetylcholinesterase inhibitors is caused by an accumulation of the ACh released from the nerve ending.
- Myasthenia gravis is an autoimmune disease characterized by antibodies to nicotinic ACh receptors. This results in a loss of ACh receptors and eventual loss of response at the NMJ.
- Acetylcholinesterase inhibitors are used to treat myasthenia gravis because they cause the accumulation of ACh in the synaptic cleft, prolonging stimulation of any ACh sites that remain.
- Alzheimer's disease is a progressive dementia characterized by a loss of ACh-producing neurons and ACh receptor sites in the cortex of the brain.
- Acetylcholinesterase inhibitors that cross the blood–brain barrier are used to manage Alzheimer's disease by increasing ACh levels in the brain and slowing the progression of the disease.
- Side-effects associated with the use of these drugs are related to stimulation of the PNS (bradycardia, hypotension, increased GI secretions and activity, increased bladder tone, relaxation of GI and genitourinary sphincters, bronchoconstriction, pupil constriction) and may limit the usefulness of some of these drugs.
- Nerve gases are irreversible acetylcholinesterase inhibitors that lead to toxic accumulations of ACh at cholinergic receptor sites and can cause parasympathetic crisis and muscle paralysis.
- Pralidoxime is an antidote for the irreversible acetylcholinesterase inhibitors; it frees the acetylcholinesterase that was inhibited.

CRITICAL THINKING SCENARIO 31-1

A Loss of Cognitive Function

The Situation

John, aged 78, had been finding it increasingly difficult to follow conversations. This had occasionally led to embarrassment when John was socializing with friends. Noting these changes in her father, his daughter encouraged him to consult his general practitioner (GP), whom John had known for many years. After consultation with his GP, John was referred to a specialist clinic. John attended the clinic with his daughter where a series of tests were performed, including a mini-mental state examination (MMSE), to assess John's cognitive function. John achieved a score of 18 out of a total of 30 points. Following further discussion with John's daughter, he was prescribed galantamine and requested to return for a reassessment in 3 months' time.

Critical Thinking

- What could be responsible for John's symptoms?
- What is the content of a MMSE?
- Consider the reasons why John's daughter was consulted prior to prescribing galantamine.
- What are the potential side-effects to consider when giving an indirectly acting cholinergic drug?
- Why is it necessary for John to return to the clinic in 3 months' time for reassessment of his cognitive function?
- What are the long-term considerations for both John and his daughter?

Discussion

Galantamine is one of the recommended treatments for mild-to-moderate dementia in Alzheimer's disease. Alzheimer's disease is a neurodegenerative disease characterized by a loss of cholinergic neurons particularly in the cerebral cortex. Prior to his referral to the clinic, John's GP would have carried out a thorough history taking and examination. As John was a regular attendee at this surgery, it is possible that his GP was also able to note the deterioration in John's cognitive function. The clinic John was referred to would be a specialist centre for the diagnosis of dementia. Here, a number of tests would be conducted to assess John's cognitive function and behaviour, including the MMSE. An MMSE asks patients a series of questions, for example the time, day, date, month and year (Folstein *et al.*, 1975). A score of 20 to 24 points usually indicates mild Alzheimer's, a score of 10 to 20 points suggests moderate Alzheimer's and those scoring below 10 points are considered to have severe Alzheimer's. As John was accompanied by his daughter, she may have been able to provide a greater insight into the way John's daily life has been affected by the dementia and also an appraisal of whether John will be able to comply to his treatment regimen. Galantamine is administered twice daily; however, if John's memory is severely affected, he may not remember to take his medication.

John was prescribed this drug based on the results of his examination at the clinic specializing in the diagnosis of dementia. Patients achieving a score between 10 and 20 points in an MMSE can be prescribed galantamine, donezepil, rivastigmine or memantine (NICE, 2007). Galantamine is a cholinesterase inhibitor which increases the level of ACh to compensate for the loss of neurons. This drug cannot reverse Alzheimer's disease; however, galantamine can slow the progression of cognitive decline in some patients. Patients are usually reassessed 3 months after treatment commences to assess the patients' response to the drug; the drug treatment is stopped if patients fail to respond. Drug treatment will only continue if the patient's MMSE score stays above 10 points, and their carer and specialist believe the drug is having a positive effect.

Alzheimer's disease is a progressive disease, and John and his daughter will have to consider how John will cope on a day-to-day basis in the future. Patients will require full-time support, and this role often falls to the relatives to fulfil. Relatives need to ensure they receive appropriate support and respite care.

Nursing Care Guide for John: Cholinergic Drugs for Alzheimer's Disease

Assessment: History and Examination

Assess history of allergies to galantamine as well as history of cardiovascular disease including conduction abnormalities, unstable angina and congestive heart failure; peptic ulcers; respiratory disease including asthma and chronic obstructive pulmonary disease; hepatic or renal dysfunction (creatinine clearance must be >9 ml per minute); bowel obstruction or urinary retention and concurrent use of other cholinergic drugs.

A Loss of Cognitive Function *(continued)*

Focus the physical examination on the following:

- CV: blood pressure, pulse rate, peripheral perfusion, ECG
- CNS: orientation, affect, reflexes, vision
- GU: urinary output, bladder tone (e.g. where possible, any patient observed changes in bladder activity – frequency of urination; colour, smell or amount of urine)
- GI: abdominal examination
- Respiratory: respirations, adventitious sounds
- Temperatures

Nursing Diagnoses

- Acute pain related to GI and CNS effects
- Impaired CNS function including confusion and depression
- Deficient knowledge regarding drug therapy
- Decreased cardiac output related to arrhythmias or myocardial infarction

Implementation

- Ensure safe and appropriate administration of drug.
- Provide comfort and safety measures (e.g. physical assistance); temperature control; pain relief; small, frequent meals.
- Monitor cardiac status and urine output throughout drug therapy.
- Provide support and reassurance to deal with side-effects, discomfort and GI effects.
- Provide patient and carer education regarding drug name, dosage, side-effects, precautions and warning signs of serious adverse effects to report.

Evaluation

- Evaluate drug effects: slowing of cognitive decline.
- Monitor for adverse effects: GI effects (nausea, vomiting, diarrhoea and abdominal pain); CNS effects (fainting or syncope, tremor, depression, fatigue); fever; urinary problems; GI effects; respiratory problems.
- Monitor for drug–drug interactions.
- Evaluate effectiveness of patient education programme and comfort and safety measures.

Patient Education for John & his Daughter

☐ The drug that was prescribed for you is called galantamine. It is called a cholinergic or a parasympathomimetic drug because it mimics the effects of the parasympathetic division of the nervous system.

☐ This drug has been prescribed for you to reduce your memory loss.

☐ Some of the following side-effects may occur:

- *Nausea, vomiting, diarrhoea*: it is wise to be near bathroom facilities after taking your drug. If these symptoms become too severe, consult your health care provider.
- *Anorexia and weight loss*: although you may not feel very hungry while taking this drug, it is important to maintain a balanced diet. Small, frequent meals might be beneficial.
- *Headache*: aspirin or other headache medication (if not contraindicated in your particular case) will help to alleviate this pain.
- *Light-headed*: you should lie down if you feel dizzy or faint. Get up slowly when you feel ready to do so.
- *Depression*: this is a side-effect that his carer should monitor.
- Report any of the following to your health care provider: *light-headedness, fainting, abdominal cramping or pain, weakness or confusion, feelings of indigestion (dyspepsia).*

☐ Tell any doctor, nurse or other health care provider involved in your care that you are taking these drugs. Patients are advised to wear or carry MedicAlert identification.

☐ It is important that you consult your prescriber before you take over-the-counter products or herbal treatments.

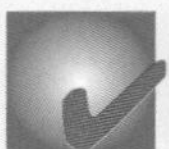

CHECK YOUR UNDERSTANDING

Answers to the questions in this chapter may be found in the Answer Key in the back of the book.

Multiple Choice

Select the best answer to the following.

1. Indirect-acting cholinergic drugs
   a. bind to acetylcholine receptor sites on the membranes of effector cells.
   b. react chemically with acetylcholinesterase to increase acetylcholine concentrations around effector cell receptor sites.
   c. are used to increase bladder tone and urinary excretion.
   d. should be given with food to decrease nausea.

2. Pilocarpine is indicated for the treatment of
   a. myasthenia gravis.
   b. neurogenic bladder.
   c. glaucoma.
   d. Alzheimer's disease.

3. Myasthenia gravis is treated with indirect-acting cholinergic agents that
   a. lead to accumulation of acetylcholine in the synaptic cleft and eventual stimulation of the muscle.
   b. block the GI effects of the disease.
   c. directly stimulate the remaining acetylcholine receptors.
   d. can be given only by injection.

4. The cholinergic drug of choice for a patient with myasthenia gravis who is no longer able to swallow would be
   a. neostigmine.
   b. distigmine.
   c. pyridostigmine.
   d. edrophonium.

5. Alzheimer's disease is marked by a progressive loss of memory and is associated with
   a. degeneration of dopamine-producing cells in the basal ganglia.
   b. loss of acetylcholine-producing neurons and their target neurons in the CNS.
   c. loss of acetylcholine receptor sites in the parasympathetic division of the nervous system.
   d. increased levels of acetylcholinesterase in the CNS.

6. Galantamine would be the Alzheimer's disease drug of choice for a patient who
   a. cannot remember family members' names.
   b. is mildly inhibited and can still follow medical dosing regimens.
   c. is unable to carry on normal activities of daily living.
   d. has memory problems and would benefit from once-a-day dosing.

7. Adverse effects associated with the use of cholinergic drugs would include
   a. constipation and insomnia.
   b. diarrhoea and urinary urgency.
   c. tachycardia and hypertension.
   d. dry mouth and tachycardia.

8. Nerve gas is an irreversible acetylcholinesterase inhibitor that can cause muscle paralysis and death. An antidote to such an agent is
   a. atropine.
   b. propranolol.
   c. pralidoxime.
   d. neostigmine.

Extended Matching Questions

Select **all** that apply.

1. A nurse is explaining myasthenia gravis to a family. Which of the following points would be included in the explanation?
   a. It is thought to be an autoimmune disease.
   b. It is associated with destruction of acetylcholine receptor sites.
   c. It is best treated with potent antibiotics.
   d. It is a chronic and progressive muscular disease.
   e. It is caused by demyelination of the nerve fibre.
   f. Once diagnosed, there is a 5-year survival rate.

2. A nurse would question an order for a cholinergic drug if the patient was also taking which of the following?
   a. Theophylline
   b. NSAIDs
   c. Cephalosporin
   d. Atropine
   e. Propranolol
   f. Memantine

Matching

Match the drug with its usual indication. Some drugs may have more than one indication.

1. ____________________ pilocarpine
2. ____________________ neostigmine
3. ____________________ pyridostigmine

4. ____________________edrophonium
5. ____________________rivastigmine
6. ____________________donepezil

A. Diagnosis of myasthenia gravis
B. Treatment of myasthenia gravis
C. Antidote for NMJ blockers
D. Glaucoma, miosis
E. Alzheimer's disease

Fill in the Blanks

1. Cholinergic drugs are chemicals that act at the same site as the neurotransmitter____________ .

2. Cholinergic drugs are often also called_____________ drugs because their action mimics the action of the parasympathetic nervous system.

3. ____________________cholinergic drugs act at acetylcholine receptor sites to cause the same reaction as acetylcholine would cause.

4. Cholinergic agents that prevent the breakdown of acetylcholine by blocking acetylcholinesterase are called___________________ cholinergic drugs.

5. ____________________is a progressive neurological condition that is marked by loss of the acetylcholine-producing neurons in the cerebral cortex.

6. ________________________________is a chronic muscular disease that is caused by a defect in neuromuscular transmission; cholinergic drugs help patients with this disease.

7. Common adverse effects in the GI tract seen with cholinergic drugs include _________________ and___________ .

8. Cardiovascular effects that are often seen with cholinergic drugs include_________________, _________________ and___________ .

Bibliography and References

British Medical Association and Royal Pharmaceutical Society of Great Britain. (2008). *British National Formulary*. London: BMJ & RPS Publishing. *This publication is updated biannually: it is imperative that the most recent edition is consulted.*

British Medical Association and Royal Pharmaceutical Society of Great Britain. (2008). *British National Formulary for Children*. London: BMJ & RPS Publishing. *This publication is updated annually: it is imperative that the most recent edition is consulted.*

Folstein, M. F., Folstein, S. E., & McHough, P. R. (1975). Mini-mental state: a practical method for grading the cognitive state of patients for the clinician. *Journal of Psychiatric Research, 12*, 189–198.

Ganong, W. (2005). *Review of medical physiology* (22nd ed.). New York: McGraw-Hill.

Howland, R. D., & Mycek, M. J. (2005). *Pharmacology* (3rd ed.). Philadelphia: Lippincott Williams & Wilkins.

Marieb, E. N., & Hoehn, K. (2009). *Human anatomy & physiology* (8th ed.). San Francisco: Pearson Benjamin Cummings.

National Institute for Health and Clinical Excellence. (2007). Donezepil, galantamine, rivastigmine, and memantine for Alzheimer's disease. Available from http://www.nice.org.uk

Porth, C. M., & Matfin, G. (2008). *Pathophysiology: Concepts of altered health states* (8th ed.). Philadelphia: Lippincott Williams & Wilkins.

Rafii, M. S., & Aisen, P. S. (2009). Recent developments in Alzheimer's disease therapeutics. *BioMed Central Medicine, 7*, 7.

Simonsen, T., Aarbakke, J., Kay, I., Coleman, I., Sinnott, P., & Lysaa, R. (2006). *Illustrated pharmacology for nurses*. London: Hodder Arnold.

Welsh-Bohmer, K. A., & White III, C. L. (2009). Alzheimer disease: what changes in the brain cause dementia? *Neurology, 72*(4), 354–360.

CHAPTER 32

Antimuscarinic Agents

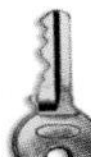

KEY TERMS

antimuscarinic

cycloplegia

mydriasis

parasympatholytic

LEARNING OBJECTIVES

Upon completion of the chapter, you will be able to:

1. Define antimuscarinic agents.
2. Describe the therapeutic actions, indications, pharmacokinetics, contraindications, most common adverse reactions and important drug–drug interactions of atropine.
3. Discuss the use of atropine across the lifespan.
4. Compare and contrast the key drug atropine with other antimuscarinic agents.
5. Outline the nursing considerations, including important teaching points, for patients receiving antimuscarinic agents.

ANTIMUSCARINIC AGENTS/ PARASYMPATHOLYTICS

atropine
benzatropine
cyclopentolate
darifenacin
dicycloverine
flavoxate
glycopyrronium
homatropine
hyoscyine
ipratropium
orphenadrine
oxybutynin
procyclidine
propantheline
solifenacin
tolterodine
trihexyphenidyl
tropicamide
trospium

Acetylcholine (ACh) is a neurotransmitter used by both the somatic (or voluntary) and autonomic divisions of the nervous system. There are two main types of ACh receptors: nicotinic and muscarinic. The nicotinic receptors are located on the pre- and postganglionic cells of the sympathetic and parasympathetic divisions of the autonomic nervous system. Nicotinic receptors are also located at the neuromuscular junction in skeletal muscle which when stimulated result in contraction. Muscarinic receptors are found in a variety of locations including the heart, exocrine glands and smooth muscle. These receptors are either stimulated (e.g. exocrine glands) or inhibited (e.g. heart) when ACh is released by the parasympathetic division of the autonomic nervous system. Although the sympathetic division acts via adrenergic receptors, the sympathetic receptors on the sweat glands are muscarinic.

Drugs that are used to block the effects of ACh target either muscarinic or nicotinic ACh receptors. The drugs inhibiting nicotinic receptors are known as neuromuscular blocking agents and are discussed in Chapter 24. Drugs acting as antagonists at muscarinic receptors are generally known as anticholinergic drugs but are more correctly known as **antimuscarinic** drugs. They are also known as **parasympatholytic** agents because they block the effects of the parasympathetic nervous system.

This class of drugs has a number of uses: (1) to dilate the bronchioles in a severe acute asthma attack, (2) to dilate the pupils and increase the area of the fundus that is visible during an eye examination, (3) as an antiarrhythmic to reverse the bradycardia associated with a myocardial infarction, (4) as a surgical premedication to reduce glandular secretions, (5) to prevent motion sickness, (6) to manage urinary incontinence and (7) to decrease gastrointestinal (GI) smooth muscle spasms, for example in irritable bowel syndrome. In some clinical situations, antimuscarinic drugs have been superseded by other more specific drugs, for example, antimuscarinics are no longer used to reduce gastric secretion and treat gastric and duodenal ulcers and have been replaced by more specific drugs such as histamine H_2-receptor antagonists. The use of antimuscarinic agents with various age groups is discussed in Box 32.1.

Antimuscarinics

Atropine, derived from the plant belladonna, was first used many centuries ago by ancient Egyptian women to dilate their pupils in an effort to make them more innocent looking and alluring. Atropine and other antimuscarinic drugs exert their therapeutic effects through the competitive inhibition of ACh at muscarinic receptor sites that are responsible for mediating the effects of the parasympathetic postganglionic impulses (Figure 32.1). Antimuscarinics also inhibit the few cholinergic receptors in the sympathetic nervous system (SNS), such as those that control sweating. These

BOX 32.1 DRUG THERAPY ACROSS THE LIFESPAN

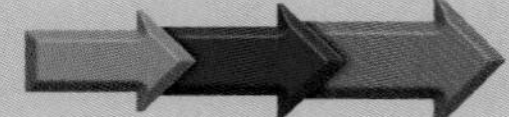

Antimuscarinic Drugs

CHILDREN

Antimuscarinic drugs are most likely to be prescribed to children to treat nocturnal enuresis (bedwetting); however, alternative measures should be the first approach rather than drug therapy. Children are often more sensitive to the adverse effects of these drugs, including constipation, urinary retention, heat intolerance and confusion. If a child is given one of these drugs, they should be closely monitored for adverse effects, and appropriate supportive measures should be instituted. All antimuscarinic drugs should be used with caution in children and young adults with Down's syndrome who are more sensitive to the adverse effects associated with these drugs.

When administering any drug to children, always consult the most recent edition of the British National Formulary for Children.

ADULTS

Adults need to be made aware of the potential for adverse effects associated with the use of these drugs. They should be encouraged to void before taking the medication if urinary retention or hesitancy is a problem. They should be encouraged to drink plenty of fluids and to avoid hot temperatures, because heat intolerance can occur and it will be important to maintain hydration should this happen. Safety precautions may be needed if blurred vision and dizziness occur. The patient should be urged not to drive or perform tasks that require concentration and coordination.

With the exception of ipratropium and some of the topically applied drugs, manufacturers recommend pregnant women either avoid taking antimuscarinic drugs unless the drug is essential and the benefit to the mother clearly outweighs the potential risk to the foetus, or they should be used with caution. Similarly, nursing mothers are advised to either avoid these drugs or take with caution because of the potential for serious adverse effects on the baby.

OLDER ADULTS

Older adults are more likely to experience the adverse effects associated with these drugs; dosage should be reduced, and the patient should be monitored closely. Older patients are more susceptible to heat intolerance owing to decreased body fluid and decreased sweating; therefore, caution should be used when an antimuscarinic drug is given. The patient should be urged to drink plenty of fluids and to avoid extremes of temperature or exertion in warm temperatures. Safety precautions may be needed if central nervous system (CNS) effects are severe. The older adult is more likely to experience confusion, hallucinations and psychotic syndromes when taking an antimuscarinic drug. Older adults may also have renal impairment, making them more likely to have problems excreting these drugs. Further reduction in dosage may be needed in patients with renal dysfunction. Men with benign prostatic hypertrophy may have increased difficulty with urination.

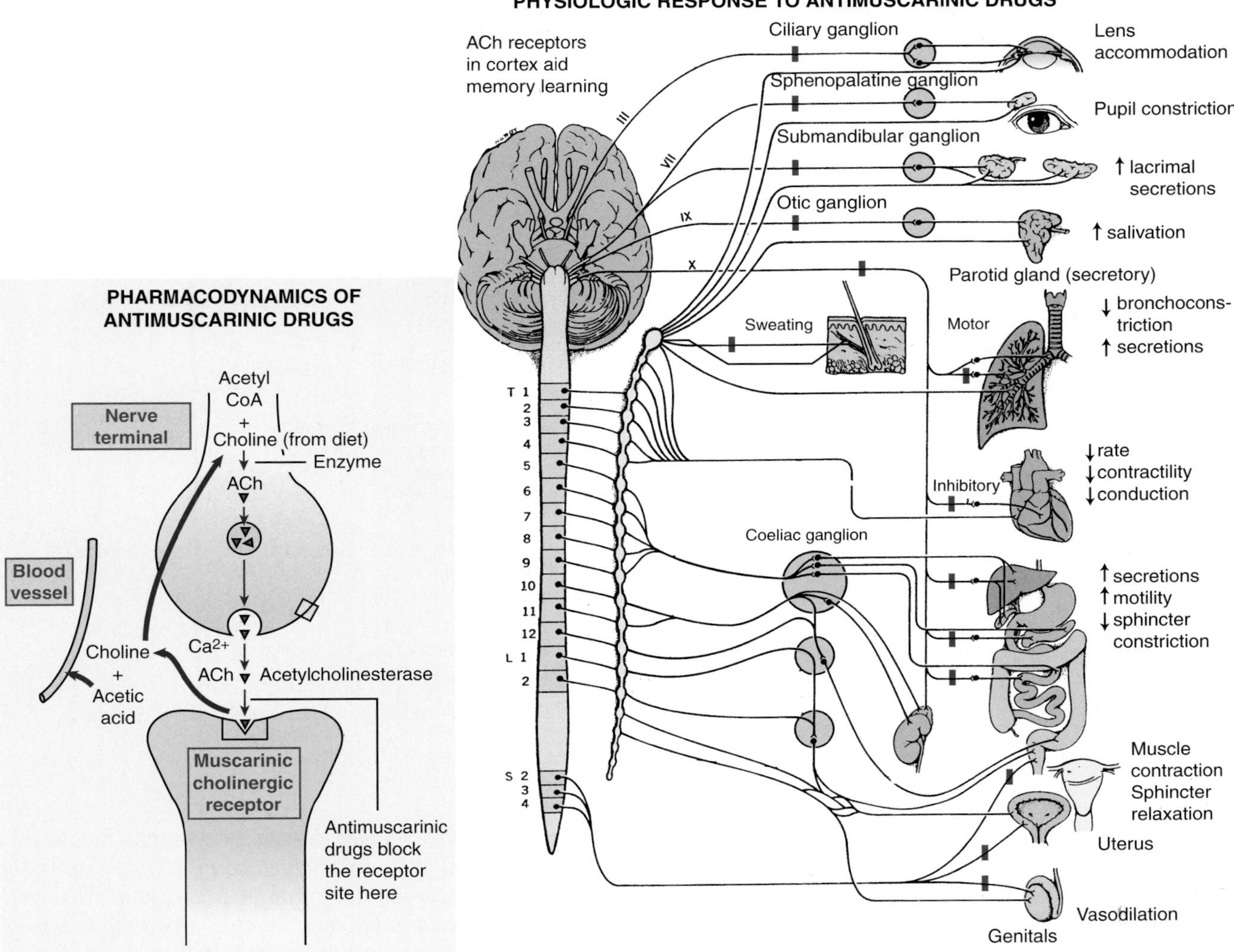

FIGURE 32.1 Pharmacodynamics of antimuscarinic drugs and associated physiologic responses. A red bar indicates blockade of that activity. For example, blocking the inhibitory effect on the heart will cause an increase in heart rate.

drugs compete with ACh for muscarinic ACh receptor sites and have no effect on the nicotinic receptors at the neuromuscular junction or between pre- and postganglionic autonomic neurons. Table 32.1 highlights the physiological consequences of parasympathetic inhibition and the drugs used to elicit these effects.

Therapeutic Actions and Indications

By competitively blocking the action of ACh at muscarinic cholinergic receptor sites in the peripheral nervous system and CNS, antimuscarinic drugs are used to manage a number of diseases or clinical situations:

- depress salivation and bronchial secretions before anaesthesia and to dilate the bronchi during an asthma attack;
- inhibit parasympathetic stimulation of the heart and restore heart rate after vagal stimulation during surgery, for example;
- relaxation of the GI tract in the management of irritable bowel syndrome;
- relaxation of bladder detrusor muscles and tightening of bladder sphincters in the treatment of urinary incontinence;
- **mydriasis** or relaxation of the muscles surrounding the pupil of the eye (also called a mydriatic effect) and **cycloplegia** or inhibition of the ability of the lens in the eye to accommodate to near vision (also called a cycloplegic effect);
- block the effects of ACh in the CNS to treat the involuntary movement and rigidity associated with parkinsonism and also as an antiemetic;
- as an antidote for poisoning by cholinergic drugs.

Many of the antimuscarinic drugs listed in Table 32.1 have very specific indications that are discussed elsewhere in relation to the systems they affect, for example benzatropine, orphenadrine, procyclidine and trihexyphenidyl

Table 32.1 Effects of Parasympathetic Inhibition and Associated Therapeutic Uses

Physiological Effect	Therapeutic Uses	Drug Example
Gastrointestinal Smooth muscle: blocks spasm, blocks peristalsis Secretory glands: decreases acid and digestive enzyme production	Decreases motility and secretory activity in peptic ulcer, gastritis, cardiospasm, pylorospasm, enteritis, diarrhoea, hypertonic constipation	Atropine, dicycloverine, hyoscine, propantheline
Urinary tract Decreases tone and motility in the ureters and fundus of the bladder; increases tone in the bladder sphincter	Increases bladder capacity in children with enuresis and paraplegics, decreases urinary urgency and frequency, antispasmodic in renal colic and to counteract bladder spasm caused by morphine	Darifenacin, flavoxate, oxybutynin, propantheline, propiverine, solifenacin, tolterodine, trospium
Bronchial smooth muscle Weakly relaxes smooth muscle	May be used during a severe asthma attack in nebulizer form	Ipratropium
Cardiovascular system Increases heart rate (may decrease heart rate at very low doses)	Counteracts bradycardia caused by vagal stimulation, surgical procedures, used to overcome heart blocks following myocardial infarction, used to counteract bradycardia associated with cholinergic drugs or in overdosage with beta-blockers.	Atropine
Ocular effects Pupil dilation, cycloplegia	Allows ophthalmological examination of the retina, optic disk, relaxes ocular muscles and decreases inflammation in the anterior segment of the eye in front of the iris	Atropine, cyclopentolate, homatropine, tropicamide
Secretions Reduces sweating, salivation, respiratory tract secretions	Preoperatively before inhalation anaesthesia; reduces nasal secretions in rhinitis, hay fever; may be used to reduce excessive sweating in hyperhidrosis	Atropine, glycopyrrolate, hyoscine, ipratropium
Central nervous system Decreases extrapyramidal motor activity	Decreases tremor in parkinsonism, helps to prevent motion sickness	Benzatropine, hyoscine, orphenadrine, procyclidine, trihexyphenidyl

(Chapter 23); flavoxate and trospium (Chapter 51); ipratropium (Chapter 54) and hyoscine (Chapter 58).

Pharmacokinetics

Antimuscarinics are well absorbed after administration and widely distributed throughout the body including the brain. Their half-lives vary according to the route of administration and the drug. They are excreted in the urine. These drugs should be used in pregnancy and lactation only if the benefit clearly outweighs the potential risk to the foetus or baby. Nursing mothers are advised to either find another way of feeding the baby or take these drugs with caution.

Contraindications and Cautions

Antimuscarinics are contraindicated in the presence of known allergy to any of these drugs. They are also contraindicated with any condition that could be exacerbated by blocking the parasympathetic nervous system. These conditions include glaucoma *because of the possibility of increased ocular pressure with pupil dilation*; stenosing peptic ulcer, intestinal atony, paralytic ileus, GI obstruction, severe ulcerative colitis and megacolon (dilation of the colon leading to constipation and obstruction), *all of which could be intensified with a further slowing of GI activity*; prostatic hypertrophy and bladder obstruction, *which could be further compounded by inhibiting bladder muscle activity and inhibiting sphincter relaxation in the bladder*; cardiac arrhythmias, tachycardia and myocardial ischaemia, *which could be exacerbated by the increased sympathetic influence in association with decreased parasympathetic influence, including tachycardia*; impaired liver or kidney function, *which could alter the metabolism and excretion of the drug*; hyperthyroidism and myasthenia gravis, *which could deteriorate with blocking of the cholinergic receptors*.

Caution should be used in patients who are breast-feeding *because of possible suppression of lactation.*

Adverse Effects

The adverse effects associated with the use of antimuscarinic drugs are caused by the systemic blockade of cholinergic receptors. What are adverse effects in some cases may be the desired therapeutic effects in others. The intensity of adverse effects is related to drug dosage: the more of the drug in the system, the greater the systemic effects. These adverse effects could include the CNS effects of blurred vision, pupil dilation and resultant photophobia, cycloplegia and increased intraocular pressure, all of which are related to the blocking of the parasympathetic effects in the eye. Care must be taken in administering antimuscarinics to patients with darkly pigmented irises as these patients are often more resistant to pupillary dilation and may require either a higher concentration of the mydriatic or more frequent administration of the drug, which could lead to overdose.

Weakness, dizziness, insomnia, mental confusion and agitation are effects related to the blocking of the cholinergic receptors within the CNS. Dry mouth results from decreasing salivary gland secretion. Altered taste perception, nausea, heartburn, constipation, bloated feelings and paralytic ileus are related to decreased GI peristaltic activity. Tachycardia and palpitations are possible effects related to inhibiting parasympathetic effects on the heart. Urinary hesitancy and retention are related to the inhibition of bladder muscle activity and relaxation of the sphincter. When given as a surgical premedication, antimuscarinics can thicken respiratory secretions potentially causing obstruction of the airways. Decreased sweating and an increased predisposition to heat stroke are related to the inability to cool the body by sweating, a result of blocking of the sympathetic cholinergic receptors responsible for sweating. Suppression of lactation is related to antimuscarinic effects in the breasts and in the CNS.

Clinically Important Drug–Drug Interactions

It is of paramount importance that the nurse establishes which other drug(s) the patient is currently taking. This includes prescription drugs, over-the-counter products and herbal treatments. The incidence of antimuscarinic effects increases if these drugs are combined with any other drugs with muscarinic-like activity, including antihistamines, antiparkinsonism drugs, monoamine oxidase inhibitors (MAOIs) and tricyclic antidepressants (TCAs). If such combinations must be used, the patient should be monitored closely and dosage adjustments made. Patients should be advised to avoid over-the-counter products that contain these drugs. The effectiveness of phenothiazines decreases if they are combined with antimuscarinic drugs and the risk of antimuscarinic side-effects increase.

Always consult a current copy of the British National Formulary for further guidance.

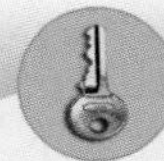

Key Drug Summary: *Atropine*

Indications: To decrease bronchial and salivary secretions before surgery, relief of bradycardia and hypotension following either a myocardial infarction or overdose with β-blockers, relaxation of the GI smooth muscle spasms, mydriasis and cycloplegia, antidote for poisoning with nerve agents and insecticides

Actions: Competitively blocks muscarinic ACh receptors, blocking the effects of the parasympathetic division of the nervous system

Pharmacokinetics:

Route	Onset	Peak	Duration
IM	10–15 min	30 min	4 h
IV	Immediate	2–4 min	4 h
Sub-cut	Varies	1–2 h	4 h
Topical	5–10 min	30–40 min	7–14 days

$T_{1/2}$: 2.5 hours, partly via liver metabolism and the remainder excreted unchanged in the urine

Adverse effects: Blurred vision, mydriasis, cycloplegia, photophobia, palpitations, transient bradycardia followed by tachycardia, dry mouth, difficulty in micturition, reduced bronchial secretions, decreased sweating, flushing and predisposition to heat prostration

FOCUS ON **PATIENT SAFETY**

Atropine Toxicity

Atropine is used in a variety of clinical settings to:

- Decrease bronchial and salivary secretions, as a preoperative agent
- Restore cardiac rate and arterial pressure during general anaesthesia when increased vagal stimulation causes a rapid parasympathetic response
- Relieve bradycardia and hypotension following myocardial infarction
- Relax GI smooth muscle spasms
- Reverse poisoning with nerve agents and insecticides
- Induce mydriasis for ophthalmic procedures

Atropine can cause poisoning, particularly following ingestion of the plants deadly nightshade and henbane. Atropine toxicity should also be considered whenever a patient receiving an antimuscarinic drug presents with a sudden onset of bizarre mental and neurological symptoms. Toxicity is dose-related and usually progresses as follows:

0.5 mg atropine – slight cardiac slowing (paradoxical bradycardia), dryness of mouth, inhibition of sweating

1 mg atropine – definite mouth and throat dryness, thirst, tachycardia, pupil dilation

2 mg atropine – tachycardia, palpitations; marked mouth dryness; dilated pupils; some blurring of vision

5 mg atropine – all of the above and marked speech disturbances; difficulty swallowing; restlessness, fatigue, headache; dry and hot skin; difficulty voiding; reduced intestinal peristalsis

10 mg atropine – all of the above symptoms, more marked; pulse rapid and weak; a barely visible iris as a result of pupil dilation; vision blurred; skin flushed, hot, dry and scarlet; ataxia; restlessness and excitement; hallucinations; delirium and coma

Treatment is as follows. If the poison was taken orally, gastric lavage should only be considered if a life-threatening amount of atropine was consumed in the previous hour. Activated charcoal is given orally to adsorb the poison before the atropine is absorbed across the GI wall. The charcoal may be effective for longer than 1 hour after ingestion. Sponging with cool water may relieve the fever and hot skin. It is important to remember that the half-life of atropine is 2.5 hours; at extremely high doses, several hours may be needed to clear the atropine from the body.

Nursing Considerations for Patients Receiving Antimuscarinic Agents

Assessment: History and Examination

Screen for the following conditions, *which could be cautions or contraindications to use of the drug*: any known allergies to these drugs; glaucoma; stenosing peptic ulcer, intestinal atony, paralytic ileus, GI obstruction, severe ulcerative colitis and megacolon; prostatic hypertrophy and bladder obstruction; cardiac arrhythmias and tachycardia, *all could be exacerbated by parasympathetic blockade*; impaired liver or kidney function, *which could alter the metabolism and excretion of the drug*; hyperthyroidism and myasthenia gravis, *which could become much worse with further blocking of cholinergic receptors* and lactation, *because of possible suppression of lactation.* Establish if patient is currently taking other medications or herbal therapies which may potentially interact with the antimuscarinic drug.

Include screening *for baseline status before beginning therapy and for any potential adverse effects*: skin colour, temperature; orientation, pupil response; pulse, blood pressure, electrocardiogram (ECG); urine output, bladder tone (e.g. any patient observed changes in bladder activity – frequency of urination; colour, smell or amount of urine) and bowel movements (e.g. frequency of passing stools) and abdominal examination.

Nursing Diagnoses

The patient receiving antimuscarinic drugs may have the following nursing diagnoses related to drug therapy:

- Acute pain related to GI, CNS and genitourinary effects
- Constipation, related to GI effects
- Urinary retention
- Mood alteration related to CNS effects
- Inadequate nutrition related to dry mouth and constipation
- Noncompliance related to adverse drug effects
- Deficient knowledge regarding drug therapy

Implementation With Rationale

- Ensure proper administration of the drug *to ensure effective use and decrease the risk of adverse effects.*
- Ensure adequate hydration and temperature control *to prevent hyperpyrexia.*
- Provide comfort measures *to help the patient tolerate drug effects*: frequent mouth care *to alleviate problems associated with dry mouth*; lighting control *to alleviate photophobia*; small and frequent meals *to alleviate GI discomfort*; bowel programme *to alleviate constipation*; safety precautions *to prevent injury if CNS effects are severe*; analgesics *to relieve pain if headaches occur*; and emptying bladder before taking medication *if urinary retention is a problem* (commonly occurs with benign prostatic hyperplasia) and postoperatively if atropine has been used in anaesthesia.
- Monitor patient response closely (blood pressure, ECG, urine output) *in order to arrange to adjust dosage accordingly to ensure benefit with the least amount of toxicity.*
- Provide thorough patient teaching, including measures to avoid adverse effects, warning signs of problems, and the need for monitoring and evaluation, *to enhance patient knowledge about drug therapy and to promote compliance.*
- Offer support and encouragement *to help the patient deal with the drug regimen.*

Evaluation

- Monitor patient response to the drug (improvement in disorder being treated).
- Monitor for adverse effects (cardiovascular changes, GI problems, CNS effects, urinary hesitancy and retention, pupil dilation and photophobia, decrease in sweating and heat intolerance).
- Evaluate the effectiveness of the teaching plan (patient can name drug, dosage, adverse effects to watch for, specific measures to avoid adverse effects, proper administration of ophthalmic drugs).
- Monitor the effectiveness of comfort measures and compliance with the regimen.

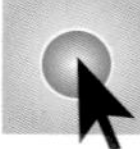

WEB LINK

Health care providers and patients may want to consult the following Internet sources:

http://bnfc.org The BNF for Children provides UK health care professionals with authoritative and practical information on the selection and clinical use of medicines in children.

http://cks.library.nhs.uk The National Health Service Clinical Knowledge Summaries provide evidence-based practical information on the common conditions observed in primary care.

http://www.bnf.org.uk The BNF provides UK health care professionals with authoritative and practical information on the selection and clinical use of medicines.

http://www.nhsdirect.nhs.uk The National Health Service Direct service provides patients with information and advice about health, illness and health services.

Points to Remember

- Antimuscarinic drugs block the effects of ACh at muscarinic ACh receptor sites.
- Antimuscarinic drugs are also called parasympatholytic drugs because they block the effects of the parasympathetic nervous system.
- Blocking of the parasympathetic nervous system causes an increase in heart rate, decrease in GI activity, decrease in urinary bladder tone and function, pupil dilation and cycloplegia (paralysis of the ciliary muscles resulting in blurred vision).
- These drugs also block muscarinic receptors in the CNS and sympathetic postganglionic cholinergic receptors, including those that cause sweating.
- Many systemic adverse effects are associated with the use of antimuscarinic drugs; they are caused by the systemic cholinergic blocking effects that can also produce the desired therapeutic effect.
- Patients receiving antimuscarinic drugs must be monitored for dry mouth, difficulty swallowing, constipation, urinary retention, tachycardia, pupil dilation and photophobia, cycloplegia resulting in blurred vision and heat intolerance caused by a decrease in sweating.

CRITICAL THINKING SCENARIO 32-1

Antimuscarinic Drugs and Heart Disease

The Situation

Erica, a 64-year-old woman with a long history of heart disease, has suffered from urinary incontinence for several years. Pelvic floor exercises and bladder training were of some benefit but did not completely reverse the problem. She was prescribed oxybutinin to relax her urinary smooth muscle. Within the next few days, she plans to travel to the Caribbean for the winter and wants any information that she should have before she goes.

Critical Thinking

- Erica presents a number of nursing care problems. What are the implications of giving an antimuscarinic drug to a person with a long history of heart disease?
- Erica is about to leave for her winter home in the sun; what information will be essential for her if she is taking an antimuscarinic when she leaves?
- What medical problems can arise with people who live in different areas at different times of the year?
- What written information should Erica take with her as she travels?

Discussion

Erica is doing well in managing her cardiac problems at the moment, but she could develop problems as a result of the prescribed antimuscarinic drug. The possible adverse effect of tachycardia and arrhythmias could tip the balance in a compensated heart, leading to congestive heart failure or oxygen delivery problems. She will need to be carefully evaluated for the status of her heart disease and potential problems.

Erica should also be evaluated to establish a baseline for vision, GI problems, etc. She should receive thorough teaching about her oxybutinin, especially adverse effects to anticipate, safety measures to take if vision changes occur and a bowel programme that she can follow to avoid constipation.

As Erica is leaving a cold climate and travelling to a warm climate, she will need to be warned that oxybutinin decreases sweating. This means that she may

(continued)

Antimuscarinic Drugs and Heart Disease *(continued)*

be susceptible to heat stroke and should be encouraged to take precautions to avoid these problems.

Antimuscarinic therapy should be reviewed after 3 to 6 months of treatment, and it will be difficult to monitor Erica while she is away. It should be anticipated that patients, such as Erica, might have two sets of health care providers who may not communicate with each other. It is important to give Erica written information about her current diagnosis, including test results; details about her drugs, including dosages; information about the adverse effects she may experience and ways to deal with them. It may be useful to include a telephone number or means of contact that Erica can use or can give to her health care provider to use if further tests or follow-up is indicated.

Nursing Care Guide for Erica: Heart Disease

Assessment: History and Examination

Assess for a history of allergy to antimuscarinic drugs, myasthenia gravis, angle-closure glaucoma (an increased intraocular pressure associated with glaucoma), bowel or urinary obstruction, severe ulcerative colitis or GI obstruction and tachycardia.

Focus the physical examination on the following:

- CV: blood pressure, pulse rate, peripheral perfusion, ECG
- CNS: orientation, effect, vision
- Skin: colour, texture, sweating
- GU: urinary output, bladder tone
- GI: abdominal examination

Nursing Diagnoses

- Constipation related to GI effects
- Acute pain related to GI, GU, CNS effects
- Poor nutrition due to dry mouth and constipation
- Heat intolerance due to decreased sweating
- Deficient knowledge regarding drug therapy
- Noncompliance related to adverse effects

Implementation

- Ensure safe and appropriate administration of drug.
- Provide comfort measures, including temperature control; dark glasses; fluids; mouth care; bowel programme.
- Provide support and reassurance to deal with drug effects, discomfort and GI effects.
- Provide patient teaching regarding drug name, dosage, adverse effects, precautions and warnings to report.
- Monitor blood pressure and pulse rate and adjust dosage as needed.

Evaluation

- Evaluate drug effects: pupil dilation, decrease in signs and symptoms being treated.
- Monitor for adverse effects: Cardiovascular effects – tachycardia, palpitations, arrhythmias; CNS – disorientation, restlessness; difficulty in micturition; GI effects – constipation and blurred vision and photophobia.
- Monitor for drug–drug interactions as indicated for each drug.
- Evaluate effectiveness of patient-teaching programme and comfort and safety measures.

Patient Teaching for Erica

- ☐ Antimuscarinics or parasympatholytics block or stop the actions of a group of nerves that are part of the parasympathetic nervous system. These drugs may decrease the activity of your GI tract, dilate your pupils or speed up your heart.
- ☐ Some of the following adverse effects may occur:
  - *Dry mouth, difficulty swallowing*: Frequent mouth care will help to remove dried secretions and keep the mouth fresh. Taking lots of fluids with meals (unless you are on fluid restriction) will help swallowing.
  - *Blurred vision, sensitivity to light*: If your vision is blurred, avoid driving, operating hazardous machinery, or doing close work that requires attention to detail until your vision returns to normal. Dark glasses will help protect your eyes from the light.
  - *Retention of urine*: Take the drug just after you have emptied your bladder. Moderate your fluid intake while the drug's effects are the highest; if possible, take the drug before bedtime, when this effect will not be a problem.
  - *Constipation*: Include fluid and fibre in your diet. Monitor your bowel movements so that appropriate laxatives can be taken if necessary.
  - *Flushing, intolerance to heat, decreased sweating*: This drug blocks sweating, which is your body's way

Antimuscarinic Drugs and Heart Disease *(continued)*

of cooling off. This places you at increased risk of heat stroke. Avoid extremes of temperature, dress coolly on very warm days and avoid exercise as much as possible.

- Report any of the following to your health care provider: *eye pain, skin rash, fever, rapid heart beat, chest pain, difficulty breathing and agitation or mood changes* (a dosage adjustment may help alleviate this problem).

☐ Avoid the use of over-the-counter medications, especially for sleep; avoid antihistamines. These products may contain drugs that cause similar antimuscarinic effects, which could cause a severe reaction. Consult with your health care provider if you feel that you need medication for symptomatic relief.

☐ Tell any doctor, nurse or other health care provider involved in your care that you are taking these drugs.

☐ Keep this drug, and all medications, out of the reach of children. Do not share these drugs with other people.

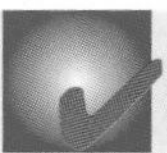

CHECK YOUR UNDERSTANDING

Answers to the questions in this chapter may be found in the Answer Key in the back of the book.

Multiple Choice

Select the most appropriate answer to the following.

1. Antimuscarinic drugs are used
   a. to block the parasympathetic system to allow the sympathetic system to dominate.
   b. to block the parasympathetic system, which is commonly hyperactive.
   c. as the drugs of choice for treating ulcers.
   d. to stimulate GI activity.

2. Atropine and hyoscine work by blocking
   a. nicotinic receptors only.
   b. muscarinic and nicotinic receptors.
   c. muscarinic receptors only.
   d. adrenergic receptors to allow cholinergic receptors to dominate.

3. Teaching patients who are taking antimuscarinic drugs would *not* include
   a. encouraging the patient to void before dosing.
   b. a bowel programme to deal with constipation.
   c. encouragement to suck ice to avoid the discomfort of dry mouth.
   d. exercise measures to increase the heart rate.

Extended Matching Questions

Select **all** that apply.

1. A nurse would expect atropine to be used for which of the following?
   a. To depress salivation
   b. To dry up bronchial secretions
   c. To increase the heart rate
   d. To promote uterine contractions
   e. To treat myasthenia gravis
   f. To treat Alzheimer's disease

2. Remembering that antimuscarinics block the effects of the parasympathetic nervous system, the nurse would question an order for an antimuscarinic drug for patients with which of the following conditions?
   a. Ulcerative colitis
   b. Asthma
   c. Bradycardia
   d. Inner ear imbalance
   e. Angle-closure glaucoma
   f. Prostatic hyperplasia

Fill in the Blanks

1. Antimuscarinic drugs block the effects of _______________ at cholinergic receptor sites.

2. Antimuscarinic drugs are also called _______________ drugs because they block the effects of the parasympathetic nervous system.

3. Blocking the parasympathetic system causes the following effects: ____________________ in heart rate, ____________________ in GI activity and in urinary bladder tone and function, pupil dilation and cycloplegia.

4. These drugs also block cholinergic receptors in the CNS and those sympathetic postganglionic receptors that are cholinergic, including those that cause ____.

5. ______________ is the prevention of accommodation of the lens for near vision.

6. Relaxation of the pupil of the eye is called a(n) ______________ effect.

7. Patients receiving antimuscarinic drugs must be monitored for problems related to eating because of the adverse effects of ______________________ and ______________________.

Bibliography

British Medical Association and Royal Pharmaceutical Society of Great Britain. (2008). *British National Formulary*. London: BMJ & RPS Publishing. *This publication is updated biannually: it is imperative that the most recent edition is consulted.*

British Medical Association and Royal Pharmaceutical Society of Great Britain. (2008). *British National Formulary for Children*. London: BMJ & RPS Publishing. *This publication is updated annually: it is imperative that the most recent edition is consulted.*

Ganong, W. (2005). *Review of medical physiology* (22nd ed.). New York: McGraw-Hill.

Howland, R. D., & Mycek, M. J. (2005). *Pharmacology* (3rd ed.). Philadelphia: Lippincott Williams & Wilkins.

Marieb, E. N., & Hoehn, K. (2009). *Human anatomy & histology* (8th ed.). San Francisco: Pearson.

Porth, C. M., & Matfin, G. (2008). *Pathophysiology: Concepts of altered health states* (8th ed.). Philadelphia: Lippincott Williams & Wilkins.

Rang, H. P., Dale, M. M., Ritter, J. M., & Flower, R. J. (2007). *Rang and Dale's pharmacology* (6th ed.). Philadelphia: Churchill Livingstone.

Simonsen, T., Aarbakke, J., Kay, I., Coleman, I., Sinnott, P., & Lysaa, R. (2006). *Illustrated pharmacology for nurses.* London: Hodder Arnold.

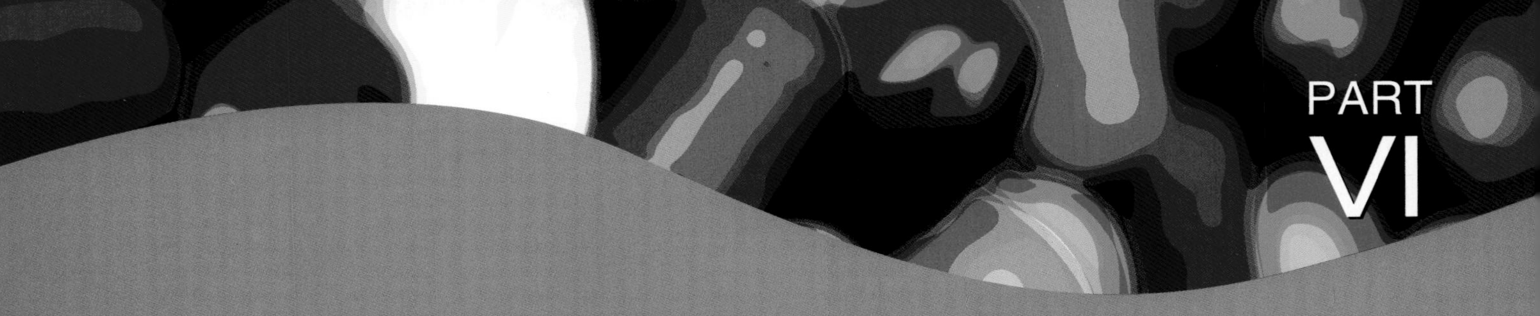

PART VI

Drugs Acting on the Endocrine System

CHAPTER 33

Introduction to the Endocrine System

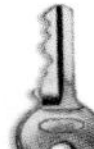

KEY TERMS

anterior pituitary
diurnal rhythm
hormones
hypothalamic–pituitary axis (HPA)
hypothalamus
inhibiting hormones
negative feedback
neuroendocrine system
pituitary gland
positive feedback
posterior pituitary
releasing hormones

LEARNING OBJECTIVES

Upon completion of this chapter, you will be able to:

1. Label a diagram showing the glands of the traditional endocrine system and list the hormones produced by each.
2. Describe mechanisms of hormone action.
3. Discuss the role of the hypothalamus as the master gland of the endocrine system, including influences on the actions of the hypothalamus.
4. Outline a negative feedback system within the endocrine system and explain the ways by which this system controls hormone levels in the body and compare this with a positive feedback mechanism.
5. Describe the hypothalamic–pituitary axis (HPA) and what would happen if a hormone level were altered within the HPA.

The nervous system and the endocrine system work together to maintain internal homeostasis and to integrate the body's response to the external and internal environments. Their activities and functions are so closely related that they are often referred to as the **neuroendocrine system**. However, this section deals with drugs affecting the 'traditional' endocrine system, which includes glands that secrete **hormones**, or chemical messengers, directly into the bloodstream to communicate with other tissues in the body. Some hormones that influence body functioning are not secreted by endocrine glands, and many tissues in the body produce hormones. For example, prostaglandins are produced in various tissues and have effects at their local site. Neurotransmitters, such as noradrenaline and dopamine, are catecholamines that are often referred to as hormones because they are secreted directly from the adrenal medulla into the bloodstream for distribution throughout the body. There are also many gastrointestinal (GI) hormones that are produced in enteroendocrine cells and act locally.

Hormones

Hormones are chemical messengers that are produced in the body and have the following characteristics; they:

- are produced in very small amounts.
- are secreted into the extracellular fluid either around cells or into the bloodstream.
- travel via the blood and act on specific receptor sites on cells or in cells throughout the body or they may act on cells in the local environment.
- act to increase or decrease the normal metabolic processes of cells when they react with their specific receptor sites.

There are three types of hormones: amino acid based such as thyroxine and peptides or proteins such as insulin, steroids such as oestrogen and lipids such as prostaglandins. Each type acts on the cell in a slightly different way to exert its actions. Peptide hormones act on specific receptors on the cell membrane to stimulate the nucleotide cyclic adenosine monophosphate (cAMP) within the cell to cause an effect. For example, insulin reacts with an insulin receptor site, it activates intracellular enzymes that cause many effects, including changing the cell membrane's permeability to glucose. Hormones such as insulin that do not enter the cell act very quickly, often within seconds, to produce an effect.

Steroid hormones, such as oestrogen, made from cholesterol, can pass through the cell membrane and actually enter the cell. They react with a cytoplasmic or nuclear receptor inside the cell to turn genes on or off and affect the cellular function. These hormones are slower acting and they may take hours/days or even longer to produce an effect. For example, the full effects of oestrogen may not be seen for months to years, as evidenced by the changes that occur at puberty. Amine hormones such as thyroxine act in a similar way to peptide and steroid hormones, some amines act on cell membrane receptors, others may act on cytoplasmic receptors or in the mitochondria. The neuroendocrine system tightly regulates the body's processes within a narrow range of normal limits; overproduction or underproduction of any hormone can affect the body's activities and other hormones within the system.

The Hypothalamus

The **hypothalamus** is responsible for coordinating the nervous and endocrine responses to internal and external stimuli. The hypothalamus constantly monitors the body's homeostasis by analysing input from the periphery and the central nervous system (CNS) and coordinating responses through the autonomic, endocrine and nervous systems. It can be as seen the 'master gland' of the neuroendocrine system.

Situated at the base of the forebrain, the hypothalamus receives input from virtually all other areas of the brain, including the limbic system and the cerebral cortex. The hypothalamus is located in an area of the brain that is poorly protected by the blood–brain barrier, so it is able to act as a sensor to various electrolytes, chemicals and hormones that are in circulation and do not affect other areas of the brain. The hypothalamus has various neurological centres that regulate a number of body functions, including body temperature, thirst, hunger, water retention, sleep and waking, blood pressure, respiration, reproduction and emotional reactions.

The hypothalamus maintains internal homeostasis by sensing blood composition and by stimulating or suppressing endocrine, autonomic and CNS activity. In essence, it can turn the autonomic nervous system and its effects on or off. The hypothalamus also produces and secretes a number of **releasing hormones or factors** that stimulate the anterior pituitary gland to release hormones stimulating other endocrine glands throughout the body (Figure 33.1). These releasing hormones include growth hormone-releasing hormone (GHRH), thyrotrophic-releasing hormone (TRH), gonadotrophic-releasing hormone (GnRH), corticotrophic-releasing hormone (CRH) and prolactin (PRL)-releasing hormone (PRH). The hypothalamus also produces two **inhibiting hormones** that act as regulators to prevent the production of hormones when levels become too high: GH release-inhibiting hormone (somatostatin) and PRL-inhibiting hormone (PIH) (Table 33.1).

The hypothalamus produces two other hormones, antidiuretic hormone (ADH – *also known as vasopressin*) and oxytocin, which are stored in the posterior pituitary gland to be released when stimulated by the hypothalamus. The hypothalamus is connected to the pituitary gland by two networks: a vascular network carries the hypothalamic

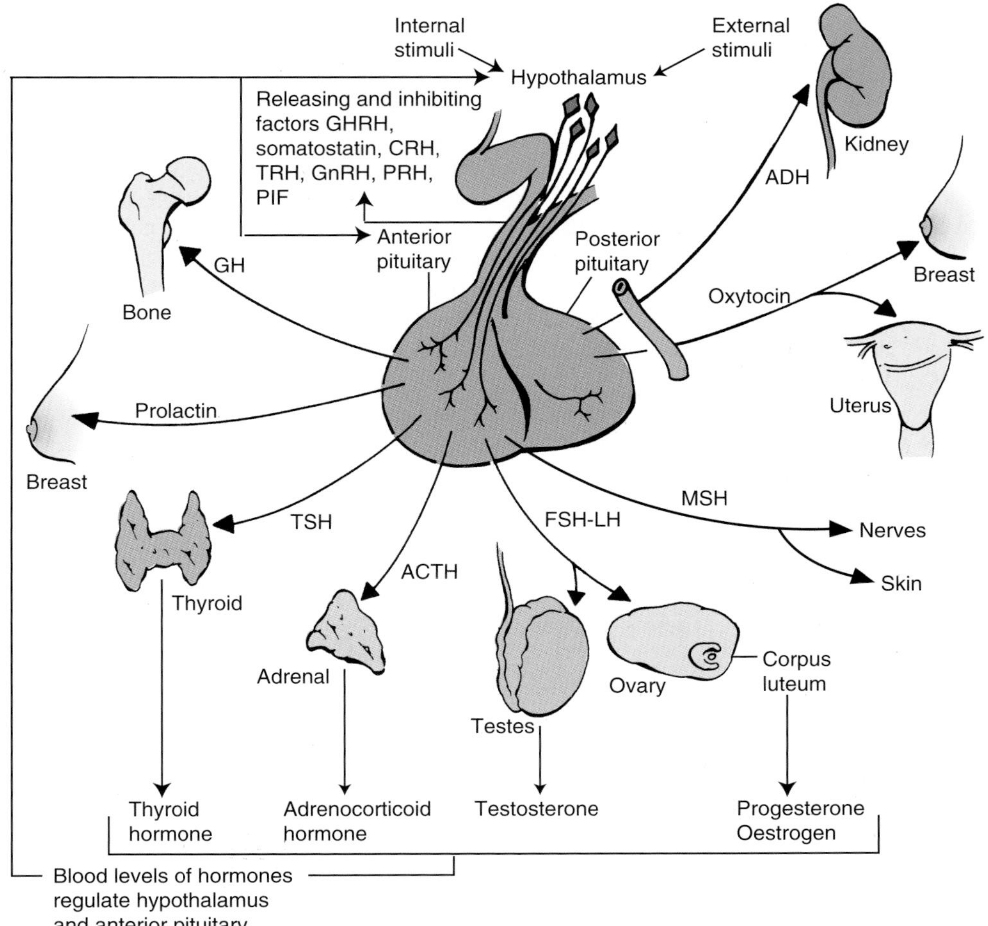

FIGURE 33.1 The traditional endocrine system.

Table 33.1 DRUGS IN FOCUS

Hypothalamic Releasing and Inhibiting Hormones and Associated Anterior Pituitary and Endocrine Gland Response

Hypothalamus Hormones	Anterior Pituitary Hormones	Target Organ Response
Stimulating Hormones		
Corticotrophin-releasing hormone (CRH)	Adrenocorticotrophic hormone (ACTH)	Adrenal corticosteroid hormones
Thyroid-releasing hormone (TRH)	TSH (thyroid-stimulating hormone)	Thyroid hormone
Growth hormone-releasing hormone (GHRH)	GH (growth hormone)	Cell growth
Gonadotrophic-releasing hormone (GnRH)	LH and FSH (luteinizing hormone, follicle-stimulating hormone)	Oestrogen and progesterone (females) testosterone (males)
Prolactin-releasing hormone (PRH)	Prolactin	Milk production
Inhibiting Hormones		
Somatostatin (growth hormone-inhibiting factor)		Stops release of GH
Prolactin-inhibiting factors (PIF)		Stops release of prolactin

releasing factors directly into the anterior pituitary, and a neurological network delivers ADH and oxytocin to the posterior pituitary gland to be stored.

The Pituitary Gland

The **pituitary gland** is located below the hypothalamus, is divided into three lobes: an anterior lobe, a posterior lobe and an intermediate lobe.

The Anterior Pituitary Gland or Adenohypophysis

The **anterior pituitary gland** produces a number of hormones. These include GH, adrenocorticotrophic hormone (ACTH), follicle-stimulating hormone (FSH), luteinizing hormone (LH), PRL and thyroid-stimulating hormone (TSH) – see Figure 33.1. These hormones are essential for the regulation of growth, reproduction and some metabolic processes. Deficiency or overproduction of these hormones disrupts this regulation.

The anterior pituitary hormones are released in a rhythmic manner into the bloodstream. Their secretion varies with time of day (often referred to as **diurnal rhythm**) or with physiological conditions such as exercise or sleep. Their release is affected by activity in the CNS, by hypothalamic hormones, by hormones of the peripheral endocrine glands, by certain diseases that can alter endocrine functioning and by a variety of drugs, which can directly or indirectly upset the homeostasis in the body and cause an endocrine response.

The anterior pituitary gland also produces melanocyte-stimulating hormones (MSHs) and lipotropins. MSH plays an important role in animals that use skin colour changes as an adaptive mechanism. It also might be important for nerve growth and development in humans and can cause skin to darken and play a role in appetite control. Lipotropins stimulate fat mobilization but have not been clearly isolated in humans.

The Posterior Pituitary Gland: Neurohypophysis

The **posterior pituitary** stores two hormones that are produced by the hypothalamus and deposited in the posterior lobe in the endings of the nerve axons where they are produced. These two hormones are ADH, also referred to as vasopressin, and oxytocin. ADH is directly released in response to increased plasma osmolarity or decreased blood volume (which often results in increased osmolarity). The osmoreceptors in the hypothalamus stimulate the release of ADH. ADH also causes vasoconstriction of the blood vessels. Oxytocin stimulates smooth muscle in the uterus resulting in the birth of a baby and in the breast causing milk ejection in lactating women.

The Intermediate Lobe

In humans, the intermediate lobe of the pituitary gland is not a distinct lobe. It consists of some cells at the borders of the anterior and posterior lobes. These cells produce endorphins and enkephalins, which are released in response to severe pain or stress and which occupy specific endorphin receptor sites in the brainstem to block the perception of pain. Nerve cells releasing endogenous opiates are not restricted to the pituitary gland but are widespread throughout the nervous system. These hormones are also produced in tissues in the periphery and in other areas of the brain. They are released in response to overactivity of pain nerves, sympathetic stimulation, transcutaneous stimulation (TENS) and vigorous exercise.

Controls

Hypothalamic–Pituitary Axis

The hypothalamus and the pituitary glands function closely to maintain endocrine activity along what is called the **hypothalamic–pituitary axis (HPA)** using a series of **negative feedback** systems.

When the hypothalamus senses a need for a particular hormone, for example thyroid hormone, it secretes the thyrotropin-releasing hormone TRH into a capillary portal system connected to the anterior pituitary. In response to the TRH, the anterior pituitary secretes TSH, which in turn stimulates the thyroid gland to produce thyroid hormone. When the hypothalamus senses the rising levels of thyroid hormone in the blood, it stops secreting TRH, resulting in decreased TSH production and subsequently reduced thyroid hormone levels. The hypothalamus, sensing the falling thyroid hormone levels, secretes TRH again. The negative feedback system continues in this fashion, maintaining the levels of thyroid hormone within a relatively narrow range of normal levels (Figure 33.2).

Two of the anterior pituitary hormones (GH and PRL) are not regulated by the same type of feedback mechanism. GH release and PRL release are directly inhibited by the hypothalamic inhibiting hormones somatostatin and PRL inhibiting factor PIH, respectively. The hypothalamus may be stimulated to release inhibiting factors by increased circulating levels of hormones or by mediating factors that are stimulated by these hormones. The HPA functions constantly to keep these particular hormones regulated.

Both PRL and GH are regulated by inhibiting and releasing factors. The only known role for PRL in humans is to stimulate the production of milk in the breast.

Other Controls

Hormones, other than stimulating hormones, are also released in response to stimuli. For example, the endocrine

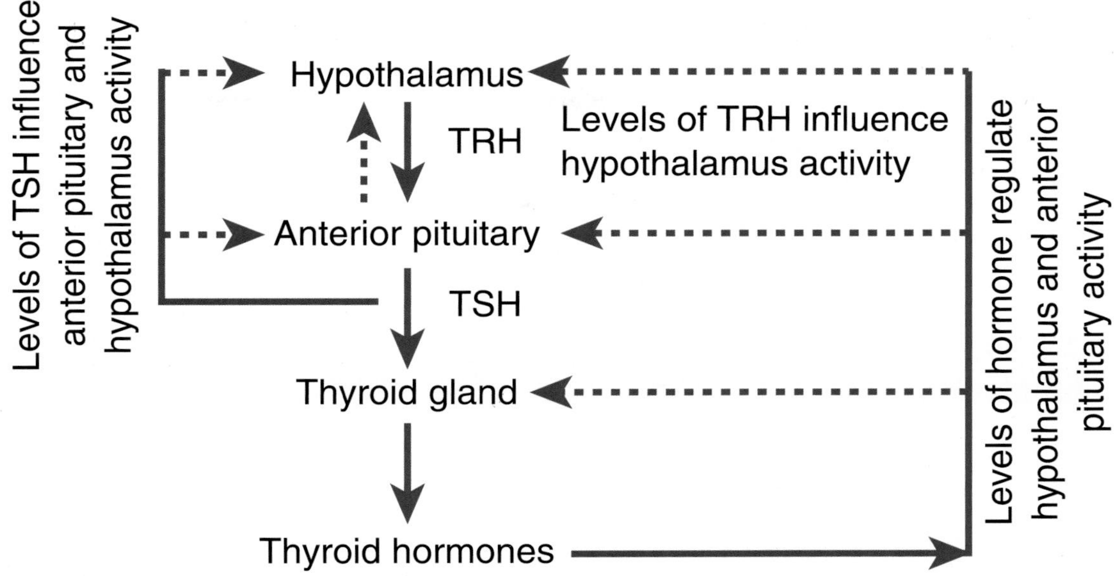

FIGURE 33.2 Negative feedback system. Thyroid hormone levels are regulated by a series of negative feedback systems influencing thyrotropin-releasing hormone (TRH), thyrotropin (TSH) and thyroid hormone levels.

pancreas produces and releases insulin, glucagon and somatostatin from different cells in response to varying blood glucose levels. The parathyroid glands release parathyroid hormone (PTH) in response to calcium levels in the blood. The juxta glomerular cells in the kidney release erythropoietin EPO in response to decreased pressure or decreased oxygenation of the blood flowing into the glomerulus. GI hormones are released in response to local stimuli in the area, such as acid, proteins or calcium or food. The thyroid gland produces and secretes another hormone, called calcitonin, in direct response to serum calcium levels. Many different prostaglandins are released throughout the body in response to local stimuli in the tissues that produce them. Activation of the sympathetic nervous system directly causes release of ACTH and the adrenal hormones to prepare the body for fight or flight. Aldosterone, an adrenocorticoid hormone, is released in response to ACTH but also is released directly in response to low sodium or high potassium levels.

A few situations such as the birth of a baby, breast-feeding and blood clotting are regulated by **positive feedback**. In positive feedback, the end result, for example pressure of the baby's head on the cervix during birth, increases the stimulus from the hypothalamus. Positive feedback moves the body away from homeostasis, so, apart from these examples, positive feedback generally has a deleterious effect on the body, for example untreated shock is an example of positive feedback.

When administering any drug that affects the endocrine or nervous systems, it is important for the nurse to remember how closely related all of these activities are. Expected or unexpected adverse effects involving areas of the endocrine and nervous systems can occur frequently.

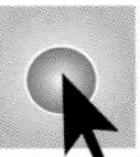

WEB LINK

Health care providers and patients may want to consult the following Internet sources:

http://www.nice.org.uk The National Institute for Health and Clinical Excellence (NICE) is an independent organization responsible for providing national guidance on promoting good health and preventing and treating ill health.

Points to Remember

- The endocrine system is a regulatory system that communicates through the use of hormones.
- The endocrine and nervous systems are connected in the regulation of body homeostasis; they are often referred to as the neuroendocrine system.
- A hormone is a chemical messenger that is produced within the body, is needed in only small amounts and travels to specific receptor sites to cause an increase or decrease in cellular activity.
- The action of hormones may last minutes to days.
- The hypothalamus can be called the 'master gland' of the neuroendocrine system. It helps regulate the central and autonomic nervous systems and the endocrine system to maintain homeostasis.
- The pituitary is made up of two lobes: anterior and posterior. The anterior lobe produces stimulating hormones in response to hypothalamic stimulation. The posterior lobe stores two hormones produced by the hypothalamus, ADH and oxytocin. The cells inbetween,

which form the intermediate lobe in some animals, produce a large precursor molecule from which ACTH, the MSHs form as well as endorphins and enkephalins that modulate pain perception.

- The hypothalamus and pituitary operate by a series of negative feedback mechanisms called the HPA. The hypothalamus secretes releasing hormones to cause the anterior pituitary gland to release stimulating hormones; this stimulation shuts down the production of releasing factors, which leads to decreased stimulating factors and, subsequently, decreased hormone release.
- Some hormones are not influenced by the HPA and are released in response to direct, local stimulation.
- When any drug that affects either the endocrine or the nervous system is given, adverse effects may occur throughout both systems because they are closely interrelated.

CHECK YOUR UNDERSTANDING

Answers to the questions in this chapter may be found in the Answer Key in the back of the book.

Multiple Choice

Select the most appropriate response to the following.

1. Aldosterone
   a. causes the loss of sodium and water from the renal tubules.
   b. is under direct hormonal control from the hypothalamus.
   c. is released into the bloodstream in response to angiotensin I.
   d. is released into the bloodstream in response to low sodium levels.

2. Antidiuretic hormone (ADH)
   a. is produced by the anterior pituitary.
   b. causes the retention of water by the kidneys.
   c. is released by the hypothalamus.
   d. causes the retention of sodium by the kidneys.

3. The endocrine glands
   a. form part of the communication system of the body.
   b. cannot be stimulated by hormones circulating in the blood.
   c. are always controlled by the autonomic nervous system.
   d. are all controlled by the hypothalamus.

4. The hypothalamus maintains internal homeostasis and could be considered the master endocrine gland because
   a. it releases stimulating hormones that cause endocrine glands to inhibit release of their hormones.
   b. no hormone-releasing gland responds unless stimulated by the hypothalamus.
   c. it secretes releasing hormones that are an important part of the hypothalamic–pituitary axis that finely regulates the traditional endocrine system.
   d. it regulates urination and bladder control as well as hormone release.

5. The posterior lobe of the pituitary gland
   a. secretes a number of stimulating hormones.
   b. produces endorphins to modulate pain perception.
   c. has no function that has yet been identified.
   d. stores ADH and oxytocin, which are produced in the hypothalamus.

6. An example of a negative feedback system would be
   a. blood clotting.
   b. PRL control.
   c. MSH control.
   d. thyroid hormone control.

7. Internal body homeostasis and communication are regulated by the
   a. cardiovascular and respiratory systems.
   b. nervous and cardiovascular systems.
   c. endocrine and nervous systems.
   d. endocrine and cardiovascular systems.

Extended Matching Questions

Select all that apply.

1. Hormones exert their influence on human cells by influencing which of the following?
   a. Enzyme-controlled reactions.
   b. Messenger RNA.
   c. Lysosome activity.
   d. Transcription RNA.
   e. Cellular DNA.
   f. Cyclic AMP activity.

2. The specific criteria that define a hormone would include which of the following?
   a. It is produced in very small amounts.
   b. It is secreted directly into the extracellular fluid.
   c. It is slowly metabolized in the liver and lungs.
   d. It reacts with a very specific receptor set on a target cell.
   e. A mechanism is always available to immediately destroy it.
   f. It can change a cell's basic function.

3. Some endocrine glands do not respond to the hypothalamic–pituitary axis. These glands would include the
   a. thyroid gland.
   b. ovaries.
   c. parathyroid glands.
   d. adrenal cortex.
   e. endocrine pancreas.
   f. GI gastrin-secreting cells.

Matching

Match the anterior pituitary hormone with the endocrine response it elicits.

1. ____________________ACTH
2. ____________________GH
3. ____________________PRL
4. ____________________TSH
5. ____________________FSH
6. ____________________LH
7. ____________________MSH
8. ____________________lipoproteins

A. Production of thyroid hormone
B. Stimulation of fat mobilization
C. Stimulation of ovulation
D. Release of cortisol, aldosterone
E. Nerve growth and development
F. Milk production in the mammary glands
G. Stimulation of follicle development in the ovaries
H. Protein catabolism and cell growth

Bibliography

British Medical Association and Royal Pharmaceutical Society of Great Britain. (2008). *British National Formulary*. London: BMJ & RPS Publishing. *This publication is updated biannually: it is imperative that the most recent edition is consulted.*

Ganong, W. (2005). *Review of medical physiology* (22nd ed.). New York: McGraw-Hill.

Howland, R. D., & Mycek, M. J. (2005). *Pharmacology* (3rd ed.). Philadelphia: Lippincott Williams & Wilkins.

Marieb, E. N., & Hoehn, K. (2007). *Human anatomy & physiology* (7th ed.). San Francisco: Pearson Benjamin Cummings.

Porth, C. M., & Matfin, G. (2008). *Pathophysiology: Concepts of altered health states* (8th ed.). Philadelphia: Lippincott Williams & Wilkins.

CHAPTER 34

Hypothalamic and Pituitary Agents

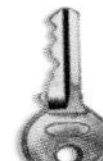

KEY TERMS

acromegaly
diabetes insipidus
gigantism
hypopituitarism

LEARNING OBJECTIVES

Upon completion of this chapter, you will be able to:

1. Describe the anatomical and physiological relationship between the hypothalamus and the pituitary gland and list the hormones produced by each.
2. Describe the therapeutic actions, indications, pharmacokinetics associated with the hypothalamic and pituitary agents.
3. Describe the contraindications, most common adverse reactions and important drug–drug interactions associated with the hypothalamic and pituitary agents.
4. Discuss the use of hypothalamic and pituitary agents across the lifespan.
5. Compare and contrast the key drugs somatropin and vasopressin with other hypothalamic and pituitary agents.
6. Outline the nursing considerations, including important teaching points, for patients receiving a hypothalamic or pituitary agent.

HYPOTHALAMIC RELEASING HORMONES

ganirelix
gonadorelin
goserelin
nafarelin

ANTERIOR PITUITARY HORMONES

chorionic gonadotrophin
corticotrophin
menotropins
somatropin
thyrotropin

GROWTH HORMONE ANTAGONISTS

bromocriptine
pegvisomant

DOPAMINERGIC DRUGS

octreotide acetate

POSTERIOR PITUITARY HORMONES

desmopressin
vasopressin (ADH)
oxytocin

The function of the endocrine system is to maintain homeostasis. This is achieved through a complex balance of glandular activities that either stimulate or suppress hormone release. Too much or too little hormone release can lead to various disorders and interfere with the normal functioning of other endocrine glands. The drugs presented in this chapter are those used to either replace or interact with the hormones produced by the hypothalamus and pituitary gland.

Hypothalamic Releasing Hormones

The hypothalamus produces a number of releasing hormones to stimulate or inhibit the release of hormones from the anterior pituitary. These releasing hormones are:

- Growth hormone-releasing hormone (GHRH)
- Thyrotrophin-releasing hormone (TRH)
- Gonadotrophin-releasing hormone (GnRH)
- Corticotrophin-releasing hormone (CRH)
- Prolactin-releasing hormone (PRH).

The hypothalamus also releases two inhibiting hormones:

- Somatostatin (GH-inhibiting hormone) and
- Prolactin-inhibiting hormone (PIH).

Note: not all of the hypothalamic hormones are used as pharmacological agents.

CRH stimulates the release of adrenocorticotrophic hormone (ACTH) from the anterior pituitary and is used to diagnose Cushing's disease (a condition characterized by hypersecretion of adrenocortical hormones in response to excessive ACTH release or a tumour of the adrenal cortex where ACTH levels would be low). Gonadorelin is a GnRH analogue that is used for diagnostic purposes to assess pituitary function. It may also be used in the treatment of endometriosis and infertility.

Goserelin is also an analogue of GnRH. After an initial burst of follicle-stimulating hormone (FSH) and luteinizing hormone (LH) release, goserelin inhibits pituitary gonadotrophin secretion with a resultant drop in the production of the sex hormones. This drug currently is used as an antineoplastic agent to treat prostatic cancers.

Ganirelix is an example of a GnRH antagonist. Therefore, it inhibits the release of LH and FSH. It is used during fertility treatment in women undergoing controlled ovarian stimulation.

Nafarelin is a potent agonist of GnRH and is used to decrease the production of hormones from the gonads through repeated stimulation of their receptor sites. After about 4 weeks of therapy, gonadal hormone levels fall. This drug is used to treat endometriosis and precocious puberty. It is also used before the induction of ovulation for in vitro fertilization (IVF) treatment.

BOX 34.1 DRUG THERAPY ACROSS THE LIFESPAN

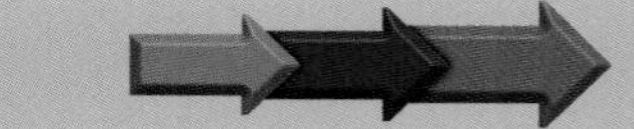

Hypothalamic and Pituitary Agents

CHILDREN

Children who receive any of the hypothalamic or pituitary agents need to be monitored closely for adverse effects associated with changes in overall endocrine function, particularly growth and development and metabolism. Periodic radiograph of the long bones as well as monitoring of blood glucose levels and electrolytes should be a standard part of the treatment plan. Children receiving GH pose many challenges. Children who are using desmopressin for diabetes insipidus need to have the administration technique monitored and should have an adult responsible for the overall treatment protocol.

When administering any drug to children, always consult the most recent edition of the British National Formulary (BNF) for Children

ADULTS

Adults also need frequent monitoring of electrolytes and blood sugar levels when receiving any of these agents. Adults using nasal forms of desmopressin to control diabetes insipidus should review the proper administration of the drug with the primary care provider periodically; inappropriate administration can lead to complications and lack of therapeutic effect. Adults receiving regular injections of these drugs should learn the proper storage, preparation and administration of the drug, including rotation of injection sites.

These drugs should not be used during pregnancy or lactation unless the benefit to the mother clearly outweighs any risk to the foetus or neonate.

OLDER ADULTS

Older adults may be more susceptible to the imbalances associated with alterations in the endocrine system. They should be evaluated periodically during treatment for hydration and nutrition as well as for electrolyte balance. Proper administration technique should be reviewed, and nasal mucus membranes should be evaluated regularly, because older patients are more apt to develop dehydrated membranes and possibly ulceration, leading to improper dosing of drugs delivered nasally.

Sermorelin (GHRH) stimulates the production of GH by the anterior pituitary. It is used for diagnostic purposes in children with short stature to determine the presence of hypothalamic or pituitary dysfunction. It is also used to evaluate the therapeutic response in patients undergoing surgery or irradiation and to treat idiopathic GH deficiency in children less than 8 years of age. It may be used with gonadotrophin to induce ovulation and to treat cachexia associated with acquired immune deficiency syndrome (AIDS).

Nursing Considerations for Patients Receiving Hypothalamic Releasing Factors

The specific nursing care of the patient who is receiving a hypothalamic releasing hormone is related to the hormone (or hormones) that the drug is affecting (see Chapter 35 for adrenocorticoid hormones, Chapter 36 for thyroid hormones and Chapters 39 and 40 for sex hormones).

Establish if patient is currently taking other medications or herbal therapies which may potentially interact with hypothalamic releasing factors.

Anterior Pituitary Hormones

Agents that affect pituitary function are used mainly to mimic or antagonize the effects of specific pituitary hormones. They may be used either as replacement therapy for conditions resulting from a hypoactive pituitary or for diagnostic purposes.

Chorionic gonadotrophin acts like LH and stimulates the production of testosterone and progesterone. It is used to treat hypogonadism in males, to induce ovulation in females with functioning ovaries and to treat prepubertal cryptorchism (*undescended testes*) when there is no anatomical obstruction to testicular movement.

- Corticotropin or ACTH is used for diagnostic purposes to test adrenal function and responsiveness. It stimulates steroid release from the adrenal cortex and therefore has anti-inflammatory effects; it also is used to treat various inflammatory disorders.
- Menotropins is a purified preparation of gonadotrophins. It is used as a fertility drug to stimulate ovulation in women and spermatogenesis in men. It contains a mixture of LH and FSH in a ratio of 1:1.
- Somatropin is a synthesized GH that is produced with the use of recombinant DNA technology. It is used in the treatment of children with growth failure, girls with Turner's syndrome and cachexia associated with AIDS and GH deficiency in adults.
- Thyrotropin is equivalent to TSH and is used as a diagnostic agent to evaluate thyroid function.

In clinical practice, the agent that is used purely as a replacement for anterior pituitary hormones is that acting as GH – somatropin.

Growth Hormone

GH is responsible for linear skeletal growth, the growth of internal organs and protein synthesis. **Hypopituitarism** is often seen as GH deficiency before any other signs and symptoms occur. Hypopituitarism may occur as a result of developmental abnormalities or congenital defects of the pituitary, circulatory disturbances (e.g. haemorrhage, infarction), acute or chronic inflammation of the pituitary and pituitary tumours. GH deficiency in children results in short stature. Adults with somatropin deficiency syndrome (SDS) may have hypopituitarism as a result of pituitary tumours or trauma, or they may have been treated for GH deficiency as children, resulting in a shutdown of the pituitary production of somatotropin.

GH deficiency was once treated with GH injections extracted from the pituitary glands of cadavers. The supply of GH was therefore rather limited and costly and dangerous. Synthetic human GH is now available from recombinant DNA sources using genetic engineering. Synthetic GH is expensive, but it is thought to be safer than cadaver GH and is being used increasingly to treat GH deficiencies. Somatropin is the only GH replacement drug in use today.

Therapeutic Actions and Indications

As noted, somatropin is a hormone of recombinant DNA origin that is equivalent to human GH. Somatropin is indicated for the treatment of growth failure due to lack of GH or due to chronic renal failure for long-term treatment of growth failure in children born small for gestational age who do not achieve catch-up growth by 2 years of age and for the treatment of short stature associated with Turner's syndrome, a genetic disorder affecting the X chromosome. It is also approved to increase protein production and growth in various AIDS-related states.

Pharmacokinetics

Somatropin is injected and reaches peak levels within 7 hours. It is widely distributed in the body and localizes in highly perfused tissues, particularly the liver and kidney. Excretion occurs through the urine and faeces. Patients with liver or renal dysfunction may experience reduced clearance and increased concentrations of the drug. This drug should be avoided in pregnancy and lactation because of the potential for adverse effects on the foetus or neonate.

Contraindications and Cautions

Somatropin is contraindicated with any known allergy to the drug or ingredients in the drug. It is also contraindicated in the presence of closed epiphyses or with underlying cranial lesions.

Always consult the most recent edition of the BNF for all contraindications and interactions.

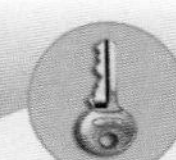

Key Drug Summary: *Somatropin*

Indications: Long-term treatment of children with growth failure associated with various deficiencies, girls with Turner's syndrome, AIDS wasting and cachexia, severe GH deficiency in adults; treatment of growth failure in children of small gestational age who do not achieve catch-up growth by 2 years of age

Actions: Replaces human GH; stimulates skeletal growth, growth of internal organs and protein synthesis

Pharmacokinetics:

Route	Onset	Peak
IM, Subcut	Varies	5–7.5 h

$T_{1/2}$: 15–50 min; metabolized in the liver and excreted in the urine and faeces

Adverse effects: Development of antibodies to GH, insulin resistance, swelling, joint pain, headache, injection site pain and breakdown of subcutaneous tissue at injection site.

Adverse Effects

The adverse effects that most often occur when using GH include breakdown of the subcutaneous tissue resulting in skin depressions at injection sites, the development of antibodies to GH and subsequent signs of inflammation and autoimmune-type reactions; swelling and joint pain and the endocrine reactions of hypothyroidism and insulin resistance (see Box 34.2).

BOX 34.2 FOCUS ON **PATIENT SAFETY**

Growth Hormone Therapy

GH can be used to treat growth failure caused either by lack of GH or by renal failure. It also can help children with normal GH levels and who are just genetically small. Before the drug is prescribed, the child must undergo screening procedures and specific testing (including radiographs and blood tests) and must display a willingness to have regular injections.

The child's family or caregivers will need instructions on the following points:

- Storage of the drug (refrigeration is required)
- Preparation of the drug (the reconstitution procedure varies depending on the brandname product used)
- Administration of the drug (sterile technique, need to rotate injection sites and need to monitor injection sites for atrophy)

They also must be advised to report any lack of growth as well as signs of glucose intolerance (thirst, hunger, voiding pattern changes) or thyroid dysfunction (fatigue, thinning hair, slow pulse, puffy skin, intolerance to the cold).

Nursing Considerations for Patients Receiving Growth Hormone

Assessment: History and Examination

Screen for possible contraindications to the use of the drug:

- History of allergy to any GH analogue or binder
- Closed epiphyseal plates
- Underlying intracranial lesions

Include screening for baseline status;

- Height/weight
- Thyroid function tests
- Glucose tolerance tests
- GH levels

Establish if patient is currently taking other medications or herbal therapies which may potentially interact with GH.

Nursing Diagnoses

The patient receiving any GH may have the following nursing diagnoses related to drug therapy:

- Imbalanced nutrition: related to metabolic changes
- Deficient knowledge regarding drug therapy

Implementation With Rationale

- Reconstitute the drug as per manufacturer's instructions and administer intramuscularly or subcutaneously
- Monitor response carefully when beginning therapy so appropriate dosage adjustments of drug can be made if required.
- Monitor patient for any adverse effects to the drug.
- Monitor thyroid function, glucose tolerance and GH levels.
- Provide patient education, including measures to avoid adverse effects, warning signs of problems and the need for regular evaluation (including blood tests) to promote compliance.
- Instruct patient, family member or caregiver in proper preparation and administration techniques.
- As pain is common at injection sites, advice may be given on how to reduce pain, for example inject slowly, and put ice on area first.

Evaluation

- Monitor patient response to the drug (return of GH levels to normal; growth and development).
- Monitor for adverse effects (hypothyroidism, glucose intolerance, nutritional imbalance).
- Evaluate the effectiveness of the teaching plan (patient can name drug, dosage, adverse effects to watch for and specific measures to avoid adverse effects; ensure patient or family member can demonstrate proper technique for preparation and administration of drug.

Growth Hormone Antagonists

GH hypersecretion can occur at any time of life. This is often referred to as hyperpituitarism. If it occurs before the epiphyseal plates of the long bones fuse, it causes acceleration in linear skeletal growth, producing **gigantism** of 7 to 8 feet in height with fairly normal body proportions. In adults after epiphyseal closure, linear growth is impossible. Instead, hypersecretion of GH causes enlargement in the peripheral parts of the body, such as the hands and feet and the internal organs, especially the heart. **Acromegaly** is the term used to describe the onset of excessive GH secretion that occurs after puberty and epiphyseal plate closure.

Most conditions of GH hypersecretion are caused by pituitary tumours and are treated by radiation therapy or surgery. Drug therapy for GH excess can be used for those patients who are not candidates for surgery or radiation therapy. The drugs used to treat GH excess include a somatostatin (GHIH) analogue, octreotide acetate, a GH analogue: pegvisomant and a dopamine agonist: bromocriptine (see Figure 34.1).

Therapeutic Actions and Indications

Somatostatin is an inhibitory hormone released from the hypothalamus. It is not used to decrease GH levels, although it does do that very effectively. It has multiple effects on many secretory systems (e.g. it inhibits release of gastrin, glucagon and insulin) and a short duration of action: it is not desirable as a therapeutic agent. An analogue of somatostatin, octreotide acetate, is considerably more potent in inhibiting GH release with less of an inhibitory effect on insulin release. Consequently, it is used instead of somatostatin.

Bromocriptine is a dopamine agonist frequently used to treat acromegaly. It may be used alone or as an adjunct to irradiation. Dopamine agonists inhibit GH secretion in some patients with acromegaly; the opposite effect occurs in normal individuals. Bromocriptine's GH-inhibiting effect may be explained by the fact that dopamine increases somatostatin release from the hypothalamus.

Pegvisomant is a GH analogue used for the treatment of acromegaly in patients who do not respond to other therapies. It binds to GH receptors on cells, inhibiting GH effects. It must be given by daily subcutaneous injections.

Pharmacokinetics

Octreotide is rapidly absorbed and widely distributed throughout the body. It is metabolized in the tissues, and about 30% is excreted unchanged in the urine. Patients with renal dysfunction may accumulate higher levels of the drug. There are no adequate studies of effects in pregnancy and during lactation and its use should be reserved for situations in which the benefits to the mother clearly outweigh any potential risks to the foetus or neonate.

Bromocriptine is effectively absorbed from the gastrointestinal (GI) tract and undergoes extensive first-pass metabolism in the liver. It is primarily excreted in the bile. The drug should not be used during pregnancy or lactation because of effects on the foetus and because it blocks lactation.

Pegvisomant is slowly absorbed from the subcutaneous tissue, reaching peak effects in 33 to 77 hours. It is cleared from the body slowly, with a half-life of 6 days. The drug is excreted in the urine. There are no well-controlled studies in pregnancy, and pegvisomant should be used during pregnancy only if the benefit clearly outweighs the potential risk to the foetus. It is not known if pegvisomant crosses into breast milk.

Contraindications and Cautions

These drugs should be used cautiously in the presence of any other endocrine disorder (e.g. diabetes, thyroid dysfunction) and in pregnancy or lactation.

Adverse Effects

Octreotide is associated with many GI complaints because of its effects on the GI tract. Constipation or diarrhoea, flatulence and nausea are not uncommon. Octreotide has also been associated with the development of acute cholecystitis, cholestatic jaundice, biliary tract obstruction and pancreatitis. Patients must be assessed for the possible development of any of these problems. Other, less common adverse effects include headache, sinus bradycardia or other cardiac dysrhythmias and decreased glucose tolerance. Octreotide must be administered subcutaneously, and it can be associated with discomfort and/or inflammation at injection sites.

Bromocriptine is given orally and is also associated with GI disturbances. It may cause drowsiness and postural hypotension because of its dopamine-blocking effects.

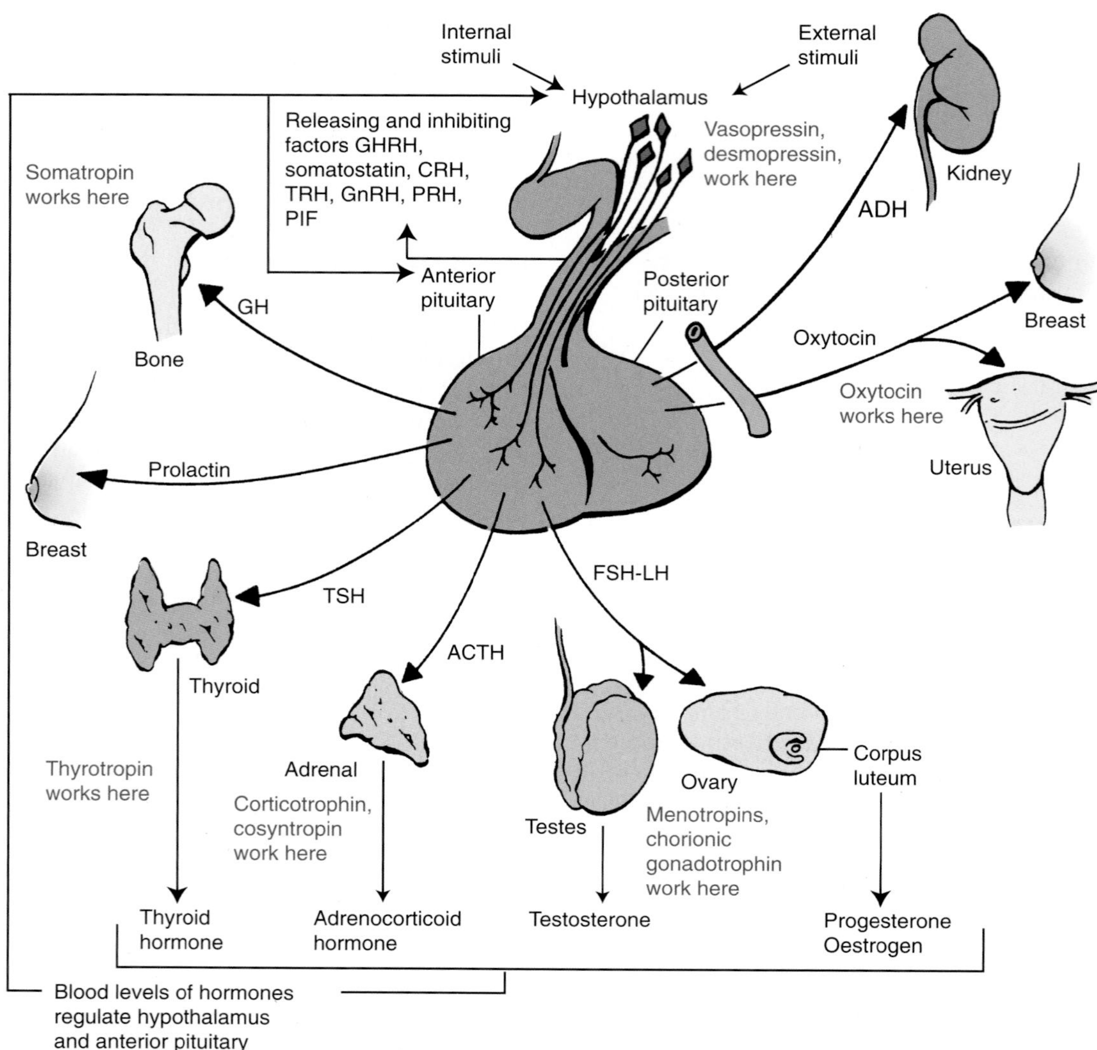

FIGURE 34.1 Sites of action of hypothalamic/pituitary agents.

It blocks lactation and should not be used by nursing mothers.

Pegvisomant is given by subcutaneous injection. Pain and inflammation at the injection site are common effects. Increased incidence of infection, nausea and diarrhoea and changes in liver function may also occur.

Clinically Important Drug–Drug Interactions

Increased serum bromocriptine levels and increased toxicity occur if this drug is combined with erythromycin. This combination should be avoided.

The effectiveness of bromocriptine may decrease if it is combined with phenothiazines. If this combination is used, the patient should be monitored carefully.

Patients receiving pegvisomant may require higher dosages to receive adequate GH suppression if they are also taking opioids. The mechanism of action of this interaction is not understood.

Always consult the most recent edition of the BNF for all contraindications and interactions.

Nursing Considerations for Patients Receiving Growth Hormone Antagonists

Assessment: History and Examination

Screen for contraindications to use of the drug:

- History of allergy
- Endocrine disturbances

- Pregnancy and lactation

Include screening for baseline status:

- Orientation, affect and reflexes
- Blood pressure, pulse and orthostatic blood pressure
- Glucose tolerance tests
- GH levels

Establish if patient is currently taking other medications or herbal therapies which may potentially interact with GH antagonists.

Nursing Diagnoses

The patient receiving any GH antagonist may have the following nursing diagnoses related to drug therapy:

- Imbalanced nutrition, related to metabolic changes
- Acute pain related to injections (octreotide, pegvisomant)
- Deficient knowledge regarding drug therapy

Implementation With Rationale

- Reconstitute octreotide and pegvisomant as per manufacturer's directions; administer these drugs subcutaneously and rotate injection sites regularly to prevent skin breakdown.
- Monitor thyroid function, glucose tolerance and GH levels.
- Arrange for baseline and periodic ultrasound evaluation of the gallbladder if using octreotide to detect any development of gallstones.
- Provide thorough patient education, including measures to avoid adverse effects, warning signs of problems and need for regular evaluation (including blood tests).
- Instruct a family member in proper preparation and administration techniques to ensure that there is another responsible person to administer the drug if needed.

Evaluation

- Monitor patient response to the drug (return of GH levels to normal, growth and development).
- Monitor for adverse effects (hypothyroidism, glucose intolerance, nutritional imbalance, GI disturbances, headache, dizziness, cholecystitis).
- Evaluate the effectiveness of the teaching plan (patient can name drug, dosage, adverse effects to watch for and specific measures to avoid adverse effects; family member can demonstrate proper technique for preparation and administration of drug).
- Monitor the effectiveness of comfort measures and concordance with the regimen.

Posterior Pituitary Hormones

The posterior pituitary stores two hormones produced in the hypothalamus: antidiuretic hormone (ADH, also known as vasopressin) and oxytocin. Oxytocin stimulates milk ejection in lactating women and stimulates uterine contractions during labour. In pharmacological doses, as syntocin, it can be used to initiate or improve uterine contractions in labour (see Chapter 39).

ADH possesses antidiuretic, vasopressor and, in very high doses, haemostatic properties. Posterior pituitary disorders that are seen clinically involve ADH release and include **diabetes insipidus**, which results from insufficient secretion and syndrome of inappropriate antidiuretic hormone (SIADH), which occurs with excessive secretion of ADH. Diabetes insipidus is characterized by the production of a large amount of dilute urine. Blood glucose levels are higher than normal, and the body responds with polyuria (increased urine production), polydipsia (increased thirst) and dehydration. Diabetes insipidus is caused by a deficiency in the amount of posterior pituitary ADH and may result from pituitary disease or injury (e.g. head trauma, surgery and tumour). The condition can be acute and short in duration, or it can be a chronic, lifelong problem.

Therapeutic Actions and Indications

ADH itself is never used as therapy for diabetes insipidus. Instead, synthetic preparations of ADH, which are purer and have fewer adverse effects, are used. The ADH preparations that are available include vasopressin, which is available in parenteral and nasal spray forms (Box 34.3) and desmopressin (see Figure 34.1). The drug of choice depends on the individual response to the drug and the patient's ability or willingness to use a particular dosage form.

ADH is released in response to an increase in plasma osmolality and/or decrease in blood volume. It produces its antidiuretic activity in the kidneys, causing the cortical and medullary parts of the collecting duct to become permeable to water, thereby increasing water reabsorption into the

BOX 34.3 FOCUS ON **CLINICAL SKILLS**

Administering a Nasal Spray

Instruct the patient to sit upright and press a finger over one nostril to close it. Then, with the spray bottle held upright, have the patient place the tip of the bottle about 1.5 cm into the open nostril. A firm squeeze should deliver the drug to the desired mucosal area for absorption. Caution the patient not to use excessive force and not to tip the head back because these actions could result in ineffective administration.

circulation and decreasing urine formation. These activities reduce plasma osmolality and increase blood volume.

The ADH preparations that are available are indicated for the treatment of neurogenic diabetes insipidus. Desmopressin is also indicated for the treatment of haemophilia A and von Willebrand's disease and it is used as a nasal spray for the treatment of nocturnal enuresis (bed wetting).

Pharmacokinetics

Synthetic preparations of these drugs are rapidly absorbed and metabolized; they are excreted in the liver and kidneys. The effects of these drugs during lactation are not clear, so caution should be used with nursing mothers (see Box 34.1).

Contraindications and Cautions

Caution should be used with any known vascular disease *because of its effects on vascular smooth muscle*, epilepsy, asthma and pregnancy or lactation.

Always consult the most recent edition of the BNF for all contraindications and interactions.

Adverse Effects

The adverse effects associated with the use of ADH preparations include water intoxication (drowsiness, light-headedness, headache, convulsions, coma) related to the shift to water retention; tremor, sweating, vertigo and headache related to water retention; abdominal cramps, flatulence, nausea and vomiting related to stimulation of GI motility and local nasal irritation related to nasal administration. Hypersensitivity reactions have also been reported, ranging from rash to bronchial constriction.

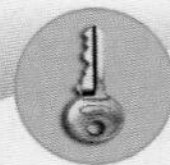

Key Drug Summary: *Vasopressin*

Indications: Treatment of diabetes insipidus, prevention and treatment of postoperative abdominal distension, to dispel gas interfering with abdominal X-ray

Actions: Vasopressor and antidiuretic effects; increases GI motility

Pharmacokinetics:

Route	Onset	Peak	Duration
IM, Sub-Cut	Varies	Unknown	2–8 h

$T_{1/2}$: 10–20 min; metabolized in the liver and excreted in the urine

Adverse effects: Tremor, sweating, vertigo, abdominal cramps, hypersensitivity reactions, water intoxication (drowsiness, light-headedness, headache, convulsions, coma)

Nursing Considerations for Patients Receiving Posterior Pituitary Hormones

Assessment: History and Examination

Screen for the following conditions which could be contraindications to use of the drug

- History of allergy
- Vascular diseases
- Epilepsy
- Renal dysfunction
- Pregnancy and lactation

Include screening for baseline status

- Skin and lesions
- Orientation and reflexes
- Blood pressure and pulse
- Respiration and abnormal chest sounds
- Abdominal examination
- Renal function tests
- Serum electrolytes

Establish if patient is currently taking other medications or herbal therapies which may potentially interact with posterior pituitary hormones.

Nursing Diagnoses

The patient receiving any posterior pituitary hormone may have the following nursing diagnoses related to drug therapy:

- Deficient knowledge regarding drug therapy
- Potential for confusion related to water intoxication due to excess ADH
- Potential for shock due to excess water loss (if drug not taken correctly)

Implementation With Rationale

- Monitor patient fluid intake/output.
- Monitor patients with vascular disease for any sign of exacerbation.
- Monitor condition of nasal passages if given intranasally to observe for nasal ulceration.
- Provide thorough patient education, including measures to avoid adverse effects, warning signs of problems and the need for regular evaluation, including blood tests, to promote concordance.

Evaluation

- Monitor patient response to the drug (maintenance of fluid balance).

- Monitor for adverse effects (GI problems, water intoxication, headache, skin rash).
- Evaluate the effectiveness of the teaching plan (patient can name drug, dosage, adverse effects to watch for and specific measures to avoid adverse effects; patient can demonstrate proper administration of nasal preparations).
- Monitor the effectiveness of comfort measures and compliance with the regimen.

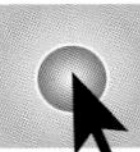

WEB LINKS

Health care providers and patients may want to consult the following Internet sources:

http://cks.library.nhs.uk The National Health Service Clinical Knowledge Summaries provides evidence-based practical information on the common conditions observed in primary care.

http://www.bnf.org.uk The BNF provides UK health care professionals with authoritative and practical information on the selection and clinical use of medicines.

http://www.nice.org.uk The National Institute for Health and Clinical Excellence (NICE) is an independent organization responsible for providing national guidance on promoting good health and preventing and treating ill health.

http://www.nhsdirect.nhs.uk The National Health Service Direct service provides patients with information and advice about health, illness and health services.

Points to Remember

- Hypothalamic releasing hormones stimulate the anterior pituitary gland to release its hormones.
- The hypothalamic releasing factors are used mostly for diagnostic testing and for treating some forms of cancer.
- Anterior pituitary hormones stimulate endocrine glands or general cell metabolism.
- GH deficiency can cause short stature in children and severe SDS in adults.
- GH replacement is done with drugs produced by recombinant DNA processes; these agents are more reliable and cause fewer problems than drugs used in the past although there may be small variations between batches.
- GH excess causes extreme height in patients whose epiphyseal plates have not closed and acromegaly in patients with closed epiphyseal plates.
- GH antagonists include octreotide and bromocriptine. Inhibition of other endocrine activity may occur when these drugs are used.
- Posterior pituitary hormones are produced in the hypothalamus and stored in the posterior pituitary gland. They include oxytocin and ADH.
- Lack of ADH produces diabetes insipidus, which is characterized by large amounts of dilute urine and excessive thirst and vascular collapse if left untreated.
- ADH replacement uses analogues of ADH and can be administered parenterally or intranasally.
- Fluid balance needs to be monitored when patients are taking ADH replacement drugs because water intoxication and dilution of essential electrolytes can occur.

CRITICAL THINKING SCENARIO 34-1

Diabetes Insipidus and Posterior Pituitary Hormones (Vasopressin)

The Situation

Jean is a 56-year-old teacher with diabetes insipidus. Her condition was eventually regulated on desmopressin nasal spray: one or two sprays per nostril four times a day. Jean seemed highly interested in her condition and therapy and learned to control her own dosage by symptom control. For several years, her symptoms were well controlled. Then at her last clinical visit, it was noted that she had postnasal ulcerations and nasal rhinitis. She also complained of several GI symptoms, including upset stomach, abdominal cramps and diarrhoea.

Discussion

An essential aspect of the ongoing nursing process is continual evaluation of how effective the drug therapy is. An evaluation of this situation shows that Jean's postnasal mucosa was ulcerated, possibly as a result of overexposure to the vasoconstrictive properties of the drug. Jean's GI tract also seemed to show evidence of increased antidiuretic hormone effects. These factors suggest that perhaps the drug was being administered incorrectly, resulting in excessive exposure of the nasal mucosa to the drug, increased absorption and increased levels of the drug reaching the systemic circulation.

The nurse should watch Jean administer a dose of the drug and then discuss the signs and symptoms of problems that Jean should watch for. In this case, Jean remembered most of the details of her drug teaching. But when administering the drug, she tilted her head back, tipped the bottle upside down and then squirted the drug into each nostril. When the nurse questioned Jean about her technique, she explained that she had seen an advertisement on TV about nasal sprays and realized that she had been doing it wrong all these years. The nurse explained the difference in the types of nasal sprays and reviewed the entire teaching plan with Jean. The drug was discontinued and Jean was placed on subcutaneous antidiuretic hormone until the nasal ulcerations healed.

It is important to remember that patient education needs regular updating and evaluation. This point is often forgotten when dealing with patients who have been taking a drug for years. However, remembering to assess the patient's knowledge about the drug can prevent problems such as Jean's from developing.

Nursing Care Guide for Jean: Diabetes Insipidus and Posterior Pituitary Hormones

Assessment: history and examination

Focus the physical assessment on the following:

- CV: Blood pressure, pulse rate, peripheral perfusion, ECG
- CNS: Orientation, affect, reflexes, vision
- Skin: Colour, lesions, texture, sweating
- GU: Urinary output, bladder tone
- GI: Abdominal examination

Nursing diagnoses

Poor tissue perfusion, potential for fainting, etc., as a result of decreased cardiac output potential for pain related to GI, GU, CNS, CV effects

Constipation/bloating related to GI effects

Lack of knowledge regarding correct use of nasal spray resulting in adverse drug effects

Implementation

Ensure safe and appropriate administration of drug.

Provide comfort and safety measures, such as physical assistance if Jean is hospitalized, temperature control, small frequent meals, fluids, mouth care and bowel programme.

Provide support and reassurance to deal with drug effects, discomfort and GI effects.

Teach patient about drug therapy, including drug name, dosage, adverse effects and precautions and warning signs of serious adverse effects to report.

Monitor her fluid status, intake output and specific gravity of urine.

Evaluation

Evaluate drug effects, including decrease in signs and symptoms being treated.

Monitor for drug–drug interactions as indicated for each drug.

Evaluate effectiveness of patient education programme and comfort and safety measures.

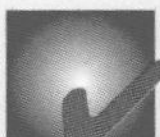

CHECK YOUR UNDERSTANDING

Answers to the questions in this chapter may be found in the Answer Key in the back of the book.

Multiple Choice

Select the most appropriate response to the following.

1. Hypothalamic hormones are normally present in very small amounts. When used therapeutically, their main indication is
   a. diagnosis of endocrine disorders and treatment of specific cancers.
   b. treatment of multiple endocrine disorders.
   c. treatment of CNS-related abnormalities.
   d. treatment of autoimmune-related problems.

2. Somatropin is a genetically engineered growth hormone that is used to
   a. diagnose hypothalamic failure.
   b. treat precocious puberty.
   c. treat children with growth failure.
   d. stimulate pituitary response.

3. Growth hormone deficiencies
   a. occur only in children.
   b. always result in reduced stature.
   c. are treated only in children because GH is usually produced only until puberty.
   d. can occur in adults as well as children.

4. Patients who are receiving growth hormone replacement therapy must be monitored very closely. Routine follow-up examinations would include
   a. a bowel programme to deal with constipation.
   b. tests of thyroid function and glucose tolerance.
   c. a calorie check to control weight gain.
   d. tests of adrenal hormone levels

5. Acromegaly and gigantism are both conditions related to excessive secretion of
   a. thyroid hormone.
   b. melanocyte-stimulating hormone.
   c. growth hormone.
   d. oxytocin

6. Diabetes insipidus is a relatively rare disease characterized by
   a. excessive secretion of ADH.
   b. renal damage.
   c. the production of large amounts of dilute urine containing no glucose.
   d. insufficient pancreatic activity.

7. Treatment with ADH preparations is associated with adverse effects including
   a. constipation.
   b. cholecystitis and bile obstruction.
   c. nocturia and bed wetting.
   d. headache, sweating and tremors.

8. A patient who is receiving an ADH preparation for diabetes insipidus may need instruction in administering the drug
   a. orally or intramuscularly.
   b. orally or intranasally.
   c. rectally or orally.
   d. intranasally or by dermal patch.

Extended Matching Questions

Select all that apply.

1. Octreotide would be the drug of choice in the treatment of acromegaly in a client with which of the following conditions?
   a. Diabetes
   b. Gallbladder disease
   c. Adrenal insufficiency
   d. Hypothalamic lesions
   e. Intolerance to other therapies
   f. Acromegaly in a client over the age of 18 years

2. A father brought his 15-year-old son to the endocrine clinic because the boy was only 5 feet tall. He wanted his son to receive growth hormone therapy because short stature would be a real detriment to his success as an adult. The boy would be considered for this therapy if:
   a. he was against the use of cadaver parts
   b. his epiphyses were closed
   c. his GH levels were very low
   d. he were also diabetic
   e. he had chronic renal failure
   f. he had hypothyroidism

References and Bibliography

British Medical Association and Royal Pharmaceutical Society of Great Britain. (2008). *British National Formulary*. London: BMJ & RPS Publishing. *This publication is updated biannually: it is imperative that the most recent edition is consulted.*

British Medical Association and Royal Pharmaceutical Society of Great Britain. (2008). *British National Formulary for Children*. London: BMJ & RPS Publishing. *This publication is updated annually: it is imperative that the most recent edition is consulted.*

Ganong, W. (2005). *Review of medical physiology* (22nd ed.). New York: McGraw-Hill.

Girard, J. (1991). *Endocrinology of puberty*. Farmington, Connecticut: Karger.

Howland, R. D. & Mycek, M. J. (2005). *Pharmacology* (3rd ed.). Philadelphia: Lippincott Williams & Wilkins.

Marieb, E. N., & Hoehn, K. (2007). *Human anatomy & physiology* (7th ed.). San Francisco: Pearson Benjamin Cummings.

North, W. G., Moses, A. M., & Shafe, L. (Eds.). (1993). The neurohypophysis: a window on brain function. Proceedings of the 5th International Conference on Neurohypophysis. *Annals of the New York Academy of Sciences, 689*, 1–706.

Porth, C. M., & Matfin G. (2008). *Pathophysiology: concepts of altered health states* (8th ed.). Philadelphia: Lippincott Williams & Wilkins.

Simonsen, T., Aarbakke, J., Kay, I., Coleman, I., Sinnott, P., & Lysaa, R. (2006). *Illustrated pharmacology for nurses.* London: Hodder Arnold.

CHAPTER 35

Adrenocortical Agents

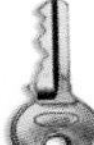

KEY TERMS

adrenal cortex
adrenal medulla
corticosteroids
diurnal rhythm
glucocorticoids
mineralocorticoids

LEARNING OBJECTIVES

Upon completion of this chapter, you will be able to:

1. Explain the control of the synthesis and secretion of the adrenocortical hormones and the physiological effects of these hormones.
2. Describe the therapeutic actions, indications, pharmacokinetics, contraindications and most common adverse reactions associated with the adrenocortical agents
3. Describe the important drug–drug interactions associated with the adrenocortical agents.
4. Discuss the use of adrenocortical agents across the lifespan.
5. Compare and contrast the key drugs, prednisolone and fludrocortisone, with other adrenocortical agents.
6. Outline the nursing considerations for patients receiving an adrenocortical agent.

GLUCOCORTICOIDS

beclometasone
betamethasone
budesonide
cortisone*
dexamethasone
flunicolide
hydrocortisone*
methylprednisolone
prednisolone
triamcinolone

MINERALOCORTICOIDS

cortisone*
fludrocortisone

*note hydrocortisone has both glucocorticoid and mineralocorticoid properties.

Adrenocortical agents are widely used to suppress the immune system. These drugs, however, do not cure any inflammatory disorders. Once widely used to treat a number of chronic problems, adrenocortical agents are now reserved for short-term use to relieve inflammation during acute stages of illness.

The Adrenal Glands

The two adrenal glands are flattened bodies that sit on top of each kidney; they are sometimes referred to as the suprarenal glands because of this positioning. Each gland is made up of an inner core called the **adrenal medulla** and an outer shell called the **adrenal cortex**.

The adrenal medulla is actually part of the sympathetic nervous system (SNS). It is a ganglion of neurons that releases the neurotransmitters noradrenaline and adrenaline into circulation when the SNS is stimulated. The secretion of these neurotransmitters directly into the bloodstream also allows them to act as hormones, travelling from the adrenal medulla to interact with specific receptor sites throughout the body. These receptors are known as adrenoceptors and can be categorized into α and β receptors. This action supports the fight-or-flight response.

The adrenal cortex surrounds the medulla and consists of three layers of cells, each of which synthesizes chemically different types of steroid hormones that exert physiological effects throughout the body. The adrenal cortex produces hormones called **corticosteroids**. There are three types of corticosteroids: androgens, glucocorticoids and mineralocorticoids. Box 35.1 discusses their use in different age groups.

Androgens (male and female sex hormones) actually have little effect compared with the sex hormones produced by the testes and ovaries. However, they are able to maintain a certain level of cellular stimulation and can contribute to cell-sensitive growth in some forms of cancers, particularly prostate, breast and ovarian cancers. These drugs are addressed in Part VII: Drugs Acting on the Reproductive System.

Glucocorticoids are so named because they stimulate an increase in glucose levels for energy. They also increase the rate of protein breakdown and decrease the rate of protein formation from amino acids, as another way of preserving energy. Glucocorticoids also cause lipogenesis or the

BOX 35.1 **DRUG THERAPY ACROSS THE LIFESPAN**

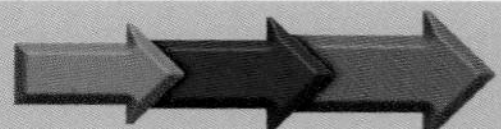

Corticosteroids

CHILDREN

Corticosteroids are used in children for the same indications as in adults. The dosage for children is determined by the severity of the condition being treated and the response to the drug, not by a weight or age formula.

Children need to be monitored closely for any effects on growth and development, and dosage adjustments should be made or drug discontinued if growth is severely retarded.

Topical use of corticosteroids should be limited in children; because their body surface area is comparatively large, the amount of the drug absorbed in relation to weight is greater than in an adult. Apply sparingly and do not use in the presence of open lesions. Do not occlude treated areas with dressings or nappies, which may increase the risk of systemic absorption.

Children need to be supervised when using nasal sprays or respiratory inhalants to ensure that the proper technique is being used.

Children receiving long-term therapy should be protected from exposure to infection, and special precautions should be established to avoid injury. If injuries or infections do occur, the child should be seen by a primary care provider as soon as possible.

When administering any drug to children, always consult the most recent edition of the British National Formulary (BNF) for Children.

ADULTS

Adults should be reminded of the importance of taking these drugs in the morning to approximate diurnal rhythm.

They should also be cautioned about the importance of tapering the drug, rather than stopping abruptly as to prevent adrenal insufficiency.

Several over-the-counter topical preparations contain corticosteroids, and adults should be cautioned to avoid combining these preparations with prescription of topical corticosteroids. They should also be cautioned to apply any of these sparingly and to avoid applying them to open lesions.

With long-term therapy, the importance of avoiding exposure to infection, crowded areas, people with colds or the flu, activities associated with injury should be stressed. If an injury or infection should occur, the patient should be encouraged to seek medical advice. Monitoring blood glucose levels should be done regularly.

These drugs should not be used during pregnancy because they cross the placenta and could cause adverse effects on the foetus. If the benefit to the mother clearly outweighs the potential risk to the foetus, they should be used with caution. Nursing mothers should find another method of feeding the baby if corticosteroids are needed, because of the potential for serious adverse effects on the baby.

OLDER ADULTS

Older adults are more likely to experience the adverse effects associated with these drugs and the dosage should be reduced and the patient monitored very closely. Older adults are more likely to have hepatic and/or renal impairment, which could lead to accumulation of drug and resultant toxic effects. They are also more likely to have medical conditions that could be imbalanced by changes in fluid and electrolytes, metabolism changes and other drug effects. Such conditions include diabetes, congestive heart failure, osteoporosis, coronary artery disease and immune suppression. Careful monitoring of drug dosage and response to the drug should be done on a regular basis.

formation and storage of fat in the body. This stored fat is then available to be broken down for energy when needed.

Mineralocorticoids affect electrolyte levels and homeostasis. These steroid hormones, such as aldosterone, directly affect the levels of electrolytes in the body: aldosterone causes potassium loss and sodium retention at the kidney nephron.

Control and Regulation

The adrenocortical hormones are normally secreted in a daily cycle known as the **diurnal rhythm** (see Box 35.2) in response to adrenocorticotropic hormone (ACTH) release from the anterior pituitary gland (see Figure 35.1). Activation of the stress reaction through the SNS bypasses the usual diurnal rhythm. The stress response is activated with cellular injury or when a person perceives fear or feels anxious. These hormones have many actions, including the following:

- Increasing the blood volume (aldosterone effect)
- Causing the release of glucose for energy
- Slowing the rate of protein production (which reserves energy)
- Blocking the activities of the inflammatory and immune systems (which reserves a great deal of energy)

These actions are important during an acute stress situation, but they can cause adverse reactions in periods of extreme or prolonged stress. For instance, a postoperative patient who is very fearful and stressed may not heal well because protein formation is blocked; infections may be hard to treat in such a patient because the inflammatory and immune systems are not functioning adequately.

Aldosterone is also released without ACTH stimulation when the blood surrounding the adrenal gland is high in potassium and low in sodium because high potassium or low sodium is a direct stimulus for aldosterone release. Aldosterone causes the kidneys to excrete potassium and retain sodium in order to restore homeostasis.

BOX 35.2 FOCUS ON THE **EVIDENCE**

Diurnal Rhythm

Research over the years has shown that the adrenocortical hormones are released in a pattern called the diurnal rhythm. The secretions of corticotropic-releasing hormone (CRH), adrenocorticotropic hormone (ACTH) and cortisol are high in the morning in day-oriented people (those who have a regular cycle of wakefulness during the day and sleep during the night). In such individuals, the peak levels of cortisol usually come between 6 and 8 a.m.. The levels then fall off slowly (with periodic spurts) and reach a low in the late evening, with lowest levels around midnight. It is thought that this cycle is related to the effects of sleeping on the hypothalamus and that the hypothalamus is regulating its stimulation of the anterior pituitary in relation to sleep and activity. The cycle may also be connected to the hypothalamic response to light. This is important to keep in mind when treating patients with corticosteroids. In order to mimic the normal diurnal pattern, corticosteroids should be taken immediately on awakening in the morning.

Complications to this pattern arise, however, when patients work shifts or change their sleeping patterns. In response, the hypothalamus shifts its release of CRH to correspond to the new cycle. For instance, if a person works all night and goes to bed at 8 a.m., arising at 3 p.m. to carry on the day's activities before going to work at 11 p.m., the hypothalamus will release CRH at about 3 p.m. in accordance with the new sleep–wake cycle. It usually takes 2 or 3 days for the hypothalamus to readjust. A patient on this schedule who is taking replacement corticosteroids would then need to take them at 3 p.m. or on arising. Patients who work several different shifts in a single week may not have time to readjust their hypothalamus, and the corticosteroid cycle may be thrown off. Patients who have to change their sleep patterns repeatedly often complain about feeling weak, being more susceptible to illness, or having trouble concentrating.

In nursing practice, it is a challenge to help patients understand how the body works and to offer ways to decrease the stress of changing sleep patterns – especially if the nurse is also working several different shifts. Many employers are willing to have employees work several days of the same shift before switching back, mainly because they have noticed an increase in productivity and a decrease in absences when employees have enough time to allow their bodies to adjust to the new shift.

Adrenal Insufficiency

Some patients experience a shortage of adrenocortical hormones and develop signs of adrenal insufficiency. This can occur for several reasons: when a patient does not produce enough ACTH, when the adrenal glands are not able to respond to ACTH, when an adrenal gland is damaged and cannot produce enough hormones (as in Addison's disease), or secondary to surgical removal of the glands.

A more common cause of adrenal insufficiency is prolonged use of corticosteroid hormones. When exogenous corticosteroids are used, they act to interrupt the regular feedback systems (Figure 35.2). The adrenal glands begin to atrophy because ACTH release is suppressed by the exogenous hormones, so the glands are no longer stimulated to produce or secrete hormones. It takes several weeks to recover from the atrophy caused by this lack of stimulation. Therefore, to prevent this from happening, patients should only receive short-term steroid therapy and should be weaned off the treatment slowly so that the adrenal glands have time to recover and start producing hormones again.

Adrenal Crisis

Patients who have an adrenal insufficiency may do quite well until they experience a period of extreme stress. They enter what is known as an adrenal crisis, which can include physiological exhaustion, hypotension, fluid shift, shock and even death, as they are not able to supplement

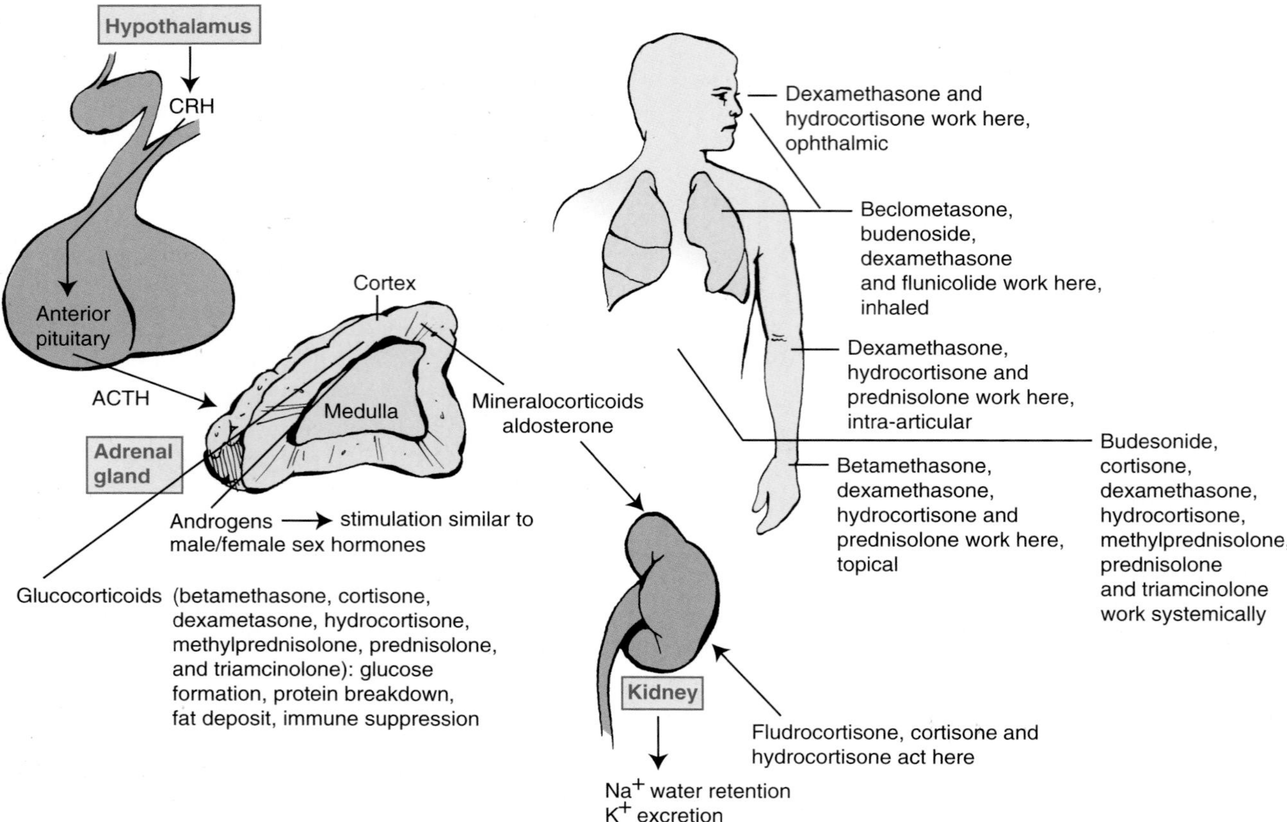

FIGURE 35.1 Sites of action of the adrenocortical agents.

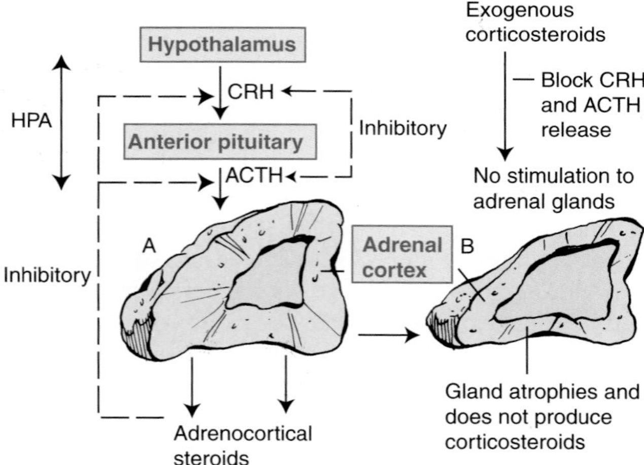

FIGURE 35.2 **(A)** Normal controls of adrenal gland. The hypothalamus releases corticotropin-releasing hormone (CRH), which causes release of corticotropin (ACTH) from the anterior pituitary. ACTH stimulates the adrenal cortex to produce and release corticosteroids. Increasing levels of corticosteroids inhibit the release of CRH and ACTH. **(B)** Exogenous corticosteroids act to inhibit CRH and ACTH release; the adrenal cortex is no longer stimulated and atrophies. Sudden stopping of steroids results in a crisis of adrenal hypofunction until hypothalamic-pituitary axis (HPA) controls stimulate the adrenal gland again.

the energy-consuming effects of the sympathetic reaction. Patients in adrenal crisis are treated with massive infusion of replacement steroids, constant monitoring and life-support procedures.

Glucocorticoids

Several glucocorticoids are available for pharmacological use .They differ mainly by route of administration and duration of action. Examples include:

- Beclometasone is available as a respiratory inhalant (inhaler) and nasal spray to block inflammation locally in the respiratory tract.
- Betamethasone is a long-acting steroid. It is available for systemic, parenteral use in acute situations. It is also available orally for short-term relief of inflammation and as a topical application for local inflammatory conditions.
- Budesonide is a relatively new steroid for intranasal use. It relieves the signs and symptoms of allergic or seasonal rhinitis with few side-effects. It is an oral agent for the treatment of mild-to-moderate active Crohn's disease.
- Cortisone was one of the first corticosteroids to be made available. It is used orally and parenterally for

replacement therapy in adrenal insufficiency, as well as acute inflammatory situations.

- Dexamethasone is widely used and available in multiple forms for dermatological, ophthalmological, intra-articular, parenteral and inhalational uses. It peaks quickly and effects can last for 2 to 3 days.
- Hydrocortisone is a powerful corticosteroid that has both glucocorticoid and mineralocorticoid activity. For that reason, it is used as replacement therapy in patients with adrenal insufficiency. It has largely been replaced for other uses (e.g. intra-articular, intravenous) by other steroid hormones with less mineralocorticoid effect. It may be preferred for use as a topical or ophthalmic agent.
- Methylprednisolone has little mineralocorticoid activity at therapeutic doses. It is the drug of choice for inflammatory and immune disorders because it has significant anti-inflammatory and immunosuppressive effects. It is available in multiple forms, including oral, parenteral, intra-articular and retention enema preparations.
- Prednisolone is an intermediate-acting corticosteroid with effects lasting only a day or so. It is used for intralesional and intra-articular injection and is also available in oral and topical forms (see critical thinking scenario 35.1).
- Triamcinolone is available in many forms for use in acute inflammatory conditions. It has been used to treat adrenal insufficiency when combined with a mineralocorticoid.

Therapeutic Actions and Indications

Glucocorticoids enter target cells and bind to cytoplasmic receptors, initiating many complex reactions that are responsible for anti-inflammatory and immunosuppressive effects. Hydrocortisone and cortisone also have some mineralocorticoid activity and affect potassium, sodium and water levels in the body (Table 35.1).

Glucocorticoids are indicated for the short-term treatment of many inflammatory disorders to relieve discomfort and to give the body a chance to heal from the effects of inflammation. They block the actions of arachidonic acid, which leads to a decrease in the formation of prostaglandins and leukotrienes. Without these chemicals, the normal inflammatory reaction is blocked. They also impair the ability of phagocytes to leave the bloodstream and move to injured tissues and they inhibit the ability of lymphocytes to act within the immune system, including a blocking of the production of antibodies. They can be used to treat local inflammation as topical agents, intranasal or inhaled agents, intra-articular injections and ophthalmic agents. Systemic use is indicated for the treatment of some cancers, hypercalcaemia associated with cancer, haematological disorders and some neurological infections. When combined with mineralocorticoids, some of these drugs can be used in replacement therapy for adrenal insufficiency.

Pharmacokinetics

These drugs are absorbed well from many sites. They are metabolized mostly within the liver and are excreted in the urine. The glucocorticoids are known to cross the placenta and to enter breast milk; they should be used during pregnancy and lactation only if the benefits to the mother clearly outweigh the potential risks to the foetus or neonate.

Contraindications and Cautions

These drugs are contraindicated in the presence of any known allergy to any steroid preparation, in the presence of an acute infection *which could become serious or even fatal if the immune and inflammatory responses are blocked* and with lactation *because the anti-inflammatory and immunosuppressive actions could be passed to the baby.*

Table 35.1 Selected Corticosteroids: Equivalent Strength, Glucocorticoid and Mineralocorticoid Effects and Duration of Effects

Drug	Equivalent Dose (mg)	Glucocorticoid Effects	Mineralocorticoid Effects	Duration of Effects
Short-acting Corticosteroids				
Cortisone	25	+	++++	8–12 h
Hydrocortisone	20	+	++++	8–12 h
Intermediate-acting Corticosteroids				
Prednisolone	5	++++	++	18–36 h
Triamcinolone	4	+++++	—	18–36 h
Methylprednisolone	4	+++++	—	18–36 h
Long-acting Corticosteroids				
Dexamethasone	0.75	+++++++++	—	36–54 h
Betamethasone	0.75	+++++++++	—	35–54 h

Caution should be used in patients with diabetes *because the glucose-elevating effects disrupt glucose control*; acute peptic ulcers *because steroid use is associated with the development of ulcers*; other endocrine disorders *which could be sent into imbalance; or pregnancy.*

Always check the latest edition of the BNF for guidance.

Adverse Effects

The adverse effects associated with the glucocorticoids are related to the route of administration used. Systemic use is associated with endocrine disorders, fluid retention and potential congestive heart failure (CHF), increased appetite and weight gain, fragile skin and loss of hair, weakness and muscle atrophy as protein breakdown occurs and protein is not replaced and increased susceptibility to infections and the development of cancers (with long-term use). Children are at risk for growth retardation associated with suppression of the hypothalamic–pituitary system. Local use is associated with local inflammations and infections, as well as burning and stinging sensations (Box 35.3).

Clinically Important Drug–Drug Interactions

Therapeutic and toxic effects increase if corticosteroids are given with erythromycin, ketoconazole or troleandomycin. Serum levels and effectiveness may decrease if corticosteroids are combined with salicylates, barbiturates, phenytoin or rifampin.

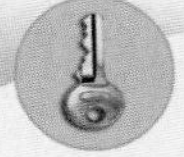

Key Drug Summary: *Fludrocortisone*

Indications: Partial replacement therapy in cortical insufficiency conditions, treatment of salt-losing adrenogenital syndrome; unlabeled use: treatment of hypotension

Actions: Increases sodium reabsorption in the renal tubules and increases potassium and hydrogen excretion, leading to water and sodium retention

Pharmacokinetics:

Route	Onset	Peak	Duration
PO	Gradual	1.7 h	18–36 h

$T_{1/2}$: 3.5 hours; metabolized in the liver and excreted in the urine

Adverse effects: Frontal and occipital headaches, joint pain, weakness, increased blood volume, oedema, hypertension, CHF, rash, anaphylaxis

BOX 35.3 Adverse Effects of Corticosteroid Use Associated With Varying Routes of Administration

Systemic: Systemic effects are most likely to occur when the corticosteroid is given by the oral, intravenous, intramuscular or subcutaneous route. Systemic absorption is possible, however, if other routes of administration are not used correctly or if tissue breakdown or injury allows direct absorption.

- Central nervous system: vertigo, headache, paresthesias, insomnia, convulsions, psychosis
- Gastrointestinal: peptic or oesophageal ulcers, pancreatitis, abdominal distension, nausea, vomiting, increased appetite, weight gain
- Cardiovascular: hypotension, shock, congestive heart failure secondary to fluid retention, thromboembolism, thrombophlebitis, fat embolism, arrhythmias secondary to electrolyte disturbances
- Haematological: sodium and fluid retention, hypokalaemia, hypocalcaemia, increased blood sugar, increased serum cholesterol, decreased thyroid hormone levels
- Musculoskeletal: muscle weakness, steroid myopathy, loss of muscle mass, osteoporosis, spontaneous fractures
- Eyes, ears, nose and throat: cataracts, glaucoma
- Dermatological: frail skin, petechiae, ecchymoses, purpura, striae, subcutaneous fat atrophy
- Endocrine: amenorrhoea, irregular menses, growth retardation, decreased carbohydrate tolerance, diabetes
- Other: immunosuppression, aggravation or masking of infections, impaired wound healing, suppression of hypothalamic–pituitary axis

Intramuscular repository injections: atrophy at the injection site
Retention enema: local pain, burning; rectal bleeding
Intra-articular injection: osteonecrosis, tendon rupture, infection
Intraspinal: meningitis, adhesive arachnoiditis, *conus medullaris* syndrome
Intrathecal administration: arachnoiditis
Topical: local burning, irritation, acneform lesions, striae, skin atrophy
Respiratory inhalant: oral, laryngeal and pharyngeal irritation; fungal infections
Intranasal: headache, nausea, nasal irritation, fungal infections, epistaxis, rebound congestion, perforation of the nasal septum, anosmia, urticaria
Ophthalmic: infections, glaucoma, cataracts
Intralesional: blindness when used on the face and head (rare)

Nursing Considerations for Patients Receiving Mineralocorticoids

Assessment: History and Examination

Screen for the following conditions, *which could be cautions or contraindications to use of the drug*: allergy to these drugs; history of CHF, hypertension or infections; high sodium intake; lactation and pregnancy.

Include screening *for baseline status before beginning therapy and for any potential adverse effects*: blood pressure, pulse and adventitious breath sounds; weight and temperature; tissue turgor; reflexes and bilateral grip strength and serum electrolyte levels.

Establish if patient is currently taking other medications or herbal therapies which may potentially interact with the mineralocorticoids.

Nursing Diagnoses

The patient receiving any mineralocorticoid may have the following nursing diagnoses related to drug therapy:

- Imbalanced nutrition: more than body requirements, related to metabolic changes
- Excess fluid volume related to sodium retention
- Impaired urinary elimination related to sodium retention
- Deficient knowledge regarding drug therapy

Implementation With Rationale

- Use only in conjunction with appropriate glucocorticoids *to maintain control of electrolyte balance.*
- Increase dosage in times of stress *to prevent adrenal insufficiency and to meet increased demands for corticosteroids under stress.*
- Monitor for hypokalaemia (weakness, serum electrolytes) *to detect the loss early and treat appropriately.*
- Discontinue if signs of overdose (excessive weight gain, oedema, hypertension and cardiomegaly) occur *to prevent the development of more severe toxicity.*
- Provide thorough patient education, including measures to avoid adverse effects; warning signs of problems; and the need for regular evaluation, including blood tests, *to enhance patient knowledge about drug therapy and promote compliance.*

Evaluation

- Monitor patient response to the drug (maintenance of electrolyte balance).
- Monitor for adverse effects (fluid retention, oedema, hypokalaemia and headache).
- Evaluate the effectiveness of the teaching plan (patient can name drug, dosage, adverse effects to watch for, specific measures to avoid adverse effects).
- Monitor the effectiveness of comfort measures and compliance with the regimen.
- Physiological effects: they include immunosuppression, peptic ulcer formation, fluid retention and oedema.
- Corticosteroids are used topically and locally to achieve the desired anti-inflammatory effects at a particular site without the systemic adverse effects that limit the usefulness of the drugs.

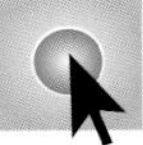

WEB LINKS

Health care providers and patients may want to consult the following Internet sources:

http://cks.library.nhs.uk The National Health Service Clinical Knowledge Summaries provides evidence-based practical information on the common conditions observed in primary care.

http://www.bnf.org.uk The BNF provides UK health care professionals with authoritative and practical information on the selection and clinical use of medicines.

http://www.nhsdirect.nhs.uk The National Health Service Direct service provides patients with information and advice about health, illness and health services.

http://www.nice.org.uk The National Institute for Health and Clinical Excellence (NICE) is an independent organization responsible for providing national guidance on promoting good health and preventing and treating ill health.

Points to Remember

- There are two adrenal glands situated superior to each kidney.
- Each adrenal gland is composed of the adrenal medulla and the adrenal cortex. The adrenal medulla is basically a sympathetic nerve ganglion that releases noradrenaline and adrenaline into the bloodstream in response to sympathetic stimulation.

- The adrenal cortex produces three types of corticosteroids: androgens (male and female sex hormones), glucocorticoids and mineralocorticoids.
- The corticosteroids are released normally in a diurnal rhythm, with the hypothalamus producing peak levels of CRH around midnight; peak adrenal response occurs around 9 a.m.. The steroid levels drop slowly during the day to reach low levels in the evening, when the hypothalamus begins CRH secretion; with peak levels again occurring around midnight. Corticosteroids are also released as part of the sympathetic stress reaction to help the body conserve energy for the fight-or-flight response.
- Prolonged use of corticosteroids suppresses the normal hypothalamic–pituitary axis and leads to adrenal atrophy from lack of stimulation. Corticosteroids need to be tapered slowly after prolonged use to allow the adrenals to resume steroid production.
- The glucocorticoids increase glucose production, stimulate fat deposition and protein breakdown and inhibit protein formation. They are used clinically to block inflammation and the immune response and in conjunction with mineralocorticoids to treat adrenal insufficiency.
- The mineralocorticoids stimulate retention of sodium and water and excretion of potassium. They are used therapeutically in conjunction with glucocorticoids to treat adrenal insufficiency.
- Adverse effects of corticosteroids are related to exaggeration of the physiological effects; they include immunosuppression, peptic ulcer formation, fluid retention and oedema.
- Corticosteroids are used topically and locally to achieve the desired anti-inflammatory effects at a particular site without the systemic adverse affects that limit the usefulness of the drugs.

CRITICAL THINKING SCENARIO 35-1

Adrenocorticosteroids

The Situation

Mel, a 48-year-old woman, was diagnosed with severe rheumatoid arthritis 7 years ago. She has retired early on ill health grounds from her job as an art teacher in the local secondary school. She now receives disability allowance. Her pain is no longer controlled by aspirin, and her doctor ordered 5 mg prednisolone (t.d.s). Over the next 4 weeks, Mel's symptoms were noticeably relieved; she was able to start painting again, and she became much more mobile. She also noticed that for the first time in years she felt 'really good'. Her appetite increased, she was no longer fatigued and her outlook on life improved. At her follow-up appointment, Mel had gained 4 kg; she had slight oedema in both ankles and her blood pressure was 150/92 mmHg. An inflamed, oozing wound was found on her right hand, which she said became infected a few weeks ago after she cut her hand, although her range of motion and joints were improved. The physician decided that Mel was past her crisis, and the prednisolone should be tapered to 5 mg/day over a 4-week period.

Critical Thinking

- Think about the pathophysiology of rheumatoid arthritis. What effects did the prednisolone have on the process at work in Mel's joints?
- What effects does the steroid have on the rest of Mel's body?
- What can be expected to occur when a patient is on prednisolone for a month?
- What precautions should be taken?
- What nursing interventions are appropriate for Mel?

Discussion

The most urgent problem for Mel at this time is the infected wound on her hand.

Steroids interfere with the normal inflammatory and immune response to infection, and, therefore, the lesion could progress to a very serious problem. The lesion should be cultured, cleaned and dressed. Mel should be instructed in how to care for her hand and how to protect it from water or further injury. An antibiotic might be prescribed and then evaluated for its appropriateness when the culture report comes back.

The real nursing challenge with Mel will be helping her to cope with and understand the need to reduce her prednisolone. Teaching about prednisolone for Mel should be thoroughly reviewed with her pointing out the side effects of drug therapy that she is already experiencing and explaining, again, the effect that prednisolone has on her body. It usually progresses from 5 mg b.d. for 2 weeks to 5 mg/day. Mel will need a great deal of encouragement and support to cope with the decrease in therapeutic benefit caused by the need to reduce the prednisolone dosage. She has felt so much

Adrenocorticosteroids *(continued)*

better while receiving the drug that she may have a real dread of losing those benefits. She should be encouraged to discuss her concerns and to call in for support if she needs it. Mel should be given an appointment for a return visit in 1 week to evaluate the wound on her hand and to check her progress in the altered dosage of the drug. She should be urged to call if the wound becomes worse to her or if she has any difficulties with her drug therapy.

Mel's case is a common example of the clinical problems that are encountered when a patient with a chronic inflammatory condition begins steroid therapy. These patients require strong nursing support and continual teaching.

Nursing Care Guide for Mel: Adrenocorticosteroids

Assessment: History and Examination

Assess for allergies to any steroids and for heart failure, pregnancy, hypertension, acute infection, peptic ulcer, vaccination with a live virus or endocrine disorders.

Also assess for concurrent use of ketoconazole, troleandomycin, oestrogens, barbiturates, phenytoin, rifampicin or salicylates.

Focus the physical examination on the following:

- Neurological: orientation, reflexes, effect
- CV: pulse, cardiac auscultation, blood pressure, oedema
- Respiratory: respiratory rate, adventitious sounds
- Laboratory tests: urinalysis, blood glucose level, renal function tests, culture and sensitivity of wound specimen
- General: temperature, site of hand infection

Nursing Diagnoses

- Decreased cardiac output related to fluid retention
- Disturbed sensory perception related to CNS effects
- Risk for infection related to immunosuppression
- Ineffective coping related to body changes caused by drug
- Excess fluid volume related to water retention
- Deficient knowledge regarding drug therapy

Implementation

- Administer around 9 a.m. to mimic normal diurnal rhythm.
- Use minimal dose for minimal period of time dosage is needed.
- Arrange for increased doses during times of stress.
- Taper gradually to allow adrenal glands to recover and produce own steroids.
- Protect patient from unnecessary exposure to infection.
- Provide support and reassurance to deal with drug therapy.
- Provide patient education regarding drug name, dosage, adverse effects, precautions and warning signs to report.

Evaluation

- Evaluate drug effects: relief of signs and symptoms of inflammation.
- Monitor for adverse effects: infection, peptic ulcer, fluid retention, hypertension, electrolyte imbalance or endocrine changes.
- Monitor for drug–drug interactions as listed.
- Evaluate effectiveness of patient education programme.
- Evaluate effectiveness of comfort and safety measures and support offered.

Patient Education for Mel

- The drug that has been prescribed for you is called prednisolone. This drug is from a class of drugs called corticosteroids, which are similar to steroids produced naturally in your body. They affect a number of bodily functions, including your body's glucose levels, blocking your body's inflammatory and immune responses and slowing the healing process.
- You should never stop taking your drug suddenly. If your prescription is low or you are unable to take the medication for any reason, notify your health care provider.

Some of the following adverse effects may occur:

- *Increased appetite*: This may be a welcome change, but if you notice a continual weight gain, you may want to watch your calories.
- *Restlessness, trouble sleeping*: Some people experience elation and a feeling of new energy; frequent rest periods should be taken.
- *Increased susceptibility to infection*: the body's normal defences will be decreased. If you notice any signs of illness or infection, notify your health care provider at once.
- Report any of the following to your health care provider: *sudden weight gain; fever or sore throat; black, tarry stools; swelling of the hands or feet; any signs of infection; or easy bruising.*

(continued)

Adrenocorticosteroids *(continued)*

- Avoid the use of any over-the-counter medication without first checking with your health care provider. Several of these medications can interfere with the effectiveness of this drug.
- Tell any doctor, nurse or other health care provider involved in your care that you are taking this drug.
- This drug affects your body's natural defences; therefore, you will need special care during any stressful situations. You may want to wear or carry medical identification showing that you are taking this medication
- It is important to have regular medical follow-up. If your drug dosage is being reduced, notify your health care provider if any of the following occur: fatigue, nausea, vomiting, diarrhoea, weight loss, weakness or dizziness.
- Keep this drug out of the reach of children. Do not give this medication to anyone else or take any similar medication that has not been prescribed for you.

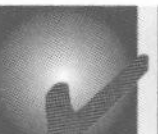

CHECK YOUR UNDERSTANDING

Answers to the questions in this chapter may be found in the Answer Key in the back of the book.

Multiple Choice

Select the most appropriate response.

1. Adrenocortical agents are widely used
   a. to cure chronic inflammatory disorders.
   b. for short-term treatment to relieve inflammation.
   c. for long-term treatment of chronic disorders.
   d. to relieve minor aches and pains and to make people feel better.

2. The adrenal medulla
   a. is the outer core of the adrenal gland.
   b. is the site of production of aldosterone and corticosteroids.
   c. is actually a neural ganglion of the SNS.
   d. consists of three layers of cells that produce different hormones.

3. Glucocorticoids are hormones that
   a. are released in response to high glucose levels.
   b. help to regulate electrolyte levels.
   c. help to regulate water balance in the body.
   d. promote the preservation of energy through increased glucose levels, protein breakdown and fat formation.

4. Diurnal rhythm in a person with a regular sleep cycle would show
   a. high levels of ACTH during the night while sleeping.
   b. rising levels of corticosteroids throughout the day.
   c. peak levels of ACTH and corticosteroids early in the morning.
   d. hypothalamic stimulation to release CRH around noon.

5. Patients who have been receiving corticosteroid therapy for a prolonged period and suddenly stop the drug will experience an adrenal crisis because their own adrenal glands will not be producing any adrenal hormones. Your assessment of a patient for the possibility of adrenal crisis may include
   a. physiological exhaustion, shock and fluid shift.
   b. acne development and hypertension.
   c. water retention and increased speed of healing.
   d. hyperglycaemia and water retention.

6. A patient is started on a regimen of prednisolone because of a crisis in her ulcerative colitis. Nursing care of this patient would need to include
   a. immunizations to prevent infections.
   b. increased calories to deal with metabolic changes.
   c. fluid restriction to decrease water retention.
   d. administration of the drug around 8 or 9 a.m. to mimic normal diurnal rhythm.

7. A patient who is taking corticosteroids is at increased risk for infection and should
   a. be protected from exposure to infections and invasive procedures.
   b. take anti-inflammatory agents regularly throughout the day.
   c. receive live virus vaccine to protect him/her from infection.
   d. be at no risk if elective surgery is needed.

8. Mineralocorticoids are used to maintain electrolyte balance in situations of adrenal insufficiency. They
   a. are usually given alone.
   b. can be given only intravenously.
   c. are always given in conjunction with appropriate glucocorticoids.
   d. are separate in their function from the glucocorticoids.

Extended Matching Questions

Select **all** that apply.

1. Patients who are taking corticosteroids would be expected to report which of the following?
   a. Weight gain
   b. Round or 'moon face' appearance
   c. Feeling of well-being
   d. Weight loss
   e. Excessive hair growth
   f. Fragile skin

2. Corticosteroid hormones are released during a sympathetic stress reaction. They would act to do which of the following?
   a. Increase blood volume
   b. Cause the release of glucose for energy
   c. Increase the rate of protein production
   d. Block the effects of the inflammatory and immune systems
   e. Store glucose to preserve energy
   f. Block protein production to save energy

True or False

Indicate whether the following statements are true (T) or false (F).

_____ 1. There are two adrenal glands, one on either side of the kidney.

_____ 2. The adrenal cortex is basically a sympathetic nerve ganglia that releases noradrenaline and adrenaline into the bloodstream in response to sympathetic stimulation.

_____ 3. The adrenal medulla produces three corticosteroids: androgens (male and female sex hormones), glucocorticoids and mineralocorticoids.

_____ 4. The corticosteroids are released normally in a diurnal rhythm.

_____ 5. Prolonged use of corticosteroids will suppress the normal hypothalamic–pituitary axis and lead to adrenal atrophy from lack of stimulation.

_____ 6. The glucocorticoids decrease glucose production, stimulate fat deposition and protein breakdown and increase protein formation.

_____ 7. The mineralocorticoids stimulate sodium and water excretion and potassium retention.

_____ 8. Adverse effects of corticosteroids are related to exaggeration of their physiological effects, including immunosuppression, peptic ulcer formation, fluid retention and oedema.

_____ 9. Corticosteroids are used topically and locally to achieve the desired anti-inflammatory effects.

_____10. Glucocorticoids are used in conjunction with mineralocorticoids to treat adrenal insufficiency.

Bibliography and References

British Medical Association and Royal Pharmaceutical Society of Great Britain. (2008). *British National Formulary*. London: BMJ & RPS Publishing. *This publication is updated biannually: it is imperative that the most recent edition is consulted.*

British Medical Association and Royal Pharmaceutical Society of Great Britain. (2008). *British National Formulary for Children*. London: BMJ & RPS Publishing. *This publication is updated annually: it is imperative that the most recent edition is consulted.*

Ganong, W. (2005). *Review of medical physiology* (22nd ed.). New York: McGraw-Hill.

Howland, R. D., & Mycek, M. J. (2005). *Pharmacology* (3rd ed.). Philadelphia: Lippincott Williams & Wilkins.

Marieb, E. N., & Hoehn, K. (2005). *Human anatomy & physiology* (7th ed.). San Francisco: Pearson Benjamin Cummings.

Porth, C. M., & Matfin G. (2008). *Pathophysiology: Concepts of altered health states* (8th ed.). Philadelphia: Lippincott Williams & Wilkins.

Simonsen, T., Aarbakke, J., Kay, I., Coleman, I., Sinnott, P., & Lysaa, R. (2006). *Illustrated pharmacology for nurses*. London: Hodder Arnold.

CHAPTER 36

Thyroid and Parathyroid Agents

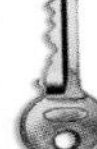

KEY TERMS

bisphosphonates
calcitonin
follicles
hypercalcaemia
hyperparathyroidism
hyperthyroidism
hypocalcaemia
hypoparathyroidism
hypothyroidism
iodine
metabolism
myxoedema
Paget's disease
parathyroid hormone (PTH)
postmenopausal osteoporosis
thioeylenes
thyroxine

LEARNING OBJECTIVES

Upon completion of this chapter, you will be able to:

1. Explain the control of the synthesis and secretion of thyroid hormones and parathyroid hormones.
2. Describe the therapeutic actions, indications, pharmacokinetics associated with thyroid, antithyroid, antihypocalcaemic and antihypocalcaemic agents.
3. Describe the contraindications, most common adverse reactions and important drug–drug interactions associated with thyroid, antithyroid, antihypocalcaemic and antihypocalcaemic agents.
4. Discuss the use of thyroid, antithyroid and calcium-regulating drugs across the lifespan.
5. Compare and contrast the key drugs levothyroxine, propylthiouracil, iodine products, calcitriol, alendronate and calcitonin with thyroid or parathyroid agents in their class.
6. Outline the nursing considerations, including important teaching points, for patients receiving drugs used to affect thyroid or parathyroid function.

THYROID HORMONE REPLACEMENTS

levothyroxine
liothyronine

ANTI-THYROID AGENTS

Thioeylenes

propylthiouracil
carbimazole

Iodides and Iodines

radioactive iodide I[13]
potassium iodide

ANTIHYPOCALCAEMIC AGENTS

calcitriol dihydrotachysterol

ANTIHYPOCALCAEMIC AGENTS

Bisphosphonates

etidronate
ibandronate
pamidronate
risedronate
tiludronate
zoledronic acid

Calcitonins

calcitonin

This chapter reviews drugs that are used to affect the function of the thyroid and parathyroid glands. These glands are closely situated in the centre of the neck and share a common goal of calcium homeostasis. In most respects, however, these glands are very different in structure and function.

The Thyroid Gland

Structure

The thyroid gland is located in the neck and lies inferior to the larynx, where it surrounds the trachea like a shield (Figure 36.1). The thyroid is a vascular gland with two lobes, one on each side of the trachea and a small isthmus connecting the lobes. The gland is made up of cells arranged in circular **follicles** known as follicular cells. The centre of each follicle is composed of colloid tissue, where the thyroid hormones are produced and stored.

The thyroid gland produces two slightly different thyroid hormones from iodine in the diet. The two hormones are tetraiodothyronine (T_4 as it contains four iodine atoms) and triiodothyronine (T_3), so named because it contains three iodine atoms. Tetraiodothyronine is commonly known as thyroxine. The thyroid cells take up **iodine** from the blood, concentrate it and prepare it for attachment to tyrosine, an amino acid. Dietary iodine is essential to produce the thyroid hormones.

When thyroid hormone is needed, the stored thyroid hormones are absorbed into the thyroid cells, where the T_3 and T_4 are broken off from thyroglobulin and released into circulation. These hormones are carried on plasma proteins, which can be measured as protein-bound iodine (PBI) levels. The thyroid gland produces more T_4 than T_3. More T_4 is released into circulation, but T_3 is more active than T_4. Most T_4 (with a half-life of about 12 hours) is converted to T_3 (with a half-life of about 1 week) at the tissue level.

Control

Thyroid hormone production and release are regulated by the anterior pituitary hormone called thyroid-stimulating hormone (TSH) or thyrotropin. The secretion of TSH is regulated by thyrotropin-releasing hormone (TRH), released from the hypothalamus. A delicate balance exists among the

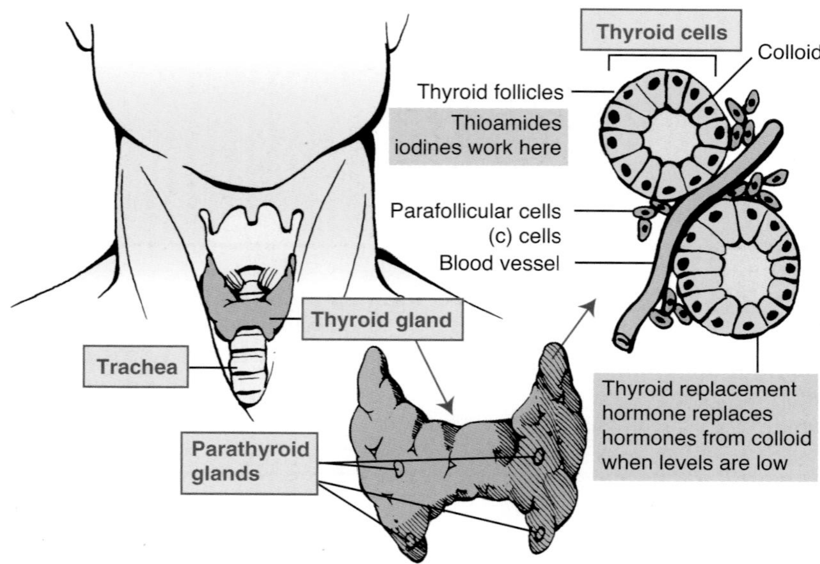

FIGURE 36.1 The thyroid and parathyroid glands. The basic unit of the thyroid gland is the follicle.

thyroid, pituitary and hypothalamus in regulating the levels of thyroid hormone in the body. The thyroid gland produces increased thyroid hormones in response to increased levels of TSH. The increased levels of thyroid hormones send a negative feedback message to the pituitary to decrease TSH release and, at the same time, to the hypothalamus to decrease TRH release. A drop in TRH levels subsequently results in a drop in TSH levels, which in turn leads to a drop in thyroid hormone levels. In response to low blood serum levels of thyroid hormone, the hypothalamus sends TRH to the anterior pituitary, which responds by releasing TSH, which in turn stimulates the thyroid gland to again produce and release thyroid hormone. The rising levels of thyroid hormone are sensed by the hypothalamus, and the cycle begins again. This intricate series of negative feedback mechanisms keeps the level of thyroid hormone within a narrow normal range (Figure 36.2).

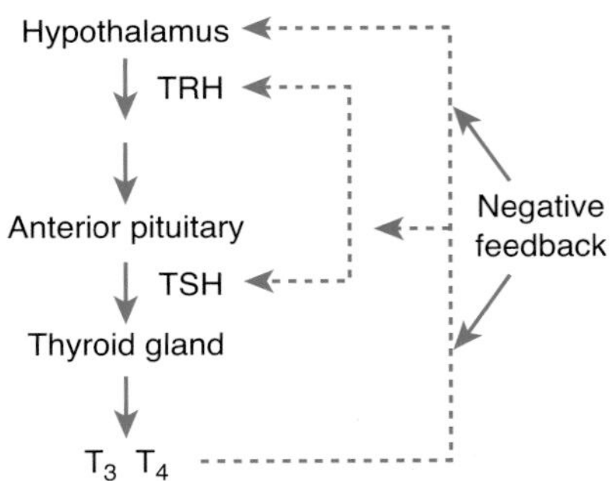

FIGURE 36.2 In response to low blood serum levels of thyroid hormone, the hypothalamus sends the thyrotropin-releasing hormone (TRH) to the anterior pituitary, which responds by releasing the thyroid-stimulating hormone (TSH) to the thyroid gland; it, in turn, responds by releasing the thyroid hormone (T_3 and T_4) into the bloodstream. The anterior pituitary is also sensitive to the increase in blood serum levels of the thyroid hormone and responds by decreasing production and release of TSH. As thyroid hormone production and release subside, the hypothalamus senses the lower serum levels and the process is repeated by the release of TRH again. This intricate series of negative feedback mechanisms keeps the level of thyroid hormone within normal limits.

Function

Thyroid hormone regulates the rate of **metabolism**; that is, the rate at which energy is burned in almost all the cells of the body. The thyroid hormones affect heat production and body temperature, oxygen consumption and cardiac output, blood volume, enzyme system activity and metabolism of carbohydrates, fats and proteins. Thyroid hormone is also an important regulator of growth and development, especially within the reproductive and nervous systems. As the thyroid has such widespread effects throughout the body, any dysfunction of the thyroid gland will have numerous systemic effects.

Cells found around the follicle of the thyroid gland, called parafollicular or C cells, produce another hormone, **calcitonin**. This hormone affects calcium levels in the plasma and acts to balance the effects of parathyroid hormone. The release of calcitonin is not controlled by the hypothalamic-pituitary axis but is regulated locally at the cellular level. The cells release calcitonin when the concentration of calcium around them rises. The calcitonin released into the bloodstream works to reduce calcium levels, by blocking bone resorption and enhancing bone formation, pulling calcium out of the serum for deposit into bone (Figure 36.3).

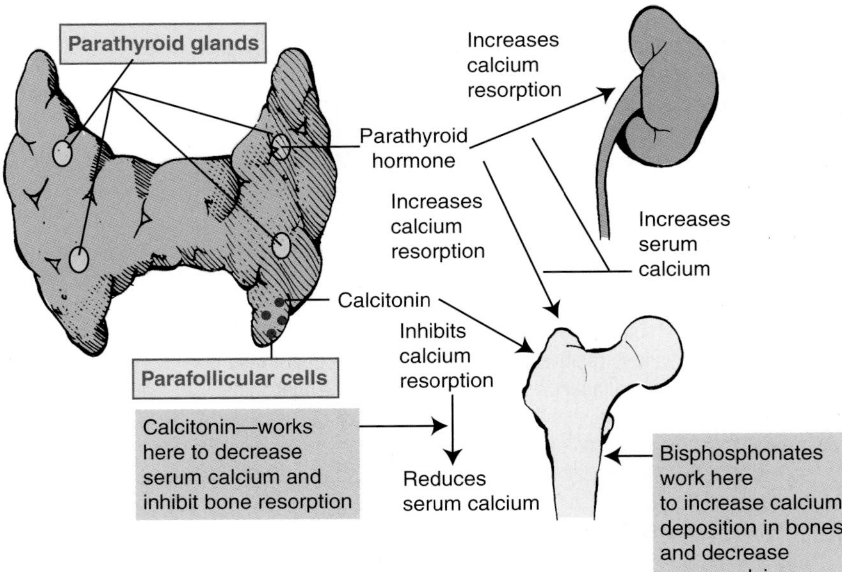

FIGURE 36.3 Calcium control. Parathyroid hormone and calcitonin work to maintain calcium homeo-stasis in the body. Calcium level surrounding the cells falls, they will no longer produce calcitonin.

Thyroid Dysfunction

Thyroid dysfunction involves either under activity, called **hypothyroidism**, or over activity, called **hyperthyroidism**. This dysfunction can affect any age group (Box 36.1).

Hypothyroidism

Hypothyroidism is a lack of sufficient levels of thyroid hormones to maintain normal metabolism. This condition occurs in a number of pathophysiological states:

- Absence of the thyroid gland
- Lack of sufficient iodine in the diet to produce the needed level of thyroid hormone
- Lack of sufficient functioning thyroid tissue due to tumour or autoimmune disorders
- Lack of TSH due to pituitary disease
- Lack of TRH related to a tumour or disorder of the hypothalamus

Hypothyroidism is the most common type of thyroid dysfunction. It is estimated that it affects approximately 5% to 10% of women over 50 years worldwide. The symptoms of hypothyroidism can be varied and vague and are frequently overlooked. The signs and symptoms of hypothyroidism, including obesity, are often mistaken for signs of normal ageing. Goitre or enlargement of the thyroid gland can be present in over and underactive glands. Goitre usually occurs when the thyroid gland is either being overstimulated by TSH (overactive), or when it is not getting enough iodine (underactive).

If untreated in childhood, these children will have short statue and they may have developmental disabilities because of the lack of thyroid hormone stimulation. Severe adult hypothyroidism is called **myxoedema**. Myxoedema usually develops gradually as the thyroid slowly stops functioning. It can develop as a result of autoimmune thyroid disease (Hashimoto's disease), viral infection, or over treatment with antithyroid drugs or because of surgical removal or irradiation of the thyroid gland. Patients with myxoedema exhibit many signs and symptoms of decreased metabolism, including lethargy, hyporeflexia, hypotension, bradycardia, pale and coarse skin, loss of hair, intolerance to the cold, decreased appetite, decreased body temperature, thickening of the tongue and vocal cords, decreased sexual function and constipation. The treatment for patients with hypothyroidism is thyroid hormone replacement therapy.

Hyperthyroidism

Hyperthyroidism (thyrotoxicosis) occurs when excessive amounts of thyroid hormones are produced and released into the circulation. Graves' disease is the most common cause of hyperthyroidism. This is an autoimmune disease

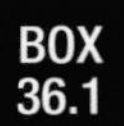

DRUG THERAPY ACROSS THE LIFESPAN

Thyroid and Parathyroid Agents

CHILDREN

Thyroid replacement therapy is required when a child is hypothyroid. Levothyroxine is the drug of choice in children. Dosage is determined based on serum thyroid hormone levels and the response of the child, including growth and development. Dosage in children tends to be higher than in adults because of the higher metabolic rate of the growing child. Usually the starting dose to consider is 10 to 15 μg/kg per day.

Regular monitoring, including growth records, is necessary to determine the accurate dosage as the child grows. Maintenance levels at the adult dosage usually occurs after puberty and when active growing stops.

If an antithyroid agent is needed, propylthiouracil is the drug of choice because it is less toxic. Radioactive agents are not used in children, unless other agents are ineffective, because of the effects of radiation on chromosomes and developing cells.

Hypercalcaemia is relatively rare in children, although it may be seen with certain malignancies. If a child develops a malignancy-related hypercalcaemia, the bisphosphonates may be used, with dosage adjustments based on age and weight. Serum calcium levels should be monitored very closely in the child and dosage adjustments made as necessary.

When administering any drug to children, always consult the most recent edition of the British National Formulary for Children.

ADULTS

Adults who require thyroid replacement therapy need to understand that this will be a lifelong replacement need. An established routine of taking the tablet first thing in the morning, with a full glass of water, may help the patient comply with the drug regimen. Levothyroxine is the drug of choice for replacement, but in some cases other agents may be needed. Periodic monitoring of thyroid hormone levels is necessary to ensure that dosage needs do not change.

OLDER ADULTS

The signs and symptoms of thyroid disease mimic many other problems that are common to older adults – hair loss, slurred speech, fluid retention, congestive heart failure and so on – it is important to screen older adults for thyroid disease carefully before beginning any therapy. The dosage should be started at a very low level and increased based on the patient response. Levothyroxine is the drug of choice for hypothyroidism. Periodic monitoring of thyroid hormone levels as well as cardiac and other responses is essential with this age group.

If antithyroid agents are needed, radioactive iodine may be the drug of choice because it has fewer adverse effects than the other agents and surgery. The patient should be monitored closely for the development of hypothyroidism, which usually occurs within a year after initiation of antithyroid therapy.

Table 36.1 Signs and Symptoms of Thyroid Dysfunction

System	Hypothyroidism	Hyperthyroidism
Central nervous system	Depressed – hypoactive reflexes, lethargy, sleepiness, slow speech, emotional dullness	Stimulated – hyperactive reflexes, anxiety, nervousness, insomnia, tremors, restlessness
Cardiovascular	Depressed – bradycardia, hypotension, anaemia, oliguria, decreased sensitivity to catecholamines	Stimulated – tachycardia, palpitations, increased pulse pressure, systolic hypertension, increased sensitivity to catecholamines
Skin, hair, nails	Pale, coarse, dry, thickened; puffy eyes and eyelids; hair coarse and thin; nails thick and hard	Flushed, warm, thin, moist, sweating; hair fine and soft; nails soft and thin
Metabolic rate	Decreased – lower body temperature; intolerance to cold; decreased appetite, higher levels of fat and cholesterol, weight gain and hypercholesterolemia	Increased – low-grade fever; intolerance to heat; increased appetite with weight loss; muscle wasting and weakness, thyroid myopathy
Generalized myxoedema	Accumulation of mucopolysaccharides in the heart, tongue, vocal cords; periorbital oedema, cardiomyopathy, hoarseness and thickened speech	Localized with accumulation of mucopolysaccharides in eyeballs, ocular muscles; periorbital oedema, lid lag, exophthalmos; pretibial oedema
Ovaries	Decreased function – menorrhagia, habitual abortion, sterility	Altered; tendency towards oligomenorrhoea, amenorrhoea
Goitre	Rare; simple nontoxic type may occur	Diffuse, highly vascular; very frequent

where an individual produces antibodies which stimulate the TSH receptors, causing an increase in thyroid gland size and function. Patients with hyperthyroidism may exhibit many signs and symptoms of overactive cellular metabolism, including increased body temperature, tachycardia, palpitations, hypertension, flushing, thin skin, an intolerance to heat, amenorrhoea, weight loss and goitre. Treatment of hyperthyroidism may involve surgical removal of the gland or portions of the gland, treatment with radiation to destroy parts or the entire gland or drug treatment to block the production of **thyroxine** in the thyroid gland. The metabolism of these patients then must be regulated with replacement thyroid hormone therapy. Table 36.1 outlines the signs and symptoms of thyroid dysfunction. Hyperthyroidism also increases a patient's risk of developing osteoporosis.

Thyroid Hormone Replacements

Several replacement hormone products are available for treating hypothyroidism. These products contain both natural and synthetic thyroid hormone. Replacement hormones act to replace low or absent levels of the thyroid hormones and to suppress overproduction of TSH by the pituitary (see Figure 36.1). Levothyroxine, a synthetic salt of T_4, is the most frequently used replacement hormone because of its predictable bioavailability and reliability.

Therapeutic Actions and Indications

The thyroid replacement hormones increase the metabolic rate of body tissues, increasing oxygen consumption, respiration, heart rate, growth and maturation and the metabolism of fats, carbohydrates and proteins. They are indicated for replacement therapy in hypothyroid states, treatment of myxoedema coma, suppression of TSH in the treatment and prevention of goitres and management of thyroid cancer. In conjunction with antithyroid drugs, they are also indicated to treat thyroid toxicity and to prevent goitre formation during thyroid over-stimulation

Pharmacokinetics

These drugs are well absorbed from the gastrointestinal (GI) tract and bound to serum proteins. De-iodination of the drugs (to convert it to its active form), occurs at several sites, including the liver, kidney and other body tissues. Elimination is primarily in the bile. Thyroid hormone does not cross the placenta and seems to have no effect on the foetus. Thyroid replacement therapy should not be discontinued during pregnancy and the need for thyroid replacement often becomes apparent during pregnancy. Thyroid hormone does enter breast milk in small amounts. Caution should be used during lactation as this could suppress the infant's thyroid function.

Adverse Effects

When the correct dosage of the replacement therapy is used, few if any adverse effects are associated with these drugs. Skin reactions and loss of hair are sometimes seen, especially during the first few months of treatment in children. Symptoms of hyperthyroidism may occur as the drug dose is regulated. Some of the less predictable effects are associated with cardiac stimulation (arrhythmias, hypertension), CNS effects (anxiety, sleeplessness and headache) and difficulty swallowing (taking the drug with a full glass of water may help).

Clinically Important Drug–Drug Interactions

Decreased absorption of the thyroid hormones occurs if they are taken concurrently with cholestyramine. If this combination is needed, the drugs should be taken 2 hours apart.

The action of oral anticoagulants is increased if they are combined with thyroid hormone. As this may lead to increased bleeding, the dosage of the oral anticoagulant should be reduced and the bleeding time checked periodically.

Decreased action of *digitalis* glycosides can occur when these drugs are combined. Consequently, *digitalis* levels should be monitored and increased dosage may be required.

Theophylline clearance is decreased in hypothyroid states. As the patient approaches normal thyroid function, theophylline dosage may need to be adjusted frequently.

Always consult a current copy of the British National Formulary for further guidance.

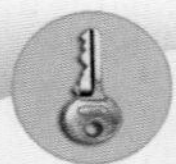

Key Drug Summary: *Levothyroxine*

Indications: Replacement therapy in hypothyroidism, pituitary TSH suppression in the treatment of simple nontoxic goitres and in the management of thyroid cancer, thyrotoxicosis in conjunction with other therapy

Actions: Increases the metabolic rate of body tissues, increasing oxygen consumption, respiration and heart rate; the rate of fat, protein and carbohydrate metabolism and growth and maturation

Pharmacokinetics:

Route	Onset	Peak	Duration
PO	Slow	1–3 wk	1–3 wk
IV	6–8 h	24–48 h	unknown

$T_{1/2}$: 6–7 days; metabolized in the liver and excreted in the bile

Adverse effects: Tremors, headache, nervousness, palpitations, tachycardia, allergic skin reactions, loss of hair in the first few months of therapy in children, diarrhoea, nausea, vomiting

Nursing Considerations for Patients Receiving Thyroid Hormones

Assessment: History and Examination

Screen for the following conditions, *which could be contraindications or cautions to use of the drug*: history of allergy to any thyroid hormone replacement, Addison's disease, acute myocardial infarction not complicated by hypothyroidism and thyrotoxicosis.

Include screening *for baseline status before beginning therapy and for any potential adverse effects* orientation; baseline pulse, blood pressure and electrocardiogram (ECG); respiration and thyroid function tests.

Establish if patient is currently taking other medications or herbal therapies which may potentially interact with the thyroid hormones.

Nursing Diagnoses

The patient receiving any thyroid hormone may have the following nursing diagnoses related to drug therapy:

- Effect of decreased cardiac output related to cardiac effects
- Imbalanced nutrition: less than body requirements related to changes in metabolism
- Deficient knowledge regarding drug therapy

Implementation With Rationale

- Administer a single daily dose before breakfast each day *to ensure consistent therapeutic levels.*
- Administer with a full glass of water *to help prevent difficulty swallowing.*
- Monitor response carefully when beginning therapy *to adjust dosage according to patient response.*
- Monitor pulse rate, BP and ECG *to detect cardiac adverse effects.*
- Assess the patient carefully *to detect any potential drug–drug interactions if giving thyroid hormone in combination with other drugs.*
- Arrange for periodic blood tests of thyroid function *to monitor the effectiveness of the therapy.*
- Provide thorough patient teaching, warning signs of problems and the need for regular evaluation if used for longer than recommended *to enhance patient knowledge of drug therapy and promote compliance.*

Evaluation

- Monitor patient response to the drug (return of metabolism to normal, prevention of goitre).

- Monitor for adverse effects (tachycardia, hypertension, anxiety, skin rash).
- Evaluate the effectiveness of the teaching plan (patient can name drug, dosage, adverse effects to watch for and specific measures to avoid adverse effects).
- Monitor the effectiveness of comfort measures and compliance to the regimen (see Critical Thinking Scenario 36-1).

Anti-thyroid Agents

Drugs used to block production of thyroid hormone and to treat hyperthyroidism include carbimazole and the **thioeylenes** and iodide solutions. Although these groups of drugs are not chemically related, they both block the formation of thyroid hormones within the thyroid gland (see Figure 36.1).

The Thioeylenes

Propylthiouracil is the most frequently used thioeylenes; but it is associated with several GI effects.

Therapeutic Actions and Indications

The thioeylenes possibly prevent the formation of thyroid hormone within the thyroid cells, lowering the serum levels of thyroid hormone. They also partially inhibit the conversion of T_4 to T_3 at the cellular level. Thioeylenes are indicated for the treatment of hyperthyroidism.

Pharmacokinetics

These drugs are well absorbed from the GI tract and are then concentrated in the thyroid gland. Some excretion can be detected in the urine. If an antithyroid drug is needed during pregnancy, propylthiouracil is the drug of choice, but caution should still be used.

Contraindications and Cautions

All patients on carbimazole should be advised to report any soreness of the throat immediately due to the rare complication of agranulocytosis due to bone marrow suppression.

Adverse Effects

The adverse effects most commonly seen with these drugs are the effects of thyroid suppression, for example: drowsiness, lethargy, bradycardia, nausea, skin rash. Other side-effects include nausea, vomiting and GI complaints. Both carbimazole and propylthiouracil are associated with bone marrow suppression, so patients using these drugs must have frequent blood tests to monitor these effects.

Clinically Important Drug–Drug Interactions

An increased risk for bleeding exists when propylthiouracil is administered with oral anticoagulants. Changes in serum levels of theophylline, metoprolol, propranolol and digitalis may lead to changes in the effects of propylthiouracil as the patient moves from hyperthyroid to euthyroid state.

Always consult a current copy of the British National Formulary for further guidance.

Iodine Solutions

Low doses of iodine are needed in the body for the formation of thyroid hormones. High doses, however, temporarily block thyroid function. Therefore, iodine preparations are sometimes used to treat hyperthyroidism. Radioactive iodine (I^{131}) is sometimes used as a diagnostic agent or to destroy thyroid tissue in cases of severe Graves' disease or carcinoma of the thyroid gland in preparation for surgery. It is usually reserved for use in patients who are older than 30 years of age because of the adverse effects associated with the radioactivity. Strong iodine products, potassium iodide and sodium iodide are taken orally and have a rapid onset of action, with effects seen within 24 hours and peak effects seen in 10 to 15 days. The effects are short-lived and may even precipitate further thyroid enlargement and dysfunction. For this reason and because of the availability of the more predictable thioeylenes, iodides are not used as often as they once were in the clinical setting but are usually reserved for the treatment of thyroid crisis (extreme hyperthyroidism).

Therapeutic Actions and Indications

It is postulated that these drugs cause the thyroid cells to become oversaturated with iodine and stop producing thyroid hormone. In some cases, the thyroid cells are actually destroyed. The strong iodine products are reserved for presurgical suppression of the thyroid gland, for treatment of acute thyrotoxicosis until thioeylene levels can take effect or for thyroid blocking during radiation therapy.

The strong iodine products are also used to block thyroid function in radiation emergencies. Radioactive iodine is taken up into the thyroid cells, which are then destroyed by the beta-radiation given off by the radioactive iodine. Except during radiation emergencies, it may be used to shrink the gland before surgery to reduce the risk of bleeding in women who cannot become pregnant and in elderly patients with such severe, complicating conditions that immediate thyroid destruction is needed.

Contraindications and Cautions

The use of strong iodine products is contraindicated in the presence of pregnancy, *because of the effect on the thyroid glands of the mother and the foetus*.

Adverse Effects

The most common adverse effect of these drugs is hypothyroidism; the patient will need to be started on replacement thyroid hormone to maintain homeostasis. Other adverse effects include iodism (metallic taste and burning in the mouth, sore teeth and gums, diarrhoea, cold symptoms and stomach upset), staining of teeth, skin rash and the development of goitre.

Clinically Important Drug–Drug Interactions

The use of drugs to destroy thyroid function may cause the patient to become hypothyroid. Patients who are taking drugs that are metabolized differently in hypothyroid and hyperthyroid states or drugs that have a small margin of safety that could be altered by the change in thyroid function should be monitored closely. These drugs include anticoagulants, theophylline, digoxin, metoprolol and propranolol.

Always consult a current copy of the British National Formulary for further guidance.

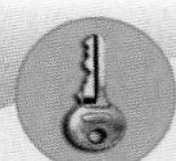

Key Drug Summary: Propylthiouracil

Indications: Treatment of hyperthyroidism

Actions: Inhibits the synthesis of thyroid hormones, partially inhibits the peripheral conversion of T_4 to T_3

Pharmacokinetics:

Route	Onset
Oral	Varies

$T_{1/2}$: 1–2 hours; metabolized in the liver and excreted in the urine

Nursing Considerations for Patients Receiving Anti-thyroid Agents

Assessment: History and Examination

Screen for the following conditions, *which could be cautions or contraindications to use of the drug*: history of allergy to any antithyroid drug, pregnancy and lactation.

Include screening *for baseline status before beginning therapy and for any potential adverse effects*: skin; orientation; pulse, blood pressure and ECG; respiration and adventitious sounds and thyroid function tests, that is TSH is measured in case the problem is pituitary based.

Nursing Diagnoses

The patient receiving any antithyroid drug may have the following nursing diagnoses related to drug therapy:

- Imbalanced nutrition: more than body requirements related to changes in metabolism
- Risk for bleeding/infection related to bone marrow suppression
- Deficient knowledge regarding drug therapy

Implementation With Rationale

- Administer propylthiouracil at regular intervals three times a day *to ensure consistent therapeutic levels.*
- Give iodine solution through a straw *to decrease staining of teeth*; tablets can be crushed.
- Monitor response carefully and arrange for periodic blood tests *to assess patient response and to monitor for adverse effects.*
- Monitor patients receiving iodine solution for any sign of iodism, *so the drug can be stopped immediately if such signs appear.*
- Provide thorough patient education, including measures to avoid adverse effects, warning signs of problems and the need for regular evaluation if used for longer than recommended, *to enhance patient knowledge of drug therapy and promote compliance.*

Evaluation

- Monitor patient response to the drug (lowering of thyroid hormone levels).
- Monitor for adverse effects (bradycardia, anxiety, skin rash).
- Evaluate the effectiveness of the teaching plan (patient can name drug, dosage, adverse effects to watch for, specific measures to avoid adverse effects).
- Monitor the effectiveness of comfort measures and compliance to the regimen.

The Parathyroid Glands

Structure and Function

The parathyroid glands are four (usually) very small groups of glandular tissue located on the back of the thyroid gland. These cells produce **parathyroid hormone** (PTH). PTH is the most important regulator of serum calcium levels in the body and has many actions, including:

- Stimulation of osteoclasts or bone cells to release calcium from the bone
- Increased intestinal absorption of calcium
- Increased calcium resorption from the kidneys
- Stimulation of cells in the kidney to produce calcitriol, the active form of vitamin D, which stimulates the uptake of calcium from the intestines, kidney tubules into the blood

Control

Calcium (Ca^{2+}) is an electrolyte that is used in many metabolic processes in the body. These processes include membrane transport systems, conduction of nerve impulses, muscle contraction and blood clotting. For these to occur, serum levels of calcium must be maintained between 2.2 and 2.6 mmol/l. This is achieved through regulation of serum calcium by two hormones: PTH and calcitonin (Figure 36.4).

Calcitonin is released when serum calcium levels rise. Calcitonin, produced in the C cells of the thyroid gland, works to reduce calcium levels by blocking bone resorption and enhancing bone formation. This action extracts calcium from the serum for depositing into the bone. PTH secretion is also directly regulated by serum calcium levels. When serum calcium levels are low, PTH release is stimulated. When serum calcium levels are high, PTH release is blocked.

Another electrolyte, magnesium (Mg^{2+}), also affects PTH secretion by mobilizing calcium and inhibiting the release of PTH when concentrations rise above or fall below normal. An increased serum phosphate level indirectly stimulates parathyroid activity. Renal tubular phosphate reabsorption is balanced by calcium secretion into the urine, which causes a drop in serum calcium, stimulating PTH secretion. The hormones PTH and calcitonin work together to maintain the delicate balance of serum calcium levels in the body and to keep serum calcium levels within the normal range.

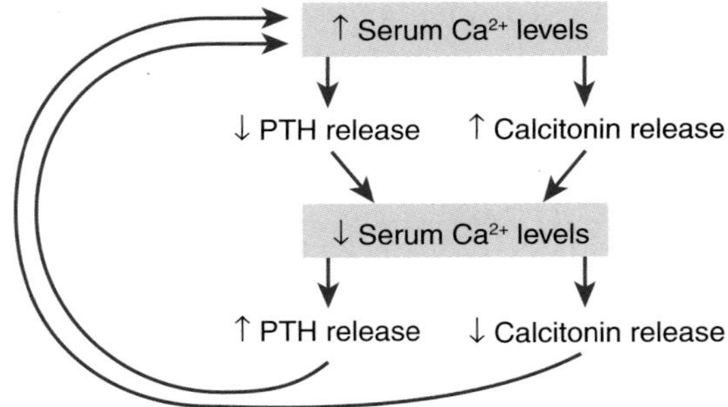

FIGURE 36.4 Control of serum Ca^{2+} levels by parathormone (PTH) and calcitonin, showing the negative feedback cycle in effect.

Parathyroid Dysfunction and Related Disorders

The absence of PTH, a condition called **hypoparathyroidism**, is relatively rare. It is most likely to occur with the accidental removal of the parathyroid glands during thyroid surgery. The treatment of hypoparathyroidism consists of calcium and vitamin D therapy to increase serum calcium levels. There is currently no replacement of PTH available.

The excessive production of PTH, called **hyperparathyroidism**, can occur as a result of parathyroid tumour or certain genetic disorders. Patients with hyperparathyroidism may present with decalcification of bone and deposits of calcium in body tissues including the kidney, resulting in kidney stones. Primary hyperparathyroidism occurs more often in women in their 60s and 70s. Secondary hyperparathyroidism occurs most frequently in patients with chronic renal failure (see Box 36.2 for more information).

The genetically linked disorder **Paget's disease** is a condition of overactive osteoclasts that are eventually replaced by enlarged and softened bony structures. Patients with this disease complain of deep bone pain, headaches and hearing loss and usually have cardiac failure and bone malformation.

Postmenopausal osteoporosis can occur when oestrogen levels fall allowing calcium to be removed from bone, resulting in weakened and honeycombed bone structure (Box 36.3). Oestrogen causes calcium to be deposited in the bone; osteoporosis is one of the many complications that accompany the loss of oestrogen at menopause.

BOX 36.2 Treatments for Secondary Hyperparathyroidism

Cinacalcet hydrochloride is used for treatment of secondary hyperparathyroidism in patients undergoing dialysis for end-stage kidney disease and for treatment of hypercalcaemia in patients with parathyroid carcinoma. Cinacalcet is a calcimimetic drug that increases the sensitivity of the calcium-sensing receptor to activation by extracellular calcium. In increasing the receptors' sensitivity, cinacalcet lowers parathyroid hormone (PTH) levels, causing a concomitant decrease in serum calcium levels.

The usual initial adult dose for secondary hyperparathyroidism is 30 mg/day PO, after which PTH, serum calcium and serum phosphorus levels are monitored to achieve the desired therapeutic effect. The drug must be used in combination with vitamin D and/or phosphate binders.

For parathyroid carcinoma, the initial dosage is 30 mg BD orally every 2 to 4 weeks to maintain serum calcium levels within a normal range; 30 to 90 mg BD up to 90 mg three to four times daily may be needed. Side-effects that the patient may experience include nausea, vomiting, diarrhoea and dizziness.

BOX 36.3 Sex Considerations: Osteoporosis

Osteoporosis is the most common bone disease found in adults. It results from a lack of bone-building cell (osteoblast) activity and a decrease in bone matrix and mass, with less calcium and phosphorus being deposited in the bone. This can occur at any age, but there is an increased risk of developing osteoporosis with advancing age, when the endocrine system is less responsive and the stimulation to build bone is absent, with menopause, when the calcium-depositing effects of oestrogen are lost, with malnutrition states, when vitamin C and proteins essential for bone production are absent from the diet and with a lack of physical stress on the bones from lack of activity, which promotes calcium removal and does not stimulate osteoclasts activity. The inactive, elderly, postmenopausal woman with those with a poor diet is a prime candidate for osteoporosis, although osteoporosis can occur in younger women and men. Fractured hips and wrists, shrinking size and curvature of the spine are all evidence of osteoporosis in patients. A patient can live with osteoporosis for many years, but often it is not diagnosed until later in life or following a fracture. Steroid use can predispose patients to osteoporosis – therefore younger people are also at risk. In addition to the use of bisphosphonates to encourage calcium deposition in the bone, several other interventions can help prevent severe osteoporosis in people with similar risk factors.

- *Aerobic exercise*: walking, even 10 minutes a day, has been shown to help increase osteoclast activity.
- *Proper diet*: calcium and proteins are essential for bone growth. Those at risk of osteoporosis could benefit from calcium supplements and encouragement to eat protein at least two to three times a week. Weight loss can also help to improve activity and decrease pressure on bones at rest.
- *Hormone replacement therapy (HRT)*: HRT has been very successful in decreasing the progression of osteoporosis. This can be given in combination with bisphosphonates.

The risk of osteoporosis should be taken into consideration as part of the health care regimen for all people as they age. Prevention can save a great deal of pain and debilitation in the long run.

Anti-hypercalcaemic Agents

Drugs used to treat PTH excess or high levels of serum calcium (**hypercalcaemia**) include the **bisphosphonates** and calcitonin (human and salmon). These drugs act on the serum levels of calcium and not directly on the parathyroid gland or PTH.

Bisphosphonates

The bisphosphonates include etidronate, ibandronate, pamidronate, risedronate, tiludronate, alendronate and zoledronic acid. These drugs act to slow or block bone resorption; by doing this, they help to lower serum calcium levels.

Therapeutic Actions and Indications

The bisphosphonates slow normal and abnormal bone reabsorption but do not inhibit normal bone formation and mineralization. These drugs are used in the treatment of Paget's disease and in postmenopausal osteoporosis. Alendronate is used to treat osteoporosis in men.

- Pamidronate, etidronate and zoledronic acid are also used for the treatment of hypercalcaemia of malignancy and of osteolytic bone lesions in certain cancer patients.
- Ibandronate is approved only for the prevention and treatment of postmenopausal osteoporosis and is available in a once-a-month dose form.
- Tiludronate is reserved for use in the treatment of Paget's disease if there is no response to other therapy
- Risedronate is used daily for 2 months to treat Paget's disease in symptomatic people who are at risk for complications
- Alendronate and risedronate are the most commonly used drugs for osteoporosis and hypercalcaemia

Serum calcium levels need to be monitored carefully with any of the drugs that affect calcium levels. Patients should be encouraged to take calcium and vitamin D in their diet or as supplements in cases of hypocalcaemia and also for prevention and treatment of osteoporosis.

Pharmacokinetics

These drugs are well absorbed in the small intestine and do not undergo metabolism. They are excreted relatively unchanged in the urine. Patients with renal dysfunction may experience toxic levels of the drug and should be evaluated for a dosage reduction. Foetal abnormalities have been associated with these drugs in animal trials, and they should not be used during pregnancy unless the benefit to the mother clearly outweighs the potential risk to the foetus. Extreme caution should be used when nursing because of the potential for adverse effects on the baby. Alendronate should not be used by nursing mothers.

Contraindications and Cautions

These drugs should not be used in hypocalcaemia, *which could be made worse by lowering calcium levels*, during pregnancy or lactation, *because of the potential for adverse effects on the foetus or neonate*, or with a history of any allergy to bisphosphonates.

Caution should be used in patients with renal dysfunction, *which could interfere with excretion of the drug*, or with upper GI disease, *which could be aggravated by the drug*. Alendronate and risedronate should not be given to anyone who is unable to remain upright for 30 minutes after taking the drug, *because serious oesophageal erosion can occur*. Taking the drug with a full glass of water and remaining upright for at least 30 minutes facilitates delivery of the drug to the stomach. Zoledronic acid should be used cautiously in aspirin-sensitive asthmatic patients. Alendronate and risedronate are now available in a once-a-week formulation to decrease the number of times the patient must take the drug, which should increase compliance with the drug regimen.

Older adults may have dietary deficiencies related to calcium and vitamin D. They should be encouraged to eat dairy products and foods high in calcium and to supplement their diet if necessary. Postmenopausal women, who are prone to develop osteoporosis, may want to consider hormone replacement therapy and calcium supplements to prevent osteoporosis. Many postmenopausal women and some older men respond well to the effect of bisphosphonates in moving calcium back into the bone. They need specific instructions on the proper way to take these drugs and may not be able to comply with the restrictions about staying upright and swallowing the tablet with a full glass of water and not eating within ½ hour of taking the medication as food prevents proper absorption.

Older adults have a greater incidence of renal and kidney impairment, and the function of both should be evaluated before starting any of these drugs. Bisphosphonates should be used in lower doses in patients with moderate renal impairment and are not recommended for those who have severe renal impairment. With any of these drugs, patients have two yearly bone scans to determine bone density and a proper calcium and vitamin D supplement as calcium is poorly absorbed.

Adverse Effects

The most common adverse effects seen with bisphosphonates are headache, nausea and diarrhoea. There is also an increase in bone pain in patients with Paget's disease, but this effect usually passes after a few days to a few weeks. Oesophageal erosion has been associated with alendronate, ibandronate and risedronate if the patient has not remained upright for at least 30 minutes after taking the tablets.

Clinically Important Drug–Drug Interactions

Oral absorption of bisphosphonates is decreased if taken with food, so no food should be taken half an hour after taking these drugs.

GI distress may increase if bisphosphonates are combined with aspirin; this combination should be avoided if possible.

Always consult a current copy of the British National Formulary for further guidance

Nursing Considerations for Patients Receiving Anti-hypercalcaemia Agents

Assessment: History and Examination

Screen for the following conditions, *which could be cautions or contraindications to use of the drug*: history of allergy to vitamin D, hypercalcaemia, vitamin toxicity, renal colic and pregnancy or lactation.

Include screening *for baseline status before beginning therapy and for any potential adverse effects*: the presence of any skin rash; orientation and effect; liver evaluation; serum calcium, magnesium and alkaline phosphate levels and radiographs of bones as appropriate.

Establish if patient is currently taking other medications or herbal therapies which may potentially interact with the antihypocalcaemia agents.

Nursing Diagnoses

The patient receiving any antihypocalcaemic drug may have the following nursing diagnoses related to drug therapy:

- Acute pain related to GI or CNS effects
- Imbalanced nutrition: less than body requirements related to GI effects
- Deficient knowledge regarding drug therapy

Implementation With Rationale

- Monitor serum calcium concentration before and periodically during treatment *to allow for adjustment of dosage to maintain calcium levels within normal limits.*
- Provide supportive measures *to help the patient deal with GI and CNS effects of the drug* (analgesics, small and frequent meals, help with activities of daily living).
- Arrange for a nutritional consultation if GI effects are severe *to ensure nutritional balance.*
- Provide thorough patient education, including measures to avoid adverse effects, warning signs of problems and the need for regular evaluation, *to enhance the patient's knowledge about drug therapy and promote compliance.*

Evaluation

- Monitor patient response to the drug (return of serum calcium levels to normal).
- Monitor for adverse effects (weakness, headache, GI effects).
- Evaluate the effectiveness of the teaching plan (patient can name drug, dosage, adverse effects to watch for and specific measures to avoid adverse effects).
- Monitor the effectiveness of comfort measures and compliance to the regimen.

Anti-hypocalcaemic Agents

Deficient levels of PTH result in **hypocalcaemia** or calcium deficiency. Vitamin D stimulates calcium absorption from the intestine and kidney tubules and restores the serum calcium to normal levels. Hypoparathyroidism is treated primarily with vitamin D and, if necessary, dietary supplements of calcium. Calcitriol is the most commonly used form of vitamin D. Dihydrotachysterol is also used.

Therapeutic Actions and Indications

Vitamin D compounds work with PTH and calcitonin to regulate calcium homeostasis; vitamin D actually functions as a prehormone. Use of these agents is indicated for the management of hypocalcaemia in patients undergoing chronic renal dialysis and for the treatment of hypoparathyroidism.

Pharmacokinetics

Antihypocalcaemic agents are well absorbed from the GI tract and widely distributed throughout the body. They are stored in the liver, fat, muscle, skin and bones. After being metabolized in the liver, they are primarily excreted in the urine. Patients with liver or renal dysfunction may experience increased levels of the drugs and/or toxic effects. At therapeutic levels, these drugs should be used during pregnancy only if the benefit to the mother clearly outweighs the potential for adverse effects on the foetus. Calcitriol has been associated with hypercalcaemia in the baby when used by nursing mothers. Another method of feeding the baby should be used if these drugs are needed during lactation.

Contraindications and Cautions

These drugs should not be used in the presence of any known allergy to vitamin D, hypercalcaemia, vitamin D toxicity or pregnancy. Caution should be used with a history of renal colic or during lactation, *when high calcium levels could cause problems.*

Adverse Effects

The adverse effects most commonly seen with these drugs are related to GI effects: metallic taste, nausea, vomiting, dry mouth, constipation and anorexia. CNS effects such as weakness, headache, somnolence and irritability may also occur. These are possibly related to the changes in electrolytes that occur with these drugs.

Clinically Important Drug–Drug Interactions

The risk of high plasma magnesium levels increases if these drugs are taken with magnesium-containing antacids. This combination should be avoided.

Reduced absorption of these compounds may occur if they are taken with cholestyramine or mineral oil, because they are fat-soluble vitamins. If this combination is used, the drugs should be separated by at least 2 hours.

It should be noted that calcium interacts with a number of foods.

Always consult a current copy of the British National Formulary (BNF) for further guidance

Calcitonins

Calcitonin is a hormone secreted by the thyroid gland to balance the effects of PTH. They are available as synthetic human calcitonin or salmon calcitonin.

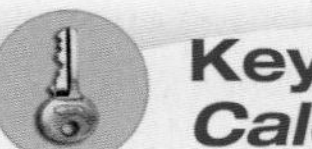

Key Drug Summary: *Calcitriol*

Indications: Management of hypocalcaemia in patients on chronic renal dialysis, management of hypocalcaemia associated with hypoparathyroidism

Actions: A vitamin D compound that regulates the absorption of calcium and phosphate from the small intestine, mineral reabsorption in bone and reabsorption of phosphate and calcium from the renal tubules, increasing the serum calcium level

Pharmacokinetics:

Route	Onset	Peak	Duration
Oral	Slow	4 h	3–5 days

$T_{1/2}$: 5–8 hours; metabolized in the liver and excreted in the bile

Adverse effects: Weakness, headache, nausea, vomiting, dry mouth, constipation, muscle pain, bone pain, metallic taste

Nursing Considerations for Patients Receiving Antihypocalcaemic Agents

Assessment: History and Examination

Screen for the following conditions, *which could be cautions or contraindications to use of the drug*: history of allergy to any of these products or to fish products with salmon calcitonin, pregnancy or lactation, hypocalcaemia and renal dysfunction.

Include screening *for baseline status before beginning therapy and for any potential adverse effects*: presence of any skin lesions, orientation and affect, abdominal examination, serum electrolytes and renal function tests. Patients with suspected osteoporosis should have a bone scan.

Establish if patient is currently taking other medications or herbal therapies which may potentially interact with the antihypocalcaemic agents.

Nursing Diagnoses

The patient receiving any antihypocalcaemic agent may have the following nursing diagnoses related to drug therapy:

- Acute pain related to GI effects
- Imbalanced nutrition: less than body requirements related to GI effects
- Deficient knowledge regarding drug therapy
- Anxiety related to the need for parenterally administered injections (specific drugs)

Implementation With Rationale

- Ensure adequate hydration with any of these agents *to reduce risk of renal complications.*
- Arrange for concomitant vitamin D, calcium supplements and hormone replacement therapy *if used to treat postmenopausal osteoporosis.*
- Rotate injection sites and monitor for inflammation if using calcitonin *to prevent tissue breakdown and irritation.*
- Assess the patient carefully for any potential drug–drug interactions if giving in combination with other drugs *to prevent serious effects.*
- Provide comfort measures and analgesics *to relieve bone pain if it returns as treatment begins.*
- Provide thorough patient education, including measures to avoid adverse effects, warning signs of problems, highlight the need for regular evaluation if used for longer than recommended and proper administration of nasal spray *to enhance patient knowledge about drug therapy and promote compliance.*

Evaluation

- Monitor patient response to the drug (return of calcium levels to normal; prevention of complications of osteoporosis, control of Paget's disease).
- Monitor for adverse effects (skin rash, nausea and vomiting, hypocalcaemia, renal dysfunction).
- Evaluate the effectiveness of the teaching plan (patient can name drug, dosage, adverse effects to watch for, specific measures to avoid adverse effects).
- Monitor the effectiveness of comfort measures and compliance to the regimen.

Therapeutic Actions and Indications

These hormones inhibit bone reabsorption, lower serum calcium levels in children and patients with Paget's disease and increase the excretion of phosphate, calcium and sodium from the kidney. Human calcitonin produced by genetic engineering is now approved in treating Paget's disease in some cases. Salmon calcitonin, which has a longer duration of action, has more approved uses. For example, it is recommended for the treatment of Paget's disease, for the treatment of postmenopausal osteoporosis in conjunction with vitamin D and calcium supplements and for the emergency treatment of hypercalcaemia. Human calcitonin can be given only by injection. Salmon calcitonin can be given by injection and most recently as a nasal spray.

Pharmacokinetics

These drugs are metabolized to inactive fragments in body tissues, these fragments are excreted by the kidney. Which are excreted by the kidney. They cross the placenta and have been associated with adverse effects on the foetus in animal studies. They should be used in pregnancy only if the benefit to the mother clearly outweighs the potential risk to the foetus. It is not known whether they are excreted in breast milk.

Contraindications and Cautions

These drugs should not be used during lactation, *because the calcium-lowering effects could cause problems for the baby.* Salmon calcitonin should not be used with a known allergy to salmon or fish products. Caution should be used in patients with renal dysfunction or pernicious anaemia, *which could be exacerbated by these drugs.*

Always consult a current copy of the British National Formulary for further guidance.

Adverse Effects

The most common adverse effects seen with these drugs are flushing of the face and hands, skin rash, nausea and vomiting, urinary frequency and local inflammation at the site of injection. Many of these side-effects lessen with time, the time varying with each individual patient.

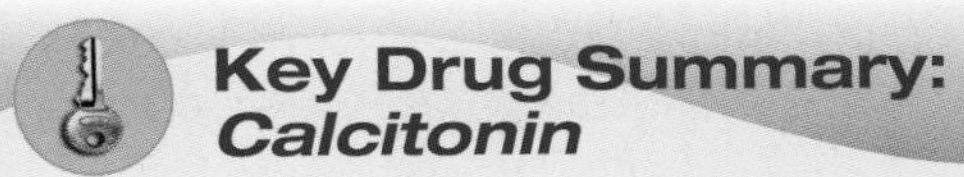

Key Drug Summary: *Calcitonin*

Indications: Paget's disease, postmenopausal osteoporosis, emergency treatment of hypercalcaemia

Actions: Inhibits bone resorption; lowers elevated serum calcium in children and patients with Paget's disease; increases the excretion of filtered phosphate, calcium and sodium by the kidney

Pharmacokinetics:

Route	Onset	Peak	Duration
IM, Sub-cut	15 min	3–4 h	8–24 h
Nasal	Rapid	31–39 min	8–24 h

$T_{1/2}$: 1.5 hours; metabolized in the kidneys and excreted in urine
Adverse effects: Flushing of face and hands, nausea, vomiting, local inflammatory reactions at and pain at injection site, nasal irritation if nasal form is used

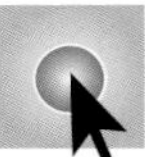

WEB LINKS

Health care providers and patients may want to consult the following Internet sources:

http://cks.library.nhs.uk The National Health Service Clinical Knowledge Summaries provides evidence-based practical information on the common conditions observed in primary care.

http://thyroid-disease.org.uk on endocrine diseases, screening and treatment.

http://www.bnf.org.uk The BNF provides UK health care professionals with authoritative and practical information on the selection and clinical use of medicines.

http://www.british-thyroid-association.org/guidelines.htm Information on thyroid diseases, support groups, treatments and research.

http://hcd2.bupa.co.uk/fact_sheets/html/osteoporosis.html Information on osteoporosis and support groups, screening, treatment and research.

http://www.nhsdirect.nhs.uk The National Health Service Direct service provides patients with information and advice about health, illness and health services.

http://www.nice.org.uk The National Institute for Health and Clinical Excellence (NICE) is an independent organization responsible for providing national guidance on promoting good health and preventing and treating ill health.

http://www.thyroiduk.org Information on thyroid diseases, support groups, treatments and research.

Points to Remember

- The thyroid gland uses iodine to produce thyroid hormones. Thyroid hormones control the rate at which most body cells use energy (metabolism).
- Control of the thyroid gland is an intricate balance between TRH, released by the hypothalamus, TSH, released by the anterior pituitary, and circulating levels of thyroid hormones.
- Hypothyroidism, or lower-than-normal levels of thyroid hormones, is treated with replacement thyroid hormone.
- Hyperthyroidism, or higher-than-normal levels of thyroid hormone, is treated with thioeylenes, which block the thyroid from producing thyroid hormone, or with iodine, which prevents thyroid hormone production or destroy parts of the gland.
- The parathyroid glands are located behind the thyroid gland and produce PTH, which works with calcitonin, produced by thyroid cells, to maintain the calcium balance in the body.
- Hypocalcaemia, or low levels of calcium, is treated with vitamin D products and calcium replacement therapy.
- Hypercalcaemia and hypercalcaemic states are related to malignancy.
- Hypercalcaemia is treated with bisphosphonates or calcitonin. Bisphosphonates slow or block bone resorption, which lowers serum calcium levels. Calcitonin inhibits bone resorption, lowers serum calcium levels in children and patients with Paget's disease and increases the excretion of phosphate, calcium and sodium from the kidney.

CRITICAL THINKING SCENARIO 36-1

Hypothyroidism

The Situation

Helen, a 38-year-old woman, complains of 'exhaustion, lethargy and sleepiness'. Her past history is vague and it is noted that her speech seems slurred and her attention span is limited. Her husband reports feeling frustrated with Helen, stating that she has become increasingly lethargic, disorganized and uninvolved at home. He also notes that she has gained weight and lost interest in her appearance. Physical examination reveals the following: pulse rate, 52 bpm; blood pressure, 90/62 mmHg; she is

Hypothyroidism *(continued)*

apyrexial; her skin is pale, dry and thick; she has peri-orbital oedema and a thick and asymmetric tongue; her height, 1.65 m and she weights 78 kg. The immediate impression is that of hypothyroidism. Laboratory tests confirm this, revealing elevated TSH and very low levels of triiodothyronine (T_3) and thyroxine (T_4). 100 μg q.d.s oral levothyroxine is prescribed.

Critical Thinking

- What teaching plans should be developed for this patient?
- What interventions would be appropriate in helping Helen and her husband accept the diagnosis and the pathophysiological basis for Helen's complaints and problems?
- What body image changes will Helen experience as her body adjusts to the thyroid therapy?
- How can Helen be helped to adjust to these changes and re-establish her body image and self-concept?

Discussion

Hypothyroidism develops slowly and it presents with fatigue, lethargy and lack of emotional response, all symptoms that result in the patient's losing interest in appearance, activities and responsibilities. If left untreated, the patient could develop myxoedema coma and die.

The teaching plan should include information about the function of the thyroid gland and the anticipated changes that will be occurring to Helen over the next week and beyond. The importance of taking the medication daily should be emphasized. The need to return for follow-up to evaluate the effectiveness of the medication and the effects on her body should also be stressed. Both Helen and her husband will need support and encouragement to deal with past frustrations and the return to normal. Lifelong therapy will probably be needed, so further teaching will be important once things have stabilized.

Nursing Care Guide for Helen: Thyroid Hormone

Assessment: History and Examination

Review the patient's history for, Addison's disease, past history of myocardial infarction (not complicated by hypothyroidism), lactation and thyrotoxicosis.

Focus the physical examination on the following:

- Neurological: orientation and effect
- Skin: colour and lesions
- CV: pulse, cardiac auscultation, blood pressure and ECG findings
- Respiratory: respirations, adventitious sounds
- Haematological: thyroid function tests

Patient Education for Helen

- ☐ This hormone is designed to replace the thyroid hormone that your body is not able to produce. The thyroid hormone is responsible for regulating your body's metabolism or the speed with which your body's cells burn energy. Thyroid hormone actions affect many body systems; so it is very important that you take this medication only as prescribed.
- ☐ Never stop taking this drug without consulting with your health care provider. The drug is used to replace a very important hormone and will probably have to be taken for life. Stopping the medication can lead to serious problems.
- ☐ Take this drug before breakfast each day with a full glass of water.
- ☐ Thyroid hormone usually causes no adverse effects. You may notice a slight skin rash or hair loss in the first few months of therapy. You should notice the signs and symptoms of your thyroid deficiency subsiding and you will feel 'back to normal'.
- ☐ Report any of the following to your health care provider: chest pain, difficulty breathing, sore throat, fever, chills, weight gain, sleeplessness, nervousness, unusual sweating or intolerance to heat.
- ☐ Avoid taking any over-the-counter medication without first checking with your health care provider because several medications can interfere with the effectiveness of this drug.
- ☐ Tell any doctor, nurse or other health care provider involved in your care that you are taking this drug. While you are taking this drug, you will need regular medical follow-up, including blood tests to check the activity of your thyroid gland, to evaluate your response to the drug and any possible underlying problems.
- ☐ Keep this drug and all medications out of the reach of children.
- ☐ Do not give this medication to anyone else or take any similar medication that has not been prescribed for you.

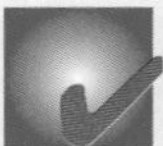

CHECK YOUR UNDERSTANDING

Answers to the questions in this chapter may be found in the Answer Key in the back of the book.

Multiple Choice

Select the most appropriate response to the following.

1. The thyroid gland produces the thyroid hormones T_3 and T_4, which are dependent on the availability of
   a. iodine produced in the liver.
   b. iodine found in the diet.
   c. iron absorbed from the gastrointestinal tract.
   d. parathyroid hormone to promote iodine binding.

2. The thyroid gland is dependent on the hypothalamic-pituitary axis for regulation. Increasing the levels of thyroid hormone (by taking replacement thyroid hormone) would
   a. increase hypothalamic release of TRH.
   b. increase pituitary release of TSH.
   c. suppress hypothalamic release of TRH.
   d. stimulate the thyroid gland to produce more T_3 and T_4.

3. Thyroid replacement therapy is indicated for the treatment of
   a. obesity.
   b. myxoedema.
   c. Graves' disease.
   d. acute thyrotoxicosis.

4. Administration of propylthiouracil would include giving the drug
   a. once a day in the morning.
   b. several times a day to assure therapeutic levels.
   c. once a day at bedtime to decrease adverse effects.
   d. if the patient is experiencing slow heart rate, skin rash or excessive bleeding.

5. The parathyroid glands produce PTH, which is important in the body as
   a. a modulator of thyroid hormone.
   b. a regulator of potassium.
   c. a regulator of calcium.
   d. an activator of vitamin D.

Extended Matching Question

Select **all** that apply.

1. A patient who is receiving a bisphosphonate for the treatment of postmenopausal osteoporosis should be taught to
   a. also take vitamin D, calcium and hormone replacement.
   b. restrict fluids as much as possible.
   c. take the drug with water before any food and wait at least half an hour before having food
   d. stay upright for at least one-half hour after taking the drug.
   e. take the drug with meals to avoid GI upset.
   f. avoid exercise to prevent bone fractures.
   g. refrain from food for ½ hour after taking drug

2. Hypothyroidism is a very common and often missed disorder. Signs and symptoms of hypothyroidism include:
   a. increased body temperature.
   b. thickening of the tongue.
   c. bradycardia.
   d. loss of hair.
   e. excessive weight loss.
   f. oily skin.

Matching

Match the following words with the appropriate choice.

1. ______________ iodine
2. ______________ thyroxine
3. ______________ liothyronine
4. ______________ calcitonin
5. ______________ hypothyroidism
6. ______________ developmental delay
7. ______________ myxoedema
8. ______________ hyperthyroidism
9. ______________ thioeylenes
10. ______________ Paget's disease

A. T_4
B. Hormone produced by the thyroid gland C cells
C. Lack of thyroid hormone in the infant
D. Excess levels of thyroid hormone
E. Dietary element used to produce thyroid hormone
F. T_3
G. Drugs used to prevent the formation of thyroid hormone
H. Severe lack of thyroid hormone in adults
I. Disorder of overactive osteoclasts
J. Lack of sufficient thyroid hormone to maintain metabolism

Bibliography

British Medical Association and Royal Pharmaceutical Society of Great Britain. (2008). *British National Formulary*. London: BMJ & RPS Publishing. *This publication is updated biannually: it is imperative that the most recent edition is consulted.*

British Medical Association and Royal Pharmaceutical Society of Great Britain. (2008). *British National Formulary for Children*. London: BMJ & RPS Publishing. *This publication is updated annually: it is imperative that the most recent edition is consulted.*

Ganong, W. (2005). *Review of medical physiology* (22nd ed.). New York: McGraw-Hill.

Howland, R. D., & Mycek, M. J. (2005). *Pharmacology* (3rd ed.). Philadelphia: Lippincott Williams & Wilkins.

Marieb, E. N., & Hoehn, K. (2004). *Human anatomy & physiology* (7th ed.). San Francisco: Pearson Benjamin Cummings.

Porth, C. M., & Matfin, G. (2008). *Pathophysiology: Concepts of altered health states* (8th ed.). Philadelphia: Lippincott Williams & Wilkins.

Simonsen, T., Aarbakke, J., Kay, I., Coleman, I., Sinnott, P., & Lysaa, R. (2006). *Illustrated pharmacology for nurses.* London: Hodder Arnold.

CHAPTER

37

Antidiabetic Agents

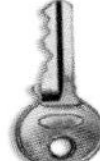

KEY TERMS

diabetes mellitus
endocrine
exocrine
glycogen
glycosuria
hyperglycaemia
hypoglycaemia
insulin
ketoacidosis
polydipsia
polyphagia
sulphonylureas
type 1 insulin-dependent diabetes mellitus (IDDM)
type 2 non-insulin-dependent diabetes mellitus (NIDDM)

LEARNING OBJECTIVES

Upon completion of this chapter, you will be able to:

1. Describe the pathophysiology of diabetes mellitus, including alterations in metabolic pathways and changes to basement membranes.
2. Describe the therapeutic actions, indications and pharmacokinetics associated with insulin and other antidiabetic and glucose-elevating agents.
3. Describe the contraindications, most common adverse reactions and important drug–drug interactions associated with insulin and other antidiabetic and glucose-elevating agents.
4. Discuss the use of antidiabetic and glucose-elevating agents across the lifespan.
5. Compare and contrast the key drugs insulin, tolbutamide and metformin with other antidiabetic agents in their class.
6. Outline the nursing considerations, including important teaching points, for patients receiving antidiabetic or glucose-elevating agents.

REPLACEMENT INSULIN

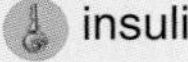 insulin

SULPHONYLUREAS

Long acting:
chlorpropamide
glibenclamide
Shorter acting:
gliclazide
glimepiride
glipizide
gliquidone
tolbutamide

BIGUANIDES

metformin

OTHER ANTIDIABETIC AGENTS

acarbose
exenatide
nateglinide
pioglitazone
repaglinide
rosiglitazone
sitagliptin

GLUCOSE-ELEVATING AGENTS

diazoxide
glucagons

Diabetes mellitus (literally, 'honey urine') is the most common of all metabolic disorders. It is estimated that 2 million people in the United Kingdom have been diagnosed with diabetes mellitus, and a further half a million people have undiagnosed diabetes mellitus (Diabetes UK, 2008). Diabetes is a complicated disorder that affects many organs and causes numerous clinical complications. Currently, treatment of diabetes is aimed at tightly regulating the blood sugar level through the use of insulin or insulin-stimulating drugs.

Glucose Regulation

Glucose is the leading energy source for the human body. It is stored in the body for rapid release and utilized in times of stress so that the serum concentration of glucose is maintained at a level that provides a constant supply of glucose to the neurons. The minute-to-minute control of glucose levels is the function of the endocrine pancreas gland.

The Pancreas and Insulin

The pancreas is both an **exocrine** and an **endocrine** gland. The exocrine function involves the release of sodium bicarbonate and pancreatic enzymes directly into the common bile duct, which is then released into the small intestine. These neutralize the acid chyme from the stomach and aid digestion, respectively. The endocrine part of the pancreas produces hormones in specialized cells called the islets of Langerhans. These islets contain endocrine cells that produce specific hormones. The alpha (α) cells release the hormone *glucagon* in response to low glucose levels, and beta (β) cells release *insulin* in response to high glucose levels. Delta (δ) cells produce somatostatin, which blocks the secretion of insulin and glucagon. These hormones work together to maintain the serum glucose level within normal limits of 3.5 to 8 mmol/l.

Insulin is the hormone released into circulation when the levels of glucose around the pancreatic beta cells rise. Insulin circulates throughout the body and binds to specific insulin receptor sites on cell membranes, stimulating the transport of glucose into the cells by facilitated diffusion. Insulin also stimulates the synthesis of **glycogen** (glucose stored for immediate release during times of stress or low glucose): the conversion of lipids into fat stored in the form of adipose tissue and the synthesis of needed proteins from amino acids.

Insulin is released after a meal when the blood glucose levels rise. It affects metabolism, allowing the body to either store or use the nutrients from the meal effectively. As insulin is released, blood glucose levels fall and insulin release is then reduced.

When an insufficient amount of insulin is released, several metabolic changes occur, beginning with **hyperglycaemia** or increased blood sugar. Hyperglycaemia results in **glycosuria**: sugar spills into the urine because the concentration of glucose in the blood is too high for complete reabsorption. The glucose transporters in the kidney nephron become saturated, and the renal threshold is reached. The sugar-rich urine is an ideal environment for bacteria; therefore, cystitis is common in hyperglycaemic patients. The patient experiences fatigue because the body's cells cannot use the glucose that is present; they need insulin to facilitate transport of the glucose into the cells. **Polyphagia** (increased hunger) occurs because the hypothalamic centres cannot take in glucose and sense that they are starving. **Polydipsia** (increased thirst) occurs because the tonicity of the blood is increased owing to the increased glucose and waste products in the blood and the loss of fluid with glucose in the urine. The hypothalamic cells that are sensitive to fluid levels sense a need to increase fluid in the system, and the patient will feel thirsty.

Lipolysis, or fat breakdown, occurs as the body breaks down stored fat for energy because the glucose present cannot be used. The patient experiences **ketoacidosis** as metabolism shifts to the use of fat, and the ketone wastes cannot be removed effectively. Acidosis also occurs because the liver cannot remove all of the waste products (acid being a primary waste product) that result from the breakdown of glucose, fat and proteins. Muscle tissues start to break down because proteins are no longer synthesized and also because the body requires the essential amino acids contained in the proteins. The breakdown of proteins results in an increase in nitrogen wastes, which manifests as an elevated blood urea nitrogen concentration and sometimes protein in the urine. Patients with hyperglycaemia have slowed wound healing because of this breakdown of proteins and the lack of a stimulus to build proteins. All these actions eventually contribute to development of the complications associated with chronic hyperglycaemia or diabetes mellitus.

Diabetes Mellitus

Diabetes mellitus is characterized by complex disturbances in metabolism. The most frequently recognized clinical signs of diabetes are hyperglycaemia (fasting blood sugar level greater than 11 mmol/l) and glycosuria (the presence of glucose in the urine). The alterations in the body's ability to effectively deal with carbohydrate, fat and protein metabolism over the long term result in a thickening of the basement membrane (a thin layer of collagen lying just below the endothelial lining of blood vessels) in large and small blood vessels. This thickening leads to changes in oxygenation of the lining of the vessel, damage to the vessel lining, which leads to narrowing and decreased blood flow through the vessel, and an inability of oxygen to rapidly diffuse across the membrane to the tissues. These changes result in an increased incidence of a number of disorders, including:

- *Atherosclerosis*: Heart attacks and strokes related to the development of atherosclerotic plaques in the vessel lining.
- *Retinopathy*: With resultant loss of vision as tiny vessels in the eye are narrowed and closed.
- *Neuropathies*: With motor and sensory changes in the feet and legs and progressive changes in other nerves as the oxygen supply to these nerves is slowly cut off.
- *Nephropathy*: With renal dysfunction related to changes in the basement membrane of the glomerulus.

The overall metabolic disturbances associated with diabetes are thought to be caused by a lack of insulin or its actions. This may occur because the:

- pancreas cannot produce enough insulin,
- insulin receptor sites have lost their sensitivity to insulin or
- person does not have enough receptor sites to support his or her body size. This may occur in obesity.

Replacement or stimulation of insulin release is the foundation of diabetes mellitus treatment. Box 37.1 describes the treatment of diabetes for all age groups. The diagnosis of diabetes mellitus involves the monitoring of fasting blood glucose levels and sometimes challenging the system with glucose for a glucose tolerance test.

Diabetes mellitus is classified as **type 1, which used to be called insulin-dependent diabetes mellitus (IDDM)**, or **type 2, which used to be called noninsulin-dependent diabetes mellitus (NIDDM)**. Type 1 diabetes is usually associated with rapid onset, mostly in younger people and is connected in many cases to viral destruction of the pancreatic beta cells. Type 1 diabetes always requires insulin replacement (see Critical Thinking Scenario 37-1, for an example of managing this type of diabetes.) Some patients have undergone islet cell transplantations where islet cells from either living or dead donors are implanted. Many of these patients either became totally independent of insulin supplements or were able to reduce their insulin dose and avoid hypoglycaemic 'lows'. However, islet cell transplantation is still at an experimental stage, and the long-term effects of remaining on immunosuppressant drugs are of concern (Bromberg *et al.*, 2007).

BOX 37.1 **DRUG THERAPY ACROSS THE LIFESPAN**

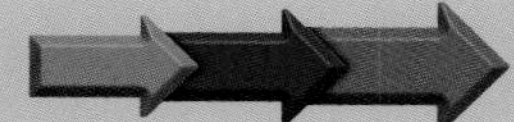

Antidiabetic Agents

CHILDREN

Treatment of diabetes in children is a difficult challenge of balancing diet, activity, growth and stress needs and insulin requirements. Children need to be carefully monitored for any sign of hypoglycaemia or hyperglycaemia and treated quickly because their fast metabolism and lack of body reserves can push them into a severe state quickly.

Teenage children often present a real challenge for diabetes management. The desire to be 'normal' often leads to a resistance to dietary restrictions and insulin injections. The metabolism of the teenager is also in flux, leading to complications in regulating insulin dosage. A collective approach, including the child, family members, teachers and even friends, may be the best way to help the child deal with the disease and the required therapy. New delivery methods for insulin may help this age group cope with drug therapy.

When administering any drug to children, always consult the most recent edition of the British National Formulary for Children.

ADULTS

Adults need extensive education about the disease as well as the drug therapy. Adults maintained on oral agents need to be monitored for changes in response to the drugs. Often additional drugs are added or dosages are changed as the disease progresses over time.

Exercise and diet should always be emphasized as the factors in dealing with diabetes. Adults need to be cautioned about the use of over-the-counter and herbal or alternative therapies. Many of these products contain agents that alter blood glucose levels and will change insulin or oral agent requirements.

Insulin therapy is the best choice for patients with diabetes during pregnancy and lactation, times of high stress and metabolic demands. Needs may change on a daily basis, and the mother should receive support and teaching about what to do if hypoglycaemia or hyperglycaemia occurs. Labour and delivery is often a critical time in diabetes management because of the stress and sudden changes in body fluid volume and hormone levels.

OLDER ADULTS

Older adults can have many underlying problems that complicate diabetic therapy. Poor vision and/or coordination may make it difficult to prepare a syringe.

Dietary deficiencies related to changes in taste, absorption or attitude may lead to wide fluctuations in blood sugar levels, making it difficult to control diabetes. Many areas offer nutritional assistance programmes for older adults (e.g. Meals on Wheels) or can refer patients to appropriate agencies that might be able to offer assistance.

Older adults have a greater incidence of renal or hepatic impairment, and kidney and liver function should be evaluated before starting any of these drugs. Combinations of oral agents may not be feasible with severe dysfunction, and the patient may need to use insulin to control blood glucose levels.

The older patient is also more likely to experience organ damage related to the diabetes – loss of vision, kidney problems, coronary artery disease, infections – and the drug regimen of these patients can become quite complex. Careful screening for drug interactions is an important aspect of the assessment of these patients.

Type 2 diabetes usually occurs in mature adults and has a slow and progressive onset. However, the incidence of type 2 diabetes in teenagers and young adults has increasing markedly (Gale, 2002). Questions are being raised about the impact of early high calorific diet and lack of exercise in contributing to this new increase in type 2 diabetes in young people. The treatment of type 2 diabetes usually begins with changes in diet and exercise. Dieting controls the amount and timing of glucose introduction into the body, and weight loss decreases the number of insulin receptor sites that need to be stimulated. Exercise increases the movement of glucose into the cells by activation of the sympathetic nervous system (SNS) and by the increase of potassium in the blood that occurs directly after exercising. Potassium acts as part of a polarizing system during exercise that pushes glucose into the cells. Clinical studies have shown that controlling serum glucose levels can decrease the risk of complications, for example macro- and microvascular complications (American Diabetes Association 2002).

When diet and exercise no longer work, oral agents (discussed later) are tried to stimulate the production of insulin in the pancreas, increase the sensitivity of the insulin receptor sites or control the entry of glucose into the system. Injection of insulin may eventually be needed to replace the missing insulin. This concept is often confusing to patients who are learning about diabetes. Type 2 diabetes often evolves until insulin is needed. Timing of the injections of insulin is correlated with food intake and anticipated increases in blood glucose levels as well as exercise levels and anticipated stress. See Box 37.2 for more information about managing glucose levels during stress.

Hyperglycaemia

Hyperglycaemia, or high blood sugar, results when there is insufficient insulin to deal with the glucose in the system. Clinical signs and symptoms of hyperglycaemia include fatigue, lethargy, irritation, glycosuria, polyphagia, polydipsia and itchy skin (from accumulation of wastes that the liver cannot clear). If the hyperglycaemia goes unchecked, the patient will experience ketoacidosis and central nervous system (CNS) changes that can progress to coma. Signs of impending dangerous complications of hyperglycaemia include:

- Fruity breath ('pear drops') as the ketones build up in the system and are excreted via the lungs.
- Dehydration as fluid and important electrolytes are lost through the kidneys.
- Slow, deep respirations (Kussmaul's respirations) as the body tries to rid itself of CO_2 and thus reduce high acid levels.
- Loss of orientation and coma.

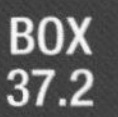

FOCUS ON THE **EVIDENCE**

Managing Glucose Levels during Stress

The body has many compensatory mechanisms for ensuring that blood glucose levels stay within a safe range. The sympathetic stress reaction elevates blood glucose levels to provide ready energy for 'fight or flight' (see Chapter 28). The stress reaction causes the breakdown of glycogen to release glucose and the breakdown of fat and proteins to release other energy forms.

Stress Reactions

The stress reaction elevates the blood glucose concentration above the normal range. In severe stress situations, such as an acute myocardial infarction or a car accident, the blood glucose level can be very high (16–24 mmol/l). The body uses that energy to fight the insult or flee from the stressor.

Nurses in acute care situations need to be aware of this reflex elevation in glucose when caring for patients in acute stress, especially patients in emergency situations, whose medical history is unknown. The usual medical response to a blood glucose concentration of 24 mmol/l would be the administration of insulin. In many situations, that is exactly what is done, especially if the patient's history is not known, and the effects of such a high glucose level could cause severe systemic reactions. Insulin administration causes a drop in the blood glucose level as glucose enters cells to be either used for energy or converted to glycogen for storage.

However, a problem may arise in the acute care setting, particularly, in a nondiabetic patient. Relieving the stress reaction can also drop glucose levels as the stimulus to increase these levels is lost, and the glucose that was there is used for energy. A patient in this situation, who has been treated with insulin, is at risk of developing potentially severe hypoglycaemia. The body's response to low glucose levels is a sympathetic stress reaction, which again elevates the blood glucose concentration. If treated, the patient can potentially enter a cycle of high and low glucose levels.

Best Nursing Practice

Nurses are often the ones in closest contact with the highly stressed patient in Accident and Emergency (A&E), the intensive care unit or the postanaesthesia room and should be constantly aware of the normal and reflex changes in blood glucose that accompany stress. Careful monitoring, with awareness of stress and the relief of stress, can prevent a prolonged treatment programme to maintain blood glucose levels within the range of normal, a situation that is not 'normal' during a stress reaction.

Diabetic patients who are in severe stress situations require changes in their insulin dosages. They should be allowed some elevation of blood glucose, even though their inability to produce sufficient insulin will make it difficult for their cells to make effective use of the increased glucose levels. It is a clinical challenge to balance glucose levels with the needs of the patient because so many factors can affect the plasma glucose level.

Table 37.1 Signs and Symptoms of Hypoglycaemia and Hyperglycaemia

System	Hypoglycaemia	Hyperglycaemia
Central nervous system	Headache, blurred vision, diplopia; drowsiness progressing to coma; ataxia; hyperactive reflexes	Decreased level of consciousness, sluggishness progressing to coma; hypoactive reflexes
Neuromuscular	Paresthesias; weakness; muscle spasms; twitching progressing to seizures	Weakness, lethargy
Cardiovascular	Tachycardia; palpitations; normal to high blood pressure	Tachycardia; hypotension
Respiratory	Rapid, shallow respirations	Rapid, deep respirations (Kussmaul's); acetone-like or fruity breath
Gastrointestinal	Hunger, nausea	Nausea; vomiting; thirst
Other	Diaphoresis; cool and clammy skin; normal eyeballs	Dry, warm, flushed skin; soft eyeballs
Laboratory tests	Urine glucose – negative; blood glucose low	Urine glucose – trongly positive; urine ketone levels – positive; blood glucose levels – high
Onset	Sudden; patient appears anxious, drunk; associated with overdose of insulin, missing a meal, increased stress	Gradual; patient is slow and sluggish; associated with lack of insulin, increased stress

This level of hyperglycaemia needs to be treated immediately with insulin.

Hypoglycaemia

Hypoglycaemia, or a blood sugar concentration lower than 3 mmol/l; occurs in a number of clinical situations, including starvation and if treatment of hyperglycaemia with insulin or oral agents lowers the blood sugar too far. The body immediately reacts to lowered blood sugar because the cells require glucose to survive, the neurons being among the cells most sensitive to the lack of glucose. The initial reaction to falling blood sugar is parasympathetic stimulation: increased gastrointestinal (GI) activity to increase digestion and absorption. Rather rapidly, the SNS responds by increasing blood glucose levels through initiating the breakdown of fat and glycogen to release glucose for rapid energy. The pancreas releases glucagon, a hormone that counters the effects of insulin and works to increase glucose levels. In many cases, the response to the hypoglycaemic state causes a hyperglycaemic state. Balancing the body's responses to glucose is sometimes difficult when one is trying to treat and control diabetes. Table 37.1 offers a comparison of the signs and symptoms of hyperglycaemia and hypoglycaemia.

Replacement Insulin

As described above, insulin promotes storage of the body's fuels, facilitates the transport of various metabolites and ions across cell membranes and stimulates the synthesis of glycogen from glucose, of fats from lipids and of proteins from amino acids. Insulin achieves this by reacting with specific receptor sites on the cell. Figure 37.1 shows the sites of action of replacement insulin and other drugs used to treat diabetic conditions.

There are several ways patients can monitor their blood glucose levels once treatment has commenced. First, using a urine dipstick to measure glucose levels in the urine. Patients should note that urine glucose levels will lag behind blood glucose levels. Alternatively, patients can measure their blood glucose levels using finger-prick blood samples and adjust their insulin dose when necessary. Although it is well known that self-monitoring is a successful way of achieving glycaemic control, the efficacy of self-monitoring has been questioned recently. Recent studies have shown that diabetic patients who did not monitor their blood glucose levels several times each week were able to control their glucose levels to the same extent as those diabetic patients who did (O'Kane *et al.*, 2008). A separate study found that self-monitoring reduced the quality of life of diabetic patients and was not cost-effective (Simon *et al.*, 2008). Patients should take the decision to stop self-monitoring only after consultation with their doctor; for some patients, self-monitoring is still beneficial.

Glycosylated haemoglobin levels, or an HbA1c test, can provide a 3-month average of glucose levels. Red blood cells are freely permeable to glucose, and a covalent bond can form between the glucose molecule and the haemoglobin molecule. The rate at which this bond forms depends on the glucose concentration. This test gives an average range of glucose exposure over the life of the red blood cell, about 120 days. This test does not require fasting before blood is drawn or the oral intake of glucose before testing. Once a baseline is established, the goal of therapy for a diabetic patient is an HbA1c level less than 7.5%, which will help to reduce the risk of long-term vascular complications. Certain conditions, for example blood loss, can affect the average lifespan of an erythrocyte. Therefore, the HbA1c levels should not be used as a diagnostic or screening test for diabetes mellitus as this test is dependent on the assumption that all erythrocytes survive for 120 days (Reynolds *et al.*, 2006).

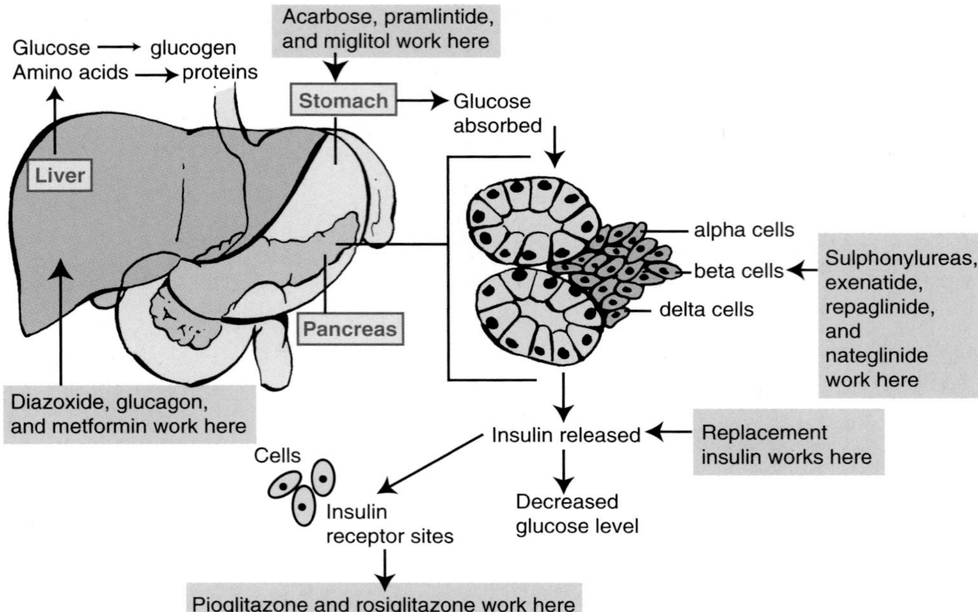

FIGURE 37.1 Sites of action of drugs used to treat diabetic conditions.

Therapeutic Actions and Indications

Replacement insulin is used to treat type 1 diabetes mellitus, type 2 diabetes mellitus in patients whose diabetes cannot be controlled by diet or other agents, severe ketoacidosis or diabetic coma and hyperkalaemia with infusion of glucose to produce a shift of potassium into the cells (polarizing solution). It is also used for short courses of therapy during periods of stress (e.g. surgery, disease) in type 2 patients with diabetes, for the stabilization of newly diagnosed patients, for patients with poor control of glucose levels and for patients with gestational diabetes.

Originally, insulin was prepared from the pancreas of cows and pigs. This has now largely been replaced by insulin prepared using recombinant DNA technology and genetically altered yeast or bacteria cells. Various preparations of insulin are available to provide short and long-term coverage. Frequently, patients use more than one preparation to provide insulin coverage at different times during the day. The most common way of administering insulin is via subcutaneous injection (Boxes 37.3 and 37.4).

Pharmacokinetics

Synthetic insulin is processed within the body in the same way as endogenous insulin. The peak, onset and duration of the different preparations vary with each type of insulin because of the placement or addition of glycine and/or arginine chains. Insulin does not cross the placenta, and it is the drug of choice for managing diabetes during pregnancy. Insulin does enter breast milk, but it is destroyed in

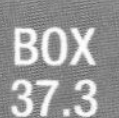

BOX 37.3

Insulin Delivery: Past, Present and Future

Past

Subcutaneous (Sub-Cut) injection: the delivery of insulin by subcutaneous injection was first introduced in the 1920s and changed the way that diabetic patients were managed clinically, giving them a chance of a normal lifestyle.

Present

Subcutaneous injection: this remains the primary delivery system.

Insulin pen: this syringe-like device resembles a pen. It has a small needle at the tip and a barrel that holds insulin. The patient 'dials' the amount of insulin to be given and injects the insulin subcutaneously by pressing on the top of the pen. This is advantageous for people who need insulin two or three times during the day but cannot easily transport syringes and needles. It is a subtle way to give insulin and is popular with students and people on the go. It is important to rotate the syringe 15 to 20 times before injecting the insulin, to disperse it. Patients often forget this point after using the pens for a while and, as a result, may inject far too much or too little insulin when it is needed. Periodic reinforcement of the administration instructions is important.

External insulin pump: this pump device can be worn on a belt or hidden in a pocket and is attached to a small tube inserted into the subcutaneous tissue of the abdomen. The device slowly leaks a base rate of insulin into the abdomen all day; the patient can pump or inject booster doses throughout the day to correspond with meals and activity. The device does have several disadvantages; for example it is awkward and the tubing poses an increased risk of infection and requires frequent changing and the patient has to frequently check blood glucose levels throughout the day to monitor response.

Inhaled insulin: the lung tissue is one of the best sites for insulin absorption. An aerosol delivery system has been developed that delivers a powdered insulin formulation directly into the lungs. The National Institute for Health and Clinical Excellence (NICE) allow patients with poor control of blood glucose or those with a diagnosed phobia of injections to use inhaled insulin.

Future

Implantable insulin pump: this pump is surgically implanted into the abdomen and delivers base insulin as well as insulin boluses as needed directly into the abdomen to be absorbed by the liver, just as pancreatic insulin is. The disadvantages are risk of infection, mechanical problems with the pump and lack of long-term data on its effectiveness.

Insulin patch: the patch is placed on the skin and delivers a constant low dose of insulin. When the patient eats a meal, tabs are pulled on the patch to release more insulin. The problem with this delivery method is that insulin does not readily pass through the skin, so there is tremendous variability in its effects. This route is not yet commercially available.

BOX 37.4 FOCUS ON **CLINICAL SKILLS**

Insulin is usually given by subcutaneous injection. Using an insulin syringe, for example with a 5, 6, 8 and 12 mm needle, inject the insulin into the loose connective tissue underneath the skin. The areas of the body that can be easily pinched to access this tissue are the abdomen, the upper thigh and the upper arm. Insert the needle at a 90 degree. Rotate sites regularly to prevent tissue damage.

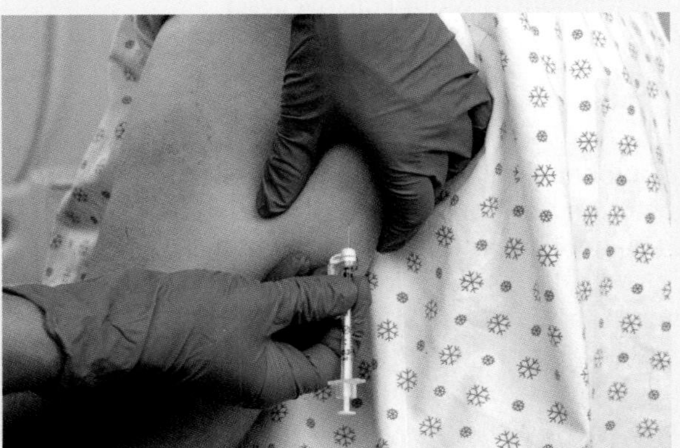

Insert the needle at a 45-degree angle. (Photo by Rick Brady, with permission from Taylor, C, Lillis, C, and LeMone, P. (2005). *Fundamentals of nursing: The art and science of nursing care* (5th ed.). Philadelphia: Lippincott Williams & Wilkins.

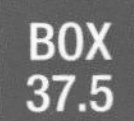

BOX 37.5 HERBAL AND ALTERNATIVE THERAPIES

Patients treated with antidiabetic therapies are at an increased risk of developing hypoglycaemia if they use juniper berries, ginseng, garlic, fenugreek, coriander, dandelion root or celery. If a patient uses these therapies, blood glucose levels should be monitored closely and appropriate dosage adjustment made in their prescribed drug.

the GI tract and does not affect the nursing baby. Insulin-dependent mothers may have inhibited milk production, however, and the effectiveness of nursing should be evaluated periodically.

Adverse Effects

The most common adverse effects to insulin use are hypoglycaemia and ketoacidosis, which can be controlled with proper dosage adjustments, and local reactions at injection sites.

Clinically Important Drug–Drug Interactions

Caution should be used when giving a patient stabilized on insulin any drug that decreases glucose levels (e.g. monoamine oxidase inhibitors, β-blockers, salicylates, alcohol). Dosage adjustments are needed when any of these drugs are added or removed. Care should also be taken when combining insulin with any β-blocker. The blocking of the SNS also blocks many of the signs and symptoms of hypoglycaemia, hindering the patient's ability to recognize problems. Patients taking β-blockers need to learn other ways to recognize hypoglycaemia. Patients should also be warned about possible interactions with various herbal therapies (Box 37.5).

Always consult a current copy of the British National Formulary for further guidance.

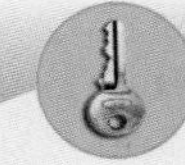

Key Drug Summary: *Insulin*

Indications: Treatment of type 1 diabetes; treatment of type 2 diabetes when other agents have failed; short-term treatment of type 2 diabetes during periods of stress; management of diabetic ketoacidosis, hyperkalaemia, marked insulin resistance

$T_{1/2}$: Varies with each preparation; metabolized at the cellular level

Adverse effects: Hypersensitivity reaction, local reactions at injection site, hypoglycaemia, ketoacidosis

Nursing Considerations for Patients Taking Insulin

Assessment: History and Examination

Screen for history of allergy to any insulin and for pregnancy or lactation *so that appropriate monitoring and dosage adjustments can be completed.* Include screening for baseline status before beginning therapy and for any potential adverse effects: presence of any skin lesions, orientation, baseline pulse and blood pressure, respiration and urinalysis and blood glucose level.

Establish if patient is currently taking other medications or herbal therapies which may potentially interact with insulin.

Nursing Diagnoses

The patient receiving insulin may have the following nursing diagnoses related to drug therapy:

- Imbalanced nutrition: less than body requirements, related to metabolic effects
- Disturbed sensory perception (kinaesthetic, visual, auditory) related to glucose levels
- Risk of infection and poor wound healing related to injections and disease process, respectively
- Ineffective coping related to diagnosis and injection therapy
- Deficient knowledge regarding drug therapy

Implementation With Rationale

- Gently rotate vial and avoid vigorous shaking *to ensure uniform suspension of insulin.*
- Give maintenance doses by the subcutaneous route only (Box 37.4) and rotate injection sites regularly *to avoid damage to muscles and to prevent subcutaneous atrophy.* Give regular insulin intramuscularly or intravenously in emergency situations.
- Monitor response carefully *to avoid adverse effects;* self-monitor blood glucose levels if appropriate.
- Store insulin in a cool place (preferably a fridge) away from direct sunlight. Predrawn syringes are stable for 1 week if refrigerated; *they offer a good way to ensure the proper dosage for patients who have limited vision.*
- Monitor patients during times of trauma or severe stress *for potential dosage adjustment needs.*

Evaluation

- Monitor patient response to the drug (stabilization of blood glucose levels).
- Monitor for adverse effects (hypoglycaemia, ketoacidosis and injection site irritation).
- Evaluate the effectiveness of the teaching plan (patient can name drug, dosage, adverse effects to watch for, specific measures to avoid adverse effects, proper administration technique).
- Monitor the effectiveness of comfort measures and compliance to the regimen.
- Instruct patients who are also receiving β-blockers about ways to monitor glucose levels and signs and symptoms of glucose abnormalities *to prevent hypoglycaemic and hyperglycaemic episodes when SNS and warning signs are blocked.*
- Provide thorough patient education, including measures to avoid adverse effects, warning signs of problems, proper administration techniques and the need to monitor disease status, *to enhance patient knowledge about drug therapy and promote compliance.*

Oral Antidiabetic Agents

Oral drugs are successful in controlling type 2 diabetes in patients who still have a functioning pancreas. These drugs should only be used if the patient fails to respond to attempts to control glucose levels through dietary restrictions and increased exercise.

The **sulphonylureas** were the first oral agents introduced and to stimulate the pancreas to release insulin. Other oral agents, including the biguanides, have been introduced more recently and decrease insulin resistance or alter glucose absorption and uptake. They are often combined with a sulphonylurea for effectiveness.

Sulphonylureas

The sulphonylureas are not effective for all patients with diabetes and may lose their effectiveness over time. All of the sulphonylureas can cause hypoglycaemia.

The older sulphonylureas (often termed first-generation) include chlorpropamide and tolbutamide. There are more side-effects associated with chlorpropamide than the other sulphonylureas, and its use is no longer recommended. Tolbutamide is cleared more easily from the body than chlorpropamide and is preferred for patients with renal dysfunction. Tolbutamide is sometimes used in combination with insulin to reduce the insulin dosage and decrease the risk of hypoglycaemia in certain type 2 patients with diabetes who have begun to use insulin to control their blood glucose level.

Newer drugs such as glipizide and glibebencalmide have several advantages over the older sulphonylureas, including:

- Excretion via urine and bile, making them safer for patients with renal dysfunction.
- They do not interact with as many protein-bound drugs as the earlier drugs.
- They have a longer duration of action, making it possible to take them only once or twice a day, thus increasing compliance.

Therapeutic Actions and Indications

The sulphonylureas close potassium channels on pancreatic beta cells and cause membrane depolarization. As the membrane depolarizes, calcium enters the cell and signals the exocytosis of insulin (see Figure 37.1). They also improve insulin binding to insulin receptors. They are also known to increase the effect of antidiuretic hormone on renal cells. They are indicated as an adjunct to diet and exercise to lower blood glucose levels in type 2 diabetes mellitus.

Pharmacokinetics

These drugs are rapidly absorbed from the GI tract and undergo hepatic metabolism. They are excreted in the urine. The peak effects and duration of effects differ because of the activity of various metabolites of the different drugs. These drugs are not for use during pregnancy. Insulin should be used if an antidiabetic agent is needed during pregnancy. Some of these drugs cross into breast milk, and adequate studies are not available on others. As there is a risk of hypoglycaemic effects in the baby, these drugs should not be used during lactation. Another method of feeding the baby should be used.

Contraindications and Cautions

Sulphonylureas are contraindicated in the presence of known allergy to any sulphonylureas and in diabetes complicated by fever, severe infection, severe trauma, major surgery, ketoacidosis, severe renal or hepatic disease, pregnancy or lactation. These drugs are also contraindicated for use in type 1 patients with diabetes.

Adverse Effects

The most common adverse effects related to the sulphonylureas are hypoglycaemia (caused by an imbalance in levels of glucose and insulin) and GI distress, including nausea, vomiting, epigastric discomfort, heartburn and anorexia (anorexia should be monitored, because affected patients may not eat after taking the sulphonylurea, which could lead to hypoglycaemia). Allergic skin reactions have been reported with some of these drugs.

Clinically Important Drug–Drug Interactions

Care should be taken with any drug that acidifies the urine, because excretion of the sulphonylurea may be decreased. Caution should also be used with β-blockers, which may mask the signs of hypoglycaemia, and with alcohol, which can lead to altered glucose levels when combined with sulphonylureas. The safety and efficacy of these drugs for use in children have not been established.

Always consult a current copy of the British National Formulary for further guidance.

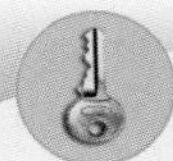

Key Drug Summary: *Tolbutamide*

Indications: Adjunct to diet and exercise to lower blood glucose level in type 2 patients with diabetes

Actions: Stimulates the release of insulin from functioning cells in the pancreas, may improve binding of insulin to insulin receptor sites

Pharmacokinetics:

Route	Onset	Peak	Duration
Oral	20 min	3–4 h	24 h

$T_{1/2}$: 4–7 hours; metabolized by the liver and largely excreted in the urine

Adverse effects: vomiting, nausea, diarrhoea, constipation, tinnitus, headache

Nursing Considerations for Patients Taking Oral Antidiabetic Agents

Assessment: History and Examination

Screen for the following conditions, *which could be cautions or contraindications to use of the drug*: history of allergy to any of the oral agents, severe renal or hepatic dysfunction and pregnancy or lactation.

Include screening for baseline status before beginning therapy and for any potential adverse effects: presence of any skin lesions, orientation and reflexes, baseline pulse and blood pressure, adventitious breath sounds, abdominal sounds and function, urinalysis and blood glucose levels, renal and liver function tests.

Establish if patient is currently taking other medications or herbal therapies which may potentially interact with the oral antidiabetic agents.

Nursing Diagnoses

The patient receiving oral antidiabetic agents may have the following nursing diagnoses related to drug therapy:

- Imbalanced nutrition: less than body requirements, related to metabolic effects
- Disturbed sensory perception (kinaesthetic, visual, auditory) related to glucose levels
- Ineffective coping related to diagnosis and therapy
- Deficient knowledge regarding drug therapy

Implementation With Rationale

- Administer the drug as prescribed in the appropriate relationship to meals *to ensure therapeutic effectiveness.*
- Monitor nutritional status *to provide nutritional consultation as needed.*
- Monitor response carefully, self-monitor blood glucose levels if appropriate.
- Monitor liver enzymes of patients very carefully *to avoid liver toxicity*, arrange to discontinue a drug *to avoid serious liver damage if liver toxicity develops.*
- Monitor patients during times of trauma, pregnancy or severe stress and *arrange alterations of insulin doses as needed.*
- Provide thorough patient education, including measures to avoid adverse effects, warning signs of problems, proper administration technique and the need to monitor disease status, *to enhance patient knowledge of drug therapy and promote compliance.*

Evaluation

- Monitor patient response to the drug (stabilization of blood glucose levels).
- Monitor for adverse effects (hypoglycaemia, GI distress).
- Evaluate the effectiveness of the teaching plan (patient can name drug, dosage, adverse effects to watch for, specific measures to avoid adverse effects).
- Monitor the effectiveness of comfort measures and compliance to the regimen.

Biguanides and Other Oral Antidiabetic Drugs

These oral agents are proven to be effective when used in combination with sulphonylureas or insulin. These drugs include:

- *Metformin*, a biguanide, increases the uptake of glucose by skeletal muscle and decreases the production of glucose by the liver. It is effective in lowering blood glucose levels and does not cause hypoglycaemia as the sulphonylureas. Common side-effects include GI disturbances. On rare occasions, metformin can cause lactic acidosis and should not be used by patients with renal dysfunction.
- *Acarbose* is an inhibitor of the intestinal enzyme alpha-glucosidase which breaks down glucose and delays glucose absorption. This drug has only a mild effect on glucose levels and is associated with flatulence and other GI disturbances, and rarely hepatic toxicity. Acarbose can be used in combination with other oral agents for patients whose glucose levels cannot be controlled with a single agent.
- *Nateglidine* and *repaglinide* stimulate insulin secretion in the same way as the sulphonylureas. These are rapid-acting drugs with a very short half-life. They are used just before meals to lower postprandial glucose levels. These drugs can be used in combination with metformin.
- The thiazolidinediones, *pioglitazone* and *rosiglitazone*, decrease insulin resistance and are used in combination with sulphonylureas or metformin to treat patients with type 2 diabetes. Patients should be monitored for any change in liver function while they are taking pioglitazone.
- Exenatide is an incretin mimetic: incretins are hormones that increase insulin release and inhibit glucagons release. This drug is used in combination with metformin or one of the sulphonylureas.
- *Sitagliptin* increases insulin secretion through the inhibition of dipeptidylpeptidase-4 which slows the inactivation of incretin hormones.

Therapeutic actions and indications, pharmacokinetics, contraindications and cautions, adverse effects and clinically important drug–drug interactions for these drugs are essentially the same as for the sulphonylureas. The safety and efficacy of these drugs for use in children have not been established.

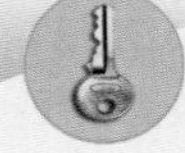

Key Drug Summary: *Metformin*

Indications: Adjunct to diet and exercise for the treatment of type 2 patients with diabetes over 10 years of age

Actions: Increases the peripheral use of glucose and decreases hepatic glucose production

Pharmacokinetics:

Route	Onset	Peak	Duration
Oral	Slow	2–2.5 h	10–16 h

$T_{1/2}$: 6.2 and then 17 hours; excreted unchanged in the urine

Adverse effects: Hypoglycaemia, lactic acidosis, GI upset, nausea, anorexia, diarrhoea, heartburn, allergic skin reaction

Glucose-elevating Agents

Some adverse conditions are associated with hypoglycaemia, or abnormally low blood sugar levels (less than 2 mmol/l), including pancreatic disorders, kidney disease, certain cancers, disorders of the anterior pituitary and unbalanced treatment of diabetes mellitus (which can occur if the patient takes the wrong dose of insulin or oral agents or if something interferes with food intake or changes stress or exercise levels). Two agents are used to elevate glucose in these conditions: diazoxide, which can be taken orally, and glucagon, the hormone produced by the alpha cells of the pancreas to elevate glucose levels. Glucagon can only be given parenterally and is preferred for emergency situations. Pure glucose can also be given orally or intravenously to increase glucose levels. Oral glucose tablets or gels are available over the counter for patients to keep on hand for management of moderate hypoglycaemic episodes.

Therapeutic Actions and Indications

These agents increase the blood glucose level by decreasing insulin release and accelerating the breakdown of glycogen in the liver to release glucose. They are indicated for the treatment of hypoglycaemic reactions related to insulin or oral antidiabetic agents, treatment of hypoglycaemia related to pancreatic or other cancers and short-term treatment of acute hypoglycaemia related to anterior pituitary dysfunction.

Pharmacokinetics

Glucagon and diazoxide are rapidly absorbed and widely distributed throughout the body. They are excreted in the urine. Diazoxide has been associated with adverse effects on the foetus and should not be used during pregnancy. There are no adequate studies on glucagon and pregnancy, so use should be reserved for those situations in which the benefits to the mother outweigh any potential risks to the foetus. Caution should be used during lactation, because these drugs may have hyperglycaemic effects on the baby.

Contraindications and Cautions

Diazoxide is contraindicated with known allergies to sulphonamides or thiazides. Both drugs are contraindicated for use during pregnancy and lactation. Caution should be used in patients with renal or hepatic dysfunction or cardiovascular disease.

Adverse Effects

Glucagon is associated with GI upset, nausea and vomiting. Diazoxide has been associated with vascular effects including hypotension, headache, cerebral ischaemia, weakness, congestive heart failure and arrhythmias; these reactions are associated with diazoxide's ability to relax arteriolar smooth muscle.

Clinically Important Drug–Drug Interactions

Taking diazoxide in combination with thiazide diuretics causes an increased risk of toxicity, because diazoxide is structurally similar to these diuretics.

Increased anticoagulation effects have been noted when glucagon is combined with oral anticoagulants. If this combination is needed, the dosage should be adjusted.

Always consult a current copy of the British National Formulary for further guidance.

Nursing Considerations for Patients Taking Glucose-elevating Agents

Assessment: History and Examination

Screen for the following conditions, *which could be cautions or contraindications to use of the drug*: history of allergy to thiazides if using diazoxide; severe renal or hepatic dysfunction, cardiovascular disease and pregnancy or lactation.

Physical assessment should include screening *for baseline status before beginning therapy and for any potential adverse effects*: orientation and reflexes; baseline pulse, blood pressure and adventitious sounds; abdominal sounds and function; urinalysis and blood glucose level renal and liver function tests.

Establish if patient is currently taking other medications or herbal therapies which may potentially interact with the glucose-elevating agents.

Nursing Diagnoses

The patient receiving glucose-elevating agents may have the following nursing diagnoses related to drug therapy:

- Imbalanced nutrition: more than body requirements, related to metabolic effects and less than body requirements, related to GI upset

- Disturbed sensory perception (kinaesthetic, visual, auditory) related to glucose levels
- Deficient knowledge regarding drug therapy

Implementation With Rationale

- Monitor blood glucose levels on a regular basis *to evaluate the effectiveness of the drug.*
- Have insulin on standby during emergency use *to treat severe hyperglycaemia if it occurs.*
- Monitor nutritional status *to provide nutritional consultation as needed.*
- Monitor patients receiving diazoxide for potential cardiovascular effects, including blood pressure.
- Monitor cardiac rhythm and output, weight changes *to avert serious adverse reactions.*
- Provide thorough patient education, including measures to avoid adverse effects, warning signs of problems, proper administration technique and the need to monitor glucose levels daily, *to enhance patient knowledge of drug therapy and promote compliance.*

Evaluation

- Monitor patient response to the drug (stabilization of blood glucose levels).
- Monitor for adverse effects (hyperglycaemia, GI distress).
- Evaluate the effectiveness of the teaching plan (patient can name drug, dosage, adverse effects to watch for, specific measures to avoid adverse effects).
- Monitor the effectiveness of comfort measures and compliance to the regimen.

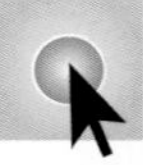

WEB LINKS

Health care providers and patients may want to consult the following Internet sources:

http://cks.library.nhs.uk The National Health Service Clinical Knowledge Summaries provide evidence-based practical information on the common conditions observed in primary care.

http://www.bnf.org.uk The BNF provides UK health care professionals with authoritative and practical information on the selection and clinical use of medicines.

http://www.diabetes.org.uk Diabetes UK is a charitable organization providing information to diabetic patients on treatment and care.

http://www.nhsdirect.nhs.uk The National Health Service Direct service provides patients with information and advice about health, illness and health services.

http://www.nice.org.uk The NICE provides guidance on best practise.

Points to Remember

- Diabetes mellitus is the most common metabolic disorder. It is characterized by high blood glucose levels and alterations in the metabolism of fats, proteins and glucose.
- Diabetes mellitus is complicated by many organ problems. These are related to thickening of basement membranes and the resultant decrease in blood flow to these areas.
- Treatment of diabetes involves tight control of blood glucose levels using diet and exercise, a combination of oral agents to stimulate insulin release or alter glucose absorption or the injection of replacement insulin.
- The amount and type of insulin given must be regulated daily. Patients taking insulin must learn to inject the drug to test their own blood (if appropriate) and to recognize the signs of hypo- and hyperglycaemia.
- Insulin is used for type 1 patients with diabetes and for type 2 patients with diabetes in times of stress or when other therapies have failed.
- Other antidiabetic agents include sulphonylureas, which stimulate the pancreas to release insulin, and other agents that alter glucose absorption, decrease insulin resistance or decrease the formation of glucose. These agents are often used in combination to achieve effective control of blood glucose levels.
- Glucose-elevating agents are used to increase glucose when levels become dangerously low. Imbalanced glucose levels while taking insulin or oral agents is a common cause of hypoglycaemia.

CRITICAL THINKING SCENARIO 37-1

Type 1 Diabetes Mellitus

THE SITUATION

Adele is an 18-year-old woman who has newly diagnosed type 1 diabetes mellitus. She was stabilized on insulin while hospitalized for diagnosis and management. One week after discharge, Adele experienced nausea and anorexia. She was unable to eat, but she took her insulin as usual in the morning. That afternoon, she experienced profuse sweating and started feeling very apprehensive, so she went to A&E. The initial diagnosis was hypoglycaemia due to taking insulin and not eating, combined with the stress of her GI distress. Adele was treated with intravenous glucose. After she had rested and her glucose levels had returned to normal, she was discharged home.

CRITICAL THINKING

- What instructions should Adele receive before she leaves?
- Consider the stress that a newly diagnosed type 1 diabetic patient undergoes while trying to cope with the diagnosis and learn self-injection.
- Think about complications of the disease that may arise in the future.
- What teaching could help Adele to reduce her stress and to effectively plan her medical regimen? *Think about the ways that stress can alter the blood glucose levels.*
- What sort of support would be useful for Adele as she adjusts to her new life?

DISCUSSION

The diagnosis of type 1 diabetes is a life-changing event. Adele had to learn about the disease and how to test her own blood and give herself injections, manage a new diet and exercise programme and cope with the knowledge that the long-term complications of diabetes can be devastating. Many patients, who are regulated on insulin in the hospital, experience a change in insulin demand after discharge. The SNS is active in the hospital and one of the effects of SNS activity is increased glucose levels, preparing the body for fight or flight. For some patients, returning home eases the stress that activated the SNS and glucose levels fall. If the patient continues to use the same insulin dose, hypoglycaemia can occur. Other patients may feel protected in the hospital and experience stress when they are sent home. They may feel anxious about taking care of themselves while coping with everyday problems and tensions. These patients may need an increased insulin dose because their stress reaction intensifies when they get home, driving their blood glucose level up.

Patients are taught how to measure their own blood glucose levels before they leave the hospital. After they get used to doing this and regulating their own insulin based on glucose concentrations, they usually manage well. The first few weeks are often the hardest. The nurse should review with Adele how to test her glucose, draw up her insulin and regulate the dose.

In addition, the nurse should give Adele a chance to talk about her diagnosis and her future. Support and encouragement will be crucial in helping Adele adjust to her disease and her drug therapy.

NURSING CARE GUIDE FOR ADELE: TYPE 1 DIABETES MELLITUS

Assessment: History and Examination

Review the patient's history for allergies to drug products, pregnancy, breast-feeding and other drugs in current use.

Focus the physical examination on the following:

- Neurological: orientation, reflexes
- Skin: colouration and/or lesions; perfusion
- CV: pulse, blood pressure
- Respiratory: respiratory rate, auscultation of chest
- Lab tests: urinalysis, blood glucose level

Nursing Diagnoses

- Imbalanced nutrition: less than body requirements, related to metabolic effects
- Disturbed sensory perception (kinaesthetic, visual, auditory, tactile) related to effects on glucose levels
- Risk of infection related to injections and disease process
- Patient not coping with the diagnosis and injections
- Deficient knowledge regarding drug therapy

Implementation

- Provide patient education regarding drug name, dosage, adverse effects, precautions, warning signs to report and proper administration technique.

(continued)

Type 1 Diabetes Mellitus *(continued)*

- Help Adele to restore blood glucose to normal levels by using insulin and constant monitoring of blood glucose levels during the day and during times of stress and trauma so that insulin dosage can be adjusted to needed amount.
- Review proper subcutaneous injection technique and site rotation.
- Provide support and reassurance to help Adele deal with drug injections, this hypoglycaemic episode and her lifetime need for insulin.
- Teach Adele how to store insulin in cool place away from light and to use caution when mixing insulin types.

Evaluation

- Evaluate drug effects: glucose levels return to normal and remain stable.
- Monitor for adverse effects: hypoglycaemia and/or injection site reaction.
- Monitor for drug–drug interactions as indicated for insulin.
- Evaluate effectiveness of patient education programme and comfort and safety measures.

Patient Education for Adele

- ☐ Insulin is a hormone that is normally produced by your pancreas. It helps to regulate your energy balance by affecting the way the body uses sugar and fats. The lack of insulin produces a disease called diabetes mellitus. By injecting insulin each day, you can help your body use the sugars and fats in your food effectively.
- ☐ Check the expiry date on your insulin. Store the insulin in a cool place (preferably a fridge) and avoid extremes of heat and light. Although Adele should be advised that she doesn't need to refrigerate the vial that she is using as it will last for up to 1 month at room temperature. It should certainly be out of the fridge for at least an hour before injecting. Cold insulin increases the pain of injection and slows down absorption.
- ☐ Gently rotate the vial between your palms before use to dispense any crystals that may have formed. Do not shake the vial because vigorous shaking can inactivate the drug.
- ☐ A prescription is required to get the syringes that you will need to administer your insulin. Keep the syringes sealed until ready to use and dispose of them appropriately. Rotate your injection sites regularly to prevent tissue damage and to ensure that the proper amount of insulin is absorbed.
- ☐ You should be aware of the signs and symptoms of hypoglycaemia (too much insulin). If any of these occur, eat or drink something high in sugar, such as orange juice, honey or boiled sweets.
- ☐ The signs and symptoms of hypoglycaemia include the following: nervousness, anxiety, sweating, pale and cool skin, headache, nausea, hunger, shakiness. These may happen if you skip a meal, exercise too much, or experience extreme stress. If these symptoms are happening on a regular basis, notify your health care provider.
- ☐ Avoid the use of any over-the-counter medications or herbal therapies without first checking with your health care provider. Several of these medications and many commonly used herbs can interfere with the effectiveness of insulin. Avoid the use of alcohol, because it increases the chances of having hypoglycaemic attacks.
- ☐ Tell any doctor, nurse or other health care provider involved in your care that you are taking this drug. You may want to wear or carry a MedicAlert tag showing that you are on this medication. This would alert any medical personnel taking care of you in an emergency to the fact that you are taking this drug.
- ☐ Report any of the following to your health care provider: loss of appetite, blurred vision, fruity odour to your breath, increased urination, increased thirst, nausea, vomiting.
- ☐ While you are taking this drug, it is important to have regular medical follow-up, including blood tests to monitor your blood glucose levels, to evaluate you for any adverse effects of your diabetes.

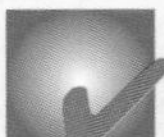

CHECK YOUR UNDERSTANDING

Answers to the questions in this chapter may be found in the answer key in the back of the book.

Multiple Choice

Select the most appropriate response to the following:

1. Currently the medical management of diabetes mellitus is aimed at
   a. controlling calorie intake.
   b. increasing exercise levels.
   c. tightly regulating blood sugar levels.
   d. decreasing fluid loss.

2. The HbA1c blood test is a good measure of overall glucose control because
   a. it reflects the level of glucose after a meal.
   b. the patient needs to fast for 8 hours before having the test done, ensuring an accurate level.
   c. it reflects a 3-month average glucose level in the body.
   d. the test can be affected by the glucose challenge.

3. A patient with hyperglycaemia will present with
   a. polyuria, polydipsia and polyphagia.
   b. polycythaemia, polyuria and polyphagia.
   c. polyadenitis, polyuria and polydipsia.
   d. polydipsia, polycythaemia and polyarteritis.

4. The long-term alterations in fat, carbohydrate and protein metabolism associated with diabetes mellitus result in
   a. obesity.
   b. thickening of the capillary basement membrane and end-organ damage.
   c. chronic obstructive pulmonary disease.
   d. lactose intolerance.

5. Insulin is available in several forms or suspensions, which differ in their
   a. effect on the pancreas.
   b. onset of action and duration of action.
   c. means of administration.
   d. tendency to cause adverse effects.

6. Teaching subjects for the patient with diabetes should include
   a. diet, exercise, hygiene and lifestyle changes that are needed.
   b. the importance of avoiding exercise, which could alter blood glucose.
   c. the need for protection from exposure to any infection.
   d. the importance of avoiding pregnancy.

Extended Matching Questions

Select **all** that apply.

1. Treatment of diabetes may include which of the following?
   a. Replacement therapy with insulin
   b. Control of glucose absorption through the GI tract
   c. Drugs that stimulate insulin release or increase sensitivity of insulin receptor sites
   d. Surgical clearing of the capillary basement membranes
   e. Slowing of gastric emptying
   f. Diet and exercise programmes

2. A client is recently diagnosed with diabetes. In reviewing his past history, which of the following would be early indicators of the problem?
   a. Lethargy
   b. Fruity smelling breath
   c. Boundless energy
   d. Weight loss
   e. Increased sweating
   f. Often getting up at night to go to the toilet

Fill in the Blanks

1. The pancreas produces three different hormones, all related to glucose control. These three hormones are __________, ____________ and _____________.

2. Insulin stimulates the synthesis of ______________ (stored glucose for immediate release during times of stress or low glucose), the conversion of ________________ into fat stored in the form of adipose tissue and the synthesis of needed __________________ from amino acids.

3. Hyperglycaemia results in ____________________ as the renal threshold for glucose is reached.

4. Hyperglycaemias will also cause _________________ (increased eating) because the hypothalamic centres cannot take in glucose and sense that they are starving.

5. ___________________ (increased thirst) occurs with hyperglycaemia. This is due to the increase in the osmolality of the blood as glucose and waste products build up and fluid is lost with glucose in the urine.

6. When a person with diabetes mellitus needs to break down fats for energy, he or she will experience ____________________ as the metabolism shifts from using sugar to the use of fat.

7. The ____________________ were the first oral antidiabetic agents. They stimulate the pancreas to produce more insulin.

8. ____________________ is an oral antidiabetic agent that decreases the production of glucose and increases its uptake into cells.

Bibliography and References

American Diabetes Association. (2002). Standards of medical care for patients with diabetes mellitus. *Diabetes Care, 25,* 213–229.

British Medical Association and Royal Pharmaceutical Society of Great Britain. (2008). *British National Formulary*. London: BMJ & RPS Publishing. *This publication is updated biannually: it is imperative that the most recent edition is consulted.*

British Medical Association and Royal Pharmaceutical Society of Great Britain. (2008). *British National Formulary for Children*. London: BMJ & RPS Publishing. *This publication is updated annually: it is imperative that the most recent edition is consulted.*

Bromberg, J. S., Kaplan, B., Halloran, P. F., & Robertson, R. P. (2007). The islet transplant experiment: time for a reassessment. *American Journal of Transplantation, 7,* 2217–2218.

Gale, E. A. M. (2002). The rise of childhood type 2 diabetes in the 20th century. *Diabetes, 51,* 3353–3361.

Ganong, W. (2005). *Review of medical physiology* (22nd ed.). New York: McGraw-Hill.

Howland, R. D., & Mycek, M. J. (2005). *Pharmacology* (3rd ed.). Philadelphia: Lippincott Williams & Wilkins.

Marieb, E. N., & Hoehn, K. (2004). *Human anatomy & physiology* (7th ed.). San Francisco: Pearson Benjamin Cummings.

NICE. (2002). Management of type 2 diabetes – managing blood glucose levels. Available from http://www.nice.org.uk.

NICE. (2004). CG15 Diagnosis and management of type 1 diabetes in children, young people and adults. Available from http://www.nice.org.uk.

O'Kane, M. J., Bunting, B., Copeland, M., & Coates, V. E. (2008). Efficacy of self monitoring blood glucose in patients with newly diagnosed type 2 diabetes (ESMON study): randomised controlled trial. *British Medical Journal, 336*(7654), 1174–1177.

Porth, C. M., & Matfin G. (2008). *Pathophysiology: Concepts of altered health states* (8th ed.). Philadelphia: Lippincott Williams & Wilkins.

Reynolds, T. M., Smellie, W. S., and Twomey, P. J. (2006). Glycated haemoglobin (HBA1c) monitoring. *British Medical Journal, 333,* 586–588.

Simon, J., Gray, A., Clarke, P., Wade, A., & Neil, A. (2008). Cost effectiveness of self monitoring of blood glucose in patients with non-insulin treated type 2 diabetes: economic evaluation of data from the DiGem trial. *British Medical Journal, 336*(7654), 1177–1180.

Simonsen, T., Aarbakke, J., Kay, I., Coleman, I., Sinnott, P., & Lysaa, R. (2006). *Illustrated pharmacology for nurses*. London: Hodder Arnold.

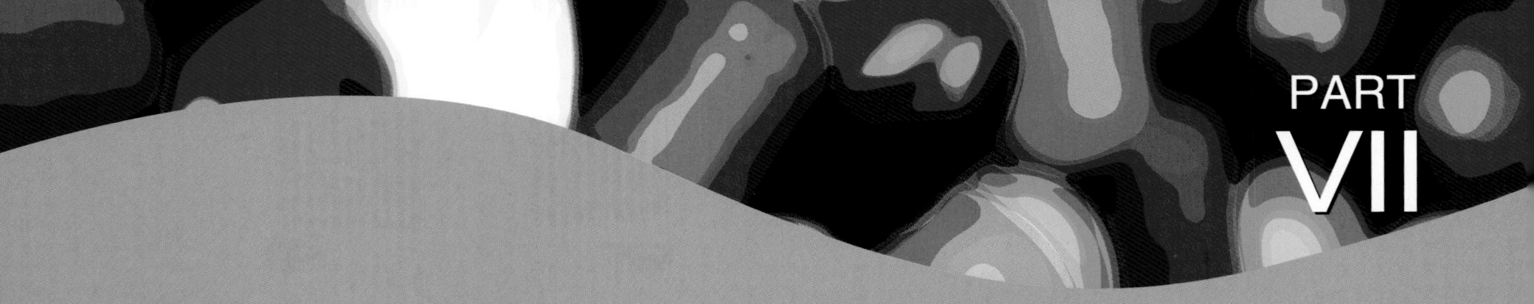

Drugs Acting on the Reproductive System

CHAPTER 38

Introduction to the Reproductive System

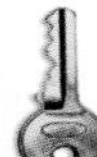

KEY TERMS

corpus luteum
follicle
glycogenolysis
inhibin
interstitial or Leydig cells
menopause
menstrual cycle
oestrogen
ova
ovaries
progesterone
puberty
seminiferous tubules
Sertoli cells
sperm
testes
testosterone
uterus

LEARNING OBJECTIVES

Upon completion of this chapter, you will be able to:

1. Label a diagram of the parts of the female and male reproductive systems and explain the function of each part.
2. Outline the controls of the male and female reproductive systems and use this outline to explain the cyclical nature of the female reproductive system.
3. List five effects of each of the sex hormones: oestrogen, progesterone and testosterone.
4. Describe the changes that occur to the female body during pregnancy.
5. Describe the phases of the human sexual response and briefly describe the clinical presentation of each stage.

The glands that produce sexual hormones (gonads) originate from the same foetal cells in both males and females. In the female, those cells stay in the abdomen and develop into the **ovaries**. In the male, the cells migrate out of the abdomen to form the **testes**, which are suspended from the body in the scrotum. Both male and female glands respond to follicle-stimulating hormone (FSH) and luteinizing hormone (LH), which are released from the anterior pituitary in response to stimulation from gonadotrophin-releasing hormone (GnRH) released from the hypothalamus.

Female Reproductive System

The female reproductive system is composed of (i) two ovaries, which store the **ova** or eggs; and which act as endocrine glands that produce **oestrogen** and **progesterone**; (ii) the **uterus**, which is the womb for the developing embryo and foetus; and (iii) the fallopian tubes, which provide a pathway for released ova from the ovaries to the uterus. Accessory parts include the vagina, clitoris, labia and breast tissue (Figure 38.1).

Ovaries

At birth, the ovaries contain all of the ova that a woman will release over her lifetime. The ova slowly degenerate over time or are released for possible fertilization. Each ovum is contained in a storage site called a **follicle**, which produces the female sex hormones, oestrogen and progesterone. The primary goal of these hormones is to prepare the body for pregnancy and to maintain the pregnancy until delivery.

In a nonpregnant woman, the levels of these hormones fluctuate in a cyclical fashion until all of the ova are gone and **menopause**, the cessation of menses, occurs. In a pregnant woman, the placenta takes over production of oestrogen and progesterone and high levels of both hormones help to maintain the pregnancy. The adrenal glands also produce small amounts of androgens, including testosterone and some oestrogens.

Controls

The developing hypothalamus is sensitive to the androgens released by the adrenal glands and does not release GnRH during childhood. As the hypothalamus matures, it loses its sensitivity to the androgens and starts to release GnRH. This occurs at **puberty**, or sexual development. The onset of puberty leads to a number of hormonal changes.

To begin with, GnRH stimulates the anterior pituitary to release FSH and LH. FSH and LH stimulate the follicles on the outer surface of the ovary to grow and develop. These follicles are called Graafian follicles; they produce progesterone, which is retained in the follicle and oestrogen, which is released into the circulation. When the circulating oestrogen level rises high enough, it stimulates a massive release

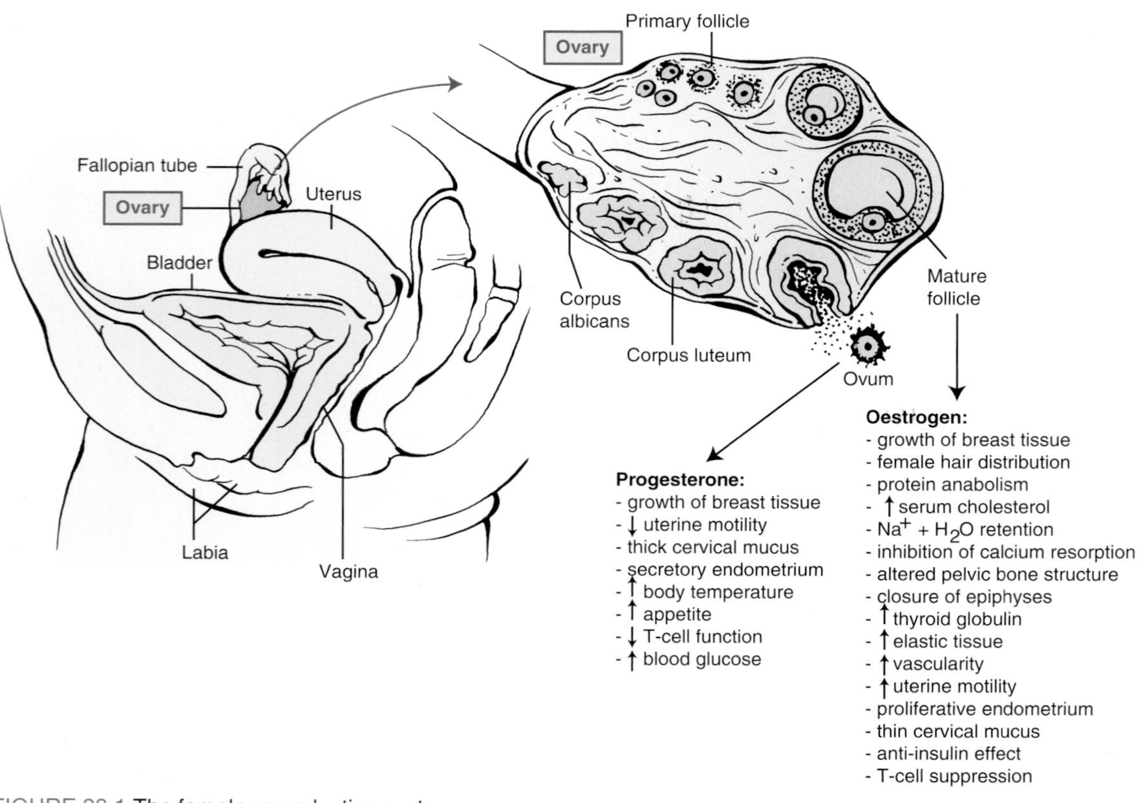

FIGURE 38.1 The female reproductive system.

of LH from the anterior pituitary known as the 'LH surge'. This causes one of the developing follicles to burst, release the ovum and all the hormones that are inside the follicle into the system. LH also causes the rest of the developing follicles to regress and eventually disappear. The release of an ovum from the follicle is called **ovulation**.

The ovum is released into the abdomen near the open end of one of the fallopian tubes (fimbriae-finger-like projections), and the constant movement of cilia within the tube helps to propel the ovum along the tube and into the uterus. The ruptured follicle becomes a functioning endocrine gland called the ***corpus luteum***. It will continue to produce oestrogen and progesterone for 10 to 14 days unless pregnancy occurs. If the ovum is fertilized and implants in the uterine wall, one of the first hormones that is produced by the junction of the fertilized embryo with the uterine wall is human chorionic gonadotrophin (HCG). This hormone stimulates the *corpus luteum* to continue to produce oestrogen and progesterone until placental levels of these hormones are high enough to sustain pregnancy.

If pregnancy does not occur, the *corpus luteum* regresses to become the *corpus albicans*. Initially, the rising levels of oestrogen and progesterone produced by the *corpus luteum* act as a negative feedback system to the hypothalamus and the pituitary, stopping the production and secretion of GnRH, FSH and LH. Later in the cycle, the *corpus luteum* atrophies, the falling levels of oestrogen and progesterone stimulate the hypothalamus to release GnRH and the cycle begins again.

After all of the follicles are used up, the ovaries no longer produce oestrogen and progesterone and menopause occurs. The hypothalamus and pituitary produce increased levels of GnRH, FSH and LH for a while in an attempt to stimulate the ovaries to produce oestrogen and progesterone. If that does not happen, the levels of these hormones fall back within a normal range in response to their own negative feedback systems. The signs and symptoms of menopause (osteoporosis, increased serum lipid levels and degeneration of secondary sex characteristics, vaginal dryness, hot flushes, moodiness, loss of bone density, increased risk of cardiovascular disease and somnolence) are related to the loss of oestrogen and progesterone effects on the body.

The hypothalamus is influenced by many internal and external factors, for example high levels of stress can disrupt the reproductive cycle. Large amounts of energy are expended in reproduction and if the body needs energy for fight-or-flight, the hypothalamus shuts down reproductive activities. In addition to stress, starvation, extreme exercise and emotional problems are all associated with a decrease in fertility.

Light has been found to have an influence on the functioning of the hypothalamus. Increased light levels boost the release of FSH and LH and increase the release of oestrogen and progesterone. Longer and earlier exposure to light leads to earlier GnRH release by the hypothalamus and earlier sexual development and is thought to contribute to the early sexual maturation of girls near the equator.

Hormones

Oestrogen and progesterone affect many other body systems while preparing the body for pregnancy or maintenance of pregnancy.

Oestrogen

Oestrogens are steroid hormones and include oestradiol, oestrone and oestriol. The oestrogens enter cells and bind to receptors within the cytoplasm to promote messenger RNA (mRNA) activity, which results in the production of specific proteins for cell activity or structure. The effects of oestrogens on the body are summarized in Box 38.1. Many of these effects are first noticed at the onset of the menstrual cycle, when the hormones begin cycling for the first time.

Progesterone

Progesterone is released into circulation after ovulation. Its effects are summarized in Box 38.2. Progesterone's effects on body temperature can be monitored in the 'rhythm method' of birth control to indicate that ovulation has just occurred.

The Menstrual Cycle

The cyclic effects of the female sex hormones on the body produce the **menstrual cycle**. The onset of the menstrual cycle at puberty is called the menarche. Each cycle starts with release of FSH and LH and stimulation of the follicles on the ovary. For about the next 14 days, the developing follicles release oestrogen into the body. The many effects of oestrogen may be noticed by the woman; for example breast tenderness, water retention, thin cervical mucosa, increased susceptibility to infections and the development of a secretory endometrium.

By about day 14, the oestrogen levels have caused the LH surge and ovulation occurs. The woman may experience an increase in body temperature, increased appetite, breast tenderness, bloating and abdominal fullness, and constipation; these are all the effects associated with progesterone. As the cycle progresses, the uterus becomes thicker and more vascular developing a proliferative endometrium. After ovulation, the lining of the uterus begins to produce glucose and other nutrients that would nurture a growing embryo; this is called a secretory endometrium. If pregnancy does not occur, after about 14 days the *corpus luteum* regresses and the levels of oestrogen and progesterone decline (Figure 38.2).

The declining levels of oestrogen and progesterone trigger the release of FSH and LH again, along with the start of another menstrual cycle. Lowered hormone levels also cause the endometrium (inner lining of the uterus) to slough off because it is no longer stimulated by the hormones. High levels of plasminogen in the uterus prevent clotting as the

BOX 38.1 Clinical Assessment of the Effects of Oestrogen

- Growth of female genitalia (in preparation for childbirth)
- Growth of breast tissue (in preparation for pregnancy and lactation)
- Characteristic female pubic hair distribution (a triangle)
- Stimulation of protein building (important for the developing foetus)
- Increased total blood cholesterol (for energy for the mother as well as the developing foetus) with an increase in high-density lipoprotein levels ('good' cholesterol, which serves to protect the female blood vessels against atherosclerosis)
- Retention of sodium and water (to provide cooling for the heat generated by the developing foetus and to increase diffusion of sodium and water to the foetus through the placenta)
- Inhibition of calcium resorption from the bones (helps to deposit calcium in the foetal bone structure; when this property is lost at menopause, osteoporosis or loss of calcium from the bone is common)
- Alteration of pelvic bone structure to a wider and flaring pelvis (to promote easier delivery)
- Closure of the epiphyses (to conserve energy for the foetus by halting growth of the mother)
- Increased thyroid hormone globulin (metabolism needs to be increased greatly during pregnancy and the increase in thyroid hormone facilitates this)
- Increased elastic tissue of the skin (to allow for the tremendous stretch of the abdominal skin during pregnancy)
- Increased vasculature of the skin (to allow for radiation loss of heat generated by the developing foetus)
- Increased uterine motility (oestrogen is high when the ovum first leaves the ovary and increased uterine motility helps to move the ovum towards the uterus and to propel the sperm towards the ovum)
- Thin, clear cervical mucus (allows easy penetration of the sperm into the uterus as ovulation occurs; used in fertility programmes as an indication that ovulation will soon occur)
- Proliferative endometrium (to prepare the lining of the uterus for implantation with the fertilized egg)
- Anti-insulin effect with increased glucose levels (to allow increased diffusion of glucose to the developing foetus)
- T-cell inhibition (to protect the 'nonself'-cells of the embryo from the immune surveillance of the mother)

spiral vessels supplying the endometrium constrict, causing ischaemia and the endometrium to shear off. Prostaglandins in the uterus stimulate uterine contraction to clamp off vessels as the lining is lost. This can cause menstrual cramps, which can be very uncomfortable for some women. This loss of the uterine lining, called menstruation, repeats approximately every 28 days. Figure 38.3 displays the various phases of the menstrual cycle.

BOX 38.2 Clinical Assessment of the Effects of Progesterone

- Decreased uterine motility (to provide increased chance that implantation can occur)
- Development of a secretory endometrium (to provide glucose and a rich blood supply for the developing placenta and embryo)
- Thickened cervical mucus (to protect the developing embryo and keep out bacteria and other pathogens; this is lost at the beginning of labour as the mucous plug)
- Breast growth (to prepare for lactation)
- Increased body temperature (a direct hypothalamic response to progesterone, which stimulates metabolism and promotes activities for the developing embryo; this increase in temperature is monitored in the 'rhythm method' of birth control to indicate that ovulation has occurred)
- Increased appetite (this is a direct effect on the satiety centres of the hypothalamus and results in increased nutrients for the developing embryo).
- Depressed T-cell function (again, this protects the nonself-cells of the developing embryo from the immune system)
- Anti-insulin effect (to generate a higher blood glucose concentration to allow rapid diffusion of glucose to the developing embryo)

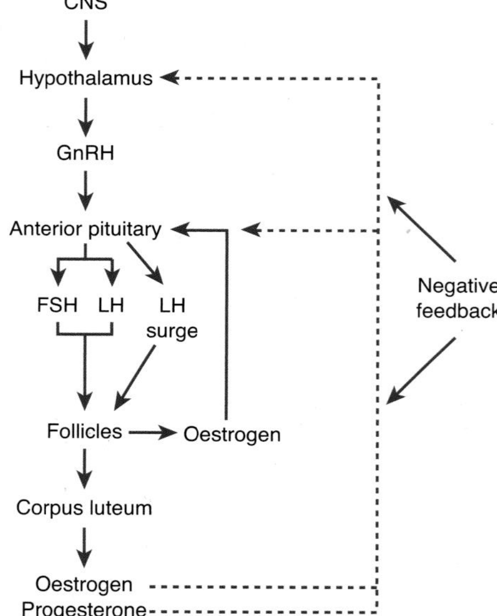

FIGURE 38.2 Interaction of the hypothalamic, pituitary, and ovarian hormones that underlies the menstrual cycle of the female. Dotted lines indicate negative feedback surge. CNS, central nervous system; FSH, follicle-stimulating hormone; GnRH, gonadotropin-releasing hormone; LH, luteinizing hormone.

Pregnancy

When the ovum is fertilized by a sperm, a new cell is produced that rapidly divides to produce the embryo. The embryo implants in the wall of the uterus and the interface between the foetal cells and the uterus produces the placenta, a large,

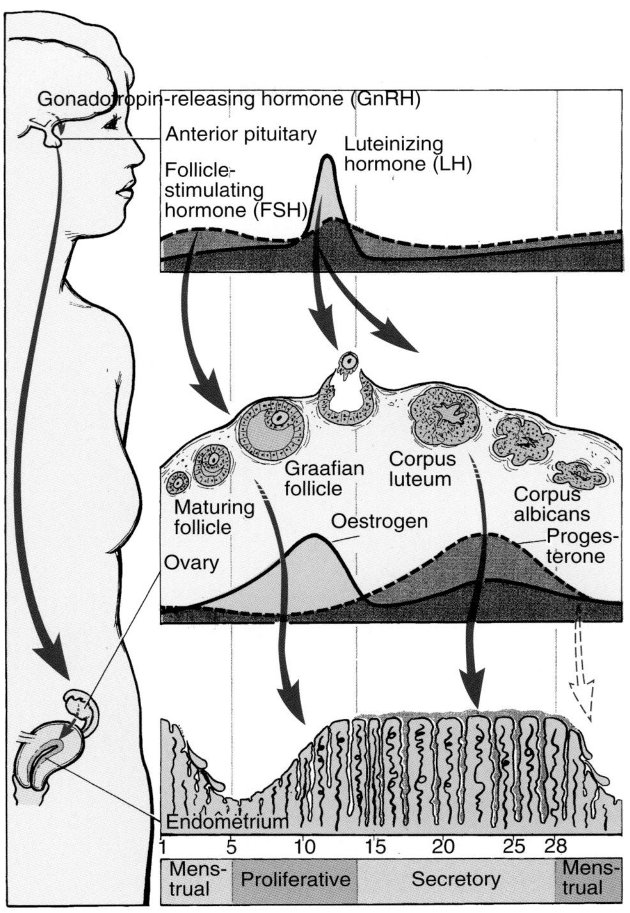

FIGURE 38.3 Relation of pituitary and ovarian hormone levels to the menstrual cycle and to ovarian and endometrial function. GnRH, gonadotropin-releasing hormone; LH, luteinizing hormone.

vascular organ that serves as an endocrine gland and a transfer point for nutrients from the mother to the foetus. The placenta maintains high levels of oestrogens and progesterone to support the uterus and the developing foetus. As the placenta develops, the levels of progesterone and oestrogens plateau.

Eventually, the tendency to block uterine activity (an effect of progesterone) is overcome by the stimulation to increase uterine activity caused by oxytocin (a hypothalamic hormone stored in the posterior pituitary). At this point, local prostaglandins stimulate uterine contraction and the onset of labour. Once the foetus and the placenta have been expelled from the uterus, the hormone levels plummet towards the nonpregnant state. This is a time of considerable adjustment for the body as it tries to reachieve homeostasis.

Male Reproductive System

The two endocrine glands that develop in the male are called the testes. The testes continually produce **sperm** as well as the hormone **testosterone**. The other parts of the male reproductive system include (i) the *vas deferens*, which stores produced sperm and carries sperm from the testes to be ejaculated from the body; (ii) the prostate gland, which produces enzymes to stimulate sperm maturation as well as an alkaline lubricating fluid; (iii) the penis, which includes two structures, the *corpus cavernosum* and *corpus spongiosum*, that allow increased blood flow and erection; (iv) the urethra, through which urine as well as the sperm and seminal fluid are delivered and (v) other glands and ducts that promote sperm and seminal fluid development (Figure 38.4).

Testes

During foetal development, the testes migrate down the abdomen and descend into the scrotum outside the body. There they are protected from the heat of the body to prevent injury to the sperm-producing cells. The testes are made up of two distinct parts: the **seminiferous tubules**, which produce sperm; and the **interstitial** or **Leydig cells**, which produce the steroid hormone testosterone.

Controls

The activity of the male sex glands is not thought to be cyclical like that of the female. The hypothalamus in the male child is also sensitive to circulating levels of adrenal androgens and suppresses GnRH release. After the hypothalamus matures, this sensitivity is lost and the hypothalamus releases GnRH. This in turn stimulates the anterior pituitary to release FSH and LH. FSH directly stimulates the seminiferous tubules to produce sperm, a process called spermatogenesis. FSH also stimulates the **Sertoli cells** in the seminiferous tubules to produce oestrogens, which provide negative feedback to the pituitary and hypothalamus to cause a decrease in the release of GnRH, FSH and LH.

The Sertoli cells support spermatogenesis. They secrete androgen-binding proteins as well as a substance called **inhibin** (an oestrogen-like molecule). Inhibin is sensed by the hypothalamus and anterior pituitary and a negative feedback response occurs, decreasing the circulating level of FSH. When the FSH level falls low enough, the hypothalamus is stimulated to again release GnRH to stimulate FSH release. This feedback system prevents overproduction of sperm in the testes (Figure 38.5). Inhibin has been investigated for many years as a possible male birth control drug, because it is thought to affect only sperm production.

The LH stimulates the interstitial (Leydig) cells to produce testosterone. The concentration of testosterone acts in a similar negative feedback system with the hypothalamus. When the concentration is high enough, the hypothalamus decreases GnRH release, leading to a subsequent decrease in FSH and LH release. The levels

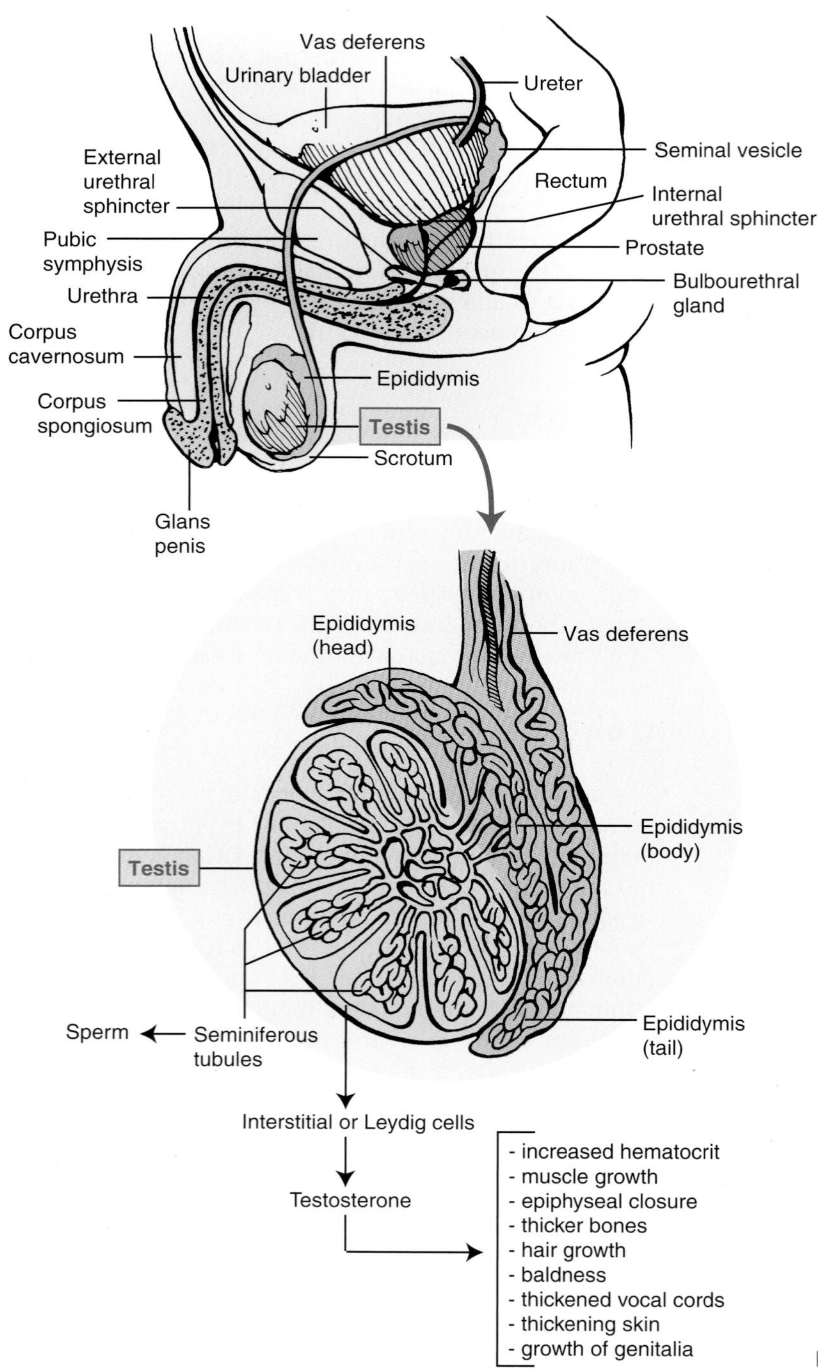

FIGURE 38.4 The male reproductive system.

of testosterone are thought to remain within a fairly well defined range of normal.

With age, the seminiferous tubules and interstitial cells atrophy and the male climacteric, a period of lessened sexual activity, occurs. This is similar to female menopause and the hypothalamus and anterior pituitary put out larger amounts of GnRH, FSH and LH in an attempt to stimulate the gland. If no increase in testosterone or inhibin occurs, the levels of GnRH, FSH and LH eventually return to normal levels.

Hormones

Testosterone is responsible for many sexual and metabolic effects in the male. Like oestrogen, testosterone is a steroid; it enters the cell and reacts with a cytoplasmic receptor site to influence mRNA activity, resulting in the production of proteins for cell structure or function. The effects of testosterone on the body are summarized in Box 38.3. Once puberty and the physical changes brought about by

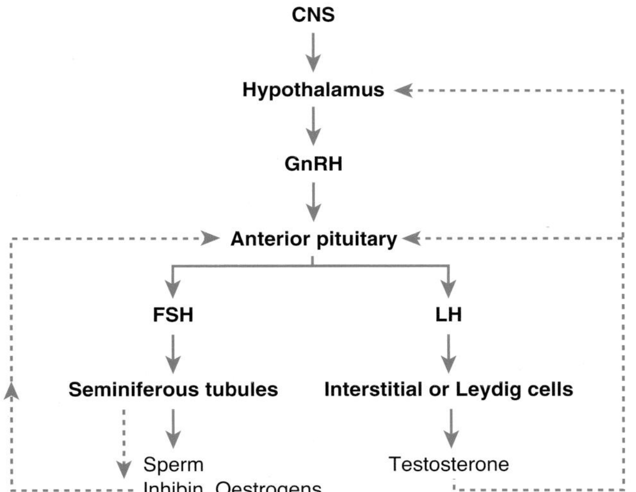

FIGURE 38.5 Interaction of the hypothalamic, pituitary, and tes-ticular hormones that underlies the male sexual hormone system. CNS, central nervous system; FSH, follicle-stimulating hormone; GnRH, gonadotropin-releasing hormone; LH, luteinizing hormone.

BOX 38.3 Clinical Assessment of the Effects of Testosterone

- Growth of male and sexual accessory organs (penis, prostate gland, seminal vesicles, vas deferens)
- Growth of testes and scrotal sac
- Thickening of vocal cords, producing the deep, male voice
- Hair growth on the face, body, arms, legs and trunk
- Male-pattern baldness
- Increased protein anabolism and decreased protein catabolism (this causes larger and more powerful muscle development)
- Increased bone growth in length and width, which ends when the testosterone stimulates closure of the epiphyses
- Thickening of the cartilage and skin, leading to the male gait
- Vascular thickening
- Increased haematocrit

testosterone have occurred, the androgens released by the adrenal glands are sufficient to sustain the male characteristics. This is important information for adult patients undergoing testicular surgery.

The Human Sexual Response

Humans and ferrets are the only animals known to be sexually stimulated and responsive at will. Many animals require particular endocrine stimuli, called an oestrous cycle, for sexual response to occur. Humans can be sexually stimulated by thoughts, sights, touch or a variety of combined stimuli. The human sexual response consists of four phases:

- A period of stimulation with mild increases in sensitivity and beginning stimulation of the sympathetic nervous system
- A plateau stage when stimulation levels off
- A climax, which results from massive sympathetic stimulation of the body
- A period of recovery or resolution, when the effects of the sympathetic stimulation are resolved.

It was once believed that male and female responses were very different, but it is now thought that the physiology of the responses is quite similar. Sexual stimulation and activity are a normal response and, in healthy individuals, are probably necessary for complete health of the body's systems. The sympathetic stimulation causes increased heart rate, increased blood pressure, sweating, pupil dilation, **glycogenolysis** (breakdown of stored glycogen to glucose for energy) and other sympathetic responses. This stimulation could be dangerous in some cardiovascular conditions that could be exacerbated by the sympathetic effects. In the male, the increased blood flow to the penis causes erection, which is necessary for penetration of the female and deposition of the sperm. Any drug therapy or disease process that interferes with the sympathetic response or the innervation of the sexual organs will change the person's ability to experience the human sexual response. This is important to keep in mind when patient education and when evaluating the effects of a drug.

Points to Remember

- Male and female reproductive systems arise from the same foetal cells.
- The female ovaries store ova and produce the sex hormones oestrogen and progesterone.
- The male testes produce sperm and the sex hormone testosterone.
- The hypothalamus releases GnRH at puberty to stimulate the anterior pituitary release of FSH and LH, thus stimulating the production and release of the sex hormones. Levels are controlled by a series of negative feedback systems.
- Female sex hormones are released in a cyclical fashion. Male sex hormones are released in a steadier fashion.
- Ovulation is the release of an egg for possible fertilization. Female sex hormones prepare the body for pregnancy and the maintenance of the pregnancy.
- If pregnancy does not occur, the prepared inner lining of the uterus is lost during menstruation in the menstrual cycle, so that the lining can be prepared again when ovulation reoccurs.

- Menopause in women and the male climacteric in men occur when the body can no longer produce sex hormones; the hypothalamus and anterior pituitary respond by releasing increasing levels of GnRH, FSH and LH in an attempt to achieve higher levels of sex hormones.
- The testes produce sperm in the seminiferous tubules, in response to FSH stimulation and testosterone in the interstitial cells, in response to LH stimulation.
- Testosterone is responsible for the development of male sex characteristics. These characteristics can be maintained by the androgens from the adrenal gland once the body has undergone the changes of puberty.

CHECK YOUR UNDERSTANDING

Answers to the questions in this chapter may be found in the answer key in the back of the book.

Multiple Choice

Select the most appropriate response to the following.

1. In a nonpregnant woman, the levels of the sex hormones fluctuate in a cyclical fashion until
   a. all of the ova are gone and menopause occurs.
   b. the FSH and LH are depleted.
   c. the hypothalamus no longer senses FSH and LH.
   d. the menarche, when the hypothalamus becomes more sensitive.

2. Ova, or eggs, are created and develop in the ovaries
   a. continually until menopause.
   b. during foetal life.
   c. until menopause.
   d. starting with puberty

3. The release of GnRH from the hypothalamus controlling the cycling of female sex hormones, may be affected by
   a. heat.
   b. stress or emotional problems.
   c. cold.
   d. androgen release.

4. The rhythm method of birth control depends on the effects of progesterone to
   a. increase uterine motility.
   b. decrease and thicken cervical secretions.
   c. elevate body temperature.
   d. depress appetite.

5. The menstrual cycle
   a. always repeats itself every 28 days.
   b. is associated with the cyclical effects of the changing hormone levels.
   c. is necessary for a human sexual response.
   d. cannot occur if ovulation does not occur.

6. In the male reproductive system the
   a. seminiferous tubules produce sperm and testosterone.
   b. interstitial cells produce sperm.
   c. seminiferous tubules produce sperm and the interstitial cells produce testosterone.
   d. interstitial cells produce sperm and testosterone.

Extended Matching Questions

Select **all** that apply.

1. Oestrogen has many effects on the body. Oestrogenic effects would include
   a. increased levels of high-density lipoproteins.
   b. increased calcium density in the bone.
   c. closing of the epiphyses.
   d. development of a thick cervical plug.
   e. increased body temperature.
   f. triangle-shaped body hair distribution.

2. Testosterone has many effects on the body. Testosterone effects would include
   a. thickening of skin and vocal cords.
   b. development of a wide and flat pelvis.
   c. development of facial hair.
   d. closure of the epiphyses.
   e. increased haematocrit.
   f. increased aggression.

Indicate whether the following statements are true (T) or false (F).

_____ 1. Male and female reproductive systems arise from different foetal cells.

_____ 2. The male testes store sperm and produce the sex hormone testosterone.

_____ 3. The hypothalamus releases GnRH at puberty to stimulate the anterior pituitary release of FSH and LH, thus stimulating the production and release of the sex hormones.

_____ 4. Levels of sex hormones are controlled by local response to specific hormone stimulation.

_____ 5. Ovulation is the release of an ovum.

_____ 6. Menopause in women and the male climacteric in men occur when the body no longer responds to the circulating sex hormones.

_____ 7. The testes produce sperm in the seminiferous tubules, in response to LH stimulation and testosterone in the interstitial cells, in response to FSH stimulation.

_____ 8. Testosterone is responsible for the development of male sex characteristics, which can be maintained by the androgens from the adrenal gland once the body has undergone the changes of puberty.

Bibliography and References

British Medical Association and Royal Pharmaceutical Society of Great Britain. (2008). British National Formulary. London: BMJ & RPS Publishing. *This publication is updated biannually: it is imperative that the most recent edition is consulted.*

British Medical Association and Royal Pharmaceutical Society of Great Britain. (2008). British National Formulary for Children. London: BMJ & RPS Publishing. *This publication is updated annually: it is imperative that the most recent edition is consulted.*

Ganong, W. (2005). *Review of medical physiology* (22nd ed.). New York: McGraw-Hill.

Howland, R. D., & Mycek, M. J. (2005). *Pharmacology* (3rd ed.). Philadelphia: Lippincott Williams & Wilkins.

Marieb, E. N., & Hoehn, K. (2004). *Human anatomy & physiology* (7th ed.). San Francisco: Pearson Benjamin Cummings.

Porth, C. M., & Matfin G. (2008). *Pathophysiology: Concepts of altered health states* (8th ed). Philadelphia: Lippincott Williams & Wilkins.

Simonsen, T., Aarbakke, J., Kay, I., Coleman, I., Sinnott, P. & Lysaa, R. (2006). *Illustrated pharmacology for nurses*. London: Hodder Arnold.

CHAPTER 39

Drugs Affecting the Female Reproductive System

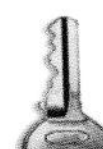

KEY TERMS

fertility drugs
myometrial relaxants
oxytocics
progestogens

LEARNING OBJECTIVES

Upon completion of this chapter, you will be able to:

1. Discuss the effects of oestrogen and progesterone on the female body and explain the therapeutic and adverse effects of these agents when used clinically.
2. Describe the therapeutic actions, indications and pharmacokinetics associated with the oestrogens, oestrogen receptor modulators, progestogens, fertility drugs and oxytocics.
3. Describe the contraindications, most common adverse reactions and important drug–drug interactions associated with the oestrogens, oestrogen receptor modulators, progestogens, fertility drugs and oxytocics.
4. Discuss the use of drugs that affect the female reproductive system across the lifespan.
5. Compare and contrast the key drugs oestradiol, raloxifene, norethisterone, clomiphene, oxytocin and dinoprostone with other agents in their class.
6. Outline the nursing considerations, including important teaching points to stress to patients receiving drugs used to affect the female reproductive system.

OESTROGENS

ethinylestradiol
oestradiol

OESTROGEN RECEPTOR MODULATORS

 raloxifene

PROGESTOGENS

medroxyprogesterone
norgestrel
norethistrone
progesterone

MYOMETRIAL RELAXANTS

atosiban
ritodrine
terbutaline
salbutamol

FERTILITY DRUGS
cetrorelix
chorionic gonadotrophin (HCG)
choriogonadotropin α
clomifene
follitropin α
follitropin β
ganirelix
urofollitropin

OXYTOCICS/ LABOUR INDUCERS
carboprost
ergometrine maleate
dinoprostone
gemeprost
mifepristone
oxytocin

EMERGENCY CONTRACEPTION
levonorgestrel

The female reproductive system uses a cycling nature to maintain homeostasis. Changing any factor in the system can have a wide variety of effects on the entire body. Drugs that are used to affect the female reproductive system include the female steroid hormones oestrogens and **progestogens** (the endogenous female hormone progesterone and its various derivatives). Others include oestrogen receptor modulators, which are not hormones but affect specific oestrogen receptor sites; **fertility drugs**, which stimulate the female reproductive system; **oxytocics**, which stimulate uterine contractions and assist labour and **myometrial relaxants**, which are used to relax the uterus to prolong pregnancy (Figure 39.1). Box 39.1 discusses the effects of these drugs across the lifespan.

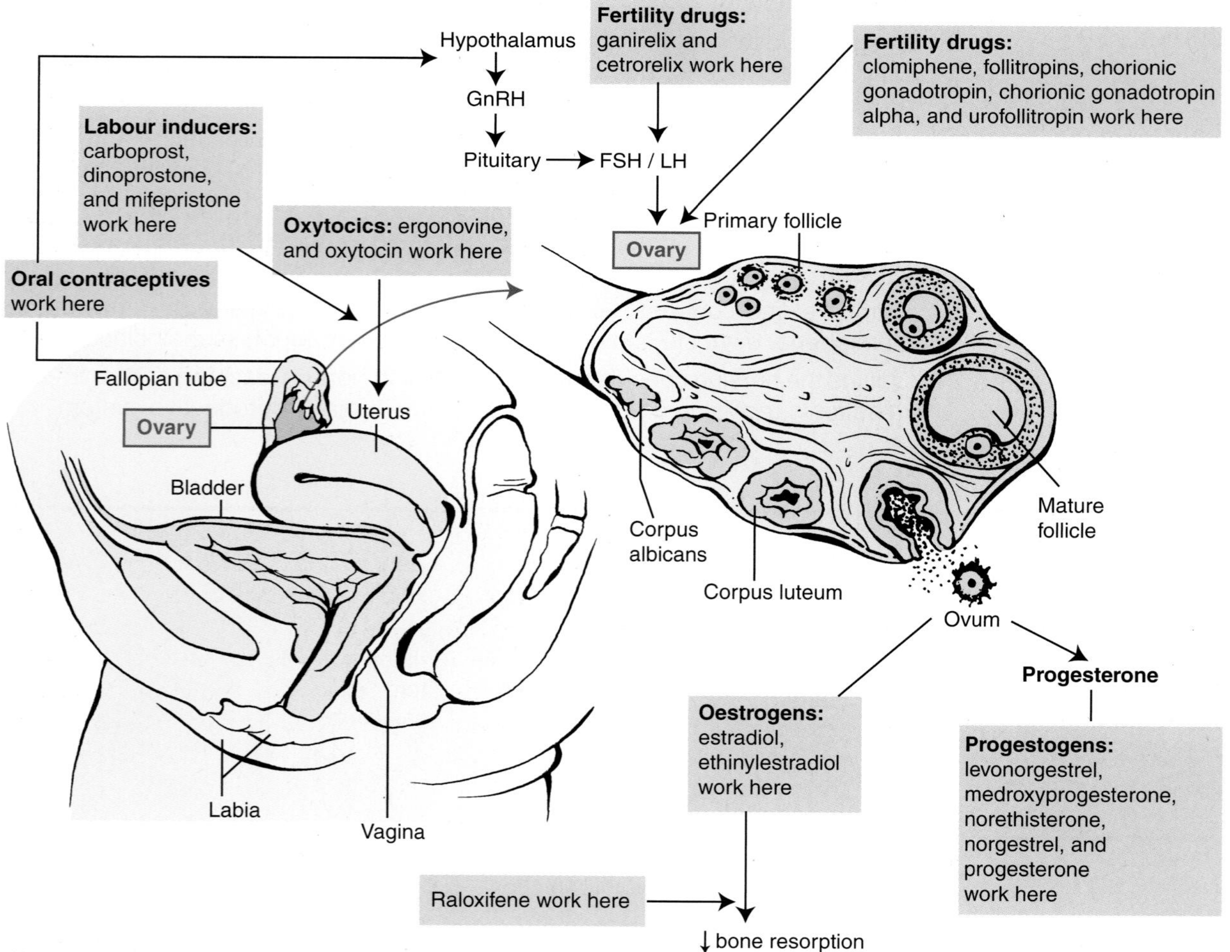

FIGURE 39.1 Sites of action of drugs affecting the female reproductive system.

BOX 39.1 **DRUG THERAPY ACROSS THE LIFESPAN**

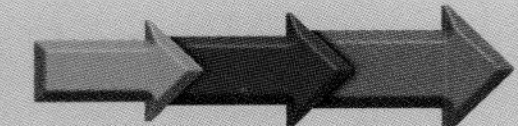

Drugs Affecting the Female Reproductive System

CHILDREN

The oestrogens and progestogens have undergone little testing in children. They should be used only with great caution in growing children.

If OCs are prescribed for teenage girls, the smallest dose possible should be used and the child should be monitored carefully for metabolic and other effects.

When administering drugs to children always consult the most up-to-date copy of the BNF for children.

ADULTS

Women who are receiving any of these drugs should receive an annual medical examination, including breast examination and Pap smear testing to monitor for adverse effects. The potential for adverse effects should be discussed and comfort measures provided. Women taking oestrogen should be advised not to smoke because of the increased risk of thrombotic events.

When combinations of these hormones are used as part of fertility programmes, women need a great deal of psychological support and comfort measures to cope with the many adverse effects associated with these drugs. The risk of multiple births should be explained, as should the need for frequent monitoring.

These agents are not for use during pregnancy or lactation because of the potential for adverse effects on the foetus or neonate.

OLDER ADULTS

HRT is no longer routinely used by postmenopausal women.

If patients are using alternative therapies, their effects on the HRT and other possible prescription drugs need to be carefully evaluated.

Oestrogens

Oestrogens are used in many clinical situations; for example in small doses, they are used for hormone replacement therapy (HRT) when ovarian activity is blocked or absent. The main oestrogen that is widely used and is found in combination form as an oral contraceptive (OC) is oestradiol.

Oestrogens are also used less often for palliative and preventive therapy during menopause, when many of the beneficial effects of oestrogen are lost. Oestrogens produce a wide variety of systemic effects, including protecting the heart from atherosclerosis; retaining calcium in the bones and maintaining the secondary female sex characteristics. Research findings suggest HRT may have its own risks (Box 39.2).

Oestrogens are indicated for the following conditions (Figure 39.2):

1. Palliation of moderate-to-severe vasomotor symptoms, atrophic vaginitis and kraurosis vulvae (atrophy of the female genitalia) associated with menopause.
2. Treatment of female hypogonadism, female castration and primary ovarian failure.
3. Prevention of postpartum breast engorgement.
4. As an oral contraceptive (OC) when used in combination with progestogens or as an emergency contraception (morning after pill) when taken in a particular sequence.
5. Retardation of osteoporosis in postmenopausal women.
6. Slow the progression of certain types of prostatic and mammary cancers.

Pharmacokinetics

Oral oestrogens are well absorbed through the gastrointestinal (GI) tract and undergo extensive hepatic metabolism. They are excreted in the urine. Oestrogens cross the placenta and enter breast milk. They should not be used during pregnancy or breast-feeding because of associated adverse effects on the foetus and neonate.

Contraindications and Cautions

Oestrogens are contraindicated in the presence of any known allergies to oestrogens and in patients with pregnancy, idiopathic vaginal bleeding; breast cancer; any oestrogen-dependent cancer and history of thromboembolic disorders. Oestrogens should be used with caution during breast-feeding, *because of possible effects on the neonate*; with metabolic bone disease, *because of the bone-conserving effect of oestrogen*; with renal insufficiency, *because of the effect on fluid and electrolytes and because oestrogens are excreted in the urine*; and with hepatic impairment, *because of the many effects on the liver and GI tract and because oestrogens are metabolized in the liver.*

Adverse Effects

Include breakthrough bleeding, menstrual irregularities, dysmenorrhoea, amenorrhoea and changes in libido. Other effects can result from the systemic effects of oestrogens, including fluid retention, electrolyte disturbances, headache, dizziness, mental changes, weight changes and oedema, premenstrual-like syndrome. GI effects also are common and include nausea, vomiting, abdominal cramps and bloating. Glucose intolerance and altered blood lipids, which may lead to acute pancreatitis and cholestatic jaundice, have been reported with the use of oestrogens.

Clinically Important Drug–Drug Interactions

If oestrogens are given in combination with drugs that enhance hepatic metabolism (e.g. barbiturates, rifampin,

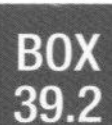

BOX 39.2 FOCUS ON THE **EVIDENCE**

Menopause and HRT—The Women's Health Initiative

Women experience the menarche (onset of the menstrual cycle) in adolescence and menopause (cessation of the menstrual cycle) in midlife. The exact age at which a woman experiences menopause or 'the change' of life varies. The family history of onset of menopause is a good guide for when the effects can be expected. Just as the physical changes associated with puberty can take a few years to be accomplished, so too can the changes associated with menopause. The signs and symptoms of menopause (vaginal dryness, hot flushes, moodiness, loss of bone density, increased risk of cardiovascular disease and somnolence) are related to the loss of oestrogen and progesterone effects on the body.

HRT or Not?

For centuries, women have proceeded through this time in their lives without pharmacological intervention, although many herbal and alternative therapies may be helpful to ease the transition through menopause. Women who rely on these therapies need to be cautioned about potential drug–drug interactions and advised to always report the use of these agents to their health care providers. Today, with more research and safer drugs available to counteract some of the effects of menopause, many women choose to use HRT if the adverse effects of menopause become too uncomfortable or difficult to tolerate. The use of HRT can decrease the discomforts associated with menopause; however, various forms of HRT have been associated with increased risks of breast, ovarian, endometrial and cervical cancer, venous thromboembolism, stroke and coronary heart disease. Many women are reluctant to consider HRT because of these risks. The newer drugs used in HRT have been shown to be associated with only a possible increase in risk of breast and cervical cancer, but with long-term use, are associated with an increased risk of cardiovascular events. Patients with many risk factors for developing these cancers are at greater risk than patients with no risk factors. Other drugs, the oestrogen receptor modulators, have antioestrogen effects on the breast and may remove the cancer risk. But these drugs may be less reliable in their management of the signs and symptoms of menopause and have not been correlated with a reduction in the risk of coronary artery disease. The Centre for Statistics in Medicine (CSM) advises that the minimum effective dose should be used for the shortest duration and treatments should be reviewed annually.

Always consult the most up-to-date edition of the British National Formulary (BNF) for current guidelines.

Many studies (Neves-e-Castro, 2003) have been conducted examining the effects of hormones on menopausal women. Initial studies suggested that HRT for postmenopausal was protective in many ways. It seemed that women using HRT had decreased coronary artery disease and cardiovascular events, decreased osteoporosis and bone fractures, decreased breast and colon cancer and improved memory. HRT was then being prescribed to prevent a number of these chronic conditions. However, more recent studies (Lowe, 2004) suggested that women using HRT for 5 or more years had an increased incidence cardiovascular disease, strokes, blood clots, gallstones and ovarian cancer. HRT is now prescribed for postmenopausal women with more caution.

Applying the Evidence

The woman who is entering menopause should have all of the information available before deciding whether HRT is for her. This can be a very difficult decision for many women, because the risks involved may outweigh the benefits or vice-versa. The nurse is often in the best position to provide information, listen to concerns and help the patient decide what is best for her.

A complete family and personal history of cancer and coronary artery disease risk factors should be completed to help the patient balance the benefits versus the risks of this therapy. If the decision is made to use HRT, the patient may need support in dealing with the effects of the drugs and may have to try several different preparations before the one best suited to her is found. As researchers continue to study women's health issues, better therapies may be developed to help women through this transition in life. Keeping up with the research as it is reported can be a difficult task, but if you work with women in clinical practice it is a necessity.

tetracyclines, phenytoin), serum oestrogen levels may decrease. Whenever a drug is added to or removed from a drug regimen that contains oestrogens, the nurse should evaluate that drug for possible interactions and either apply the appropriate dosage adjustments if prescribing or consult with the prescriber.

Smoking while taking oestrogens should be strongly discouraged, because the combination with nicotine increases the risk for development of thrombi and emboli.

Grapefruit juice can inhibit the metabolism of oestrogens leading to increased serum levels. Patients should be discouraged from drinking large quantities of grapefruit juice.

Always check the most up-to-date copy of the British National Formulary (BNF) for interactions and contraindications

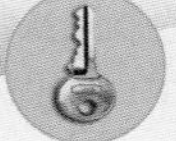

Key Drug Summary: *Oestradiol (used as HRT)*

Indications: Palliation of moderate-to-severe vasomotor symptoms associated with menopause; prevention of postmenopausal osteoporosis; treatment of female hypogonadism, female ovarian failure; palliation of inoperable and progressing breast cancer and inoperable prostatic cancer. *Oestradiol is usually given with a cyclical progestogen in women with an intact uterus.*

Actions: Most potent endogenous female sex hormone, responsible for oestrogen effects on the body

Pharmacokinetics:

Route	Onset	Peak	Duration
PO	Slow	Days	Unknown

Topical preparations are not generally absorbed systemically.

$T_{1/2}$: Not known; with hepatic metabolism and excretion in the urine

Adverse effects: Corneal changes, photosensitivity, peripheral oedema, hepatic adenoma, nausea, vomiting, abdominal cramps, bloating, breakthrough bleeding, change in menstrual flow, dysmenorrhoea, premenstrual-like syndrome

Please refer to the most up-to-date version of the British National Formulary (BNF) for further details.

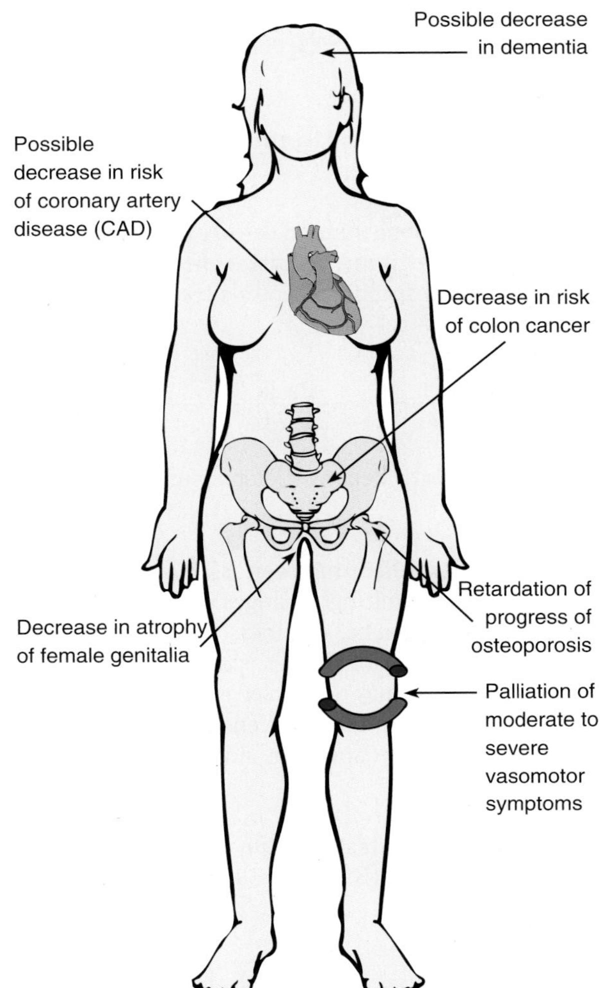

FIGURE 39.2 Sites of action of the oestrogens.

Oestrogen Receptor Modulators

Oestrogen receptor modulators were developed to produce some of the positive effects of oestrogen replacement, yet limit the adverse effects. The main oestrogen receptor modulator that is currently available is raloxifene, which is used to prevent and treat osteoporosis.

Therapeutic Actions and Indications

Raloxifene has modulating effects on oestrogen receptor sites, stimulating some and blocking others. It is used therapeutically to stimulate specific oestrogen receptor sites so as to increase bone mineral density without stimulating the endometrium. It is indicated for the treatment of postmenopausal osteoporosis, although it has no effect on menopausal vasomotor symptoms.

Pharmacokinetics

Raloxifene is well absorbed from the GI tract and is metabolized in the liver. Excretion occurs through the faeces. It is known to cross the placenta and enter into breast milk, so it should not be used during pregnancy or lactation.

Contraindications and Cautions

Raloxifene may have a role in oestrogen receptor positive breast cancer. It is contraindicated in the presence of any known allergy to raloxifene and in pregnancy and lactation, *because of potential effects on the foetus or neonate*. Caution should be used in patients with a history of venous thrombosis or smoking, *because of an increased risk of blood clot formation if smoking and oestrogen are combined.*

Always check the latest edition of the British National Formulary (BNF) for interactions and contraindications.

Clinically Important Drug–Drug Interactions

Cholestyramine reduces the absorption of raloxifene. Highly protein-bound drugs, such as diazepam ibuprofen, indomethacin may interfere with binding sites. Warfarin taken with raloxifene may decrease the prothrombin time (PT); patients using this combination must be monitored closely.

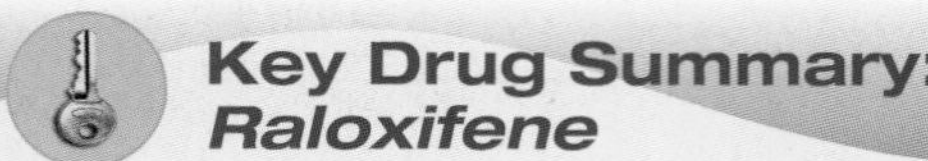

Key Drug Summary: *Raloxifene*

Indications: Prevention and treatment of osteoporosis in postmenopausal women

Actions: Increases bone mineral density without stimulating the endometrium; modulates effects of endogenous oestrogen at specific receptor sites

Pharmacokinetics:

Route	Onset	Peak	Duration
PO	Varies	4–7 h	24 h

$T_{1/2}$: 27.7 hours, with hepatic metabolism and excretion in the faeces

Adverse effects: Raloxifene has been associated with GI upset, nausea and vomiting. Changes in fluid balance may also cause headache, dizziness, visual changes and mental changes. Hot flushes, skin rash, oedema and vaginal bleeding may occur, secondary to specific oestrogen receptor stimulation. Venous thromboembolism is a potentially dangerous side-effect that has been reported

Always check the latest edition of the British National Formulary (BNF) for interactions and contraindications.

Progestogens

Progestogens are compounds that mimic the naturally occurring hormone progesterone. They can be categorized into progesterone (and its derivatives) and testosterone analogues. They are used as contraceptives, most effectively in combination with oestrogens to treat amenorrhoea and functional uterine bleeding, and as part of fertility programmes. Like the oestrogens, some progestogens are useful in treating specific cancers with specific receptor site sensitivity (see Chapter 13). Medroxyprogesterone, a progesterone is available orally for treatment of amenorrhoea, endometriosis and for cancer palliation therapy. Norethisterone and norgestrel are both testosterone analogues. Norethisterone is used in combination OCs and alone for the treatment of amenorrhoea. Norgestrel is an OC that is most effective when used in combination form. Levonorgestrel a newer form of norgestrel is much more potent. It was once available as an implant system to prevent pregnancy but now is available only in combination form OCs or as a uterine insert this is also used as the 'morning after' pill (Levonelle).

For a full list of the available female sex hormones always check the latest edition of the BNF.

Therapeutic Actions and Indications

The progestogens have many therapeutic actions, for example they transform the proliferative endometrium into a secretory endometrium, inhibit the secretion of follicle-stimulating hormone (FSH) and luteinizing hormone (LH), prevent follicle maturation and ovulation, inhibit uterine contractions and may have some anabolic and oestrogenic effects. When they are used as contraceptives, the exact mechanism of action is not known, but it is thought that circulating progestogens and oestrogens 'deceive' the hypothalamus and pituitary and prevent the release of gonadotropin-releasing hormone (GnRH), FSH and LH, thus preventing follicle development and ovulation. The low levels of these hormones do not produce an abundant endometrium that is receptive to implantation and if ovulation and fertilization were to occur, the chances of implantation would be remote.

Pharmacokinetics

The progestogens are well absorbed, undergo hepatic metabolism and are excreted in the urine. They are known to cross the placenta and to enter breast milk. They are not to be used during pregnancy or breast-feeding, because of the potential for adverse effects on the foetus or neonate.

Contraindications and Cautions

Progestogens should be used with caution in patients suffering from; pregnancy *(serious foetal defects have occurred)*; idiopathic vaginal bleeding; breast cancer or genital cancer; history of thromboembolic disorders, including cerebrovascular accident, *because of the increased risk of thrombus and embolus development*; hepatic dysfunction (or a history of liver tumours), *because of the effects of* progestogens *on the liver function*; pelvic inflammatory disease (PID), sexually transmitted diseases, endometriosis, or pelvic surgery, *because of the effects of* progestogens *on the uterus*; and breast-feeding, *because of potential effects on the neonate.*

Progestogens should be used with caution in patients with epilepsy, migraine headaches, asthma, cardiac or renal dysfunction, *because of the potential exacerbation of these conditions.*

Adverse Effects

Adverse effects associated with progestogens vary with the administration route used. OCs are associated with thromboembolic disorders (particularly when combined with nicotine), increased blood pressure, weight gain and headache. Dermal patch contraceptives are associated with the same systemic effects as well as local skin irritation. Vaginal gel use is associated with headache,nervousness, constipation, breast enlargement and perineal pain. Intrauterine systems are associated with abdominal pain, endometriosis, abortion, PID and expulsion of the intrauterine device. Vaginal use is associated with local irritation and swelling. Parenteral routes are associated with breakthrough bleeding, spotting, changes in the menstrual cycle, breast tenderness, thrombophlebitis, vision changes, weight gain and fluid retention and pain at the injection site.

Clinically Important Drug–Drug Interactions

Interaction with barbiturates, carbamazepine, phenytoin or rifampin may reduce the effect of progestogens.

Always check the most up-to-date copy of the British National Formulary (BNF) for interactions and contraindications

Nursing Considerations for Patients Receiving Oestrogens/ Oestrogen Receptor Modulators or Progestogens.

Assessment: History and Examination

Screen for the following conditions which could be contraindications to use of the drug

- History of allergy
- Pregnancy and breast-feeding
- Hepatic dysfunction
- Cardiovascular disease
- Breast or genital cancer
- Renal disease
- Metabolic bone disease
- History of thromboembolism
- Smoking
- Idiopathic vaginal bleeding.

Include screening for baseline status

- Skin colour (lesions/texture)
- Orientation, mental status
- Blood pressure, pulse, cardiac auscultation
- Perfusion
- Abdominal examination
- Liver examination
- Pelvic examination (Pap smear, urinalysis)
- Breast examination
- Ophthalmic examination (particularly if the patient wears contact lenses).

Establish if patient is currently taking other medications or herbal therapies which may potentially interact with the oestrogens/oestrogen receptor modulators or progestogens.

Nursing Diagnoses

The patient receiving oestrogens or oestrogen receptor modulators may have the following nursing diagnoses related to drug therapy:

- Excess fluid volume related to fluid retention
- Acute pain related to systemic side-effects
- Ineffective tissue perfusion (cerebral, cardiopulmonary, peripheral)
- Deficient knowledge regarding drug therapy

Implementation With Rationale

- Administer drug as prescribed, *to prevent adverse effects;* administer with food if GI upset is severe, or *to relieve GI distress.*
- Provide analgesics *for relief of headache as appropriate.*
- Arrange for at least an annual physical examination, including pelvic examination, Pap smear *and* breast examination, *to avert adverse effects and monitor drug effects.*
- Monitor liver function periodically for the patient on long-term therapy, *to ensure that the drug is discontinued at any sign of hepatic dysfunction.*
- Provide support and reassurance *to deal with the drug and drug effects.*
- Provide thorough patient education, including measures to avoid adverse effects, warning signs of problems *and* the need for regular evaluation, *to enhance patient knowledge about drug therapy and to promote concordance*

Evaluation

- Monitor patient response to the drug (palliation of signs and symptoms of menopause, prevention of pregnancy, decreased risk factors for coronary artery disease, palliation of certain cancers).
- Monitor for adverse effects (liver changes, GI upset, oedema, changes in secondary sex characteristics, headaches, thromboembolic episodes, breakthrough bleeding).
- Monitor for potential drug–drug interactions as indicated.
- Evaluate the effectiveness of the teaching plan: patient can name drug, dosage, adverse effects

to watch for, specific measures to avoid adverse effects.

- Monitor the effectiveness of comfort measures and compliance to the regimen.

Fertility Drugs

Women without primary ovarian failure who cannot get pregnant after 1 year of trying may be candidates for the use of fertility drugs. These drugs act to stimulate follicle development and ovulation in functioning ovaries and are combined with human chorionic gonadotropin (HCG) to maintain the follicles once ovulation has occurred.

Chorionic gonadotropin is an injected drug that is used to stimulate ovulation by acting like GnRH and affecting FSH and LH release. Chorionic gonadotropin α is an injected drug that stimulates final follicular development and ovulation in infertile women. Clomifene is a commonly used oral agent that is also used for the treatment of male infertility. Follitropin α and follitropin β are FSH molecules produced by recombinant DNA technology; they are injected to stimulate follicular development in infertility and for harvesting of ova for in vitro fertilization. Ganirelix is an injected drug that inhibits premature LH surges in women undergoing controlled ovarian hyperstimulation as part of a fertility programme.

Therapeutic Actions and Indications

Fertility drugs work either directly or by stimulating the hypothalamus to increase FSH and LH levels, leading to ovarian follicular development and maturation of ova. Given in sequence with HCG to maintain the follicle and hormone production, these drugs are used to treat infertility in women with functioning ovaries whose partners are fertile. Fertility drugs also may be used to stimulate multiple follicle development for the harvesting of ova for in vitro fertilization.

Pharmacokinetics

These drugs are well absorbed and are treated like endogenous hormones within the body, undergoing hepatic metabolism and renal excretion. They should not be used during pregnancy or lactation because of the potential for adverse hormonal effects on the foetus or neonate.

Contraindications and Cautions

These drugs are contraindicated in the presence of primary ovarian failure *(they only work to stimulate functioning ovaries)*; thyroid or adrenal dysfunction, *because of the effects on the hypothalamic-pituitary axis*; ovarian cysts; pregnancy *(serious foetal defects have occurred)*; idiopathic uterine bleeding and known allergy to any fertility drug.

Caution should be used in women who are breast-feeding and in those with thromboembolic diseases, *because of the risk of increased thrombus formation*; and in women with respiratory diseases, *because of alterations in fluid volume and blood flow.*

Adverse Effects

Adverse effects associated with fertility drugs include a greatly increased risk of multiple births and birth defects; ovarian overstimulation (abdominal pain, distension, ascites, pleural effusion) and headache, fluid retention, nausea, bloating, uterine bleeding, ovarian enlargement, gynecomastia and febrile reactions (possibly due to stimulation of progesterone release).

Always check the most up-to-date copy of the British National Formulary (BNF) for interactions and contraindications

Therapeutic Actions and Indications

Oestrogens are important for the development of the female reproductive system and secondary sex characteristics. They affect the release of pituitary FSH and LH; cause capillary dilatation, fluid retention, protein anabolism and thinning the cervical mucus; conservation of calcium and phosphorus and they encourage bone formation. When given artificially oestrogens can inhibit ovulation and prevent postpartum breast discomfort. Oestrogens also are responsible for the proliferation of the endometrial lining. An absence or decrease in oestrogen produces the signs and symptoms of menopause in the uterus, vagina, breasts and cervix. Oestrogens are known to compete with androgens for receptor sites; this trait makes them beneficial in certain androgen-dependent prostate cancers.

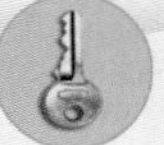

Key Drug Summary: *Clomiphene*

Indications: Treatment of ovarian failure in patients with normal liver function and normal endogenous oestrogens; unlabelled use: treatment of male sterility

Actions: Binds to oestrogen receptors, decreasing the number of available oestrogen receptors, which gives the hypothalamus the false signal to increase FSH and LH secretion, leading to ovarian stimulation

Pharmacokinetics:

Route	Onset	Peak	Duration
PO	5–8 days	Unknown	6 wk

$T_{1/2}$: 5 days, with hepatic metabolism and excretion in the faeces

Adverse effects: Vasomotor flushing, visual changes, abdominal discomfort, distension and bloating, nausea, vomiting, ovarian enlargement, breast tenderness, ovarian over stimulation, multiple pregnancies

Please check the latest edition of the British National Formulary(BNF) for interactions and contraindications.

Nursing Considerations for Patients Receiving Fertility Drugs

Assessment: History and Examination

Screen for the following conditions, *which could be cautions or contraindications to use of the drug*: history of allergy to any fertility drug, pregnancy, lactation, ovarian failure, thyroid or adrenal dysfunction, ovarian cysts, idiopathic uterine bleeding, thromboembolic diseases *and* respiratory diseases.

Include screening *for baseline status before beginning therapy and for any potential adverse effects*: skin, lesions; orientation, affect, reflexes; blood pressure, pulse; respiration, adventitious sounds; hormone levels, Pap smear, breast examination.

Establish if patient is currently taking other medications or herbal therapies which may potentially interact with the fertility drugs.

Nursing Diagnoses

The patient receiving fertility drugs may have the following nursing diagnoses related to drug therapy:

- Disturbed body image related to drug treatment and diagnosis
- Acute pain related to headache, fluid retention, GI upset
- Sexual dysfunction
- Deficient knowledge regarding drug therapy

Implementation With Rationale

- Assess the cause of dysfunction before beginning therapy, *to ensure appropriate use of the drug.*
- Complete a pelvic examination before each cycle of drug therapy, *to rule out ovarian enlargement, pregnancy, or uterine problems.*
- Check urine oestrogen and oestradiol levels before beginning therapy, *to verify ovarian function.*
- Administer with an appropriate dosage of HCG as indicated, *to ensure beneficial effects.*
- Discontinue the drug at any sign of ovarian overstimulation *and* arrange for hospitalization *to monitor and support patient* if this occurs.
- Provide women with a calendar of treatment days, explanations of adverse effects to anticipate *and* instructions on when intercourse should occur, *to increase the therapeutic effectiveness of the drug.*
- Provide warnings about the risk and hazards of multiple births, *so the patient can make informed decisions about drug therapy.*
- Provide thorough patient education, including measures to avoid adverse effects, warning signs of problems *and* the need for regular evaluation *to enhance patient knowledge about drug therapy and to promote compliance.*

Evaluation

- Monitor patient response to the drug (ovulation).
- Monitor for adverse effects (abdominal bloating, weight gain, ovarian overstimulation, multiple births).
- Evaluate the effectiveness of the teaching plan (patient can name drug, dosage, adverse effects to watch for, specific measures to avoid adverse effects).
- Monitor the effectiveness of comfort measures and compliance with the regimen.

Oxytocics

Oxytocic drugs are used to stimulate contraction of the uterus, much like the action of the hypothalamic hormone oxytocin, which is stored in the posterior pituitary. These drugs include ergonovine which is given intramuscularly or intravenously and is used to prevent and treat postpartum and postabortion uterine atony, and oxytocin which is used to induce labour and to promote uterine contractions after labour. Oxytocin is also available in a nasal form to stimulate milk 'let down' in lactating women.

Therapeutic Actions and Indications

The oxytocics directly affect neuroreceptor sites to stimulate contraction of the uterus. They are especially effective in the gravid uterus. Oxytocin, a synthetic form of the hypothalamic hormone, also stimulates the lacteal glands in the breast to contract, promoting milk ejection in lactating women.

Oxytocics are indicated for the prevention and treatment of uterine atony after delivery. This is important to prevent postpartum haemorrhage. Ergonovine is being investigated for use in diagnostic tests for angina during arteriography studies because it has been shown to induce coronary artery contraction.

Pharmacokinetics

The oxytocics are rapidly absorbed, metabolized in the liver and excreted in urine and faeces. They cross the placenta and enter breast milk. They are not used during pregnancy because of their effects on the uterus. Oxytocin is used during lactation because of its effects on milk ejection, but the baby should be evaluated for any adverse effects associated with the hormone.

Contraindications and Cautions

Oxytocics are contraindicated with cephalopelvic disproportion, unfavourable foetal position, complete uterine atony or early pregnancy. Caution should be used in patients with coronary disease, hypertension, lactation or previous caesarean section *because of the effects on artery contraction and uterine contraction.*

Adverse Effects

The adverse effects most often associated with the oxytocics are related to excessive effects (e.g., uterine hypertonicity and spasm, uterine rupture, postpartum haemorrhage, decreased foetal heart rate). GI upset, nausea, headache and dizziness are not uncommon. Ergonovine and methylergonovine can produce ergotism (e.g., nausea, blood pressure changes, weak pulse, dyspnea, chest pain, numbness and coldness in extremities, confusion, excitement, delirium, convulsions and even coma). Oxytocin has caused severe water intoxication with coma and even maternal death when used for a prolonged period. This is thought to occur because of related effects of antidiuretic hormone (ADH), which is also stored in the posterior pituitary and may be released in response to oxytocin activity, causing water retention in the kidney.

Always check the most up-to-date copy of the British National Formulary(BNF) for interactions and contraindications.

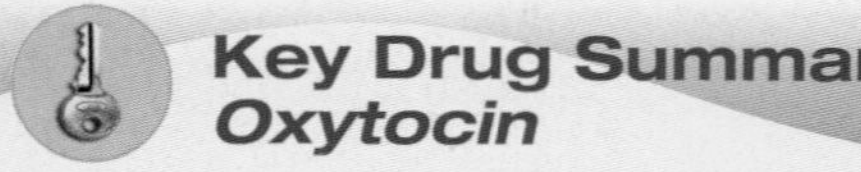

Key Drug Summary: *Oxytocin*

Indications: To initiate or improve uterine contractions for early vaginal delivery; to stimulate or reinforce labour in selected cases of uterine inertia; to manage inevitable or incomplete abortion; second-trimester abortion; to control postpartum bleeding or haemorrhage; to treat lactation deficiency

Actions: Synthetic form stimulates the uterus, especially the gravid uterus; causes myoepithelium of the lacteal glands to contract, resulting in milk ejection in lactating women

Pharmacokinetics:

Route	Onset	Peak	Duration
IV	Immediate	Unknown	60 min
IM	3–5 min	Unknown	2–3 h

$T_{1/2}$: 1–6 min, with tissue metabolism and excretion in the urine

Adverse effects: Cardiac arrhythmias, hypertension, foetal bradycardia, nausea, vomiting, uterine rupture, pelvic haematoma, uterine hypertonicity, severe water intoxication, anaphylactic reaction

Nursing Considerations for Patients Receiving Oxytocics

Assessment: History and Examination

Screen for the following conditions, *which could be cautions or contraindications to use of the drug*: history of allergy to any labour inducer or prostaglandin preparation; active PID; cardiac, hepatic, pulmonary or renal disease; history of asthma and hypotension, hypertension, epilepsy, scarred uterus or acute vaginitis.

Include screening *for baseline status before beginning therapy and for any potential adverse effects*: skin, lesions; orientation, affect; blood pressure, pulse; respiration, adventitious sounds; vaginal discharge, pelvic examination, uterine tone and liver and renal function tests, leukocyte count and urinalysis.

Establish if patient is currently taking other medications or herbal therapies which may potentially interact with the oxytocics.

Nursing Diagnoses

The patient receiving abortifacients may have the following nursing diagnoses related to drug therapy:

- Acute pain related to uterine contractions, headache, fluid retention, GI upset

- Ineffective coping related to abortion or foetal death
- Deficient knowledge regarding drug therapy

Implementation With Rationale

- Administer via route indicated, following the manufacturer's directions for storage and preparation, *to ensure safe and therapeutic use of the drug.*
- Confirm the age of the pregnancy before administering the drug, *to ensure appropriate use of the drug.*
- Confirm that abortion or uterine evacuation is complete, *to avoid potential bleeding problems;* prepare for dilation and curettage (D&C) if necessary.
- Monitor blood pressure periodically during and after administration, *to assess for adverse effects;* discontinue the drug if blood pressure rises dramatically.
- Monitor uterine tone and involution and the amount of bleeding during and for several days after use of the drug, *to ensure appropriate response and recovery from the drug.*
- Provide support and appropriate referrals, *to help the patient deal with abortion or foetal death.*
- Provide thorough patient education, including measures to avoid adverse effects and warning signs of problems to report, *to enhance patient knowledge about drug therapy and to promote concordance.*

Evaluation

- Monitor patient response to the drug (evacuation of uterus).
- Monitor for adverse effects (GI upset, nausea, blood pressure changes, haemorrhage, uterine rupture).
- Evaluate the effectiveness of the teaching plan (patient can name drug, dosage, adverse effects to watch for, specific measures to avoid adverse effects).
- Monitor the effectiveness of comfort measures and compliance to the regimen.

Labour inducers

Labour inducers are drugs that can be used to bring on labour if the pregnancy over runs or if the pregnancy is terminated. These drugs stimulate intense uterine contractions. Carboprost is an intramuscular drug used to terminate early pregnancy, evacuate a missed abortion or control postpartum haemorrhage. Gemeprost, a similar drug is the preferred prostaglandin treatment for the induction of an abortion; it is given by vaginal suppository. Dinoprostone is also a prostaglandin that stimulates uterine contractions; it is given by intravaginal suppository, vaginal tablets or gels. In addition to evacuating the uterus, it is also used to stimulate cervical ripening before labour.

Therapeutic Actions and Indications

The labour inducers stimulate uterine activity, dislodging any implanted trophoblast (early embryonic stages) and preventing implantation of any fertilized egg. These drugs are approved for use to terminate pregnancy 12 to 20 weeks from the date of the last menstrual period. Mifepristone is approved for use during the first 49 days of the pregnancy. Carboprost and dinoprostone are also approved for use to evacuate the uterus after a missed abortion or foetal death. Carboprost also is used to treat postpartum haemorrhage that is not responsive to the usual therapy.

Pharmacokinetics

These drugs are well absorbed, metabolized in the liver and excreted in the urine. These drugs are only used during pregnancy to end the pregnancy, because of their effects on the uterus. They are not recommended for use during lactation because of the potential for serious effects on the neonate. If these drugs are to be used by a lactating mother, another method of feeding the baby should be used.

Contraindications and Cautions

Labour inducers when used as an abortifactant should not be used with any known allergy to the drugs or prostaglandins; after 20 weeks from the last menstrual period or with active PID or acute cardiovascular, hepatic, renal or pulmonary disease.

Caution should be used with any history of asthma, hypertension or adrenal disease and with acute vaginitis (inflammation of the vagina) or scarred uterus.

Adverse Effects

Adverse effects associated with labour inducers include abdominal cramping, heavy uterine bleeding, perforated uterus and uterine rupture, all of which are related to exaggeration of the desired effects of the drug. Other side-effects include headache, nausea and vomiting, diarrhoea, diaphoresis (sweating), backache and rash.

Always check the most up-to-date copy of the British National Formulary (BNF) for interactions and contraindications

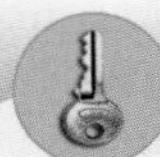

Key Drug Summary: *Dinoprostone*

Indications: Termination of pregnancy 12 to 20 weeks from the first day of the last menstrual period; evacuation of the uterus (D&C) in the management of missed abortion or intrauterine foetal death; management of nonmetastatic gestational trophoblastic disease; initiation of cervical ripening

Actions: Stimulates the myometrium of the pregnant uterus to contract, evacuating the contents of the uterus

Pharmacokinetics:

Route	Onset	Peak	Duration
Intravaginal	10 min	15 min	2–3 h

$T_{1/2}$: 5–10 hours, with tissue metabolism and excretion in the urine

Adverse effects: Headache, paresthesias, hypotension, vomiting, diarrhoea, nausea, uterine rupture, uterine or vaginal pain, chills, diaphoresis, backache, fever

Myometrial relaxants

Uterine contractions that become strong before term can lead to premature labour and delivery, which can have detrimental effects on the neonate. Drugs used to relax the uterine smooth muscle and prevent contractions leading to premature labour and delivery are called tocolytics. They are usually reserved for use after 20 weeks of gestation, when the neonate has a chance of survival outside the uterus. If premature contractions occur, atosiban an oxytocin antagonist or terbutaline, a β_2-selective adrenergic agonist may be given.

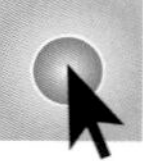

WEB LINKS

Health care providers and patients may want to consult the following Internet sources:

http://cks.library.nhs.uk The National Health Service Clinical Knowledge Summaries provides evidence-based practical information on the common conditions observed in primary care.

http://www.bnf.org.uk The BNF provides UK health care professionals with authoritative and practical information on the selection and clinical use of medicines.

http://www.nhsdirect.nhs.uk The National Health Service Direct service provides patients with information and advice about health, illness and health services.

www.fpa.org.uk Family Planning Association is the UK's leading sexual health charity. Whose purpose is to enable people in the United Kingdom to make informed choices about sex and to enjoy sexual health.

http://www.nice.org.uk National Institute for Health and Clinical Excellence is an independent organization responsible for providing national guidance on promoting good health and preventing and treating ill health.

Points to Remember

- Oestrogens are female sex hormones that are important in the development of the female reproductive system and secondary sex characteristics.
- Oestrogens are used pharmacologically mainly to replace hormones lost at menopause so as to prevent many of the signs and symptoms associated with menopause, including the development of coronary artery disease; to stimulate ovulation in woman with hypogonadism; and in combination with progestogens for OCs.
- Progestogens are female sex hormones that are responsible for maintenance of a pregnancy and for the development of some secondary sex characteristics.
- Progestogens are used in combination with oestrogens for contraception, to treat uterine bleeding and for palliation in certain cancers with sensitive receptor sites.
- Fertility drugs stimulate FSH and LH in women with functioning ovaries to increase follicle development and improve the chances for pregnancy.
- A major adverse effect of fertility drugs is multiple births and birth defects.
- Oxytocic drugs act like the hypothalamic hormone oxytocin to stimulate uterine contractions and induce or speed up labour. They are most frequently used to control bleeding and promote postpartum involution of the uterus.
- Labour inducers are drugs that stimulate uterine activity to cause uterine evacuation. These drugs can be used to induce abortion in early pregnancy or to promote uterine evacuation after intrauterine foetal death.
- Tocolytics are drugs that relax the uterine smooth muscle; they are used to stop premature labour in patients after 20 weeks' gestation.

CRITICAL THINKING SCENARIO 39-1

Birth Control

The Situation

Jill is a 25-year-old woman who is being seen in her practice nurse for a routine annual physical examination and Pap smear test. Jill reports that she has just become sexually active and would like to start using contraceptives. She has some concerns about stories she has heard about 'the pill' and would like to know the safest and most effective birth control to use.

Discussion

This appointment presents a good opportunity for the health care provider to allow Jill to discuss this new aspect of her life. She may have questions about the experience and about things she should be doing or should be questioning. The risk of sexually transmitted diseases as well as pregnancy can be discussed. Jill needs comprehensive information about the various forms of birth control that are available for use. Nonpharmacological measures, such as condoms *and* the rhythm method *and* their reliability can be discussed.

The use of hormones for birth control should then be explained, including the 96% to 98% reliability of these methods when used correctly. The numerous delivery methods for these hormones should be outlined. A variety of possibilities exist, from the transdermal patch to injection to the vaginal ring to the traditional tablet. Jill elected to go with an OC. Jill will need teaching about drug and herbal interactions with the OC and will need to have written instructions on what to do if a dose is missed. The action that should be taken if a dose is missed can be very complicated and involves knowing on which day in the cycle the dose was missed.

It is also important to stress that the OC will not protect Jill from sexually transmitted diseases and that precautions will need to be taken to avoid exposure to these diseases. She should also be advised not to smoke, because smoking combined with OC use increases the risk for emboli. The adverse effects that she might experience should be reviewed and the importance of an annual pelvic examination and Pap test should be stressed. A trusting nurse-patient relationship is important at this time so that Jill can feel free to call with questions or problems in the future.

Nursing Care Guide for Jill: Oral Contraceptives

Assessment: History and Examination

Assess the patient's health history for allergies, pregnancy, lactation; breast or genital cancer; hepatic dysfunction; coronary artery disease; thromboembolic disease; renal disease; idiopathic vaginal bleeding; metabolic bone disease; diabetes

Focus the physical examination on the following:

- CV: pulse, cardiac auscultation, blood pressure, oedema, perfusion
- GI: abdominal examination, liver examination
- GU: pelvic examination, Pap smear, urinalysis
- Eye: ophthalmologic examination

Nursing Diagnoses

- Excess fluid volume related to fluid retention
- Acute pain related to systemic side-effects
- Ineffective tissue perfusion (oedema/ poor circulation)

Implementation

- Administer medication as prescribed.
- Arrange at least annual physical examination, including Pap smear and breast examination.
- Provide patient education regarding drug name, dosage, adverse effects, precautions, warnings to report, safe administration.

Evaluation

Evaluate drug effects: prevention of pregnancy; relief of signs and symptoms of menopause; decreased risk of coronary artery disease.

Monitor for adverse effects: signs of liver dysfunction; GI upset; oedema; changes in secondary sex characteristics; headaches; thromboembolic episodes; breakthrough bleeding.

Monitor for drug–drug interactions as indicated for each drug.

Evaluate effectiveness of patient education programme and comfort and safety measures.

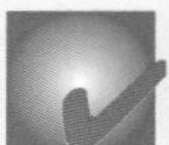

CHECK YOUR UNDERSTANDING

Answers to the questions in this chapter may be found in the answer key in the back of the book.

Multiple Choice

Select the most appropriate response to the following.

1. A postmenopausal woman is started on oestrogens to control her unpleasant menopausal symptoms. She should be instructed that, as a result of the drug therapy, she may experience
   a. constipation.
   b. breakthrough bleeding.
   c. weight loss.
   d. persistently elevated body temperature.

2. An oestrogen receptor modulator might be the drug of choice in the treatment of postmenopausal osteoporosis in a patient with a family history of breast or uterine cancer. She should be taught that she might experience.
   a. constipation and dry, itchy skin.
   b. flushing and dry vaginal mucosa.
   c. hot flushes and vaginal bleeding.
   d. no associated adverse effects.

3. Combination oestrogens and progestogens are commonly used as OCs. It is thought that this combination has its effect by
   a. acting like circulating oestrogen and progesterone to block the hypothalamic release of FSH and LH.
   b. preventing follicle development and ovulation.
   c. directly suppressing the ovaries and preventing ovulation.
   d. keeping the endometrium constantly lush and blood filled.
   e. preventing menstruation, which prevents pregnancy.

4. Any patient who is taking oestrogens, progestogens, or combination products should be cautioned to avoid smoking because
   a. nicotine increases the metabolism of the hormones and they may not be effective.
   b. the combination leads to an increased risk of potentially dangerous thromboembolic episodes.
   c. nicotine amplifies the adverse effects of the hormones.
   d. nicotine blocks hormone receptor sites and they may no longer be effective.

5. A synthetic form of oxytocin is used to
   a. induce abortion.
   b. stimulate milk 'let down' in the lactating woman.
   c. increase fertility and the chance of conception.
   d. relax the gravid uterus and prevent preterm labour.

6. The use of a labour inducer as an abortifacient drug would be contraindicated in a woman who
   a. is 15 weeks pregnant.
   b. is older than 50 years of age.
   c. has had four caesarean sections in the past.
   d. is 10 weeks pregnant.

Extended Matching Questions

Select **all** that apply.

1. Oestrogens produce a wide variety of systemic effects. Effects attributed to oestrogen include
   a. protecting the heart from atherosclerosis.
   b. retaining calcium in the bones.
   c. maintaining the secondary female sex characteristics.
   d. relaxing the gravid uterus to prolong pregnancy.
   e. stimulating the uterus to increase the chances of conception.
   f. relaxing blood vessels.

2. A client is taking clomiphene after 6 years of inability to conceive a child. The client will need to be informed about the
   a. need for a complete physical and pelvic examination before each course of drug therapy
   b. risks and hazards of multiple births
   c. importance of scheduling treatments and intercourse to increase the chance of conception
   d. need to avoid intercourse during drug therapy
   e. need to report blurred vision
   f. light-headedness, dizziness and drowsiness are common side-effects

3. A client is receiving an oxytocic drug to stimulate labour. The nursing care of this client would include which of the following?
   a. Monitoring of foetal heart beat during labour
   b. Regulation of drug delivery between contractions
   c. Administration of blood pressure-lowering drugs to balance hypertensive effects
   d. Monitoring of maternal blood pressure periodically during and after administration
   e. Close monitoring of maternal blood loss following delivery
   f. Isolation of mother and newborn to prevent infection

Fill in the Blanks

1. Drugs that stimulate uterine contractions are called ________________.
2. Drugs that are used to relax the gravid uterus to prolong pregnancy are referred to as ____________.
3. Loss of oestrogen is associated with many problems at menopause, including ________________ or a loss of calcium from the bones, ______________________ associated with vascular spasms and an increased risk of __________________, the leading cause of death among women.
4. Women are strongly discouraged from smoking when taking oestrogen replacement therapy because of an increased risk of __________________ and __________________ development.
5. ____________________ is an oestrogen receptor modulator, stimulating some receptors and blocking others.
6. Medroxyprogesterone is available *as depo-provera*, a form of birth control that is delivered every 3 months by __________________________.
7. Women without primary ovarian failure who cannot become pregnant after a year of trying may be candidates for the use of __________________.
8. Drugs that can be used to induce abortion in early pregnancy or to promote uterine evacuation after intrauterine foetal death are called __________________.

Bibliography and References

British Medical Association and Royal Pharmaceutical Society of Great Britain. (2008). *British National Formulary*. London: BMJ & RPS Publishing. *This publication is updated biannually: it is imperative that the most recent edition is consulted.*

British Medical Association and Royal Pharmaceutical Society of Great Britain. (2008). *British National Formulary for Children*. London: BMJ & RPS Publishing. *This publication is updated annually: it is imperative that the most recent edition is consulted.*

Brunton, L., Lazo, J. S., Parker, K., Goodman, L. S., & Gilman, A. G. (2005). *Goodman and Gilman's the pharmacological basis of therapeutics* (11th ed.). London: McGraw-Hill.

Daly, E., Roche, M., Barlow, D., Gray, A., McPherson, K., & Vessey, M. (1992). HRT: An analysis benefits, risks and costs. *British Medical Bulletin, 48*, 368–400.

Ganong, W. (2005). *Review of medical physiology* (22nd ed.). New York: McGraw-Hill.

Howland, R. D., & Mycek, M. J. (2005). *Pharmacology* (3rd ed.). Philadelphia: Lippincott Williams & Wilkins.

Kendall, A., Folkerd, E. J., & Dowsett, M. (2007). Influences on circulating oestrogens in postmenopausal women: Relationship with breast cancer. *Journal of Steroid Biochemistry and Molecular Biology, 103*(2), 99–109.

Karch, A. M. (2006). *2007 Lippincott's nursing drug guide*. Philadelphia: Lippincott Williams & Wilkins.

Lowe, G. D. O. (2004). HRT & CV disease. Increase risk of venous thromboembolism, stroke and no protection from coronary disease. *Journal of Internal Medicine, 256*(5), 361–374.

Marieb, E. N., & Hoehn, K. (2004). *Human anatomy & physiology* (7th ed.). San Francisco: Pearson Benjamin Cummings.

Nelson, H. D. (2008). Menopause. *The Lancet, 371*, 760–770.

Neves-e-Castro, M. (2003). Menopause in crisis post-Women's Health Initiative? *Human Reproduction, 18*, 2512–2518.

Porth, C. M., & Matfin G. (2008). *Pathophysiology: Concepts of altered health states* (8th ed.). Philadelphia, PA: Lippincott Williams & Wilkins.

Simonsen, T., Aarbakke, J., Kay, I., Coleman, I., Sinnott, P., & Lysaa, R. (2006). *Illustrated pharmacology for nurses*. London: Hodder Arnold.

CHAPTER 40

Drugs Affecting the Male Reproductive System

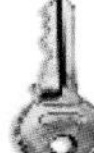

KEY TERMS

anabolic steroids

androgenic effects

androgens

cyclic guanosine mono-phosphate (cGMP)

hirsutism

hypogonadism

penile erectile dysfunction

LEARNING OBJECTIVES

Upon completion of this chapter, you will be able to:

1. Discuss the effects of testosterone and other androgens on the male body and use this information to explain the therapeutic and adverse effects of these agents when used clinically.
2. Describe the therapeutic actions, indications, pharmacokinetics associated with androgens, anabolic steroids and drugs used to treat erectile dysfunction.
3. Describe the contraindications, most common adverse reactions and important drug–drug interactions associated with androgens, anabolic steroids and drugs used to treat erectile dysfunction.
4. Discuss the use of drugs that affect the male reproductive system across the lifespan.
5. Compare and contrast the key drugs testosterone and sildenafil with other agents in their classes.
6. Outline the nursing considerations, including important teaching points, for patients receiving drugs used to affect the male reproductive system.

ANDROGENS

 testosterone

ANABOLIC STEROIDS

nandrolone

DRUGS FOR TREATING PENILE ERECTILE DYSFUNCTION

alprostadil

sildenafil

tadalafil

Drugs that are used to affect the male reproductive system include male steroid hormones or **androgens**, which act like the male sex hormone, testosterone. Others include **anabolic steroids**, which are synthetic testosterone preparations that have more anabolic (tissue-building) effects than **androgenic effects** (effects associated with development of male sexual characteristics), and drugs that act to improve penile dysfunction. This last group includes alprostadil, which is a prostaglandin and sildenafil and tadalafil which are selective inhibitors of **cyclic guanosine mono-phosphate** (cGMP), a reactive tissue enzyme inhibitor) that increase nitric oxide in the corpus cavernosum to improve erection (Figure 40.1). Box 40.1 describes the effect of these drugs across the lifespan.

Androgens

The primary natural androgen is testosterone is used for replacement therapy in cases of **hypogonadism** (underdeveloped testes) and to treat certain breast cancers.

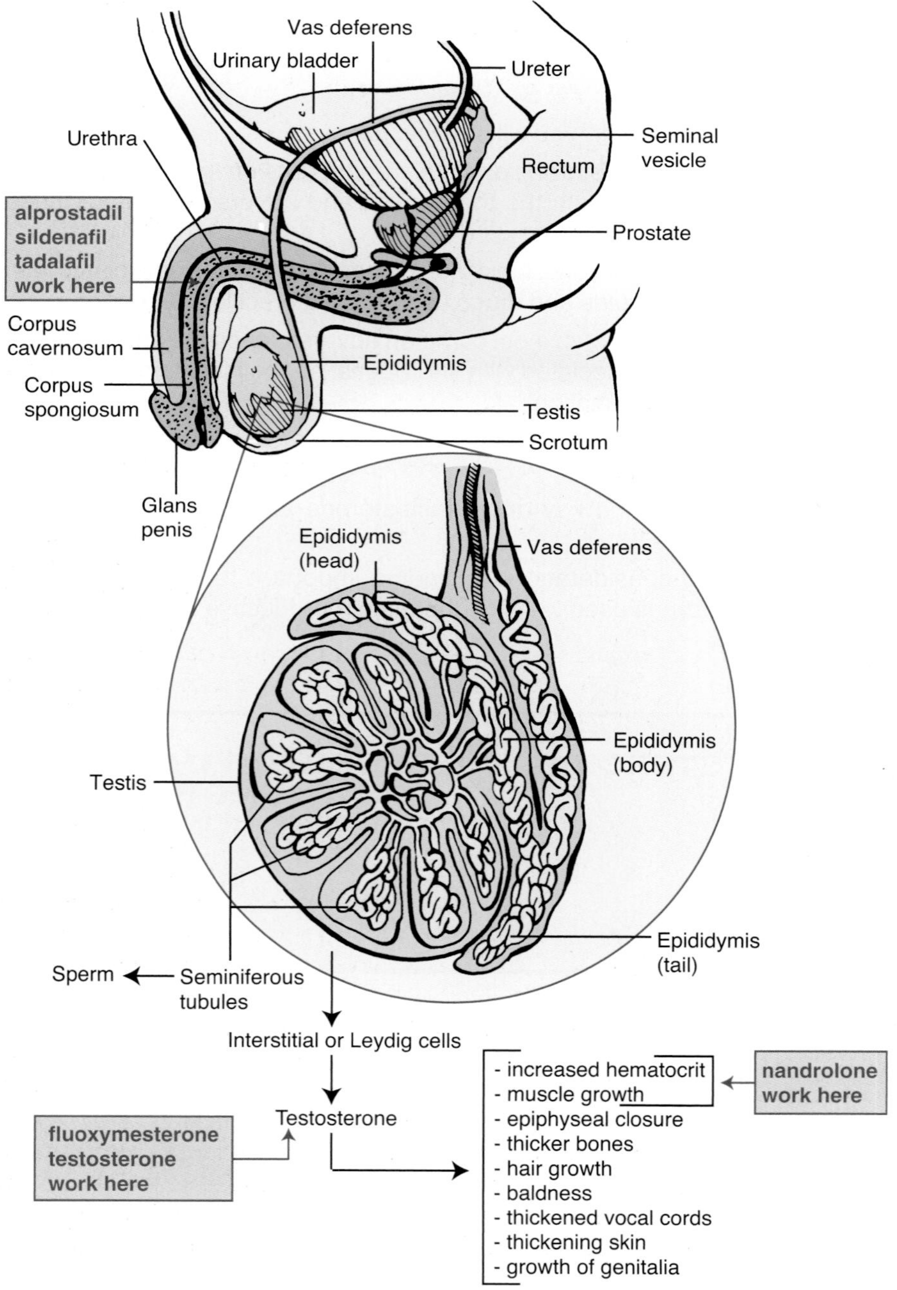

FIGURE 40.1 Sites of action of drugs affecting the male reproductive system.

BOX 40.1 DRUG THERAPY ACROSS THE LIFESPAN

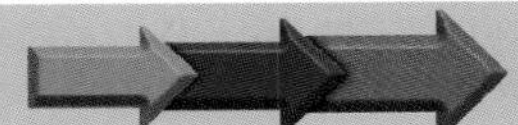

Drugs Affecting the Male Reproductive System

CHILDREN

These drugs are used in children as replacement therapy and to increase red blood cell production in renal failure. As these hormones effect epiphyseal closure, children should be closely monitored with hand and wrist radiographs pretreatment and every 6 months. If precocious puberty occurs, the drug should be stopped.

Adolescents who are prescribed androgens should be alerted to the potential for increased acne and other effects.

Adolescent athletes need education about the risks associated with the use of anabolic steroids to improve athletic performance and the lack of scientific evidence of to support its beneficial effects.

When administering or prescribing any drug to children, always consult the most recent edition of the British National Formulary for Children

ADULTS

Adults also need reinforcement of the information about anabolic steroid use and athletics.

Men who are receiving these drugs for replacement therapy may need to learn self-injection technique. Women who are prescribed these drugs may experience masculinization effects and may need support in coping with these body changes.

Periodic liver function tests are important in monitoring the effects of these drugs on the liver.

These drugs are not indicated for use in pregnancy or lactation because of the potential for serious effects on the foetus or neonate.

OLDER ADULTS

Older adults may have problems with androgen therapy because of underlying conditions that are aggravated by the drug effects. Hypertension, congestive heart failure and coronary artery disease may be aggravated by the fluid retention associated with these drugs. Benign prostatic hyperplasia, a common problem in older men, may be aggravated by androgenic effects that may enlarge the prostate further, leading to urinary difficulties and increased risk of prostate cancer.

Many older adults have hepatic dysfunction and these drugs can be hepatotoxic. Older patients should be monitored very carefully and dosage should be reduced. If signs of liver failure or hepatitis occur, the drug should be stopped immediately.

Therapeutic Actions and Indications

The androgens are forms of testosterone. They are responsible for the growth and development of male sex organs and the maintenance of secondary sex characteristics (see Figure 40.1). They act to increase the retention of nitrogen, sodium, potassium and phosphorus and to decrease the urinary excretion of calcium. Testosterones increase protein anabolism and decrease protein catabolism (breakdown). They also increase the production of red blood cells.

Androgens can be indicated for the treatment of hypogonadism and delayed puberty in male patients. They are also indicated for the treatment of certain breast cancers in postmenopausal women, for the prevention of ovulation to treat endometriosis, for the prevention of postpartum breast engorgement (testosterone) and for the treatment of hereditary angio-oedema. Testosterone is long-acting and is available in several forms, including tablet, implant (deep, slow-release) IM injections and a dermal patch.

Pharmacokinetics

The androgens are well absorbed and widely distributed throughout the body. They are metabolized in the liver and excreted in the urine. Androgens are contraindicated for use in pregnancy because of adverse effects on the foetus. It is not known whether androgens enter breast milk, but because of the potential for adverse effects, another method of feeding the baby should be used if these drugs are needed during lactation.

Contraindications and Cautions

These drugs are contraindicated with any known allergy to the drug or ingredients in the drug; during pregnancy and lactation, *because of potential effects on the neonate*; and in the presence of prostate or breast cancer in men. They should be used cautiously in the presence of any liver dysfunction or cardiovascular disease, *because these disorders could be exacerbated by the effects of the hormones.*

Adverse Effects

Androgenic effects include acne, oedema, **hirsutism** (increased hair distribution), deepening of the voice, oily skin and hair, weight gain, decrease in breast size and testicular atrophy. Antioestrogen effects – flushing, sweating, vaginitis, nervousness and emotional lability – can be anticipated when these drugs are used with women. Other common effects include headache (possibly related to fluid and electrolyte changes), dizziness, sleep disorders and fatigue, rash and altered serum electrolytes. A potentially life-threatening effect that has been documented is hepatocellular cancer. This may occur because of the effect of testosterone on hepatic cells. Patients on long-term therapy should have hepatic function tests monitored regularly – before beginning therapy and every 6 months during therapy.

Always consult a current copy of the British National Formulary for further guidance

Clinically Significant Drug–Laboratory Test Interferences

While a patient is taking androgens, there may be a decrease in thyroid function as well as increased creatinine clearance, results that are not associated with disease states. These effects can last up to 2 weeks after the discontinuation of therapy.

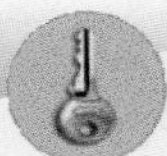

Key Drug Summary: *Testosterone*

Indications: Replacement therapy in hypogonadism, inoperable breast cancer

Actions: Primary natural androgen, responsible for growth and development of male sex organs and maintenance of secondary sex characteristics; increases the retention of nitrogen, sodium, potassium and phosphorus; decreases urinary excretion of calcium; increases protein anabolism; stimulates red blood cell production

Pharmacokinetics:

Route	Onset	Peak
IM	Slow	1–3 days
Dermal	Rapid	24 h

$T_{1/2}$: 10–100 minutes, with hepatic metabolism and excretion in the urine and faeces

Adverse effects: Dizziness, headache, sleep disorders, fatigue, rash androgenic effects (acne, deepening voice, oily skin), hypoestrogenic effects (flushing, sweating, vaginitis), polycythaemia, nausea, hepatocellular carcinoma

Anabolic Steroids

The anabolic steroids are analogues of testosterone that have been developed to produce the tissue-building effects of testosterone with less androgenic effect. These are controlled substances that are known to be used illegally for the enhancement of athletic performance through increased muscle mass, increased haematocrit and, theoretically, an increase in strength and endurance. The adverse effects of these drugs can be deadly when they are used in the amounts needed for enhanced athletic performance. Cardiomyopathy, hepatic carcinoma, personality changes and sexual dysfunction are all associated with the excessive and nonindicated use of anabolic steroids.

Nandrolone is an anabolic steroid indicated for the treatment of anaemia associated with chronic renal failure; however, it is infamous as an agent used illegally by athletes to improve performance.

Therapeutic Actions and Indications

Anabolic steroids promote body tissue-building processes, reverse catabolic or tissue-destroying processes and increase haemoglobin and red blood cell production.

Indications for particular anabolic steroids vary with the drug. They can be used to treat anaemias, certain cancers and angio-oedema. They also promote weight gain and tissue repair in debilitated patients and protein anabolism in patients who are receiving long-term corticosteroid therapy.

Pharmacokinetics

Like the androgens, the anabolic steroids are well absorbed and widely distributed throughout the body. They are metabolized in the liver and excreted in the urine. Anabolic steroids are contraindicated for use in pregnancy because of adverse effects to the foetus. It is not known whether anabolic steroids enter breast milk, but because of the potential for adverse effects, another method of feeding the baby should be used if these drugs are needed during lactation.

Contraindications and Cautions

These drugs are contraindicated in the presence of any known allergy to anabolic steroids; during pregnancy and lactation, *because of potential masculinization in the neonate*; and in the presence of liver dysfunction *(because these drugs are metabolized in the liver and are known to cause liver toxicity)*, coronary disease *(because of cholesterol-raising effects through effects on the liver)*, or prostate or breast cancer in males.

Adverse Effects

In prepubertal males, adverse effects include virilization (e.g. phallic enlargement, hirsutism, increased skin pigmentation). Postpubertal males may experience inhibition of testicular function, gynecomastia, testicular atrophy, priapism (a painful and continual erection of the penis), baldness and change in libido (increased or decreased). There is an increased risk of prostate problems, especially in older patients. Women may experience hirsutism, hoarseness, deepening of the voice, clitoral enlargement, baldness and menstrual irregularities. As with the androgens, serum electrolyte changes, liver dysfunction (including life-threatening hepatitis), insomnia and weight gain may occur.

Clinically Important Drug–Drug Interactions

Anabolic steroids affect the liver, therefore there is a potential for interaction with oral anticoagulants and a potentially decreased need for antidiabetic agents, which may not be metabolized normally. Patients should be monitored closely and appropriate dosage adjustments made.

Always refer to the latest edition of the British National Formulary for contraindications and interactions.

Nursing Considerations for Patients Receiving Androgens or Anabolic Steroids

Assessment: History and Examination

Screen for the following conditions which could be cautions or contraindications to use of the drug: history of allergy to any testosterone or androgen, pregnancy, lactation, hepatic dysfunction, cardiovascular disease and breast or prostate cancer in men.

Include screening for baseline status before beginning therapy and for any potential adverse effects: skin colour, hair distribution, peripheral sensation; abdominal examination; serum electrolytes, serum cholesterol and liver function tests; and radiographs of the long bones in children

Establish if patient is currently taking other medications or herbal therapies which may potentially interact with the androgens or anabolic steroids.

Nursing Diagnoses

The patient receiving an anabolic steroid may have the following nursing diagnoses related to drug therapy:

- Disturbed body image related to systemic effects
- Acute pain related to injection site, GI disturbances, central nervous system effects
- Deficient knowledge regarding drug therapy

Implementation With Rationale

- Administer with food if GI effects are severe, to relieve GI distress.
- Monitor endocrine function, hepatic function and serum electrolytes before and periodically during therapy, so that dosage can be adjusted appropriately and severe adverse effects can be avoided.
- Arrange for radiographs of the long bones of children every 3 to 6 months, so that the drug can be discontinued if bone growth reaches the norm for the child's age.
- Provide thorough patient education, including measures to avoid adverse effects and warning signs of problems, as well as the need for regular evaluation including blood tests, to enhance patient knowledge about drug therapy and to promote compliance with drug regimen.

Evaluation

- Monitor patient response to the drug (increase in haematocrit, protein anabolism).
- Monitor for adverse effects (androgenic effects, serum electrolyte disturbances, epiphyseal closure in paediatrics, hepatic dysfunction, personality changes and cardiac effects).
- Evaluate the effectiveness of the teaching plan (patient can name drug, dosage, adverse effects to watch for, specific measures to avoid adverse effects).
- Monitor the effectiveness of comfort measures and compliance to the regimen.

Drugs for Treating Penile Erectile Dysfunction

Two very different drugs are approved for the treatment of **penile erectile dysfunction**, a condition in which the corpus cavernosum does not fill with blood to allow for penile erection. Penile erection can be compromised by the ageing process and by vascular and neurological conditions. Alprostadil is a prostaglandin that relaxes vascular smooth muscle and allows filling of the corpus cavernosum when it is injected directly into the cavernosum. Sildenafil *(Viagra)* and tadalafil, selectively inhibit the phosphodiesterase type 5 receptors (PDE5) receptors and increase nitrous oxide levels, allowing blood flow into the *corpus cavernosum*. These drugs have the advantage of being oral drugs that can be timed in coordination with sexual activity, based on the drug's onset.

Therapeutic Actions and Indications

The prostaglandin alprostadil and the PDE5 inhibitors are indicated for the treatment of penile erectile dysfunction.

The prostaglandin alprostadil is injected and acts locally to relax vascular smooth muscle and promote blood flow into the corpus cavernosum, causing penile erection. Alprostadil is metabolized to inactive compounds in the lungs and excreted in the urine. As the effects on pregnancy are not known, if alprostadil is being used, condoms should be used during intercourse with a pregnant woman.

The PDE5 inhibitors are taken orally and act to increase nitrous oxide levels in the corpus cavernosum. Nitrous oxide activates the enzyme cGMP, which causes smooth muscle relaxation, allowing the flow of blood into the corpus cavernosum. They prevent the breakdown of cGMP by phosphodiesterase, leading to increased cGMP levels and prolonged smooth muscle relaxation, thus promoting the flow of blood into the corpus cavernosum, resulting in penile erection. Sildenafil is also approved for the treatment of pulmonary arterial hypertension. By relaxing smooth muscle, the pulmonary artery relaxes and there is less resistance and pressure in the pulmonary bed. All these drugs are well absorbed from the gastrointestinal (GI) tract, they undergo metabolism in the liver and are excreted in the faeces. The differences among the three drugs lie in their onset and duration of action. Sildenafil has an approximate onset of 27 minutes and duration of approximately 4 hours. Patients are encouraged to take the drug 1 hour before anticipated sexual stimulation. Tadalafil has an onset of action of 45 minutes and duration of 36 hours. A patient might select this drug if the timing of sexual stimulation is not known and may be several hours away. None of these drugs is indicated for use in women, so no adequate studies have been done during pregnancy and lactation.

Contraindications and Cautions

These drugs are contraindicated in the presence of any anatomical obstruction or condition that might predispose to priapism. They cannot be used with penile implants and they are not indicated for use in women. However, sildenafil is used in women for the treatment of pulmonary arterial hypertension.

Caution should be used in patients with bleeding disorders. The PDE5 inhibitors should also be used cautiously in those patients with coronary artery disease, active peptic ulcer, retinitis pigmentosa, optic neuropathy, hypotension or severe hypertension, congenital prolonged QT interval or severe hepatic or renal disorders, *because of the risk of exacerbating these diseases.*

Adverse Effects

Adverse effects associated with alprostadil are local effects such as pain at the injection site, infection, priapism, fibrosis and rash. The PDE5 inhibitors are associated with more systemic effects, including headache, flushing (related to relaxation of vascular smooth muscle), dyspepsia, urinary tract infection, diarrhoea, dizziness, rash and possible optic neuropathy.

Clinically Important Drug–Drug Interactions

The PDE5 inhibitors cannot be taken in combination with any organic nitrates or α-adrenergic blockers; serious cardiovascular effects, including death, have occurred. There is also a possibility of increased tadalafil levels and effects if PDE5 inhibitors are taken with drugs such as erythromycin; the patients should be monitored and dosage reduced as needed.

Always refer to the latest edition of the British National Formulary for contraindications and interactions.

FOCUS ON **PATIENT SAFETY**

Patients who are using PDE5 inhibitors need to be advised to avoid drinking grapefruit juice while using the drug. Grapefruit juice can cause a decrease in the metabolism of the PDE5 inhibitor, leading to increased serum levels and a risk of toxicity. They should also be advised to avoid taking the drug with or just after a high-fat meal. The presence of fat in the GI tract will delay the absorption and onset of action of the drug, which could cause problems for patients who are timing onset of action with their sexual activity.

The use of these drugs is not without risks. Deaths have been reported when these drugs were combined with nitrates (e.g. GTN) or α-adrenergic blockers. Headache, flushing, stomach upset and urinary tract infections may occur. These drugs can be used only once daily and they do not work without sexual stimulation. The adverse effects, timing of administration and drug combinations to avoid should be discussed with the patient before the drug is prescribed. Patients also should be reminded that they need to use protection against sexually transmitted diseases.

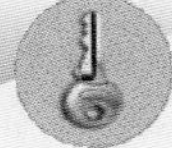

Key Drug Summary: *Sildenafil*

Indications: Treatment of erectile dysfunction in the presence of sexual stimulation; treatment of pulmonary arterial hypertension

Actions: Inhibits PDE5 receptors, leading to a release of nitrous oxide, which activates cGMP to cause a prolonged smooth muscle relaxation, allowing the flow of blood into the corpus cavernosum and facilitating erection

Pharmacokinetics:

Route	Onset	Peak	Duration
PO	15–30 min	30–120 min	4 h

$T_{1/2}$: 4 hours, with hepatic metabolism and excretion in the faeces and urine

Adverse effects: Headache, abnormal vision, flushing, dyspepsia, urinary tract infection, rash

Nursing Considerations for Patients Receiving Drugs to Treat Penile Erectile Dysfunction

Assessment: History and Examination

Screen for the following conditions, which could be cautions or contraindications to the use of the drug: history of allergy to any of the preparations, penile structural abnormalities, penile implants, bleeding disorders, active peptic ulcer, coronary artery disease, hypotension or severe hypertension, congenital prolonged QT interval, or severe hepatic or renal disorders.

An appropriate patient assessment including a thorough history should be taken. Specific questions about the following conditions should be asked; history of allergy to any of the preparations, penile structural abnormalities, penile implants, bleeding disorders, active peptic ulcer, coronary artery disease, hypotension or severe hypertension, congenital prolonged QT interval or severe hepatic or renal disorders. Include screening for baseline status before beginning therapy and for any potential adverse effects: blood pressure, pulse; respiration, electrocardiogram liver function tests, international normalized ratio (INR-coagulation) screen, and local inspection of penis.

Establish if patient is currently taking other medications or herbal therapies which may potentially interact with the drugs to treat penile erectile dysfunction.

Nursing Diagnoses

The patient receiving drugs for treating penile dysfunction may have the following nursing diagnoses related to drug therapy:

- Acute pain related to injection of alprostadil
- Sexual dysfunction
- Deficient knowledge regarding drug therapy

Implementation With Rationale

- Assess the cause of dysfunction before beginning therapy, to ensure appropriate use of these drugs.
- Monitor patients with vascular disease for any sign of exacerbation, so that the drug can be discontinued or the drug dose reduced before severe adverse effects occur.
- Instruct the patient in the injection of alprostadil, storage of the drug, filling of the syringe, sterile technique, site rotation and proper disposal of needles, to ensure safe and proper administration of the drug.
- Carefully monitor patients who are taking PDE5 inhibitors for use of nitrates or α-blockers, to avert potentially serious cardiovascular drug–drug interactions.
- Provide thorough patient education including measures to avoid adverse effects and warning signs of problems, as well as the need for regular evaluation, to enhance patient knowledge about drug therapy and to promote compliance with the drug regimen.

Evaluation

- Monitor patient response to the drug (improvement in penile erection).
- Monitor for adverse effects (dizziness, flushing, local inflammation or infection, fibrosis, diarrhoea, dyspepsia).
- Evaluate the effectiveness of the teaching plan (patient can name drug, dosage, adverse effects to watch for, specific measures to avoid adverse effects; patient can demonstrate proper administration of injected drug).
- Monitor the effectiveness of comfort measures and compliance to the regimen.

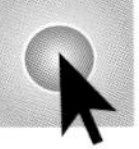

WEB LINKS

Health care providers and patients may want to consult the following Internet sources:

http://cks.library.nhs.uk The National Health Service Clinical Knowledge Summaries provides evidence-based practical information on the common conditions observed in primary care.

http://www.bnf.org.uk The BNF provides UK health care professionals with authoritative and practical information on the selection and clinical use of medicines.

http://www.nhsdirect.nhs.uk The National Health Service Direct service provides patients with information and advice about health, illness and health services.

http://www.nice.org.uk National Institute for Health and Clinical Excellence is an independent organization responsible for providing national guidance on promoting good health and preventing and treating ill health.

Points to Remember

- Androgens are male sex hormones, specifically testosterone or testosterone-like compounds.
- Androgens are responsible for the development and maintenance of male sex characteristics and secondary sex characteristics or androgenic effects.

- Side-effects related to androgen use involve excess of the desired effects as well as potentially deadly hepatocellular carcinoma.
- Androgens can be used for replacement therapy or to block other hormone effects, as is seen with their use in the treatment of specific breast cancers.
- Anabolic steroids are analogues of testosterone that have been developed to have more anabolic or protein-building effects than androgenic effects.
- Anabolic steroids have been abused to enhance muscle development and athletic performance, often with deadly effects.
- Anabolic steroids are used to increase haematocrit and improve protein anabolism in certain depleted states.
- Penile erectile dysfunction can inhibit erection and male sexual function.
- Alprostadil, a prostaglandin, can be injected into the penis to stimulate erection.
- The PDE5 inhibitors are oral agents that act quickly to promote vascular filling of the corpus cavernosum and promote penile erection. They differ in duration and time of onset. They are effective only in the presence of sexual stimulation.
- Dangerous cardiovascular effects, including death, have occurred when the PDE5 inhibitors are combined with organic nitrates or α-blockers. Careful patient education is very important to avoid this drug–drug interaction.

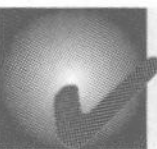

CHECK YOUR UNDERSTANDING

Answers to the questions in this chapter may be found in the answer key in the back of the book.

Multiple Choice

Select the most appropriate response to the following:

1. Testosterone is approved for use in
   a. treatment of breast cancers.
   b. increasing muscle strength in athletes.
   c. oral contraceptives.
   d. increasing hair distribution in male pattern baldness.

2. Illegal use of large quantities of unprescribed anabolic steroids to enhance athletic performance has been associated with
   a. increased sexual ability.
   b. muscle rupture from overexpansion.
   c. development of chronic obstructive pulmonary disease.
   d. cardiomyopathy and liver cancers.

3. Anabolic steroids would be indicated for the treatment of
   a. anaemia.
   b. angio-oedema.
   c. debilitation and severe weight loss.
   d. breast cancers in males.

4. Erectile penile dysfunction is a condition in which
   a. problems with childhood authority figures prevent a male erection.
   b. the corpus cavernosum does not fill with blood to allow for penile erection.
   c. the sympathetic nervous system fails to function.
   d. past exposure to sexually transmitted disease causes physical damage within the penis.

5. A potentially deadly drug–drug interaction can occur if a PDE5 inhibitor, sildenafil, tadalafil, is combined with
   a. corticosteroids.
   b. oral contraceptives.
   c. organic nitrates.
   d. halothane anaesthetics.

6. To achieve erection, a patient taking sildenafil would require
   a. sexual stimulation of the penis.
   b. no additional stimulation.
   c. privacy.
   d. 10 to 15 minutes after taking the oral drug.

Extended Matching questions

Select **all** that apply.

1. In assessing a client for androgenic effects, you would expect to find which of the following?
   a. Hirsutism
   b. Deepening of the voice
   c. Testicular enlargement
   d. Acne
   e. Elevated body temperature
   f. Sudden growth

2. A child treated with anabolic steroids because of anaemia associated with renal disease will need
   a. early sex education classes because of the effects of the drug.

b. X-rays of the long bones every 3 to 6 months so the drug can be stopped when the bone size is appropriate to the child's age.
c. to learn to shave.
d. to learn to cope with an altered body image.
e. regular monitoring of liver function tests.
f. monitoring for the development of oedema.

True or False

Indicate whether the following statements are true (T) or false (F).

_____ 1. Androgens are male sex hormones, specifically testosterone or testosterone-like compounds.

_____ 2. Androgens are responsible for the development and maintenance of male sex characteristics and secondary sex characteristics or oestrogenic effects.

_____ 3. Adverse effects related to androgen use involve potentially deadly hepatocellular carcinoma.

_____ 4. Androgens can be used for replacement therapy or to block other hormone effects.

_____ 5. Anabolic steroids are analogues of oestrogen that have been developed to have protein-building effects.

_____ 6. Anabolic steroids are used pharmacologically to enhance muscle development and athletic performance, often with deadly effects.

_____ 7. Anabolic steroids are used to increase haematocrit and improve protein anabolism in certain depleted states.

_____ 8. Erectile penile dysfunction can inhibit erection and male sexual function.

_____ 9. Alprostadil, a prostaglandin, is an oral agent used to stimulate penile erection.

_____10. Sildenafil is an injected agent that acts quickly to promote vascular filling of the corpus cavernosum and promote penile erection.

Fill in the Blanks

1. ____________________ effects are associated with development of male sexual characteristics.

2. ____________________ effects are tissue-building effects associated with androgen use.

3. ____________________ is the primary natural androgen.

4. ____________________ is a condition in which the corpus cavernosum does not fill with blood to allow for penile erection.

5. Alprostadil is a ____________________ that relaxes vascular smooth muscle and allows filling of the corpus cavernosum when ____________________ directly into the cavernosum.

6. ____________________ is taken orally and acts to increase nitrous oxide levels in the corpus cavernosum.

Bibliography

Abramowicz, M. (Ed.). (2003). Tadalafil for erectile dysfunction. *The Medical Letter on Drugs and Therapeutics, 45*, 101–102.

British Medical Association and Royal Pharmaceutical Society of Great Britain. (2008). *British National Formulary*. London: BMJ & RPS Publishing. *This publication is updated biannually: it is imperative that the most recent edition is consulted.*

British Medical Association and Royal Pharmaceutical Society of Great Britain. (2008). *British National Formulary for Children*. London: BMJ & RPS Publishing. *This publication is updated annually: it is imperative that the most recent edition is consulted.*

Davis, S. R., & Burger, H. G. (1996). Androgens and postmenopausal women. *Journal of Endocrinology and Metabolism, 81*, 2759–2763.

Ganong, W. (2005). *Review of medical physiology* (22nd ed.). New York: McGraw-Hill.

Guyton, A., & Hall, J. (2005). *Textbook of medical physiology* (11th ed.). Philadelphia: W. B. Saunders.

Howland, R. D., & Mycek, M. J. (2005). *Pharmacology* (3rd ed.). Philadelphia: Lippincott Williams & Wilkins.

Marieb, E. N., & Hoehn, K. (2004). *Human anatomy & physiology* (7th ed.). San Francisco: Pearson Benjamin Cummings.

Porth, C. M., & Matfin G. (2008). *Pathophysiology: Concepts of altered health states* (8th ed). Philadelphia: Lippincott Williams & Wilkins.

Simonsen, T., Aarbakke, J., Kay, I., Coleman, I., Sinnott, P., & Lysaa, R. (2006). *Illustrated pharmacology for nurses.* London: Hodder Arnold.

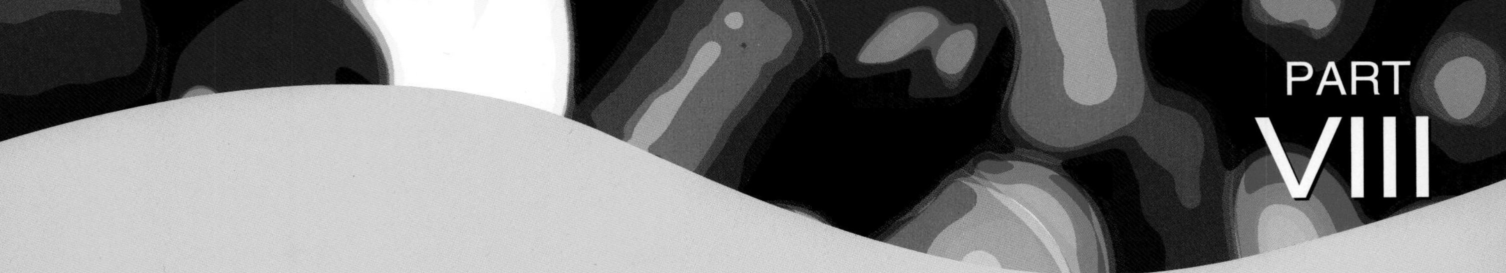

PART VIII

Drugs Acting on the Cardiovascular System

CHAPTER 41

Introduction to the Cardiovascular System

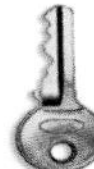

KEY TERMS

absolute refractory period
actin
aldosterone
arrhythmia
arteries
atrium
auricle
automaticity
baroreceptors
bradycardia
capillary
capacitance (venous) system
cardiac cycle
conductivity
depolarization
diastole
dysrhythmia
ectopic focus
electrocardiogram (ECG)
fibrillation
hypertension
mitral
myocardium
myosin
oncotic pressure
parasympathetic
pulse pressure
repolarization
renin–angiotensin
resistance system
sarcomere
sinoatrial (SA) node
sinus rhythm
Starling's law of the heart
sympathetic
syncytia
systole
tachycardia
troponin
vagus
veins
ventricle
vena cava

LEARNING OBJECTIVES

Upon completion of this chapter, you will be able to:

1. Label a diagram of the heart, including all chambers, valves, great vessels, coronary vessels and the conduction system.
2. Describe the flow of blood during the cardiac cycle, including flow to the cardiac muscle.
3. Outline the conduction system of the heart and correlate the normal ECG pattern with the underlying electrical activity in the heart.
4. Discuss the long and short-term regulation of blood pressure control.
5. Describe the capillary fluid shift, including factors that influence the movement of fluid between fluid compartments in clinical situations.

The cardiovascular system is responsible for delivering oxygen and nutrients to all of the cells of the body and for removing waste products for excretion. The cardiovascular system consists of a pump – the heart – and an interconnected series of tubes that continually move blood throughout the body – the circulation.

The Heart

The heart is a hollow, muscular organ that is divided into four chambers. It consists of two upper chambers known as the atria and two lower known as the **ventricles**. Attached to each **atrium** is an appendage called the auricle; here, blood collects before being forced into the ventricles by atrial contraction. Between the atria and ventricles are two cardiac valves. The valve on the right side of the heart is called the tricuspid valve because it is composed of three leaflets or cusps (see Figure 41.1). The valve on the left side of the heart, called the mitral or bicuspid valve, is composed of two leaflets or cusps (see Figure 41.1). A partition called a septum separates the right half of the heart from the left. The right half receives reduced oxygenated blood from everywhere in the body through the veins (vessels that carry blood toward the heart) and directs that blood into the lungs. The ventricles pump blood out of the heart. The right ventricle pumps blood into the pulmonary artery, which takes blood to the lungs, whereas the left ventricle pumps blood into the aorta, which supplies blood to the rest of the body. The left half of the heart receives the now oxygenated blood from the lungs and directs it into the aorta. The aorta delivers blood into the systemic circulation by way of arteries (vessels that carry blood away from the heart) (Figure 41.1).

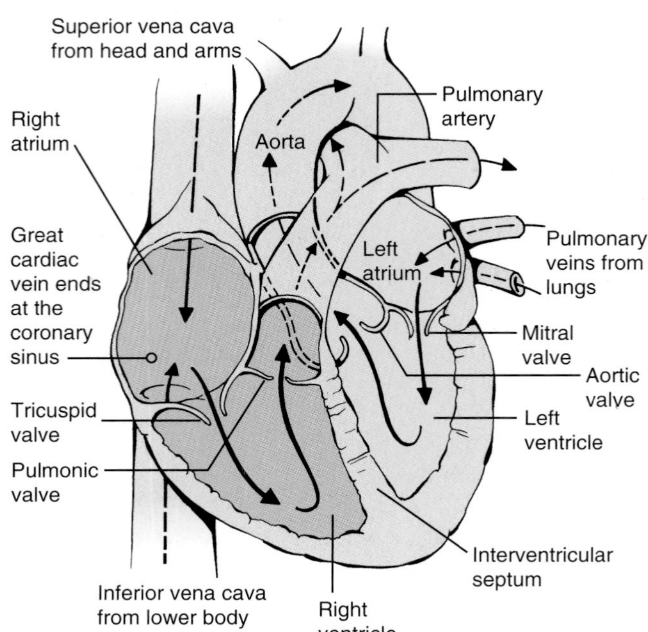

FIGURE 41.1 Blood flow into and out of the heart. Deoxygenated blood enters the right atrium from the great cardiac vein and the superior and inferior venae cavae and falls through the tricuspid valve into the right ventricle, which contracts and sends the blood through the pulmonic valve into the pulmonary artery and to the lungs. Oxygenated blood from the lungs enters the left atrium through the pulmonary veins and passes through the mitral valve into the left ventricle, which contracts and ejects the blood through the aortic valve into the aorta and out to the systemic circulation.

The Cardiac Cycle

The heart possesses structural and functional properties that are different from those of other muscles. The fibres of the cardiac muscle, or myocardium, form two intertwining networks called the atrial and ventricular syncytia. These interlacing structures enable first the atria and then the ventricles to contract synchronously when excited by the same stimulus.

Simultaneous contraction is a necessary property for a muscle that acts as a pump. A hollow pumping mechanism must also pause long enough in the pumping cycle to allow the chambers to fill with blood. Heart muscle relaxes long enough to ensure adequate filling; the more completely it fills, the stronger is the subsequent contraction. This occurs because the muscle fibres of the heart, stretched by the increased volume of blood that has returned to them, spring back to normal size. This is similar to stretching an elastic band, which returns to its normal size after it is stretched – the further it is stretched, the stronger it springs back to normal. This property is defined in the **Starling's law of the heart**.

During **diastole**, the period of cardiac muscle relaxation, blood returns to the heart from the systemic and pulmonary veins, which flow into the right and left atria, respectively. When the pressure generated by the blood volume in the atria is greater than the pressure in the ventricles, blood flows through the atrioventricular (AV) valves into the ventricles. Just before the ventricles are stimulated to contract, the atria contract, pushing a small amount of blood into each ventricle. The much more powerful ventricles then contract, pumping blood out to the lungs through the pulmonary valve or out to the aorta through the aortic valve and into the systemic circulation. The contraction of the ventricles is referred to as **systole**. Each period of systole followed by a period of **diastole** is called a **cardiac cycle**. The series of one-way valves within the heart keep the blood flowing in the correct direction, as follows (see Figure 41.1):

- *Deoxygenated blood: through the superior and inferior vena cava,* right atrium, through tricuspid valve to right ventricle, through pulmonary valve to the lungs.
- *Oxygenated blood:* Through the pulmonary veins to the left atrium, through the mitral valve to the left ventricle, through the aortic valve to the aorta.

The AV valves close very tightly when the ventricles contract, preventing blood from flowing backward into the atria and keeping it moving forward through the system. The pulmonary and aortic valves open with the pressure of ventricular contraction and close tightly during diastole, keeping blood from flowing backward into the ventricles. The proper functioning of the cardiac valves is important in maintaining the functioning of the cardiovascular system.

Conduction System of the Heart

Each cycle of cardiac contraction and relaxation is controlled by impulses that arise spontaneously in specialized pacemaker cells of the **sinoatrial (SA) node** of the heart. These impulses are conducted from the pacemaker cells by a specialized conducting system that spreads throughout the heart muscle almost simultaneously. These continuous, rhythmic contractions are controlled by the heart itself; the brain does not stimulate the heart to beat. This safety feature allows the heart to beat as long as it has enough nutrients and oxygen to survive, regardless of the status of the rest of the body.

The conduction system of the heart consists of the SA node, atrial bundles, AV node, bundle of His, bundle branches and Purkinje fibres (Figure 41.2). The SA node located at the top of the right atrium acts as the pacemaker of the heart. Atrial bundles conduct the impulse through the atrial muscle. The AV node slows the impulse, allowing for the delay needed for ventricular filling and sends it from the atria into the ventricles by way of the bundle of His. This enters the septum and then divides into three bundle branches. These bundle branches, which conduct the impulses through the ventricles, break into a fine network of conducting fibres called the Purkinje fibres, which deliver the impulse to the ventricular cells.

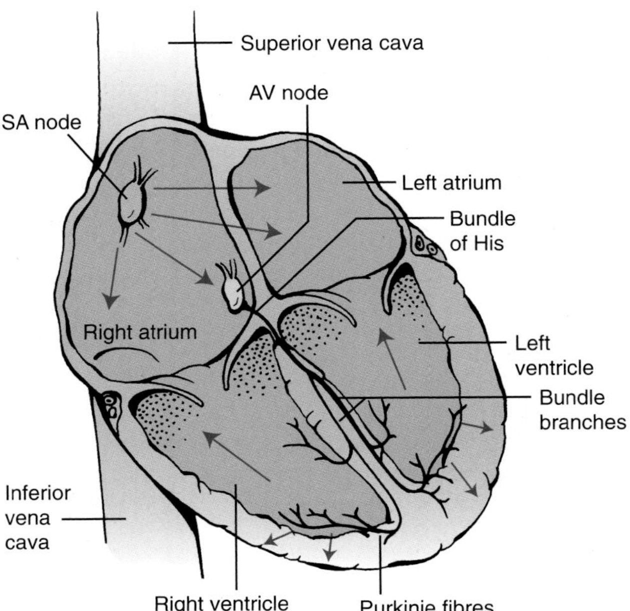

FIGURE 41.2 The conducting system of the heart. Impulses originating in the sinoatrial (SA) node are transmitted through the atrial bundles to the atrioventricular (AV) node and down the bundle of His and the bundle branches by way of the Purkinje fibers through the ventricles.

Automaticity

The pacemaker cells can generate action potentials or electrical impulses without being excited by external stimuli (nerve supply or hormones). This property is called **automaticity**.

All cardiac cells possess some degree of automaticity. During diastole or rest, these cells undergo a spontaneous depolarization because sodium leaks into the cell and there is a decrease in the flow of potassium ions out of the cell. This causes an action potential to be generated. This action potential is basically the same as the action potential of the neuron (see Chapter 18). However, the action potential of the cardiac muscle cell consists of five phases (see Figure 41.3):

- *Phase 0* occurs when the cell reaches a point of stimulation. The sodium channels open along the cell membrane and sodium rushes into the cell, resulting in a positive flow of ions into the cell – an electrical potential – therefore **depolarization**.

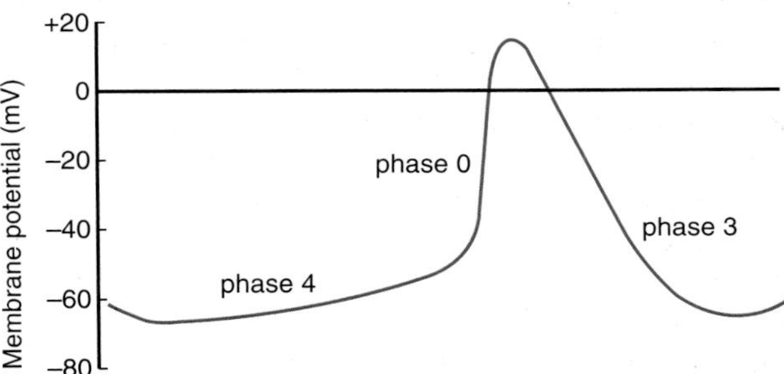

A SA node action potential

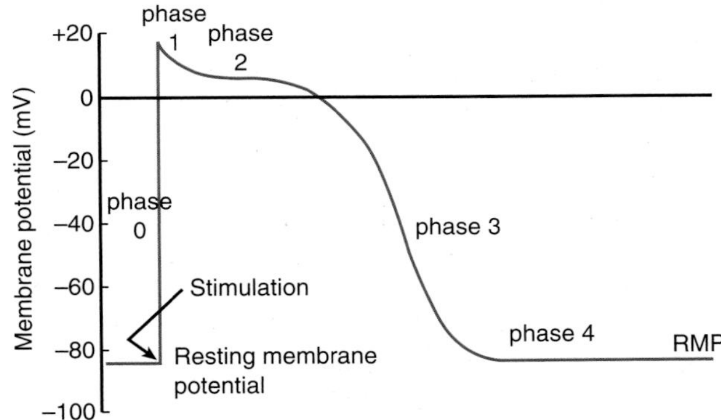

B Ventricular muscle cell action potential

FIGURE 41.3 Action potentials recorded from a cell in the sinoatrial (SA) node (A) showing diastolic depolarization in phase 4, and recorded from a ventricular muscle cell (B). In *phase 0,* the cell is stimulated, sodium rushes into the cell, and the cell is depolarized. In *phase 1,* sodium levels equalize. In *phase 2,* the plateau phase, calcium enters the cell (the slow current), and potassium and sodium leave. In *phase 3,* the slow current stops, and sodium and potassium leave the cell. In *phase 4,* the resting membrane potential (RMP) returns and the pacemaker potential begins in the SA node cell.

- *Phase 1* is the very short period when the sodium ion concentrations are equal inside and outside the cell.
- *Phase 2*, or the plateau stage, occurs as the cell membrane becomes less permeable to sodium. Calcium slowly enters the cell, and potassium begins to leave the cell. The cell membrane is trying to return to its resting state – therefore **repolarization**.
- *Phase 3* is a period of rapid repolarization, as the sodium gates are closed and potassium rapidly moves out of the cell.
- *Phase 4* occurs when the cell comes to rest as the sodium–potassium pump returns the membrane to its previous state, with a high concentration of sodium outside the cell and a high concentration of potassium inside the cell. Spontaneous depolarization begins again.

Conductivity

Normally, the SA node sets the pace for the heart rate because it depolarizes faster than any cell in the heart. However, the other cells in the heart are capable of generating an impulse if anything happens to the SA node; this is another protective feature of the heart. When the SA node sets the pace for the heart rate, the person is said to be in sinus rhythm.

The specialized cells of the heart can conduct an impulse rapidly through the system so that the muscle cells of the heart are stimulated at approximately the same time. This property of cardiac cells is called **conductivity**.

A delay in conduction at the AV node, between the atria and the ventricles, accounts for the fact that the atria contract for a fraction of a second before the ventricles contract. This allows extra time for the ventricles to fill completely before they contract. The almost simultaneous spread of the impulse through the Purkinje fibres permits a simultaneous and powerful contraction of the ventricle muscles, making them an effective pump.

After a cell membrane has conducted an action potential, there is a span of time in which it is impossible to stimulate that area of membrane; this is called the **absolute refractory period**. The absolute refractory period is the minimal amount of time that must elapse between two stimuli applied at one site in the heart for each of these stimuli to cause an action potential. This time reflects the responsiveness of the heart cells to stimuli. *Cardiac drugs may affect the refractory period of the cells to make the heart more or less responsive.*

Autonomic Influences

The autonomic nervous system (see Chapter 28) can influence the heart rate and rhythm and the strength of contraction. The two branches of the autonomic nervous system work together to help the heart meet the body's demands. The **parasympathetic** nerves, primarily the **vagus** nerve (tenth cranial nerve), can slow the heart rate and decrease the speed of conduction through the AV node. This allows the heart to rest and conserve its strength. The parasympathetic influence on the SA node is the dominant influence most of the time, usually keeping the resting heart rate at 70 to 80 beats per minute (bpm).

The **sympathetic** nervous system stimulates the heart to beat faster; it speeds conduction through the AV node and causes the heart muscle to contract harder. This action is important during exercise or stress, when the body's cells need to have more oxygen. Drugs can be used to influence either of these branches of the autonomic nervous system and are therefore said to have autonomic effects on the heart (see Chapters 28–32).

Mechanical Activity

The end result of the electrical stimulation of the heart cells is the unified contraction of the atria and ventricles, which moves the blood throughout the vascular system. The basic unit of the cardiac muscle is the **sarcomere**. A sarcomere is made up of two contractile proteins: **actin**, a thin filament, and **myosin**, a thick filament with small projections on it. These proteins readily react with each other, but at rest, they are kept apart by the protein **troponin** (Figure 41.4).

When a cardiac muscle cell is stimulated, calcium from the extracellular fluid enters the cell through channels in the cell membrane. Calcium is also released from storage sites within the cell. This occurs during the action potential, when the cell is starting to repolarize. The calcium reacts with the troponin and inactivates it. This action allows the actin and myosin proteins to react with each other, forming actin and myosin cross-bridges. These bridges then break quickly, and the myosin slides along to form new bridges. The contraction process requires energy and oxygen for the chemical reaction that allows the formation of the cross-bridges. Calcium is also essential to allow the bridge formation to occur.

As long as calcium is present, the actin–myosin bridges continue to form. This action slides the proteins together, shortening or contracting the sarcomere. Cardiac muscle cells are linked together by desmosomes, gap junctions and intercalated discs; when one cell is stimulated to contract, all the cells are stimulated to contract. As the cell reaches its depolarized state, calcium is removed from the cell by

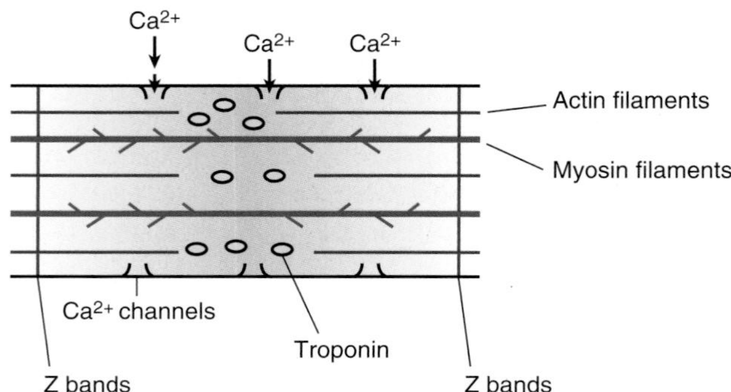

FIGURE 41.4 A sarcomere, the functioning unit of cardiac muscle.

the sodium–calcium pump and calcium returns to storage sites within the cell.

The degree of shortening (the strength of contraction) is determined by the amount of calcium present – the more calcium is present, the more bridges will be formed – and by the stretch of the sarcomere before contraction begins. The further apart the actin and myosin proteins are before the cell is stimulated, the more bridges will be formed and the stronger the contraction will be. This correlates with the **Starling's law of the heart** – the more the cardiac muscle is stretched, the greater the contraction will be; therefore, the more blood you put into the heart, the greater the contraction will be to empty the heart, up to a point. However, if the bridges are stretched too far apart, they will not be able to reach each other to form the actin–myosin bridges and no contraction will occur (see Figure 41.4).

Cardiac Arrhythmias

Various factors, such as drugs, acidosis, decreased oxygen levels, changes in the electrolytes in the area and the build up of waste products, can change the cardiac rate and rhythm. A disruption in cardiac rate or rhythm is called an **arrhythmia** or a **dysrhythmia**. Arrhythmias interfere with the work of the heart and can disrupt cardiac output, which will affect every cell in the body. Arrhythmias can arise because of changes in the automaticity or conductivity of the heart cells. Some arrhythmias occur when there is a shift in the pacemaker of the heart from the SA node to some other site; this is called an **ectopic focus**. This occurs most frequently with damage to the heart muscle and can be seen in the form of premature contractions. These premature beats may be unimportant and sporadic, but in some cases, they can be the prelude to more serious or even fatal arrhythmias if the coordinated pumping action of the muscle is lost.

A reduction in conductivity through the AV node produces a condition called heart block. In first-degree heart block, all of the impulses from the SA node arrive in the ventricles, but take a longer time than normal. In second-degree heart block, some of the impulses are lost and do not get through to the ventricles, resulting in a slow rate of ventricular contraction. In third-degree or complete heart block, no impulses from the SA node get through to the ventricles and the much slower ventricular automaticity takes over. Very serious arrhythmias arise when the combination of ectopic foci and altered conduction set off an irregular, uncoordinated twitching of the atrial or ventricular muscle, called **fibrillation**. In this situation, the pumping action of the heart is lost, and the cardiac output falls. Individuals can live quite normally with atrial fibrillation, but if the ventricles fibrillate (ventricular fibrillation-VF), there is total loss of cardiac output, and death can occur if treatment is not initiated quickly. Treatment involves defibrillating (stopping the heart by passing a high voltage across it), and hopefully, normal rhythm resumes as the SA node begins to act as a pacemaker again.

The Electrocardiogram

The patterns of electrical impulses as they move through the heart can be recorded by a process know as electrocardiography. The electrical activity can be detected by surface electrodes placed on the patient's skin. This is possible because the extracellular fluid acts as a good conductor of this electrical activity. The activity recorded is known as an **electrocardiogram (ECG)**.

The normal ECG wave pattern is made up of:

- the **P** wave, which is formed as impulses originating in the SA node or pacemaker pass through the atrial tissues and corresponds to atrial depolarization or contraction,
- the **QRS** complex, which represents depolarization of the bundle of His (Q) and the ventricles (**RS**),
- the **T** wave, which represents repolarization of the ventricles (Figure 41.5).

The P wave immediately precedes the contraction of the atria. The QRS complex immediately precedes the contraction of the ventricles and then relaxation of the ventricles during the T wave. The repolarization of the atria occurs at the same time as the QRS complex and is masked by this activity; therefore, it is not usually seen on an ECG.

The critical points of the ECG are as follows:

P–R interval: Reflects the normal delay of conduction at the AV node

Q–T interval: Reflects the critical timing of repolarization of the ventricles

S–T segment: Reflects important information about the repolarization of the ventricles

Abnormalities in the shape or timing of each part of an ECG tracing reveal the presence of particular cardiac disorders. A person with a normal ECG pattern and a heart rate within the normal range for that person's age group is said to be in **normal sinus rhythm**.

Types of Arrhythmias

Sinus Arrhythmias

The SA node is influenced by the autonomic nervous system to change the rate of firing in order to meet the body's demands for oxygen. A faster-than-normal heart rate, usually anything faster than 100 bpm **in** an adult, with a normal-appearing ECG pattern is called **sinus tachycardia**. **Sinus bradycardia** is a slower-than-normal heart rate (usually less than 60 bpm) with a normal-appearing ECG pattern.

Supraventricular Arrhythmias

Arrhythmias that originate above the ventricles but not in the SA node are called supraventricular arrhythmias. These arrhythmias feature an abnormally shaped P wave because the site of origin is not the sinus node; however, they show normal QRS complexes because the ventricles are still conducting impulses normally. Supraventricular arrhythmias include the following:

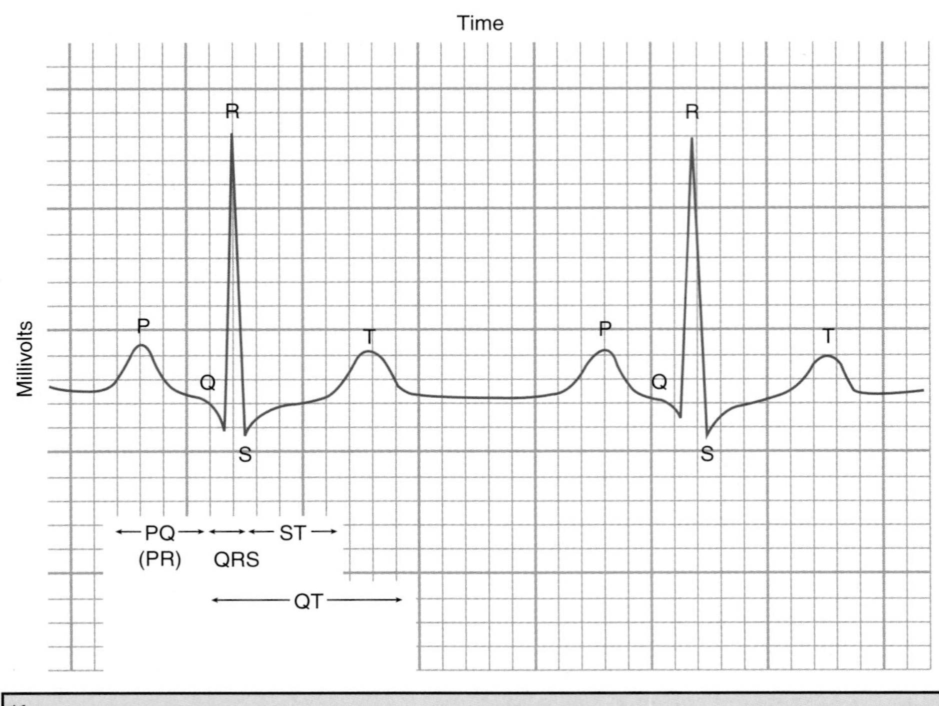

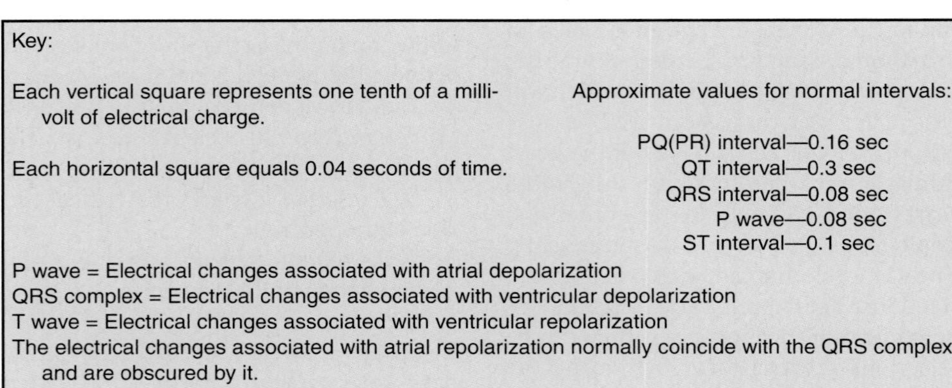

FIGURE 41.5 The normal electrocardiogram pattern.

- *Premature atrial contractions (PACs),* which reflect an ectopic focus in the atria that is generating an impulse out of the normal rhythm.
- *Paroxysmal atrial tachycardia (PAT),* sporadically occurring runs of rapid heart rate originating in the atria.
- *Atrial flutter,* characterized by sawtooth-shaped P waves reflecting a single ectopic focus that is generating a regular, fast atrial depolarization.
- *Atrial fibrillation,* with irregular P waves representing many ectopic foci firing in an uncoordinated manner through the atria.

Atrioventricular Block

First-degree heart block is characterized on the ECG by a lengthening of the P–R interval beyond the normal 0.16 to 0.20 seconds. Each P wave is followed by a QRS complex. In second-degree heart block, a QRS complex may follow one, two, three or four P waves. Third-degree heart block, or complete heart block, shows a total dissociation of P waves from QRS complexes and T waves. As the P waves can come at any time, the P–R interval is not constant. The QRS complexes appear at a very slow rate and may not be sufficient to meet the body's needs.

Ventricular Arrhythmias

Impulses that originate below the AV node originate from ectopic foci that do not use the normal conduction pathways. The QRS complexes appear wide and prolonged, and the T waves are inverted, reflecting the slower conduction across cardiac tissue that is not part of the rapid conduction system. Ventricular fibrillation is seen as a bizarre, irregular, distorted wave. It is potentially fatal because it reflects a lack of any coordinated stimulation of the ventricles; this leads to an inability to contract in a coordinated manner, resulting in no blood pumped to the body or the brain.

The Cardiovascular System

The purpose of the heart's continual pumping action is to keep blood flowing to and from all of the body's tissues. Blood delivers oxygen and much-needed nutrients to the cells for producing energy, and it carries away carbon dioxide and other waste products of metabolism. The steady circulation of blood is essential for the proper functioning of all of the body's organs, including the heart itself.

Circulation

The circulation of the blood follows two courses:

- *Pulmonary circulation:* The right side of the heart sends blood to the lungs, where carbon dioxide and some waste products are removed from the blood and oxygen is picked up by the red blood cells.
- *Systemic circulation:* The left side of the heart sends oxygenated blood out to all of the cells in the body.

The blood moves through the circulatory system from areas of high pressure to areas of lower pressure. The system is a 'closed' system, that is, it has no openings or holes that would allow blood to leak out. The closed nature of the system is what keeps the pressure differences in the proper relationship so that blood always flows in the direction in which it is intended to flow (Figure 41.6).

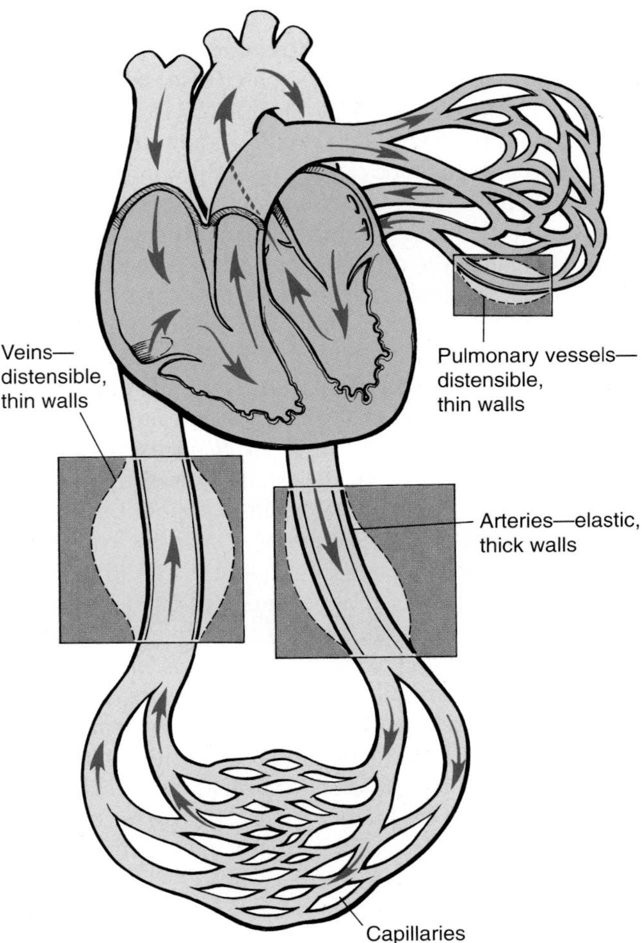

FIGURE 41.6 Blood flow through the systemic and pulmonary vasculature circuits.

Pulmonary and Systemic Circulation

All of the deoxygenated blood from the body flows into the right atrium from the **inferior** and **superior vena cava** (see Figure 41.1) and from the great cardiac vein, which returns deoxygenated blood from the heart muscle. The right atrium is a very low-pressure area in the cardiovascular system. As the blood flows into the atrium, the pressure increases. When the pressure becomes greater than the pressure in the right ventricle, most of the blood flows into the right ventricle; this is called the rapid-filling phase. At this point in the cardiac cycle, the atrium is stimulated to contract and pushes the remaining blood into the right ventricle. The ventricle is then stimulated to contract; it generates pressure that pushes open the semilunar or pulmonary valves (see Figure 41.1) and sends blood into the pulmonary artery, which takes the blood into the lungs, a very low-pressure area. The blood then circulates around the alveoli of the lungs, picking up oxygen and getting rid of carbon dioxide, flows through pulmonary capillaries (the tiny blood vessels that connect arteries and veins) into the pulmonary veins and then flows into the left atrium. When the pressure of blood volume in the left atrium is greater than the pressure in the large left ventricle, this oxygenated blood flows into the left ventricle. The left atrium contracts and pushes any remaining blood into the left ventricle. The left ventricle is stimulated to contract and generates high pressure to push the blood out of the aorta through the aortic valves to supply all the tissues throughout the body.

In a normal heart, the right and left atria contract simultaneously, as do the right and left ventricles.

Arteries, Capillaries and Veins

The aorta and other large arteries have thick, muscular walls. The entire arterial system contains muscles in the walls of the vessels all the way to the terminal branches or arterioles, which consist of fragments of muscle and endothelial cells. These muscles offer resistance to the blood that is sent pumping into the arterial system by the left ventricle, generating pressure. The arterial system is referred to as a **resistance system**. The vessels can either constrict or dilate, increasing or decreasing resistance, based on the needs of the body. The arterioles are able to completely shut off blood flow to some areas of the body, that is, they can shunt blood to another area where it is needed more. The arterioles, because of their ability to increase or decrease resistance in the system, are one of the main regulators of blood pressure.

Blood from the tiny arterioles flows into the **capillary** system, which connects the arterial and venous systems. These microscopic vessels are composed of loosely connected endothelial cells. Oxygen, fluid and nutrients are able to pass through the arterial end of the capillaries and enter the interstitial area between tissue cells. Fluid at the venous end of the capillary is drawn back into the vessel and contains carbon dioxide and other waste products. This shifting of fluid in the capillaries, called the capillary fluid shift, is carefully regulated by a balance between hydrostatic (fluid pressure) forces on the arterial end of the capillary and **oncotic pressure** (the pulling pressure of the large, vascular proteins) on the venous end of the capillary. In a normal situation, the higher pressure at the arterial end of a capillary forces fluid out of the vessel and into the tissue, and the now-concentrated proteins (which are too large to leave the capillary) exert a pull on the fluid at the venous end of the capillary to pull it back in. A disruption in the hydrostatic pressure or in the concentration of proteins in the capillary can lead to accumulation of interstitial fluid referred to as **oedema**. The capillaries merge into venules, which merge into veins, which are responsible for returning the blood to the heart (Figure 41.7).

The veins are thin-walled, elastic, low-pressure vessels. The venous system is referred to as a **capacitance system** because the veins have the capacity to hold large quantities of fluid as they distend with fluid volume. These capacitance vessels have a great deal of influence on the venous return to the heart, the amount of blood that is delivered to the right atrium.

Coronary Circulation

The heart muscle requires a constant supply of oxygenated blood to keep contracting. The myocardium receives blood through two main coronary arteries that branch off the base of the aorta from an area called the sinuses of Valsalva. These arteries encircle the heart in a pattern resembling a crown, which is why they are called the coronary arteries.

The artery arising from the left side of the aorta bifurcates, or divides, into two large vessels called the left circumflex artery (which travels down the left side of the heart and supplies most of the left ventricle) and the left anterior descending coronary artery (which travels down the front of the heart and supplies the septum and anterior areas, including much of the conduction system). The artery arising from the right side of the aorta supplies most of the right side of the heart, including the SA node.

The coronary arteries receive blood during diastole, when the muscle is relaxed so that blood can flow freely down into the muscle. When the ventricle contracts, it forces the aortic valve open and the cusps of the valve cover the openings of the coronary arteries. When the ventricles relax, the blood is no longer pumped forward and starts to flow back toward the ventricle. The blood flowing down the sides of the aorta closes the aortic valve and fills up the coronary arteries.

The pressure that fills the coronary arteries is the difference between the systolic ejection pressure and the diastolic resting pressure. This is called the **pulse pressure** (systolic

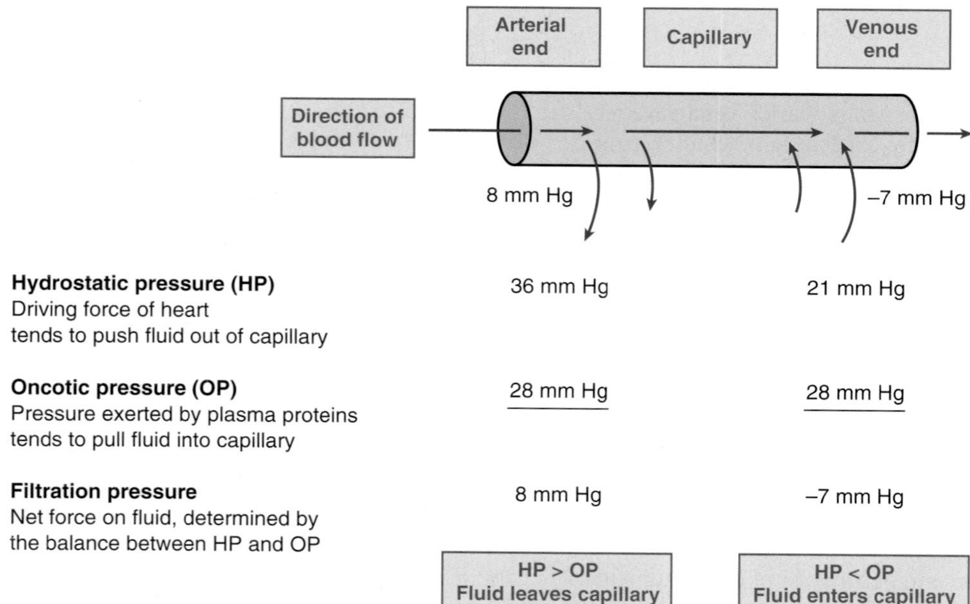

FIGURE 41.7 The net shift of fluid out of and into the capillary is determined by the balance between the hydrostatic pressure (HP) and the oncotic pressure (OP). HP tends to push fluid out of the capillary, and the OP tends to pull it back into the capillary. At the arterial end of the capillary bed, the blood pressure is higher than at the venous end. At the arterial end, HP exceeds OP, and fluid filters out. At the venous end, HP has fallen and HP is less than OP; fluid is pulled back into the capillary from the surrounding tissue. The lymphatic system also returns fluids and substances from the tissues to the circulation.

minus diastolic blood pressure readings). The pulse pressure is monitored clinically to evaluate the filling pressure of the coronary arteries. The oxygenated blood that is fed into the heart by the coronary circulation reaches every cardiac muscle fibre as the vessels divide and subdivide throughout the myocardium (Figure 41.8).

The heart's supply of and demand for oxygen is met by changes in the delivery of oxygen through the coronary system. Problems can arise, however, when an imbalance develops between the supply of oxygen delivered to the heart muscle and the myocardial demand for oxygen.

The main forces that determine the heart's use of oxygen or oxygen consumption are as follows:

- *Heart rate:* The more the heart has to pump, the more oxygen it will require.
- *Preload (amount of blood that is brought back to the heart to be pumped around):* The more blood that is returned to the heart, the harder it will have to work to pump the blood around. The volume of blood in the system is a determinant of preload.
- *Afterload (resistance against which the heart has to beat):* The higher the resistance in the system, the harder the heart will have to contract to force open the valves and pump the blood along. Blood pressure is a measure of afterload.
- *Stretch on the ventricles:* If the ventricular muscle is stretched before it is stimulated to contract, more actin–myosin bridges will be formed (which will take more energy), or if the muscle is stimulated to contract harder than usual (which happens with sympathetic stimulation), more bridges will be formed, which will require more energy.

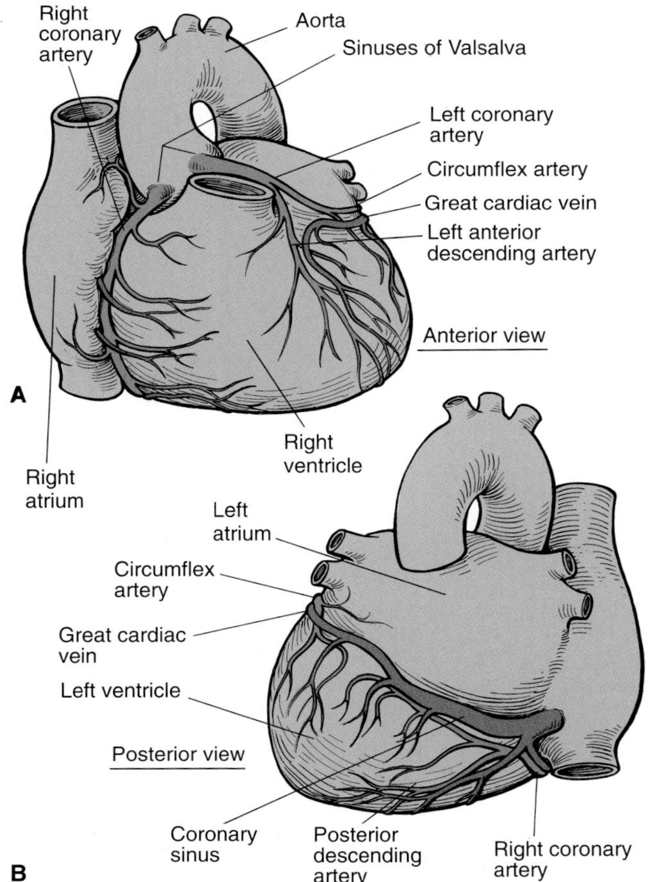

FIGURE 41.8 Coronary arteries and veins. **(A)** Anterior view; **(B)** posterior view.

The muscle can be stretched, for example, in ventricular hypertrophy (related to chronic hypertension) or cardiac muscle damage, or in heart failure when the ventricle does not empty completely and blood backs up in the system.

The supply of blood to the myocardium can be altered if the heart fails to pump effectively and cannot deliver blood to the coronary arteries. This happens in congestive heart failure (CHF) and cases of hypotension. The supply is most frequently altered, however, when the coronary vessels become narrowed and unresponsive to stimuli to dilate and deliver more blood. This happens in atherosclerosis or coronary artery disease. The end result of this narrowing can be a total blockage of a coronary artery, leading to hypoxia and eventual death of the cells that depend on that vessel for oxygen. This is called a **myocardial infarction** (MI). This is the leading cause of death in the United Kingdom and accounts for over 208,000 deaths each year (BHF.org 2005).

Note: The umbrella term *'Acute Coronary Syndrome'* is commonly used in clinical practice to include: angina (stable and unstable) and MI [ST elevation MI (STEMI) and non-ST elevation MI (non-STEMI)].

The contraction of the left ventricle, which sends blood surging out into the aorta, creates a pressure that continues to force blood into all of the branches of the aorta. This pressure against arterial walls is greatest during systole (cardiac contraction) and falls to its lowest level during diastole. Measurement of both the systolic and the diastolic pressure indicates both the pumping pressure of the ventricle and the generalized pressure in the system, or the pressure the ventricle has to overcome to pump blood out of the heart.

Hypotension

The pressure in the arteries needs to remain relatively high to ensure that blood is delivered to every cell in the body and to keep the blood flowing from high-pressure to low-pressure areas. Hypotension can occur if the blood pressure falls dramatically, either from loss of blood volume or from failure of the heart muscle to pump effectively. Severe hypotension can progress to shock and even death as cells fail to receive an oxygen supply.

Hypertension

Constant, excessive high blood pressure, called **hypertension**, can damage the fragile inner lining (endothelium) of blood vessels and cause a disruption of blood flow to the tissues. It also puts a tremendous strain on the heart muscle, increasing myocardial oxygen consumption and putting the heart muscle at risk of damage. Hypertension can be caused by neurostimulation of the blood vessels, causing them to constrict (increasing total peripheral resistance) and raising blood pressure, or by increased fluid volume in the system. In most cases, the cause of hypertension is not known (this is called essential or primary hypertension), and drug therapy to correct it is aimed at changing one or more of the normal reflexes that control vascular resistance or the force of cardiac muscle contraction.

BP = Cardiac Output × Total Peripheral Resistance.

Vasomotor Tone

The smooth muscles in the walls of the arteries receive constant input from nerve fibres of the sympathetic nervous system. These impulses work to dilate the vessels if more blood flow is needed in an area, to constrict vessels if increased pressure is needed in the system and to maintain muscle tone so that the vessel remains patent and responsive.

The coordination of these impulses is regulated through the medulla in an area called the cardiovascular centre. If increased pressure is needed, this centre increases sympathetic flow to the vessels. If pressure rises too high, this is sensed by pressure receptors called **baroreceptors** in the aortic arch and carotid sinus, and the sympathetic flow is decreased. Chapter 42 discusses the drugs that are used to influence the stimulation of vessels to alter blood pressure.

Renin–Angiotensin System

Another determinant of blood pressure is the **renin–angiotensin** system (see Figure 41.9). This system is activated when blood flow to the kidneys is decreased. Cells in the kidney release an enzyme called renin. Renin is transported to the liver, where it converts angiotensinogen (produced in the liver) to angiotensin I. Angiotensin I travels to the lungs, where it is converted by angiotensin-converting enzyme (ACE) to angiotensin II. Angiotensin II travels through the body and reacts with angiotensin II receptor sites on blood vessels to cause a severe vasoconstriction. This increases blood pressure and should increase blood flow to the kidneys to decrease the release of renin. Angiotensin II also causes the release of **aldosterone** from the adrenal cortex, which is a steroid hormone, which causes retention of sodium and water. This also leads to the release of antidiuretic hormone (ADH) to retain water and increase blood volume and in turn increase blood pressure.

Venous Pressure

Pressure in the veins may also increase. This can happen if the heart is not pumping effectively and cannot pump out all of the blood that is trying to return to it. This results in a back up or congestion of blood waiting to enter the heart. Pressure rises in the right atrium and then in the veins that are trying to return blood to the heart as they encounter resistance. The venous system begins to back up or become congested with blood.

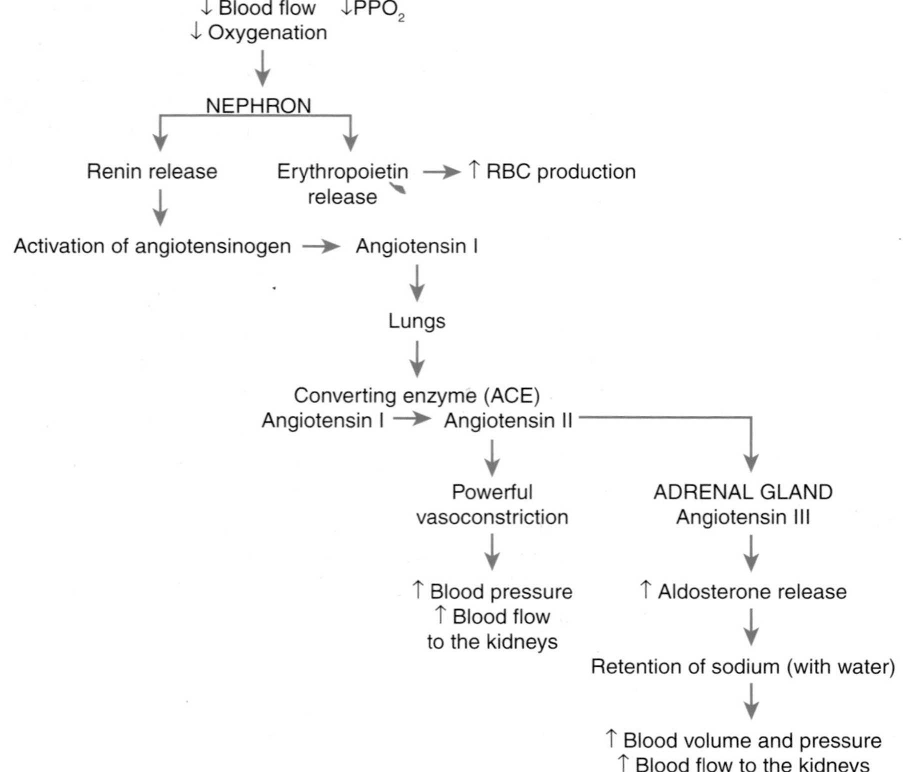

FIGURE 41.9 The renin-angiotensin system for reflex maintenance of blood pressure control.

Congestive Heart Failure and Oedema

If the heart muscle is failing to do its job of effectively pumping blood through the system, blood backs up and the system becomes congested. This is called CHF. The rise in venous pressure that results from this back up of blood increases the hydrostatic pressure on the venous end of the capillaries. The hydrostatic pressure pushing fluid out of the capillary is soon higher than the oncotic pressure that is trying to pull the fluid back into the vessel, causing fluid to collect in the interstitial space. This shift of fluid accounts for the oedema seen with CHF. Pulmonary oedema results when the left side of the heart is failing (fluid collects in the pulmonary system); peripheral, abdominal and liver oedema occur when the right side of the heart is failing (fluid accumulates in the systemic system).

Other factors that can contribute to this loss of fluid in the tissues include protein loss and fluid retention. Protein loss can lead to a fall in oncotic pressure and an inability to pull fluid back into the vascular system. Protein levels fall in renal failure, when protein is lost in the urine, and in liver failure, when the liver is no longer able to produce plasma proteins. Fluid retention, which often is stimulated by aldosterone and ADH as described earlier, can increase the hydrostatic pressure so much that fluid is pushed out under higher pressure and the balancing pressure to pull it back into the vessel is not sufficient. Drugs that are used to treat CHF may affect the vascular system at any of these areas in an attempt to return a balance to the pressures in the system.

Points to Remember

- The heart is a hollow muscle that is divided into a right and a left side by a thick septum and into four chambers – the two upper atria and the two lower ventricles.
- The heart is responsible for pumping oxygenated blood to every cell in the body and for picking up waste products from the tissues.
- The cardiac cycle consists of a period of rest, or **diastole**, when blood is returned to the heart by veins, and a period of contraction, or **systole**, when the blood is pumped out of the heart.
- The right side of the heart receives all of the deoxygenated blood from the body through the veins and directs it into the lungs.
- The left side of the heart receives oxygenated blood from the lungs and pumps it out to every cell in the body through the arteries.
- The heart muscle possesses the properties of automaticity (the ability to generate an action potential in the absence of stimulation) and conductivity (the ability to rapidly transmit an action potential).
- The heart muscle is stimulated to contract by impulses generated in the heart, not by stimuli from the brain. The autonomic nervous system can affect the heart to increase (sympathetic) or decrease (parasympathetic) activity.
- The normal conduction or stimulatory system of the heart consists of the SA node, the atrial bundles, the AV node, the bundle of His, the bundle branches and the Purkinje fibres.
- In normal sinus rhythm, cells in the SA node generate an impulse that is transmitted through the atrial bundles and delayed slightly at the AV node before being sent down the bundle of His into the ventricles. When cardiac muscle cells are stimulated, they contract.
- Alterations in the generation of conduction of impulses in the heart cause arrhythmias (dysrhythmias), which can upset the normal balance in the cardiovascular system and lead to a decrease in cardiac output, affecting all of the cells of the body.
- Heart muscle contracts by the sliding of actin and myosin filaments in a functioning unit called a sarcomere. Contraction requires energy and calcium to allow the filaments to react with each other and slide together.
- The heart muscle needs a constant supply of blood, which is furnished by the coronary arteries. Increase in demand for oxygen can occur with changes in heart rate, preload, afterload or a stretch on the muscle.
- The cardiovascular system is a closed pressure system that uses arteries (muscular, pressure or resistance tubes) to carry blood from the heart, veins (flexible, distensible capacitance vessels) to return blood to the heart and capillaries (which connect arteries to veins) to keep blood flowing from areas of high pressure to areas of low pressure.
- Blood pressure is maintained by a stimulus from the sympathetic system and reflex control of blood volume and pressure by the renin–angiotensin system and the aldosterone–ADH system. Alterations in blood pressure (hypotension or hypertension) can upset the balance of the cardiovascular system and lead to problems in blood delivery.
- Fluid shifts out of the blood at the arterial ends of capillaries to deliver oxygen and nutrients to the tissues. It is pushed out of the vessel by the hydrostatic or fluid pressure in the arterial side of the system. Fluid returns to the system at the venous end of the capillaries because of the oncotic pull of proteins in the vessels. Disruptions in these pressures can lead to oedema or loss of fluid in the tissues.

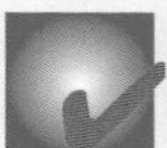

CHECK YOUR UNDERSTANDING

Answers to the questions in this chapter may be found in the answer key at the back of the book.

Multiple Choice

Select the most appropriate response to the following.

1. When referring to the heart valves,
   a. the closing of the AV valves is what is responsible for heart sounds.
   b. small muscles attached to the AV valves are responsible for opening and closing of the valves with each cycle's contraction.
   c. the aortic valve opens when the pressure in the left ventricle becomes slightly greater than the pressure in the aorta.
   d. the valves leading to the great vessels are called cuspid valves.

2. In the heart,
   a. the ventricles will not contract unless they are stimulated by action potentials arising from the SA node in the right atrium.
   b. fibrillation of the atria will cause blood pressure to fall to zero.
   c. spontaneous depolarization of the muscle membrane can occur in the absence of nerve stimulation.
   d. the muscle can continue to contract for a long period of time in the absence of oxygen through the use of anaerobic glycolysis to synthesize adenosine triphosphate (ATP).

3. The activity of the heart depends on both the inherent properties of the cardiac muscle cells and the activity of the autonomic nerves to the heart. Therefore,
   a. cutting all of the autonomic nerves to the heart will produce a decrease in heart rate.
   b. blocking the parasympathetic nerves to the heart decreases the heart rate.
   c. stimulating the sympathetic nerves to the heart increases the time available to fill the ventricles during diastole.
   d. dehydration leads to an increase in heart rate.

4. A heart transplantation patient has no nerve connections to the transplanted heart. In such an individual, one would expect to find
   a. a slower than normal resting heart rate.
   b. atria that contract at a different rate than ventricles.
   c. an increase in heart rate during emotional stress.
   d. inability to exercise because there is no way to increase heart rate or force of contraction to increase cardiac output.

5. The baroreceptors in the carotid sinus and aortic arch
   a. are in appropriate position to protect the brain from sudden changes in blood pressure.
   b. decrease the frequency of impulses sent to the cardiovascular centre when arterial blood pressure is increased.
   c. monitor the magnitude of concentration of oxygen in the vessels.
   d. react to high levels of carbon dioxide.

6. Cardiac cells differ from skeletal muscle cells in that
   a. they contain actin and myosin.
   b. they possess automaticity and conductivity.
   c. calcium must be present for muscle contraction to occur.
   d. they do not require oxygen to survive.

7. Clinically, dysrhythmias or arrhythmias cause
   a. alterations in cardiac output that could affect all cells.
   b. changes in capillary filling pressures.
   c. alterations in osmotic pressure.
   d. valve dysfunction.

8. A client is brought into Accident and Emergency (A&E) with a suspected MI. The client is very upset because he had just had an ECG in his doctor's office and it was fine. The explanation of this common phenomenon would include the fact that the ECG
   a. only reflects changes in cardiac output.
   b. is not a very accurate test.
   c. only measures the flow of electrical current through the heart and does not indicate mechanical activity or blood flow to the muscle.
   d. is not related to the heart problems.

9. Blood flow to the myocardium differs from blood flow to the rest of the cells of the body in that
   a. blood perfuses the myocardium during systole.
   b. blood flow is determined by many local factors including build up of acid.
   c. blood perfuses the myocardium during diastole.
   d. oxygenated blood flows to the myocardium via veins.

Extended Matching Questions

Select all that apply.

1. During diastole, which of the following would occur?
   a. Opening of the AV valves
   b. Relaxation of the myocardial muscle
   c. Flow of blood from the atria to the ventricles
   d. Contraction of the ventricles

e. Closing of the semilunar valves
f. Filling of the coronary arteries

2. The sympathetic nervous system would be expected to have which of the following effects?
a. Stimulate the heart to beat faster
b. Speed conduction through the AV node
c. Cause the heart muscle to contract harder
d. Slow conduction through the AV node
e. Decrease overall vascular volume
f. Increase total peripheral resistance

Definitions

Define the following terms.

1. troponin ____________________
2. actin ____________________
3. myosin ____________________
4. arrhythmia ____________________
5. Starling's law of the heart ____________________
6. fibrillation ____________________
7. capillary ____________________
8. resistance system ____________________

Matching

Match the word with the appropriate definition.

1. ____________________ atrium
2. ____________________ ventricle
3. ____________________ auricle
4. ____________________ vein
5. ____________________ artery
6. ____________________ myocardium
7. ____________________ syncytia
8. ____________________ diastole
9. ____________________ systole
10. ____________________ automaticity
11. ____________________ conductivity
12. ____________________ pulse pressure

A. Resting phase of the heart
B. Reflects the filling pressure of the coronary arteries
C. Bottom chamber of the heart
D. Vessel that takes blood away from the heart
E. Vessel that returns blood to the heart
F. Appendage on the atria of the heart
G. Property of heart cells to generate an action potential
H. Top chamber of the heart
I. Property of heart cells to rapidly conduct an action potential of electrical impulse
J. Intertwining network of muscle fibres
K. Contracting phase of the heart
L. Muscle of the heart

Bibliography

British Medical Association and Royal Pharmaceutical Society of Great Britain. (2008). *British National Formulary*. London: BMJ & RPS Publishing. *This publication is updated biannually: it is imperative that the most recent edition is consulted.*

British Medical Association and Royal Pharmaceutical Society of Great Britain. (2008). *British National Formulary for Children*. London: BMJ & RPS Publishing. *This publication is updated annually: it is imperative that the most recent edition is consulted.*

Ganong, W. (2005). *Review of medical physiology* (22nd ed.). New York: McGraw-Hill.

Howland, R. D., & Mycek, M. J. (2005). *Pharmacology* (3rd ed.). Philadelphia: Lippincott Williams & Wilkins.

Marieb, E. N., & Hoehn, K. (2004). *Human anatomy & physiology* (7th ed.). San Francisco: Pearson Benjamin Cummings.

Porth, C. M., & Matfin, G. (2008). *Pathophysiology: Concepts of altered health states* (8th ed.). Philadelphia: Lippincott Williams & Wilkins.

Simonsen, T., Aarbakke, J., Kay, I., Coleman, I., Sinnott, P., & Lysaa, R. (2006). *Illustrated pharmacology for nurses*. London: Hodder Arnold.

CHAPTER 42

Drugs Affecting Blood Pressure

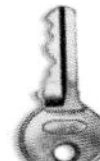

KEY TERMS

ACE inhibitor
angiotensin II receptors
baroreceptor
cardiovascular (vasomotor) centre
essential hypertension
hypotension
peripheral resistance
renin
renin–angiotensin system
shock
stroke volume

LEARNING OBJECTIVES

Upon completion of this chapter, you should be able to:

1. Outline the normal physiological controls of blood pressure and explain how the various drugs used to treat hypertension or hypotension affect these controls.
2. Describe the therapeutic actions, indications, pharmacokinetics and contraindications associated with the angiotensin-converting inhibitors, angiotensin II receptor antagonists, calcium channel antagonists and vasodilators.
3. Describe the most common adverse reactions and important drug–drug interactions associated with the angiotensin-converting inhibitors, angiotensin II receptor antagonists, calcium channel antagonists and vasodilators.
4. Discuss the use of drugs that affect blood pressure across the lifespan.
5. Compare and contrast the key drugs captopril, losartan, diltiazem and nitroprusside with other agents in their class and with other agents used to affect blood pressure.
6. Outline the nursing considerations, including important teaching points, for patients receiving drugs used to treat hypertension.

ANTIHYPERTENSIVE AGENTS

Angiotensin-Converting Enzyme Inhibitors

captopril
enalapril
lisinopril
moexipril
perindopril
quinapril
ramipril
trandolapril

Angiotensin II Receptor Antagonists

candesartan
eprosartan
irbesartan
losartan
olmesartan
telmisartan
valsartan

Calcium Channel Antagonists

amlodipine
diltiazem
felodipine
isradipine
nicardipine
nifedipine
nisoldipine
verapamil

Vasodilators

diazoxide
hydralazine
minoxidil
nitroprusside

The cardiovascular system is a closed system of blood vessels responsible for delivering oxygenated blood to the tissues and removing waste products from the tissues. The blood in this system flows from areas of higher pressure to areas of lower pressure. The area of highest pressure in the system is always the left ventricle during systole. The pressure in this area propels the blood out of the aorta and into the system of arteries. The lowest pressure is in the right atrium, which collects all of the reduced oxygenated blood from the body. The maintenance of this pressure system is controlled by specific areas of the brain and various hormones. If the pressure becomes too high, the person is said to be hypertensive. If the pressure becomes too low and blood cannot be delivered effectively, the person is said to be hypotensive. Helping the patient to maintain their blood pressure within normal limits is the goal when drug therapy is introduced.

Blood Pressure Control

The pressure in the cardiovascular system is determined by three elements:

- Heart rate,
- **Stroke volume** or the amount of blood that is pumped out of the ventricle with each heartbeat (primarily determined by the volume of blood in the system),
- Total **peripheral resistance** (TPR) or the resistance of the muscular arteries to the blood being pumped through.

The small arterioles are thought to be the most important sites in determining peripheral resistance. These vessels with muscular walls and small diameter lumens are able to almost stop blood flow into capillary beds when they constrict, building up tremendous pressure in the arteries behind them as they prevent the blood from flowing through. The arterioles are very responsive to stimulation from the sympathetic nervous system; they constrict when the sympathetic system is stimulated (via α_1 adrenoreceptors), increasing TPR and blood pressure. The body uses this responsiveness to regulate blood pressure on a minute-to-minute basis to ensure that there is enough pressure in the system to deliver sufficient blood to the brain.

Baroreceptors

As the blood leaves the left ventricle through the aorta, it influences specialized cells in the arch of the aorta called **baroreceptors** (pressure receptors which respond to stretch). Similar cells are located in the carotid arteries, which deliver blood to the brain. If there is sufficient pressure in these vessels, the baroreceptors are stimulated, sending that information to the brain. If the pressure falls, the stimulation of the baroreceptors falls off. That information is also sent to the brain.

The sensory input from the baroreceptors is received in the medulla oblongata, in an area called the **cardiovascular (vasomotor) centre**. If the pressure is high, the medulla stimulates vasodilation and a decrease in cardiac rate and output, causing the pressure in the system to drop. If the pressure is low, the medulla directly stimulates an increase in cardiac rate and output and vasoconstriction; this increases TPR and raises the blood pressure. The medulla mediates these effects through the autonomic nervous system (see Chapter 28).

The baroreceptor reflex continually functions to maintain blood pressure within a predetermined range of normal. For example, if you have been lying down flat and suddenly stand up, the blood pools in your lower limbs (an effect of gravity), so venous return falls. You may even feel light-headed or dizzy for a short time. When you stand and the blood flow drops, the baroreceptors are not stretched. The medulla oblongata senses this drop and stimulates a rise in heart rate, cardiac output and a generalized vasoconstriction, which increases TPR, and all these factors increase blood pressure. These increases should raise pressure in the system, which restores blood flow to the brain and stimulates the baroreceptors. The stimulation of the baroreceptors leads to a decrease in stimulatory impulses from the medulla and the blood pressure falls back within normal limits (Figure 42.1).

Renin–Angiotensin System

Another compensatory system is activated when the blood pressure within the kidneys falls. As the kidneys require a constant perfusion to function properly, they have a compensatory mechanism to help ensure that blood flow is maintained. This mechanism is called the **renin–angiotensin system** (it is sometimes referred to as the renin–angiotensin–aldosterone system).

Low blood pressure or poor oxygenation of the nephrons in the kidneys causes the release of **renin** from the juxtaglomerular cells, a group of cells that monitor blood pressure and blood flow into the glomerulus. Renin is released into the bloodstream and arrives in the liver to convert the compound angiotensinogen (produced in the liver) to angiotensin I. Angiotensin I travels in the bloodstream to the lungs, where the metabolic cells of the alveoli and bronchial mucosa use angiotensin-converting enzyme (ACE) to convert angiotensin I to angiotensin II. Angiotensin II reacts with specific angiotensin II receptor sites on blood vessels to cause intense vasoconstriction. This effect raises the TPR and raises the blood pressure, restoring blood flow to the kidneys and decreasing the release of renin.

Angiotensin II also stimulates the adrenal cortex to release aldosterone. Aldosterone acts on the nephrons to cause the retention of sodium and water. This effect increases blood volume, which should also contribute to increasing blood pressure. The sodium-rich blood stimulates the osmoreceptors in the hypothalamus to cause

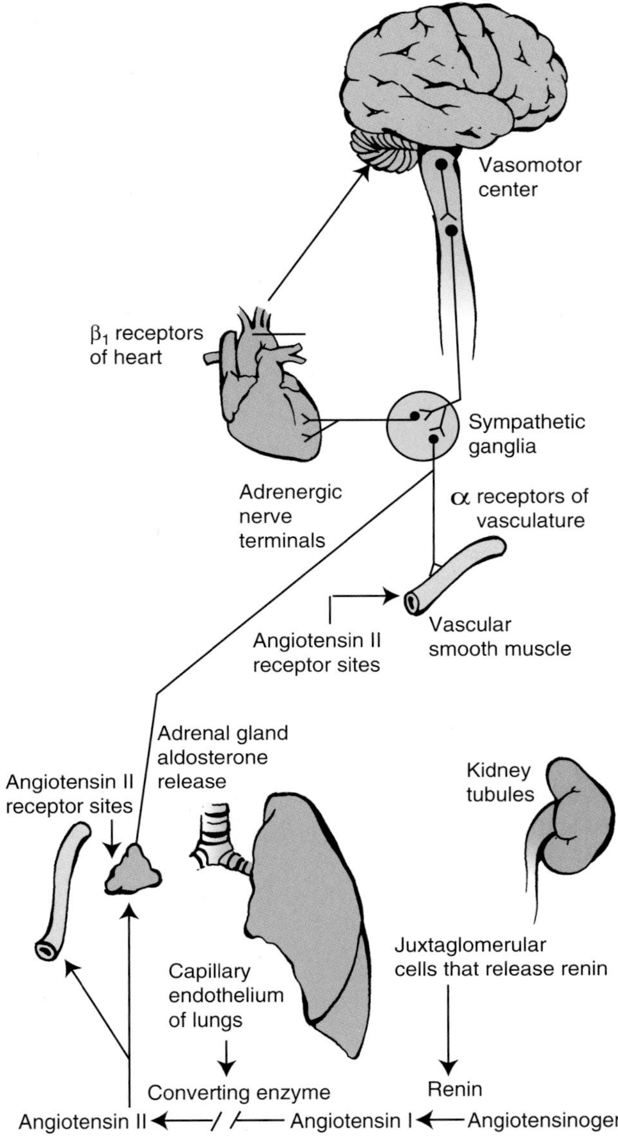

FIGURE 42.1 Control of blood pressure. The vasomotor center in the medulla responds to stimuli from aortic and carotid baroreceptors to cause sympathetic stimulation. The kidneys release renin to activate the renin-angiotensin system, causing vasoconstriction and increased blood volume.

the release of antidiuretic hormone, which in turn causes retention of water in the nephrons, further increasing the blood volume. This increase in blood volume increases the blood pressure, which should increase blood flow to the kidneys. This should lead to a decrease in the release of renin, thus causing the compensatory mechanisms to stop (Figure 42.2).

Hypertension

When a person's blood pressure is above 'normal' limits (see Table 42.1) for a sustained period, a diagnosis of hypertension is made. It is estimated that at least 40% of adults in England and Wales have hypertension and many are unaware of it (BHF 2006).

Table 42.1 Categories Rating the Severity of Hypertension

Blood Pressure (BP) Classification	Systolic Blood Pressure (mmHg)	Diastolic Blood Pressure (mmHg)
Optimal BP	<120	<80
Normal BP	<130	<85
High–normal BP	130–139	85–89
Grade 1 hypertension (mild)	140–159	90–99
Grade 2 hypertension (moderate)	160–179	100–109
Grade 3 hypertension (severe)	≥180	≥110

Source: Guidelines for management of hypertension: report of the fourth Working Party of the British Hypertension Society, 2004 BHS IV

B. Williams et al.: Journal of Human Hypertension, 2004, 18, 139–185. www.nice.org.uk/CG034NICEguideline

Ninety percent of the people with hypertension have what is called **essential hypertension** or hypertension with no known cause. People with essential hypertension usually have elevated TPR due to atherosclerosis or persistent activation of the sympathetic nervous system. Their organs are perfused effectively and they usually display no symptoms. A few people develop secondary hypertension or high blood pressure resulting from a known cause, for instance, kidney problems or a tumour in the adrenal medulla, called a phaeochromocytoma; in this case, hypertension usually resolves after the tumour is removed.

The underlying danger of hypertension of any type is the prolonged force on the vessels of the vascular system. The muscles in the arterial system eventually thicken, leading to a loss of responsiveness in the system. The left ventricle thickens (hypertrophy) because the muscle must constantly work hard to expel blood at a greater force. The thickening of the heart muscle and the increased pressure that the muscle has to generate increases the workload of the heart and the risk of coronary artery disease (CAD). The hydrostatic force of the blood being forced through arteries damages the lining of endothelial cells, making these vessels susceptible to atherosclerosis and to narrowing of the lumen of the vessels (see Chapter 46). Tiny vessels can be damaged and destroyed, leading to loss of vision (if the vessels are in the retina), kidney function (if the vessels include the glomeruli in the nephrons) or cerebral function (if the vessels are small and fragile in the brain).

Untreated hypertension increases the risk for the following conditions: CAD and cardiac death, stroke, renal failure and loss of vision. As hypertension has no symptoms, it is difficult to diagnose and treat and it is often called the 'silent killer'. Most of the drugs used to treat hypertension have adverse effects, many of which are seen as unacceptable by otherwise healthy people. Nurses face a difficult challenge trying to

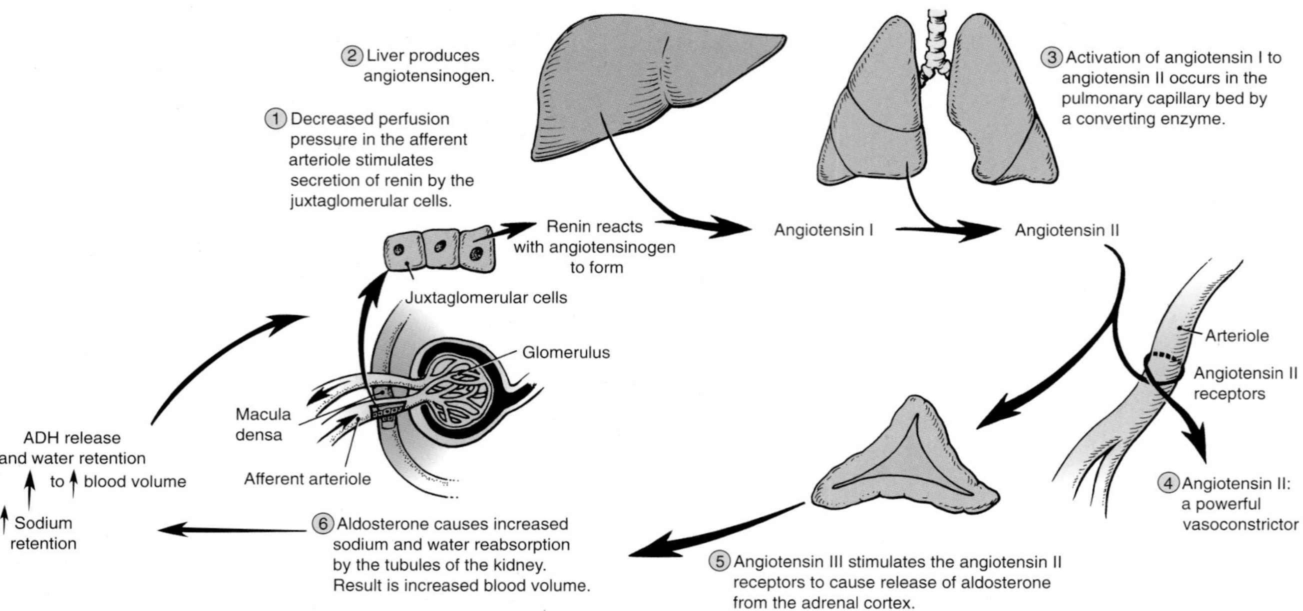

FIGURE 42.2 The renin-angiotensin system.

convince patients to comply with their drug regimens when they experience adverse effects and do not see any positive effects of the drugs. Research into the cause of hypertension is ongoing and many theories have been proposed for the cause of the disorder. Factors that are known to increase blood pressure in some people include high levels of psychological stress, exposure to high-frequency noise, a high-salt diet, lack of rest and genetic predisposition (see Box 42.1).

BOX 42.1 FOCUS ON THE **EVIDENCE**

'White Coat' Hypertension

The diagnosis of hypertension is accompanied by the impact of serious ramifications such as increased risk for numerous diseases and cardiovascular death, the potential need for significant lifestyle changes and the potential need for drug therapy, which may include many unpleasant adverse effects. Consequently, it is important that a patient be correctly diagnosed before being labelled hypertensive.

Researchers in the 1990s discovered that some patients were hypertensive only when they were in their doctor's clinic having their blood pressure measured. This was correlated to a sympathetic stress reaction (which elevates systolic blood pressure) and a tendency to tighten the muscles (isometric exercise, which elevates diastolic blood pressure) while waiting to be seen and during the blood pressure measurement. The researchers labelled this phenomenon 'white coat' hypertension.

The British Heart Foundation (BHF) has put forward guidelines for the diagnosis and treatment of hypertension. A patient should have three consecutive blood pressure readings above normal, when taken by a clinician, over a period of 2 to 3 weeks. These guidelines point out the importance of using the correct technique when taking a patient's blood pressure, especially because the results can have such a tremendous impact on a patient. It is good practice to periodically review the process for performing this routine task. For example, the nurse should

- Select a cuff that is the correct size for the patient's arm (a cuff that is too small may give a high reading; a cuff that is too large may give a lower reading).
- Try to put the patient at ease, make them sit in a comfortable position and reassure them.
- Ensure that the arm that will be used is supported.
- Palpate the brachial artery before beginning.
- Identify the radial or radial artery and note pulse.
- Place the cuff over the brachial artery directly onto the patient's skin instead of on top of clothing and palpating the radial pulse, inflate the cuff until the pulse can be no longer palpated. Continue to increase the pressure by 30 mmHg then deflate the cuff noting when the pulse could be felt again, this is an estimation of the systolic blood pressure.
- Deflate the cuff, place the stethoscope over the brachial artery and reinflate the cuff again, 30 mmHg above the point where the pulse reappeared.
- Listen carefully and record the first sound heard (systolic) and the absence of sound (the diastolic).

Nurses are the health care providers most likely to be taking and recording blood pressure, so it is important to always use the proper technique and to make accurate recordings.

Hypotension

If blood pressure becomes too low, the vital centres in the brain as well as the rest of the tissues of the body may not receive enough oxygenated blood to continue functioning. **Hypotension** can progress to **shock**, when waste products accumulate and cells begin to die from lack of oxygen. Hypotensive states can occur in the following situations:

- When the heart muscle is damaged and unable to pump effectively.
- With severe blood loss, when volume drops dramatically.
- When there is extreme stress and the body's levels of adrenaline are depleted, leaving the body unable to respond to stimuli to raise blood pressure.

Antihypertensive Agents

As an underlying cause of hypertension is usually unknown, altering the body's regulatory mechanisms is the best treatment currently available. Drugs used to treat hypertension work to alter the normal reflexes that control blood pressure. Treatment for essential hypertension does not cure the disease but is aimed at maintaining the blood pressure within normal (accepted) limits to prevent the damage that hypertension can cause. Not all patients respond the same way to antihypertensive drugs because different factors may contribute to each person's hypertension. Patients may have complicating conditions such as diabetes or acute myocardial infarction (MI) that makes it unwise to use certain drugs (see Box 42.2).

Several different types of drugs, which affect different areas of blood pressure control, may need to be used in combination to actually maintain a patient's blood pressure within normal limits. Trials of drugs and combinations of drugs are often needed to develop an individual regimen that is effective without producing adverse effects that are unacceptable to the patient. For current NICE guidelines on drug treatment for patients newly diagnosed with hypertension (see Figure 42.4).

Research is ongoing into the treatment of more specific hypertensions (e.g. pulmonary hypertension). The development of drugs that target specific blood vessel sites and chemicals could lead to a new approach to the treatment of essential hypertension in the future. For antihypertensive drug use across the life span (see Box 42.4).

BOX 42.2 CULTURAL CONSIDERATIONS FOR DRUG THERAPY

Antihypertensive Therapy

Taking medication to reduce raised blood pressure can decrease the risk of coronary disease, renal impairment, stroke and heart failure. The ideal threshold is systolic blood pressure less than 140 mmHg and diastolic blood pressure of less than 90 mmHg; however, the thresholds and targets for treatment may vary depending on the patient's age, pre-existing conditions and ethnic background. The current guidelines for the treatment of hypertension can be found summarized in the most recent edition of the British National Formulary (BNF). In addition, the National Institute for Health and Clinical Excellence (NICE) guidelines on the treatment, goals and targets for hypertension are available from the NICE website: www.nice.org.uk.

The choice of antihypertensive drug will depend upon the relevant indications and contraindications for the individual patient.

Stepped-Care Approach to Treating Hypertension

The importance of treating hypertension has been proven in numerous research studies. If hypertension is controlled, the patient's risk of cardiovascular death and disease is reduced. The risk of developing cardiovascular complications is directly related to the patient's degree of hypertension (see Table 42.1). Lowering the degree of hypertension lowers the risk.

The British Hypertension Society in conjunction with the NICE provides updated guidelines and recommendations to tackle hypertension in England and Wales (www.nice.org.uk/CG034guidance). Currently, the guidelines recommend:

Step1 Lifestyle modifications are instituted. These include weight reduction, smoking cessation, reduction in the use of alcohol and salt in the diet (all of these conditions have been shown to increase blood pressure) and an increase in physical exercise (which has been shown to decrease blood pressure and improve cardiovascular tone and reserve).

Step2 In hypertensive patients below the age of 55 years, the first choice of initial therapy should be an ACE inhibitor. If this is not tolerated by the patient, then an angiotensin receptor blocker (ARB) should be used.

Step3 In hypertensive patients of 55 years or older or black patients (African or Caribbean decent) of any age, first choice initial therapy should be a calcium channel blocker or a thiazide (thiazide-like) diuretic

Step4 If the initial therapy was using a calcium channel blocker or a thiazide diuretic and a further drug is required, an ACE inhibitor (or an ARB, if an ACE inhibitor cannot be tolerated) should be used. If an ACE inhibitor was used as an initial therapy then a calcium channel blocker or thiazide diuretic can be added to the regimen.

Step5 If three drugs are required then a combination of ACE inhibitor (or an ARB, if an ACE inhibitor cannot be tolerated), a thiazide-like diuretic and a calcium channel blocker is recommended

The current decision of not to recommend β-blockers for first-line therapy is based on research evidence that they perform less well as antihypertensives and that carry an increased risk of patients developing type 2 diabetes.

Angiotensin-Converting Enzyme Inhibitors

The **ACE inhibitors** block the conversion of angiotensin I to angiotensin II in the lungs (see Figure 42.2), as angiotensin II is a powerful vasoconstrictor, and these drugs stop the renin–angiotensin system, preventing vasoconstriction and aldosterone release. The ACE inhibitors may be used as a monotherapy for hypertension management or they may be combined with diuretics. ACE inhibitors that are used include the following agents:

- **Captopril** is indicated for use in hypertension and in treating congestive heart failure (CHF), diabetic nephropathy and left ventricular dysfunction after MI. It has been associated with a sometimes fatal pancytopenia (abnormal depression of all the cellular elements of the blood), a persistent dry cough and unpleasant gastrointestinal (GI) distress.
- **Enalapril** is used for the treatment of hypertension, CHF and left ventricular dysfunction; it has the advantage of parenteral use (if oral use is not feasible or rapid onset is desirable).
- **Lisinopril** is an oral drug used in treating hypertension and CHF and is used in stable patients within 24 hours after acute MI to improve the likelihood of survival.
- **Moexipril** is a less well-tolerated oral drug used in the treatment of hypertension; it is associated with many unpleasant GI and skin effects, cough and cardiac arrhythmias. Fatal MI and pancytopenia have sometimes been associated with this drug.
- **Perindopril** is an oral drug that is used alone or in combination with other antihypertensive agents to control blood pressure. It is associated with a sometimes fatal pancytopenia as well as a serious-to-fatal airway obstruction, mood and sleep disturbances.
- **Quinapril** is used orally for the treatment of hypertension and as an adjunct treatment of CHF; it is not associated with as many adverse effects as some of the other agents.
- **Ramipril** is used orally for the treatment of mild-to-moderate hypertension and as an adjunct treatment of CHF; it is not associated with as many adverse effects as some of the other agents.
- **Trandolapril** is used orally for the treatment of hypertension and for CHF after an acute MI and left ventricular dysfunction. It is fairly well tolerated.

Therapeutic Actions and Indications

The actions of ACE inhibitors include a decrease in blood pressure and in aldosterone secretion, with a resultant slight increase in serum potassium and a loss of serum sodium and fluid.

These drugs are indicated for the treatment of hypertension, alone or in combination with other drugs. They are also used in conjunction with digoxin and diuretics for the treatment of CHF and left ventricular dysfunction. Their therapeutic effect in these cases is thought to be related to a decrease in cardiac workload associated with the decrease in peripheral resistance and blood volume.

Pharmacokinetics

These drugs are well absorbed, widely distributed, metabolized in the liver and excreted in the urine and faeces. They are known to cross the placenta and have been associated with serious foetal abnormalities. These drugs should not be used during pregnancy. Several of these drugs have been detected in breast milk. As there is a potential for serious adverse effects in the neonate, another method of feeding the baby should be used during lactation or another antihypertensive should be chosen.

Contraindications and Cautions

ACE inhibitors reduce or abolish glomerular filtration and are likely to cause severe and progressive renal failure; therefore, ACE inhibitors are used with caution for patients with impaired renal function, as this could be exacerbated by the effects of this drug in decreasing renal blood flow, with pregnancy, because of the potential for adverse effects on the foetus and amniotic fluid production, and during lactation, because of potential decrease in milk production and effects on the neonate.

Adverse Effects

The adverse effects associated with the ACE inhibitors are related to the effects of vasodilation and alterations in blood flow. Such effects include reflex tachycardia, chest pain, angina, CHF and cardiac arrhythmias; GI irritation, ulcers, constipation and liver injury; renal insufficiency, renal failure and proteinuria; and rash, alopecia, dermatitis and photosensitivity. Many of these drugs cause an unrelenting cough thought to be related to the accumulation of bradykinin in the bronchial mucosa, where the ACE is inhibited. This may lead patients to discontinue the drug treatment. Some of these drugs have been associated with fatal pancytopenia and MI.

Always consult a current copy of the BNF for further guidance

Clinically Important Drug–Drug Interactions

The risk of hypersensitivity reactions increases if these drugs are taken with allopurinol.

Clinically Important Drug–Food Interactions

Absorption of oral ACE inhibitors decreases if they are taken with food. They should be taken on an empty stomach, 1 hour before or 2 hours after meals.

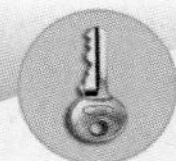

Key Drug Summary: *Ramipril*

Indications: Severe hypertension resistant to other therapy, CHF, diabetic nephropathy, left ventricular dysfunction after an MI

Actions: Blocks ACE from converting angiotensin I to angiotensin II, leading to a decrease in blood pressure, a decrease in aldosterone production and a small increase in serum potassium levels along with sodium and fluid loss

Pharmacokinetics:

Route	Onset	Peak
Oral	15 min	30–90 min

$T_{1/2}$: 2 hours; excreted in urine

Adverse effects: Cough, tachycardia, MI, rash, pruritus, gastric irritation, aphthous ulcers, peptic ulcers, proteinuria and bone marrow suppression.

Nursing Considerations for Patients Receiving ACE Inhibitors

Assessment: History and Examination

Screen for the following conditions, *which could be cautions or contraindications to use of the drug*: any known allergies to these drugs, impaired kidney function, *which could be exacerbated by these drugs*, *pregnancy* or lactation, *because of the potential adverse effects on the foetus or neonate*, salt/volume depletion, *which could be exacerbated by these drugs*, and CHF.

Include screening *for baseline status before beginning therapy and for any potential adverse effects*. Assess the following: body temperature and weight; skin colour, lesions and temperature; pulse, blood pressure, baseline ECG and perfusion; respirations and adventitious breath sounds; bowel sounds and abdominal examination; and renal function tests, complete blood count with differential and serum electrolytes.

Establish if patient is currently taking other medications or herbal therapies, which may potentially interact with the ACE inhibitors.

Nursing Diagnoses

The patient receiving an ACE inhibitor may have the following nursing diagnoses related to drug therapy:

- Ineffective tissue perfusion (total body) related to changes in cardiac output.
- Impaired skin integrity related to dermatological effects.
- Acute pain related to GI distress and cough.
- Deficient knowledge regarding drug therapy.

Implementation With Rationale

- Encourage the patient to implement lifestyle changes, including weight loss, smoking cessation, decreased alcohol and salt in the diet and increased exercise, *to increase the effectiveness of antihypertensive therapy*.
- Administer on an empty stomach, 1 hour before or 2 hours after meals, *to ensure proper absorption of drug*.
- Inform the surgeon of the patient's medication if the patient is to undergo surgery, *to alert medical personnel that the blockage of compensatory angiotensin II could result in hypotension after surgery that would need to be reversed with volume expansion*.
- Give parenteral forms only if an oral form is not feasible and transfer to an oral form as soon as possible, *to avert an increased risk of adverse effects*.
- Consult with the prescriber to reduce dosage in patients with renal failure, *to account for their decreased production of renin and lower-than-normal levels of angiotensin II*.
- Monitor the patient carefully in any situation that might lead to a drop in fluid volume (e.g. excessive sweating, vomiting, diarrhoea and dehydration), *to detect and treat excessive hypotension that may occur*.
- Provide comfort measures *to help the patient tolerate drug effects*. These include small, frequent meals; environmental controls; safety precautions and appropriate skin care as needed.
- Provide thorough patient education, including the name of the drug, dosage prescribed, measures to avoid adverse effects, warning signs of problems

and the need for periodic monitoring and evaluation, *to enhance patient knowledge about drug therapy and to promote compliance.*
- Offer support and encouragement, *to help the patient deal with the diagnosis and the drug regimen.*

Evaluation

- Arrange for regular review of the patient to allow monitoring of the patient response to the drug (maintenance of blood pressure within normal limits and stable urea and electrolytes (U&E's)).
- Monitor for adverse effects (hypotension, cardiac arrhythmias, renal dysfunction, skin reactions, dry cough, pancytopenia and CHF).
- Evaluate the effectiveness of the teaching plan (patient can name drug, dosage, adverse effects to watch for, specific measures to avoid adverse effects and the importance of continued follow-up).
- Monitor the effectiveness of comfort measures and compliance with the treatment regimen.

Angiotensin II Receptor Antagonists

The ARBs selectively bind to **angiotensin II receptors** in blood vessels to prevent vasoconstriction and in the adrenal cortex to prevent the release of aldosterone that is caused by reaction of these receptors with angiotensin II. These actions lead to a decrease in blood pressure caused by a decrease in TPR and blood volume. The ARBs include the following drugs:

- **Candesartan** is used alone or as part of combination therapy to treat hypertension.
- **Eprosartan** is used alone or as part of combination therapy to treat hypertension in adults.
- **Irbesartan** is used as monotherapy in the treatment of hypertension but can be combined with other antihypertensives if needed. It is also used to slow the progression of kidney disease in patients with hypertension and type 2 diabetes.
- **Losartan** can be used alone or as part of combination therapy for hypertension, as well as for treatment of diabetic neuropathy with an elevated serum creatinine and proteinuria in patients with hypertension and type 2 diabetes.
- **Olmesartan** is used alone or as part of combination therapy to treat hypertension. This is the newest angiotensin II receptor blocker.
- **Telmisartan** is used alone or as part of combination therapy to treat hypertension.
- **Valsartan** can be used alone or as part of combination therapy for hypertension and for the treatment of heart failure in patients who are intolerant to ACE inhibitors.

Therapeutic Actions and Indications

The ARBs selectively bind to angiotensin II receptor sites in vascular smooth muscle and in the adrenal gland to block vasoconstriction and the release of aldosterone. These actions block the blood pressure-raising effects of the renin–angiotensin system and lower blood pressure. They are indicated to be used alone or in combination therapy for the treatment of hypertension and for the treatment of CHF in patients who are intolerant to ACE inhibitors. Recently, they were also found to slow the progression of renal disease in patients with hypertension and type 2 diabetes. This action is thought to be related to the effects of blocking angiotensin receptors in the vascular endothelium. Unlike ACE inhibitors, they do not inhibit the breakdown of bradykinin and other kinins, and are thus unlikely to cause the persistent dry cough, which complicates ACE inhibitor therapy. They are, therefore, a useful alternative for patients who have to discontinue an ACE inhibitor because of a persistent cough.

Pharmacokinetics

These agents are well absorbed and undergo metabolism in the liver by the cytochrome P450 system. They are excreted in faeces and in urine. Known to cross the placenta, the ARBs have been associated with serious foetal abnormalities and even stillbirth when given in the second or third trimester. Women of childbearing age should be advised to use barrier contraceptives to avoid pregnancy; if a pregnancy does occur, the ARB should be discontinued immediately. Candesartan, eprosartan, irbesartan, olmesartan and telmisartan should not be used during the second or third trimester of pregnancy because of associated foetal abnormalities and death. Losartan and valsartan should not be used at any time during pregnancy. It is not known whether the ARBs enter breast milk during lactation; however, because of the potential for serious adverse effects in the neonate, these drugs should not be used in lactating women.

Contraindications and Cautions

The ARBs are contraindicated in the presence of allergy to any of these drugs, during pregnancy, *because of associated foetal death and severe abnormalities*, and during lactation, *because of potential adverse effects on the neonate.* Caution should be used in the presence of hepatic or renal dysfunction, *which could alter the metabolism and excretion of these drugs*; *and* with hypovolaemia, *because of the blocking of potentially life-saving compensatory mechanisms*.

These drugs should not be prescribed to patients with renal disease as they reduce renal blood flow and may reduce GFR in patients with already compromised renal function.

Adverse Effects

The adverse effects most commonly associated with ARBs include the following: headache, dizziness, syncope and weakness, which could be associated with drops in blood pressure; hypotension; GI complaints including diarrhoea, abdominal pain, nausea, dry mouth and tooth pain; symptoms of upper respiratory tract infections; rash, dry skin and alopecia. Hyperkalaemia occurs occasionally; angioedema has also been reported with some angiotensin II receptor antagonists.

Clinically Important Drug–Drug Interactions

The risk of decreased serum levels and loss of effectiveness increases if the ARB is taken in combination with phenobarbital. If this combination is used, the patient should be closely monitored and dosage adjustments made.

Always consult the most recent edition of the BNF.

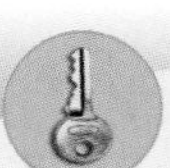

Key Drug Summary: *Losartan*

Indications: Alone or as part of combination therapy for the treatment of hypertension; treatment of diabetic nephropathy with an elevated serum creatinine and proteinuria in patients with type 2 diabetes and hypertension

Actions: Selectively blocks the binding of angiotensin II to specific tissue receptors found in the vascular smooth muscle and adrenal glands and blocks the vasoconstriction and release of aldosterone associated with the renin–angiotensin system

Pharmacokinetics:

Route	Onset	Peak	Duration
Oral	Varies	1–3 h	24 h

$T_{1/2}$: 2 hours, then for the metabolites 6 to 9 hours; metabolized in the liver and excreted in urine and faeces

Adverse effects: Dizziness, headache, diarrhoea, abdominal pain, symptoms of upper respiratory tract infection, cough, back pain, fever, muscle weakness and hypotension

Calcium Channel Antagonists

The calcium channel antagonists prevent the movement of calcium into the cardiac and smooth muscle cells when the cells are stimulated. This blocking of calcium interferes with the muscle cell's ability to contract, leading to a loss of smooth muscle tone, vasodilation and a decrease in peripheral resistance. These effects decrease blood pressure, cardiac workload and myocardial oxygen consumption. Calcium channel antagonists are very effective in the treatment of angina (see Chapter 45) because they decrease the cardiac workload (see Critical Thinking Scenario 42-1).

Not all calcium channel antagonists are used to treat hypertension. Some are considered safe and effective in treating hypertension only if they are given as sustained-release or extended-release preparations. The calcium channel antagonists used in treating hypertension include the following:

- **Amlodipine** an oral drug that may be used alone or in combination with other agents to treat hypertension. It is also is used for angina.
- **Diltiazem** is a sustained-release preparation recommended for the treatment of hypertension.
- **Felodipine** is indicated alone or in combination with other agents for the treatment of hypertension. This drug may be used as a prophylaxis for angina.
- **Isradipin**e is not used for angina but is indicated alone or in combination with thiazide diuretics for the treatment of hypertension.
- **Nicardipine** is used alone or in combination with other agents to treat hypertension and as a prophylaxis for angina. It is also available in intravenous form for short-term use when oral administration is not feasible.
- **Nifedipine** is indicated for the treatment of hypertension, prophylaxis of angina and Raynaud's phenomenon.
- **Nisoldipine** comes in extended-release tablets and is indicated for the treatment of hypertension as monotherapy or as part of combination therapy and for the prophylaxis of angina.
- **Verapamil** comes in extended-release tablets and is indicated for the treatment of essential hypertension; other preparations are used for angina and treating various arrhythmias. This drug should not be given by injection to patients on β-blockers due to the risk of hypotension and asystole.

Therapeutic Actions and Indications

Calcium channel antagonists inhibit the movement of calcium ions across the membranes of myocardial and arterial muscle cells, altering the action potential and blocking muscle cell contraction. This effect depresses myocardial contractility, slows cardiac impulse formation in the conductive tissues, reduces vascular tone as it relaxes and dilates arteries, causing a fall in blood pressure and a decrease in venous return.

Pharmacokinetics

These drugs are generally well absorbed, metabolized in the liver and excreted in the urine. These drugs cross the placenta and enter breast milk. Foetal toxicity has been reported in animal studies, and, although there are no well-defined studies about effects during human pregnancy, they should not be used during pregnancy unless the benefit to the mother clearly outweighs any potential risk to the foetus.

Contraindications and Cautions

These drugs are contraindicated in patients with heart block or sick sinus syndrome, *which could be exacerbated by the conduction-slowing effects of these drugs*, with renal or hepatic dysfunction, *which could alter the metabolism and excretion of these drugs*, and with pregnancy or lactation, *because of the potential for adverse effects on the foetus or neonate*.

Adverse Effects

The adverse effects associated with these drugs relate to their effects on cardiac output and on smooth muscle. Central nervous system (CNS) effects include dizziness, light-headedness, headache and fatigue. GI problems include nausea and hepatic injury related to direct toxic effects on hepatic cells. Cardiovascular effects include hypotension, bradycardia, peripheral oedema and heart block. Skin flushing and rash may also occur.

For further information and guidance, always consult the most recent edition of the BNF.

Clinically Important Drug–Drug Interactions

Drug–drug interactions vary with each of the calcium channel antagonists used to treat hypertension. A potentially serious effect to note is an increase in serum levels and toxicity of cyclosporine if taken with diltiazem.

FOCUS ON **PATIENT SAFETY**

The calcium channel antagonists are a class of drugs that interact with grapefruit juice. When grapefruit juice is present in the body, the concentrations of calcium channel antagonists sometimes increase to toxic levels. Advise patients to avoid the use of grapefruit juice if they are taking a calcium channel blocker.

Diuretics

Diuretics are drugs that increase the excretion of sodium and hence water from the kidney (see Chapter 50 and Figure 42.3). These drugs are often the first agents tried in mild hypertension; they affect blood sodium levels and blood volume.

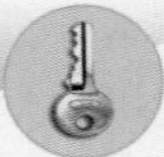

Key Drug Summary: *Diltiazem*

Indications: Treatment of essential hypertension in the extended-release form. Prophylaxis and treatment of angina.

Actions: Inhibits the movement of calcium ions across the membranes of cardiac and arterial muscle cells, depressing the impulse and leading to slowed conduction, decreased myocardial contractility and dilation of arterioles, which lowers blood pressure and decreases myocardial oxygen consumption

Pharmacokinetics:

Route	Onset	Peak	Duration
Oral	30–60 min	6–11 h	12 h

$T_{1/2}$: 5 to 7 hours; metabolized in the liver and excreted in urine

Adverse effects: Dizziness, light-headedness, headache, peripheral oedema, bradycardia, atrioventricular block, flushing and nausea

Nursing Considerations for Patients Receiving Angiotensin II Receptor Antagonists, vasodilators and Calcium Channel Antagonists

Assessment: History and Examination

Screen for the following conditions, *which could be cautions or contraindications to use of the drug:* any known allergies to these drugs, impaired kidney or liver function, *which could be exacerbated by these drugs*, pregnancy and lactation, *because of the potential adverse effects on the foetus and neonate*, and hypovolaemia, *which could potentiate the blood pressure-lowering effects*.

Include screening *for baseline status before beginning therapy and for any potential adverse effects*. Assess the following: body temperature and weight; skin colour, lesions and temperature; pulse, blood pressure, baseline electrocardiogram (ECG) and perfusion; respirations and adventitious breath sounds; bowel sounds and abdominal examination; and renal and liver function tests.

Establish if patient is currently taking other medications or herbal therapies, which may potentially interact with the angiotensin II receptor antagonists, vasodilators and calcium channel antagonists.

Nursing Diagnoses

The patient receiving an ARB, vasodilator antagonists or calcium channel may have the following nursing diagnoses related to drug therapy:

- Ineffective tissue perfusion (total body) related to changes in cardiac output.
- Impaired skin integrity related to dermatological effects.
- Acute pain related to GI distress, cough, skin effects and headache.
- Deficient knowledge regarding drug therapy.

Implementation With Rationale

- Encourage the patient to implement lifestyle changes, where appropriate, for example, weight loss, smoking cessation, decreased alcohol and salt in the diet and increased exercise, *to increase the effectiveness of antihypertensive therapy*.
- Administer with food, *to decrease GI distress if needed*.
- Alert the surgeon and mark the patient's chart prominently if the patient is to undergo surgery, *to notify medical personnel that the blockage of compensatory angiotensin II could result in hypotension after surgery that would need to be reversed with volume expansion*.
- Ensure that the female patient is not pregnant before beginning therapy and suggest the use of barrier contraceptives while she is taking this drug, *to avert potential foetal abnormalities and foetal death, which have been associated with these drugs*.
- Find an alternative method of feeding the baby if the patient is nursing, *to prevent the potentially dangerous blockade of the renin–angiotensin system in the neonate*.
- Monitor the patient carefully in any situation that might lead to a drop in fluid volume (e.g. excessive sweating, vomiting, diarrhoea and dehydration), *to detect and treat excessive hypotension that may occur*.
- Provide comfort measures, *to help the patient tolerate drug effects*, including small, frequent meals; access to bathroom facilities; safety precautions if CNS effects occur; environmental controls; appropriate skin care as needed and analgesics as needed.
- Provide thorough patient teaching (education), including the name of the drug, dosage prescribed, measures to avoid adverse effects, warning signs of problems and the need for periodic monitoring and evaluation, *to enhance patient knowledge about drug therapy and to promote concordance*.
- Offer support and encouragement, *to help the patient deal with the diagnosis and the drug regimen*.

Evaluation

- Arrange for regular review of the patient to allow monitoring of the patient and their response to the drug (maintenance of blood pressure within normal limits).
- Monitor for adverse effects (hypotension, GI distress, skin reactions, cough, headache and dizziness). Evaluate effectiveness of the teaching plan (patient can name drug, dosage, adverse effects to watch for, measures to avoid adverse effects and the importance of continued follow-up).
- Monitor the effectiveness of comfort measures and compliance to the regimen.

Other Antihypertensive Agents

Sympathetic Nervous System Antagonists

Drugs that block the effects of the sympathetic nervous system (see Chapter 30) are useful in blocking many of the compensatory effects of the sympathetic nervous system (see Figure 42.3).

- **β-adrenergic antagonists** block vasoconstriction, decrease heart rate, decrease cardiac muscle contraction and tend to increase blood flow to the kidneys, leading to a decrease in the release of renin. These drugs have many adverse effects and are not recommended for all people. They are often used as monotherapy in step 2 treatment, and in some patients, they control blood pressure adequately.
- **α and β-adrenergic antagonists** are useful in conjunction with other agents and tend to be somewhat more powerful, blocking all of the receptors in the sympathetic system. Patients often complain of fatigue, loss of libido, inability to sleep and GI and genitourinary disturbances, and they may be unwilling to continue taking these drugs.
- **α-adrenergic antagonists** inhibit the postsynaptic α_1-adrenergic receptors, decreasing sympathetic tone in the vasculature and causing vasodilation, which leads to a lowering of blood pressure. However, these drugs also block presynaptic α_2-receptors, preventing the feedback

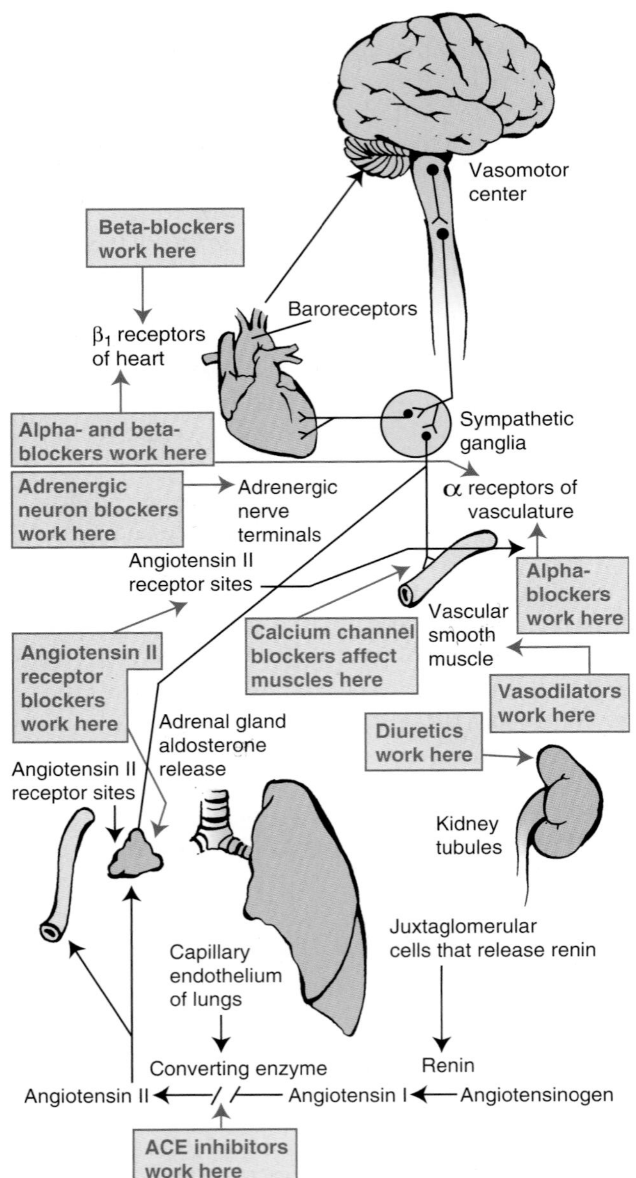

FIGURE 42.3 Sites of action of antihypertensive drugs.

control of adrenaline release. The result is an increase in the reflex tachycardia that occurs when blood pressure decreases. These drugs are used to diagnose and manage episodes of phaeochromocytoma, but they have limited usefulness in essential hypertension because of the associated adverse effects.

- **α_1-adrenergic antagonists** are used to treat hypertension because of their ability to block the postsynaptic α_1-receptor sites. This decreases vascular tone and promotes vasodilation, leading to a fall in blood pressure. These drugs do not block the presynaptic α_2-receptor sites and therefore the reflex tachycardia that accompanies a fall in blood pressure does not occur.
- **α_2-adrenergic agonists** stimulate the α_2-receptors in the CNS and inhibit the cardiovascular centres, leading to a decrease in sympathetic outflow from the CNS and a resultant drop in blood pressure. These drugs are associated with many adverse CNS and GI effects as well as cardiac dysrhythmias.

Vasodilators

If other drug therapies do not achieve the desired reduction in blood pressure, it is sometimes necessary to use a direct vasodilator. Vasodilators produce relaxation of the vascular smooth muscle, decreasing peripheral resistance and reducing blood pressure. They do not block the reflex tachycardia that occurs when blood pressure drops. Most of the vasodilators are reserved for use in severe hypertension or hypertensive emergencies. They are potent drugs, especially when used in combination with a β-blocker and a thiazide. The vasodilators that might be used to treat severe hypertension include the following:

- **Diazoxide** is used as an intravenous drug in hospitalized patients with severe hypertension. This drug also increases blood glucose levels by blocking insulin release, so it must be used with extreme caution with functional hypoglycaemia.
- **Hydralazine** is available for oral, intravenous and intramuscular use for the treatment of severe hypertension. It is thought to maintain or increase renal blood flow while relaxing smooth muscle.
- **Minoxidil** is an oral agent used only for the treatment of severe and unresponsive hypertension. It is associated with reflex tachycardia and increased renin release leading to volume increase (the oral drug is associated with changes in body hair growth and distribution, which led to a topical preparation for the treatment of baldness).
- **Sodium nitroprusside** is used intravenously for the treatment of hypertensive crisis and to maintain controlled hypotension during surgery; toxic levels cause cyanide toxicity.

Pharmacokinetics

These drugs are rapidly absorbed and widely distributed. They are metabolized in the liver and primarily excreted in urine. They cross the placenta and enter breast milk. They should not be used during pregnancy unless the benefit to the mother clearly outweighs the potential risk to the foetus. Do not use these drugs during lactation. If they are needed by a nursing mother, then another method of feeding the baby should be selected.

Contraindications and Cautions

The vasodilators are contraindicated in the presence of known allergy to the drug; with pregnancy and lactation, *because of the potential for adverse effects on the foetus or neonate* and with any condition that could be exacerbated by a sudden fall in blood pressure such as cerebral insufficiency. Caution should be used in patients with peripheral vascular disease, CAD, CHF or tachycardia, *all of which could be exacerbated by the fall in blood pressure.*

Adverse Effects

The adverse effects most frequently seen with these drugs are related to the changes in blood pressure. These include dizziness, anxiety and headache; reflex tachycardia, CHF, chest pain, oedema; skin rash and lesions (abnormal hair growth with minoxidil); and GI upset, nausea and vomiting. Cyanide toxicity (dyspnoea, headache, vomiting, dizziness, ataxia and loss of consciousness, imperceptible pulse, absent reflexes, dilated pupils, pink colour, distant heart sounds and shallow breathing) may occur with nitroprusside, which is metabolized to cyanide and which also suppresses iodine uptake and can cause hypothyroidism.

Clinically Important Drug–Drug Interactions

Each of these drugs works differently in the body, so before use, each drug should be checked for potential drug–drug interactions in the latest edition of the BNF.

Sympathetic Adrenergic Agonists

Sympathomimetic drugs bind to sympathetic adrenergic receptors to cause the following effects of a sympathetic stress response: increased blood pressure, increased blood volume

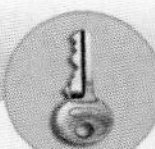

Key Drug Summary: *Sodium Nitroprusside*

Indications: Hypertensive crisis, maintenance of controlled hypotension during anaesthesia, acute or chronic CHF

Actions: Acts directly on vascular smooth muscle to cause vasodilation and drop of blood pressure, does not inhibit cardiovascular reflexes and tachycardia, renin release will occur

Pharmacokinetics:

Route	Onset	Peak	Duration
Intravenous	1–2 min	rapid	1–10 min

$T_{1/2}$: 2 minutes; metabolized in the liver and excretion in urine

Adverse effects: Associated with over rapid reduction in blood pressure. Apprehension, headache, retrosternal pressure, palpitations, cyanide toxicity, diaphoresis, nausea, vomiting, abdominal pain and irritation at the injection site

Abbreviations:
A = ACE inhibitor
(consider angiotensin-II receptor antagonist if ACE intolerant)
C = calcium-channel blocker
D = thiazide-type diuretic

Black patients are those of African or Caribbean descent, and not mixed-race, Asian or Chinese patients

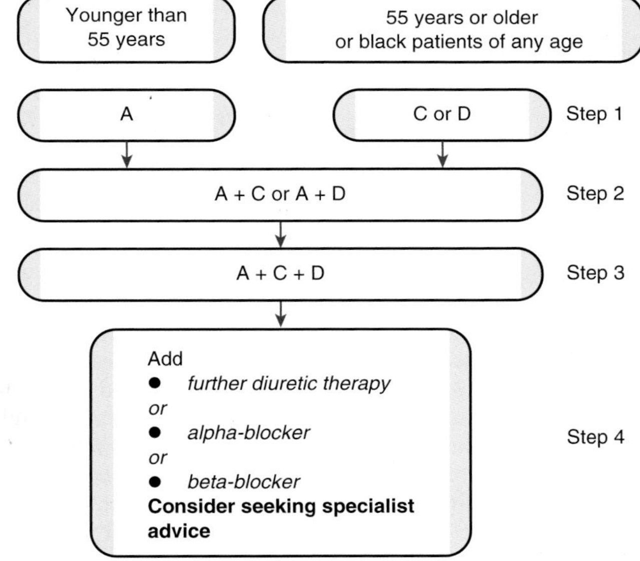

NHS
National Institute for Health and Clinical Excellence

FIGURE 42.4 Current guidelines on drug treatment for patients newly diagnosed with hypertension. Reproduced with permission from http://www.nice.org.uk

and increased strength of cardiac muscle contraction. These actions increase blood pressure and may restore balance to the cardiovascular system while the underlying cause of the shock (e.g. volume depletion and blood loss) is treated. The sympathomimetic drugs are discussed in Chapter 29 (see Box 42.3).

Adverse Effects

The most common adverse effects associated with this drug are related to the stimulation of α-receptors and include piloerection, chills and rash; hypertension and bradycardia; dizziness, vision changes, vertigo and headache; and problems with urination.

Clinically Important Drug–Drug Interactions

There is a risk of increased effects and toxicity of cardiac glycosides, β-antagonists, α-adrenergic agents and corticosteroids if they are taken with midodrine. Patients who are receiving any of these combinations should be monitored carefully for the need for a dosage adjustment.

BOX 42.3 Sympathomimetic Drugs Used to Treat Severe Hypotension and Shock

Sympathomimetic Drugs (see Chapter 29)

- dobutamine
- dopamine
- ephedrine
- epinephrine
- isoproterenol
- metaraminol

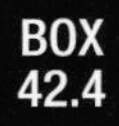

BOX 42.4 DRUG THERAPY ACROSS THE LIFESPAN

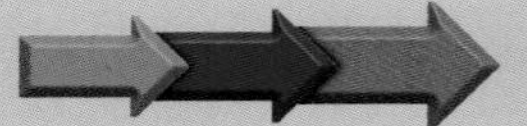

Drugs Affecting Blood Pressure

CHILDREN

National standards for determining normal levels of blood pressure in children are quite new. It has been determined that hypertension may start as a childhood disease and more screening studies are being done to establish normal values for each age group.

Children are thought to be more likely to have secondary hypertension caused by renal disease or congenital problems such as coarctation of the aorta.

Treatment of childhood hypertension should be done very cautiously because the long-term effects of the antihypertensive agents are not known. Lifestyle changes should be instituted before drug therapy if at all possible. Weight loss and increased activity may bring an elevated blood pressure back to normal in many children.

If drug therapy is used, a mild diuretic may be tried first, with monitoring of blood glucose and electrolyte levels on a regular basis. β-antagonists have been used with success in some children; adverse effects may limit their usefulness in others. The safety and efficacy of the ACE inhibitors and the ARBs have not been established in children. Calcium channel antagonists have been used to treat hypertension in children and may be a first consideration if drug therapy is needed. Careful follow-up of the growing child is essential to monitor for changes in blood pressure as well as adverse effects.

When administering any drug to children, always consult the most recent edition of the BNF for Children.

ADULTS

Adults receiving any of these drugs need to be instructed about adverse reactions that should be reported immediately. They need to be reminded of safety precautions that may be needed in hot weather or with conditions that cause fluid depletion (e.g. diarrhoea and vomiting). If they are taking any other drugs, the interacting effects of the various drugs should be evaluated. The importance of other measures to help lower blood pressure – weight loss, smoking cessation and increased activity – should be emphasized.

The safety for the use of these drugs during pregnancy has not been established. ACE inhibitors and ARBs should not be used during pregnancy and women of childbearing age should be advised to use barrier contraceptives to prevent pregnancy while taking these drugs. Calcium channel antagonists and vasodilators should not be used in pregnancy unless the benefit to the mother clearly outweighs the potential risk to the foetus. The drugs do enter breast milk and can have serious adverse effects on the baby. Caution should be used or another method of feeding the baby should be used if one of these drugs is needed during lactation. The main treatment for hypertension during pregnancy is the β-adrenoceptor blocking agent, labetalol; this drug also has arteriolar vasodilating action, which lowers TPR.

OLDER ADULTS

Older adults are frequently prescribed one of these drugs. They are more susceptible to the toxic effects of the drugs and are more likely to have underlying conditions that could interfere with drug metabolism and excretion. Renal or hepatic impairment can lead to accumulation of the drugs in the body. If the patient has renal or hepatic dysfunction, the dosage should be reduced and the patient monitored very closely.

The total drug regimen of the older patient should be co-ordinated, with careful attention to interactions among drugs and alternative therapies.

Older adults need to use special caution in any situation that could lead to a fall in blood pressure such as loss of fluids from diarrhoea or vomiting, lack of fluid intake or excessive heat with decreased sweating that comes with age. Dizziness, falls or syncope can occur if the blood pressure falls too far in these situations. The blood pressure should always be taken immediately before an antihypertensive is administered to an older adult to avoid excessive lowering of blood pressure.

Older patients should be especially cautioned about sustained-release antihypertensives that cannot be cut, crushed or chewed to avoid the potential for excessive dosing if these drugs are inappropriately cut.

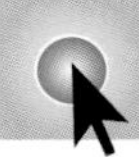

WEB LINKS

Health care providers and patients may want to consult the following Internet sources:

http://cks.library.nhs.uk The National Health Service Clinical Knowledge Summaries provides evidence-based practical information on the common conditions observed in primary care.

http://www.bhf.org.uk Patient information, support groups, diet, exercise and research information on hypertension and other cardiovascular diseases.

http://www.bnf.org.uk The BNF provides UK health care professionals with authoritative and practical information on the selection and clinical use of medicines.

http://www.nhsdirect.nhs.uk The National Health Service Direct service provides patients with information and advice about health, illness and health services.

http://www.nice.org.uk The National Institute for Health and Clinical Excellence provide guidelines and recommendations for tackling hypertension in England and Wales.

http://www.medscape.com Specific information on the care of the paediatric hypertensive patient; enter 'paediatric hypertension' in the search box.

Points to Remember

- The cardiovascular system is a closed system that depends on pressure differences to ensure the delivery of blood to the tissues and the return of that blood to the heart.
- Blood pressure is related to heart rate, stroke volume and the TPR against which the heart has to push the blood.
- Peripheral resistance is primarily controlled by constriction or relaxation of the arterioles. Constricted arterioles raise the pressure, whereas dilated arterioles lower the pressure.
- Control of blood pressure involves baroreceptor (pressure receptor) stimulation of the medulla to activate the sympathetic nervous system, which causes vasoconstriction and increased fluid retention when pressure is low in the aorta and carotid arteries and vasodilation and loss of fluid when pressure is too high.
- The kidneys activate the renin–angiotensin system when blood flow to the kidneys is decreased.
- Renin activates conversion of angiotensinogen to angiotensin I in the liver; angiotensin I is converted by ACE to angiotensin II in the lungs; angiotensin II then reacts with specific receptor sites on blood vessels to cause vasoconstriction to raise blood pressure and in the adrenal gland to cause release of aldosterone, which leads to retention of fluid and increased blood volume.
- Hypertension is a sustained state of higher-than-normal blood pressure that can lead to damage to blood vessels, increased risk of atherosclerosis and damage to small vessels in end organs. Hypertension often has no signs or symptoms; therefore, it may be referred to as the silent killer.
- Essential hypertension has no underlying cause and treatment can vary widely from individual to individual. Treatment approaches include lifestyle changes first, followed by careful addition and adjustment of various antihypertensive drugs.
- Drug treatment of hypertension is aimed at altering one or more of the normal reflexes that control blood pressure: diuretics decrease sodium levels and volume; ACE inhibitors prevent the conversion of angiotensin I to angiotensin II; ARBs prevent the body from responding to angiotensin II; calcium channel antagonists interfere with the ability of muscles to contract and lead to vasodilation; and vasodilators directly cause the relaxation of vascular smooth muscle and sympathetic nervous system drugs alter the sympathetic response and lead to vascular dilation and decreased pumping power of the heart.
- Hypotension is a state of lower-than-normal blood pressure that can result in decreased oxygenation of the tissues, cell death, tissue damage and even death. Hypotension is most often treated with sympathomimetic drugs, which stimulate the sympathetic receptor sites to cause vasoconstriction, fluid retention and return of normal pressure.

CRITICAL THINKING SCENARIO 42-1

Initiating Antihypertensive Therapy

The Situation

Clive a 65-year-old man was attending his general practitioner for a routine medical check-up. His examination was normal except for a blood pressure reading of 164/102 mmHg. He was also approximately 9 kg overweight. Urinalysis and blood results were all within normal limits. He was given a 1200-calorie-per-day diet to follow and was encouraged to reduce his salt and alcohol intake, start exercising and stop smoking. He was asked to return in 3 weeks for a follow-up appointment (step 1). Three weeks later, Clive returned with a 3.2 kg weight loss and an average blood pressure reading (of three readings) of 145/92 mm Hg. Discussion was held about starting Clive on a diuretic (step 2) in addition to the lifestyle changes that Clive was undertaking. He was reluctant to take a diuretic and after much discussion, was prescribed a calcium channel antagonist. Clive asked for a couple of more weeks to try to bring his blood pressure down with lifestyle changes before starting the drug.

Critical Thinking

- What nursing interventions should be done at this point? *Consider the risk factors that* Clive *has for hypertension and the damage that hypertension can cause.*
- What are the chances that Clive can bring his blood pressure within a normal range with lifestyle changes alone?
- What additional teaching points should be covered with Clive before a treatment decision is made?
- What effects could diuretic therapy have on Clive's day-to-day life?

Discussion

Clive was asked to change many things in his life over the last 3 weeks. These changes themselves can be stressful and can increase a person's blood pressure. Clive's reluctance to take a diuretic is understandable for a busy man who might not want his day interrupted by many bathroom stops. This may have an impact on Clive's work and home life. The decision to use a calcium channel antagonist may decrease some of the stress Clive was feeling about the diuretic.

Clive may benefit from trying for a couple more weeks to make lifestyle changes that will help bring his blood pressure into normal range. He will then feel that he has some control and input into the situation and if drug therapy is needed, he may be more willing to comply with the prescribed treatment. The diagnosis of hypertension may be delayed for these 2 weeks while Clive changes his lifestyle. Such a diagnosis should be made only after three consecutive blood pressure readings in the high range are recorded. Clive may be able to have his blood pressure checked at work in a comfortable environment, which will improve the accuracy of the reading.

Clive must receive regular follow-up and frequent blood pressure checks; it may be a good idea to allow him to take some control and continue lifestyle changes. If at the end of the 2 weeks no further progress has been made or Clive's blood pressure has risen, drug therapy should be considered. Teaching should be aimed at helping Clive to incorporate the drug effects into his lifestyle, to improve his compliance and tolerance of the therapy.

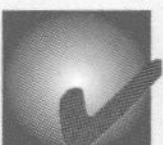

CHECK YOUR UNDERSTANDING

Answers to the questions in this chapter may be found in the Answer Key in the back of the book.

Multiple Choice

Select the most appropriate response to the following:

1. The baroreceptors are the most important factor in minute-to-minute control of blood pressure. The baroreceptors
   a. are evenly distributed throughout the body to maintain pressure in the system.
   b. sense pressure and immediately send that information to the medulla in the brain.
   c. are directly connected to the sympathetic nervous system.
   d. are as sensitive to oxygen levels as to pressure changes.

2. Essential hypertension is the most commonly diagnosed form of high blood pressure. It is usually
   a. caused by a tumour in the adrenal gland.
   b. associated with no known cause.
   c. related to renal disease.
   d. caused by liver dysfunction.

3. Hypertension is associated with
   a. loss of vision.
   b. strokes.
   c. atherosclerosis.
   d. all of the above.

4. The stepped-care approach to the treatment of hypertension would include
   a. lifestyle modification, including exercise, diet and decreased smoking and alcohol intake.
   b. use of a diuretic, beta-blocker, or ACE inhibitor to supplement lifestyle changes.
   c. a combination of antihypertensive drug classes to achieve desired control.
   d. all of the above.

5. ACE inhibitors work on the renin–angiotensin system to prevent the conversion of angiotensin I to angiotensin II. Because this blocking occurs in the cells in the lung, which is usually the site of this conversion, use of ACE inhibitors often results in
   a. spontaneous pneumothorax.
   b. pneumonia.
   c. unrelenting cough.
   d. respiratory depression.

6. A client taking an ACE inhibitor is scheduled for surgery. The nurse should
   a. stop the drug.
   b. alert the surgeon and mark the client's chart prominently, because the blockage of compensatory angiotensin II could result in hypotension after surgery that would need to be reversed with volume expansion.
   c. cancel the surgery and consult with the prescriber.
   d. monitor fluid levels and make the sure the fluids are restricted before surgery.

7. A patient who is hypertensive becomes pregnant. The drug of choice for this patient would be
   a. an angiotensin II receptor blocker.
   b. an ACE inhibitor.
   c. a diuretic.
   d. a calcium channel blocker.

Extending Matching Questions

Select all that apply.

1. Pressure within the vascular system is determined by which of the following?
   a. Peripheral resistance
   b. Stroke volume
   c. Sodium load
   d. Heart rate
   e. Total intravascular volume
   f. Rate of erythropoietin release

2. The renin–angiotensin system is associated with which of the following?
   a. Intense vasoconstriction and blood pressure elevation
   b. Blood flow through the kidneys
   c. Production of surfactant in the lungs
   d. Release of aldosterone from the adrenal cortex
   e. Retention of sodium and water in the kidneys
   f. Liver production of fibrinogen

Matching

Match the following drugs with their appropriate class of antihypertensive agents. (Some classes may be used more than once.)

1. ____________________ candesartan
2. ____________________ quinapril
3. ____________________ losartan
4. ____________________ nitroprusside
5. ____________________ lisinopril
6. ____________________ valsartan

7. ____________________ nicardipine
8. ____________________ minoxidil
9. ____________________ amlodipine

A. ACE inhibitor
B. Angiotensin II receptor antagonist
C. Calcium channel antagonist
D. Vasodilator
E. Ganglionic antagonist

True or False

Indicate whether the following statements are true (T) or false (F).

_____ 1. The cardiovascular system is an open system that depends on pressure differences to ensure the delivery of blood.

_____ 2. Blood pressure is related to heart rate, stroke volume and the TPR.

_____ 3. Constricted arterioles lower pressure; dilated arterioles raise pressure.

_____ 4. Control of blood pressure involves baroreceptor (pressure receptor) stimulation of the medulla to activate the parasympathetic nervous system.

_____ 5. The kidneys activate the renin–angiotensin system when blood flow to the kidneys is decreased.

_____ 6. Renin activates angiotensinogen to angiotensin I in the lung using ACE.

_____ 7. Hypertension is a sustained state of higher-than-normal blood pressure.

_____ 8. Essential hypertension has no underlying cause and treatment can vary widely.

_____ 9. Angiotensin II receptor antagonists prevent the body from responding to angiotensin II and blocking calcium channels.

_____ 10. Hypotension can result in decreased oxygenation of the tissues, cell death, tissue damage and even death.

Bibliography and References

British Medical Association and Royal Pharmaceutical Society of Great Britain. (2008). *British National Formulary*. London: BMJ & RPS Publishing. *This publication is updated biannually, it is imperative that the most recent edition is consulted.*

British Medical Association and Royal Pharmaceutical Society of Great Britain. (2008). *British National Formulary for Children*. London: BMJ & RPS Publishing. *This publication is updated annually, it is imperative that the most recent edition is consulted.*

Ganong, W. (2005). *Review of medical physiology* (22nd ed.). New York: McGraw-Hill.

Howland, R. D., & Mycek, M. J. (2005). *Pharmacology* (3rd ed.). Philadelphia: Lippincott Williams & Wilkins.

Marieb, E. N., & Hoehn, K. (2004). *Human anatomy & physiology* (7th ed.). San Francisco: Pearson Benjamin Cummings.

Porth, C. M., & Matfin G. (2008). *Pathophysiology: concepts of altered health states* (8th ed.). Philadelphia: Lippincott Williams & Wilkins.

Simonsen, T., Aarbakke, J., Kay, I., Coleman, I., Sinnott, P., & Lysaa, R. (2006). *Illustrated pharmacology for nurses.* London: Hodder Arnold.

CHAPTER 43

Inotropic Agents

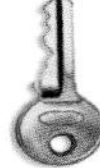

KEY TERMS

actin
baroreceptor
cardiomegaly
cardiomyopathy
congestive heart failure (CHF)
dyspnoea
haemoptysis
myosin
nocturia
orthopnoea
positive inotropic
pulmonary oedema
tachypnoea
troponin

LEARNING OBJECTIVES

Upon completion of this chapter, you will be able to:

1. Describe the pathophysiological process of heart failure and the resultant clinical signs.
2. Explain the body's compensatory mechanisms when heart failure occurs.
3. Describe the therapeutic actions, indications and pharmacokinetics associated with the cardiac glycosides, the phosphodiesterase inhibitors and the digoxin antidote.
4. Describe the contraindications, most common adverse reactions and important drug–drug interactions associated with the cardiac glycosides, the phosphodiesterase inhibitors and the digoxin antidote.
5. Discuss the use of inotropic agents across the lifespan.
6. Compare and contrast the key drugs digoxin and enoximone and digoxin-specific antibody fragments.
7. Outline the nursing considerations, including important teaching points, for patients receiving inotropic agents.

CARDIAC GLYCOSIDES

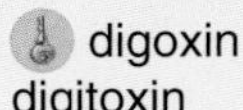

digoxin
digitoxin

PHOSPHODIESTERASE INHIBITORS

enoximone
milrinone

DIGOXIN ANTIDOTE

digoxin-specific antibody fragments

Congestive heart failure (CHF) is an 'umbrella term' used to describe conditions in which the heart fails to effectively pump blood around the body. The cardiac cycle normally involves a tight balance between the pumping of the right and left sides of the heart. Any failure of the muscle to pump blood out of either side of the heart will result in an inadequate perfusion of the body's tissues, and the cells become deprived of oxygen and nutrients and waste products build up in the tissues. The primary treatment for CHF involves helping the heart muscle to contract more efficiently to bring the system back into balance. A diagnosis of 'heart failure (HF)' can be associated with a 50% mortality rate over 5 years (Levy *et al.*, 2002).

Review of Cardiac Muscle Function

The underlying problem in CHF usually involves muscle function:

(1) the muscle could be damaged by atherosclerosis or **cardiomyopathy** (a disease of the heart muscle that leads to an enlarged heart and eventually to complete muscle failure and death);

(2) the muscle could be forced to work too hard to maintain an efficient output, as with hypertension or valvular disease;

(3) the structure of the heart could be abnormal, as with congenital cardiac defects.

The basic unit of the heart muscle, the sarcomere, contains two contractile proteins, **actin** and **myosin**, which are highly reactive with each other but at rest are kept apart by **troponin**. When a cardiac muscle cell is stimulated, calcium enters the cell and inactivates the troponin, allowing the actin and myosin to form actomyosin bridges. The formation of these bridges allows the muscle fibres to slide together or contract (Figure 43.1) (see Chapter 41 for a review of heart muscle contraction processes).

The contraction process requires energy, oxygen and calcium to allow the formation of the actin–myosin bridges. The degree of shortening, or the strength of contraction, is determined by the amount of calcium present (the more calcium present, the more bridges will be formed) and by the stretch of the sarcomere before contraction begins (the further apart the actin and myosin proteins are before the cell is stimulated, the more bridges will be formed and the stronger the contraction will be). This correlates with Starling's law of the heart: *the more the cardiac muscle is stretched,*

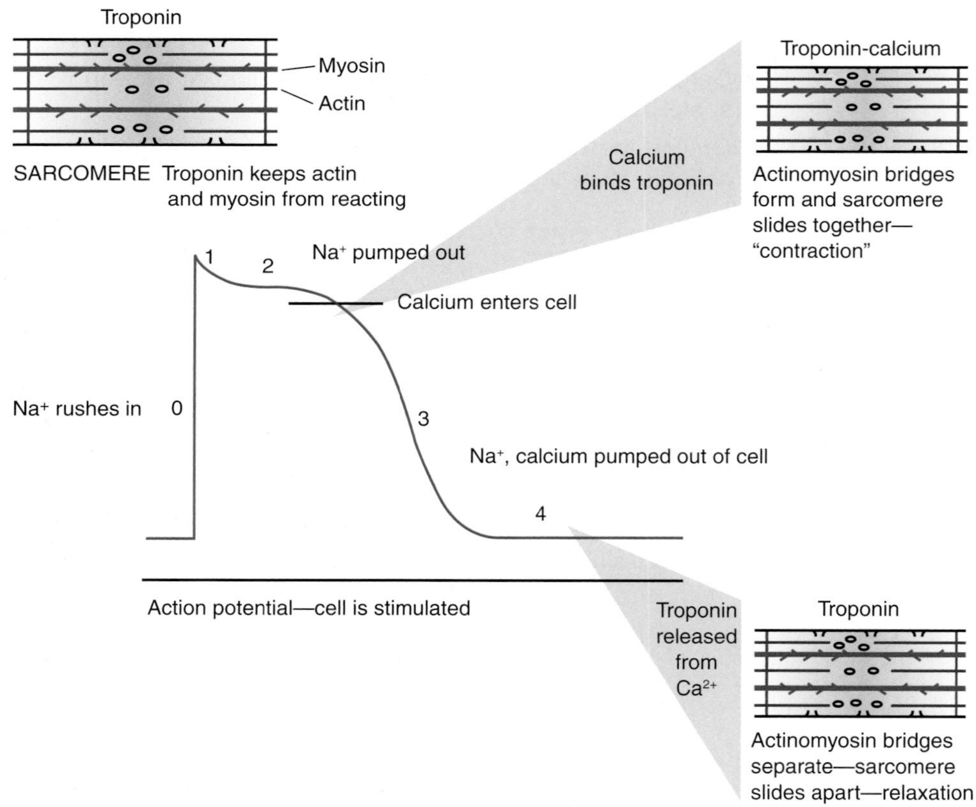

FIGURE 43.1 The sliding filaments of myocardial muscles. Calcium entering the cell deactivates troponin and allows actin and myosin to react, causing contraction. Calcium pumped out of the cell frees troponin to separate actin and myosin; the sarcomere filament slides apart and the cell relaxes.

the greater the contraction will be. The more blood you put into the heart, the greater the contraction will be to empty the heart, up to a point. If the bridges are stretched too far apart, they will not be able to reach each other to form the actin–myosin bridges, and no contraction will occur. This extreme response can be seen with severe cardiomyopathy: the muscle cells are stretched and distorted and eventually stop contracting because they can no longer respond.

Congestive Heart Failure

CHF is a condition that can occur with any of the disorders that damage or overwork the heart muscle.

- Coronary artery disease (CAD) is the leading cause of CHF in the UK, accounting for approximately 70% (National HF audit 2008; see Chapter 46 for a discussion of CAD). CAD results in an insufficient supply of blood to meet the oxygen demands of the myocardium. Consequently, the muscles become hypoxic and can no longer function efficiently. When CAD evolves into a myocardial infarction (MI), muscle cells die or are damaged, leading to an inefficient pumping effort.
- Cardiomyopathy can occur as a result of a viral infection, alcoholism, postpartum, anabolic steroid abuse or a collagen disorder. It causes muscle alterations and ineffective contraction and pumping.
- Hypertension eventually leads to an enlarged cardiac muscle because the heart has to work harder than normal to pump against the high pressure in the arteries. Hypertension puts constant, increased demands for oxygen on the system because the heart is pumping so hard all the time.
- Valvular heart disease leads to an overload of the ventricles because the valves do not close tightly, which allows blood to leak backward into the ventricles. This overloading causes muscle stretching and increased demand for oxygen and energy as the heart muscle has to constantly contract harder (valvular heart disease is rarely seen today owing to the success of cardiac surgery and effective treatment for rheumatic fever).

The end result of all of these conditions is that the heart muscle cannot pump blood effectively throughout the vascular system.

- If the left ventricle pumps inefficiently, blood backs up into the lungs, causing pulmonary vessel congestion and fluid leakage into the alveoli and lung tissue. In severe cases, **pulmonary oedema** [wheezes, blood-tinged sputum, low oxygenation, development of a third heart sound (S3)] can occur.
- If the right side of the heart is the primary problem, blood backs up in the venous system leading to the right side of the heart. Liver congestion and oedema of the legs and feet reflect right-sided failure. As the cardiovascular system works as a closed system, one-sided failure, if left untreated, eventually leads to failure of both sides, and the signs and symptoms of total CHF occur.

Compensatory Mechanisms in Congestive Heart Failure

The body has several compensatory mechanisms that function if the heart muscle starts to fail (Figure 43.2). Decreased cardiac output stimulates the **baroreceptors** in the aortic arch and the carotid sinus arteries, causing sympathetic stimulation (see Chapter 28). This sympathetic stimulation causes an increase in heart rate, blood pressure and rate and depth of respirations, as well as a **positive inotropic** effect (increased force of contraction) on the heart and an increase in blood volume (through the release of aldosterone). The decrease in cardiac output also stimulates the release of renin from the kidneys and activates the renin–angiotensin system, which further increases blood pressure and blood volume.

If these compensatory mechanisms are working effectively, the patient may have no signs or symptoms of CHF and is said to be compensated. Over time, however, all of these effects increase the workload of the heart, contributing to further development of CHF. Eventually, the heart muscle stretches from overwork and the chambers of the

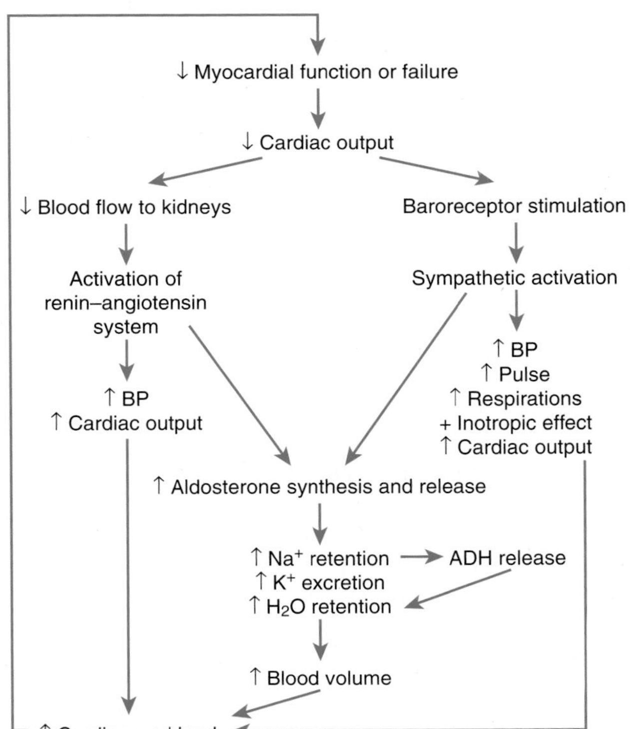

FIGURE 43.2 Compensatory mechanisms in congestive heart failure (CHF), which lead to increased cardiac workload and further CHF. ADH, antidiuretic hormone; BP, blood pressure; P, pulse.

heart dilate secondary to the increased blood volume that they have to handle. This hypertrophy (enlargement) of the heart muscle leads to inefficient pumping and eventually to an increased CHF.

Cellular Changes in Congestive Heart Failure

The function of myocardial cells is affected with prolonged CHF. Unlike healthy heart cells, the cells of the failing heart seem to lack the ability to produce energy and use it for effective contractions. They are no longer able to effectively move calcium ions into and out of the cell. This defect in the calcium movement process may lead to further deterioration because the muscle contracts ineffectively and is unable to deliver blood to the cardiac muscle itself.

Signs and Symptoms of Congestive Heart Failure

Hypertrophy of the heart muscle can be detected using radiography, electrocardiography or direct percussion and palpation. The heart rate will be rapid secondary to sympathetic stimulation, and the patient may develop atrial flutter or fibrillation as atrial cells are stretched and damaged. Anxiety often occurs as the body stimulates the sympathetic stress reaction. Heart murmurs may develop when the muscle is no longer able to support the papillary muscles or the annuli supporting the cardiac valves. Peripheral congestion and oedema occur as the blood starts to engorge vessels as it waits to be pumped through the heart. The result is an enlarged liver (hepatomegaly), enlarged spleen (splenomegaly), decreased blood flow to the gastrointestinal (GI) tract causing feelings of nausea and abdominal pain, swollen legs and feet and dependent oedema in the coccyx or other dependent areas, with decreased peripheral pulses and hypoxia of those tissues. With left-sided failure, oedema of the lungs reflected in engorged vessels and increased hydrostatic pressure throughout the cardiovascular system are also seen. **Cardiomegaly** or enlargement of the heart may occur as the heart muscle increases in size to accommodate the increase in hydrostatic pressure (Figure 43.3).

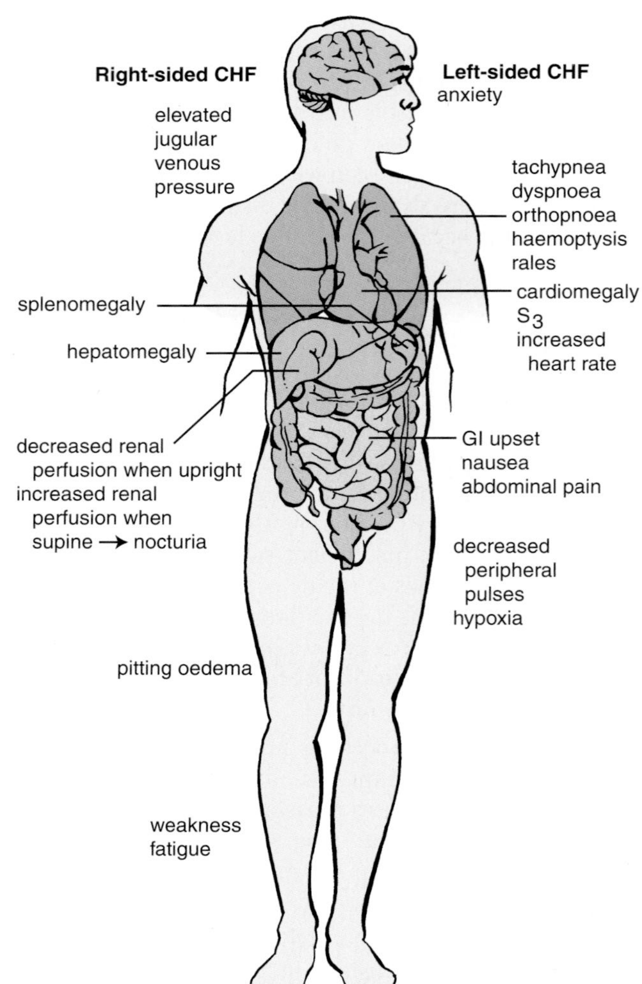

FIGURE 43.3 Signs and symptoms of congestive heart failure (CHF).

Left-Sided Congestive Heart Failure

Left-sided CHF reflects engorgement of the pulmonary veins, which eventually leads to difficulty in breathing. Patients complain of **tachypnoea** (rapid, shallow respiration), **dyspnoea** (discomfort with breathing often accompanied by a panicked feeling of being unable to breathe); and **orthopnoea** (increased difficulty in breathing when lying down). Orthopnoea occurs in the supine position, as the fluid in the lungs will affect a greater surface area of lung tissue (due to gravity) impairing gaseous exchange (Figure 43.4). Orthopnoea is usually relieved when the patient sits up, thereby reducing the blood flow through the lungs. The degree of CHF is often calculated by the number of pillows required to get relief (e.g. one-pillow, two-pillow or three-pillow orthopnoea).

The patient with left-sided CHF may also experience coughing and **haemoptysis** (coughing up of the blood).

Right-sided Congestive Heart Failure

Right-sided CHF usually occurs as a result of chronic obstructive pulmonary disease (COPD) or other lung diseases that elevate the pulmonary pressure. It often results when the right side of the heart, normally a very low-pressure system, must generate more and more force to move the blood into the lungs (Figure 43.5).

In right-sided CHF, venous return to the heart is decreased because of the increased pressure in the right side of the heart. This causes a congestion and backup of blood in the systemic system. Jugular venous pressure (JVP) rises and can be seen in distended neck veins, reflecting increased central venous pressure (CVP). The liver enlarges and becomes congested with blood, which

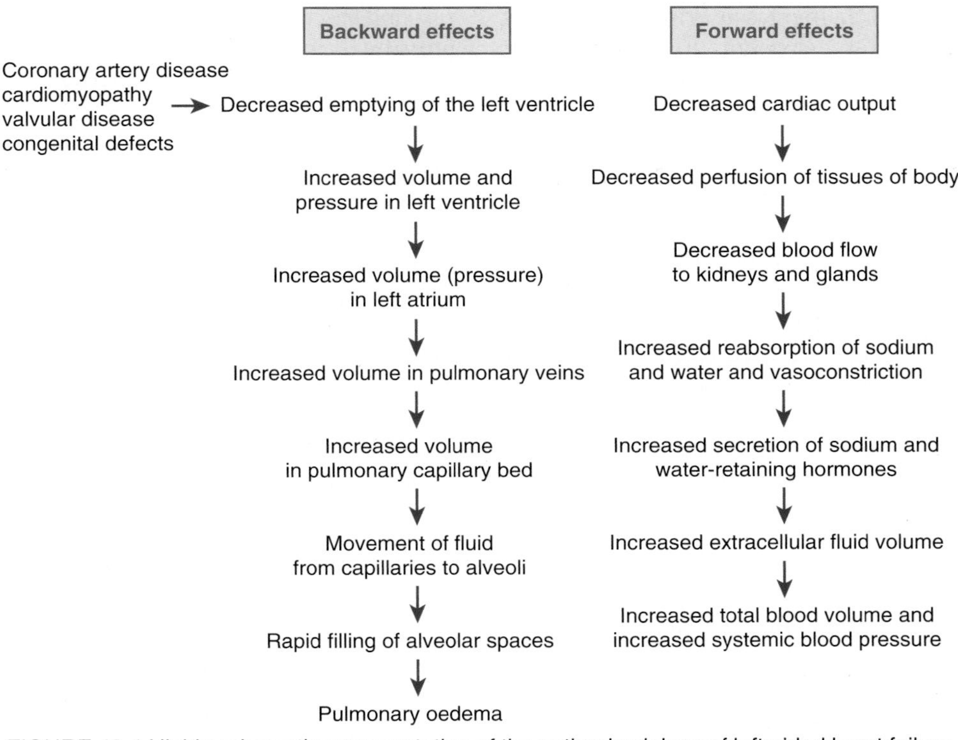

FIGURE 43.4 Highly schematic representation of the pathophysiology of left-sided heart failure.

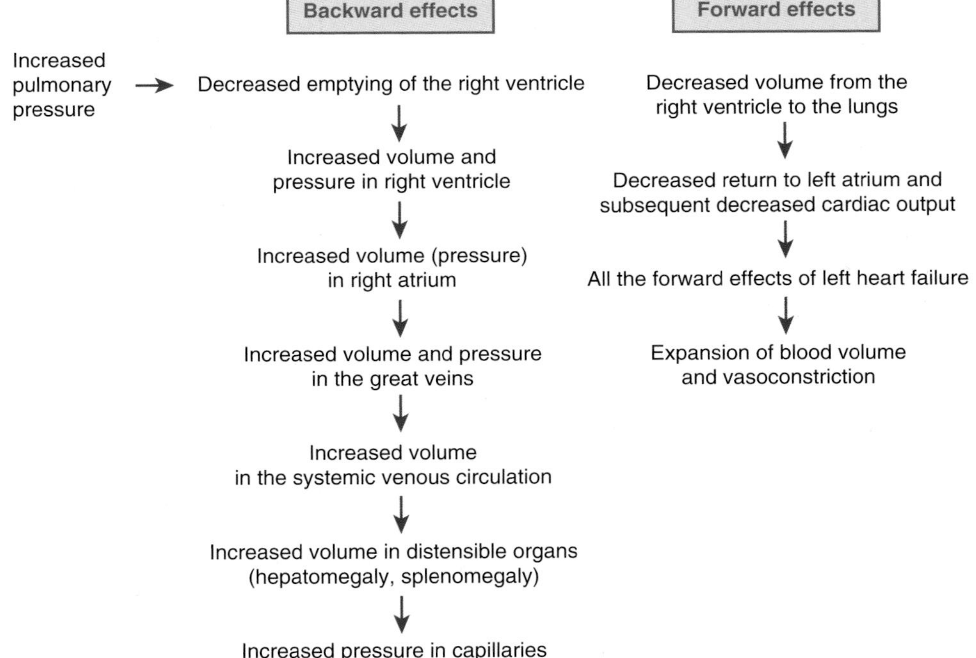

FIGURE 43.5 Highly schematic representation of the pathophysiology of right-sided heart failure.

leads initially to pain and tenderness and eventually to liver dysfunction and jaundice.

Dependent areas develop oedema or swelling of the tissues as fluid leaves the congested blood vessels and pools in the tissues. Pitting oedema in the legs is a common finding, reflecting a pool of fluid in the tissues. When the patient with right-sided CHF changes position and the legs are no longer dependent, for example, the fluid will be pulled back into circulation and returned to the heart. This increase in cardiovascular volume increases blood flow to the kidneys, causing increased urine output. This is often seen as **nocturia** (excessive micturition during the night) in a person who is up and around during the day and supine at night. The person may need to get up during the night to eliminate all the urine produced as a result of the fluid shift.

Treatments for Congestive Heart Failure

Several different approaches are used to treat CHF. This chapter focuses on the inotropic drugs (also called **positive inotropic drugs**) that work to directly increase the force of cardiac muscle contraction. Other drug therapies used to treat CHF are discussed in other chapters and are only briefly mentioned here.

Vasodilators

Vasodilators [angiotensin-converting enzyme (ACE) inhibitors and nitrates] are used to treat CHF because they can decrease the workload of the overworked cardiac muscle. By relaxing vascular smooth muscle, these drugs decrease the pressure the heart has to pump against (afterload). They also cause a pooling of blood in stretchable veins (usually the large capacitance vessels in the legs) when the vessels relax, decreasing the venous return to the heart and decreasing the preload on the heart muscle.

ACE inhibitors block the enzyme that converts angiotensin I to angiotensin II in the lungs, thus blocking the vasoconstriction and the release of aldosterone from the adrenal gland caused by angiotensin II (Figure 43.6). This in turn decreases the afterload by relieving vasoconstriction and by reducing blood volume through its effects on decreasing the release of aldosterone, which also decreases the afterload. ACE inhibitors are the vasodilators of choice in treating CHF. They are most effective in mild CHF and in patients who are at high risk of developing of CHF or who have only initial signs and symptoms.

Nitrates directly relax vascular muscle (by the production of nitric oxide) and cause a decrease in blood pressure and a pooling of blood in the veins (see Figure 43.6). These two actions also decrease preload and afterload. Nitrates are often used to treat more severe CHF (see Chapters 42 and 45 for additional information).

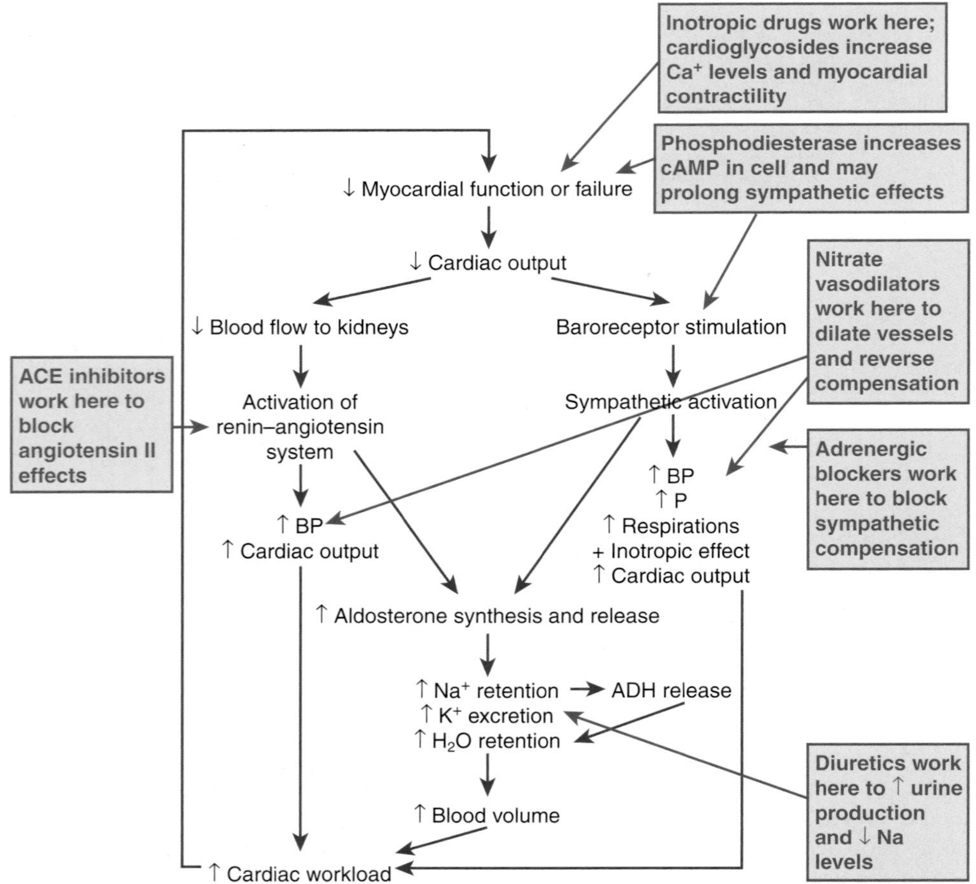

FIGURE 43.6 Sites of action of drugs used to treat congestive heart failure (CHF).

Diuretics

Diuretics are used to decrease blood volume, which decreases venous return and blood pressure (see Figure 43.6). The end result is a decrease in afterload and preload and a decrease in the heart's workload. Diuretics are available in mild-to-potent compounds and are frequently used as adjunctive therapy in the treatment of all degrees of CHF (see Chapter 50 for additional information.)

β-Adrenergic Agonists

β-Adrenergic agonists stimulate the β-adrenoceptors in the sympathetic nervous system, increasing calcium flow into the myocardial cells and causing increased contraction, a positive inotropic effect (see Figure 43.6). Other sympathetic stimulation effects can cause increased CHF because the heart's workload is increased by most sympathetic activity. Dobutamine is the β-agonist most frequently used to treat CHF. However, it must be given by intravenous infusion in an acute care setting and it is usually reserved for treatment of acute CHF (see Chapter 29 for additional information).

Inotropic Drugs

Inotropic drugs affect the intracellular calcium levels in the heart muscle, leading to increased contractility. This increase in contraction strength leads to increased cardiac output, which causes increased renal blood flow and increased urine production. Increased renal blood flow decreases renin release, reducing the effects of the renin–angiotensin system and increasing urine output, leading to decreased blood volume. Together, these effects decrease the heart's workload and help to relieve CHF. Two types of inotropic drugs are used: the classic cardiac glycosides, which have been used for hundreds of years and the newer phosphodiesterase inhibitors. See Box 43.1 for the use of inotropic drugs in different age groups.

Cardiac Glycosides

The cardiac glycosides were originally derived from the foxglove or digitalis plant. Today, digoxin is the drug most often used to treat CHF; it has a very rapid onset of action and is available for parenteral and oral use. It is excreted unchanged in the urine, making it a safe drug for patients

BOX 43.1 DRUG THERAPY ACROSS THE LIFESPAN

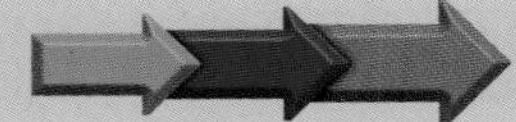

Inotropic Agents

CHILDREN

Paediatric and older adult patients are at increased risk for digoxin toxicity. Individuals in both of these groups have body masses that are smaller than the average adult body mass and they may have immature or ageing kidneys. Digoxin is excreted unchanged in the kidneys, so any change in kidney function can result in increased serum digoxin levels and subsequent digoxin toxicity. Extreme care should be taken when administering digoxin to patients in either of these age groups.

Digoxin is used widely in children with heart defects and related cardiac problems. The margin of safety for the dosage of the drug is very small with children. The dosage needs to be very carefully calculated and should be double-checked by another nurse before administration. Children should be monitored closely for any sign of impending digitalis toxicity and should have serum digoxin levels monitored

The phosphodiesterase inhibitors are not recommended for use in children.

When administering any drug to children, always consult the most recent edition of the British National Formulary for Children.

ADULTS

Adults receiving any of these drugs need to be taught to identify adverse reactions and instructed as to what adverse reactions to report immediately. They should learn to take their own pulse and should be encouraged to keep track of rate and regularity on a calendar. They may be asked to weigh themselves in the same clothing and at the same time of the day to monitor for fluid retention. Any changes in diet, gastrointestinal activity or medications should be reported to the health care provider because of the potential for altering serum levels and causing toxic reactions or ineffective dosing. Adults should also be monitored for digoxin toxicity.

Patients should be advised against switching between brands of digoxin because there have been reports of different bioavailabilities, leading to toxic reactions.

The safety of these drugs during pregnancy has not been established. They should not be used in pregnancy unless the benefit to the mother clearly outweighs the potential risk to the foetus. The drugs do enter breast milk, but they have not been associated with any adverse effects in the neonate.

OLDER ADULTS

Older adults are frequently prescribed one of these drugs. They are more susceptible to the toxic effects of the drugs and are more likely to have underlying conditions that could interfere with their metabolism and excretion.

Renal impairment can lead to accumulation of digoxin in the body. If renal dysfunction is present, the dosage needs to be reduced and the patient monitored very closely for signs of digoxin toxicity.

The total drug regimen of the older patient should be coordinated, with careful attention to interacting drugs or alternative therapies.

As a precaution, in situations of stress or illness, a significant other person should be instructed in how to take the patient's pulse and the adverse effects to watch for while the patient is taking this drug.

BOX 43.2 Digoxin Antidote: Digoxin-specific Antibody Fragments

Digoxin is an antigen-binding fragment derived from specific antidigoxin antibodies. These antibodies bind molecules of digoxin, making them unavailable at their site of action. The digoxin antibody–antigen complexes accumulate in the blood and are excreted through the kidney. Digoxin-specific antibody fragments are used for the treatment of life-threatening digoxin intoxication (serum levels >10 ng/ml with serum potassium >5 mEq/l in a setting of digoxin intoxication) and potential life-threatening digoxin overdose.

The amount of digoxin-specific antibody fragments that is infused intravenously is determined by the amount of digoxin ingested or by the serum digoxin level if the ingested amount is unknown. The patient's cardiac status should be monitored continually while the drug is given and for several hours after the infusion is finished. There is a risk of hypersensitivity reaction to the infused protein; therefore life-support equipment should be on standby.

Serum digoxin levels will be very high and unreliable for about 3 days after the digoxin-specific antibody fragments infusion because of the high levels of digoxin in the blood. The patient should not be re-treated with digoxin for several days to 1 week after digoxin-specific antibody fragments has been used because of the potential of remaining fragments in the blood.

with liver dysfunction. Digoxin is the most important of the cardiac glycosides. Used in HF, particularly where it is associated with atrial fibrillation. Digoxin has a very narrow therapeutic window (meaning that the therapeutic dose is very close to the toxic dose), so extreme care must be taken when using this drug. Digoxin toxicity is a real possibility in clinical practice because of the narrow margin of safety. A digoxin antidote, digoxin-specific antibody fragments, has been developed to rapidly treat digoxin toxicity (see Box 43.2).

Therapeutic Actions and Indications

Digoxin increases intracellular calcium and allows more calcium to enter myocardial cells during depolarization (see Figure 43.6). The change in ion movements, coupled with effects on the autonomic nervous system, accounts for changes to the function of the heart's conduction system. The cardiac glycosides enhance parasympathetic stimulation of the heart. The outcome, in terms of cardiac function, is that the rate of impulse generation by the sinoatrial node is decreased. Any change in heart rate is known as a chronotrophic effect; a decreased rate is a negative chronotrophic effect. Such an effect is desirable because the excessive sympathetic stimulation characterizing CHF causes a rapid irregular pulse. The conduction velocity through the atrioventricular (AV) node and ventricles decreases as does the number of impulses transmitted through the former. This, in effect, means that the interval between contraction of the atria and contraction of the ventricles increases. An increase in this interval allows more time for the ventricles to fill with blood (Galbraith *et al.*, 1997).

In summary, the cardiac glycosides will cause the following effects:

- Increased force of myocardial contraction (a positive inotropic effect).
- Increased cardiac output and renal perfusion (which has a diuretic effect, increasing urine output and decreasing blood volume while decreasing renin release and activation of the renin–angiotensin system).
- Slowed heart rate, owing to slowing of the rate of cellular repolarization (a negative chronotrophic effect).
- Decreased conduction velocity through the AV node.

The overall effect is a decrease in the myocardial workload and relief of CHF. The cardiac glycosides are indicated for the treatment of advanced CHF, atrial flutter, atrial fibrillation and paroxysmal atrial tachycardia. Digoxin improves symptoms of HF and exercise tolerance and reduces hospitalization due to acute exacerbations but it does not reduce mortality. Digoxin is reserved for patients with atrial fibrillation and also for selected patients in sinus rhythm who remain symptomatic despite treatment with an ACE inhibitor, a β-blocker, and a diuretic

Pharmacokinetics

Digoxin is rapidly absorbed and widely distributed throughout the body. Digoxin is primarily excreted unchanged in the urine. Caution should be used in the presence of renal impairment because the drug may not be excreted and could accumulate, causing toxicity. It is not known whether digoxin causes foetal toxicity; it should be given during pregnancy only if the benefit to the mother clearly outweighs the risk to the foetus. Digoxin does enter breast milk, but it has not been shown to cause problems for the neonate. However, caution should be taken, during lactation.

Contraindications and Cautions

Cardiac glycosides are also contraindicated in the following conditions: ventricular tachycardia or fibrillation, *which are potentially fatal arrhythmias and should be treated with other drugs*; heart block or sick sinus syndrome, *which could be made worse by slowing of conduction through the AV node*; idiopathic hypertrophic subaortic stenosis (IHSS), *because the increase in force of contraction could obstruct the outflow tract to the aorta and cause severe problems*; acute MI, *because the increase in force of contraction could cause more muscle damage and infarct*; renal insufficiency, *because the drug is excreted through the kidneys and toxic levels could develop* and electrolyte abnormalities (e.g. increased calcium, decreased potassium, decreased magnesium), *which could alter the action potential and change the effects of the drug.*

Cardiac glycosides should be used cautiously in patients who are pregnant or lactating *because of the potential for adverse effects on the foetus or neonate, expert advice should always be sought.* Paediatric and older adult patients are also at higher risk (see Box 43.1).

Adverse Effects

The adverse effects most frequently seen with the cardiac glycosides include headache, weakness, drowsiness and vision changes (a yellow aura around objects is often reported with digoxin toxicity). GI upset and anorexia also commonly occur. A risk of developing arrhythmia exists because the glycosides affect the action potential and conduction system of the heart.

Always consult a current copy of the British National Formulary for further guidance.

Clinically Important Drug–Drug Interactions

There is a risk of increased therapeutic effects and toxic effects of digoxin if it is taken with verapamil, amiodarone, quinidine, quinine, erythromycin, tetracycline or cyclosporine. If digoxin is combined with any of these drugs, it may be necessary to decrease the digoxin dose to prevent toxicity. If one of these drugs has been part of a medical regimen with digoxin and is discontinued, the digoxin dose may need to be increased. The risk of cardiac arrhythmias could increase if these drugs are taken with potassium-losing diuretics. If this combination is used, the patient's potassium levels should be checked regularly and appropriate replacement done. Digoxin may be less effective if it is combined with thyroid hormones or penicillamine, and increased digoxin dosage may be needed.

Absorption of oral digoxin may be decreased if it is taken with cholestyramine, charcoal, colestipol, bleomycin or methotrexate. If it is used in combination with any of these agents, the drugs should not be taken at the same time, but should be administered 2 to 4 hours apart. See Box 43.3 for information about the interactions between digoxin and common herbal remedies.

Always consult a current copy of the British National Formulary for further guidance.

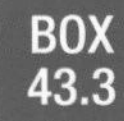

HERBAL AND ALTERNATIVE THERAPIES

St. John's wort and psyllium have been shown to decrease the effectiveness of digoxin; this combination should be avoided. Increased digoxin toxicity has been reported with ginseng, hawthorn and liquorice. Patients should be advised to avoid these combinations.

Phosphodiesterase Inhibitors

The phosphodiesterase inhibitors belong to a second class of drugs that act as inotropic (cardiotonic) agents. Milrinone is available only for intravenous use for the short-term management of CHF in patients unresponsive to conventional maintenance therapy, who are receiving digoxin and diuretics. Enoximone is also used to treat CHF. It is used when cardiac output is reduced and filling pressures are increased. These drugs have been associated with the development of potentially fatal ventricular arrhythmias; therefore, their use is limited to severe situations.

Therapeutic Actions and Indications

The phosphodiesterase inhibitors block the enzyme phosphodiesterase. This blocking effect leads to an increase in myocardial cell cyclic adenosine monophosphate (cAMP), which increases calcium levels in the cell (see Figure 43.6). Increased cellular calcium causes a stronger contraction and prolongs the effects of sympathetic stimulation, which can lead to vasodilation, increased oxygen consumption and arrhythmias. These drugs are indicated for the short-term treatment of CHF that has not responded to digoxin or diuretics alone or that has had a poor response to digoxin, diuretics and vasodilators.

Pharmacokinetics

These drugs are widely distributed after injection. They are metabolized in the liver and excreted primarily in the urine. There are no adequate studies about the effects of these drugs during pregnancy and their use should be reserved for situations in which the benefit to the mother clearly outweighs the potential risk to the foetus. It is not known whether these drugs enter breast milk, so caution should be used if patient is breast-feeding.

Contraindications and Cautions

Phosphodiesterase inhibitors are contraindicated in the presence of allergy to either of these drugs or to bisulphites. They are also contraindicated in the following conditions: severe aortic or pulmonary valvular disease, *which could be exacerbated by increased contraction*; acute MI, *which could be exacerbated by increased oxygen consumption and increased force of contraction;* fluid volume deficit, *which could be made worse by increased renal perfusion* and ventricular arrhythmias, *which could be exacerbated by these drugs.*

Adverse Effects

The adverse effects most frequently seen with these drugs are ventricular arrhythmias (which can progress to fatal ventricular fibrillation), hypotension and chest pain. GI effects include nausea, vomiting, anorexia and abdominal pain. Thrombocytopaenia can occur with milrinone. Hypersensitivity reactions associated with these drugs include vasculitis, pericarditis, pleuritis and ascites. Burning at the injection site is also a frequent adverse effect.

Clinically Important Drug–Drug Interactions

Precipitates form when these drugs are given in solution with furosemide. Avoid this combination in solution. Use alternate lines if both of these drugs are being given intravenously.

Always consult a current copy of the British National Formulary for further guidance.

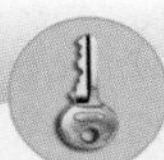

Key Drug Summary: *Digoxin*

Indications: Treatment of advanced CHF who remain symptomatic with optimal other HF medication, atrial fibrillation.

Actions: Increases intracellular calcium and allows more calcium to enter the myocardial cell during depolarization; this causes a positive inotropic effect (increased force of contraction), increased renal perfusion with a diuretic effect and decrease in renin release, a negative chronotrophic effect (slower heart rate) and slowed conduction through the AV node

Pharmacokinetics:

Route	Onset	Peak
Oral	30–120 min	2–6 h
Intravenous	5–30 min	1–5 h

$T_{1/2}$: 30–40 hours; largely excreted unchanged in the urine. According to the laws of pharmacokinetics, it takes approximately five half-lives to reach the plateau in the plasma. With constant dosing of digoxin, this would take more than a week of therapy. If the therapeutic effects are required more quickly, then a dosing regimen of a large loading dose followed by a smaller maintenance dose can be implemented.

The long half-life of the drug means that when toxic reactions occur, they will persist for a long time (Galbraith *et al.*, 1997).

Adverse effects usually associated with excessive dosing include: headache, weakness, drowsiness, visual disturbances, arrhythmias, GI upset, hallucinations, depression and arrhythmias.

Nursing Considerations for Patients Receiving Cardiac Glycosides

Assessment: History and Examination

Screening for the following conditions, *which could be cautions or contraindications to use of the drug*: known allergies to any digitalis product; impaired kidney function, *which could alter the excretion of the drug*; ventricular tachycardia or fibrillation; heart block or sick sinus syndrome; acute MI; electrolyte abnormalities (increased calcium, decreased potassium or decreased magnesium), *which could increase the toxicity of the drug* and pregnancy or lactation *because of the potential adverse effects on the foetus or neonate.*

Include screening *for baseline status before beginning therapy and for any potential adverse effects.* Assess the following: weight, skin colour and perfusion, orientation and reflexes; pulse, blood pressure, electrocardiogram (ECG) and cardiac auscultation; respiratory rate and adventitious sounds; renal function tests and serum electrolyte levels.

Establish if patient is currently taking other medications or herbal therapies, which may potentially interact with cardiac glycosides.

Nursing Diagnoses

The patient receiving a cardiac glycoside may have the following nursing diagnoses related to drug therapy:

- Poor tissue perfusion (total body) due to reduction in cardiac output.
- Impaired gas exchange related to reduction in cardiac output.
- Deficient knowledge regarding drug therapy.
- Poor recall due to reduced cardiac output.

Implementation With Rationale

- Consult with the prescriber about the need for a loading dose when beginning therapy, *to achieve therapeutic effect as soon as possible.*
- Monitor pulse for 1 full minute before administering the drug, *to monitor for adverse effects.* With hold the dose if the pulse is less than 60 beats/minute in an adult or less than 90 beats/minute in an infant (age); retake pulse in 1 hour. If pulse remains low, document pulse, withhold the drug and notify the prescriber *because the pulse rate could indicate digoxin toxicity, consider checking digoxin levels?*

- Monitor pulse for any change in quality or rhythm, *to detect arrhythmias or early signs of toxicity.*
- Check the dosage and preparation carefully, *because digoxin has a very small margin of safety,* and *inadvertent drug errors can cause serious problems.*
- Check paediatric dosage with extreme care, *because children are more likely to develop digoxin toxicity.* Have the dosage double-checked by another nurse before administration.
- Follow dilution instructions carefully for intravenous use; use promptly *to avoid drug degradation.*
- Maintain emergency equipment on standby: potassium salts, phenytoin (*for treatment of seizures*), atropine (*to increase heart rate*) and a cardiac monitor, *in case severe toxicity should occur. In acute setting.*
- Administer intravenous doses very slowly over at least 5 minutes, *to avoid cardiac arrhythmias and adverse effects.*
- Arrange for the patient to be weighed at the same time each day, in the same clothes, *to monitor for fluid retention and CHF.*
- Avoid administering the oral drug with food or antacids, *to avoid delays in absorption.*
- Monitor the patient for therapeutic digoxin levels, *to evaluate therapeutic dosing and to monitor for the development of toxicity.*
- Provide comfort measures? *To help the patient tolerate drug effects.*
- Provide thorough patient education, including the name of the drug, dosage prescribed, proper administration, measures to avoid adverse effects, warning signs of problems and the need for periodic monitoring and evaluation, *to enhance patient knowledge about drug therapy and to promote compliance* (see Critical Thinking Scenario 43-1).
- Offer support and encouragement, *to help the patient deal with the diagnosis and the drug regimen.*

Evaluation

- Monitor patient response to the drug (improvement in signs and symptoms of CHF, resolution of atrial arrhythmias and serum digoxin level).
- Monitor for adverse effects (vision changes, arrhythmias, CHF, headache, dizziness, drowsiness, GI upset and nausea).
- Evaluate the effectiveness of the teaching plan (patient can name drug, dosage, proper administration, adverse effects to watch for, specific measures to avoid adverse effects and the importance of continued follow-up).
- Monitor the effectiveness of comfort measures and compliance to the regimen.

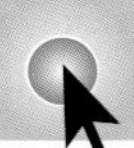

WEB LINKS

Health care providers and patients may want to consult the following Internet sources:

http://cks.library.nhs.uk The National Health Service Clinical Knowledge Summaries provide evidence-based practical information on the common conditions observed in primary care.

http://www.bnf.org.uk The British National Formulary provides UK health care professionals with authoritative and practical information on the selection and clinical use of medicines.

http://www.nhsdirect.nhs.uk The National Health Service Direct service provides patients with information and advice about health, illness and health services.

http://www.nice.org.uk National Institute for Health and Clinical Excellence is an independent organization responsible for providing national guidance on promoting good health and preventing and treating ill health.

Points to Remember

- CHF is a condition in which the heart muscle fails to effectively pump blood through the cardiovascular system, leading to a build up of blood or congestion in the system.
- CHF can be the result of a damaged heart muscle and increased demand to work harder secondary to CAD, hypertension, cardiomyopathy, valvular disease or congenital heart abnormalities.
- The sarcomere, the functioning unit of the heart muscle, is made up of protein fibres, —thin actin fibres and thick myosin fibres.
- Actin and myosin fibres connect with each other and slide over one another, contracting the sarcomere, when calcium is present to inactivate troponin.
- Troponin is an inhibitory compound that prevents this reaction. This sliding action requires the use of energy.
- Calcium enters the cell during the action potential after the cell has been stimulated. It gains entrance to the cell through calcium channels in the cell membrane and from storage sites within the cell.

- Failing cardiac muscle cells lose the ability to effectively use energy to move calcium into the cell and contractions become weak and ineffective.
- Treatment for CHF can include the use of vasodilators (to reduce the heart's workload), diuretics (to reduce blood volume and the heart's workload), β-blockers (which decrease the heart's workload precipitated by the activation of the sympathetic reaction) and inotropic agents (which directly stimulate the muscle to contract more effectively).
- Signs and symptoms of CHF reflect the backup of blood in the vascular system and the loss of fluid in the tissues. Oedema, associated weight gain, liver congestion, elevated JVP and nocturia reflect right-sided CHF. Tachypnoea, fatigue, dyspnoea, orthopnoea, haemoptysis, anxiety and low blood oxygenation reflect left-sided CHF.
- Cardiac glycosides increase the movement of calcium into the heart muscle. This results in increased force of contraction, which increases blood flow to the kidneys (causing a diuretic effect), slows the heart rate and slows conduction through the AV node. All of these effects decrease the heart's workload, helping to bring the system back into balance or compensation.
- Phosphodiesterase inhibitors block the breakdown of cAMP in the cardiac muscle. This allows more calcium to enter the cell (leading to more intense contraction) and increases the effects of sympathetic stimulation (which can lead to vasodilation but also can increase pulse, blood pressure and workload on the heart). These drugs are associated with severe effects and are reserved for use in extreme situations.

CRITICAL THINKING SCENARIO 43-1

Inadequate Digoxin Absorption

The Situation

Betty is an 82-year-old woman with a 50-year history of rheumatic mitral valve disease. She has been stabilized on digoxin for 10 years in a compensated state of CHF. Betty recently moved into a nursing home because she was having difficulty caring for herself. She was examined by a doctor at the nursing home and was found to be stable. It was noted that Betty had an irregular pulse of 76 beats/minute and an ECG was performed as documentation of her chronic atrial fibrillation.

Three weeks after her arrival at the nursing home, Betty began to develop progressive weakness, dyspnoea on exertion, two-pillow orthopnoea and peripheral 2+ pitting oedema. These signs and symptoms became progressively worse. Betty was admitted to the hospital with a diagnosis of CHF. Physical examination revealed a heart rate of 96 beats/minute with atrial fibrillation, third heart sound, wheezes, 2+ pitting oedema bilaterally up to the knees, elevated JVP, cardiomegaly, weak pulses and poor peripheral perfusion. Betty's serum digoxin level was 0.12 ng/ml (therapeutic range, 0.5–2 ng/ml). She was treated with diuretics and was given digoxin in the hospital with close cardiac monitoring.

After her condition stabilized, Betty reported that she knew she had been taking digoxin every day because she recognized the pill. The only difference she could identify was that she was given the pill in the afternoon with her dinner, while at home she always took it on an empty stomach first thing in the morning. The nursing home staff confirmed that Betty had received the drug daily in the afternoon and that it was the same brand name she had used at home.

Critical Thinking

- What nursing interventions should be done at this point? *Think about the signs and symptoms of CHF and how they show the progression of the HF.*
- How could the change in the timing of drug administration be related to the decreased serum digoxin levels noted on Betty's admission?
- Consider the factors that affect absorption of a drug. What alterations in dosing could be suggested that would prevent this from happening to Betty again?
- What potential problems with trust could develop for Betty on her return to the nursing home? Suggest an explanation for what happened to Betty and possible ways that this problem could have been avoided.

Discussion

Betty's immediate needs involve trying to alleviate the alteration to her cardiac output that occurred when she lost the therapeutic effects of digoxin. Positioning, cool environment, small and frequent meals and rest periods can help to decrease the workload on her heart. Digoxin has a small margin of safety and requires an adequate serum level to be therapeutic. Betty was

Inadequate Digoxin Absorption *(continued)*

not absorbing enough digoxin to achieve a therapeutic serum level; consequently, her body began to go through the progression of CHF, first right-sided and then left-sided.

Nursing Care Guide for Betty: Digoxin

Assessment: History and Examination

Assess the patient's health history for allergies to any digitalis product, renal dysfunction, IHSS, arrhythmias, heart block and electrolyte abnormalities

Focus the physical examination on the following areas:

- Cardiovascular: blood pressure, pulse, perfusion and ECG.
- Neurological (central nervous system): orientation, reflexes and vision.
- Skin: colour and perfusion.
- Respiratory: respiratory rate and character and adventitious sounds.
- GI: abdominal examination and bowel sounds.
- Laboratory tests: serum electrolytes.
- Body weight.

Nursing Diagnoses

- Decreased cardiac output related to cardiac effect.
- Deficient fluid volume related to diuretic effects.
- Ineffective tissue perfusion related to changes in cardiac output.
- Impaired gas exchange related to changes in cardiac output.
- Deficient knowledge regarding drug therapy.

Implementation

- Administer a loading dose to provide rapid therapeutic effects.
- Monitor apical pulse for 1 full minute before administering to assess for adverse and therapeutic effects.
- Check dosage very carefully.
- Provide comfort and safety measures: give small, frequent meals.
- Administer intravenously over 5 minutes; keep emergency equipment on standby.
- Provide support and reassurance to deal with drug effects.
- Provide patient education regarding drug, dosage, adverse effects, what to report and safety precautions.

Evaluation

- Evaluate drug effects: relief of signs and symptoms of CHF, resolution of atrial arrhythmias, serum digoxin levels 0.5 to 2 ng/ml.
- Monitor for adverse effects, including arrhythmias, vision changes (yellow halo), GI upset, headache and drowsiness.
- Monitor for drug–drug interactions as indicated for each drug.
- Evaluate effectiveness of patient education programme.
- Evaluate effectiveness of comfort and safety measures.

Patient Education for Betty

- Digoxin is a digitalis preparation. Digitalis has many helpful effects on the heart, for example, it helps the heart to beat more slowly and efficiently. These effects promote better circulation and should help to reduce the swelling in your ankles or legs. It also should increase the amount of urine that you produce every day.
- Digoxin is a very powerful drug and must be taken exactly as prescribed. It is important to have regular medical checkups to ensure that the dosage of the drug is correct for you and that it is having the desired effect on your heart.
- Do not stop taking this drug without consulting your health care provider. Never skip doses and never try to 'catch up' any missed doses because serious adverse effects could occur.
- Learn to take your own pulse. Take it each morning before engaging in any activity. Write your pulse rate on a calendar so you will be aware of any changes and can notify your health care provider if the rate or rhythm of your pulse shows a consistent change.
- Your normal pulse rate is _________.
- Try to monitor your weight fairly closely. Weigh yourself every day, at the same time of the day and in the same amount of clothing. Record your weight on your calendar for easy reference. If you gain or lose 1 kg or more in 1 day, it may indicate a problem with your drug. Consult your health care provider.

(continued)

Inadequate Digoxin Absorption *(continued)*

Some of the following adverse effects may occur:

- *Dizziness, drowsiness and headache:* Avoid driving or performing hazardous tasks or delicate tasks that require concentration if these occur. Consult your health care provider for an appropriate analgesic if the headache is a problem.
- *Nausea, gastrointestinal upset and loss of appetite:* Small, frequent meals may help; monitor your weight loss; if it becomes severe, consult your health care provider.
- *Vision changes, 'yellow' halos around objects:* These effects may pass with time. Take extra care in your activities for the first few days. If these reactions do not go away after 3 to 4 days, consult with your health care provider.
- Report any of the following to your health care provider: *unusually slow or irregular pulse; rapid weight gain; 'yellow vision'; unusual tiredness or weakness; skin rash or hives; swelling of the ankles, legs or fingers and difficulty in breathing.*
- Tell any doctor, nurse, dentist or other health care provider that you are taking this drug.
- Keep this drug and all medications, out of the reach of children.
- Avoid the use of over-the-counter medications while you are taking this drug. If you think that you need one of these, consult with your health care provider for the best choice. Many of these drugs contain ingredients that could interfere with your digoxin.
- Consider wearing or carrying a medical identification to alert any medical personnel who might take care of you in an emergency that you are taking this drug.
- Schedule regular medical checkups to evaluate the actions of the drug and to adjust the dosage if necessary.

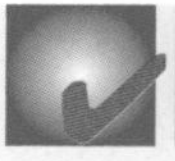

CHECK YOUR UNDERSTANDING

Answers to the questions in this chapter may be found in the Answer Key in the back of the book.

Multiple Choice

Select the most appropriate response to the following.

1. Patients with CHF present clinically with
   a. cardiac arrest.
   b. congestion of blood vessels.
   c. an MI.
   d. a pulmonary embolism.

2. Calcium is needed in the cardiac muscle to
   a. break apart actin–myosin bridges.
   b. activate troponin.
   c. allow actin–myosin bridges to form, causing contraction.
   d. maintain the electrical rhythm.

3. A patient with right-sided CHF might exhibit oedema
   a. in any gravity-dependent areas.
   b. in the hands and fingers.
   c. around the eyes.
   d. when lying down.

4. ACE inhibitors and other vasodilators are used in the early treatment of CHF. They act to
   a. cause loss of volume.
   b. increase arterial pressure and perfusion.
   c. cause pooling of the blood and decreased venous return to the heart, decreasing the workload of the muscle.
   d. increase the release of aldosterone and improve fluid balance.

5. Inotropic drugs are drugs that
   a. block the sympathetic nervous system.
   b. block the renin–angiotensin system.
   c. block the parasympathetic influence on the heart muscle.
   d. affect intracellular calcium levels in the heart muscle, leading to increased contractility.

6. A patient taking digoxin for the treatment of CHF would be advised to
   a. make up any missed doses the next day.
   b. report changes in vision or in heart rate.
   c. avoid exposure to the sun.
   d. switch to generic tablets if they are less expensive.

7. A nurse is about to administer *digoxin* to a patient whose apical pulse is 48 beats/minute. She should
   a. give the drug and notify the prescriber.
   b. Withhold the drug retake the pulse in 15 minutes and give the drug if the pulse has not changed.
   c. Withhold the drug retake the pulse in 1 hour and withhold the drug if the pulse is still less than 60 beats/minutes.
   d. withhold the drug and notify the prescriber.

8. Before giving digoxin to an infant, the nurse would
   a. notify the prescriber that the dose is about to be given.
   b. check the apical pulse and have another nurse double-check the dose.
   c. make sure the infant has eaten and has a full stomach.
   d. check the pulse and give the drug very slowly.

Extending Matching Questions

Select **all** that apply.

1. CHF occurs when the heart fails to pump effectively. Which of the following could cause CHF?
   a. CAD
   b. Chronic hypertension
   c. Cardiomyopathy
   d. Fluid overload
   e. Pneumonia
   f. Cirrhosis

2. A client develops left-sided CHF after an MI. Which of the following would the nurse expect during the client assessment?
   a. Orthopnoea
   b. Polyuria
   c. Tachypnoea
   d. Dyspnoea
   e. Blood-tinged sputum
   f. Swollen ankles

Bibliography and References

British Medical Association and Royal Pharmaceutical Society of Great Britain. (2008). *British National Formulary*. London: BMJ & RPS Publishing. *This publication is updated biannually: it is imperative that the most recent edition is consulted.*

British Medical Association and Royal Pharmaceutical Society of Great Britain. (2008). *British National Formulary for Children*. London: BMJ & RPS Publishing. *This publication is updated annually: it is imperative that the most recent edition is consulted.*

Galbraith, A., Bullock, S., Manias, E., Hunt, B., & Richards, A. (1997). *Fundamentals of pharmacology. A text for nurses and health professionals.* Harlow, England: Pearson, Prentice Hall.

Ganong, W. (2005). *Review of medical physiology* (22nd ed.). New York: McGraw-Hill.

Howland, R. D., & Mycek, M. J. (2005). *Pharmacology* (3rd ed.). Philadelphia: Lippincott Williams & Wilkins.

Levy, D., Kenchaiah, S., Larson, M. G., Benjamin, E. J., Kupka, M. J., Ho, K. L., Murabito, J., & Vasan, R. S. (2002) *Long-term trends in the incidence of and survival with heart failure.* The New England Journal of Medicine, *347*(18), 1397–1402.

Marieb, E. N., & Hoehn, K. (2004). *Human anatomy & physiology* (7th ed.). San Francisco: Pearson Benjamin Cummings.

Porth, C. M., & Matfin, G. (2008). *Pathophysiology: concepts of altered health states* (8th ed.). Philadelphia: Lippincott Williams & Wilkins.

Simonsen, T., Aarbakke, J., Kay, I., Coleman, I., Sinnott, P., & Lysaa, R. (2006). *Illustrated pharmacology for nurses.* London: Hodder Arnold.

CHAPTER 44

Antiarrhythmic Agents

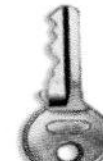

KEY TERMS

antiarrhythmics
bradycardia
cardiac output
heart block
haemodynamics
premature ventricular contraction (PVC)
premature atrial contraction (PAC)
tachycardia
supraventricular arrhythmias

LEARNING OBJECTIVES

Upon completion of this chapter, you will be able to:

1. Describe the cardiac action potential and the processes, which occur during each phase and use this information to explain the changes made by each class of antiarrhythmic agents.
2. Describe the therapeutic actions, indications, pharmacokinetics, contraindications, most common adverse reactions and important drug–drug interactions associated with antiarrhythmic agents.
3. Discuss the use of antiarrhythmic agents across the lifespan.
4. Compare and contrast the key drugs lidocaine, propranolol, sotalol and diltiazem with other agents in their class and with other classes of antiarrhythmics.
5. Outline the nursing considerations, including important teaching points, for patients receiving antiarrhythmic agents.

CLASS IA ANTIARRHYTHMICS

disopyramide
procainamide
quinidine

CLASS IB ANTIARRHYTHMICS

lidocaine
mexiletine

CLASS IC ANTIARRHYTHMICS

flecainide
propafenone

CLASS II ANTIARRHYTHMIC

(β-blockers)
acebutolol
atenolol
esmolol
propranolol

CLASS III ANTIARRHYTHMICS

amiodarone
sotalol

CLASS IV ANTIARRHYTHMICS

(Calcium channel blockers)
diltiazem
verapamil

OTHER

adenosine
digoxin

Arrhythmias are caused by disruptions in cardiac impulse formation and in the conduction of impulses through the myocardium. Disruptions in the normal rhythm of the heart can interfere with myocardial contractions and affect the amount of blood pumped with each beat known as the **cardiac output**. Arrhythmias that seriously disrupt cardiac output can be fatal. Drugs used to treat arrhythmias suppress automaticity or alter the conductivity of the heart. Generally, antiarrthymic agents act by impeding the movement of ions across the membrane of myocardial cells. This affects the characteristics of the cardiac action potential. Antiarrthymic agents are best suited to the treatment of ectopic beats and increases in heart rate because they act to stabilize the excitable myocardial tissue. The means by which the various drug categories achieve this can be by suppressing automaticity, by depressing the rate of depolarization, by slowing impulse conduction through the tissue, by prolonging the action potential and by increasing the refractory period. The net result is that the number of action potentials, and consequently, the number of myocardial contractions, in a given time interval, are reduced (Galbraith *et al.*, 1997).

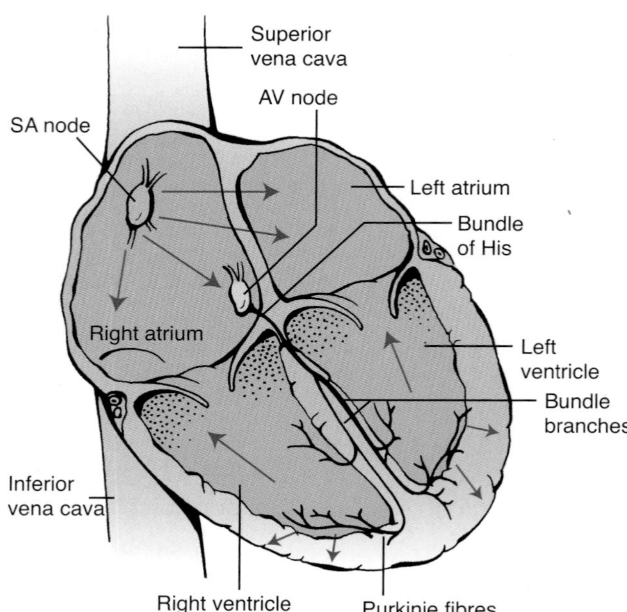

FIGURE 44.1 The conducting system of the heart. Impulses originating in the sinoatrial (SA) node are transmitted through the atrial bundles to the atrioventricular (AV) node and down the bundle of His and the bundle branches by way of the Purkinje fibers through the ventricles.

Review of Cardiac Conduction

As discussed in Chapter 41, each cycle of cardiac contraction and relaxation is controlled by impulses that arise spontaneously in the sinoatrial (SA) node of the heart. These impulses are conducted from the pacemaker cells by a specialized conducting system that activates all parts of the heart muscle almost simultaneously. These continuous and rhythmic contractions are controlled by the heart itself. This property allows the heart to beat as long as it has enough nutrients and oxygen to survive, regardless of the status of the rest of the body. The conduction system of the heart comprises the following:

- The SA node, located in the top of the right atrium, which acts as the pacemaker of the heart.
- Atrial bundles that conduct the impulse through the atrial muscle.
- The atrioventricular (AV) node, which slows the impulse and sends it from the atria into the ventricles by way of the bundle of His.
- The bundle of His, which enters the septum and then divides into three bundle branches.
- The bundle branches, which conduct the impulses through the ventricles; these branches break into a fine network of conducting fibres called the Purkinje fibres.
- The Purkinje fibres, which deliver the impulse to the ventricular cells (Figure 44.1).

Automaticity of the Heart

All cardiac cells possess some degree of automaticity, as described in Chapter 41. These cells undergo a spontaneous depolarization during diastole or rest because they decrease the flow of potassium ions out of the cell and probably leak sodium into the cell, causing an action potential. This action potential is similar to the action potential of the neuron (described in Chapter 18).

The action potential of the cardiac muscle cell consists of five phases:

Phase 0 occurs when the cell reaches a point of stimulation. The sodium channels open along the cell membrane and sodium rushes into the cell; this positive flow of electrons into the cell results in an electrical potential. This is called depolarization.

Phase 1 is a very short period during which the sodium ion concentration equalizes inside and outside of the cell.

Phase 2, or the plateau stage, occurs as the cell membrane becomes less permeable to sodium, the depolarization causes the opening of special calcium channels and calcium slowly enters the cell. The depolarization also causes the opening of voltage-sensitive potassium channels and potassium begins to leave the cell. The cell membrane is trying to return to its resting state, a process called repolarization.

Phase 3 is a time of rapid repolarization as the sodium gates are closed and potassium flows out of the cell.

Phase 4 is when the cell is at rest; the sodium–potassium pump returns the membrane to its resting membrane potential and spontaneous depolarization begins again.

Each area of the heart has a slightly different rate of rhythmicity. The SA node generates an impulse about 80 to 90 times a minute, the AV node about 40 to 50 times a minute and the complex ventricular muscle cells about 10 to 20 times a minute.

Cardiac Arrhythmias

As noted earlier, various factors can change the cardiac rate and rhythm. Arrhythmias can be caused by changes in rate [**tachycardia**, which is a faster-than-normal heart rate (between 60 and 100 beats/minute), or **bradycardia**, which is a slower-than-normal heart rate (less than 60 beats/minute)] by stimulation from an ectopic focus such as **premature atrial contractions (PACs)** or **premature ventricular contractions (PVCs)**, atrial flutter, atrial fibrillation (AF) (see Box 44.1) or ventricular fibrillation; or by alterations in conduction through the muscle such as **heart blocks** and bundle branch blocks. Figure 44.2 displays an electrocardiogram (ECG) strip showing normal sinus rhythm; Figures 44.3, 44.4, 44.5 and 44.6 are ECG strips showing various arrhythmias.

Causes of Arrhythmias

The underlying causes of arrhythmias can arise from changes to the automaticity or conductivity of the heart cells. These changes can be caused by several factors, including

- Electrolyte disturbances that alter the action potential.

BOX 44.1 Understanding Atrial Fibrillation (AF)

Atrial fibrillation (AF) is a relatively common arrhythmia of the atria. It has been associated with coronary artery disease, myocardial inflammation, valvular disease, cardiomegaly and rheumatic heart disease. The cells of the atria are connected side to side and top to bottom and are relatively simple cells. In contrast, the cells of the ventricles are connected only from top to bottom, with one cell connected only to one or two other cells. It is much easier, therefore, for an ectopic focus in the atria to spread that impulse throughout the entire atria, setting up a cycle of chaotic depolarization and repolarization. It is more difficult to stimulate fibrillation in the ventricles because one ectopic site cannot rapidly spread impulses to many other cells, only to the cells connected in its two- or three-cell set.

Fibrillation results in lack of any coordinated pumping action because the muscles are not stimulated to contract and pump out blood. In the ventricles, this is a life-threatening situation. If the ventricles do not pump blood, no blood is delivered to the brain, the tissues of the body or the heart muscle itself. However, loss of pumping action in the atria per se does not usually cause much of a problem.

Danger of Blood Clots

One of the problems with AF occurs when it exists for longer than 1 week. The auricles (those appendages hanging on the atria to collect blood; see Chapter 41) fill with blood that is not effectively pumped into the ventricles. Over time, this somewhat stagnant blood tends to clot. As the auricles are sacks of striated muscle fibres, blood clots form around these fibres. In this situation, if the atria were to contract in a coordinated manner, there is a substantial risk that those clots or emboli would be pumped into the ventricles and then into the lungs (from the right auricle), which could lead to pulmonary emboli, or to the brain or periphery (from the left auricle), which could cause a stroke or occlusion of peripheral vessels.

Treatment Choices

Treatment of AF can be complicated if the length of time the patient has been in AF is not known. If a patient goes into AF acutely, drug therapy is available for rapid conversion. Alternatively, if the patient's condition is unstable, a method of cardioversion can be used for rapid conversion. This method involves the patient been heavily sedated for a short period of time, and low voltage defibrillation is used to "shock" the heart back into a sinus rhythm. For current practice, please refer to Resuscitation Councils Advanced Life Support (ALS) Group Guidelines: http://www.resus.org.uk). Drug therapy is then utilized for long-term stabilization.

If the onset of AF is not known and it is suspected that the atria may have been fibrillating for longer than 1 week, the patient is better off staying in AF without drug therapy. Prophylactic oral anticoagulants are given to decrease the risk of clot formation and emboli being pumped into the system. Conversion in this case could result in potentially life-threatening embolism affecting the lungs, brain or other tissues.

Supraventricular tachycardia: Another Danger

The other danger of AF is rapid ventricular response to the atrial stimuli, a condition called supraventricular tachycardia (SVT). With the atria firing impulses, possibly 200 to 300 a minute, the number of stimuli conducted into the ventricles is erratic and irregular. If the ventricle is responding too rapidly – more than 120 times a minute – the filling time of the ventricles is greatly reduced, causing cardiac output to fall dramatically. In these situations and when AF is anticipated [such as with atrial flutter or paroxysmal atrial tachycardia (PAT)], drugs may be given to slow conduction and protect the ventricles from rapid rates. Adenosine is commonly used to convert rapid SVT when the patient's condition is compromised (6 mg, 6 mg, 12 mg intravenously consecutively as rapid infusion); – please refer to (ALS) Guidelines.

Esmolol, diltiazem and verapamil are used intravenously to convert SVT with rapid ventricular response, which could progress to AF.

Implications for Nurses

Careful patient assessment and monitoring is essential before beginning treatment for AF. If a history cannot be established from patient information and medical records are not available, it is usually recommended that AF be left untreated and anticoagulant therapy be started. This can pose a challenge for the nurse in trying to teach patients about why their rapid and irregular heart rate will not be treated and explaining all of the factors involved in the long-term use of oral anticoagulants.

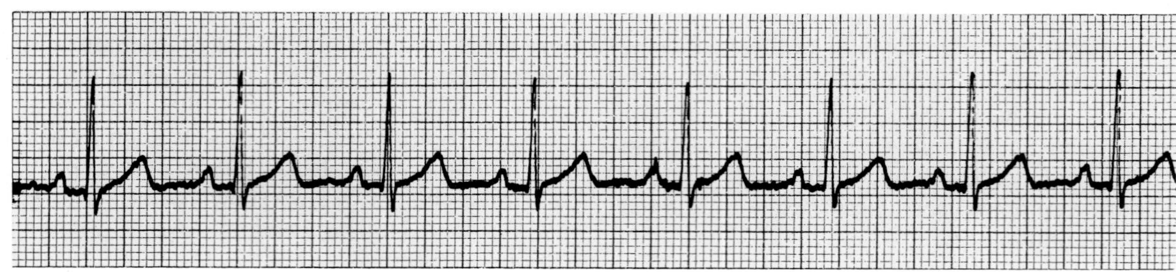

FIGURE 44.2 Normal sinus rhythm. Rhythm: regular. Rate: 60 to 100 beats/min. P–R interval: 0.12 to 0.20 s. QRS: 0.06 to 0.10 seconds.

- Decreases in oxygen delivered to the cells, which lead to hypoxia or anoxia and which change the cell's action potential and ability to maintain a membrane potential.
- Structural damage that changes the conduction pathway through the heart.
- Acidosis or accumulation of waste products that alters the action potential in that area.

In some cases, changes to the heart's automaticity or conductivity may result from drugs that alter the action potential or cardiac conduction.

Haemodynamics

The study of the forces that move blood throughout the cardiovascular system is called **haemodynamics**. The ability of the heart to effectively pump blood depends on the coordinated contraction of the atrial and ventricular muscles. The muscular walls of these chambers are activated to contract by impulses that arise at the SA node, travel through the atria, are delayed slightly at the AV node and then stimulate the bundle of His–Purkinje system through the ventricles. The conduction system is designed so that atrial stimulation is followed by total atrial contraction and ventricular stimulation is followed by total ventricular contraction.

To be an effective pump, these muscles need to contract together. If this orderly initiation and conduction of impulses is altered, the result can be a poorly coordinated contraction of the ventricles that is unable to deliver an adequate supply of oxygenated blood to the brain and other organs, including the heart muscle itself. If these haemodynamic alterations are severe, serious complications can occur. For example, lack of sufficient blood flow to the brain can cause syncope or precipitate stroke; lack of sufficient blood flow to the myocardium can exacerbate atherosclerosis and cause angina or myocardial infarction (MI).

Antiarrhythmic Drugs

Antiarrhythmics affect the action potential of the cardiac cells, altering their automaticity, conductivity or both. This effect can cause antiarrhythmic drugs to produce new arrhythmias, that is, they are **proarrhythmic**. Antiarrhythmics are used in emergency situations when the haemodynamics arising from the patient's arrhythmia are severe and could potentially be fatal. The effects of antiarrhythmic drugs across the lifespan can be see in Box 44.2.

Class I Antiarrhythmics

Class I antiarrhythmics are drugs that **block the sodium channels** in the cell membrane during an action potential (Figure 44.7). The Class I drugs are local anaesthetics or membrane-stabilizing agents. They bind more quickly to sodium channels that are open or inactive, ones that have been stimulated and are not yet recovered. This characteristic makes these drugs preferable in conditions such as tachycardia, in which the sodium gates are open frequently. The Class I antiarrhythmics are further broken down into three

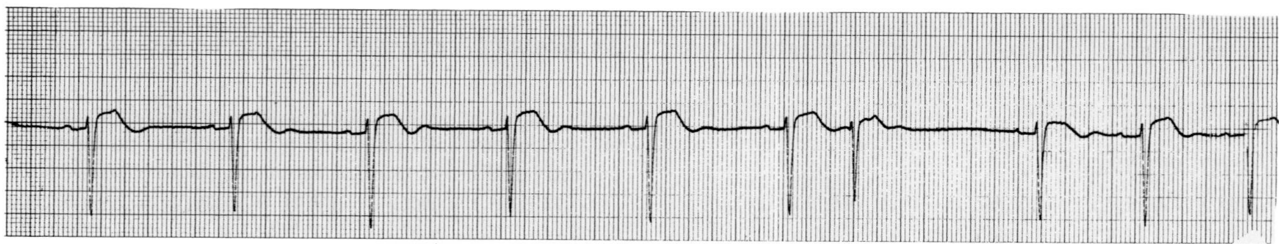

FIGURE 44.3 Premature atrial contractions (PACs). Rhythm: irregular due to the origination of a beat outside the normal conduction system (ectopic). Rate: normal sinus rate, except for PACs. P–R interval: P wave is abnormal and interval may be slightly shortened in ectopic beat. QRS: normal.

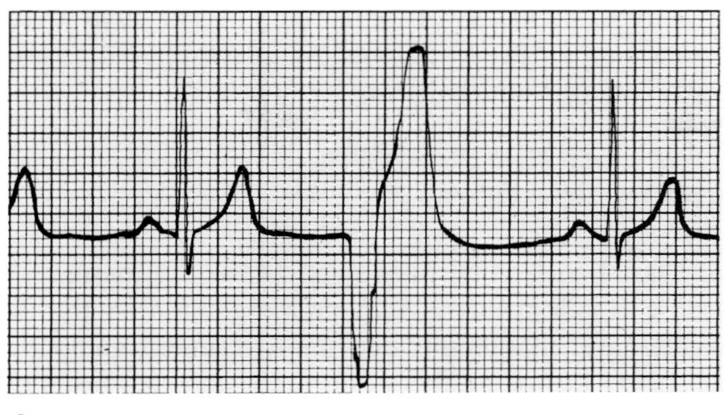

A

Premature ventricular contraction (PVC).

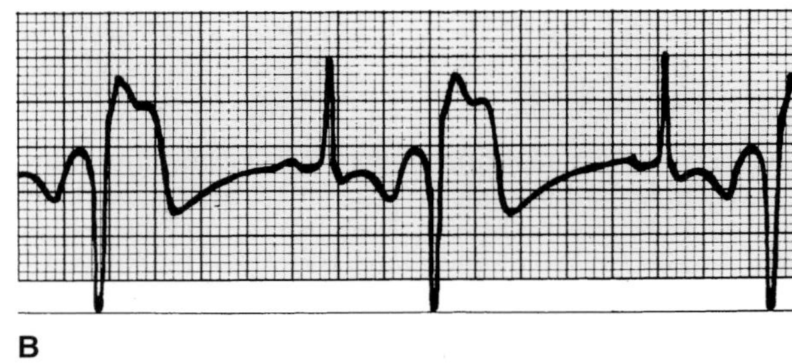

B

Ventricular bigeminy. (Every other beat is a PVC.)

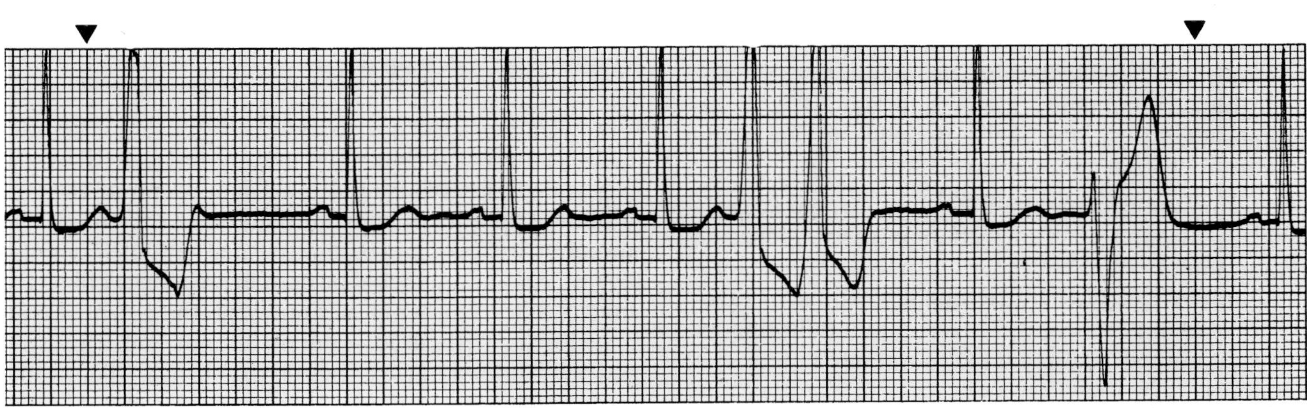

C

Multiformed PVCs.

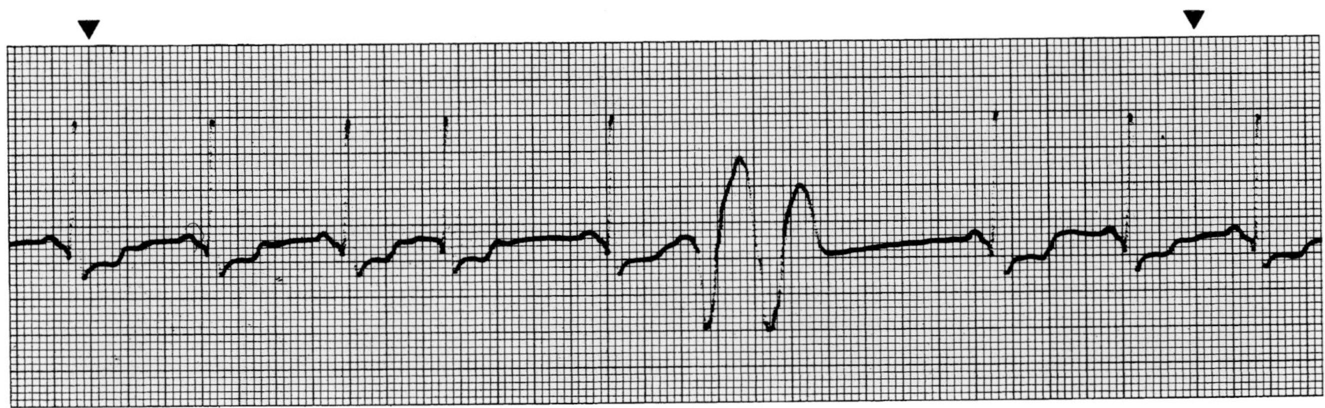

D

Heart block with PVCs.

FIGURE 44.4 Premature ventricular contractions (PVCs) or ventricular premature beats. Rhythm: irregular. Rate: variable; only interrupts the cycle of the ectopic, ventricular contraction. P–R: normal in sinus beats, not measurable in PVCs. QRS: wide, bizarre, greater than 0.12 s.

subclasses, reflecting the manner in which their blockage of sodium channels affects the action potential.

- *Class Ia drugs* depress phase 0 of the action potential and prolong the duration of the action potential.

Disopyramide is an oral drug that is available for adults and children and is recommended for the treatment of life-threatening ventricular arrhythmias. Procainamide is available in intramuscular, intravenous and oral forms,

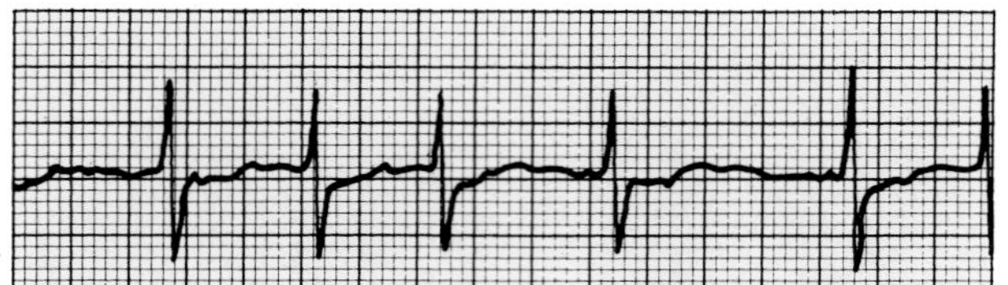

FIGURE 44.5 Atrial fibrillation. Rhythm: irregularly irregular. Rate: variable; usually rapid on initiation of rhythm; decreases when controlled by medication. P–R interval: no P waves are seen, replaced by an irregular wavy baseline. The atria are fibrillating because impulses are arising at a rate greater than 350 per min. The ventricles respond when the atrioventricular node is stimulated to threshold and can receive the impulse. QRS: normal.

making it a good drug with which to start treatment and then switch to oral therapy if possible. It is used for the treatment of documented life-threatening ventricular arrhythmias. Quinidine is available for oral, IM or intravenous administration and is especially effective in the treatment of atrial arrhythmias.

- *Class Ib drugs* depress phase 0 somewhat and actually shorten the duration of the action potential. Lidocaine (lignocaine) is the traditional but now less frequently used antiarrhythmic because of its potential to exacerbate and already unstable myocardium following an acute MI. Amiodarone is now the drug of choice and is administered by the intravenous route to manage acute ventricular arrhythmias in patients with MI or during cardiac surgery (please refer to http://www.resus.org.uk for up-to-date guidelines). Mexiletine is an oral drug that is approved only for use in life-threatening arrhythmias.
- *Class Ic drugs* markedly depress phase 0, with a resultant extreme slowing of conduction. They have little effect on the duration of the action potential. Flecainide is available as an oral drug for use in the treatment of life-threatening ventricular arrhythmias and for the prevention of PAT in symptomatic patients without structural heart disease. Propafenone is another oral Class Ic drug that can be used to treat potentially life-threatening ventricular arrhythmias and for prevention of PAT in symptomatic patients who are without structural heart defects.

Therapeutic Actions and Indications

The Class I antiarrhythmics stabilize the cell membrane by binding to sodium channels, depressing phase 0 of the action potential and changing the duration of the action potential. They have a local anaesthetic effect. These drugs are indicated for the treatment of potentially life-threatening ventricular arrhythmias and should not be used to treat other arrhythmias because of the risk of a proarrhythmic effect. Flecainide and propafenone are also used to prevent PAT in symptomatic patients who do not have structural heart defects.

Pharmacokinetics

These drugs are widely distributed after injection or after rapid absorption through the gastrointestinal (GI) tract. They undergo extensive hepatic metabolism and are excreted in urine. These drugs cross the placenta; although no specific adverse effects have been associated with their use, it is suggested that they should be used in pregnancy only if the benefits to the mother clearly outweigh the potential risks to the foetus. These drugs enter breast milk and, because of the potential for adverse effects on the neonate, they should not be used during lactation. Another method of feeding the baby should be chosen.

Contraindications and Cautions

These drugs are contraindicated with bradycardia or heart block unless an artificial pacemaker is in place, *because changes in conduction could lead to complete heart block*; with congestive heart failure (CHF), hypotension or shock, *which could be exacerbated by effects on the action potential*; with lactation, *because of the potential for adverse*

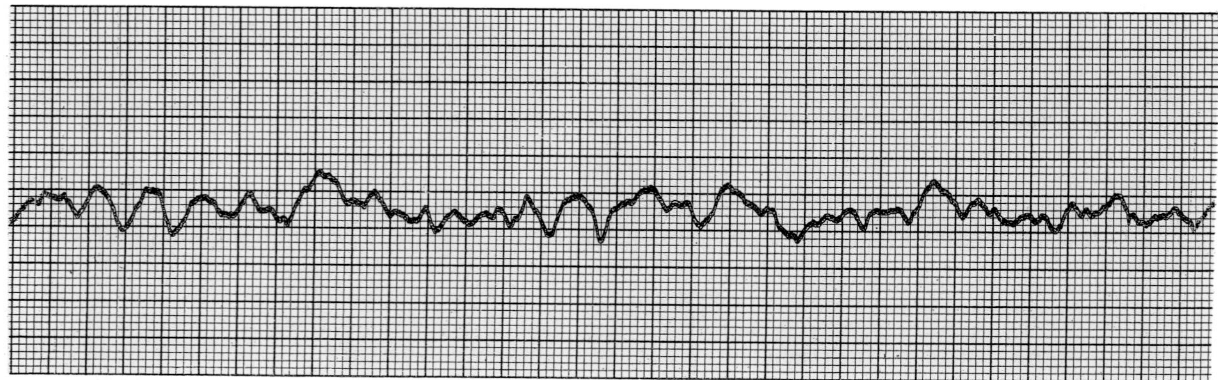

FIGURE 44.6 Ventricular fibrillation. Rhythm: irregular. Rate: not measurable. P–R interval: not measurable. QRS: not measurable, replaced by an irregular wavy baseline. No coordinated electrical or mechanical activity in the ventricle, no cardiac output.

BOX 44.2 DRUG THERAPY ACROSS THE LIFESPAN

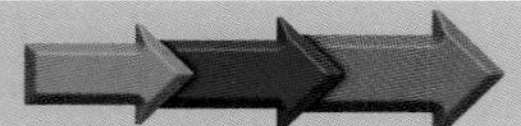

Antiarrhythmic Agents

CHILDREN

Antiarrhythmic agents are not used as often in children as they are in adults. Children, who do require these drugs after cardiac surgery or because of congenital heart problems, need to be monitored very closely to deal with the related adverse effects that can occur with these drugs.

Digoxin is approved for use in children to treat arrhythmias and has an established recommended dosage. If other antiarrhythmics are used, the dosage should be carefully calculated using weight and age and should be double-checked by another nurse before administration.

Adenosine, propranolol, procainamide and digoxin have been successfully used to treat supraventricular arrhythmias, with propranolol and digoxin being the drugs of choice for long-term management. Verapamil should be avoided in children.

Many arrhythmias in children are now treated by ablation techniques to destroy the arrhythmia-producing cells. This has been very successful in treating Wolff–Parkinson–White and related syndromes in children. The child should have continual cardiac monitoring.

When administering any drug to children, always consult the most recent edition of the British National Formulary for Children.

ADULTS

Adults receive these drugs most often as emergency measures. Patient monitoring and careful evaluation of the total drug regimen should be a routine procedure to ensure the most effective treatment with the least chance of adverse effects. Frequent monitoring and medical follow-up are very important for these patients.

The safety for the use of these drugs during pregnancy has not been established. They should not be used in pregnancy unless the benefit to the mother clearly outweighs the potential risk to the foetus. The drugs do enter breast milk and some have been associated with adverse effects on the neonate. Class I, III and IV agents should not be used during lactation; if they are needed, then another method of feeding the baby should be used.

OLDER ADULTS

Older adults are frequently prescribed one of these drugs. Older adults are more likely to develop adverse effects associated with the use of these drugs, including arrhythmias, hypotension and CHF. They are also more likely to have renal and/or hepatic impairment related to underlying medical conditions, which could interfere with the metabolism and excretion of these drugs.

The dosage for older adults should be started at a lower level than that recommended for other adults. The patient should be monitored very closely and the dosage adjusted based on patient response. If other drugs are added or removed from the drug regimen, appropriate dosage adjustments may need to be made.

effects on the neonate and with electrolyte disturbances, *which could alter the effectiveness of these drugs.* Caution should be used with renal or hepatic dysfunction, *which could interfere with the biotransformation and excretion of these drugs and* during pregnancy, *because of the potential for adverse effects on the foetus.*

Adverse Effects

The adverse effects of the Class I antiarrhythmics are associated with their membrane-stabilizing effects and effects on action potentials. Central nervous system (CNS) effects can include dizziness, drowsiness, fatigue, twitching, mouth numbness, slurred speech, vision changes and tremors that can progress to convulsions. GI symptoms include changes in taste, nausea and vomiting. Cardiovascular effects include the development of arrhythmias (including heart blocks), hypotension, vasodilation and the potential for cardiac arrest. Respiratory depression progressing to respiratory arrest can also occur. Other adverse effects include rash, hypersensitivity reactions, loss of hair and potential bone marrow depression.

Always consult a current copy of the British National Formulary for further guidance.

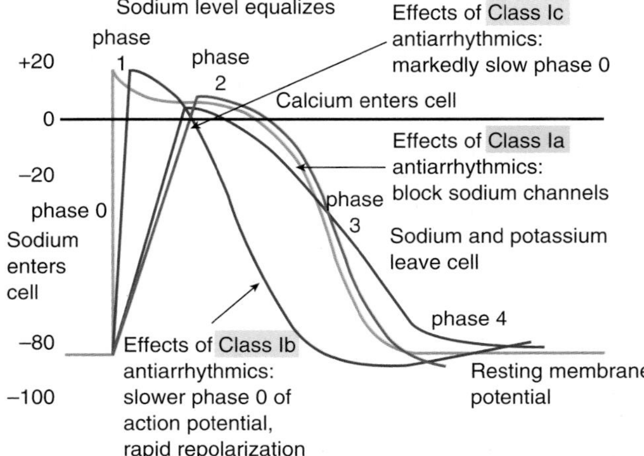

FIGURE 44.7 The cardiac action potentials, showing the effects of class Ia, Ib and Ic antiarrhythmics.

Clinically Important Drug–Drug Interactions

Several drug–drug interactions have been reported with these agents, so the possibility of an interaction should always be considered before any drug is added to a regimen containing an antiarrhythmic. The risk for arrhythmia increases if these agents are combined with other drugs that are known to cause arrhythmias such as digoxin and the β-blockers.

As captopril, amiodarone, verapamil and nifedipine compete for renal transport sites with digoxin, the combination of these drugs with digoxin can lead to increased digoxin levels and digoxin toxicity. If these drugs are used in combination, the patient's digoxin level should be monitored and appropriate dosage adjustment made. Serum levels and toxicity of the Class I antiarrhythmics increase if they are combined with cimetidine; extreme caution should be used if patients are receiving this combination.

The risk of bleeding effects of these drugs increases if they are combined with oral anticoagulants; patients receiving this combination should be monitored closely and have their anticoagulant dose reduced as needed. Check individual drug monographs for specific interactions associated with each drug.

Class II Antiarrhythmics

The Class II antiarrhythmics are β-adrenergic blockers that block β-receptors, causing a depression of phase 4 of the action potential (Figure 44.8). In this way, these drugs slow the recovery of the cells, leading to a slowing of conduction and decreased automaticity of the heart. Several β-adrenergic blockers are used as antiarrhythmics.

Acebutolol, an oral drug also used as an antihypertensive, is especially effective in the treatment of PVCs. Esmolol, an intravenous drug, is used for the short-term management of SVT and tachycardia that is not responding to other measures. Propranolol is used as an antihypertensive, antianginal and antimigraine headache drug and as an antiarrhythmic to treat SVTs caused by digoxin or catecholamines.

Therapeutic Actions and Indications

The Class II antiarrhythmics competitively block β-receptor sites in the heart and kidneys, thereby decreasing heart rate, cardiac excitability and cardiac output; slowing conduction through the AV node and decreasing the release of renin. These effects stabilize excitable cardiac tissue and decrease blood pressure, which decreases the heart's workload and may further stabilize hypoxic cardiac tissue. These drugs are indicated for the treatment of SVTs and PVCs.

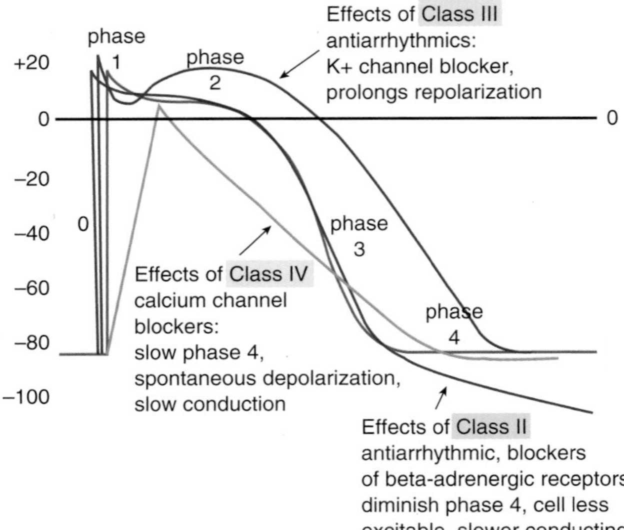

FIGURE 44.8 The cardiac action potentials, showing the effects of class II, III and IV antiarrhythmics.

Pharmacokinetics

These drugs are absorbed from the GI tract and undergo hepatic metabolism. Food has been found to increase the bioavailability of propranolol, although this effect has not been found with other β-adrenergic blocking agents. These drugs are excreted in urine; therefore, caution is required in patients with renal impairment. Teratogenic effects have occurred in animal studies with all of these drugs. The use of any β-adrenergic blocker during pregnancy should be reserved for situations in which the benefit to the mother outweighs the risk to the foetus. In general, they should not be used during lactation because of the potential for adverse effects on the baby. The safety and efficacy for use of these drugs in children has not been established.

Contraindications and Cautions

The use of these drugs is contraindicated in the presence of sinus bradycardia (rate less than 44 beats/minute) and AV block, *which could be exacerbated by the effects of these drugs*; with cardiogenic shock, CHF, asthma or respiratory depression, *which could be made worse by the blocking of β-receptors*; and with pregnancy and lactation, *because of the potential for adverse effects on the foetus or neonate*.

Caution should be used in patients with diabetes and thyroid dysfunction, *which could be altered by the blockade of the β-receptors* and with renal and hepatic dysfunction, *which could alter the metabolism and excretion of these drugs*.

Adverse Effects

The adverse effects associated with **Class II** antiarrhythmics are related to the effects of **blocking β-receptors** in the sympathetic nervous system. CNS effects include dizziness, insomnia, dreams and fatigue. Cardiovascular symptoms can include hypotension, bradycardia, AV block, arrhythmias and alterations in peripheral perfusion. Respiratory effects can include bronchospasm and dyspnoea. GI problems frequently include nausea, vomiting, anorexia, constipation and diarrhoea. Other effects to anticipate include a loss of libido, decreased exercise tolerance and alterations in blood glucose levels.

Always consult a current copy of the British National Formulary for further guidance.

Clinically Important Drug–Drug Interactions

The risk of adverse effects increases if these drugs are taken with verapamil; if this combination is used, dosage adjustment will be needed.

There is a possibility of increased hypoglycaemia if these drugs are combined with insulin; patients should be monitored closely.

Other specific drug interactions may occur with each drug; check a drug reference before combining these drugs with any others.

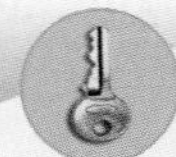

Key Drug Summary: *Propranolol*

Indications: Treatment of cardiac arrhythmias, especially SVT, treatment of ventricular tachycardia induced by digitalis or catecholamines.

Actions: Competitively blocks β-adrenergic receptors in the heart and kidney, has a membrane-stabilizing effect and decreases the influence of the sympathetic nervous system.

Pharmacokinetics:

Route	Onset	Peak	Duration
Oral	20–30 min	60–90 min	6–12 h
Intravenous	Immediate	1 min	4–6 h

$T_{1/2}$: 3 to 5 hours; metabolized in the liver and excreted in urine.

Adverse effects: Bradycardia, CHF, cardiac arrhythmias, heart blocks, cerebrovascular accident (CVA), pulmonary oedema, gastric pain, flatulence, nausea, vomiting, diarrhoea, impotence, decreased exercise tolerance and peripheral vasoconstriction. This drug can cause bronchospasm in susceptible patients; it, therefore, should not be used with patient with a history of asthma or breathing difficulties.

Class III Antiarrhythmics

The **Class III** antiarrhythmics block **potassium channels**, prolonging phase 3 of the action potential, which prolongs repolarization and slows the rate and conduction of the heart (see Figure 44.8). Class III antiarrhythmics include a number of agents.

- **Amiodarone** is available as an oral or an intravenous drug. It should be used only to treat documented life-threatening arrhythmias because it has been associated with serious and even fatal toxic reactions.
- **Sotalol** is an oral drug that is indicated for the treatment of documented life-threatening arrhythmias and for the maintenance of normal sinus rhythm after conversion of atrial arrhythmias. It is known to be proarrhythmic; therefore, patients should be monitored very closely at the initiation of therapy and periodically during therapy.

Therapeutic Actions and Indications

The Class III antiarrhythmics block potassium channels and slow the outward movement of potassium during phase 3 of the action potential. This action prolongs the action potential. All of these drugs are proarrhythmic and have the potential of inducing arrhythmias. These drugs are indicated for the treatment of life-threatening ventricular arrhythmias (amiodarone and sotalol) and for maintenance of sinus rhythm after conversion of atrial arrhythmias (sotalol).

Pharmacokinetics

These drugs are well absorbed and widely distributed. Absorption of sotalol is decreased by the presence of food. They are metabolized in the liver and excreted in urine. There are no well-controlled studies on the effects of sotalol during pregnancy, so its use during pregnancy should be limited to those situations in which the benefit to the mother far outweighs any potential risk to the foetus. There is sparse information available about its use during lactation.

DiMarco *et al.* (2005) describe the pharmacokinetics of amiodarone as quite different from other cardiovascular drugs. It can be administered orally or intravenously. The onset of action for orally administered amiodarone is slow and variable, ranging from between 2 and 21 days (Brantman and Howie, 2006). Owing to this, loading doses are recommended to obtain the necessary therapeutic tissue levels in a shorter period of time. In addition, amiodarone undergoes extensive hepatic metabolism and its main metabolite is desethylamiodarone, which has antiarrthymic properties and is not dialysable. There is minimal excretion by the kidneys and, therefore, no dose adjustment is required for those with renal disease. Amiodarone is mainly excreted through bile and faeces (O'Donovan, 2006).

In clinical situations, where a more rapid response is required, intravenous amiodarone is administered and this achieves an antiarrthymic effect in less than 30 minutes (DiMarco *et al.*, 2005; Siddoway, 2003). The half-life of amiodarone is long and variable, ranging between 25 and 110 days. The prolonged half-life is thought to be a result of its slow release from lipid-rich tissues (O'Donovan, 2006).

Contraindications and Cautions

When these drugs are used to treat life-threatening arrhythmias for which no other drug has been effective, there are no contraindications. Caution should be used with all of these drugs in the presence of shock, hypotension or respiratory depression; with a prolonged QT interval, *which could be made worse by the depressive effects on action potentials* and with renal or hepatic disease, *which could alter the biotransformation and excretion of these drugs.*

There are a number of contraindications to amiodarone, which include the following:

- Known hypersensitivity to amiodarone or iodine, active thyroid toxicosis.
- Severe sinus node dysfunction because of its negative chronotrophic and dromotropic effects, amiodarone can worsen sinus node dysfunction or any conduction abnormalities such as second- or third-degree AV block. In this situation, amiodarone may only be prescribed if the patient has a pacemaker in place (Sanofi Aventis, 2006).
- Marked bradycardia, second- or third-degree heart block.
- Cardiogenic shock or circulatory collapse; amiodarone is contraindicated because of its peripheral vasodilatory effects which may result in reduced preload and further reduced cardiac output.
- Liver cirrhosis or other forms of advanced liver disease.
- Severe pulmonary disease.

Amiodarone should not be used in pregnancy as it can interfere with the foetal thyroid gland and is, therefore, contraindicated unless in exceptional circumstances. Amiodarone is excreted in the breast milk in large quantities (Sanofi Aventis, 2006). If it is needed by a lactating mother, another method of feeding the baby should be used because of the risk of adverse effects on the neonate.

Adverse Effects

The adverse effects associated with these drugs are related to the changes that they cause in action potentials. Nausea, vomiting and GI distress; weakness and dizziness; and hypotension, CHF and arrhythmia are common. Amiodarone has been associated with a potentially fatal liver toxicity, ocular abnormalities and the development of very serious cardiac arrhythmias.

Amiodarone is distributed throughout several organs such as the liver, thyroid gland, eyes, skin and the lungs; therefore, it can be the cause of a number of adverse effects. The frequency of most adverse effects is related to the dosage and duration of treatment. Adverse effects are reported by 75% of patients but only 18% to 37% of this group need to discontinue the drug regimen (Braunwald *et al.*, 2002). Most adverse effects resolve with dose reduction, but those requiring cessation of the drug regimen include people with pulmonary toxicity and GI complaints. In addition, because of its long half-life, adverse effects are potentially more severe and difficult to manage than those of drugs with shorter half-lives (Goldschager *et al.*, 2000)

Clinically Important Drug–Drug Interactions

These drugs can cause serious toxic effects if they are combined with digoxin.

Other specific drug–drug interactions have been reported with individual drugs; for example, amiodarone can interact with several classes of drugs such as β-blockers and tricyclic antidepressants. It also interacts with warfarin, simvastatin, cyclosporin and stimulant laxatives. The most common and potentially serious interactions are with warfarin and digoxin, drugs that prolong the QT interval. A drug reference should always be consulted when adding a new drug to a regimen containing any of these agents.

Always consult a current copy of the British National Formulary for further guidance.

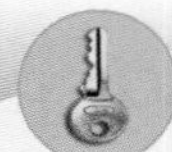

Key Drug Summary: Sotalol

Indications: Treatment of life-threatening ventricular arrhythmias; maintenance of sinus rhythm to delay the time to recurrence of AF/flutter in patients with symptomatic AF/flutter that are currently in sinus rhythm.

Actions: Blocks β-adrenergic receptors in the heart, as well as potassium channels, prolonging phase 3 of the action potential, which prolongs repolarization and slows the rate and conduction of the heart.

Pharmacokinetics:

Route	Onset	Peak	Duration
Oral	Varies	3–4 h	8–12 h

$T_{1/2}$: 12 hours; largely excreted unchanged in urine.

Adverse effects: Laryngospasm, respiratory distress, CHF, cardiac arrhythmias, heart blocks, CVA, pulmonary oedema, gastric pain, flatulence, constipation, diarrhoea, nausea, vomiting, impotence and decreased exercise tolerance.

Class IV Antiarrhythmics

The **Class IV** antiarrhythmics act to block **calcium channels** in the cell membrane, leading to a depression of depolarization and a prolongation of phases 1 and 2 of repolarization, which slows automaticity and conduction (see Figure 44.8). The calcium channel blockers are used as antihypertensives (see Chapter 42) and to treat angina (see Chapter 45). The two calcium channel blockers that seem to have special effects on the heart muscle are diltiazem, which is administered intravenously to treat paroxysmal SVT and verapamil, which is used parenterally to treat SVT and to temporarily control the rapid ventricular response to atrial flutter or fibrillation.

Therapeutic Actions and Indications

The Class IV antiarrhythmics block the movement of calcium ions across the cell membrane, delaying phases 1 and 2 of repolarization and slowing conduction through the AV node. They are indicated for the treatment of SVT and to control the ventricular response to rapid atrial rates and are usually administered by intravenous route.

Pharmacokinetics

These drugs are well absorbed, highly protein bound and metabolized in the liver. They are excreted in the urine. They cross the placenta and have been associated with foetal abnormalities in animal studies. They should not be used in pregnancy unless the benefit to the mother clearly outweighs the risk to the foetus. They enter breast milk and if they are needed by a lactating mother, another method of feeding the baby should be used because of the risk of adverse effects on the neonate.

Contraindications and Cautions

These drugs are contraindicated with sick sinus syndrome or heart block (unless an artificial pacemaker is in place), *because the block could be exacerbated by these drugs*; with pregnancy or lactation, *because of the potential for adverse effects on the foetus or neonate* and with CHF or hypotension, *because of the hypotensive effects of these drugs.* Caution should be used with idiopathic hypertrophic subaortic stenosis, *which could be exacerbated,* or with impaired renal or liver function, *which could affect the metabolism or excretion of these drugs*.

Adverse Effects

The adverse effects associated with these drugs are related to their vasodilation of blood vessels throughout the body. CNS effects include dizziness, weakness, fatigue, depression and headache. GI upset, nausea and vomiting can occur. Hypotension, CHF, shock, arrhythmias and oedema have also been reported.

Always consult a current copy of the British National Formulary for further guidance.

Clinically Important Drug–Drug Interactions

Verapamil has been associated with many drug–drug interactions, including increased risk of cardiac depression with β-blockers; additive AV slowing with digoxin; increased serum levels and toxicity of digoxin, carbamazepine and prazosin; increased respiratory depression with atracurium, gallamine, pancuronium and tubocurarine, also decreased effects if combined with calcium products or rifampin.

There is a risk of severe cardiac effects if these drugs are given intravenously within 48 hours of intravenous β-adrenergic drugs. The combination should be avoided. It may also be hazardous to give a blocker with verapamil by mouth so this too should be avoided.

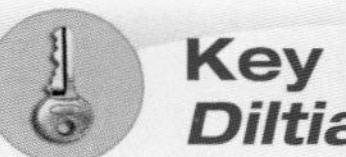

Key Drug Summary: *Diltiazem*

Indications: Treatment of paroxysmal SVT, AF and atrial flutter.

Actions: Blocks the movement of calcium ions across the cell membrane, depressing the generation of action potentials, delaying phases 1 and 2 of repolarization and slowing conduction through the AV node.

Pharmacokinetics:

Route	Onset	Peak	Duration
Oral	30–60 min	2–3 h	6–8 h
Intravenous	Immediate	2–3 min	Unknown

$T_{1/2}$: 3.5 to –6 hours; metabolized in the liver and excreted in urine.

Adverse effects: Dizziness, light-headedness, headache, asthenia, peripheral oedema, bradycardia, AV block, flushing, nausea and hepatic injury.

Other Drugs Used to Treat Arrhythmias

Adenosine is another antiarrhythmic agent that is used to convert SVT to sinus rhythm if vagal manoeuvres have been ineffective. It is often the drug of choice for terminating SVTs, including those associated with the use of alternative conduction pathways around the AV node (e.g. Wolff–Parkinson–White syndrome), for two reasons: it has a very short duration of action (about 15 seconds), after which it is picked up by circulating red blood cells and cleared through the liver; and it is associated with very few adverse effects (headache, flushing and dyspnoea of short duration). This drug slows conduction through the AV node, prolongs the refractory period and decreases automaticity in the AV node. It is given intravenously with continuous monitoring of the patient.

Digoxin (see Chapter 43) is also used at times to treat arrhythmias. This drug slows calcium from leaving the cell, prolonging the action potential and slowing conduction and heart rate. Digoxin is effective in the treatment of atrial arrhythmias. The drug is also positively inotropic, leading to increased cardiac output, which increases perfusion of the coronary arteries and may eliminate the cause of some arrhythmias as hypoxia is resolved and waste products are removed more effectively.

Nursing Considerations for Patients Receiving Antiarrhymics

Assessment: History and Examination

Screen for the following conditions, *which could be cautions or contraindications to use of the drug*; any known allergies to these drugs; impaired liver or kidney function, *which could alter the metabolism and excretion of the drug*; any condition that could be exacerbated by the depressive effects of the drugs (e.g. heart block, CHF, hypotension, shock, respiratory dysfunction and electrolyte disturbances) and pregnancy and lactation, *because of the potential for adverse effects on the foetus or neonate*.

Include screening *for baseline status before beginning therapy and for any potential adverse effects*. Assess the following: body temperature and weight; skin colour, perfusion and temperature; orientation, reflexes, pulse, blood pressure and baseline ECG; respirations and adventitious sounds; bowel sounds and abdominal examination; and renal and liver function tests.

Establish if patient is currently taking other medications or herbal therapies, which may potentially interact with the antiarrhymic drug.

Nursing Diagnoses

The patient receiving an antiarrhythmic may have the following nursing diagnoses related to drug therapy:

- Disturbed sensory perception related to CNS effects.
- Risk for injury related to CNS effects.
- Decreased cardiac output related to cardiac effects.
- Deficient knowledge regarding drug therapy.

Implementation With Rationale

- Continually monitor cardiac rhythm when initiating or changing dose, *to detect potentially serious adverse effects and to evaluate drug effectiveness*.
- Maintain life-support equipment on standby, *to treat severe adverse reactions that might occur*.
- Give parenteral forms only if the oral form is not feasible; transfer to the oral form as soon as possible, *to decrease the potential for severe adverse effects*.
- Limit the dose to the smallest amount needed to achieve control of the arrhythmia, *to decrease the risk of severe adverse effects*.
- Consult with the prescriber to reduce the dosage in patients with renal or hepatic dysfunction; reduced dosage may be needed *to ensure therapeutic effects without increased risk of toxic effects*.
- Arrange for periodic monitoring of cardiac rhythm when the patient is receiving long-term therapy, *to evaluate effects on cardiac status*.
- Provide comfort measures, *to help the patient tolerate drug effects*.
- Provide thorough patient education, including the name of the drug, dosage prescribed, measures to avoid adverse effects and warning signs of problems as well as the need for periodic monitoring and evaluation, *to enhance patient knowledge about drug therapy and promote compliance with the drug regimen*.
- Offer support and encouragement, *to help the patient deal with the diagnosis and the drug regimen*.

Evaluation

- Monitor patient response to the drug (stabilization of cardiac rhythm and output).
- Monitor for adverse effects (sedation, hypotension, cardiac arrhythmias, respiratory depression and CNS effects).
- Evaluate the effectiveness of the teaching plan (patient can name drug, dosage, adverse effects to watch for, specific measures to avoid adverse effects and the importance of continued follow-up).
- Monitor the effectiveness of comfort measures and compliance to the regimen (see Critical Thinking Scenario 44-1).

WEBLINKS

Health care providers and patients may want to consult the following Internet sources:

http://cks.library.nhs.uk The National Health Service Clinical Knowledge Summaries provides evidence-based practical information on the common conditions observed in primary care.

http://www.bhf.org.uk Patient information, support groups, research information on heart disease and scientific programmes.

http://www.bnf.org.uk The British National Formulary provides UK health care professionals with authoritative and practical information on the selection and clinical use of medicines.

http://www.nhsdirect.nhs.uk The National Health Service Direct service provides patients with information and advice about health, illness and health services.

http://www.nice.org.uk The National Institute for Health and Clinical Excellence is an independent organization responsible for providing national guidance on promoting good health and preventing and treating ill health.

http://www.resus.org.uk provides education and reference materials to health care professionals and the general public in the most effective methods of resuscitation.

Points to Remember

- Disruptions in the normal rate or rhythm of the heart are called arrhythmias (also known as dysrhythmias).
- Cardiac rate and rhythm are normally determined by the heart's specialized conduction system, starting with the SA node and progressing through the atria to the AV node, through the bundle of His into the ventricles and down the bundle branches to the fibres of the Purkinje system.
- The cardiac cells possess the property of automaticity, which allows them to generate an action potential and to stimulate the cardiac muscle without stimulation from external sources.
- Disruptions in the automaticity of the cells or in the conduction of the impulse that result in arrhythmias can be caused by changes in heart rate (tachycardia or bradycardia), stimulation from ectopic foci in the atria or ventricles that cause an uncoordinated muscle contraction or blocks in the conduction system (e.g. AV heart block and bundle branch blocks) that alter the normal movement of the impulse through the system.
- Arrhythmias can arise because of changes to the automaticity or the conductivity of the heart cells caused by electrolyte disturbances; decreases in the oxygen delivered to the cells, leading to hypoxia or anoxia; structural damage that changes the conduction pathway; acidosis or the accumulation of waste products; or drug effects.
- Arrhythmias cause problems because they alter the haemodynamics of the cardiovascular system. They can cause a decrease in cardiac output related to the uncoordinated pumping action of the irregular rhythm, leading to lack of filling time for the ventricles. Any of these effects can interfere with the delivery of blood to the brain, to other tissues, or to the heart muscle itself.
- Antiarrhythmics are drugs that alter the action potential of the heart cells and interrupt arrhythmias. The Cardiac Arrhythmia Suppression Trial study found that the long-term treatment of arrhythmias may actually cause cardiac death, so these drugs are now indicated only for the short-term treatment of potentially life-threatening ventricular arrhythmias.
- Class I antiarrhythmics block sodium channels, depress phase 0 of the action potential and generally prolong the action potential, leading to a slowing of conduction and automaticity.
- Class II antiarrhythmics are adrenergic receptor blockers that prevent sympathetic stimulation.
- Class III antiarrhythmics block potassium channels and prolong phase 3 of the action potential.
- Class IV antiarrhythmics are calcium channel blockers that shorten the action potential, disrupting ineffective rhythms and rates.
- A patient receiving an antiarrhythmic drug needs to be constantly monitored while being stabilized and during the use of the drug to detect the development of arrhythmias or other adverse effects associated with alteration of the action potentials of other muscles or nerves.

CRITICAL THINKING SCENARIO 44-1

Recognizing Digoxin Toxicity

The Situation

Ray, a 61-year-old man, began taking digoxin 2 weeks ago after being admitted to hospital with fast AF. Ray has become concerned because over the past few days he has been experiencing nausea and vomiting and episodes of confusion and forgetfulness. He is also having episodes of "blurred" vision and headaches; he feels generally unwell. Ray is concerned that his fast AF has re-occurred, so he presents at the local Accident and Emergency (A&E) department for advice. On examination, Rays pulse is 120 beats/minute and an ECG showed atrial tachycardia with AV block. His

(continued)

Recognizing Digoxin Toxicity *(continued)*

blood pressure was 90/60 mmHg. Blood tests revealed his digoxin levels to be 2.6 mg/ml.

Critical Thinking

Based on your knowledge of the drug digoxin and the symptoms reported by Ray, what do you think has happened?

What investigations will Ray require and what should be done to alleviate his signs and symptoms?

What alternative medications could be used to control Ray's condition?

Should any other problems be addressed while Ray is being evaluated at this time?

Discussion

Ray has many signs and symptoms of digoxin toxicity; atriotachycardia with AV heart block, hypotension, nausea, vomiting, dizziness, headache and confusion. The initial treatment for this condition includes withholding all medications, ordering blood drawn for a serum digoxin level determination and careful monitoring of Ray, with emergency life-support equipment on standby in case his condition deteriorates.

The signs and symptoms of digoxin toxicity should be reviewed with Ray, as well as precautionary measures that he should take. He should be told that he did the correct thing in calling and should be encouraged to do so again if he has further problems. The teaching programme should be directed at preventing future problems.

While Ray is within the health care system, it is important to offer him support and encouragement. Ray may need to ventilate his feelings and explore new ways of coping with or avoiding stressful situations. The effects of stress on the heart can be reviewed with Ray to help him realize the importance of stress management. It would also be helpful to review the problems of self-medication for various complaints while taking a prescription drug. Ray should receive all information in writing for future reference. Eventually, he may be re-evaluated to determine the actual need for continuing this medication. In the meantime, good patient education can help prevent serious complications while he is using the drug.

Patient Education for Ray

- ☐ An antiarrhythmic drug such as digoxin acts to stop irregular rhythm in the heart, helping it to beat more regularly and, therefore, more efficiently. The drug may work by making the heart less irritable and by slowing it down to a more effective rate.
- ☐ Digoxin may be taken with food if GI upset occurs.
- ☐ Some of the following adverse effects may occur:
  - *Tiredness and weakness:* Space your activities throughout the day and take periodic rest periods to help conserve your energy and rest your heart.
  - *Nausea, vomiting and loss of appetite:* These problems may pass over time; taking the drug with meals, if appropriate, or eating small, frequent meals may help.
  - *Sensitivity to light*: Avoid prolonged exposure to ultraviolet light or sunlight.
  - *Constipation or diarrhoea:* These reactions are very common; if either occurs or becomes too uncomfortable; consult your health care provider.
  - Report any of the following to your health care provider: *chest pain, difficulty in breathing, ringing in the ears, swelling in the ankles or legs, unusually slow pulse rate* (>35 beats/minute), *unusually fast pulse rate* (>15 beats/minute above your normal rate), *suddenly irregular pulse rate, fever and rash.*
  - Tell any doctor, nurse or other health care provider involved in your care that you are taking this drug.
  - Keep this drug and all medications out of the reach of children.
  - Avoid using over-the-counter medications while you are taking this drug. If you feel that you need one of these, consult with your health care provider for the best choice. Many of these drugs can interfere with the effects of your medication.
  - Schedule regular medical appointments while you are on this drug to evaluate your heart rhythm and your response to the drug.
  - Do not stop taking this medication. If you have to stop the medication for any reason, contact your health care provider immediately.

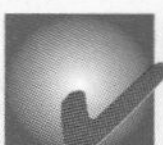

CHECK YOUR UNDERSTANDING

Answers to the questions in this chapter may be found in the Answer Key in the back of the book.

Multiple Choice

Select the most appropriate response to the following:

1. Cardiac contraction and relaxation are controlled by
   a. the brain.
   b. the sympathetic nervous system.
   c. the autonomic nervous system.
   d. impulses that arise spontaneously with the heart itself.

2. Antiarrhythmic drugs alter the action potential of the cardiac cells. As they alter the action potential, antiarrhythmic drugs often
   a. cause CHF.
   b. alter blood flow to the kidney.
   c. cause new arrhythmias.
   d. cause electrolyte disturbances.

3. The drug of choice for the treatment of a SVT associated with Wolff–Parkinson–White syndrome is
   a. digoxin.
   b. verapamil.
   c. amiodarone.
   d. adenosine.

4. A patient who is receiving an antiarrhythmic drug needs
   a. constant cardiac monitoring until stabilized.
   b. frequent blood tests including drug levels.
   c. an antidepressant drug to deal with the psychological depression.
   d. changes in diet and exercise programmes to prevent irritation of the heart muscle.

5. A client stabilized on quinidine for the regulation of AF would be cautioned to avoid foods
   a. high in potassium.
   b. high in tyrosine.
   c. high in sodium content.
   d. that alkalinize the urine.

Extended Matching Questions

Select all that apply.

1. The conduction system of the heart would include which of the following?
   a. The SA node
   b. The sinuses of Valsalva
   c. The atrial bundles
   d. The Purkinje fibres
   e. The coronary sinus
   f. The bundle of His

2. Arrhythmias or dysrhythmias can be caused by which of the following?
   a. Lack of oxygen to the heart muscle cells
   b. Acidosis near a cell
   c. Structural damage in the conduction pathway through the heart
   d. Vasodilation in the myocardial vascular bed
   e. Thyroid hormone imbalance
   f. Electrolyte imbalances

Fill in the Blanks

1. Arrhythmias can be caused by changes in heart rate, either ________________ or ________________.

2. Arrhythmias can cause a decrease in ________________ ________________ leading to a decrease in the amount of blood being pumped to the brain and periphery.

3. Antiarrhythmics alter the ________________ of the heart cells and interfere with conduction, blocking arrhythmias.

4. Cardiac cells possess the property of ________________, which allows them to generate an action potential but also makes them susceptible to arrhythmias.

5. Class II antiarrhythmics are ________________ blockers.

6. A commonly used cardiotonic agent that is used to slow the heart rate and treat atrial arrhythmias is ________________.

7. ________________ can be used to treat ventricular arrhythmias in emergency situations and is also a commonly used local anaesthetic.

Bibliography and References

Brantman L., Howie J. (2006). Use of amiodarone to prevent atrial fibrillation after cardiac surgery. *Critical Care Nurse*, 26(1), 48–59.

British Medical Association and Royal Pharmaceutical Society of Great Britain. (2008). *British National Formulary*. London: BMJ & RPS Publishing. *This publication is updated biannually; it is imperative that the most recent edition is consulted.*

British Medical Association and Royal Pharmaceutical Society of Great Britain. (2008). *British National Formulary for Children*. London: BMJ & RPS Publishing. *This publication is updated annually; it is imperative that the most recent edition is consulted.*

Brunton, L., Lazo, J. S., Parker, K., Goodman, L. S., & Gilman, A. G. (2005). *Goodman and Gilman's the pharmacological basis of therapeutics* (11th ed.). London: McGraw-Hill.

DiMarco, J. P., Gersh, B. J., & Opie, L. H. (2005). *Antiarrthymic drugs and strategies.* In: L. H. Opie (Ed.). *Drugs for the heart* (6th ed). Philadelphia: Elsevier Saunders.

Fang, M. C., Stafford, R. S., Ruskin, J. N., & Singer, D. E. (2004). National trends in antiarrhythmic and antithrombotic medication use in atrial fibrillation. *Archives of Internal Medicine*, 164(1), 55–60.

Galbraith, A., Bullock, S., Manias, E., Hunt, B., & Richards, A. (1997). *Fundamentals of pharmacology.* Harlow: Pearson Prentice Hall.

Ganong, W. (2005). *Review of medical physiology* (22nd ed.). New York: McGraw-Hill.

Goldschlager, N., Epstein, A. E., Naccarelli, G., Olshansky, B., & Singh, B. (2000). Practical guidelines for clinicians who treat patients with amiodarone. *Archives of Internal Medicine*, 160(12), 1741–1748.

Guyton, A., & Hall, J. (2005). *Textbook of medical physiology* (11th ed.). Philadelphia: W.B. Saunders.

Karch, A. M. (2006). *2007 Lippincott's nursing drug guide.* Philadelphia: Lippincott Williams & Wilkins.

Marieb, E.N., & Hoehn, K. (2007). *Human anatomy & physiology* (7th ed.). San Francisco: Pearson Benjamin Cummings.

McEvoy, B. R. (2006). *Facts and comparisons 2004.* St. Louis: Facts and Comparisons. *The medical letter on drugs and therapeutics.* New Rochelle, New York: Medical Letter.

O'Donovan, K. (2006). Amiodarone as a class III antiarrthymic drug. *British Journal of Cardiac Nursing*, 1(11), 530–539.

Porth, C. M., & Matfin, G. (2008). *Pathophysiology: concepts of altered health states* (8th ed.). Philadelphia: Lippincott Williams & Wilkins.

Resuscitation Councils Advanced Life Support guidelines. (2005). Available from http://www.resus.org.uk.

Sanofi Aventis. (2006). *Cordarone X 100, Cordarone X 200. Summary of product characteristics*. Surrey: Sanofi Aventis.

Siddoway, L.A. (2003). Amiodarone: guidelines for use and monitoring. *American Family Physician*, 68(11), 2189–2196.

CHAPTER

45

Antianginal Agents

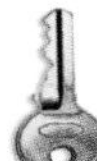

KEY TERMS

angina pectoris

atheromas

atherosclerosis

coronary artery disease (CAD)

nitrates

pulse pressure

acute coronary syndrome

- stable angina
- unstable angina
- myocardial infarction (Non-STEM1, STEM1)

LEARNING OBJECTIVES

Upon completion of this chapter, you will be able to:

1. Describe the nature of coronary artery disease the identified risk factors associated with the development of the disease and the clinical presentation of the disease.
2. Describe the therapeutic actions, indications and pharmacokinetics associated with the nitrates, β-blockers and calcium channel blockers used to treat angina.
3. Describe the contraindications, most common adverse reactions and important drug–drug interactions associated with the nitrates, β-blockers and calcium channel blockers used to treat angina.
4. Discuss the use of antianginal agents across the lifespan.
5. Compare and contrast metoprolol, atenolol and diltiazem with other agents used to treat angina.
6. Outline the nursing considerations, including important teaching points, for patients receiving drugs used to treat angina.

NITRATES

glyceryl trinitrate (GTN)
isosorbide dinitrate
isosorbide mononitrate

BETA-BLOCKERS

acebutalol
atenolol
metoprolol
nadolol
propranolol

CALCIUM CHANNEL BLOCKERS

amlodipine
diltiazem
nicardipine
nifedipine
verapamil

POTASSIUM-CHANNEL ACTIVATORS

Nicorandil

Cardiovascular disease (CVD) is the most common cause of premature death in the UK: 21% of premature deaths in men and 12% of premature deaths in women are from coronary heart disease (CHD). Nearly all deaths from CHD are because of a myocardial infarction (MI). Around 230,000 in the UK suffer an MI each year, and in 30% of these cases the patient dies. The good news is that death rates for CHD have been falling in the UK since the late 1970s. For adults under 65 years, the death rate from an MI has fallen by over 44% in the last 10 years (British Heart Foundation Statistics, 2006).

Whereas mortality from CHD is falling rapidly, morbidity from CHD and other circulatory disease appears to be rising, especially in older age groups. In those aged 65 years and older, morbidity has risen by around 20% since the late 1980s. Around 1.3 million people in the UK have had a heart attack, and approximately 2 million people are suffering from angina, the most common form of CHD (British Heart Foundation Statistics, 2006).

Despite vast development in the understanding of the contributing causes of this disease and ways to prevent it, CHD still claims more lives than any other disease (Gemmell *et al.*, 2006). The drugs discussed in this chapter are used to reduce the risk of myocardial death when the coronary vessels are already seriously damaged and are having difficulty maintaining the blood flow to the heart muscle. Chapters 45 and 46 discuss drugs that are used to prevent the occlusion of the coronary arteries before they become narrowed and damaged or to restore blood flow through narrowed vessels.

Coronary Vascular Disease

The myocardium, or heart muscle, must receive a constant supply of blood in order to have the oxygen and nutrients needed to maintain a constant pumping action. The myocardium receives all of its blood from two coronary arteries that exit the sinuses of Valsalva at the base of the aorta. These vessels divide and subdivide to form the capillaries that deliver oxygen to heart muscle fibres.

Unlike other tissues in the body, cardiac muscle receives its blood supply during diastole, while it is at rest. This is important because when the heart muscle contracts, it becomes tight and clamps the blood vessels closed, rendering them unable to receive blood during systole, which is when all other tissues receive oxygenated blood. The openings in the sinuses of Valsalva, which are the origins of the coronary arteries, are positioned so that they can be filled when the blood flows back against the aortic valve when the heart is at rest. The pressure that fills these vessels is the **pulse pressure** (the systolic pressure minus the diastolic pressure) – the pressure of the column of blood falling back onto the closed aortic valve. The heart has just finished contracting and using energy and oxygen. The acid and carbon dioxide built-up in the muscle causes a local vasodilation, and the blood flows freely through the coronary arteries and into the muscle cells.

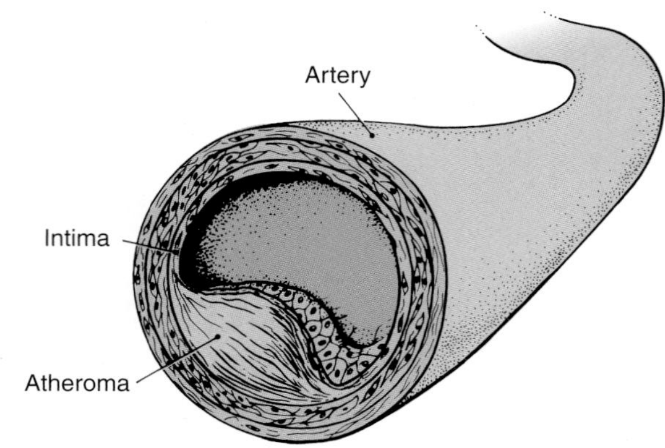

FIGURE 45.1 Schematic illustration of atheromatous plaque.

In CVD, the lumens of the blood vessels become narrowed so that blood is no longer able to flow freely to the muscle cells. The narrowing of the vessels is caused by the development of **atheromas** or fatty deposits in the intima of the vessels (Figure 45.1). This is a process called **atherosclerosis**. These fatty deposits cause damage to the intima lining of the vessels, attracting platelets and immune factors and causing swelling and the development of a larger deposit. Over time, these deposits severely decrease the lumen size of the vessel. While the vessel is being narrowed by the deposits, it is also losing its natural elasticity and becoming unable to respond to the normal stimuli to dilate or constrict to meet the needs of the tissues.

The person with atherosclerosis has a classic supply-and-demand problem. The heart may be able to meet demand until there is increased activity or other stresses that put a demand on it to beat faster or harder. The normal heart would stimulate the vessels to deliver more blood when this occurs, but the narrowed vessels are not able to respond and cannot supply the blood needed by the working heart (Figure 45.2). The heart muscle then becomes hypoxic (low oxygen levels).

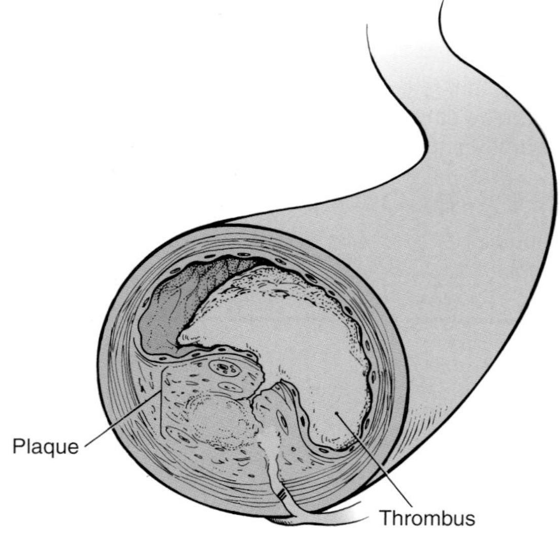

FIGURE 45.2 Thrombosis of atherosclerotic plaque. It may partially or completely occlude the lumen of the vessel.

This happens with **angina pectoris**, literally 'suffocation of the chest'. If the supply-and-demand issue becomes worse, or if a vessel becomes so narrow that it occludes, the cells in the myocardium may actually die from lack of oxygen and become necrotic. The umbrella term *'Acute Coronary Syndrome'* is commonly used in clinical practice to include: angina – (stable and unstable), **MI (ST elevation MI) (STEMI)** and non-ST elevation **MI (non-STEMI)**.

Stable Angina

The body's response to a lack of oxygen in the heart muscle is pain. Although the heart muscle does not have any pain fibres, a chemical mediator called substance P is released from ischaemic myocardial cells, and pain is felt wherever substance P reacts with pain receptors. For many people this pain is felt in the chest, while others feel referred pain in the left arm or in the jaw, teeth, shoulders and upper gastric area. The basic response to this type of pain is to stop whatever one is doing and to wait for the pain to go away. In cases of minor limitations to the blood flow through vessels, stopping activity may bring the supply and demand for blood back into balance. This condition is called **stable angina**. There is no damage to heart muscle, and the basic reflexes surrounding the pain restore blood flow to the heart muscle.

Unstable Angina

If the narrowing of the coronary arteries becomes more pronounced, the heart may experience episodes of ischaemia even when the patient is at rest. When this occurs, this condition is called **unstable angina**. Though there is still no damage to heart muscle, the person is at great risk of a complete cessation of blood flow to the heart muscle, if the heart should have to work hard or increase demand.

Acute Myocardial Infarction

If a coronary vessel becomes completely occluded and is unable to deliver blood to the cardiac muscle, the area of muscle that depends on that vessel for oxygen becomes ischaemic and then necrotic and an MI occurs. The pain associated with this event can be excruciating; nausea and a severe sympathetic stress reaction may also be present. A serious danger of an MI is that arrhythmias can develop in nearby tissue. Most of the deaths caused by MI occur as a result of fatal arrhythmias.

If the heart muscle has a chance to heal, within 6 to 10 weeks the dead area will be replaced with scar tissue, and the muscle will attempt to compensate for the injury. If the area of the muscle that is damaged is very large, the muscle may not be able to compensate for the loss and congestive heart failure (CHF) and even cardiogenic shock may occur. These conditions can be fatal or can leave a person severely limited by the weakened heart muscle.

Antianginal Drugs

In early cases of angina, avoidance of exertion or stressful situations may be sufficient to prevent anginal pain. Antianginal drugs are used to help restore the supply-and-demand ratio in oxygen/blood delivery to the myocardium when rest is not enough. These drugs can work to improve blood delivery to the heart muscle in one of two ways by:

- dilating blood vessels (i.e. increasing the supply of oxygen)
- decreasing the work of the heart (i.e. decreasing the demand for oxygen).

Nitrates, β-adrenergic blockers, calcium channel blockers and potassium channel activators are used to treat angina (Figure 45.3). They are all effective and are sometimes used in combination to achieve good control of the anginal pain. The type of drug that is best for a patient is determined by tolerance of adverse effects and response to the drug. The use of antianginal agents with different age groups is discussed in Box 45.1.

Nitrates

Nitrates are drugs that act directly on smooth muscle to cause relaxation and to depress muscle tone. The action is direct; therefore, it does not have to influence any nerve or other activity. The response to this type of drug is usually quite fast. The nitrates relax and dilate veins, arteries and capillaries, allowing increased blood flow through these vessels and lowering systemic blood pressure because of a drop in resistance. The nitrates probably have very little effect on increasing blood flow through the coronary arteries because CAD causes a stiffening and lack of responsiveness in the coronary arteries (Gatzka *et al.,* 1998); however, they do increase blood flow through healthy coronary arteries, so there will be an increased supply of blood through any healthy vessels in the heart and that could help the heart to compensate somewhat.

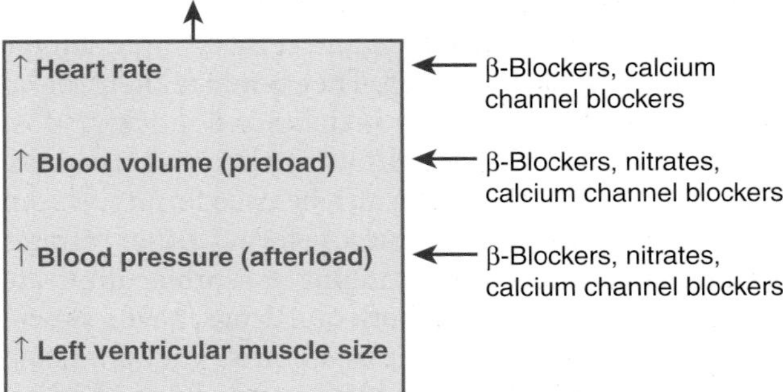

FIGURE 45.3 Factors affecting myocardial oxygen demand and points where antianginal drugs have their effects.

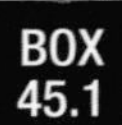

BOX 45.1 DRUG THERAPY ACROSS THE LIFESPAN

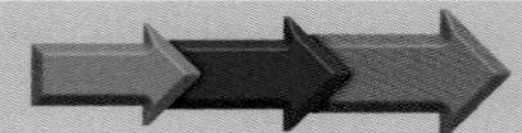

Antianginal Agents

CHILDREN

Antianginals are not indicated for any condition commonly found in children. In some situations, for example congenital heart defects or cardiac surgery, glyceryl trinitrate (GTN) may be used under specialist supervision.The dose of the drug should be determined by considering age and weight. The child should be very carefully monitored for adverse reactions, including potentially dangerous changes in blood pressure.

When administering any drug to children, always consult the most recent edition of the British National Formulary for Children.

ADULTS

Adults who receive antianginal agents should be instructed in their proper administration for example sublingual (under the tongue) as in the case of GTN. Patients should also be encouraged to determine what activities or situations tend to precipitate an anginal attack so that they can take measures to avoid those particular circumstances or take an antianginal agent before the event occurs.

Patients should know that regular medical follow-up is important and should be instructed in appropriate nonpharmacological measures – weight loss, smoking cessation, activity changes, dietary changes – that could decrease the risk of progression of their coronary artery disease and improve the effectiveness of the antianginal therapy.

The safety for the use of these drugs during pregnancy has not been established therefore, if angina occurs in pregnancy then referral to specialist care is essential. There is a significant potential for adverse effects on the foetus related to blood flow changes and direct drug effects when the drugs cross the placenta. The drugs do enter breast milk, and it is advised that another method of feeding the baby be used if one of these drugs is prescribed during lactation.

OLDER ADULTS

Older adults frequently are prescribed one or more of these drugs. Older adults are more likely to develop adverse effects associated with the use of these drugs – arrhythmias, hypotension and congestive heart disease. Safety measures may be needed if these effects occur and interfere with the patient's mobility and balance.

The older adults are also more likely to have renal and/or hepatic impairment related to underlying medical conditions, which could interfere with the metabolism and excretion of these drugs. The dosage for older adults should be started at a lower level than that recommended for younger adults. The patient should be monitored very closely and dosage adjusted based on patient response.

If other drugs are added or removed from the drug regimen, appropriate dosage adjustments should be considered

The main effect of nitrates, however, seems to be related to the drop in blood pressure that occurs. The action of nitrates is attributed to the production of nitric oxide, which is a powerful vasodilating agent. The vasodilation causes blood to pool in veins and capillaries, decreasing the volume of blood that the heart has to pump around (the preload), while the relaxation of the vessels decreases the resistance the heart has to pump against (the afterload). The combination of these effects greatly reduces the cardiac workload and the demand for oxygen, thus bringing the supply-and-demand ratio back into balance.

Sublingual GTN (see Box 45.2) is the nitrate of choice in an acute anginal attack. It can be given sublingually, as a translingual spray, intravenously (IV), transdermally, topically or as a transmucosal agent. It is very lipid soluble and therefore rapidly absorbed. They produce their therapeutic effects rapidly but are metabolized quickly. Most preparations can be carried with the patient, who can use it when the need arises. It can also be used for prevention of anginal attacks in the slow-release forms. Other nitrates are also available for treating angina. Isosorbide dinitrate and isosorbide mononitrate, both oral drugs, have a slower onset of action but may last up to 4 hours. They are taken before chest pain begins in situations in which exertion or stress can be anticipated. They are not drugs of choice during an acute attack, however, they have a more longer lasting effect than GTN, making them more suitable for prophylaxis of angina.

Therapeutic Actions and Indications

The nitrates cause direct relaxation of smooth muscle with a resultant decrease in venous return and decrease in arterial pressure, effects that reduce cardiac workload and decrease myocardial oxygen consumption. They are indicated for the prevention and treatment of attacks of angina pectoris.

Pharmacokinetics

These drugs are very rapidly absorbed, metabolized in the liver and excreted in urine. They cross the placenta and enter breast milk. They are not recommended for use during pregnancy or lactation, because of the potential for serious adverse effects related to blood flow changes on the foetus and neonate.

Contraindications and Cautions

Nitrates are contraindicated in the presence of any allergy to nitrates. These drugs also are contraindicated in the following conditions: severe anaemia, *because the decrease in cardiac output could be detrimental*; head trauma or cerebral haemorrhage, *because the relaxation of cerebral vessels could cause intracranial bleeding* and pregnancy or lactation, *because of potential adverse effects on the neonate and ineffective blood flow to the foetus.*

BOX 45.2 FOCUS ON **CLINICAL SKILLS**

Sublingual Administration of GTN

Nitrates can be given by several routes; sublingual administration is the most common. The most commonly used method of administration is the sublingual spray although sublingual tablets may still be used. One advantage the sublingual spray has over the sublingual tablet is a longer shelf life. Patients often prefer to administer the drug themselves, even in the institutional setting. It is important for the nurse to make sure that the drug is given correctly: Prior to administration, the patient's blood pressure and pulse should be checked to ensure patient is not hypotensive, bradycardic or complaining of light-headedness or dizziness.

With the spray, patients should administer one to two doses under the tongue, then close their mouth. When using sublingual tablets:

- Check under the tongue to make sure there are no lesions or abrasions that could interfere with the absorption of the drug. Encourage the patient to take a sip of water to moisten the mucous membranes so the tablet will dissolve quickly. Then instruct the patient to place the tablet under the tongue, close the mouth and wait until the tablet has dissolved.
- Caution the patient not to swallow the tablet; its effectiveness would be lost if the tablet entered the stomach. If the patient uses sublingual drugs often, encourage the patient to alternate sides of the tongue—placing it under the left side for one dose and under the right side for the other dose.
- Here's a tip to help administer sublingual medications to patients who cannot do it themselves or who cannot open their mouths: Use a tongue depressor to move the tongue aside and place the tablet under the tongue.

During an acute angina attack:

- If administering spray, check blood pressure (BP) first.
- Ask patient to open mouth and lift up tongue.
- Administer two puffs of spray under tongue
- Wait 5 minutes for spray to take effect. During these 5 minutes, recheck blood pressure and pulse. Reassess patient's pain levels (using a pain score is helpful, 0 = no pain, 5 = medium pain and 10 = severe pain.
- If pain is still present and systolic BP remains over 90 mmHg, administer a further two puffs of spray.
- Again wait 5 minutes and reassess patient as above.
- Reassess pain levels, using pain score and if pain is still present administer another two puffs of spray.

Do not exceed six puffs of spray over a 15-minute period. Six puffs is the maximum dose that can be administered if bp remains stable. Important to reassess patient's pain levels throughout.

Caution should be used in patients with hepatic or renal disease, *which could alter the metabolism and excretion of these drugs.* Caution also is required with hypotension, hypovolaemia and conditions that limit cardiac output (e.g. tamponade, low ventricular filling pressure, low pulmonary capillary wedge pressure), *because these conditions could be exacerbated, resulting in serious adverse effects.*

Adverse Effects

The adverse effects associated with these drugs are related to the vasodilation fall in blood pressure and decrease in blood flow that occurs. Common central nervous system (CNS) effects include headache, dizziness and weakness. Less common gastrointestinal (GI) symptoms can include nausea, vomiting and incontinence. Cardiovascular problems which must be monitored include hypotension, which can be severe; reflex tachycardia (that may occur when blood pressure falls); syncope and angina. Skin-related effects include flushing, pallor and increased perspiration. With the transdermal preparation, there is a risk of contact dermatitis and local hypersensitivity reactions.

Clinically Important Drug–Drug Interactions

There is a risk of hypertension and decreased antianginal effects, if these drugs are given with ergot derivatives, for example ergotamine or bromocriptine. There is also a risk of decreased therapeutic effects of heparin if these drugs are given together with heparin; if this combination is used, the patient should be monitored and appropriate dosage adjustments made.

Always consult a current copy of the British National Formulary for further guidance.

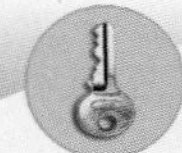

Key Drug Summary: *Glyceryl Trinitrate (GTN)*

Indications: Treatment of acute angina, prophylaxis of angina, intravenous treatment of angina unresponsive to β-blockers or organic nitrates, CHF associated with acute MI; perioperative hypertension to produce controlled hypotension during surgery

Actions: Relaxes vascular smooth muscle with a resultant decrease in venous return and decrease in arterial blood pressure, reducing (preload) the left ventricular workload and decreasing myocardial oxygen consumption. GTN will have very little, if any, dilating actions on occluded coronary arteries.

Pharmacokinetics:

Route	Onset	Duration
IV	1–2 min	3–5 min
Sublingual	1–3 min	20–30 min
Translingual spray	2 min	20–30 min
Transmucosal tablet	1–2 min	3–5 min
Oral, SR tablet	20–45 min	8–12 h
Topical ointment	30–60 min	4–8 h
Transdermal	30–60 min	24 h

$T_{1/2}$: 1–4 minutes; metabolized in the liver and excreted in urine

Adverse effects: Hypotension, headache, dizziness, tachycardia, rash, flushing, nausea, vomiting, sweating, chest pain

Nursing Considerations for Patients Receiving Nitrates

Assessment: History and Examination

A thorough patient history should be taken using a recognized systematic approach such as a specific question regarding CVD and the following should be included; impaired liver or kidney function, *which could alter the metabolism and excretion of the drug*; any condition that could be exacerbated by the hypotension and change in blood flow caused by these drugs (e.g. early MI, head trauma, cerebral haemorrhage, hypotension, hypovolaemia, anaemia, low cardiac output states); and pregnancy or lactation, *because of the potential adverse effects on the foetus or neonate.*

Include screening *for baseline status before beginning therapy and for any potential adverse effects.* Assess and record the following: pulse, blood pressure, baseline electrocardiogram (ECG), skin colour, perfusion and temperature; respirations and adventitious sounds; liver and renal function tests; full blood count including the haemoglobin level: lipids screening and other blood tests (if not already recorded).

Establish if patient is currently taking other medications or herbal therapies which may potentially interact with nitrates

Nursing Diagnoses

The patient receiving a nitrate may have the following nursing diagnoses related to drug therapy:

- Decreased cardiac output related to hypotensive effects
- Risk for injury related to CNS or cardiovascular effects and hypotensive effects
- Ineffective tissue perfusion (total body) related to hypotension or change in cardiac output
- Deficient knowledge regarding drug therapy

Implementation With Rationale

- Ask the patient if the tablet 'fizzles' or burns, which indicates potency. Always check the expiration date on the bottle and protect the medication from heat and light, *because these drugs are volatile and lose their potency.*
- Give sustained-release (SR) forms with water and caution the patient not to chew or crush them, *because these preparations need to reach the GI tract intact.*
- Rotate the sites of topical forms *to decrease the risk of skin abrasion and breakdown*; monitor for signs of skin breakdown *to arrange for appropriate skin care as needed.*
- Make sure that sublingual spray is used under the tongue and not inhaled *to ensure that the therapeutic effects are optimized.*
- Provide thorough patient education, including the name of the drug, dosage prescribed, proper administration, measures to avoid adverse effects, warning signs of problems and the importance of periodic monitoring and evaluation, *to enhance patient knowledge about drug therapy and promote compliance to the drug regimen.*
- Offer support and encouragement *to help the patient deal with the diagnosis and the drug regimen.*
- *Education, advice remanagement of side-effects* , for example *headaches*

Evaluation

- Monitor patient response to the drug (alleviation of signs and symptoms of angina, prevention of angina).
- Monitor for adverse effects (hypotension, cardiac arrhythmias, GI upset, skin reactions and headache).
- Evaluate the effectiveness of the teaching plan (patient can name drug, dosage, proper administration, adverse effects to watch for, specific measures to avoid adverse effects and the importance of continued follow-up).
- Monitor the effectiveness of comfort measures and compliance to the regimen (see Critical Thinking Scenario 45-1).

β-Blockers

As discussed in Chapter 30, β-adrenergic blockers are used to block the stimulatory effects of the sympathetic nervous system. These drugs block β-adrenergic receptors and prevent vasoconstriction (thereby stopping an increase in blood pressure), prevent an increase in heart rate and increased intensity of myocardial contraction that occurs with sympathetic stimulation such as exertion or stress. These effects decrease the cardiac workload and the demand for oxygen.

β-Blockers are sometimes used in combination with nitrates to increase exercise tolerance in patients with coronary artery disease. β-Blockers have many adverse effects associated with the blockade of the sympathetic nervous system bradycardia, hypotension and GI disturbances. The dose that is used to prevent angina is usually lower than doses used to treat hypertension, so there is a decreased incidence of adverse effects associated with this specific use of β-blockers. These drugs are not usually recommended for use in patients with peripheral vascular disease or chronic obstructive pulmonary disease (COPD), because the effects on the sympathetic nervous system could exacerbate these problems (Engred *et al.*, 2005).The β-blockers that are recommended for use in angina are metoprolol and atenolol (López-Sendó *et al.,* 2004).

Three Generations of β-blockers

First generation β-blockers like propranolol are largely nonselective β1 and β2 adrenoceptor inhibitors. Although sometimes still used, they have limited clinical use owing largely to their antagonistic effect on β2 receptors.

Second generation β-blockers, in contrast, bind preferentially to the β1 receptor and are therefore described as β-selective. Of the commonly used β-blockers, those which select the β1 receptor include bisoprolol, atenolol, metoprolol and acebutolol. Bisoprolol displays a 14-fold greater affinity for the β1 receptor than for the β2 receptor (Baker, 2005). Second generation β-blockers have limited effect on β receptors and this enables them to be used more safely in patients with asthma. Although patients have varied and unpredictable responses to these drugs, there is now increased clinical evidence that at least in cases of short-term use, β1-selective β-blockers like Bisoprolol and atenolol may be used in mild-to-moderate reversible airway disease or chronic COPD (Barnett *et al.*, 2005; Salpeter *et al.,* 2002;) (cited by Khan, 2006).

Third Generation

Third generation β-blockers possess a vasodilator effect in addition to their β-blockade effect. β selectivity of this generation varies. Carvedilol is a relatively selective (seven-fold greater) β1 antagonist especially at lower doses. It also has some effect on the β2 receptors, as well as a number of α1 receptor blockade properties, through which it mediates its vasodilator effect (Khan, 2006). Nebivolol is a novel third generation β-receptor antagonist that is highly β1 selective (significantly more than Bisoprolol). Nebivolol also has a vasodilator effect. Its vasodilator effect is mediated by nitric oxide/L-arginine dependent pathway, in a manner similar to nitrates.

Owing to their vasodilator effect, third generation β-blockers have been examined in some depth in association with heart failure (Khan, 2006).

Therapeutic Actions and Indications

The β-blockers competitively block β-adrenergic receptors in the heart and juxtaglomerular apparatus, decreasing the influence of the sympathetic nervous system on these tissues and thereby decreasing the excitability of the heart, decreasing cardiac output, decreasing cardiac oxygen compensation and lowering blood pressure. They are indicated for the long-term management of angina pectoris caused by atherosclerosis. They are not indicated for the treatment of Prinzmetal's angina, because they could cause vasospasm when they block β-receptor sites. Atenolol is generally the drug of choice if there is no evidence of heart failure; used to prevent reinfarction in stable patients 1 to 4 weeks after an MI. If left ventricular failure is present, bisoprolol or carvedilol is recommended, or metoprolol may be used as it is shorter acting.

Use of β-blockers in cardiac illness has long been recognized by a number of national and international regulating and governing bodies, including the European Cardiac Society, The British Cardiac Society, the British Hypertension Society and the American College of Cardiologists. The National Institute for Clinical Excellence (NICE) has published a number of guidelines that suggest the early introduction of β blocker therapy in heart failure and after a MI (National Institute of Health and Clinical Excellence, 2003).

Pharmacokinetics

These drugs are absorbed from the GI tract and undergo hepatic metabolism. Food has been found to increase the bioavailability of propranolol, but this effect has not been found with other β-adrenergic blocking agents. These drugs are excreted in urine, necessitating caution in patients with renal impairment. Teratogenic effects have occurred in animal studies with all of these drugs. The use of any β-adrenergic blocker during pregnancy should be reserved for situations in which the benefit to the mother outweighs the risk to the foetus. In general, they should not be used during lactation because of the potential for adverse effects on the baby. The safety and efficacy of the use of these drugs in children has not been established.

Contraindications and Cautions

The β-blockers are contraindicated in patients with uncontrolled heart failure, heart block – cardiogenic shock, asthma or COPD *because their blocking of the sympathetic response could exacerbate these diseases.* They also are contraindicated with pregnancy and lactation, *because of the potential for adverse effects on the foetus or neonate.*

Caution should be used in patients with diabetes, peripheral vascular disease or thyrotoxicosis, *because the blockade of the sympathetic response blocks normal reflexes that are necessary for maintaining homeostasis in patients with these diseases.*

Adverse Effects

Side-effects often depend on the type of drug administered and the patient's underlying pathology. Cardiac side-effects which may be expected are bradycardia and atrioventricular (AV) conduction blocks. If the patient is older, fibrosis may influence proper conduction in the heart and may further increase these risks. In such cases, β-blockers may also lead to abnormalities in the function of the SA node leading to sick-sinus syndrome (Marriott and Conovor, 1998).

The association of beta-blockade with erectile dysfunction has been widely discussed. Nebivolol is suggested to be beneficial in the presence of this side-effect, potentially owing to its nitric oxide-related vasodilator effects (Khan, 2006).

The adverse effects associated with these drugs are related to their blockade of the sympathetic nervous system. CNS effects include dizziness, fatigue, emotional depression and sleep disturbances. GI problems include gastric pain, nausea, vomiting, colitis and diarrhoea. Cardiovascular effects can include CHF, reduced cardiac output and arrhythmias. Respiratory symptoms can include bronchospasm, dyspnoea and cough. Decreased exercise tolerance malaise and cold peripheries are also common complaints.

Always consult a current copy of the British National Formulary for further guidance.

Clinically Important Drug–Drug Interactions

A paradoxical hypertension occurs when clonidine is given with β-blockers and an increased rebound hypertension with clonidine withdrawal may also occur; it is best to avoid this combination.

A decreased antihypertensive effect occurs when β-blockers are given with NSAIDs; if this combination is used, the patient should be monitored closely and a dosage adjustment made.

An initial hypertensive episode followed by bradycardia occurs if these drugs are given with adrenaline and a possibility of peripheral ischaemia exists if β-blockers are taken in combination with ergot alkaloids.

Antiarrthymics tend to increase the effect of β-blockers. The effect may be stronger with certain antiarrthymics such as sotolol. Verapamil and a β-blocker is contraindicated. Verapamil has a negative dromotropy effect (reduced conduction velocity) particularly on the AV node. Similarly, diltiazem and β-blockers are contraindicated. Diltiazem has a significant dromotropic effect on cardiac conduction (Khan, 2006).

There also is a potential for a change in blood glucose levels if these drugs are given with insulin or antidiabetic agents, and the patient will not have the usual signs and symptoms of hypoglycaemia or hyperglycaemia to alert him or her to potential problems. If this combination is used, patient education should be provided; the patient should monitor blood glucose frequently throughout the day and should be alert to new warnings about glucose imbalance.

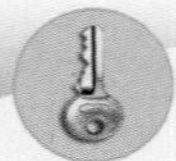

Key Drug Summary: *Metoprolol*

Indications: Treatment of stable angina pectoris; also used for treatment of hypertension, prevention of reinfarction in MI patients and treatment of stable, symptomatic CHF

Actions: Competitively blocks β-adrenergic receptors in the heart and kidneys, decreasing the influence of the sympathetic nervous system on these tissues and the excitability of the heart; decreases cardiac output and the release of renin, which results in a lowered blood pressure and decreased cardiac workload

Pharmacokinetics:

Route	Onset	Peak	Duration
Oral	15 min	90 min	15–19 h
IV	Immediate	60–90 min	15–19 h

$T_{1/2}$: 3–4 hours; metabolized in the liver and excreted in urine

Adverse effects: Dizziness, vertigo, CHF, bradycardia, arrhythmias, gastric pain, flatulence, diarrhoea, vomiting, impotence, decreased exercise tolerance, fatigue, cold peripheries

Calcium Channel Blockers

The calcium channel blockers are a group of drugs that block the calcium channels on the plasma membranes of vascular smooth muscle cells, the myocardium and SA and AV nodal cells of the cardiac conduction system. They act primarily as vasodilators and reduce peripheral vascular resistance. These effects decrease venous return (preload) and the resistance the heart muscle has to pump against (afterload), which in turn decrease cardiac workload and oxygen consumption. The drug of choice depends on the patient's diagnosis and ability to tolerate adverse drug effects.

Therapeutic Actions and Indications

The calcium channel blockers are a group of drugs that block the calcium channels on the plasma membranes of vascular smooth muscle cells, the myocardium and SA and AV nodal cells of the cardiac conduction system. They act primarily as vasodilators and reduce peripheral vascular resistance.

Calcium channel blockers inhibit the movement of calcium ions across the membranes altering the action potential and blocking muscle cell contraction. These effects depress myocardial contractility, slow cardiac impulse formation in the conductive tissues and relax and dilate arteries, causing a fall in blood pressure and a decrease in venous return. These effects decrease the workload of the heart and myocardial oxygen consumption and increase blood flow to the muscle cells. These drugs are indicated for the treatment of chronic angina, effort-associated angina and hypertension.

Pharmacokinetics

Calcium channel blockers are generally well absorbed, metabolized in the liver and excreted in urine. These drugs cross the placenta and enter breast milk. The drug is excreted through the intestines. As a result, patients with renal impairment do not require any dose adjustments (Bennett and Brown, 2003).

Foetal toxicity has been reported in animal studies. Although there are no well-defined studies about effects during pregnancy, these drugs should not be used during pregnancy unless the benefit to the mother clearly outweighs any potential risk to the foetus.

Classification

Calcium channel blockers can be subdivided into three subtypes: Dihydropyridines such as nifedipine, amlodipine; phenylalkylamines such as verapamil and benzothiazepines such as diltiazem.

The phenylalkylamines and benzothiazepines are referred to as nondihydropyridines or as heart lowering drugs (Sargent, 2006). Nondihydropyridines act on nodal tissues of the cardiac conduction system. They have the effect of lowering myocardial contractility.

Dihydropyridines exert their inhibitory effects on vascular smooth muscle. This vascular selectivity means the dihydropyridine subtype of calcium channel blockers, for example nifedipine are more suited to the treatment of hypertension and angina due to their potent arteriolar vasodilator effects.

The benzothiazepines, such as diltiazem, are more cardiac selective, and they primarily affect the smooth muscles of the coronary arteries, thus making them useful in the treatment of angina. They also have a degree of negative effect on the contractility of the myocardium as well as an antidysrhythmic effect. This vascular effect is less than that of dihydropyridines (Sargent, 2006).

The Joint Formulary Committee (2006) state that diltiazem may be used in patients with angina for whom β-blockers are contraindicated. It has similar therapeutic effects as β-blockers, such as a reduction in heart rate and myocardial contractility.

Contraindications and Cautions

Calcium channel blockers are contraindicated with heart block or sick sinus syndrome, *which could be exacerbated by the conduction-slowing effects of these drugs*; with renal or hepatic dysfunction, *which could alter the metabolism and excretion of these drugs*; and with pregnancy or lactation, *because of the potential for adverse effects on the foetus or neonate.*

Short acting calcium channel blockers such as the dihydropyridines have been shown to increase the risk of MI in patients with hypertension and ischaemic heart disease. This is because that the profound effect that these drugs have on blood pressure causes a rebound sympathetic nervous stimulation (increased heart rate and blood pressure) which subsequently increases myocardial oxygen demand and can therefore exacerbate the symptoms of people with acute coronary syndromes.

Angina symptoms can be exacerbated by calcium channel blockers when they stimulate a reflex tachycardia which increases the myocardial oxygen demand.

Adverse Effects

The adverse effects associated with these drugs are related to their effects on cardiac output and on smooth muscle. CNS effects include dizziness, light-headedness, headache and fatigue. GI effects can include nausea, constipation (especially with verapamil), hepatic injury related to direct toxic effects on hepatic cells. Cardiovascular effects include hypotension, bradycardia, peripheral oedema (particularly with amlodipine) and heart block. Skin effects include flushing and rash.

Clinically Important Drug–Drug Interactions

Drug–drug interactions vary with each of the calcium channel blockers. Potentially serious effects to keep in mind include increased serum levels and toxicity of cyclosporin if taken with diltiazem and increased risk of heart block and digoxin toxicity if combined with verapamil (because verapamil increases digoxin serum levels). Both drugs depress myocardial conduction. If any combinations of these drugs must be used, the patient should be monitored very closely and appropriate dosage adjustments made. Verapamil has also been associated with serious respiratory depression when given with general anaesthetics or as an adjunct to anaesthesia.

Always consult a current copy of the British National Formulary for further guidance.

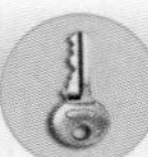

Key Drug Summary: *Diltiazem*

Indications: Treatment of effort-associated angina, chronic stable angina; also used to treat essential hypertension

Actions: Inhibits the movement of calcium ions across the membranes of myocardial and arterial muscle cells, altering the action potential and blocking muscle cell contraction, which depresses myocardial contractility; slows cardiac impulse formation in the conductive tissues and relaxes and dilates arteries, causing a fall in blood pressure and a decrease in venous return; decreases the workload of the heart and myocardial oxygen consumption and also relieves the vasospasm of the coronary artery, increasing blood flow to the muscle cells

Pharmacokinetics:

Route	Onset	Peak
Oral	30–60 min	2–3 h
SR, ER	30–60 min	6–11 h
IV	Immediate	2–3 min

$T_{1/2}$: 3.5–6 hours (sustained release), 5–7 hours (extended release) metabolized in the liver and excreted in urine

Adverse effects: Dizziness, light-headedness, headache, peripheral oedema, bradycardia, AV block, flushing, rash, nausea

Nursing Considerations for Patients Receiving Calcium Channel Blockers

Assessment: History and Examination

Screen for the following conditions, *which could be cautions or contraindications to use of the drug;* impaired liver or kidney function, *which could alter the metabolism and excretion of the drug;* heart block, *which could be exacerbated by the conduction depression of these drugs* and pregnancy or lactation, *because of the potential adverse effects on the foetus or neonate.*

Include screening *for baseline status before beginning therapy and for any potential adverse effects.* Assess the following: skin colour and temperature; orientation and reflexes; pulse, auscultation, blood pressure, perfusion and baseline ECG; respirations and adventitious sounds and liver and renal function tests.

Establish if patient is currently taking other medications or herbal therapies which may potentially interact with calcium channel blockers.

Nursing Diagnoses

The patient receiving a calcium channel blocker may have the following nursing diagnoses related to drug therapy:

- Decreased cardiac output related to hypotension
- Risk for injury related to CNS or cardiovascular effects
- Ineffective tissue perfusion (total body) related to hypotension or change in cardiac output
- Deficient knowledge regarding drug therapy

Implementation With Rationale

- Monitor the patient carefully (blood pressure, cardiac rhythm, cardiac output) while the drug is being titrated or dosage is being changed *to ensure early detection of potentially serious adverse effects.*
- Monitor blood pressure very carefully if the patient is also taking nitrates, *because there is an increased risk of hypotensive episodes.*
- Periodically monitor blood pressure and cardiac rhythm while the patient is using these drugs long term, *because of the potential for adverse cardiovascular effects.*
- Provide comfort measures *to help the patient tolerate drug effects.*
- Provide thorough patient education, including the name of the drug, dosage prescribed, proper administration, measures to avoid adverse effects, warning signs of problems and the need for periodic monitoring and evaluation, *to enhance patient knowledge about drug therapy and to promote compliance with the drug regimen.*
- Offer support and encouragement *to help the patient deal with the diagnosis and the drug regimen.*

Evaluation

- Monitor patient response to the drug (alleviation of signs and symptoms of angina, prevention of angina).
- Monitor for adverse effects (hypotension, cardiac arrhythmias, GI upset, skin reactions and headache).
- Evaluate the effectiveness of the teaching plan (patient can name drug, dosage, proper administration, adverse effects to watch for, specific measures

to avoid adverse effects and the importance of continued follow-up).

- Monitor the effectiveness of comfort measures and compliance to the regimen.

Potassium Channel Activators

Potassium channel activators may be used to treat ischaemic heart disease. These are a relatively new development and act by increasing the efflux of potassium ions in smooth muscle cells of blood vessels. This leads to hyperpolarization of vascular smooth muscle thereby reducing the excitability and bringing about vasodilation. The resulting vasodilation in coronary arterioles improves blood flow to the myocardium. This, in combination with a reduction in both afterload and preload, relieves the angina. Nicorandil is an example of a potassium channel activator. Adverse reactions are headache, dizziness and hypotension (Thorp, 2008).

Cautions include: Hypovolaemia, low systolic blood pressure, acute pulmonary oedema, acute MI with acute left ventricular failure and low filling pressures, pregnancy (British Medical Association and Royal Pharmaceutical Society of Great Britain, 2008).

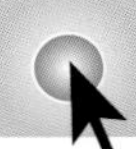

WEB LINKS

Health care providers and patients may want to consult the following Internet sources:

http://cks.library.nhs.uk The National Health Service Clinical Knowledge Summaries provide evidence-based practical information on the common conditions observed in primary care.

http://www.bhf.org.uk Patient information, support groups, research information on heart disease and scientific programmes

http://www.bnf.org.uk The BNF provides UK health care professionals with authoritative and practical information on the selection and clinical use of medicines.

http://emc.medicines.org.uk A reliable source of evidence-based information and practical 'know how' about the common conditions managed in primary care. They are aimed at health care professionals working in primary and first-contact care.

http://www.nice.org.uk The National Institute for Health and Clinical Excellence (NICE) is an independent organization responsible for providing national guidance on promoting good health and preventing and treating ill health.

http://www.nhsdirect.nhs.uk The National Health Service Direct service provides patients with information and advice about health, illness and health services.

Points to Remember

- CVD is the most common cause of premature death in the UK: 21% of premature deaths in men and 12% of premature deaths in women are from CHD (British Heart Foundation Statistics, 2006).
- CVD develops when changes in the intima of coronary vessels lead to the development of atheromas or fatty tumours, accumulation of platelets and debris and a thickening of arterial muscles, resulting in a loss of elasticity and responsiveness to normal stimuli.
- Narrowing of the coronary arteries secondary to the atheroma plaque is called atherosclerosis.
- Narrowed coronary arteries eventually become unable to deliver all the blood that is needed by the myocardial cells, causing a problem of supply and demand.
- The umbrella term *'Acute Coronary Syndrome'* is commonly used in clinical practice to include: angina – (stable and unstable), MI [ST elevation MI (STEMI)] and non-ST elevation MI (non-STEMI).
- Angina pectoris occurs when the myocardial demand for oxygen cannot be met by the narrowed vessels. Pain, anxiety and fatigue develop when the supply-and-demand ratio is upset and demand exceeds supply.
- Stable angina occurs when the heart muscle is perfused adequately except during exertion or increased demand.
- People usually respond to the pain of angina by stopping all activity and resting, which decreases the demand for oxygen and restores the supply-and-demand balance.
- Unstable angina occurs when the vessels are so narrowed that the myocardial cells are low on oxygen even at rest
- MI occurs when a coronary vessel is completely occluded and the cells that depend on that vessel for oxygen become ischaemic and die.
- Angina can be treated by drugs that either increase the supply of oxygen or decrease the heart's workload, which decreases the demand for oxygen.
- Nitrates cause vasoconstriction and β-blockers are used to prevent vasoconstriction; both decrease arterial resistance and hence venous return therefore decreasing cardiac workload and oxygen consumption.
- Calcium channel blockers block muscle contraction in smooth muscle and decrease the heart's workload, relax spasm in Prinzmetal's angina and possibly block the proliferation of the damaged endothelium in coronary vessels.

CRITICAL THINKING SCENARIO 45-1

An Angina Attack

The Situation

Stella is a 62-year-old woman with a 2-year history of angina pectoris. She was given sublingual GTN to use when she had chest pain. She has been stable for the past 6 months, experiencing mild chest pain. This morning after her exercise class, Stella had an argument with her daughter and experienced severe chest pain that was unrelieved by four GTN tablets taken over a 20-minute period. Stella's daughter rushed her to the hospital, where she was given oxygen via a nonrebreather mask, which delivers 85% oxygen, at 10 l. This is the gold standard for an acutely breathless patient, as per Resuscitation Council (2005) guidelines. She was placed on a cardiac monitor, which showed a sinus tachycardia of 110 beats/min, and all other observations were within normal limits. A 12-lead ECG showed no changes from her previous ECG of 7 months ago.

Stella did not have elevated troponin levels. The chest pain subsided within 3 minutes after she received another sublingual GTN. It was decided that Stella should stay in hospital and referred to cardiology for observation. The diagnosis of an angina attack was made.

Critical Thinking

- What nursing interventions are appropriate for Stella while she is still in Accident & Emergency (A&E)?
- What teaching points should be stressed with this patient?
- Should any further tests or treatments be performed with Stella when discussing her heart disease?
- Consider her daughter's reaction and feelings to the situation.

Discussion

Stella's vital signs should be monitored closely while she is in A&E. If her attack subsides, she will be discharged and teaching about CAD should be discussed with her. It would be a good time to discuss angina with Stella and her daughter, explaining the pathophysiology of the disease and ways to avoid upsetting the supply-and-demand ratio in the heart muscle.

They should both receive support and encouragement to cope with the angina and its implications.

Written information, including drug information, should be given to Stella once her condition is stabilized, and further investigations will be indicated to monitor the progress of her disease

Stella should be referred to a cardiologist to have an Exercise stress test (EST) performed. A further diagnostic coronary angiogram may be required pending on the results of the EST to establish the extent, prevalence of CAD. Stella is at risk of experiencing an MI. Measures should be put in place to prevent this, and an urgent referral to a cardiologist would be imperative as outlined by the National Service Framework (2005).

Nursing Care Guide for Stella: Antianginal Nitrates

Assessment: History and Examination

Assess for renal or hepatic dysfunction, pregnancy and lactation (if appropriate), hypotension or hypovolaemia

Focus the physical examination on the following areas:

- CV: measure blood pressure, pulse, ECG, monitor heart rhythm, obtain venous access, obtain bloods, FBP, U&E and troponin. Continuously assess patient's pain levels using a pain score (explained earlier).
- Neurological (CNS): orientation, affect, reflexes, vision
- Skin: colour, texture, perfusion
- Respiratory: respiratory rate and character, adventitious sounds, administer oxygen using a nonrebreather mask at 10 l.
- GI: abdominal examination, bowel sounds
- Full head-to-toe assessment, observing for rashes, bruises, any bleeding, swelling, particularly peripheral oedema, ankle oedema.
- Laboratory tests: liver and renal function tests, FBC, troponin, lipid profile, blood glucose levels

Nursing Diagnoses

- Possible decreased cardiac output related to hypotension
- Possible risk for injury related to CNS, CV effects
- Possible ineffective tissue perfusion (total body) related to CV effects
- Deficient knowledge regarding drug therapy

Implementation

Ensure proper administration of drug and protect drug from heat and light.

An Angina Attack *(continued)*

Provide comfort and safety measures:

- Ensure method of tablet administration is appropriate.
- Offer environmental control for headaches.
- Ensure referral to a cardiologist
- Give drug with food if GI upset occurs.
- Provide support and reassurance to deal with drug effects.
- Provide patient education regarding drug, dosage, adverse effects, what to report, safety precautions.

Evaluation

- Evaluate drug effects: relief of signs and symptoms of angina, prevention of angina.
- Monitor for adverse effects: headache, dizziness; arrhythmias; GI upset; skin reactions; hypotension and CV effects.
- Monitor for drug–drug interactions as indicated for each drug.
- Evaluate effectiveness of patient education programme and comfort and safety measures.

Patient Education for Stella

☐ A nitrate is given to patients with chest pain that occurs because the heart muscle is not receiving enough oxygen. The nitrates act by decreasing the heart's workload and thus its need for oxygen, which it uses for energy. This relieves the pain of angina.

☐ Besides taking the drug as prescribed, you can also help your heart by decreasing the work that it must do. For example, you can:

- Reduce weight, if necessary.
- Decrease or avoid the use of coffee, cigarettes or alcoholic beverages.
- Avoid going outside in very cold weather; if this can't be avoided, dress warmly and avoid exertion while outside.
- Learn to slow down, rest periodically throughout the day and to help you to maintain your activities without pain.

☐ GTN tablets are taken sublingually. Place one tablet under your tongue. Do not swallow until the tablet has dissolved. The tablet should 'fizzle' under your tongue; if this does not occur, the tablet is not effective and you should get a fresh supply of tablets.

☐ If Stella is prescribed GTN spray, the nurse should teach Stella the correct regimen of administering spray safely (discussed earlier).

☐ Ideally, take the GTN before your chest pain begins. If you know that a certain activity usually causes pain (e.g. eating a big meal, attending a business meeting, engaging in sexual intercourse), take the tablet before undertaking the particular activity.

☐ Dermal patches should be applied daily. They may be placed on the chest, upper arm, upper thigh or back. They should be placed on an area that is free of body hair. The site of the application should be changed slightly each day to avoid excess irritation to the skin.

☐ Some of the following adverse effects may occur:

- *Dizziness, light-headedness:* This often passes as you adjust to the drug. Use great care if you are taking sublingual forms of the drug. Sit down when taking the drug to avoid dizziness or falls. Change position slowly to help decrease the dizziness.
- *Headache:* This is a common problem. Over-the-counter headache remedies often provide no relief for the pain. Lying down in a cool environment and resting may help alleviate some of the discomfort.
- *Flushing of the face and neck:* This is usually a very minor problem that passes as the drug's effects pass.
- Report any of the following to your health care provider: *blurred vision, persistent or severe headache, and skin rash, more frequent or more severe angina attacks, fainting.*
- Sublingual GTN usually relieves chest pain within 3 to 5 minutes. If pain is not relieved within 5 minutes, take another tablet. If pain continues, take another tablet in 5 minutes. A total of three tablets may be used, spaced every 5 minutes. If the pain is not relieved after that time, go to a hospital as soon as possible.
- Tell any doctor, nurse or other health care provider involved in your care that you are taking this drug.

☐ Keep this drug and all medications out of the reach of children.

☐ Avoid taking over-the-counter medications while you are taking this drug. If you feel that you need one of these, consult with your health care provider for the best choice. Many of these drugs can change the effects of this drug and cause problems.

☐ Avoid alcohol while you are taking this drug because the combination can cause serious problems.

☐ If you are taking this drug for a prolonged period of time, do not stop taking it suddenly. Your body will need time to adjust to the loss of the drug. The dosage must be gradually reduced to prevent serious problems from developing.

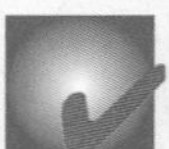

CHECK YOUR UNDERSTANDING

Answers to the questions in this chapter may be found in the answer key in the back of the book.

Multiple Choice

Select the most appropriate response to the following.

1. Coronary artery disease results in
   a. an imbalance in the supply and the demand for oxygen in the heart muscle.
   b. delivery of blood to the heart muscle during systole.
   c. increased pulse pressure.
   d. a decreased workload on the heart.

2. Angina
   a. causes death of heart muscle cells.
   b. is pain associated with lack of oxygen to heart muscle cells.
   c. only occurs with vigorous exercise.
   d. is not treatable.

3. Nitrates are commonly used antianginal drugs that act to
   a. increase the preload on the heart.
   b. increase the afterload on the heart.
   c. dilate coronary vessels to increase the delivery of oxygen through those vessels.
   d. decrease venous return to the heart, thereby decreasing the myocardial workload.

4. Calcium channel blockers are effective in treating angina because they
   a. prevent any cardiovascular exercise, preventing strain on the heart.
   b. block strong muscle contractions and cause vasodilation, decreasing the work of the heart.
   c. alter the electrolyte balance of the heart and prevent arrhythmias.
   d. increase the heart rate, making it more efficient.

5. Verapamil has been associated with potentially serious adverse effects if given with
   a. oral contraceptives.
   b. cyclosporine.
   c. digoxin.
   d. barbiturate anaesthetics.

Extended Matching Questions

Select **all** that apply.

1. Risk factors for the development of atherosclerosis would include which of the following?
   a. A high-fat diet
   b. Increasing age
   c. Female sex
   d. A sedentary lifestyle
   e. Diabetes mellitus
   f. Hypertension

2. An acute myocardial infarction is usually associated with which of the following?
   a. Permanent injury to the heart muscle
   b. Potentially serious arrhythmias
   c. Pain, nausea and sympathetic stress reaction
   d. The development of hypertension
   e. Loss of consciousness
   f. Sweating and a feeling of anxiety

3. Antianginal drugs work to do which of the following?
   a. Decrease the workload on the heart
   b. Increase the supply of oxygen to the heart
   c. Change the metabolic pathway in the heart muscle to remove the need for oxygen
   d. Restore the supply-and-demand balance of oxygen in the heart
   e. Decrease venous return to the heart
   f. Alter the coronary artery filling pathway

4. A client who has GTN to avert an acute anginal attack would need to be taught to
   a. take five or six tablets and then seek medical help if no relief occurs.
   b. buy the tablets in bulk to decrease the cost.
   c. protect tablets from light and to discard them if they do not fizzle when placed under the tongue.
   d. store the tablets in a clearly marked, clear container in open view, where they can easily be found if they are needed.
   e. use the GTN before an event or activity that will most likely precipitate an anginal attack.
   f. explain that a headache may occur after taking the GTN.

Matching

Match the word with the appropriate definition.

1. ____________________CAD
2. ____________________pulse pressure
3. ____________________atheroma
4. ____________________atherosclerosis
5. ____________________angina pectoris
6. ____________________myocardial infarction
7. ____________________nitrates

A. 'Suffocation of the chest'
B. Drop in blood flow through the coronary arteries caused by a vasospasm in the artery
C. Coronary artery disease
D. End result of vessel blockage in the heart
E. Fatty tumour in the intima of a coronary artery
F. Filling pressure of the coronary arteries
G. Narrowing of the arteries caused by the build up of atheromas
H. Drugs used to cause direct relaxation of smooth muscle

True or False

Indicate whether the following statements are true (T) or false (F).

_____ 1. Coronary artery disease (CAD) is second to cancer as the leading cause of death in most Western nations.

_____ 2. CAD develops when changes in the intima of coronary vessels lead to the development of atheromas, or fatty tumours.

_____ 3. Narrowing of the coronary arteries secondary to the atheroma build up is called angina.

_____ 4. Angina pectoris, or 'suffocation of the chest', occurs when the narrowed vessels cannot meet the myocardial demand for oxygen.

_____ 5. Stable angina occurs when the heart muscle is perfused adequately except at rest.

_____ 6. Unstable or preinfarction angina occurs when the vessels are so narrowed that the myocardial cells are low on oxygen during exertion.

_____ 7. Prinzmetal's angina occurs as a result of a spasm of a coronary vessel.

_____ 8. Myocardial infarction occurs when a coronary vessel is completely occluded.

Bibliography

British Medical Association and Royal Pharmaceutical Society of Great Britain. (2008). *British National Formulary*. London: BMJ & RPS Publishing. *This publication is updated biannually: it is imperative that the most recent edition is consulted.*

British Medical Association and Royal Pharmaceutical Society of Great Britain. (2008). *British National Formulary for Children*. London: BMJ & RPS Publishing. *This publication is updated annually: it is imperative that the most recent edition is consulted.*

Ganong, W. (2005). *Review of medical physiology* (22nd ed.). New York: McGraw-Hill.

Howland, R. D., & Mycek, M. J. (2005). *Pharmacology* (3rd ed.). Philadelphia: Lippincott Williams & Wilkins.

Marieb, E. N., & Hoehn, K. (2004). *Human anatomy & physiology* (7th ed.). San Francisco: Pearson Benjamin Cummings.

Porth, C. M., & Matfin G. (2008). *Pathophysiology: Concepts of altered health states* (8th ed.). Philadelphia: Lippincott Williams & Wilkins.

Simonsen, T., Aarbakke, J., Kay, I., Coleman, I., Sinnott, P., & Lysaa, R. (2006). *Illustrated pharmacology for nurses.* London: Hodder Arnold.

References

Baker, J. G. (2005). The selectivity of beta-adrenoreceptor antagonist at the human beta1, beta2, beta3 adrenoreceptors. *British Journal of Pharmacology,* 144, 317–322.

Barnett, M. J., Milaretz, G., & Kaboli, P. J. (2005). Beta-blocker therapy in veterans with asthma or chronic obstructive pulmonary disease *Pharmacotherapy, 25*(11), 1550–1559.

Bennett, P. N., & Brown, M. J. (2003). *Clinical pharmacology* (8th ed.) London: Churchill Livingstone.

British Heart Foundation Statistics. (2006). *2006 coronary heart disease statistics*. London: British Heart Foundation.

Engred, M., Shaw, S., Mohammad, B., Waitt, P., & Rodrigues, E. (2005). Under-use of β-blockers in patients with ischaemic heart disease and concomitant chronic obstructive pulmonary disease. *QJM: An International Journal of Medicine, 98*(7), 493–497.

Gatzka, C. D., Cameron, J. D., Kingwell, B. A., & Dart, A. M. (1998). Relation between coronary artery disease, aortic stiffness, and left ventricular structure in a population sample. *Hypertension, 32,* 575–578.

Gemmell, I., Heller, R. F., Payne, K., Edwards, R., Roland, M., & Durrington, P. (2006). Secondary prevention strategies disease in England: comparing primary and strategy for reducing the burden of coronary heart. *Quality and Safety in Health Care, 15,* 339–343.

Joint Formulary Committee. (2006). *British National Formulary* 50. London: BMJ Publishing.

Khan, E. (2006). Beta-blockers: Types and clinical implications. *British Journal of Cardiac Nursing, 1*(3), 132–136.

López-Sendó, J., Swedberg, K., McMurray, J., Tamargo, J., Aldo, P., Maggioni, A.P., et al. (2004). Expert consensus document on β-adrenergic receptor blockers. *The Task Force on β-Blockers of the European Society of Cardiology, 25,* 1341–1362.

Marriott, H. L. L., & Conover, M. B. (1998). Advanced concepts in arrthymias (3rd ed.). St Louis: Mosby.

National Institute of Health and Clinical Excellence. (2003). *NICE guidelines on prophylaxis for patients who have experienced a myocardial infarction.* Available from http://www.nice.or.uk.

Sargent, A. (2006). Understanding calcium channel blockers in hypertension, angina, and supraventricular tachycardias. *British Journal of Cardiac Nursing, 1*(5), 241–246.

Salpeter, S., Ormiston, T., & Salpeter, E. (2002). Cardio-selective beta-blockers for reversible airways disease. *Cochrane Database Systematic Review, 200*(4), CD002992.

Thorp, C. M. (2008). *Pharmacology for the health care professions*. Oxford: Wiley-Blackwell.

CHAPTER 46

Lipid-Lowering Agents

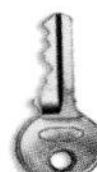

KEY TERMS

bile acids

cholesterol

chylomicron

high-density lipoprotein (HDL)

HMG-CoA reductase

hyperlipidaemia

low-density lipoprotein (LDL)

risk factors

LEARNING OBJECTIVES

Upon completion of this chapter, you will be able to:

1. Outline the mechanisms of fat metabolism in the body and discuss the role of hyperlipidaemia as a risk factor for cardiovascular disease.
2. Describe the therapeutic actions, indications, pharmacokinetics associated with agents used to lower lipid levels.
3. Describe the contraindications associated with agents used to lower lipid levels.
4. Describe the most common adverse reactions and important drug–drug interactions associated with agents used to lower lipid levels.
5. Discuss the use of drugs that lower lipid levels across the lifespan.
6. Compare and contrast the key drugs cholestyramine, atorvastatin and ezetimibe, with other agents used to lower lipid levels.
7. Outline the nursing considerations, including important teaching points, for patients receiving drugs used to lower lipid levels.

ANION-EXCHANGE RESINS

cholestyramine
colestipol

HMG-CoA REDUCTASE INHIBITORS 'STATINS'

atorvastatin
fluvastatin
pravastatin
rosuvastatin
simvastatin

CHOLESTEROL ABSORPTION INHIBITOR

ezetimibe

OTHER ANTIHYPER-LIPIDAEMIC (LIPID-LOWERING) AGENTS

fenofibrate
gemfibrozil

The drugs discussed in this chapter reduce serum levels of cholesterol and lipids. There is mounting evidence that the incidence of cardiovascular disease (CVD), the leading killer of adults in the Western world, is higher among people with high serum lipid levels. Tsiara *et al.* (2003) The Department of Health (DH) (2000) state that it is now established practice to administer statin therapy to patients with known coronary heart disease (CHD).

Cardiovascular Disease (CVD)

CVD is characterized by the progressive growth of atheromatous plaques, or atheromas, in the coronary arteries (as explained in Chapter 45). These plaques, which begin as fatty streaks in the endothelium, eventually injure the endothelial lining of the artery, causing an inflammatory reaction. This inflammatory process triggers the development of characteristic foam cells, containing fats and white blood cells that further injure the endothelial lining. Over time, platelets, fibrin and other fats collect on the injured vessel lining and cause the atheroma to grow, further narrowing the interior (lumen) of the blood vessel and limiting blood flow.

The injury to the vessel also causes scarring and a thickening of the vessel wall. As the vessel thickens, it becomes less distensible and less reactive to many neurological and chemical stimuli that would ordinarily dilate or constrict it. As a result, the coronary vessels no longer are able to balance the myocardial demand for oxygen with increased blood supply.

Risk Factors

Strong evidence exists to suggest that patients with elevated serum cholesterol and lipid levels develop atheroma more quickly than those with lower levels (Stamler *et al.*, 1986). Patients who consume high-fat diets are more likely to develop high lipid levels. However, patients without increased lipid levels can also develop atheromas leading to CVD, so other factors evidently contribute to this process. Although the exact mechanism of atherogenesis (atheroma development) is not understood, certain **risk factors** increase the likelihood that a person will develop CVD. CVD risk may be determined using the 'Cardiovascular predictor charts' issues by the Joint British Societies (Heart 2005) which are also available in the BNF.

The following is a list of unmodifiable and modifiable risk factors (see also Critical Thinking Scenario 46-1):

Unmodifiable Risk Factors for CVD

Genetic predispositions: CVD is more likely to occur in people who have a family history of the disease.

Age: The incidence of CVD increases with age.

Sex: Men are more likely than premenopausal women to have CVD; however, the incidence is almost equal in men and postmenopausal women, a possible link to a protective effect of oestrogens (see Box 46.1).

BOX 46.1 SEX CONSIDERATIONS: WOMEN AND HEART DISEASE

Women appear to have a protective hormone effect against the development of CVD until menopause, when oestrogen loss seems to rapidly increase the production of atheromas and the development of CVD. In several studies, women who received hormone replacement therapy (HRT) at menopause had a significantly reduced risk of CVD and myocardial infarction (MI) in the first few years after the onset of menopause. Research has shown, however, that after 5 years of HRT, the incidence of MI and stroke increased sharply, leading to an early closure of the study. Studies have found that women experience different symptoms of heart disease; jaw and neck pain, fatigue and insomnia and sometimes these are overlooked (Goldberg *et al.*, 1998).

HRT is not recommended as a means of reducing risk of heart disease or stroke, although women should be advised to take steps to reduce other cardiac risk factors by eating a diet low in saturated fats, exercising regularly, not smoking, controlling weight, managing stress and seeking treatment for gout, hypertension and diabetes.

Modifiable Risk Factors

High stress levels: Constant sympathetic reactions increase the myocardial oxygen demand while causing vasoconstriction and may contribute to a remodelling of the blood vessel endothelium, thus, leading to an increased susceptibility to atheroma development.

Hypertension: High pressure in the arteries causes endothelial injury and increases afterload and myocardial oxygen demand.

Cigarette smoking: Nicotine causes vasoconstriction and has an effect on the endothelium of blood vessels; over time, smoking can lower oxygen levels in the blood. Smoking increases risk of CVD, and there is a reduction in risk after stopping smoking.

Obesity: This may reflect altered fat metabolism, which increases the workload of the heart.

Diabetes: Patients with diabetes have a capillary membrane thickening, which accelerates the effects of atherosclerosis and an abnormal fat metabolism.

Sedentary lifestyle: Exercise increases the levels of chemicals that seem to protect the coronary arteries.

Gout: Increased uric acid levels seem to damage vessel walls.

Other factors that, if untreated, may contribute to CVD include bacterial infections *(Chlamydia* infections have been correlated with onset of CVD, and treatment with tetracycline has been associated with decreased incidence of CVD, indicating a possible bacterial link) and autoimmune processes (some plaques contain antibodies and other products of immune reactions, making autoimmune reactions a possibility). Different ethnic groups may also have different risk factors.

Table 46.1 Risk Factors for Coronary Artery Disease

Unmodifiable Risks	Modifiable Risks	Suggested Modifications
Family history	Sedentary lifestyle	Exercise
Age	High-fat diet	Low-fat diet (polyunsaturated and monounsaturated fats)
Gender	Smoking	Smoking cessation
	Obesity	Weight loss
	High stress levels	Stress management
	Bacterial infections	Antibiotic treatment
	Diabetes	Control of blood glucose levels
	Hypertension	Control of blood pressure
	Gout	Control of uric acid levels
	Menopause	Hormone replacement therapy (first few years of menopause only)

Treatment

An exact cause of CVD is not known, therefore, the successful treatment involves manipulating a number of these risk factors (Table 46.1). Overall treatment and prevention of CVD should include the following measures: reducing cholesterol levels (to below 5 mmol/l); decreasing dietary fats (a decrease in total fat intake and limiting saturated fats seems to have the most impact on serum lipid levels); losing weight; eliminating smoking; increasing exercise levels; decreasing stress; optimal treatment of hypertension, diabetes and gout.

Fats and Biotransformation (Metabolism)

Fats are taken into the body as dietary fat; they are then broken down in the stomach to fatty acids, lipids and cholesterol (Figure 46.1). The presence of these products in the duodenum stimulates contraction of the gallbladder and the release of bile. **Bile acids** containing high levels of cholesterol (fat) act like a detergent in the small intestine, breaking up fats. (Imagine ads for dishwashing detergents that break up the grease and fats in the dishwashing water; bile acids do much the same thing.)

Bile acids break down the fats into small units called micelles; these can be absorbed into the wall of the small intestine. The bile acids are then reabsorbed and recycled to the gallbladder, where they remain until the gallbladder is again stimulated to release them to facilitate fat absorption.

Fats and water do not mix; therefore, fats cannot be absorbed directly into the plasma but need to be transported on a plasma protein. To allow absorption, micelles are carried on a **chylomicron**, a package of fats and proteins. This packaging is done by brush border enzymes in the small intestine. The chylomicrons pass through the wall of the small intestine, where they are picked up by the lymphatic system surrounding the intestines. The chylomicrons travel through the lymphatic system to the heart, where they are distributed throughout the circulation. The proteins that are exposed on the chylomicron, called apoproteins, determine the fate of the lipids or fats being carried. For example, some of these packages are broken down in the tissues to be used for energy, some are stored in fat deposits for future use as energy and some continue to the liver, where they are further processed into lipoproteins.

The lipoproteins produced in the liver that have well-known clinical implications are the **low-density lipoproteins (LDLs)** and the **high-density lipoproteins (HDLs)**. Lipoproteins are named according to the **protein/fat ratio; therefore, LDLs have a low protein/fat ratio and HDLs have a high protein/fat ratio.**

LDLs enter circulation as tightly packed cholesterol, triglycerides and lipids, all of which are carried by proteins that enter circulation to be broken down for energy or stored for future use as energy. When an LDL package is broken down, many remnants or leftovers need to be returned to the liver for recycling. If a person has many of these remnants in the blood vessels, it is thought that the inflammatory process is initiated to help remove this debris. Some experts believe that this is the underlying process involved in atherogenesis.

HDLs enter circulation as loosely packed lipids that are used for energy and to pick up remnants of fats and cholesterol that are left in the periphery by LDL breakdown. HDLs serve a protective role in cleaning up remnants in blood vessels. It is known that HDL levels increase during exercise, which could explain why people who exercise regularly lower their risk of CVD. HDL levels also increase in response to oestrogen, which could explain some of the protective effects of oestrogen before menopause.

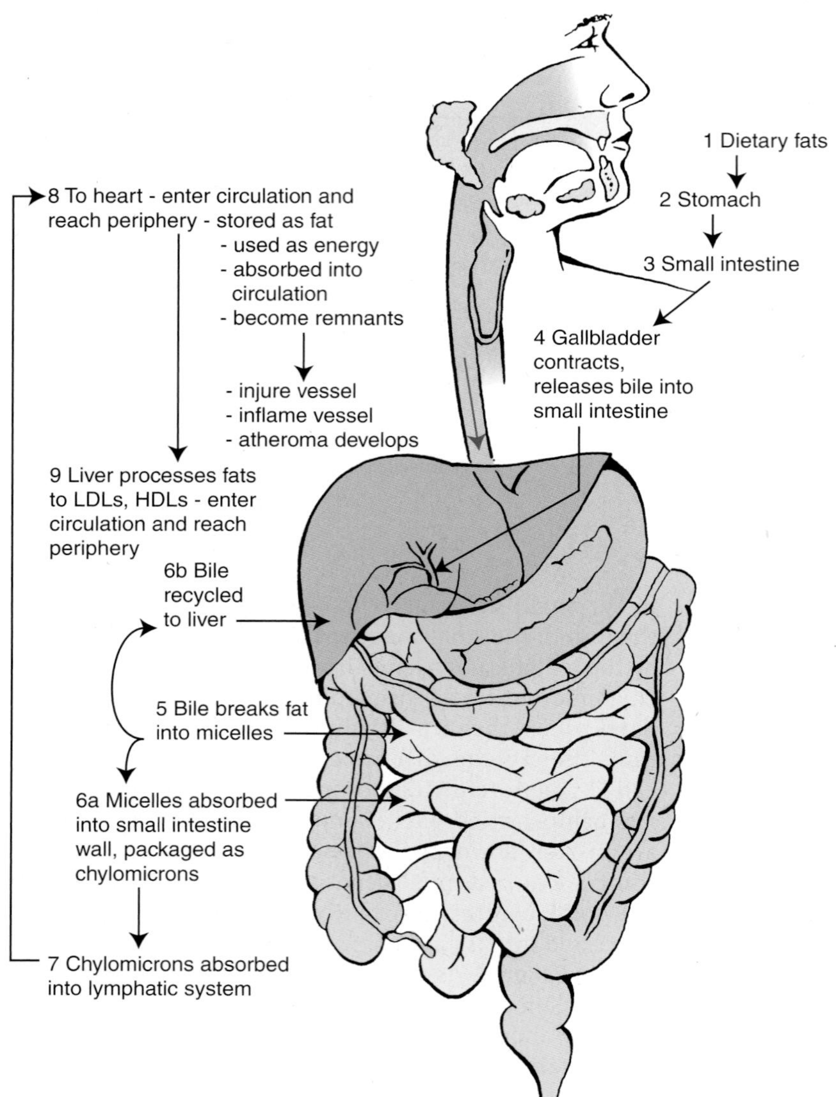

FIGURE 46.1 Metabolism of fats in the body.

Cholesterol

The body needs fats, particularly cholesterol, to maintain normal function. Cholesterol is essential for the formation of the steroid hormones (the sex hormones as well as the adrenal cortical hormones). It is also a basic unit in the formation and maintenance of cell membranes. Cholesterol is usually provided through the diet and the fat metabolism process as described earlier. If dietary cholesterol falls off, the body is prepared to produce cholesterol to ensure that the cell membranes and the endocrine system are intact. Every cell in the body has the metabolic capability of producing cholesterol. The enzyme hydroxymethylglutaryl-coenzyme-A reductase **(HMG-CoA reductase)** plays an important role in the synthesis of cholesterol within hepatocytes. If dietary cholesterol is severely limited, the cellular synthesis of cholesterol will increase (Figure 46.2).

Hyperlipidaemias

Hyperlipidaemia is raised serum cholesterol level in the blood. This increases a person's risk for the development of CVD. The exact role that lipids play is not completely

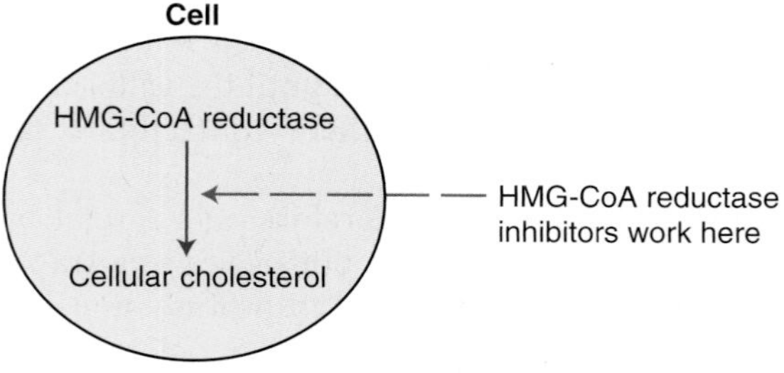

FIGURE 46.2 Cellular production of cholesterol.

understood; however, the levels of lipids that contribute to CVD risk have been established. Hyperlipidaemia can result from excessive dietary intake of fats or from genetic alterations in fat metabolism leading to a variety of elevated fats in the blood (e.g. familial hypercholesterolaemia, hypertriglyceridaemia, alterations in LDL and HDL concentrations). Dietary modifications are often successful in treating hyperlipidaemia that is caused by excessive dietary intake of fats. Drug therapy is needed if the cause is genetically linked alterations in lipid levels or if dietary limits do not decrease the serum lipid levels to an acceptable range.

Antihyperlipidaemic Agents

Drugs that are used to treat hyperlipidaemia include anion-exchange resins, HMG-CoA inhibitors (statins), cholesterol absorption inhibitors, fibrates and, in some cases, hormones (in women). These drugs are often used in combination and should be part of an overall health care regimen that includes exercise, dietary restrictions and lifestyle changes to decrease the risk of CVD. (See Box 46.2 for their use in various age groups.)

Anion-exchange resins

Anion-exchange resins bind with bile acids, leading to their excretion in the faeces. The resulting low levels of bile acids re-entering hepatic circulation stimulate the production of more bile acids in the liver. Bile acids contain cholesterol. The liver must use cholesterol to manufacture bile acids, therefore, the hepatic intracellular cholesterol level falls, leading to an increased absorption of cholesterol-containing LDL segments from circulation to replenish the cell's cholesterol. The end result is a decrease in plasma cholesterol levels. Anion-exchange resins currently in use are **cholestyramine**, a powder that must be mixed with liquids and taken up to six times a day, and colestipol, available in both powder and tablet form, is taken only four times a day.

Therapeutic Actions and Indications

Anion-exchange resins (bind with bile acids in the intestine to form a complex that is excreted in the faeces (Figure 46.3). As a result, the liver must use cholesterol to make more bile acids. The serum levels of cholesterol and LDL decrease as the circulating cholesterol is used to provide the cholesterol the liver needs to make bile acids. These drugs are used alone or in combination to reduce serum cholesterol in patients with primary hypercholesterolaemia (manifested by high cholesterol and high LDLs) as an adjunct to diet and exercise. Cholestyramine is also used to treat pruritus (itching) associated with partial biliary obstruction.

Pharmacokinetics

The anion-exchange resins are resins that bind with bile acids in the intestine to form an insoluble complex that is then excreted in faeces. These drugs are not absorbed

DRUG THERAPY ACROSS THE LIFESPAN

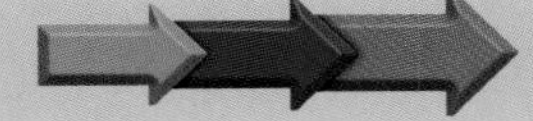

Hyperlipidaemic Agents

CHILDREN

Familial hypercholesterolaemia may be seen in children. Due to the importance of lipids in the developing nervous system, treatment is usually restricted to tight dietary restrictions to limit fats and calories. Specialist referral and management is needed. Clofibrate has been used to treat genetic hypercholesterolaemia that is unresponsive to dietary restrictions. The HMG-CoA inhibitors simvastatin and atorvastatin can be used in postmenarchal girls and boys 10 to 17 years of age for treating familial hypercholesterolaemia. Pravastatin has been approved for use in children of more than 8 years of age (Frishman *et al.*, 2005), but these children should be monitored very closely.

When administering any drug to children, always consult the most recent edition of the British National Formulary for Children.

ADULTS

Lifestyle changes including dietary restrictions, exercise, smoking cessation and stress reduction should be tried before any cholesterol-lowering drug is used.

Statins (HMG-CoA reductase inhibitors) are the first drug of choice in the treatment of hypercholesterolaemia in patients who are at risk for, or who have already developed, CVD. The drugs are well tolerated and less expensive than some of the other cholesterol-lowering drugs. Combination therapy with an anion-exchange resin, a fibrate, or niacin may be necessary if lipid levels still cannot be reduced using a statin alone.

Women of child-bearing age should not take HMG-CoA reductase inhibitors. Anion-exchange resins are the drug of choice for these women if a lipid-lowering agent is needed.

OLDER ADULTS

No outcome data are available to prove the impact of lipid-lowering agents in decreasing the incidence of myocardial infarction or cardiac death in the older population.

Lifestyle changes including dietary restrictions, exercise, smoking cessation and stress reduction should be tried before any cholesterol-lowering drug is used.

Lower doses of statins should be used in elderly patients and in any patient with renal dysfunction.

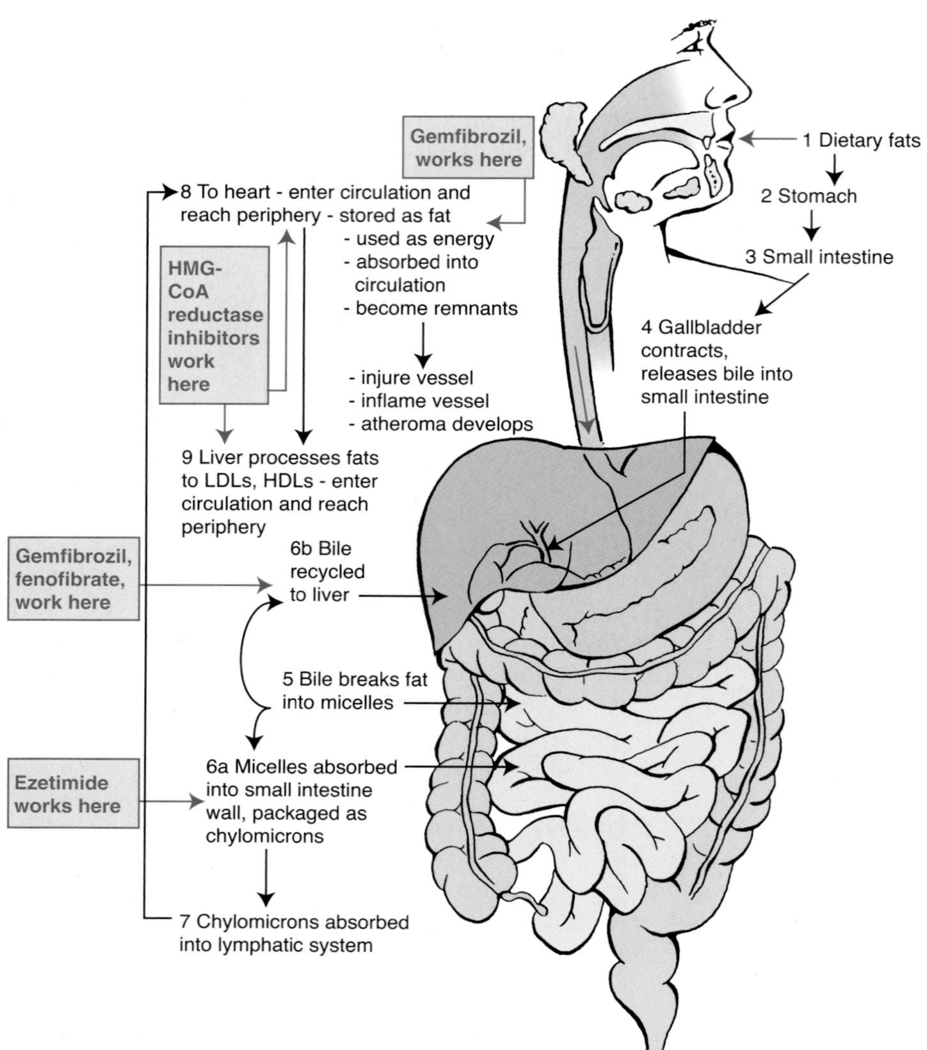

FIGURE 46.3 Sites of action of lipid-lowering agents.

systemically. Their action is limited to their effects while they are present in the intestine.

Contraindications and Cautions

Anion-exchange resins are contraindicated in the following conditions: complete biliary obstruction, *which would prevent bile from being secreted into the intestine;* abnormal intestinal function, *which could be aggravated by the presence of these drugs* and pregnancy or lactation, *because the potential decrease in the absorption of fat and fat-soluble vitamins could have a detrimental effect on the foetus or neonate.*

Adverse Effects

Adverse effects associated with the use of these drugs include headache, anxiety, fatigue and drowsiness, which could be related to changes in serum **cholesterol** levels. Direct gastrointestinal (GI) irritation, including nausea and constipation that may progress to faecal impaction and aggravation of haemorrhoids may occur. Other effects include increased bleeding times related to a decreased absorption of vitamin K and consequent decreased production of clotting factors, vitamin A and D deficiencies related to decreased absorption of fat-soluble vitamins, rash and muscle aches and pains.

Always consult the most up-to-date version of the British National Formulary (BNF) for current guidelines and information

Clinically Important Drug–Drug Interactions

Fat-soluble vitamins may be poorly absorbed when they are combined with these drugs. These drugs decrease or delay the absorption of thiazide diuretics, digoxin, warfarin, thyroid hormones and corticosteroids. Consequently, any of these drugs should be taken 1 hour before or 4 to 6 hours after the anion-exchange resin.

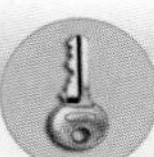

Key Drug Summary: *Cholestyramine*

Indications: Reduction of elevated serum cholesterol in patients with primary hypercholesterolaemia, pruritus associated with partial biliary obstruction

Actions: Binds bile acids in the intestine, allowing excretion in faeces instead of reabsorption, causing cholesterol to be ionized in the liver and serum cholesterol levels to fall

Pharmacokinetics: Not absorbed systemically

$T_{1/2}$: Not absorbed systemically, excreted in faeces

Adverse effects: Rash, headache, anxiety, vertigo, dizziness, constipation due to faecal impaction, exacerbation of haemorrhoids, cramps, flatulence, nausea, increased bleeding tendencies, vitamin A and D deficiencies, muscle and joint pain

Nursing Considerations for Patients Receiving Anion-exchange resins

Assessment: History and Examination

Screen for the following conditions: known allergies to these drugs; impaired intestinal function, *which could be exacerbated by these drugs;* biliary obstruction, *which could block the effectiveness of these drugs* and pregnancy and lactation, *which are contraindications.*

Include screening *for baseline status before beginning therapy and for any potential adverse effects.* Assess the following: pulse, blood pressure, skin, bowel sounds and abdominal examination and serum cholesterol and lipid levels.

Nursing Diagnoses

The patient receiving anion-exchange resins may have the following nursing diagnoses related to drug therapy:

- Acute pain related to central nervous system (CNS) and GI effects
- Constipation related to GI effects
- Decreased cardiac output related to increased bleeding
- Deficient knowledge regarding drug therapy

Implementation With Rationale

- Do not administer powdered agents in dry form; *these drugs must be mixed in fluids to be effective.* They may be mixed with fruit juices, soups, liquids, cereals or pulpy fruits. Colestipol, but not cholestyramine, may be mixed with carbonated beverages. Stir and swallow the entire dose.
- If the patient is taking tablets, ensure that tablets are not cut, chewed or crushed, *because they are designed to be broken down in the GI tract; if they are crushed, the active ingredients will not be effective.* Tablets should be swallowed whole with plenty of fluid.
- Give the drug before meals *to ensure that the drug is in the GI tract with food.*
- Administer other oral medications 1 hour before or 4 to 6 hours after the anion-exchange resin *to avoid drug–drug interactions.*
- Provide comfort measures *to help the patient tolerate the drug effects*
- Provide thorough patient education, including the name of the drug, dosage prescribed, proper administration, measures to avoid adverse effects, warning signs of problems, the importance of periodic monitoring and evaluation and the need to avoid overdose and poisoning, *to enhance patient knowledge about drug therapy and promote compliance with the drug regimen.*
- Offer support and encouragement *to help the patient deal with the diagnosis and the drug regimen and lifestyle changes that may be necessary*

Evaluation

- Monitor patient response to the drug as appropriate (reduction in serum cholesterol levels).
- Monitor for adverse effects (headache, vitamin deficiency, increased bleeding times, constipation, nausea, rash).
- Evaluate the effectiveness of the teaching plan (patient can name drug, dosage, adverse effects to watch for, specific measures to avoid adverse effects; patient understands importance of continued follow-up).
- Monitor the effectiveness of comfort measures and compliance with the regimen.

HMG-CoA Reductase Inhibitors (Statins)

If HMG-CoA reductase is blocked, serum cholesterol and LDL levels decrease, because more LDLs are absorbed by the cells for processing into cholesterol. In contrast, HDL levels increase slightly with this alteration in fat metabolism. HMG-CoA reductase inhibitors block HMG-CoA reductase from completing the synthesis of cholesterol. Most of these drugs are chemical modifications of compounds produced by fungi. As a group, they are frequently referred to as 'statins'. Overall the mode of action of HMG-CoA reductase inhibitors is that they competitively inhibit the action of this enzyme, so reducing the amount of cholesterol which is synthesized by the liver. The resulting reduction in cholesterol which is available for the synthesis of bile salts promotes a compensatory up-regulation in the number of LDL receptors on the cell surface. This increases the clearance of circulating LDL cholesterol (Khan, 2003; Prosser *et al.,* 2000; Rang *et al.,* 2003; Taylor and Reide, 2001; Waller *et al.*, 2004).

The HMG-CoA reductase inhibitors (Statins) include the following:

Atorvastatin can be used to lower cholesterol levels in children 10 to 17 years of age who meet specific criteria but it is associated with severe liver complications. **Atorvastatin** is licensed for use in the UK as an adjunct to diet for the treatment of people with primary hypercholesterolaemia, familial hypercholesterolaemia and combined hyperlipidaemia when response to diet and other nonpharmacological measures are inadequate (Walthall, 2006).

- **Fluvastatin** is actually a fungal product and should not be used with any known allergies to fungal by-products. *The Scottish Medicines Consortium* advised in February 2004 that this drug could be used following percutaneous coronary angioplasty to prevent secondary coronary events. Fluvastatin is licensed for use in the UK to slow the progression of coronary atherosclerosis in people with primary hypercholesterolaemia who do not respond adequately to diet control and for secondary prevention of coronary events after percutaneous transluminal coronary angioplasty in people with coronary heart disease
- **Simvastatin** is indicated for lowering cholesterol and preventing MI in patients with known hypercholesterolaemia and CVD; this drug is not associated with the severe liver toxicities of some of the other statins. It is also approved for use in children 10 to 17 years of age who meet specific criteria.
- **Pravastatin** is the only statin with outcome data to show that it is effective in decreasing CVD and the incidence of MI. It is used to prevent a first MI even in patients who do not have a documented increased cholesterol concentration, an effect that may be related to blocking of the formation of foam cells in injured arteries, which can decrease the risk of MI. It is also used with children 8 years of age or older who meet specific criteria. This drug is not associated with the severe liver toxicities of some of the other statins.
- **Rosuvastatin** is the newest statin. It appears to lower LDL and raise HDL slightly better than the other statins and at a lower price. Some concern has been raised that it appears to pose a higher risk for the development of rhabdomyolysis in Asian patients, so it is recommended that this drug be reserved for use in non-Asian patients.

Therapeutic Actions and Indications

HMG-CoA reductase inhibitors block the formation of cellular cholesterol, leading to a decrease in serum cholesterol and a decrease in serum LDLs, with a slight increase or no change in the levels of HDLs (see Figure 46.2). These drugs undergo a marked first-pass effect in the liver; therefore, most of their effects are seen in the liver. These drugs may also have some effects on the process that generates atheromas in vessel walls. That exact mechanism of action is not understood. These drugs are indicated as adjuncts with diet and exercise for the treatment of increased cholesterol and LDL levels that are unresponsive to dietary restrictions alone, to slow the progression of CVD in patients with documented CVD (pravastatin and simvastatin) and to prevent first MI in patients who are at risk for MI (pravastatin, atorvastatin and simvastatin).

Pharmacokinetics

The statins are all absorbed from the GI tract and undergo first-pass metabolism in the liver. They should be given orally at night. They are excreted through faeces and urine. Simvastatin is the only statin which is given in its inactive form and is then metabolized in the liver to create its active form.

Atorvastatin levels are not affected by renal disease, but patients with renal impairment who are taking other statins must be monitored closely. The peak effect of these drugs is usually attained within 2 to 4 weeks. The effects of these drugs on cholesterol pathways can cause serious harm to the developing foetus, and they should be avoided by women of child-bearing age who might become pregnant. Most of these drugs have been found to cross into breast milk and, because of their effect on cholesterol synthesis; they could pose a threat to the neonate. Nursing mothers who need this drug should find another way to feed the baby.

Contraindications and Cautions

These drugs are contraindicated in the presence of allergy to any of the statins or to fungal by-products or compounds. They also are contraindicated with active liver disease or a history of alcoholic liver disease, *which could be exacerbated, leading to severe liver failure and* with pregnancy or lactation, *because of the potential for adverse effects on the foetus or neonate.* Caution should be used in patients with impaired endocrine function *because of the potential alteration in the formation of steroid hormones.*

Adverse Effects

The most common adverse effects associated with these drugs reflect their effects on the GI system: flatulence, abdominal pain, cramps, nausea, vomiting and constipation, altered liver function. CNS effects can include headache, dizziness, blurred vision, insomnia, fatigue and cataract development and may reflect changes in the cell membrane and synthesis of cholesterol. Increased concentrations of liver enzymes commonly occur, and acute liver failure has been reported with the use of atorvastatin and fluvastatin. Reversible myositis is a rare but potentially significant side-effect of the statins.

Rhabdomyolysis, a breakdown of muscles whose waste products can injure the glomerulus and cause acute renal failure, has also occurred with the use of atorvastatin, fluvastatin and rosuvastatin. The CSM have advised that although the incidence is low, approximately, 1 in 100,000, the risk of myositis and hence rhabdomyolysis is increased in patients with renal impairment and hypothyroidism. The British National Formulary (BNF) (Joint Formulary Committee, 2006) identifies that if muscle symptoms are severe or if myopathy is suspected and creatinine kinase levels are elevated (more than five times the upper limits of normal), statin therapy should be discontinued.

Always consult the most up-to-date version of the British National Formulary (BNF) and National Institute for Health and Clinical Excellence guidelines (2006) for current guidelines and information

Clinically Important Drug–Drug Interactions

The risk of rhabdomyolysis increases if any of these drugs is combined with erythromycin, cyclosporine, gemfibrozil, niacin or antifungal drugs; such combinations should be avoided.

FOCUS ON **PATIENT SAFETY**

Patients who are taking HMG-CoA inhibitors need to be cautioned to avoid using grapefruit or grapefruit juice while taking these drugs. Grapefruit juice alters the metabolism of the drugs, leading to an increased serum level of drug and increased risk for adverse effects, such as the potentially fatal rhabdomyolysis with renal failure. The effects may last for several days, so just drinking the grapefruit juice at a different time of day does not protect the patient from risk.

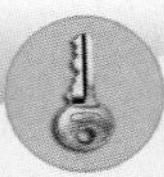

Key Drug Summary: *Simvastatin*

Indications: Adjunct to diet in the treatment of elevated cholesterol, triglycerides and LDL; to increase HDL cholesterol in patients with primary hypercholesterolaemia; treatment of boys and postmenarchal girls aged 10 to 17 years with familial hypercholesterolaemia and two or more risk factors for CVD

Actions: Inhibits HMG-CoA, causing a decrease in serum cholesterol levels, LDLs and triglycerides and an increase in HDL levels

Pharmacokinetics:

Route	Onset	Peak	Duration
Oral	Slow	1–2 h	20–30 h

$T_{1/2}$: 14 hours; metabolized in the liver and cells and excreted in bile

Adverse effects: Headache, flatulence, abdominal pain, cramps, constipation, rhabdomyolysis with acute renal failure

Increased serum levels and resultant toxicity can occur if these drugs are combined with digoxin or warfarin; if this combination is used, serum digoxin levels and/or clotting times should be monitored carefully and the prescriber consulted for appropriate dosage changes.

Increased oestrogen levels can occur if these drugs are taken with oral contraceptives; the patient should be monitored carefully if this combination is used.

Serum levels and the risk of toxicity increase if these drugs are combined with grapefruit juice; this combination should be avoided.

Nursing Considerations for Patients Receiving Statins

Assessment: History and Examination

Take an appropriate structured history from the patient using a systematic approach such as a POMR and enquire specifically about any known allergies to these drugs or to fungal by-products; active liver disease or history of alcoholic liver disease, *which could be exacerbated by the effects of these drugs;* pregnancy or lactation, *because of potential adverse effects on the foetus or neonate;* and impaired endocrine function, *which could be exacerbated by effects on steroid hormones.*

Include screening *for baseline status before beginning therapy and for any potential adverse effects.* Assess the following: body temperature and weight; skin, pulse, blood pressure and perfusion; respirations and abdominal examination; renal and liver function tests and serum lipid levels.

Nursing Diagnoses

The patient receiving an HMG-CoA reductase inhibitor may have the following nursing diagnoses related to drug therapy:

- Risk of disturbed sensory perception (visual, kinaesthetic, gustatory) related to CNS effects
- Risk for injury related to CNS, liver and renal effects
- Risk of acute pain related to headache, myalgia and GI effects
- Deficient knowledge regarding drug therapy

Implementation With Rationale

- Administer the drug at bedtime, *because the highest rates of cholesterol synthesis occur between midnight and 5 a.m.* (atorvastatin can be taken at any time during the day), and the drug should be taken when it will be most effective.
- Monitor serum cholesterol and LDL levels by blood testing before and periodically during therapy *to evaluate the effectiveness of this drug.*
- Monitor liver function tests before and periodically during therapy *to monitor for liver damage;* consult with the prescriber to discontinue the drug if the aspartate aminotransferase (AST) or alanine aminotransferase (ALT) level increases to three times normal.
- Ensure that the patient has attempted a cholesterol-lowering diet and exercise programme for at least 3 to 6 months before beginning therapy *to ensure the need for drug therapy.*
- Encourage the patient to make the lifestyle changes necessary *to decrease the risk of CVD and to increase the effectiveness of drug therapy.*
- Withhold atorvastatin, or fluvastatin, in any acute, serious medical condition (*e.g.*, infection, hypotension, major surgery or trauma, metabolic endocrine disorders, seizures) *that might suggest myopathy or serve as a risk factor for the development of renal failure.*
- Suggest the use of barrier contraceptives for women of child-bearing age, *because there is a risk of severe foetal abnormalities if these drugs are taken during pregnancy.*
- Provide comfort measures *to help the patient tolerate drug effects*
- Provide thorough patient education, including the name of the drug, dosage prescribed, measures to avoid adverse effects, warning signs of problems and the need for periodic monitoring and evaluation, *to enhance the patient's knowledge of drug therapy and to promote compliance with the drug regimen.*
- Offer support and encouragement *to help the patient deal with the diagnosis, needed lifestyle changes and the drug regimen.*

Evaluation

- Monitor patient response to the drug (lowering of serum cholesterol and LDL levels, prevention of first MI, slowing of progression of CVD).
- Encourage reporting of adverse effects (headache, dizziness, blurred vision, cataracts, GI upset, liver failure, rhabdomyolysis).
- Evaluate the effectiveness of the teaching plan (patient can name drug, dosage, adverse effects to watch for, specific measures to avoid adverse effects; patient understands importance of continued follow-up).
- Monitor the effectiveness of comfort measures and compliance with the regimen.

Nurses need to be able to interpret the patient's blood cholesterol profile and to ensure that he/she is aware of the correct recommended cholesterol levels. They should refer to the JBS 2: Joint British Societies' Guidelines on Prevention of Cardiovascular Disease in Clinical Practice for the most up-to-date advice (British Cardiac Society *et al.*, 2005).

Cholesterol Absorption Inhibitors

This class of drugs localizes in the brush border of the small intestine and inhibits the absorption of cholesterol from the small intestine. As a result, less dietary cholesterol is delivered to the liver, and the liver increases the clearance of cholesterol from the serum to make up for the drop in dietary cholesterol, causing the total serum cholesterol level to drop. Ezetimibe is the first drug of this class to be approved.

Therapeutic Actions and Indications

Ezetimibe works in the brush border of the small intestine to decrease the absorption of dietary cholesterol, leading to a drop in serum cholesterol levels. It is indicated as an adjunct to diet and exercise to lower cholesterol levels as monotherapy or as part of combination therapy with an HMG-CoA inhibitor or a anion-exchange resin, in combination with atorvastatin or simvastatin as a treatment for homozygous familial hypercholesterolaemia and as adjunctive therapy to diet for the treatment of homozygous sitosterolaemia to reduce elevated sitosterol and campesterol levels.

Pharmacokinetics

Ezetimibe is absorbed well after oral administration, reaching peak levels in 4 to 6 hours. It is metabolized in the liver and the small intestine, with a 22-hour half-life. Excretion is through faeces and urine. It is not known whether the drug crosses the placenta or enters breast milk.

Contraindications and Cautions

Ezetimibe, if used in combination with a statin, should not be used during pregnancy or lactation or with severe liver disease *because of the known effects of statins, including possible liver problems and renal failure.*

Use in pregnant or lactating women should be reserved for those situations in which the benefits outweigh any potential risk to the foetus or neonate. The drug should be used with caution as monotherapy during pregnancy or lactation, *because the effects on the foetus or neonate are not known.*

Adverse Effects

The most common adverse effects associated with ezetimibe are mild abdominal pain and diarrhoea. It is not associated with the bloating and flatulence that occurs with the anion-exchange resins and the fibrates. Other adverse effects that have been reported include headache, dizziness, fatigue, upper respiratory tract infection (URI), back pain and muscle aches and pains.

Always consult the most up-to-date version of the British National Formulary (BNF) for current guidelines and information

Clinically Important Drug–Drug Interactions

The risk of elevated serum levels of ezetimibe increases if it is given with cholestyramine, fenofibrate, gemfibrozil or antacids. If these drugs are used in combination, ezetimibe should be taken at least 2 hours before or 4 hours after the other drugs.

The risk of toxicity also increases if ezetimibe is combined with cyclosporine. If this combination cannot be avoided, the patient should be monitored very closely.

If ezetimibe is combined with any fibrate, the risk of cholethiasis increases. The patient should be monitored closely.

Warfarin levels increase in a patient who is also taking ezetimibe; if this combination is used, the patient should be monitored very closely.

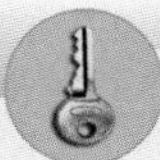

Key Drug Summary: *Ezetimibe*

Indications: Adjunct to diet and exercise to lower serum cholesterol levels, in combination with atorvastatin or simvastatin for the treatment of homozygous familial hypercholesterolaemia, with diet for the treatment of homozygous sitosterolaemia to lower sitosterol and campesterol levels

Actions: Works in the brush border of the small intestine to inhibit the absorption of cholesterol

Pharmacokinetics:

Route	Onset	Peak
Oral	Moderate	4–12 h

$T_{1/2}$: 22 hours; metabolized in the liver and small intestine and excreted in faeces and urine

Adverse effects: Headache, dizziness, GI disturbances, abdominal pain, diarrhoea, myalgia, arthralgia

Other Drugs Used to Affect Lipid Levels

Other drugs that are used to affect lipid levels do not fall into any of the classes discussed previously. They include the fibrates (derivatives of fibric acid). The fibrates stimulate the breakdown of lipoproteins from the tissues and their removal from the plasma. They lead to a decrease in lipoprotein and triglyceride synthesis and secretion. The fibrates are absorbed from the GI tract and are metabolized in the liver and excreted in urine. Fibrates in use today include the following agents:

- **Fenofibrate** inhibits triglyceride synthesis in the liver, resulting in reduction of LDL levels; increases uric acid secretion and may stimulate triglyceride breakdown. It is used for adults with very high triglyceride levels that are not responsive to strict dietary measures and who are at risk for pancreatitis. Peak effects are usually seen within 4 weeks, and the patient's serum lipid levels should be re-evaluated at that time.
- **Gemfibrozil** inhibits peripheral breakdown of lipids, reduces production of triglycerides and LDLs and increases HDL concentrations. It is associated with GI and muscle discomfort. This drug should not be combined with statins. There is an increased risk of rhabdomyolysis from 3 weeks to several months after therapy if this combination is used. If this combination cannot be avoided, the patient should be monitored very closely.

Nursing Considerations for Patients Receiving Cholesterol Absorption Inhibitors

Assessment: History and Examination

Screen for the following conditions, *which could be cautions or contraindications to use of the drug:* any known allergies to any component of the drug; pregnancy or lactation, *because the possible effects on the foetus or neonate are not known;* or liver dysfunction or advanced age, *because the processing of the drug may differ from the norm.*

Include screening *for baseline status before beginning therapy and for any potential adverse effects.* Assess the following: skin, reflexes, respirations and adventitious sounds, abdominal examination, liver function tests and serum lipid levels.

Nursing Diagnoses

The patient receiving a cholesterol absorption inhibitor may have the following nursing diagnoses related to drug therapy:

- Disturbed sensory perception (visual, kinaesthetic, gustatory) related to CNS effects

- Acute pain related to headache, myalgia and GI effects
- Deficient knowledge regarding drug therapy

Implementation With Rationale

- Monitor serum cholesterol, triglyceride and LDL levels before and periodically during therapy *to evaluate the effectiveness of this drug.*
- Monitor liver function tests before and periodically during therapy *to detect possible liver damage*; consult with the prescriber *to discontinue drug use* if the AST or ALT level increases to three times normal.
- Ensure that the patient has attempted a cholesterol-lowering diet and exercise programme for at least several months before beginning therapy *to ensure the need for drug therapy.*
- Encourage the patient to make the lifestyle changes necessary *to decrease the risk of CVD and to increase the effectiveness of drug therapy.*
- Suggest the use of barrier contraceptives for women of child-bearing age if the drug is being used in combination with a statin, *because there is a risk of severe foetal abnormalities if these drugs are taken during pregnancy.*
- Provide comfort measures *to help the patient tolerate drug effect.*
- Provide thorough patient education, including the name of the drug, dosage prescribed, measures to avoid adverse effects, warning signs of problems and the need for periodic monitoring and evaluation, *to enhance the patient's knowledge of drug therapy and to promote compliance with the drug regimen.*
- Offer support and encouragement *to help the patient deal with the diagnosis, needed lifestyle changes and drug regimen.*

Evaluation

- Monitor patient response to the drug (lowering of serum cholesterol and LDL levels).
- Monitor for adverse effects (headache, dizziness, GI pain, muscle aches and pains, URI).
- Evaluate the effectiveness of the teaching plan (patient can name drug, dosage, adverse effects to watch for, specific measures to avoid adverse effects; patient understands importance of continued follow-up).
- Monitor the effectiveness of comfort measures and compliance with the regimen.

WEB LINKS

Health care providers and patients may want to consult the following Internet sources:

http://www.bnf.org.uk The BNF provides UK health care professionals with authoritative and practical information on the selection and clinical use of medicines.

http://cks.library.nhs.uk The National Health Service Clinical Knowledge Summaries provide evidence-based practical information on the common conditions observed in primary care.

http://www.bhf.org.uk The British Heart Foundation is a charity which aims to reduce mortality due to heart disease by pioneering research, vital prevention activities and by ensuring quality care and support for people living with heart disease.

http://www.nhsdirect.nhs.uk The National Health Service Direct service provides patients with information and advice about health, illness and health services.

http://www.nice.org.uk The National Institute for Health and Clinical Excellence (NICE) is an independent organization responsible for providing national guidance on promoting good health and preventing and treating ill health.

http://www.statistics.gov.uk This site covers statistics relating to information gathered on public health, health services provided by the National Health Service (NHS), social care, and health and safety at work.

Points to Remember

- CVD is the main cause of death in the UK, accounting for four out of every 10 deaths (http://www.statistics.gov.uk).
- It is associated with the development of atheromas or plaques in arterial linings that lead to narrowing of the lumen of the artery and hardening of the artery wall, with loss of ability to distend and responsiveness to stimuli for contraction or dilation.
- The cause of CVD is not known, but many contributing risk factors have been identified, including increasing age, male sex, genetic predisposition, high-fat diet, sedentary lifestyle, smoking, obesity, high stress levels, bacterial infections, diabetes, hypertension and gout.
- Treatment and prevention of CVD is aimed at manipulating the known risk factors to decrease CVD development and progression.
- Fats are metabolized with the aid of bile acids, which act as a detergent to break fats into small molecules called micelles. Micelles are absorbed into the intestinal wall and combined with proteins to become chylomicrons, which can be transported throughout the circulatory system.
- Some fats are used immediately for energy or are stored in adipose tissue; others are processed in the liver to

LDLs, which are associated with the development of CVD. LDLs are broken down in the periphery and leave many remnants (e.g. fats) that must be removed from blood vessels. This process involves the inflammatory reaction and may initiate or contribute to atheroma production.

- Some fats are processed into HDLs, which are able to absorb fats and remnants from the periphery and offer a protective effect against the development of CVD.
- Cholesterol is an important fat that is used to make bile acids. It is the base for steroid hormones and provides necessary structure for cell membranes. All cells can produce cholesterol.
- HMG-CoA reductase is an enzyme that controls the final step in production of cellular cholesterol. Blockade of this enzyme using statin results in lower serum cholesterol levels, a resultant breakdown of LDLs and a slight increase in HDLs.
- Anion-exchange resins bind with bile acids in the intestine and lead to their excretion in faeces. This results in lower bile acid levels as the liver uses cholesterol to produce more bile acids. The end result is a decrease in serum cholesterol and LDL levels as the liver changes its metabolism of these fats to meet the need for more bile acids.
- The cholesterol absorption inhibitor, ezetimibe, works in the brush border of the small intestine to prevent the absorption of dietary cholesterol, which leads to increased clearance of cholesterol by the liver and a resultant fall in serum cholesterol.
- Overall treatment of patients taking lipid-lowering drugs should include diet, exercise and lifestyle changes to reduce the risk of CVD. Such lifestyle changes include stopping smoking; managing stress; and treating hypertension, gout, diabetes, oestrogen deficiencies and bacterial infections (particularly Chlamydia infections).

CRITICAL THINKING SCENARIO 46-1

Treating Hyperlipidaemia

The Situation

Tom is a 55-year-old businessman; he was seen for a routine medical when applying for life insurance. He was found to be obese (BMI 35) and borderline hypertensive (BP 145/92), with a nonfasting, low-density lipoprotein (LDL) level of 4 mmol/l, high-density lipoprotein (HDL) level of 1.5 mmol/l and total cholesterol level of 6.8 mmol/l. Tom admitted he smokes two packets of cigarettes a day. His family history highlighted that both of his parents died of heart attacks before age 50. He described himself as a 'workaholic' with no time to exercise and a tendency to eat most of his meals in restaurants. It was suggested to Tom that he should try to stop smoking, lose some weight and make some dietary changes to eliminate saturated fats from his diet. He was also advised to try and reduce his stress levels. On a return visit after 4 weeks, Tom had lost 2 kg and reported a decrease in smoking, but his LDL levels were unchanged. The use of a cholesterol-lowering drug was discussed.

Critical Thinking

- What nursing interventions are appropriate at this point? *Consider all of the known risk factors for CVD, then rank Tom's risk based on those factors.*
- What lifestyle changes would help Tom reduce his risk of heart disease?
- What support services could be utilized to help Tom?
- Should other tests be done before considering any drug therapy for Tom? *Think about the kind of patient education that would help Tom cope with the overwhelming lifestyle changes that have been suggested, yet remain compliant to his medical regimen.*

Discussion

Tom's description of himself as a workaholic should alert the nurse to the possibility that he will have trouble adapting to any prescribed lifestyle changes; *workaholics tend to be very organized, goal-driven and somewhat controlling individuals*. Tom should first receive extensive teaching about CVD, his risk factors and his options. The benefits of decreasing or eliminating risk factors should then be discussed. Tom may be more compliant if he has some control over his situation, so he should be invited to suggest possible lifestyle changes or adaptations. Tom also should be encouraged to set short-range goals that are achievable, to help him feel successful.

Referral to a dietician and to an exercise programme may help Tom select foods and exercises that fit into his lifestyle. A stress test, angiogram, or both, may be ordered to evaluate the actual state of Tom's coronary arteries. The results of these tests could serve as powerful teaching tools and motivator.

Tom needs to understand that statins are generally well tolerated but can cause some side-effects these include: dizziness, headaches, gastrointestinal upset and

(continued)

Treating Hyperlipidaemia *(continued)*

constipation. Tom may have trouble coping with these adverse effects because of his busy lifestyle. Tom's health care provider may need to try a variety of different drugs or combinations of drugs to find ones that are effective but do not cause unacceptable adverse effects.

Nursing Care Guide for Tom: HMG-CoA Reductase Inhibitors

Assessment: History and Examination

Assess Tom's health history for allergies to any HMG-CoA reductase0 inhibitor or fungal by-products, hepatic dysfunction and endocrine disorders.

Focus the physical examination on the following areas:

- CV: blood pressure, pulse, perfusion
- Neuro (CNS): orientation, reflexes, vision
- Skin: colour
- Resp: rate, adventitious sounds
- GI: abdominal examination
- Laboratory tests: liver and renal function tests, serum lipids

Nursing Diagnoses

- Risk of disturbed sensory perception related to CNS effects
- Risk for injury related to CNS, liver, renal effects
- Acute pain related to headache, myalgia and GI effects
- Deficient knowledge regarding drug therapy

Implementation

- Administer drug at bedtime.
- Monitor serum lipids prior to therapy.
- Provide comfort and safety measures: give small meals.
- Arrange for periodic ophthalmic exams to screen for cataracts.
- Give drug with food if GI upset occurs, if needed monitor liver function and arrange to stop drug if liver impairment occurs.
- Provide support and reassurance to deal with drug effects and need to make lifestyle, diet and exercise changes.
- Provide patient education regarding drug, dosage, adverse effects, what to report, safety precautions.

Evaluation

- Evaluate drug effects: lowering of serum cholesterol and lipid levels, prevention of first myocardial infarction, slowed progression of CVD.
- Monitor for adverse effects: sedation, dizziness, headache, cataracts, GI upset; hepatic or renal dysfunction; rhabdomyolysis.
- Monitor for drug–drug interactions as indicated for each drug.
- Evaluate effectiveness of patient education programme.
- Evaluate effectiveness of comfort and safety measures.

Patient Education for Tom

- An HMG-CoA reductase inhibitor, or 'statin', is a cholesterol-lowering agent, which means it works to decrease the levels of certain lipids, or fats, in your blood. An increase in blood lipid levels has been associated with the development of many blood vessel disorders, including CVD, which can lead to a heart attack. This drug must be used in conjunction with a low-calorie, low-saturated fat diet and an exercise programme.

Some of the following adverse effects may occur:

- *Nausea, vomiting, flatulence, constipation:* small, frequent meals may help. If constipation becomes a problem, consult with your health care provider for appropriate interventions.
- Report any of the following to your health care provider: *severe GI upset, vision changes, unusual bleeding, dark urine or light-coloured stools.*
- You will need to have regular medical examinations to monitor the effectiveness of this drug on your lipid levels and to detect any adverse effects. These examinations will include blood tests.
- *Headache, blurred vision, nervousness, insomnia: If suffering form any of these much rarer adverse effects* avoid performing hazardous or delicate tasks that require concentration; these effects may pass with time.
- Tell any doctor, nurse or other health care provider that you are taking this drug.
- Keep this drug and all medications out of the reach of children
- To help decrease your risk of heart disease, follow these guidelines: adhere to a diet that is low in calories and saturated fat, exercise regularly, stop smoking and reduce stress

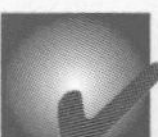

CHECK YOUR UNDERSTANDING

Answers to the questions in this chapter may be found in the answer key in the back of the book.

Multiple Choice

Select the most appropriate response the following.

1. The body uses cholesterol in many ways, including the
   a. production of water-soluble vitamins.
   b. formation of steroid hormones.
   c. mineralization of bones.
   d. development of dental plaques.

2. The formation of atheromas in blood vessels precedes the signs and symptoms of
   a. hepatitis.
   b. cardiovascular disease.
   c. diabetes mellitus.
   d. COPD.

3. High cholesterol levels are considered to be
   a. a normal finding in adult males.
   b. related to stress levels.
   c. a treatable risk factor for the development of heart disease.
   d. a side effect of cigarette smoking.

4. The anion-exchange resins
   a. are absorbed into the liver.
   b. take several weeks to show an effect.
   c. have no associated adverse effects.
   d. work in the small intestine to prevent bile salts from being reabsorbed.

5. HMG-CoA reductase works in the
   a. process of bile secretion.
   b. process of formation of cholesterol within the cell.
   c. intestinal wall to block fat absorption.
   d. kidney to block fat excretion.

6. Patients taking HMG-CoA reductase inhibitors (statins)
   a. will not have a heart attack.
   b. will not develop CVD.
   c. may develop cataracts as a result.
   d. may stop absorbing fat-soluble vitamins.

7. Rhabdomyolysis is a very serious adverse effect that can be seen with HMG-CoA reductase inhibitors; to detect it, patients taking these drugs would be monitored for
   a. flatulence and abdominal bloating.
   b. increased bleeding.
   c. the development of cataracts.
   d. muscle pain and weakness.

Extended Matching Questions

Select **all** that apply.

1. Anion-exchange resins would be a drug of choice for a client who has which of the following?
   a. A high LDL concentration
   b. A high triglyceride concentration
   c. Biliary obstruction
   d. Vitamin K deficiency
   e. A high HDL concentration
   f. Intolerance to statins

2. A client presents with high cholesterol and high LDL levels. Teaching for this client should include which of the following?
   a. The importance of exercise
   b. The need for dietary changes to alter cholesterol levels
   c. That taking a statin will allow a full, unrestricted diet
   d. That drug therapy is always needed when these levels are elevated
   e. The importance of controlling blood pressure and blood glucose levels
   f. That stopping smoking may also help lower lipid levels

Bibliography and References

Abramowicz, M. (1996). Choice of lipid-lowering drugs. *Medical Letter, 38*, 67–70.

British Medical Association and Royal Pharmaceutical Society of Great Britain. (2008). *British National Formulary*. London: BMJ & RPS Publishing. *This publication is updated biannually: it is imperative that the most recent edition is consulted.*

British Medical Association and Royal Pharmaceutical Society of Great Britain. (2008). *British National Formulary for Children*. London: BMJ & RPS Publishing. *This publication is updated annually: it is imperative that the most recent edition is consulted.*

The Joint British Societies (2005) Cardiovascular predictor charts, Heart: 91 suppl. V; v1–v52

Department of Health. (2000). *Coronary heart disease: National Service Framework for Coronary Heart Disease – Modern Standards and Service Models*. London: Department of Health.

Frishman, W. H., Cheng-Lai, A., & Nawarskas, J. (2005). Current cardiovascular drugs (4th ed.). Switzerland. Birkhäuser.

Ganong, W. (2005). *Review of medical physiology* (22nd ed.). New York: McGraw-Hill.

Goldberg, R. J., O'Donnell, C., Yarzebski, J., Bigelow, C., Savageau, J., & Gore, J. (1998). Sex differences in symptom presentation associated with acute myocardial infarction: A population-based perspective. *American Heart Journal, 136*(2), 189–195.

Howland, R. D., & Mycek, M. J. (2005). *Pharmacology* (3rd ed.). Philadelphia: Lippincott Williams & Wilkins.

JBS 2: Joint British Societies' guidelines on prevention of cardiovascular disease in clinical practice (2005); Prepared by: British Cardiac Society, British Hypertension Society, Diabetes UK, HEART UK, Primary Care Cardiovascular Society, The Stroke Association. *Heart* 91 (Supplement 5): v1–v52

Karch, A. M. (2006). *2007 Lippincott's nursing drug guide.* Philadelphia: Lippincott Williams & Wilkins.

Khan, M. G. (2003). *Cardiac drug therapy* (6th ed.) Philadelphia: Saunders.

Knopp, R. H. (1999). Drug treatment of lipid disorders. *New England Journal of Medicine, 341*, 498–511.

Marieb, E. N., & Hoehn, K. (2007). *Human anatomy & physiology* (7th ed.). San Francisco: Pearson Benjamin Cummings.

National Institute for Health and Clinical Excellence. (2006). NICE guidelines on statins for the prevention of cardiovascular events. Available from http://www.nice.org.uk

The medical letter on drugs and therapeutics. (2006). New Rochelle, New York: Medical Letter.

Porth, C. M., & Matfin, G. (2008). *Pathophysiology: Concepts of altered health states* (8th ed.). Philadelphia: Lippincott Williams & Wilkins.

Rang, H. P., Dale, M. M., Ritter, J. M., & Moore, P. K. (2003). *Pharmacology* (5th ed.) Edinburgh: Churchill Livingstone.

Simonsen, T., Aarbakke, J., Kay, I., Coleman, I., Sinnott, P., & Lysaa, R. (2006). *Illustrated pharmacology for nurses.* London: Hodder Arnold.

Stamler, J., Wentworth, D., & Neaton, J. D. (1986). Is relationship between serum cholesterol and risk of premature death from coronary heart disease continuous and graded? Findings in 356222 primary screens of the multiple risk factor intervention trial (MRFIT). *Journal of the American Medical Association, 256*(20), 2823–2828.

Tsiara, S., Eisaf, M., & Mikhaildis, D. P. (2003). Early vascular benefits of statin therapy. *Current Medical Research Opinion, 19*, 540–556.

Walthall, H. (2006). Statin therapy in cardiovascular disease. *British Journal of Cardiac Nursing, 1*(6), 270–277.

CHAPTER

47

Drugs Affecting Blood Coagulation

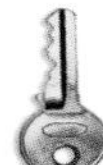

KEY TERMS

anticoagulants
clotting factors
coagulation
common pathway
extrinsic pathway
haemophilia
haemorrhagic disorders
haemostasis
intrinsic pathway
plasminogen
platelet aggregation
thrombin
thromboembolic disorders
thrombolytic drugs

LEARNING OBJECTIVES

Upon completion of this chapter, you will be able to:

1. Outline the mechanisms by which blood clots dissolve in the body and correlate this information with the actions of drugs used to affect blood clotting.
2. Describe the therapeutic actions, indications, pharmacokinetics and contraindications associated with antiplatelet agents, anticoagulants, low-molecular-weight heparins, thrombolytic agents, antihaemophilic agents and haemostatic agents.
3. Describe the most common adverse reactions and important drug–drug interactions associated with antiplatelet agents, anticoagulants, low-molecular-weight heparins, thrombolytic agents, antihaemophilic agents and haemostatic agents.
4. Discuss the use of drugs that affect blood coagulation across the lifespan.
5. Compare and contrast the key drugs aspirin, heparin, streptokinase, antihaemophilic factor with other agents used to affect blood coagulation.
6. Outline the nursing considerations, including important teaching points, for patients receiving drugs used to affect blood coagulation.

ANTICOAGULANTS

Antiplatelet Drugs

abciximab
aspirin
cilostazol
clopidogrel
dipyridamole
eptifibatide
ticlopidine
tirofiban

Anticoagulants

antithrombin
heparin
warfarin

Thrombin Inhibitor

bivalirudin
lepirudin

Low-Molecular-Weight Heparins

dalteparin
enoxaparin
tinzaparin

Anticoagulant Therapy

protamine sulphate
vitamin K

Haemorrheologic Agent

pentoxifylline

Thrombolytic Agents

alteplase (rTPA)
reteplase
streptokinase
tenecteplase
urokinase

DRUGS USED TO CONTROL BLEEDING

Antihaemophilic Agents

antihaemophilic factor
coagulation factor VIIa
factor IX complex

The cardiovascular system is a closed system, the blood is trapped in a closed space; therefore, it maintains the difference in pressures required to keep the system moving along. If the vascular system is damaged from a cut, a puncture or capillary destruction, the blood could leak out, cause the system to lose pressure and potentially shut down entirely.

Haemostasis is the process that stops bleeding. Several protective measures act to limit the blood loss from the body. These include:

- Constriction of blood vessels
- Platelet aggregation and the formation of a platelet plug
- Coagulation (the formation of fibrin)

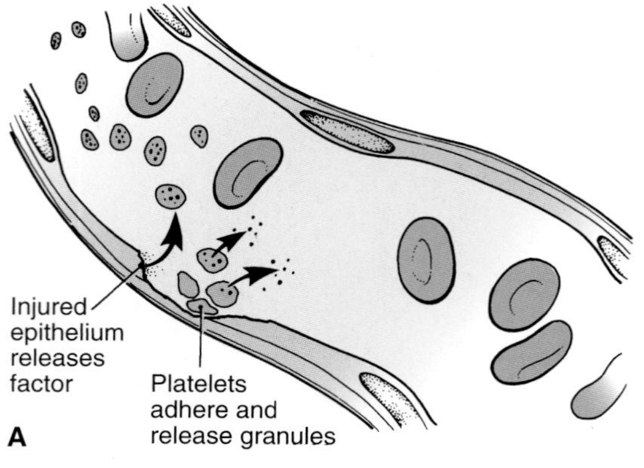

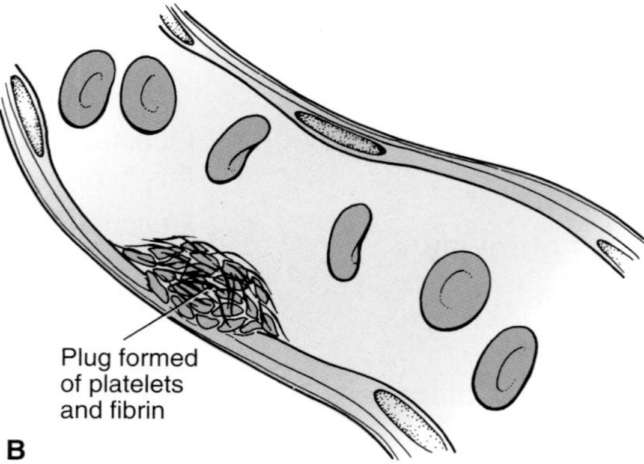

FIGURE 47.2 (A) Damaged vessel endothelium is a stimulus to circulating platelets, causing platelet adhesion. Platelets release mediators (B) and platelet aggregation results.

Vasoconstriction

The first reaction to a blood vessel injury is local vasoconstriction (Figure 47.1). If the injury to the blood vessel is very small, this vasoconstriction can seal off any break and allow the area to heal.

Platelet Aggregation

Injury to a blood vessel exposes blood to the collagen and other substances under the endothelial lining of the vessel. This exposure causes platelets in the circulating blood to stick or adhere to the site of the injury. Once they stick, the platelets release granule contents, including adenosine diphosphate (ADP) and other chemicals that attract other platelets, causing them to aggregate and to stick together. ADP is also a precursor of the prostaglandins from which thromboxane A_2 is formed. Thromboxane A_2 causes local vasoconstriction and further **platelet aggregation** and adhesion. This series of events forms a platelet plug at the site of the vessel injury. In many injuries, the combination of vasoconstriction and platelet aggregation is enough to seal off the injury and keep the cardiovascular system intact (Figure 47.2).

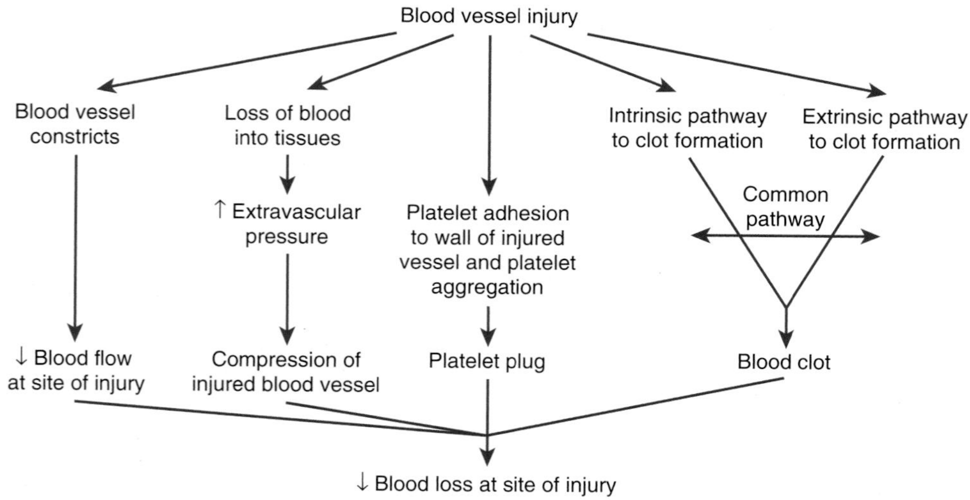

FIGURE 47.1 Process of blood coagulation.

BOX 47.1 DRUG THERAPY ACROSS THE LIFESPAN

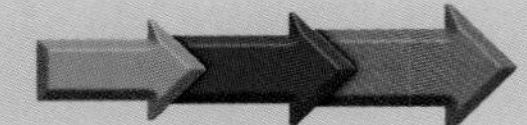

Drugs Affecting Coagulation

CHILDREN

Little research is available on the use of anticoagulants in children. If they are used, usually under specialist supervision, the child needs to be monitored very carefully to avoid excessive bleeding related to drug interactions or alterations in gastrointestinal (GI) or liver function. People who interact with the child need to understand the importance of preventing injuries and providing safety precautions and should be aware of what to do if the child is injured and begins to bleed.

If heparin is used, the dosage should be carefully calculated based on weight and age and checked by another person before the drug is administered.

Warfarin is used with children undergoing cardiac surgery. Again, the dosage must be determined based on weight and age, and the child should be monitored closely.

The safety of low-molecular-weight heparins has not been established in children.

At this time, there are no indications for the use of antiplatelet or thrombolytic drugs with children.

When administering any drug to children, always consult the most recent edition of the British National Formulary (BNF) for Children.

ADULTS

Adults receiving these drugs need to be instructed in ways to prevent injury – such as using a soft-bristled toothbrush to protect the gums, avoiding contact sports, and instructed in what to do if bleeding does occur (apply constant, firm pressure and contact a health care provider if bleeding persists). They should receive a written list of signs of bleeding to watch for and to report to their health care provider.

Many drugs and alternative therapies are known to interact with these agents (see Box 47.2); therefore, it is very important that these patients be urged to report the use of this drug to any other health care provider and to consult with one before using any over-the-counter drugs or alternative therapies.

It is prudent to advise any patient using one of these drugs in the home setting to carry or wear a MedicAlert notification in case of emergency.

The patient also needs to understand the importance of regular, periodic blood tests to monitor and evaluate the effects of the drug.

Many drugs are associated with increased bleeding or increased blood clotting during pregnancy; therefore, these drugs should not be used during pregnancy unless the benefit to the mother clearly outweighs the potential risk to the foetus and to the mother at delivery. The risk of altered blood clotting in the neonate makes these drugs generally inadvisable for use during lactation.

OLDER ADULTS

Older adults may have many underlying medical conditions that require the need for drugs that alter blood clotting [e.g. coronary artery disease (CAD), cerebrovascular accident (CVA), peripheral vascular disease, transient ischaemic attacks (TIAs)]. Statistically, older adults also take more medications, making them more likely to encounter drug interactions associated with these drugs. The older adult is also more likely to have impaired liver and kidney function, conditions that can alter the metabolism and excretion of these drugs.

The older adult should be carefully evaluated for liver and kidney function, use of other medications and ability to follow through with regular blood testing and medical evaluation before therapy begins. Therapy should be started at the lowest possible level and adjusted accordingly after the patient response has been noted.

Careful attention needs to be given to the patient's total drug regimen. Starting, stopping or changing the dosage of another drug may alter the body's metabolism of the drug that is being used to affect coagulation, leading to increased risk of bleeding or ineffective anticoagulation.

Blood Coagulation

Blood coagulation is a complex process that involves a cascade of **clotting factors** produced in the liver that eventually react to convert fibrinogen (a protein also produced in the liver) into insoluble fibrin threads and a stable clot. When a clot is formed, plasmin (another blood protein) acts to break it down.

Consequently, the system must maintain an intricate balance between the tendency to clot or form a solid state, called **coagulation**, and the need to prevent extensions of coagulation outside the site of injury and to keep the vessels open and the blood flowing. If a great deal of vascular damage occurs, such as with a major cut or incision, the balance in the area shifts to a procoagulation mode and a large clot is formed.

Drugs that affect blood coagulation work at various steps in the blood-clotting and clot-dissolving processes to restore the balance that is needed to maintain the cardiovascular system. Box 47.1 discusses the uses of these drugs in various age groups.

Intrinsic Pathway

As blood comes in contact with the exposed collagen of the injured blood vessel, one of the clotting factors, factor XII

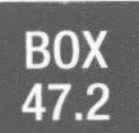

BOX 47.2 HERBAL AND ALTERNATIVE THERAPIES

Many herbal therapies can cause problems when used with drugs that affect blood coagulation. Patients taking drugs that affect blood coagulation should be advised to refrain from taking herbal or alternative therapies before discussing their effects with an appropriate healthcare professional. If a patient who is taking an anticoagulant presents with increased bleeding and no other interaction or cause is found, the patient should be questioned about the possibility of use of herbal therapies.

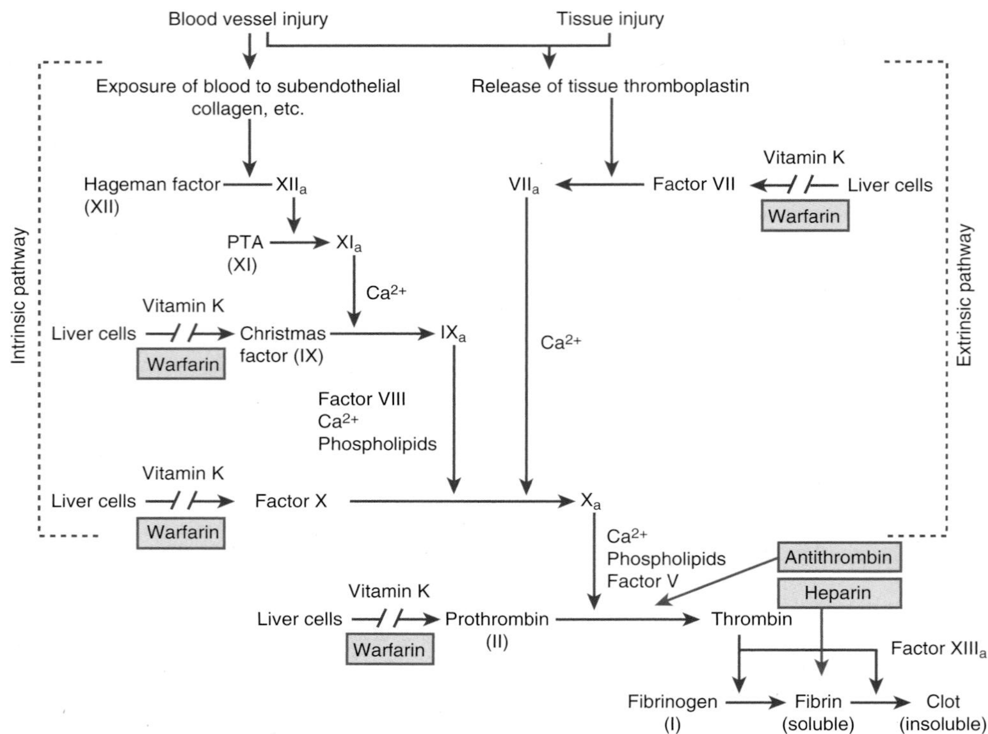

FIGURE 47.3 Details of the intrinsic and extrinsic clotting pathways. The sites of action of some of the drugs that can influence these processes are shown in red.

(also known as Hageman factor), a chemical substance that is found circulating in the blood, is activated. Clotting factors have names, but they are more commonly known by a Roman numeral. When one of these factors becomes activated, the lowercase letter 'a' is added; for example, activated factor XII is also called factor XIIa. Activation of the factors starts a number of reactions in the area: the clot formation process is activated, the clot-dissolving process is activated and the inflammatory response is started (see Chapter 14). The activation of factor XIIa first activates clotting factor XI (plasma thromboplastin antecedent or PTA) and then activates a cascading series of coagulant reactions, called the **intrinsic pathway** (Figure 47.3). Initiation of the intrinsic pathway occurs when prekallikrein, high molecular weight kininogen, factor XI and factor XII are exposed to a damaged endothelial/collagen surface. The reaction of these components ultimately results in activating factor XII and then activating factor XI (to factor XIa), factor IX to IXa which goes on to cleave factor X to its active form (factor Xa). This pathway ends with the conversion of prothrombin to **thrombin**. Activated thrombin breaks down fibrinogen to form insoluble fibrin threads, which form a clot inside the blood vessel. The clot, called a thrombus, acts to plug the injury and seal the system.

Extrinsic Pathway

While the coagulation process is going on inside the blood vessel via the intrinsic pathway, the blood that has leaked out of the vascular system and into the surrounding tissues is caused to clot by the **extrinsic pathway**. Injured cells release a substance called tissue thromboplastin, which forms a complex with factor VIIa, which goes on to activate factor X (and factor IX). This activation of clotting factors in the blood starts the clotting cascade to form a clot on the outside of the blood vessel. The injured vessel is now vasoconstricted and has a platelet plug as well as a clot on both the inside and the outside of the blood vessel in the area of the injury. These actions maintain the closed nature of the cardiovascular system (see Figure 47.3).

The common point in both these pathways is the activation of factor X to factor Xa, which converts prothrombin to thrombin, which in turn converts fibrinogen to fibrin. This is known as the **common pathway**.

Clot Resolution and Coagulation

Blood plasma also contains anticlotting substances that inhibit coagulation reactions that might otherwise lead to an obstruction of blood vessels by blood clots. For example, antithrombin III prevents the formation of **thrombin**, thus stopping the breakdown of the fibrin threads.

Another substance in the plasma, called plasmin, reduces excessive thrombus formation, whereby it dissolves clots to ensure free movement of blood through the system. Plasmin is a protein-dissolving substance that breaks down the fibrin framework of blood clots and opens up vessels. Its

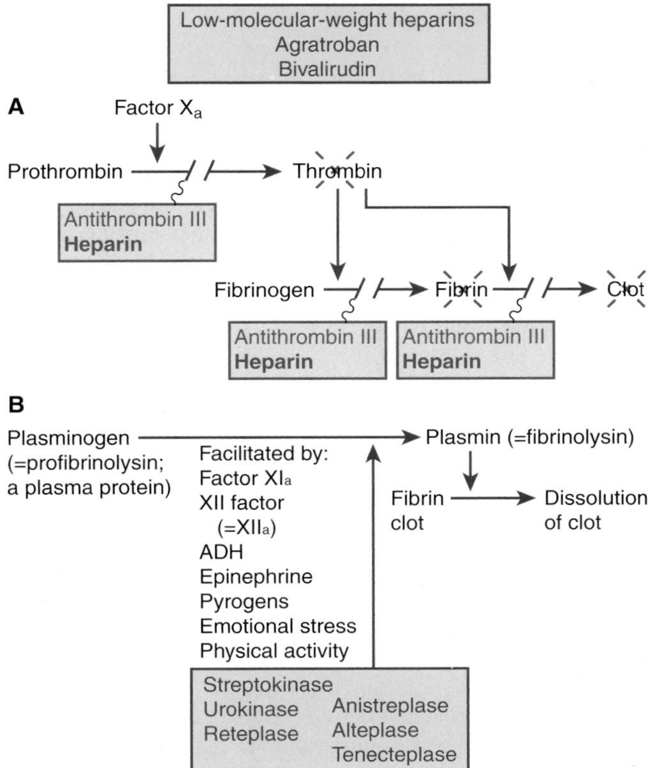

FIGURE 47.4(A) Anticlotting process. Antithrombin III (in plasma) inhibits the activity of factor Xa and thrombin; the drug, heparin, enhances the activity of antithrombin III. Steps in clot formation that are inhibited by heparin are shown in red. (B) Fibrinolytic process: Clots are dissolved. The step that is facilitated by the clot-dissolving drugs and by other agents is shown in blue.

precursor, **plasminogen**, is found in the plasma. The conversion of plasminogen to active plasmin involves tissue plasminogen activator (tPA) and urokinase. The activation of factor XII is facilitated by a number of other components, including antidiuretic hormone (ADH), adrenaline, pyrogens, emotional stress, physical activity and streptokinase. Very high levels of plasmin are found in the lungs (which contain millions of tiny, easily injured capillaries) and in the uterus (which in pregnancy must maintain a constant blood flow for the developing foetus). The action of plasmin is evident in the female menstrual flow in that clots do not form rapidly when the lining of the uterus is shed; the blood oozes slowly over a period of days (Figure 47.4).

Thromboembolic Disorders

Medical conditions that involve the formation of thrombi result in decreased blood flow through or total occlusion of a blood vessel. These conditions are marked by the signs and symptoms of hypoxia, anoxia or even necrosis in areas affected by the decreased blood flow. In some of these disorders, pieces of the thrombus, called emboli, can break off and travel through the cardiovascular system until they become lodged in a tiny vessel, plugging it and restricting blood flow.

Conditions that predispose a person to the formation of clots and emboli are called **thromboembolic disorders**. CAD involves a narrowing of the coronary arteries caused by damage to the endothelial lining of these vessels. Thrombi tend to form along the damaged endothelial lining. As the damage builds up, the lumen of the vessels become narrower and narrower. Over time, the coronary arteries are unable to deliver enough blood to meet the needs of the heart muscle and hypoxia develops. If a vessel becomes so narrow that a tiny clot occludes it completely, the blood supply to that area is cut off and anoxia occurs, followed by infarction and necrosis. With age, many of the vessels in the body can be damaged and develop similar problems with narrowing and blood delivery. These disorders are treated with drugs that interfere with the normal coagulation process to prevent the formation of clots in the system.

Haemorrhagic Disorders

Haemorrhagic disorders, in which excess bleeding occurs, are less common than thromboembolic disorders. These disorders include **haemophilia**, in which there is a genetic lack of certain clotting factors; liver disease, in which clotting factors and proteins needed for clotting are not produced; and bone marrow disorders, in which platelets are not formed in sufficient quantity to be effective. These disorders are treated with clotting factors and drugs that promote the coagulation process.

Anticoagulants

Anticoagulants are drugs that interfere with the normal coagulation process. They can affect the process at any step to slow or prevent clot formation. Anticoagulants interfere with the clotting cascade and thrombin formation. Fibrinolytic drugs act as thrombolytics by stimulating the activation of plasminogen to form plasmin; this degrades fibrin which therefore breaks up the thrombus. These drugs, for example, alteplase (rTPA), streptokinase or tenecteplase, have been shown to be of great value in improving the mortality rates following a myocardial infarction (MI).

Antiplatelet Drugs

Antiplatelet drugs decrease the formation of the platelet plug by decreasing the responsiveness of the platelets to stimuli that would cause them to stick and aggregate on a vessel wall. These drugs are used effectively to treat cardiovascular diseases that are prone to produce occluded vessels, for the maintenance of venous and arterial grafts, to prevent cerebrovascular occlusion and as adjuncts to thrombolytic therapy in the treatment of MI and the prevention of reinfarction. The prescriber's choice of drug depends on the intended use and the patient's tolerance of the associated adverse effects. ***The patient's baseline prothrombin time*** (PT), ***activated clotting time, activated partial thromboplastin time*** (*APTT*), ***platelet count and haemoglobin and haematocrit should be monitored on a regular basis.*** Antiplatelet drugs that are available for use include:

- *Abciximab* is an intravenous (IV) drug used in conjunction with heparin and aspirin to prevent acute cardiac events during transluminal coronary angioplasty and as early treatment of unstable angina and non-Q-wave MI.
- *Aspirin* is an oral drug that has been shown to be effective in decreasing the incidence of TIAs and strokes in men and in reducing the risk of death or nonfatal MI in patients with a past history of MI or with angina.
- *Cilostazol* is an oral drug that is indicated for the reduction of symptoms of intermittent claudication in individuals with peripheral vascular artery disease, allowing increased walking distance.
- *Clopidogrel* is an oral drug used in patients who are at risk for ischaemic events and in those with a history of MI, peripheral artery disease or ischaemic stroke and for the treatment of patients with acute coronary syndrome. Clopidogrel in combination with low-dose aspirin is recommended by National Institute for Health and Clinical Excellence (NICE) to treat patients at moderate-to-high risk of an MI.
- *Dipyridamole* is used orally in combination with warfarin to prevent thromboembolism in patients with artificial heart valves, as well as intravenously to aid diagnosis of CAD in patients who cannot exercise.
- *Eptifibatide* is an IV drug used to treat acute coronary syndrome and to prevent ischaemic episodes in patients undergoing percutaneous coronary interventions. This drug is usually given in conjunction with aspirin or heparin to prevent an early MI in patients with unstable angina.
- *Ticlopidine* is an oral drug used in patients who are intolerant to aspirin therapy to decrease the risk of thrombotic stroke in patients with TIAs or history of stroke.
- *Tirofiban* is an IV drug used in combination with heparin to treat acute coronary syndrome and prevent cardiac ischaemic events during percutaneous coronary intervention.

Therapeutic Actions and Indications

The antiplatelet drugs inhibit platelet adhesion and aggregation by blocking receptor sites on the platelet membrane, preventing platelet–platelet interaction or the interaction of platelets with other clotting factors. These drugs are used to decrease the risk of fatal MI, to prevent reinfarction after MI, to prevent thromboembolic stroke and to maintain the patency of grafts; in addition, an unlabelled use is the treatment of other thromboembolic disorders.

Pharmacokinetics

These drugs are generally well absorbed and highly bound to plasma proteins. They are metabolized in the liver and excreted in urine. There are no adequate studies of these drugs in pregnancy, but, because of the potential for increased bleeding, they should be used during pregnancy only if the benefits to the mother clearly outweigh the potential risks to the foetus. These drugs tend to enter breast milk. If they are needed by a breast-feeding mother, she should find another method of feeding the baby.

Contraindications and Cautions

Caution should be used in the following conditions: the presence of any known bleeding disorder, *because of the risk of excessive blood loss;* recent surgery, *because of the risk of increased bleeding in unhealed vessels* and closed head injuries, *because of the risk of bleeding from the injured vessels in the brain.*

Adverse Effects

The most common adverse effect seen with these drugs is bleeding, which often occurs as increased bruising and bleeding while brushing the teeth. Other common problems include headache, dizziness and weakness; the cause of these reactions is not understood. Nausea and GI distress may occur because of direct irritating effects of the oral drug on the GI tract. Skin rash, another common effect, may be related to direct drug effects on the dermis.

Clinically Important Drug–Drug Interactions

The risk of excessive bleeding increases if any of these drugs is combined with another drug that affects blood clotting.

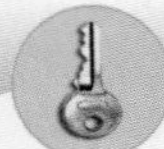

Key drug Summary: *Aspirin*

Indications: Reduction of risk of recurrent TIAs or strokes in males with a history of TIA due to fibrin or platelet emboli, reduction in the risk of death or non-fatal MI in patients with a history of infarction or unstable angina, MI prophylaxis, also used for its anti-inflammatory, analgesic and antipyretic effects,

Actions: Inhibits platelet aggregation by inhibiting platelet synthesis of thromboxane A_2

Pharmacokinetics:

Route	Onset	Peak	Duration
Oral	5–30 min	0.25–2 h	3–6 h

$T_{1/2}$: 15 minutes to 12 hours; metabolized in the liver and excreted in urine

Adverse effects: Acute aspirin toxicity with hyperpnoea, possibly leading to fever, coma and cardiovascular collapse; nausea, dyspepsia, heartburn, epigastric discomfort, GI bleeding, occult blood loss, dizziness, tinnitus, difficulty hearing, anaphylactic reaction, bronchospasm

Nursing Considerations for Patients Receiving Antiplatelet Drugs

Assessment: History and Examination

A structured systematic history should be taken; *Before beginning therapy complete the appropriate baseline observations and investigations including*: body temperature; skin colour and temperature; orientation and reflexes; pulse, blood pressure and perfusion; respirations and adventitious sounds; full blood count (FBC) and clotting studies.

Screen for the following conditions: pregnancy or lactation, *because of the potential adverse effects on the foetus or neonate*; and bleeding disorders, recent surgery or closed head injury or head injury, *because of the potential for excessive bleeding.*

Establish if patient is currently taking other medications or herbal therapies which may potentially interact with antiplatelet drugs.

Nursing Diagnoses

The patient receiving antiplatelet drugs may have the following nursing diagnoses related to drug therapy:

- Potential risk for injury related to bleeding effects or central nervous system (CNS) effects
- Potential acute pain related to GI or CNS effects
- Deficient knowledge regarding drug therapy

Implementation With Rationale

- Provide small, frequent meals *to relieve GI discomfort* if GI upset is a problem.
- Provide comfort measures and analgesia for headache *to relieve pain and improve patient compliance to the drug regimen.*
- Suggest safety measures, including the use of an electric razor and avoidance of contact sports, *to decrease the risk of bleeding.*
- Provide increased precautions against bleeding during invasive procedures, use pressure dressings and ice *to decrease excessive blood loss caused by anticoagulation.*
- Mark the chart of any patient receiving this drug *to alert medical staff that there is a potential for increased bleeding.*
- Provide thorough patient education, including the name of the drug, dosage prescribed, measures to avoid adverse effects, highlight the importance of observing for signs of bleeding, the need for periodic monitoring and evaluation and the need to wear or carry a MedicAlert notification *to enhance patient knowledge about drug therapy and to promote compliance with the drug regimen.*
- Offer support and encouragement *to help the patient deal with the diagnosis and the drug regimen.*

Evaluation

- Monitor patient response to the drug (increased bleeding time, prevention of emboli formation)
- Monitor for adverse effects (bleeding, GI upset, dizziness and headache).
- Evaluate the effectiveness of the teaching plan (patient can name drug, dosage, adverse effects to watch for, specific measures to avoid adverse effects; patient understands importance of continued follow-up).
- Monitor the effectiveness of comfort measures and compliance to the regimen.

Anticoagulants

Anticoagulants interfere with coagulation by disrupting the clotting cascade and thrombin formation. Anticoagulants do not prevent platelet plug formation nor do they breakdown clots already formed. Drugs in this class include warfarin, heparin, antithrombin and bivalirudin. These drugs can be used orally (warfarin) or parenterally (heparin, antithrombin and bivalirudin).

- *Warfarin,* an oral drug, is used to maintain a state of anticoagulation in situations in which the patient is susceptible to potentially dangerous clot formation. Warfarin works by interfering with the formation of vitamin K-dependent clotting factors in the liver (VII, IX, X and II). The eventual effect is a depletion of these clotting factors and a prolongation of clotting times. Warfarin is readily absorbed through the GI tract, metabolized in the liver and excreted in urine and faeces. The half-life of warfarin is approximately 40 hours. Warfarin's onset of action is about 3 days, and its effects last for 4 to 5 days. As there is a time delay, warfarin is not the drug of choice in an acute situation, but it is convenient and useful for prolonged effects. It is used to treat patients with atrial fibrillation (AF), artificial heart valves or valvular damage that makes them susceptible to thrombus and embolus formation. It also is used to treat and prevent venous thrombosis and embolization after acute MI or pulmonary embolism. Warfarin is not used during pregnancy as it has teratogenic effects or during lactation because of the risk of bleeding complications for the mother and the baby. Warfarin interacts with many drugs – some common interactions are listed in Table 47.1.

- *Heparin* is a naturally occurring substance that inhibits the conversion of prothrombin to thrombin, thus blocking the conversion of fibrinogen to fibrin, the final step in clot formation. It is injected IV or subcutaneously and has an almost immediate onset of action. It is excreted in urine. Heparin does not cross the placenta (although some adverse foetal effects have been reported with its use during pregnancy) and does not enter breast milk, so it would be the anticoagulant of choice if one is needed during pregnancy and lactation. Its usual indications include acute treatment and prevention of venous thrombosis and pulmonary embolism; treatment of AF with risk of an embolus, prevention of clotting in blood samples and in dialysis and venous tubing and diagnosis and treatment of disseminated intravascular coagulation (DIC; see Box 47.3). It is also used as an adjunct in the treatment of MI and stroke. Heparin must be injected; therefore, it is not often the drug of choice for outpatients, who would be responsible for injecting the drug

BOX 47.3 Understanding Disseminated Intravascular Coagulation

DIC is a syndrome in which bleeding and thrombosis are found together. It can occur as a complication of many problems, including severe infection with septic shock, traumatic childbirth or missed abortion and massive injuries. In these disorders, local tissue damage causes the release of coagulation-stimulating substances into the circulation. These substances then stimulate the coagulation process, causing fibrin clot formation in small vessels in the lungs, kidneys, brain and other organs. This continuing reaction consumes excessive amounts of fibrinogen, other clotting factors and platelets. The end result is increased bleeding. In essence, the patient clots too much, resulting in the possibility of bleeding to death.

The first step in treating this disorder is to control the problem that initially precipitated it. For example, treating the infection, performing dilation and curettage to clear the uterus or stabilizing injuries can help stop this continuing process. Whole-blood infusions, fresh-frozen plasma or the infusion of fibrinogen may be used to buy some time until the patient is stable and can form clotting factors again. There are associated problems with giving whole blood (e.g. development of hepatitis or HIV) and there is a risk that fibrinogen may set off further intravascular clotting. Paradoxically, the treatment of choice for DIC is the anticoagulant heparin. Heparin prevents the clotting phase from being completed, thus inhibiting the breakdown of fibrinogen. It may also help avoid haemorrhage by preventing the body from depleting its entire store of coagulation factors.

Heparin is usually administered to prevent blood clotting and the adverse effects that are monitored with heparin therapy include signs of bleeding; it can be a real challenge for the nursing staff to feel comfortable administering heparin to a patient who is bleeding to death. Understanding of the disease process can help alleviate any doubts about the treatment.

Table 47.1 Examples of Clinically Important Drug–Drug Interactions with Warfarin. Always consult the current edition of the British National Formulary (BNF) for a complete list of interactions.

↑Anticoagulation	↑Warfarin Metabolism (↓Anticoagulant Effect)
Tricyclic antidepressants	Barbituates
Simvastatin	Carbamazipine
Amiodarone	Phenytoin
Aspirin (↑ risk of bleeding due to antiplatelet effect)	Cimetidine
Corticosteroids	High-dose corticosteroids
Colestyramine	Colestyramine
Erythromycin	Primidone
Oestrogens	Oestrogens
Progestogens	
Cranberry juice	
Tamoxifen	
Testosterone	
Clopidogrel (↑ risk of bleeding due to antiplatelet effect)	

BOX 47.4 Lepirudin: Treating Heparin Allergy

Lepirudin is an IV drug that was developed to treat a rare allergic reaction to heparin. In some patients, an allergy to heparin precipitates a heparin-induced thrombocytopaenia with associated thromboembolic disease. Lepirudin directly inhibits thrombin, blocking the thromboembolic effects of this reaction. A 0.4 mg/kg initial IV bolus followed by a continuous infusion of 0.15 mg/kg for 2 to 10 days is the usual treatment. The patient needs to be monitored for bleeding from any site and for the development of direct hepatic injury.

several times during the day. Patients may be started on heparin in the acute situation and then switched to the oral drug warfarin. Refer to Box 47.4 for details on allergies to heparin.

- *Antithrombin III* is a naturally occurring anticoagulant. The body handles it in the same way that it handles naturally occurring antithrombin. It has been used without reported adverse effects during pregnancy and lactation. It is given IV to patients with hereditary antithrombin III deficiencies and who are undergoing surgery or obstetrical procedures that might put them at risk of thromboembolism. It also is used for replacement therapy in congenital antithrombin III deficiency.

FOCUS ON PATIENT SAFETY

Injectable vitamin K is used to reverse the effects of warfarin. Vitamin K is responsible for promoting the liver synthesis of several clotting factors. When these pathways have been inhibited by warfarin, clotting time is increased. Therefore, the patient's international normalized ratio or INR (blood test used to monitor warfarin treatment) derived from the PT will increase (normal range 0.8–1.2). If an increased level of vitamin K is provided, more of these factors are produced, and the coagulation time can be brought back within a target range. There is a delay of at least 24 hours from the time the drug is given until some change can be seen, because of the way in which vitamin K exerts its effects on clotting. This occurs because there is no direct effect on the warfarin itself but rather an increased stimulation of the liver, which must then produce the clotting factors. The usual dosage for the treatment of anticoagulant-induced prothrombin deficiency is 2.5 to 10 mg intramuscularly (IM) or subcutaneously (sub-cut) or, rarely, 25 mg IM or sub-cut. Oral doses can be used if injection is not feasible. An increased INR value within 6 to 8 hours after parenteral doses or 12 to 48 hours after oral doses will determine the need for a repeat dose. If a response is not seen and the patient is bleeding excessively, fresh-frozen plasma factor concentrates or an infusion of whole blood may be needed.

FOCUS ON PATIENT SAFETY

In cases of a heparin overdose, the antidote is protamine sulphate. This strongly basic protein drug forms stable salts with heparin as soon as the two drugs come into contact, immediately reversing heparin's anticoagulant effects. Paradoxically, if protamine is given to a patient who has not received heparin, it has anticoagulant effects. The dosage is determined by the amount of heparin that was given and the time that elapsed since then. A dose of 1 mg IV protamine neutralizes 90 units of heparin derived from lung tissue or 110 units of heparin derived from intestinal mucosa. The drug must be administered very slowly, not to exceed 50 mg IV in any 10 min period. Care must be taken to calculate the amount of heparin that has been given to the patient. Potentially fatal anaphylactic reactions have been reported with the use of protamine sulphate, so life-support equipment should be readily available when it is used.

- *Bivalirudin* is an IV drug that directly inhibits thrombin. It is used with aspirin to prevent ischaemic events in patients undergoing transluminal coronary angioplasty.

Therapeutic Actions and Indications

As noted previously, the anticoagulants interfere with the normal cascade of events involved in the clotting process. Warfarin causes a decrease in the production of vitamin K-dependent clotting factors in the liver. Heparin and bivalirudin block the formation of thrombin from prothrombin. Antithrombin interferes with the formation of thrombin from prothrombin. These drugs are used to treat thromboembolic disorders such as AF, MI, pulmonary embolus and evolving stroke and to prevent the formation of thrombi in such disorders.

Contraindications and Cautions

The anticoagulants are contraindicated in the presence of known allergy to the drugs. They also should not be used with any conditions *that could be compromised by increased bleeding tendencies,* including haemorrhagic disorders, recent trauma, spinal puncture, GI ulcers, recent surgery, intrauterine device placement, tuberculosis, presence of indwelling catheters and threatened abortion. In addition, anticoagulants are contraindicated in pregnancy, *because foetal injury and death have occurred;* in lactation (use of heparin is suggested if an anticoagulant is needed during lactation); and in renal or hepatic disease, *which could interfere with the metabolism and effectiveness of these drugs.*

Caution should be used in patients with congestive heart failure (CHF), hyperthyroidism, senility or psychosis and in those with diarrhoea or fever, *which could alter the normal clotting process by, respectively, loss of vitamin K from the intestine or activation of plasminogen.*

Adverse Effects

The most commonly encountered adverse effect of the anticoagulants is bleeding, ranging from bleeding gums with tooth brushing to severe internal haemorrhage. Clotting times should be monitored closely to avoid these problems. Nausea, GI upset, diarrhoea and hepatic dysfunction also may occur secondary to direct drug toxicity. Warfarin has been associated with alopecia and dermatitis as well as bone marrow depression and, less frequently, with prolonged and painful erections.

Clinically Important Drug–Drug Interactions

Increased bleeding can occur if heparin is combined with oral anticoagulants, salicylates, penicillins or cephalosporins. Decreased anticoagulation can occur if heparin is combined with glyceryl trinitrate (GTN).

Warfarin has documented drug–drug interactions with a vast number of other drugs (see Table 47.1 for some examples). It is wise practice never to add or take away a drug from the regimen of a patient receiving warfarin without careful patient monitoring and adjustment of the warfarin dosage to prevent serious adverse effects.

Please consult the most up-to-date version of the BNF for current guidelines and information

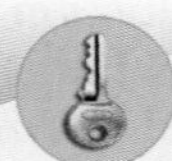

Key drug Summary: *Heparin*

Indications: Prevention and treatment of venous thrombosis and pulmonary emboli; treatment of AF with embolization; diagnosis and treatment of DIC; prevention of clotting in blood samples and heparin lock sets

Actions: Inhibits thrombus and clot production by blocking the conversion of prothrombin to thrombin and fibrinogen to fibrin

Pharmacokinetics:

Route	Onset	Peak	Duration
IV	Immediate	Min	2–6 h
Subcut	20–60	min 2–4 h	8–12 h

$T_{1/2}$: 30–180 minutes; metabolized in the cells and excreted in urine

Adverse effects: Loss of hair, bruising, fever, osteoporosis, suppression of renal function (with long-term use). Side-effects of haemorrhage, skin necrosis, thrombocytopaenia, hyperkalaemia and osteoporosis may also occur after prolonged use.

Nursing Considerations for Patients Receiving Anticoagulants

Assessment: History and Examination

Screen for any known allergies to these drugs. Also screen for conditions *that could be exacerbated by increased bleeding tendencies*, including haemorrhagic disorders, recent trauma, spinal puncture, GI ulcers, recent surgery, intrauterine device placement, tuberculosis, presence of indwelling catheters and threatened abortion. Also screen for pregnancy, *because foetal injury and death have occurred*; lactation (use of heparin is suggested if an anticoagulant is needed during lactation); renal or hepatic disease, *which could interfere with the metabolism and effectiveness of these drugs*; CHF; thyrotoxicosis; senility or psychosis, *because of the potential for unexpected effects;* and diarrhoea or fever, *which could alter the normal clotting process.*

Include screening *for baseline status before beginning therapy and for any potential adverse effects.* Assess the following: body temperature; skin colour, lesions or bruising, temperature; affect, orientation and reflexes; pulse, blood pressure and perfusion; respirations and adventitious sounds; clotting studies, renal and hepatic function tests, FBC and hidden blood in the stools (guaiac); and electrocardiogram (ECG), if appropriate.

Establish if patient is currently taking other medications or herbal therapies which may potentially interact with the anticoagulant drugs.

Nursing Diagnoses

The patient receiving an anticoagulant may have the following nursing diagnoses related to drug therapy:

- Risk for injury related to bleeding effects and bone marrow depression
- Potential disturbed body image related to alopecia and skin rash
- Potential ineffective tissue perfusion (total body) related to blood loss
- Deficient knowledge regarding drug therapy

Implementation With Rationale

- Evaluate for therapeutic effects of warfarin–PT 1.5 to 2.5 times the control value to INR of 2 to 4 *to evaluate the effectiveness of the drug dose. (This value of 2–4 depends upon the diagnosis/condition as the target INR may vary within this range, i.e. 3–4)*

- Evaluate for therapeutic effects of heparin: whole-blood-clotting time (WBCT) 2.5 to three times of control or APTT 1.5 to three times the control value *to evaluate the effectiveness of the drug dose.*
- Evaluate the patient regularly for any sign of blood loss (petechiae, bleeding gums, bruises, dark-coloured stools and dark-coloured urine) *to evaluate the effectiveness of the drug dose and to consult with the prescriber if bleeding becomes apparent.*
- Establish safety precautions *to protect the patient from injury.*
- Provide safety measures, such as use of an electric razor and avoidance of contact sports, *to decrease the risk of bleeding.*
- Provide increased precautions against bleeding during invasive procedures, use pressure dressings, avoid intramuscular injections and do not rub sub-cut injection sites, *because the state of anticoagulation increases the risk of blood loss.*
- Mark the chart of any patient receiving this drug *to alert the medical staff that there is a potential for increased bleeding.*
- Maintain antidotes on standby (protamine sulphate for heparin, vitamin K for warfarin) *in case of overdose.*
- Monitor the patient carefully when any drug is added to or withdrawn from the drug regimen of a patient taking warfarin, *because of the risk of drug–drug interactions that would change the effectiveness of the anticoagulant.*
- Make sure that the patient receives regular follow-up and monitoring, including measurement of clotting times, *to ensure maximum therapeutic effects.*
- Provide thorough patient education, including the name of the drug, dosage prescribed, measures to avoid adverse effects, warning signs of problems, the need for periodic monitoring and evaluation and the need to wear or carry a Medic-Alert notification, *to enhance patient knowledge about drug therapy and to promote compliance with the drug regimen.*
- Offer support and encouragement *to help the patient deal with the diagnosis and the drug regimen.*

Evaluation

- Monitor patient response to the drug:increased bleeding time (warfarin, PT 1.5 to 2.5 times the control value or INR ratio of 2 to 3; heparin, WBCT of 2.5 to 3 times the control value or APTT of 1.5 to 3 times control).
- Monitor for adverse effects (bleeding, bone marrow depression, alopecia, GI upset, rash).
- Evaluate the effectiveness of the teaching plan (patient can name drug, dosage, adverse effects to watch for, specific measures to avoid adverse effects; patient understands importance of continued follow-up).
- Monitor the effectiveness of comfort measures and compliance to the regimen (Critical Thinking Scenario 47-1).

Low-molecular-weight Heparins

In the late 1990s, a series of low-molecular-weight heparins were developed. These drugs inhibit thrombus and clot formation by activating antithrombin (blocking factors Xa and IIa). These drugs are indicated for very specific uses in the prevention of clots and emboli formation after certain surgeries or prolonged bed rest. They have also been found to block angiogenesis, the process that allows cancer cells to develop new blood vessels and are being studied as possible adjuncts to cancer chemotherapy.

The nursing care of a patient receiving one of these drugs is similar to that of a patient receiving heparin. The drug is given just before (or just after) the surgery and is then continued for 7 to 14 days during the postoperative recovery process. Caution must be used to avoid combining these drugs with standard heparin therapy; serious bleeding episodes and deaths have been reported when this combination was inadvertently used.

Thrombolytic Agents

If a thrombus has already formed in a vessel (*e.g.* during an acute MI), it may be necessary to dissolve that clot to open the vessel and restore blood flow to the dependent tissue. All of the drugs that are available for this purpose work to activate the natural fibrinolysis system for the conversion of plasminogen to plasmin. The activation of this system breaks down fibrin threads and dissolves any formed clot. The **thrombolytic drugs** are effective only if the patient has plasminogen in the plasma. Thrombolytic agents include the following:

- *Alteplase* is a recombinant tissue plasminogen activator, rTPA. It is used for treatment of MI, acute pulmonary embolism and acute ischaemic stroke. It is given IV, and the patient needs to be monitored closely for bleeding.
- *Reteplase* is given IV for the treatment of coronary artery thrombosis associated with an acute MI.

BOX 47.5 Specific Factor Xa Inhibitor to Prevent Deep Venous Thrombosis

Fondaparinux, a specific blocker of factor Xa, was approved in 2002 for the prevention of venous thromboembolic events in patients undergoing surgery for hip fracture, hip replacement or knee replacement. It is supplied in prefilled syringes, making it convenient for patients who will be self-administering the drug at home. As with other drugs that affect coagulation, bleeding is the most common and potentially the most serious adverse effect that can occur with the use of this drug. Patients need teaching about administration, disposal of the syringes and signs of bleeding to watch for. Periodic blood tests will be needed to assess the effects of the drug on the body.

- *Streptokinase,* although less commonly used now, is used IV to treat coronary artery thrombosis, acute MI, pulmonary embolism, DVT (see also Box 47.5 for another inhibitor of DVT) and arterial thrombosis or embolism and to open an occluded atrioventricular cannula.
- *Tenecteplase* is given IV to reduce mortality associated with acute MI. The timing of administration is critical to the success of the therapy.
- *Urokinase* is used IV to lyse pulmonary emboli, to treat coronary thrombosis and to clear occluded IV catheters.
- *Pentoxifylline* can induce haemorrhage (see Box 47.6).

Therapeutic Actions and Indications

The thrombolytic agents work by activating plasminogen to plasmin, which in turn breaks down fibrin threads in a clot to dissolve a formed clot. They are indicated for the treatment of acute MI (to dissolve the clot and prevent further tissue damage, if used within 6 hours after the onset of symptoms); to treat pulmonary emboli and ischaemic stroke and to open clotted IV catheters.

BOX 47.6 Pentoxifylline: Haemorrheologic Agent

Pentoxifylline is known as a haemorrheologic agent or a drug that can induce haemorrhage. As a xanthine, like caffeine and theophylline, it decreases platelet aggregation and decreases the fibrinogen concentration in the blood. These effects can decrease blood clot formation and increase blood flow through narrowed or damaged vessels. The mechanism of action by which pentoxifylline does these things is not known. It is one of the very few drugs found to be effective in treating intermittent claudication, a painful vascular problem of the legs.

Pentoxifylline is also associated with many cardiovascular stimulatory effects. Patients with underlying cardiovascular problems need to be monitored carefully when taking this drug. Pentoxifylline can also cause headache, dizziness, nausea and upset stomach. It is taken orally three times a day for at least 8 weeks to evaluate its effectiveness.

Pharmacokinetics

These drugs must be injected and are cleared from the body after liver metabolism. They cross the placenta and have been associated with adverse foetal effects. These drugs should not be used during pregnancy unless the benefits to the mother clearly outweigh the potential risks to the foetus. It is not known whether these drugs enter breast milk. Caution should be used during lactation because of the potential risk for bleeding effects.

Contraindications and Cautions

The use of thrombolytic agents is contraindicated in the presence of allergy to any of these drugs. They also should not be used with any condition *that could be worsened by the dissolution of clots,* including recent surgery, active internal bleeding, CVA within the last 2 months, aneurysm, obstetrical delivery, organ biopsy, recent serious GI bleeding, rupture of a noncompressible blood vessel, recent major trauma (including cardiopulmonary resuscitation); known blood-clotting defects, cerebrovascular disease, uncontrolled hypertension, liver disease *which could affect normal clotting factors and the production of plasminogen* and pregnancy or lactation *because of the possible adverse effects on the foetus or neonate.*

Adverse Effects

The most common adverse effect associated with the use of thrombolytic agents is bleeding. Patients should be monitored closely for the occurrence of cardiac arrhythmias (with coronary reperfusion) and hypotension. Hypersensitivity reactions are not uncommon; they range from rash and flushing to bronchospasm and anaphylactic reaction.

Clinically Important Drug–Drug Interactions

The risk of haemorrhage increases if thrombolytic agents are used with any anticoagulant or antiplatelet drug.

Please consult the most up-to-date version of the British National Formulary (BNF) for current guidelines and information

Nursing Considerations for Patients Receiving Thrombolytic Agents

Assessment: History and Examination

Screen for any known allergies to these drugs. Also screen for any conditions *that could be worsened by the dissolution of clots,* including recent surgery, recent head injury, active internal bleeding, CVA within the last 2 months, aneurysm, obstetrical delivery, organ biopsy, recent serious GI bleeding, rupture of a noncompressible blood vessel, recent major trauma (including cardiopulmonary resuscitation), known blood-clotting defects, cerebrovascular disease, uncontrolled hypertension, liver disease *(which could affect normal clotting factors and the production of plasminogen)* and pregnancy or lactation *(because of the possible adverse effects on the neonate)*.

Include screening *for baseline status before beginning therapy and for any potential adverse effects.* Assess the following: body temperature; skin colour, lesions and temperature; affect, orientation and reflexes; pulse, blood pressure and perfusion; respirations and adventitious sounds; and clotting studies, renal and hepatic function tests, FBC, guaiac test for occult blood in stool and ECG.

Establish if patient is currently taking other medications or herbal therapies which may potentially interact with thrombolytic agents.

Nursing Diagnoses

The patient receiving a thrombolytic drug may have the following nursing diagnoses related to drug therapy:

- Risk for injury related to clot-dissolving effects
- Ineffective tissue perfusion (total body) related to possible blood loss
- Decreased cardiac output related to bleeding and arrhythmias
- Deficient knowledge regarding drug therapy

Implementation With Rationale

- Discontinue heparin if it is being given before administration of a thrombolytic agent, unless specifically ordered for coronary artery infusion, *to prevent excessive loss of blood.*
- Evaluate the patient regularly for any sign of blood loss (petechiae, bleeding gums, bruises, dark-coloured stools, dark-coloured urine) *to evaluate drug effectiveness and to consult with the prescriber if blood loss becomes apparent.*
- Monitor coagulation studies regularly; consult with the prescriber *to adjust the drug dose appropriately.*
- Institute treatment within 6 hours after the onset of symptoms of acute MI *to achieve optimum therapeutic effectiveness.*
- Arrange to type and cross-match blood *in case of serious blood loss that requires whole-blood transfusion.*
- Monitor cardiac rhythm continuously if being given for acute MI, *because of the risk of alteration in cardiac function*; have life-support equipment on standby as needed.
- Provide increased precautions against bleeding during invasive procedures; use pressure dressings and ice; avoid intramuscular injections; and do not rub subcut injection sites, *because of the risk of increased blood loss in the anticoagulated state.*
- Mark the chart of any patient receiving this drug *to alert medical staff that there is a potential for increased bleeding.*
- Provide thorough patient education, including the name of the drug, dosage prescribed, measures to avoid adverse effects, warning signs of problems and the need for periodic monitoring and evaluation, *to enhance patient knowledge about drug therapy and to promote compliance with the drug regimen.*
- Offer support and encouragement *to help the patient deal with the diagnosis and the drug regimen.*

Evaluation

- Monitor patient response to the drug (dissolution of the clot and return of blood flow to the area).
- Monitor for adverse effects (bleeding, arrhythmias, hypotension and hypersensitivity reaction).
- Evaluate the effectiveness of the teaching plan (patient can name drug, adverse effects to watch for, specific measures to avoid adverse effects).
- Monitor the effectiveness of comfort measures and concordance with the regimen.

Drugs Used to Control Bleeding

On the other end of the spectrum of coagulation problems are various bleeding disorders. These include the following:

- *Haemophilia,* in which there is a genetic lack of certain clotting factors, leaves the patient vulnerable to excessive bleeding with any injury,
- *Liver disease,* in which clotting factors and proteins needed for clotting are not produced,
- *Bone marrow disorders,* in which platelets are not formed in sufficient quantity to be effective.

These disorders are treated with clotting factors and drugs that promote the coagulation process.

Antihaemophilic Agents

The drugs used to treat haemophilia are replacement factors for the specific clotting factors that are genetically missing in that particular type of haemophilia. These drugs include the following:

- *Antihaemophilic factor (factor VIII),* the clotting factor that is missing in classic haemophilia (haemophilia A). It is used to correct or prevent bleeding episodes or to allow necessary surgery.
- *Coagulation factor VIIa* is a preparation, made from mouse, hamster and bovine proteins, which contains variable amounts of preformed clotting factors. It is used to treat bleeding episodes in patients with haemophilia A or B.
- *Factor IX complex* contains plasma fractions of many of the clotting factors and increases blood levels of factors II, VII, IX and X. It is given intravenously to prevent or treat haemophilia B (Christmas disease, a deficiency of factor IX) to control bleeding episodes in haemophilia A and to control bleeding episodes in cases of factor VII deficiency.

Therapeutic Actions and Indications

The antihaemophilic drugs replace clotting factors that are either genetically missing or low in a particular type of haemophilia. They are used to prevent blood loss from injury or surgery and to treat bleeding episodes. The drug of choice depends on the particular haemophilia that is being treated.

Pharmacokinetics

These agents replace normal clotting factors and are processed as such by the body. They should be used during pregnancy only if the benefit to the mother clearly outweighs the potential risk to the foetus. It is recommended that another method of feeding the baby be used if these drugs are needed during lactation because of the potential for adverse effects on the baby.

Contraindications and Cautions

Antihaemophilic factor is contraindicated in the presence of known allergy to mouse proteins. Factor IX is contraindicated in the presence of liver disease with signs of intravascular coagulation or fibrinolysis. Coagulation factor VIIa is contraindicated with known allergies to mouse, hamster or bovine products. These drugs are not recommended for use during lactation, and caution should be used during pregnancy *because of the potential for adverse effects on the baby or foetus.* There are few contraindications to the use of these drugs, because they are used to prevent serious bleeding problems or to treat bleeding episodes.

Adverse Effects

The most common adverse effects associated with antihaemophilic agents involve risks associated with the use of blood products (e.g. hepatitis, HIV). Headache, flushing, chills, fever and lethargy may occur as a reaction to the injection of a foreign protein. Nausea and vomiting may also occur, as may stinging, itching and burning at the site of the injection.

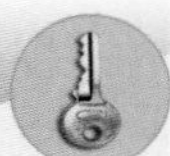

Key Drug Summary: Antihaemophilic Factor

Indications: Treatment of classic haemophilia to provide temporary replacement of clotting factors to correct or prevent bleeding episodes or to allow necessary surgery

Actions: Normal plasma protein that is needed for the transformation of prothrombin to thrombin – the final step in the clotting pathway

Pharmacokinetics:

Route	Onset	Peak	Duration
IV	Immediate	Unknown	Unknown

$T_{1/2}$: 12 hours; cleared from the body by normal protein metabolism

Adverse effects: Allergic reaction, stinging at injection site, headache, rash, chills, nausea, hepatitis, HIV (risks associated with the use of blood products).

Nursing Considerations for Patients Receiving Antihaemophilic Agents

Assessment: History and Examination

Screen for the following conditions, *which could be cautions or contraindications to use of the drug:* any known allergies to these drugs or to antihaemophilic factor, liver disease.

Include screening *for baseline status before beginning therapy and for any potential adverse effects.* Assess the following: body temperature; skin colour, lesions and temperature; affect, orientation and reflexes; pulse, blood pressure and perfusion; respirations and adventitious sounds; clotting studies; and liver function tests.

Establish if patient is currently taking other medications or herbal therapies which may potentially interact with antihaemophilic agents.

Nursing Diagnoses

The patient receiving an antihaemophilic drug may have the following nursing diagnoses related to drug therapy:

- Ineffective tissue perfusion (total body) related to changes in coagulation pale/bluish appearance – cold to touch
- Acute pain related to GI, CNS or skin effects
- Anxiety or fear related to the diagnosis and use of blood-related products
- Deficient knowledge regarding drug therapy

Implementation With Rationale

- Administer by the IV route only *to ensure therapeutic effectiveness.*
- Monitor clinical response and clotting factor levels regularly *in order to arrange to adjust dosage as needed.*
- Monitor the patient for any sign of thrombosis *to arrange to use comfort and support measures as needed*
- Decrease the rate of infusion if headache, fever or tingling occurs *to prevent severe drug reaction;* in some individuals, the drug will need to be discontinued.
- Arrange to type and cross-match blood *in case of serious blood loss that will require whole-blood transfusion.*
- Mark the chart of any patient receiving this drug *to alert medical staff that there is a potential for increased bleeding.*
- Provide thorough patient education, including the name of the drug, dosage prescribed, measures to avoid adverse effects, warning signs of problems and the need for periodic monitoring and evaluation, *to enhance patient knowledge about drug therapy and to promote compliance with the drug regimen.*
- Offer support and encouragement *to help the patient deal with the diagnosis and the drug regimen.*

Evaluation

- Monitor patient response to the drug (control of bleeding episodes, prevention of bleeding episodes).
- Monitor for adverse effects (thrombosis, CNS effects, nausea, hypersensitivity reaction, hepatitis, HIV)
- Evaluate the effectiveness of the teaching plan (patient can name drug, dosage of drug, adverse effects to watch for, specific measures to avoid adverse effects, warning signs to report).
- Monitor the effectiveness of comfort measures and compliance to the regimen.

Nursing Considerations for Patients Receiving Systemic Haemostatic Agents

Assessment: History and Examination

Screen for the following conditions, *which could be cautions or contraindications to use of the drug*: cardiac disease, *because of the risk of arrhythmias*; renal and hepatic dysfunction, *which could alter the excretion of these drugs and the normal clotting processes*; and lactation, *because of the potential for adverse effects on the neonate.*

Include screening *for baseline status before beginning therapy and for any potential adverse effects.* Assess the following: body temperature; skin colour and temperature; orientation and reflexes; pulse, blood pressure and perfusion; respirations and adventitious sounds; bowel sounds and activity; urinalysis and clotting studies; and renal and hepatic function tests.

Nursing Diagnoses

The patient receiving a systemic haemostatic drug may have the following nursing diagnoses related to drug therapy:

- Disturbed sensory perception related to CNS effects
- Potential acute pain related to GI, CNS or muscle effects
- Risk for injury related to CNS or blood-clotting effects
- Deficient knowledge regarding drug therapy

Implementation With Rationale

- Monitor clinical response and clotting factor levels regularly *in order to arrange to adjust dosage as needed.*
- Monitor the patient for any sign of thrombosis *in order to arrange to use comfort and support measures as needed* (*e.g.* support hose, positioning, ambulation and exercise).
- Orient patient and offer support and safety measures if hallucinations or psychoses occur *to prevent patient injury.*
- Offer comfort measures *to help the patient deal with the effects of the drug.* These include small, frequent meals; mouth care; environmental controls; and safety measures.
- Provide thorough patient education, including the name of the drug, dosage prescribed, measures to avoid adverse effects, warning signs of problems

and the need for periodic monitoring and evaluation, *to enhance patient knowledge about drug therapy and to promote compliance with the drug regimen.*

- Offer support and encouragement *to help the patient deal with the diagnosis and the drug regimen.*

Evaluation

- Monitor the patient response to the drug (control of bleeding episodes).
- Monitor for adverse effects (thrombosis, CNS effects, nausea and hypersensitivity reaction).
- Evaluate the effectiveness of the teaching plan (patient can name drug, dosage of drug, adverse effects to watch for, specific measures to avoid adverse effects, warning signs to report).
- Monitor the effectiveness of comfort measures and compliance to the regimen.

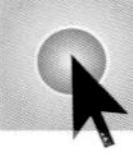

WEB LINKS

Health care providers and patients may want to consult the following Internet sources:

http://cks.library.nhs.uk The National Health Service Clinical Knowledge Summaries provide evidence-based practical information on the common conditions observed in primary care.

http://www.bnf.org.uk The BNF provides UK health care professionals with authoritative and practical information on the selection and clinical use of medicines.

http://www.medicalert.org.uk MedicAlert is a registered charity providing a life-saving identification system for individuals with hidden medical conditions and allergies.

http://www.nhsdirect.nhs.uk The National Health Service Direct service provides patients with information and advice about health, illness and health services.

http://www.nice.org.uk The NICE is an independent organization responsible for providing national guidance on promoting good health and preventing and treating ill health.

Points to Remember

- Coagulation is the transformation of fluid blood into a solid state to repair damage in the vascular system.
- Coagulation involves several processes, including vasoconstriction, platelet aggregation to form a plug and intrinsic and extrinsic pathways, to seal off any damaged area/injury.
- The final step of clot formation is the conversion of prothrombin to thrombin, which breaks down fibrinogen to form insoluble fibrin threads.
- Once a clot is formed, it must be dissolved to prevent extension beyond the site of injury, the occlusion of blood vessels and loss of blood supply to tissues.
- Plasminogen is the basis of the clot-dissolving system. It is converted to plasmin by several factors. Plasmin dissolves fibrin threads and resolves the clot.
- Anticoagulants block blood coagulation by interfering with one or more of the steps involved, such as blocking platelet aggregation or inhibiting the intrinsic or extrinsic pathways to clot formation.
- Thrombolytic drugs dissolve clots or thrombi that have formed. They activate the plasminogen system to stimulate natural clot dissolution.
- Haemostatic drugs are used to stop bleeding. They may replace missing clotting factors or prevent the plasminogen system from dissolving formed clots.
- Haemophilia, a genetic lack of certain essential clotting factors, results in excessive bleeding. It is treated by replacing missing clotting factors.

CRITICAL THINKING SCENARIO 47-1

Oral Anticoagulant Therapy

The Situation

May is a 68-year-old woman with a history of severe mitral valve disease. For the last few years, she has been able to manage her condition with digoxin and captopril. However, on a recent visit to her doctor for her regular echogram, she disclosed that she had been experiencing periods of breathlessness, palpitations and dizziness. Her 24-hour ECG showed that she was having frequent periods of AF, with a heart rate of up to 140 beats/min. Warfarin therapy was started because of the risk of emboli as a result of her valve disease and the bouts of AF.

Critical Thinking

- What nursing interventions should be done at this point?
- Why do people with mitral valve disease frequently develop AF? *Think about why emboli form when the atria fibrillate.*
- Stabilizing May on warfarin may take several weeks of blood tests and dosage adjustments. How can this process be made easier?
- What patient education points should be covered with May to ensure that she is protected from emboli and does not experience excessive bleeding?

Discussion

May's situation is complex. She has a progressive degenerative valve disease that usually leads to CHF and frequently to other complications, such as AF and emboli formation. Her digoxin and potassium levels should be checked to determine whether her CHF is stabilized or the digoxin is causing the AF because of excessive doses or potassium imbalance. If these tests are within normal limits, May might be experiencing AF because of irritation to the atrial cells caused by the damaged mitral valve and associated swelling and scarring. If this is the case, an anticoagulant will help protect her against emboli, which form in the auricles when blood pools there while the atria are fibrillating. There is less chance of emboli formation if clotting is slowed.

May will require some information about warfarin, including the need for frequent blood tests, the list of potential drug–drug interactions, the importance of being alert to the many factors that can affect dosage needs (including illness and diet) and how to monitor for subtle blood loss. This can also be a good opportunity to review teaching about valvular disease and CHF and to answer any questions that she might have about how all of these things interrelate.

Nursing Care Guide for May: Warfarin

Assessment: History and Examination

Assess health history for allergies to warfarin, subacute bacterial endocarditis (SBE), haemorrhagic disorders, tuberculosis, renal or hepatic dysfunction, gastric ulcers, thyroid disease, uncontrolled hypertension, severe trauma or a long-term indwelling catheter (which increases the risk of bleeding). Also assess concurrent use of numerous drugs and herbal therapies

Focus the physical examination on the following areas: blood pressure, pulse, perfusion, baseline ECG, orientation, affect, reflexes, vision; skin: colour, lesions, texture; respiratory rate and character, abdominal examination, guaiac stool test results (for occult blood)

Laboratory tests should include liver and renal function tests, FBC, white cell count, prothrombin time (PT) and INR.

Nursing Diagnoses

- Ineffective tissue perfusion (total body) related to alteration in clotting effects.
- Risk for injury related to anticoagulant effects.
- Disturbed body image related to potential alopecia, skin rash.
- Deficient knowledge regarding drug therapy.

Implementation

- Ensure proper administration of drug.
- Provide comfort and safety measures, such as small meals, protection from injury during invasive and other procedures, bowel programme as needed, standby antidotes (e.g. vitamin K) and careful skin care.
- Provide support and reassurance to deal with drug effects.
- Provide patient education regarding drug, dosage, adverse effects, what to report, safety precautions.

Evaluation

- Evaluate drug effects: increased bleeding times, PT 1.5 to –2.5 times control or INR of 2:3.

(continued)

Oral Anticoagulant Therapy *(continued)*

- Monitor for adverse effects: bleeding, alopecia, rash, GI upset and excessive bleeding.
- Monitor for drug–drug interactions (numerous).
- Evaluate effectiveness of patient education programme comfort and safety measures

Patient Education for May

- ☐ An anticoagulant slows the body's normal blood-clotting processes to prevent harmful blood clots from forming. This type of drug is often called a 'blood thinner;' however, it cannot dissolve any clots that have already formed.
- ☐ *Never* change any medication that you are taking such as adding or stopping another drug, taking a new over-the-counter medication or stopping one that you have been taking regularly, without consulting with your health care provider. Many other drugs affect the way that your anticoagulant works; starting or stopping another drug can cause excessive bleeding or interfere with the desired effects of the drug.
- ☐ Some of the following adverse effects may occur:
  - *Stomach bloating, cramps:* These problems often pass with time; consult your health care provider if they persist or become too uncomfortable.
  - *Loss of hair, skin rash:* These problems can be very frustrating; you may wish to discuss these with your health care provider.
  - *Orange–yellow discolouration of the urine:* This can be frightening, but it may just be an effect of the drug. If you are concerned that this might be blood, simply add vinegar to your urine; the colour should disappear. If the colour does not disappear, it may be caused by blood and you should contact your health care provider.
- ☐ Report any of the following to your health care provider: *unusual bleeding (when brushing your teeth, excessive bleeding from an injury, excessive bruising); black or tarry stools; cloudy or dark urine; sore throat, fever or chills; severe headache or dizziness.*
- ☐ Tell any doctor, nurse or other health care provider involved in your care that you are taking this drug. You should carry or wear medical identification stating that you are taking this drug to alert emergency medical personnel that you are at increased risk for bleeding.
- ☐ Avoid situations in which you could be easily injured, for example engaging in contact sports or games with children or using a straight razor.
- ☐ Keep this drug and all medications out of the reach of children.
- ☐ Arrange regular blood tests while you are taking this drug to monitor the effects of the drug on your body and adjust your dosage as needed.

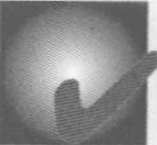

CHECK YOUR UNDERSTANDING

Answers to the questions in this chapter may be found in the Answer Key in the back of the book.

Multiple Choice

Select the most appropriate response to the following.

1. Blood coagulation is a complex reaction that involves
   a. vasoconstriction, platelet aggregation and plasminogen action.
   b. vasodilation, platelet aggregation and activation of the clotting cascade.
   c. vasoconstriction, platelet aggregation and conversion of prothrombin to thrombin.
   d. vasodilation, platelet inhibition and action of the intrinsic and extrinsic clotting cascades.

2. Warfarin, an oral anticoagulant,
   a. acts to directly prevent the conversion of prothrombin to thrombin.
   b. acts to decrease the production of vitamin K clotting factors in the liver.
   c. acts as a catalyst in the conversion of plasminogen to plasmin.
   d. is poorly absorbed through the GI tract so it is best given by IV.

3. Heparin reacts to prevent the conversion of prothrombin to thrombin. Heparin
   a. is available in oral and parenteral forms.
   b. takes about 72 hours to cause a therapeutic effect.
   c. effects are reversed with the administration of protamine sulphate.
   d. effects are reversed with the injection of vitamin K.

4. The low-molecular-weight heparin of choice for preventing deep venous thrombosis after hip replacement therapy would be
   a. tinzaparin.
   b. dalteparin.
   c. heparin.
   d. enoxaparin.

5. A thrombolytic agent could be safely used in
   a. CVA within the last 2 months.
   b. acute MI within the last 3 hours.
   c. recent, serious GI bleeding.
   d. obstetrical delivery.

6. Antihaemophilic agents are used to replace missing clotting factors to prevent severe blood loss. The most common side-effects associated with the use of these drugs are
   a. bleeding.
   b. dark stools and urine.
   c. hepatitis, AIDS/HIV
   d. constipation.

Extended Matching Questions

Select **all** that apply.

1. Factor XII (Hageman factor) is known to activate which of the following?
   a. The clotting cascade
   b. The anticlotting process
   c. The inflammatory response
   d. Platelet aggregation
   e. Thromboxane A_2
   f. Troponin coupling

2. Plasminogen is converted to plasmin, a clot-dissolving substance, by which of the following?
   a. Nicotine
   b. Factor XII
   c. Streptokinase
   d. Pyrogens
   e. Thrombin
   f. Christmas factor

3. Antiplatelet drugs block the aggregation of platelets and keep vessels open. These drugs would be useful in which of the following?
   a. Maintaining the patency of grafts
   b. Decreasing the risk of fatal MI
   c. Preventing reinfarction after MI
   d. Dissolving a pulmonary embolus and improving oxygenation
   e. Decreasing damage in a subarachnoid bleed
   f. Preventing thromboembolic strokes

4. Evaluating a client who is taking an anticoagulant for blood loss would usually include assessing for which of the following?
   a. The presence of petechiae
   b. Bleeding gums while brushing the teeth
   c. Dark-coloured urine
   d. Yellow colour to the sclera or skin
   e. The presence of ecchymotic areas
   f. Loss of hair

True or False

Indicate whether the following statements are true (T) or false (F).

_____ 1. Coagulation is the transformation of fluid blood to a solid state.

_____ 2. Coagulation involves vasodilation, platelet aggregation and intrinsic and extrinsic clot formation.

_____ 3. Coagulation is initiated by factor XII (Hageman factor) to plug up any holes in the cardiovascular system.

_____ 4. The final step of clot formation is the conversion of prothrombin to thrombin, which breaks down fibrinogen to form soluble fibrin threads.

_____ 5. Once a clot is formed, it must be dissolved to prevent the occlusion of blood vessels and loss of blood supply to tissues.

_____ 6. Plasminogen is the basis of the coagulation system.

_____ 7. Plasmin dissolves fibrin threads and resolves the clot.

_____ 8. Anticoagulants dissolve clots that have formed.

_____ 9. Thrombolytic drugs block coagulation and prevent the formation of clots.

_____ 10. Haemophilia is a genetic lack of essential clotting factors that results in excessive bleeding situations.

Bibliography

British Medical Association and Royal Pharmaceutical Society of Great Britain. (2008). *British National Formulary*. London: BMJ & RPS Publishing. *This publication is updated biannually: it is imperative that the most recent edition is consulted.*

British Medical Association and Royal Pharmaceutical Society of Great Britain. (2008). *British National Formulary for Children*. London: BMJ & RPS Publishing. *This publication is updated annually: it is imperative that the most recent edition is consulted.*

Ganong, W. (2005). *Review of medical physiology* (22nd ed.). New York: McGraw-Hill.

Howland, R. D., & Mycek, M. J. (2005). *Pharmacology* (3rd ed.). Philadelphia: Lippincott Williams & Wilkins.

Marieb, E. N., & Hoehn, K. (2004). *Human anatomy & physiology* (7th ed.). San Francisco: Pearson Benjamin Cummings.

Porth, C. M., & Matfin, G. (2008). *Pathophysiology: Concepts of altered health states* (8th ed.). Philadelphia: Lippincott Williams & Wilkins.

Simonsen, T., Aarbakke, J., Kay, I., Coleman, I., Sinnott, P., & Lysaa, R. (2006). *Illustrated pharmacology for nurses.* London: Hodder Arnold.

CHAPTER 48

Drugs Used to Treat Anaemias

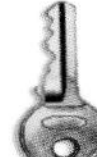

KEY TERMS

anaemia
erythrocytes
erythropoiesis
erythropoietin
intrinsic factor
iron deficiency anaemia
leucocytes
megaloblastic anaemia
pernicious anaemia
plasma
platelets
reticulocyte

LEARNING OBJECTIVES

Upon completion of this chapter, you will be able to:

1. Explain the process of erythropoiesis and use this information to discuss the development of three types of anaemias.
2. Describe the therapeutic actions, indications, pharmacokinetics and contraindications associated with erythropoietic agents, iron preparations, folic acid derivatives and vitamin B_{12}.
3. Describe the most common adverse reactions and important drug–drug interactions associated with erythropoietic agents, iron preparations, folic acid derivatives and vitamin B_{12}.
4. Discuss the use of drugs used to treat anaemias across the lifespan.
5. Compare and contrast the key drugs epoetin alfa, ferrous sulphate, folic acid and hydroxocobalamin with other agents in their class.
6. Outline the nursing considerations, including important teaching points, for patients receiving drugs used to treat anaemias.

ERYTHROPOIETIN

darbepoetin alfa
epoetin alfa

IRON PREPARATIONS

ferrous fumarate
ferrous gluconate
ferrous sulphate
iron dextran
iron sucrose

FOLIC ACID DERIVATIVES

folic acid
leucovorin

VITAMIN B_{12}

cyanocobalamin
hydroxocobalamin

The cardiovascular system exists to pump blood to all of the body's cells. Blood is essential for cell survival because it carries oxygen and nutrients and removes waste products that could be toxic to the tissues. It also contains clotting factors that help maintain the vascular system and keep it sealed. In addition, blood contains the important components of the immune system that protect the body from infection. This chapter discusses drugs that are used to treat anaemias. Anaemias are disorders where there are too few red blood cells (RBCs) or ineffective RBCs that can reduce the oxygen-carrying capacity of the blood. Galbraith *et al.* (1997) explain that anaemias result from a deficiency of normal functioning erythrocytes either due to structural abnormalities or low numbers of circulating RBCs. As a consequence, the oxygen-carrying capacity of the blood is diminished, and the function of body tissues may become compromised.

Blood Components

Blood is composed of liquid and formed elements. The liquid part of blood is called **plasma**. Plasma is mostly water, but it also contains proteins that are essential for the immune response and blood clotting. The formed elements of the blood include **leucocytes** (white blood cells), which are an important part of the immune system (see Chapter 14); **erythrocytes** (RBCs), which carry oxygen to the tissues and remove carbon dioxide for delivery to the lungs and **platelets**, which play an important role in coagulation (see Chapter 47).

Erythropoiesis

Erythropoiesis is the process of RBC production. RBCs are produced in the myeloid tissue of the bone marrow. The rate of RBC production is controlled by the hormone **erythropoietin** (EPO), which is released from the kidneys in response to low oxygen levels in the blood. Under the influence of EPO, an undifferentiated cell in the bone marrow becomes a haemocytoblast. This cell requires certain amino acids, lipids, carbohydrates, vitamin B_{12}, folic acid and iron to develop into an immature RBC. In the last phase of RBC production, the cell loses its nucleus and enters the circulation. This cell, called a **reticulocyte**, finishes its maturing process in the circulation (Figure 48.1).

As the mature RBC has no nucleus, it has a vast surface area to improve its ability to transport oxygen and carbon dioxide. The RBC cannot reproduce or maintain itself because it lacks a nucleus, so it will eventually wear out. The average lifespan of a RBC is about 120 days. The ageing or damaged RBC is lysed in the liver, spleen or bone marrow. The building blocks of the RBC (e.g. iron, vitamin B_{12}) are then recycled and returned to the bone marrow for the production of new RBCs (see Figure 48.1). The only part of the RBC that cannot be recycled is the toxic pigment bilirubin, which is conjugated in the liver, passed into the bile and excreted from the body in the faeces or urine. Bilirubin is what gives colour to both of these excretions. Erythropoiesis is a constant process, wherein about 1% of the body's RBCs are destroyed and replaced each day.

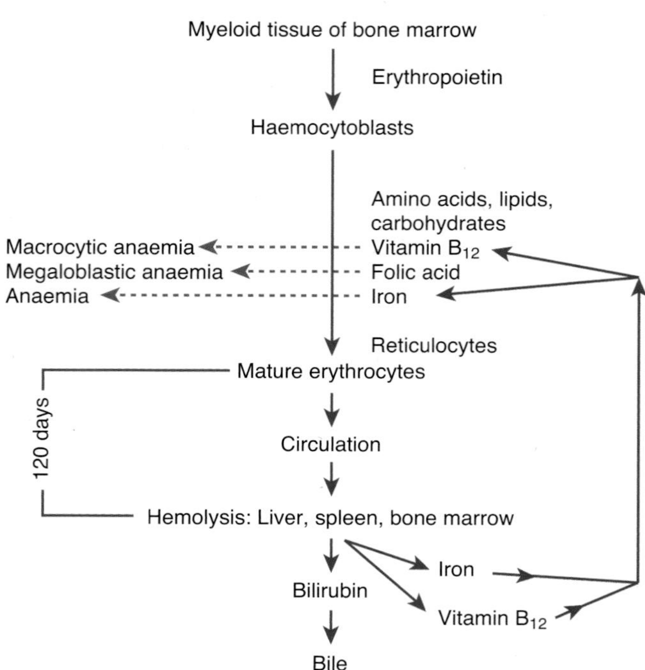

FIGURE 48.1 Erythropoiesis. Red blood cells are produced in the myeloid tissue of the bone marrow in response to the hormone erythropoietin. The hemocytoblasts require various essential factors to produce mature erythrocytes. A lack of any one of these can result in an anaemia of the type indicated opposite each factor. Mature erythrocytes survive for about 120 days and are then lysed in the liver, spleen, or bone marrow.

Anaemia

Anaemia, caused by a reduction in the number of RBCs (a decrease in the production of RBCs, an increase in the destruction of RBCs or by blood loss) or a reduction in the oxygen-carrying capacity of the blood, can occur if EPO levels are low. This is seen in renal failure, when the kidneys are no longer able to produce EPO. It can also occur if the body does not have enough of the building blocks necessary to form RBCs, for example:

- Adequate amounts of iron, which is used in forming haemoglobin to carry the oxygen;
- Vitamin B_{12} and folic acid to allow the RBCs to mature and form a strong supporting structure that can survive travelling through blood vessels for 120 days;
- Essential amino acids and carbohydrates to complete the haemoglobin rings, cell membrane and basic structure.

Anaemias can be classified by:-

- Erythrocyte morphology or size:
  - small or *microcytic* – iron deficiency anaemia;
  - normal or *normocytic* – splenic anaemia caused by enlargement of the spleen, that is in portal hypertension;
  - large or *macrocytic* due to folate or vitamin B_{12} deficiency.
- Cause:
  - *deficiency* – leading to inadequate erythropoiesis or haemoglobin synthesis caused by a deficiency in nutrition, that is iron, renal atropy or failure;
  - *Haemorrhagic* due to excess bleeding caused by trauma, diseases such as haemophilia;
  - *Haemolytic* due to erythrocyte destruction, malaria, sickle cell disease.

Normally, an individual's diet supplies adequate amounts of all of these substances, which are absorbed from the gastrointestinal (GI) tract and transported to the bone marrow. But when the diet cannot supply enough of a nutrient, or insufficient amounts of the nutrient are absorbed, the person can develop a deficiency anaemia. Fewer RBCs are produced, and the ones that are produced contain less haemoglobin and are therefore not efficient iron carriers. The person with this type of anaemia (an **iron deficiency anaemia**) may complain of being tired because there is insufficient oxygen delivery to the tissues.

Another type of anaemia is **megaloblastic anaemia**; this can also be described as a deficiency anaemia condition in which the RBCs remain large and immature as megaloblasts. There is an increase in these immature cells in circulation. Overall, fewer RBCs are produced, and those that are produced are ineffective and do not usually survive for the 120 days that is normal for the life of an RBC. Patients with megaloblastic anaemia usually have a lack of vitamin B_{12} and/or folate. (See Box 48.1 for information on sickle cell anaemia and Box 48.2 on issues involving different age groups.)

Iron Deficiency Anaemias

All cells in the body require some amount of iron; the daily requirement for iron is approximately 10 to 20 mg/day. But iron can be very toxic to cells, especially neurons. To maintain the required iron levels and avoid toxic levels, the body has developed a system for controlling the amount of iron that can enter the body through intestinal absorption. Only enough iron is absorbed to replace the amount of iron lost each day. Once iron is absorbed, it is carried by a plasma protein called transferrin, a beta-globulin. This protein carries iron to various tissues to be stored, for example, in the bone marrow and transports iron from RBC lysis back to the bone marrow for recycling. The total iron in the blood at any one time is approximately 4 mg (bound to transferrin).

BOX 48.1 CULTURAL CONSIDERATIONS FOR DRUG THERAPY

Sickle Cell Anaemia

Sickle cell anaemia is a chronic haemolytic anaemia which is currently the most common genetic disease in England affecting in the region of 12,500 people. It occurs most commonly in individuals whose families originate from areas where malaria is common (Africa, parts of the Mediterranean, Middle East and India) Haemolytic anaemias involve a losing of RBCs because of genetic factors or from exposure to toxins. Sickle cell anaemia is characterized by a genetically inherited haemoglobin S, which replaces the usual α and β globin chains and gives the RBCs a sickle-shaped appearance. The patient with sickle cell anaemia produces fewer than normal RBCs, and the RBCs produced are unable to carry oxygen efficiently.

The sickle-shaped RBCs can become lodged in tiny blood vessels, where they stack up on one another and occlude the vessel. This occlusion leads to anoxia and infarction of the tissue in that area, which is characterized by severe pain and an acute inflammatory reaction – a condition often called *sickle cell crisis*. The patient may have ulcers on the extremities as a result of such occlusions. Severe, acute episodes of sickling with vessel occlusion may be associated with acute infections and the body's reactions to the immune and inflammatory responses.

In the past, the only treatment for sickle cell anaemia was pain medication and support of the patient. Now *hydroxyurea* has been found to effectively treat this disease. Hydroxyurea is a cytotoxic antineoplastic agent that is used to treat leukaemia, ovarian cancer and melanoma. It has been shown that it increases the amount of foetal haemoglobin produced in the bone marrow and dilutes the formation of the abnormal haemoglobin S in patients with sickle cell anaemia. The process takes several months, but, once effective, it prevents the clogging of small vessels and the painful, anoxic effects of RBC sickling. This drug is associated with several uncomfortable adverse effects including GI problems, rash, headache and possible bone marrow depression; therefore, the decision to use it is not made lightly. However, it has been found to be effective in preventing the painful crises of sickle cell anaemia.

Small amounts of iron are lost each day in sweat, sloughed skin, from GI and urinary tract linings. The body is very efficient at iron recycling and so very little iron is usually needed in the diet and most diets quite adequately replace the lost iron. However, in situations in which blood is being lost, such as internal bleeding or heavy menstrual flow, a negative iron balance might occur and the patient could develop **iron deficiency anaemia**. This can also occur in certain GI diseases in which the patient is unable to absorb iron from the GI tract. These conditions are usually treated with iron replacement therapy.

Elemental iron is available in a variety of forms each containing variable amounts of the essential mineral. The form most efficiently absorbed from the gut is the ferrous ion. Salts of the ferrous ion (ferrous sulphate, gluconate or fumarate) are used as oral supplements. Ferrous sulphate contains more elemental iron than the gluconate form.

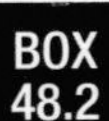

BOX 48.2 DRUG THERAPY ACROSS THE LIFESPAN

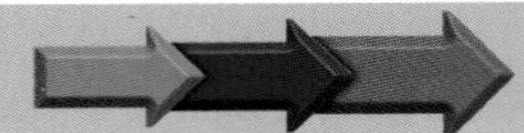

Drugs Used to Treat Anaemia

CHILDREN

Proper nutrition should be established for children to provide the essential elements needed for formation of RBCs. The cause of the anaemia should be determined to avoid prolonged problems.

Iron doses for replacement therapy are determined by age. If a liquid solution is used, the child should drink it through a straw to avoid staining of the teeth. Periodic blood counts should be performed; it may take 4 to 6 months of oral therapy to reverse an iron deficiency. Remember that iron can be toxic to children, and iron supplements should be kept out of their reach and administration monitored.

Maintenance doses for folic acid have been established for children based on age. Nutritional means should be used to establish folic acid levels whenever possible.

Children with pernicious anaemia will require a monthly injection of vitamin B_{12}; the nasal form has not been approved for use with children.

When administering any drug to children, always consult the most recent edition of the British National Formulary for Children.

ADULTS

The underlying cause of the anaemia should be established and appropriate steps taken to reverse the cause if possible. Adults receiving epoetin alfa or darbepoetin alfa should be monitored closely for response for the need for iron or other RBC building blocks and for the possibility of development of pure red cell aplasia.

Adults receiving iron replacement may experience GI upset and frequently experience constipation. Appropriate measures to maintain bowel function may be needed.

Adults also need to know that periodic blood tests will be needed to evaluate response.

Proper nutrition during pregnancy and lactation is often not adequate to meet the increased demands of those states. Prenatal vitamins contain iron and folic acid and are usually prescribed for pregnant women to prevent anaemia and neural tube defects. Use of epoetin alfa or darbepoetin alfa is not recommended during pregnancy or lactation because of the potential for adverse effects on the foetus or baby. Iron replacement is frequently needed postpartum to provide the iron lost during delivery.

Women maintained on vitamin B_{12} before pregnancy should continue the treatment during pregnancy. Increased doses may be needed due to changes associated with the pregnancy.

OLDER ADULTS

Older adults may have nutritional problems related to age and may lose more iron through cellular sloughing. Older adults should be assessed for anaemia, and possible causes should be evaluated.

Replacement therapy in the older adult can cause the same adverse effects as are seen in the younger person. Bowel training programmes, high-fibre diet and laxatives may be needed to prevent severe constipation.

Use of nasal vitamin B_{12} may not be practical. If the patient desires to use this administration technique, nasal mucous membranes should be evaluated before and periodically during treatment.

Also, supplements containing combinations of iron and folic acid are indicated for the prevention and treatment of nutritional anaemias in pregnancy. Combined supplements containing a number of vitamins (vitamin E and vitamins from the B group) involved in erythrocyte production are also available. Some preparations contain iron, others do not (Galbraith *et al.,* 1997).

Megaloblastic Anaemias

Megaloblastic anaemias occur when there is insufficient folic acid or vitamin B_{12} to adequately create the stromal structure needed in a healthy RBC. The lack of these two compounds causes impaired nuclear DNA synthesis in human cells. This effect is seen in other rapidly dividing cells, not just bone marrow cells. For example, cells in the GI tract are often affected, resulting in the appearance of a characteristic red and glossy tongue and diarrhoea.

Folic Acid Deficiency

Folic acid is essential for cell division in all types of tissue. Deficiencies in folic acid are noticed first in rapidly growing cells, such as those in cancerous tissues, in the GI tract and in the bone marrow. Most people can get all the folic acid they need from their diet. For example, folic acid is found in green leafy vegetables, milk, eggs and liver. Deficiency in folic acid may occur in certain malabsorption states, such as coeliac disease. Malnutrition that accompanies alcoholism is also a common cause of folic acid deficiency. Repeated pregnancies and extended treatment with certain antiepileptic medications can also contribute to folic acid deficiency. This disorder is treated by the administration of folic acid or folate.

Vitamin B_{12} Deficiency

Vitamin B_{12} is used in minute amounts by the body, and it is stored for use if dietary intake falls. It is necessary for the health of the RBCs and for the normal functioning of the brain and the nervous system. It is found in the diet in meats, seafood, eggs and cheese. Strict vegetarians who eat nothing but vegetables may develop a vitamin B_{12} deficiency. Such individuals with a dietary insufficiency of vitamin B_{12} typically respond to vitamin B_{12} replacement therapy to reverse their anaemia.

The most common cause of this deficiency is the inability of the GI tract to absorb the required amounts of the vitamin. Gastric parietal cells produce a substance called **intrinsic factor**, which is necessary for the absorption of vitamin B_{12} by the small intestine.

Pernicious anaemia occurs when the gastric mucosa cannot produce intrinsic factor and so vitamin B_{12} cannot be absorbed. The person with pernicious anaemia will complain of fatigue and lethargy and central nervous system (CNS) effects. Patients may complain of numbness, tingling and eventually lack of coordination and motor activity. Pernicious anaemia was once a fatal disease, but it is now treated with injections of vitamin B_{12} to replace the amount that can no longer be absorbed. In pernicious anaemia, the area of the stomach which produces intrinsic factor is either severely damaged or has been surgically removed. Therefore, for these individuals, vitamin B_{12} supplementation must be via a parenteral route (Galbraith *et al.,* 1997).

Erythropoietins

Patients who are no longer able to produce enough EPO in the kidneys may benefit from treatment with EPO, which is available as the drugs epoetin alfa and darbepoetin alfa. Epoetin alfa is used to treat anaemia associated with renal failure, including patients on dialysis. It is also used to decrease the need for blood transfusions in patients undergoing surgery and to treat anaemias related to treatment for AIDS.

It is not approved to treat severe anaemia associated with other causes, and it is not meant to replace whole blood for emergency treatment of anaemia. There is a risk of decreasing the normal levels of EPO if this drug is given to patients who have normal renal functioning and adequate levels of EPO. A negative feedback occurs with the renal cells, and less endogenous EPO is produced if exogenous EPO is given. Administration of this drug to an anaemic patient with normal renal function can actually cause a more severe anaemia if the endogenous levels fall and no longer stimulate RBC production (Figure 48.2).

Darbepoetin alfa is an EPO-like protein produced with the use of recombinant DNA technology. It is used to treat anaemia associated with chronic renal failure, including patients on dialysis and to treat cancer chemotherapy-induced anaemia. It has the advantage of once-weekly administration, compared with two to three times a week, as with epoetin alfa. This drug gained negative publicity after it was used by athletes to increase their RBC count in the hope that it would give them more endurance and strength. Many athletic groups now screen for the presence of darbepoetin among other banned drugs.

Therapeutic Actions and Indications

Epoetin alfa acts like the natural hormone EPO to stimulate the production of RBCs in the bone marrow (Figure 48.3). It is indicated in the treatment of anaemia associated with renal failure and for patients on dialysis. It is also used to decrease the need for blood transfusions in patients under-

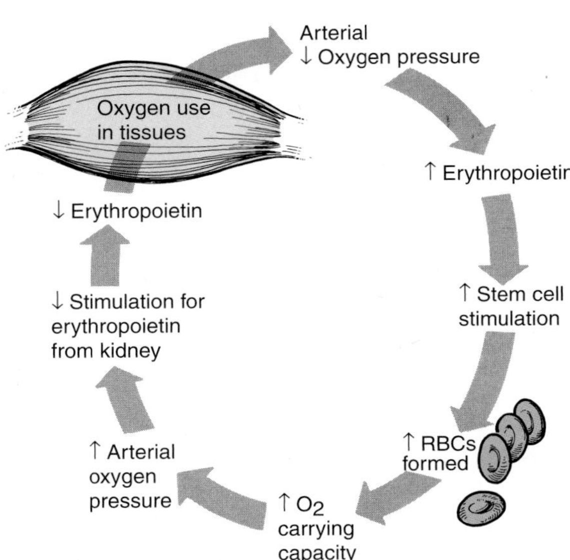

FIGURE 48.2 Erythropoiesis controls the rate of blood cell production.

going surgery for the treatment of anaemia associated with AIDS therapy and for the treatment of anaemia associated with cancer chemotherapy. Darbepoetin alfa is indicated only for the treatment of anaemia associated with chronic renal failure and for anaemia induced by cancer chemotherapy.

Pharmacokinetics

Epoetin alfa is metabolized through the normal kinetic processes with a half-life of 4 to 13 hours. Darbepoetin alfa has a half-life of 21 hours after intravenous administration or 48 hours after subcutaneous administration. There are no adequate studies in pregnancy, so use should be limited to those situations in which the benefit to the mother clearly outweighs the potential risk to the foetus. It is not known whether epoetin alfa enters into breast milk, whereas darbepoetin alfa is known to enter breast milk. Caution should be used if this drug is needed by breast-feeding women.

Contraindications and Cautions

Epoetin alfa and darbepoetin alfa are contraindicated in the presence of uncontrolled hypertension, *because of the risk of even further hypertension when RBC numbers increase and the pressure within the vascular system increases;* with allergy to mammalian cell-derived products or to human albumin; and with lactation, *because of the potential for allergic-type reactions with the neonate.*

Adverse Effects

The adverse effects most commonly associated with these drugs include the CNS effects of headache, fatigue, asthenia

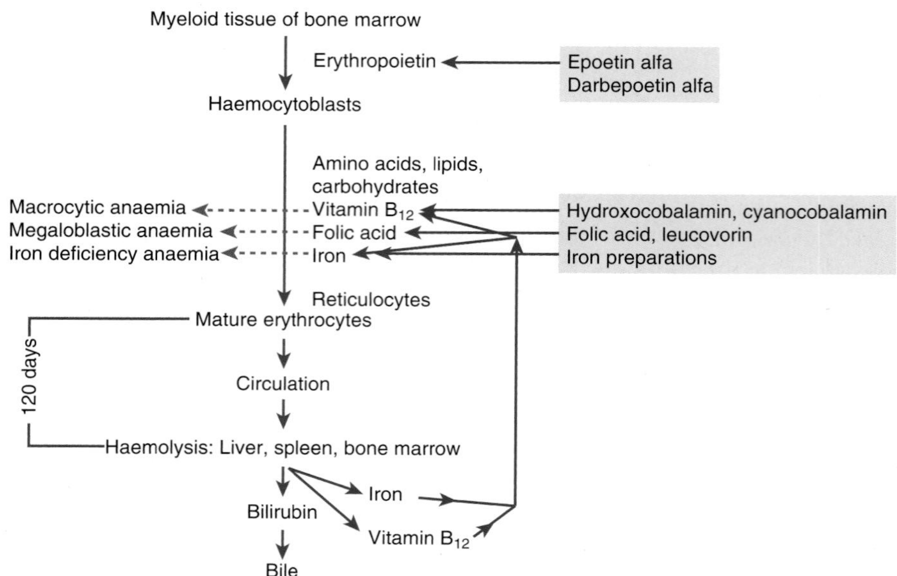

FIGURE 48.3 Sites of action of drugs used to treat anaemia.

and dizziness and the potential for serious seizures. These effects may be the result of a cellular response to the glycoprotein. Nausea, vomiting and diarrhoea are also common effects. Cardiovascular symptoms can include hypertension, oedema and possible chest pain and may be related to the increase in RBC numbers changing the balance within the cardiovascular system. Patients receiving intravenous administration must also be monitored for possible clotting of the access line related to direct cellular effects of the drug.

FOCUS ON PATIENT SAFETY

Cases of pure red cell aplasia and severe anaemias, with or without cytopenias, had been reported by users of epoetin and darbepoetin alfa. These cases were associated with the development of neutralizing antibodies to EPO. Use of any therapeutic protein brings with it the risk of antibody production. All of the erythropoietic proteins will now carry a warning about the potential for this problem. If a patient is treated with one of these drugs and develops a sudden loss of response, accompanied by severe anaemia and low reticulocyte count, the patient should be assessed for the possible causes. Assays for binding and neutralizing antibodies should be done. If an antibody-mediated anaemia is confirmed, the drug should be permanently stopped and the patient should not be switched to another erythropoietic protein because cross-reaction could occur. Most of the patients in the reported cases had chronic renal failure and were being treated with subcutaneous injections. It is now recommended that patients on haemodialysis receive the drug intravenously and not subcutaneously. If the drug is started and there is no response or if a patient fails to maintain a response, the dosage should not be increased and RBC aplasia should be suspected. The patient should be evaluated with the appropriate tests and supported.

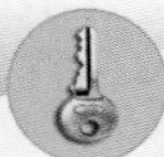

Key Drug Summary: Epoetin Alfa

Indications: Treatment of anaemia associated with chronic renal failure, related to treatment of HIV infection or to chemotherapy in cancer patients, to reduce the need for allogenic blood transfusions in surgical patients

Actions: Natural glycoprotein that stimulates RBC production in the bone marrow

Pharmacokinetics:

Route	Onset	Peak	Duration
Sub-cut	7–14 days	5–24 h	24 h

$T_{1/2}$: 4–13 hours; metabolized in serum and excreted in urine

Adverse effects: Headache, fatigue, asthenia, dizziness, hypertension, oedema, chest pain, nausea, vomiting, diarrhoea

Nursing Considerations for Patients Receiving Erythropoietin

Assessment: History and Examination

Screen for the following conditions, *which could be cautions or contraindications to use of the drug:* any known allergies to this drug, to mammalian cell-derived products or to human albumin; severe hypertension, *which could be exacerbated* and lactation, *because of potential adverse effects on the neonate.*

Include screening *for baseline status before beginning therapy and for any potential adverse effects.* Assess the following: affect, orientation and reflexes; pulse, blood pressure and perfusion; respirations and adventitious breath sounds; and renal function tests, full blood count (FBC), haematocrit, iron levels and electrolytes.

Establish if patient is currently taking other medications or herbal therapies which may potentially interact with the EPO.

Nursing Diagnoses

The patient receiving EPO may have the following nursing diagnoses related to drug therapy:

- Nausea, diarrhoea related to GI effects
- Risk for injury related to CNS effects, for example weakness, dizziness, syncope
- Risk for imbalanced fluid volume related to cardiovascular effects
- Deficient knowledge regarding drug therapy
- Ineffective tissue perfusion, related to ineffective response to drug (Adams *et al.,* 2005)
- Activity intolerance, related to RBC deficiency

Implementation With Rationale

- Confirm the chronic, renal nature of the patient's anaemia before administering the drug *to ensure proper use of the drug.*
- Do not mix with any other drug solution *to avoid potential incompatibilities.*
- Monitor access lines for clotting and *arrange to clear line as needed.*
- *Monitor vital signs especially blood pressure. (The rate of hypertension is directly related to the rate of rise of the haematocrit. Patients who have existing hypertension are at higher risk for stroke and seizures. Hypertension is also much more likely in patients with chronic renal failure.)*
- Arrange for haematocrit reading before drug administration *to determine correct dosage.* If the patient does not respond within 8 weeks, re-evaluate the cause of anaemia.
- Evaluate iron stores before and periodically during therapy *because supplemental iron may be needed as the patient makes more RBCs.*
- *Monitor for side-effects, especially symptoms of neurological or cardiovascular events.*
- Maintain seizure precautions on standby *in case seizures occur as a reaction to the drug.*
- Provide comfort measures *to help the patient tolerate the drug effects.*
- Provide thorough patient education, including the name of the drug, dosage prescribed, measures to avoid adverse effects, warning signs of problems and the need for periodic monitoring and evaluation, *to enhance patient knowledge about drug therapy and to promote compliance with the drug regimen.*
- Offer support and encouragement *to help the patient deal with the diagnosis and the drug regimen.*
- Monitor patient for signs of thrombus such as swelling, warmth and pain in an extremity *[as haematocrit rises, there is an increased chance of thrombus formation particularly for patients with chronic renal failure (Adams et al., 2005)].*

Evaluation

- Monitor dietary intake. Ensure adequate intake of all essential nutrients. Response to this medication is minimal if blood levels of iron, folic acid and vitamin B12 are deficient.
- Monitor patient response to the drug (alleviation of anaemia).
- Monitor for adverse effects (headache, hypertension, nausea, vomiting, seizures, dizziness).
- Evaluate the effectiveness of the teaching plan (patient can name drug, dosage, adverse effects to watch for, specific measures to avoid adverse effects; patient understands importance of continued follow-up).
- Monitor the effectiveness of comfort measures and compliance to the regimen.

Iron Preparations

Although most people get all the iron they need through diet, in some situations, diet alone may not be adequate. Iron deficiency anaemia is a relatively common problem in certain groups including the following:

- Menstruating women, who lose RBCs monthly;
- Pregnant and nursing women, who have increased demands for iron;
- Rapidly growing adolescents, especially those who do not have a nutritious diet;
- Persons with GI bleeding, including individuals with slow bleeding associated with use of nonsteroidal anti-inflammatory drugs (NSAIDs).

Oral iron preparations are often used to help these patients regain a positive iron balance; these preparations need to be supplemented with adequate dietary intake of iron. Ferrous fumarate, ferrous gluconate and ferrous sulphate are the oral iron preparations that are available for use. Most of the drug that is taken is lost in the faeces, but slowly some of the metal is absorbed into the intestine and transported to the bone marrow. It can take 2 to 3 weeks to see improvement and up to 6 to 10 months to return to a stable iron level once a deficiency exists or an alternative treatment must be continued for 4 to 6 months to replenish iron stores.

Iron dextran is a parenteral form of iron that may be used if the oral form cannot be given or cannot be tolerated. Patients with severe GI absorption problems may require this form of iron. If given intramuscularly, it must be given by the Z-track method, because it can stain the tissues brown and can be very painful (see Box 48.3). Patients should be switched to the oral form if at all possible. Severe hypersensitivity reactions have been associated with the parenteral form of iron. Iron sucrose is given intravenously, specifically for patients who are undergoing chronic haemodialysis or who are in renal failure but not on dialysis and who are also receiving supplemental EPO therapy.

Therapeutic Actions and Indications

Iron preparations elevate the serum iron concentration (see Figure 48.3). They are then either converted to haemoglobin or trapped in reticuloendothelial cells for storage and eventual release and conversion into a useable form of iron for RBC production. They are indicated for the treatment of iron deficiency anaemias and may also be used as adjunctive therapy in patients receiving epoetin alfa.

Pharmacokinetics

Iron is primarily absorbed from the small intestine by an active transport system. It is transported in the blood (bound to transferrin) to storage compartments and the bone marrow. Small amounts are lost daily in the sweat, urine, sloughing of skin and mucosal cells and sloughing of intestinal cells, faeces, as well as in the menstrual flow of women.

Contraindications and Cautions

These drugs are contraindicated for patients with known allergy to any of these preparations. They are also contraindicated in the following conditions: haemochromatosis (excessive iron); haemolytic anaemias, *which may increase serum iron levels and cause toxicity;* normal iron balance, *because the drug will not be absorbed and will just pass through the body* and peptic ulcer, colitis or regional enteritis, *because the drug can be directly irritating to these tissues and can cause exacerbation of the diseases.*

Adverse Effects

The most common adverse effects associated with oral iron are related to direct GI irritation; these include GI upset, anorexia, nausea, vomiting, diarrhoea, dark stools and constipation. With increasing serum levels, iron can be directly CNS toxic, causing coma and even death. (Box 48.4 discusses iron toxicity and drugs that are used to counteract this effect.) Parenteral iron is associated with severe anaphylactic reactions, local irritation, staining of the tissues and phlebitis.

Clinically Important Drug–Drug Interactions

Iron absorption decreases if iron preparations are taken with antacids, tetracyclines or cimetidine; if these drugs must be used, they should be spaced at least 2 hours apart.

Anti-infective response to ciprofloxacin, norfloxacin or ofloxacin can decrease if these drugs are taken with iron, because of a decrease in absorption; they also should be taken at least 2 hours apart.

Increased iron levels occur if iron preparations are taken with chloramphenicol; patients receiving this combination should be monitored closely for any sign of iron toxicity. The effects of levodopa may decrease if it is taken with iron preparations; patients receiving both of these drugs should take them at least 2 hours apart.

Always consult a current copy of the British National Formulary for further guidance.

BOX 48.3 FOCUS ON **CLINICAL SKILLS**

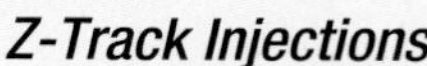

Z-Track Injections

The Z-track or zigzag method is used when injecting iron to reduce the risk of subcutaneous staining and irritation. It is a good idea to review the method of giving Z-track injections before giving one. The area to be injected is prepped for the injection. Place your gloved finger on the skin surface and pull the skin and the subcutaneous layers out of alignment with the muscle lying beneath. Try to move the skin about 1 cm. Insert the needle at a 90-degree angle at the point where you originally placed your finger. Inject the drug and then withdraw the needle. Remove your finger from the skin, which will allow the layers to slide back into their normal position. The track that the needle made when inserting into the muscle is now broken by the layers, and the drug is trapped in the muscle.

Use the Z-track technique for injections: **(A)** Normal skin and tissues. **(B)** Move the skin to one side. **(C)** Insert needle at a 90-degree angle and aspirate for blood. **(D)** Withdraw the needle and allow the displaced tissue to return to normal position, thereby keeping the solution from leaving the muscle tissue [with permission from Taylor, C., Lillis, C., & LeMone, P. (2005). *Fundamentals of nursing: The art and science of nursing care.* 5th ed. Philadelphia: Lippincott Williams & Wilkins].

BOX 48.4

Chelating Agents

Heavy metals, including iron, lead, arsenic, mercury, copper and gold, can cause toxicity in the body by their ability to tie up chemicals in living tissues that need to be free in order for the cell to function normally. When these vital substances (thiols, sulphurs, carboxyls and phosphoryls) are bound to the metal, certain cellular enzyme systems become deactivated, resulting in failure of cellular function and eventual cell death. Drugs that have been developed to counteract metal toxicity are called chelating agents.

Chelating agents grasp and hold a toxic metal so that it can be carried out of the body before it has time to harm the tissues. The chelating agent binds the molecules of the metal, preventing it from damaging the cells within the body. The complex that is formed by the chelating agent and the metal is nontoxic and is excreted by the kidneys.

Clinically Important Drug–Food Interactions

Iron is not absorbed if taken with antacids, eggs, milk, coffee or tea. These substances should not be administered concurrently.

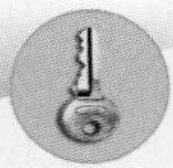

Key Drug Summary: *Ferrous Sulphate*

Indications: Prevention and treatment of iron deficiency anaemia, dietary supplement for iron

Actions: Elevates the serum iron concentration and is then converted to haemoglobin or stored for eventual conversion to a usable form of iron

Pharmacokinetics:

Route	Onset	Peak	Duration
Oral	4 days	7–10 days	2–4 months

$T_{1/2}$: Not known; recycled for use, not excreted

Adverse effects: GI upset, anorexia, nausea, vomiting, constipation, diarrhoea, CNS toxicity progressing to coma and death with overdose

Nursing Considerations for Patients Receiving Iron Preparations

Assessment: History and Examination

Screen for the following conditions, *which could be cautions or contraindications to use of the drug:* any known allergies to this drug, hyperchromatosis, colitis, enteritis, peptic ulcer and haemolytic anaemias.

Include screening *for baseline status before beginning therapy and for any potential adverse effects.* Assess the following: skin colour, gums and teeth; orientation and reflexes; pulse, blood pressure and perfusion; respirations and adventitious sounds; bowel sounds; and FBC, haematocrit, haemoglobin and serum ferritin assays.

Establish if patient is currently taking other medications or herbal therapies which may potentially interact with the iron preparations.

Nursing Diagnoses

The patient receiving iron may have the following nursing diagnoses related to drug therapy:

- Acute pain related to CNS or GI effects
- Risk for imbalanced nutrition, related to inadequate iron intake.
- Risk for impaired gas exchange, related to low RBC count resulting in decreased oxygenation.
- Disturbed body image related to drug staining
- Risk for injury related to CNS effects (weakness, dizziness, syncope)
- Deficient knowledge regarding drug therapy

Implementation With Rationale

- Confirm iron deficiency anaemia before administering drugs *to ensure proper use of the drug.*
- Consult with the doctor/clinician to arrange for investigation and treatment of the underlying cause of anaemia, if possible, *because iron replacement will not correct the cause of the iron loss.*
- Monitor vital signs especially pulse. *(Increased pulse is an indicator of decreased oxygen content in the blood.)*
- Monitor complete blood count *to evaluate effectiveness of treatment.*
- Administer with meals (avoiding eggs, milk, coffee and tea) *to reduce the risk of GI irritation.* Have patient (especially with children) drink solutions through a straw *to prevent staining of teeth.*
- Caution advise the patient that stool may become dark or green because of the iron supplements.
- Administer intramuscularly only by Z-track technique *to ensure proper administration and to avoid staining. Advise patient to report any pain or discomfort.*
- Arrange for haematocrit and haemoglobin measurements before administration and periodically during therapy *to monitor drug effectiveness.*

- Provide comfort measures *to help the patient tolerate drug effects.* These may include small, frequent meals.
- Provide thorough patient education about the purpose and actions of the drug, including the name of the drug, dosage prescribed, measures to avoid adverse effects, warning signs of problems and the need for periodic monitoring and evaluation, *to enhance patient knowledge about drug therapy and to promote compliance with drug regimen* (see Critical Thinking Scenario 48-1).
- Offer support and encouragement *to help the patient deal with the diagnosis and the drug regimen.*

Evaluation

- Monitor patient response to the drug (alleviation of anaemia).
- Advise patient to report adverse effects GI upset and reaction and monitor for signs of CNS toxicity.
- Evaluate the effectiveness of the teaching plan (patient can name drug, dosage, adverse effects to watch for, specific measures to avoid adverse effects; patient understands importance of continued follow-up).
- Monitor the effectiveness of comfort measures and compliance to the regimen.

Folic Acid Derivatives and Vitamin B_{12}

Megaloblastic anaemia is treated with folic acid and/or vitamin B_{12}. Folate deficiency usually occurs secondary to increased demand (as in pregnancy or growth spurts), as a result of absorption problems in the small intestine, because of drugs that cause folate deficiencies or secondary to the malnutrition of alcoholism. Vitamin B_{12} deficiencies can result from poor diet or increased demand, but the usual cause is lack of intrinsic factor in the stomach, which is necessary for absorption. The drugs are usually given together to ensure that the problem is addressed, and the blood cells can be formed properly.

Folic acid can be given in oral or parenteral form. The parenteral form is restricted to patients with potential absorption problems; all other patients should be given the oral form. Leucovorin is a reduced form of folic acid that is available for oral, intramuscular and intravenous use. (It is used for the 'leucovorin rescue' of patients receiving high doses of methotrexate for osteocarcinoma, allowing noncancerous cells to survive the chemotherapy. It is also used with fluorouracil for palliative treatment of colorectal cancer; see Chapter 13.)

Hydroxocobalamin is the traditional treatment for pernicious anaemia and vitamin B_{12} deficiency. It must be given intramuscularly at regular intervals. It cannot be taken orally, because the problem with pernicious anaemia is the inability to absorb vitamin B_{12} secondary to low levels of intrinsic factor. It can be used in states of increased demand (e.g. pregnancy, growth spurts), or dietary deficiency, but oral vitamins are preferred in most of those cases. Cyanocobalamin is not as tightly bound to proteins and does not last in the body as long as hydroxocobalamin.

Therapeutic Actions and Indications

Folic acid and vitamin B_{12} are essential for cell growth and division and for the production of a strong stroma in RBCs (see Figure 48.3). Vitamin B_{12} is also necessary for maintenance of the myelin sheath in nerve tissue. Both are given as replacement therapy for dietary deficiencies, as replacement in high-demand states such as pregnancy and lactation and to treat megaloblastic anaemia. Folic acid is used as a rescue drug for cells exposed to some toxic chemotherapeutic agents.

Pharmacokinetics

These vitamins are well absorbed after injection, metabolized mainly in the liver and excreted in urine. Much of the hydroxocobalamin is highly protein bound and slowly released for use in the body. Cyanocobalamin is primarily stored in the liver and slowly released as needed for metabolic functions. These vitamins are considered essential during pregnancy and lactation because of the increased demands of the mother's metabolism.

Contraindications and Cautions

These drugs are contraindicated in the presence of known allergies to these drugs or to their components. They should be used cautiously in patients who are pregnant or lactating or who have other anaemias.

Adverse Effects

These drugs have relatively few adverse effects because they are used as replacement for required chemicals. Pain and discomfort can occur at injection sites.

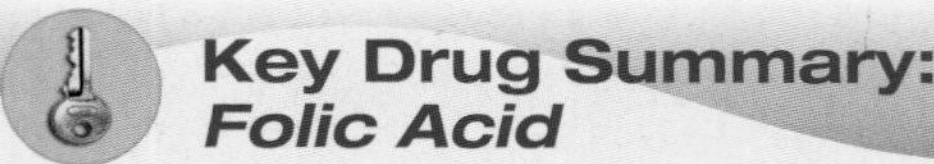

Indications: Treatment of megaloblastic anaemia due to coeliac disease, nutritional deficiency or pregnancy. Folic acid should not be used for undiagnosed megaloblastic anaemia unless prescribed with a vitamin B_{12} supplement.

Actions: Reduced form of folic acid, required for nucleoprotein synthesis and maintenance of normal erythropoiesis

Pharmacokinetics:

Route	Onset	Peak
Oral, IM, sub-cut, IV	Varies	30–60 min

$T_{1/2}$: Unknown; metabolized in the liver and excreted in urine

Adverse effects: Allergic reactions, pain and discomfort at injection site

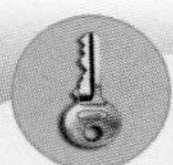

Key Drug Summary: *Hydroxocobalamin*

Indications: Treatment of vitamin B_{12} deficiency; to meet increased vitamin B_{12} requirements related to disease, pregnancy or blood loss

Actions: Essential for nucleic acid and protein synthesis; used for growth, cell reproduction, haematopoiesis and nucleoprotein and myelin synthesis

Pharmacokinetics:

Route	Onset	Peak
Oral, IM, sub-cut, IV	Intermediate	60 min

$T_{1/2}$: 24–36 hours; metabolized in the liver and excreted in urine

Adverse effects: Itching, transitory exanthema, mild diarrhoea, anaphylactic reaction, congestive heart failure, pulmonary oedema, hypokalaemia, pain at injection site

Nursing Considerations for Patients Receiving Folic Acid Derivatives or Vitamin B_{12}

Assessment: History and Examination

Screen for the following conditions, *which could be cautions or contraindications to use of the drug:* any known allergies to these drugs or drug components, other anaemias, pregnancy and lactation.

Include screening *for baseline status before beginning therapy and for any potential adverse effects.* Assess the following: affect, orientation and reflexes; pulse, blood pressure and perfusion; respirations and adventitious sounds; and renal function tests, FBC, haematocrit, iron levels and electrolytes.

Establish if patient is currently taking other medications or herbal therapies which may potentially interact with the folic acid derivatives or vitamin B_{12}.

Nursing Diagnoses

The patient receiving folic acid/vitamin B_{12} may have the following nursing diagnoses related to drug therapy:

- Acute pain related to injection
- Risk for fluid volume imbalance related to cardiovascular effects
- Deficient knowledge regarding drug therapy

Implementation With Rationale

- Confirm the nature of the megaloblastic anaemia *to ensure that the proper drug regimen is being used.*
- Give both types of drugs in cases of pernicious anaemia *to ensure therapeutic effectiveness.*
- Monitor vital signs *(altered potassium levels and overexertion may produce cardiovascular complications, especially irregular rhythm).*
- Monitor potassium levels during first 48 hours of therapy. *(Conversion to normal RBC production increases the need for potassium).*
- Parenteral vitamin B_{12} must be given intramuscularly three times a week days and then once every 3 months *if used to treat pernicious anaemia.*
- Arrange for dietician consultation *to ensure a well-balanced diet.*
- Monitor for the possibility of hypersensitivity reactions, *have life-support equipment on standby in case reactions occur.*
- Arrange for haematocrit readings before and periodically during therapy *to monitor drug effectiveness.*
- Provide comfort measures *to help the patient tolerate drug effects.* These include small, frequent meals, access to bathroom facilities and analgesia for muscle pain.
- Provide thorough patient education, including the name of the drug, dosage prescribed, measures to avoid adverse effects, warning signs of problems and the need for periodic monitoring and evaluation, *to enhance patient knowledge about drug therapy and to promote compliance with the drug regimen.*
- Offer support and encouragement *to help the patient deal with the diagnosis and the drug regimen.*

Evaluation

- Monitor patient response to the drug (alleviation of anaemia).
- Monitor for adverse effects (pain at injection site, nausea).
- Evaluate the effectiveness of the teaching plan (patient can name drug, dosage, adverse effects to watch for, specific measures to avoid adverse effects; patient understands importance of continued follow-up).
- Monitor the effectiveness of comfort measures and compliance to the regimen.

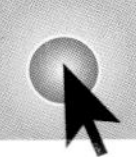

WEB LINKS

Health care providers and patients may want to consult the following Internet sources:

http://cks.library.nhs.uk The National Health Service Clinical Knowledge Summaries provide evidence-based practical information on the common conditions observed in primary care.

http://www.anaemia.com Information designed for patients and families regarding anaemias.

http://www.aplastic.org Information on various forms of anaemias: causes, characteristics, diagnosis and treatment.

http://www.bnf.org.uk The BNF provides UK health care professionals with authoritative and practical information on the selection and clinical use of medicines.

http://www.nhsdirect.nhs.uk The National Health Service Direct service provides patients with information and advice about health, illness and health services.

http://www.nice.org.uk The National Institute for Health and Clinical Excellence (NICE) is an independent organiZation responsible for providing national guidance on promoting good health and preventing and treating ill health.

Points to Remember

- The cardiovascular system exists to pump blood to all of the body's cells.
- Blood contains oxygen and nutrients that are essential for cell survival; it delivers these to the cells and removes waste products from the tissues.
- Blood is composed of liquid plasma (containing water, proteins, glucose and electrolytes) and formed components including white blood cells, RBCs and platelets.
- RBCs are produced in the bone marrow in a process called erythropoiesis, which is controlled by the hormone EPO, produced by the kidneys.
- RBCs do not have a nucleus and their lifespan is about 120 days, at which time they are lysed and their components are recycled to make new RBCs.
- The bone marrow uses iron, amino acids, carbohydrates, folic acid and vitamin B_{12} to produce healthy, efficient RBCs.
- An insufficient number or immaturity of RBCs results in low oxygen levels in the tissues, with tiredness, fatigue and loss of reserve.
- Anaemia can be caused by a decrease in the production of RBCs, an increase in the destruction of RBCs or by blood loss.
- Iron deficiency anaemia occurs when there is inadequate iron intake in the diet or an inability to absorb iron from the GI tract. Iron is needed to produce haemoglobin, which carries oxygen. Iron deficiency anaemia is treated with iron replacement.
- Iron is a very toxic mineral at high levels. The body controls the absorption of iron and carefully regulates its storage and movement in the body.
- Folic acid and vitamin B_{12} are needed to produce a strong supporting structure in the RBC so that it can survive 120 days of being propelled through the vascular system. These are usually found in adequate amounts in the diet.
- A dietary lack of or inability to absorb folic acid, vitamin B_{12}, or both will produce a megaloblastic anaemia, in which the RBCs are large and immature and have a short lifespan.
- Pernicious anaemia is a lack of vitamin B_{12}, which is also used by the body to maintain the myelin sheath on nerve axons. If vitamin B_{12} is lacking, these neurons will degenerate and cause many CNS effects.
- Pernicious anaemia is caused by the deficient production of intrinsic factor by gastric cells.
- Intrinsic factor is needed to allow the body to absorb vitamin B_{12}. If intrinsic factor is lacking, vitamin B_{12} must be prescribed.

CRITICAL THINKING SCENARIO 48-1

Iron Preparations and Toxicity

The Situation

Lisa, a 28-year-old woman, suffered a miscarriage 6 weeks ago. She lost a great deal of blood during the miscarriage and underwent a dilation and curettage to control the bleeding. On her 6-week routine follow-up visit, she was found to have recovered physically from the event but was still depressed over her loss. Her haematocrit was 31% (normal range) and she admitted feeling tired and weak. Further questioning revealed that she was stating pertinent negatives. The nurse recommended Lisa made use of the emotional support and counselling services provided by the hospital. Lisa was given a supply of ferrous sulphate tablets, with the instructions to take one tablet three times a day with food.

At home, Lisa transferred the pills to a decorative bottle that had once held vitamins and left it on her table as a reminder for her to take the tablets. The next day, she discovered her 2-year-old daughter eating the tablets. Not knowing how many the toddler had eaten, Lisa immediately took her to Accident and Emergency (A&E), taking the tablets with her. On examination, the toddler was found to have a weak, rapid pulse (156 beats/min); rapid, shallow respirations (32 per minute) and a low blood pressure (60/42 mmHg). When a diagnosis of acute iron toxicity was made, Lisa became distraught. She said she had no idea that iron could be dangerous as it can be bought over the counter (OTC) in so many preparations. She had not read the written information given to her because it was 'just iron'.

Critical Thinking

- What nursing interventions should be done at this point?
- What sort of crisis intervention would be most appropriate for Lisa? *Think about the combined depression from the miscarriage, fear and anxiety related to this crisis and Lisa's iron-depleted state.*
- What kind of reserve does she have for dealing with this crisis? Which measures would be appropriate for helping the mother cope with this crisis and for treating the toddler?

Discussion

The first priority is to support and detoxify the child in iron toxicity. Gastric lavage using a 1% sodium bicarbonate solution can be done in a controlled environment (A&E). This procedure is safe for about the first hour after ingestion. After that time, there is an increased risk of gastric erosion caused by the corrosive iron, making the lavage very dangerous. This toddler is well beyond the first hour; therefore, other measures will be needed. In severe toxicity, an iron-chelating agent such as desferrioxamine should be given intravenously. Supportive measures to deal with shock, dehydration and GI damage will be necessary.

During this crisis, Lisa will need a great deal of support (including a partner/ husband, responsible relative, friend or other person who can stay with her). She also will need reassurance and a place to rest. After the situation is stabilized, Lisa will need teaching and additional support. For example, she should be reassured that most people do not take OTC drugs seriously, and many do not even read the labels. However, the nurse can use this opportunity to stress the importance of reading all of the labels and following the directions that come with OTC drugs. Lisa also should be commended for getting medical care for the toddler quickly. Finally, she should receive a review of the iron-teaching information and be encouraged to ask questions.

Nursing Care Guide for Lisa: Iron Preparations

Assessment: History and Examination

Assess for colitis, enteritis, hepatic dysfunction, peptic ulcer. Then focus the physical examination on the following areas: blood pressure, pulse, perfusion; orientation; skin, gums, teeth; respiratory rate and adventitious sounds; abdominal examination including bowel sounds. Laboratory tests should include FBC, haemoglobin, haematocrit, serum ferritin assays.

Nursing Diagnoses

- Acute pain related to GI, CNS effects
- Risk for injury related to CNS effects
- Disturbed body image related to drug induced teeth staining
- Deficient knowledge regarding drug therapy

Implementation

- Confirm iron deficiency anaemia before administering the drug.
- Provide comfort and safety measures, for example, give small meals; ensure access to bathroom facilities; use

(continued)

Iron Preparations and Toxicity *(continued)*

Z-track method for IM injections; give drug with food if GI upset occurs and institute bowel programme as needed.

- Arrange for treatment of underlying cause of anaemia.
- Provide support and reassurance to deal with drug effects.
- Provide patient education regarding drug, dosage, adverse effects, what to report, safety precautions.

Evaluation

- Evaluate drug effects (relief of signs and symptoms of anaemia, haematocrit within normal limits).
- Monitor for adverse effects: GI upset, CNS toxicity, coma.
- Monitor haematocrit and haemoglobin periodically.
- Monitor for drug–drug interactions as indicated for each drug.
- Evaluate effectiveness of patient education programme and comfort and safety measures.

Patient Education for Lisa

- ☐ Iron is a naturally occurring mineral found in many foods. It is used by the body to make RBCs, which carry oxygen to all parts of the body. Supplemental iron needs to be taken when the body does not have enough iron available to make healthy RBCs, a condition called anaemia.
- ☐ Iron is a toxic substance if too much is taken. You must avoid self-medicating with over-the-counter preparations containing iron while you are taking this drug.
- ☐ You will need to return for regular medical checkups while taking this drug to determine its effectiveness.
- ☐ Take your medication as follows, depending on the specific iron preparation that has been prescribed:
  - Dissolve *ferrous salts* in orange juice to improve the taste.
  - Take *liquid iron preparations* with a straw to prevent the iron from staining teeth.
  - Place iron drops on the back of the tongue to prevent staining of the teeth.
- ☐ Some of the following adverse effects may occur:
  - *Dark, tarry or green stools:* The iron preparations stain the stools; the colour remains as long as you are taking the drug and should not cause concern.
  - *Constipation:* This is a common problem; if it becomes too uncomfortable, consult with your health care provider for an appropriate remedy.
  - *Nausea, indigestion, vomiting:* This problem can often be solved by taking the drug with food, making sure to avoid the foods listed earlier.
- ☐ Report any of the following to your health care provider: *severe diarrhoea, severe abdominal pain or cramping, unusual tiredness or weakness, bluish tint to the lips or finger nail beds.*
- ☐ Tell any doctor, nurse or other health care provider that you are taking this drug.
- ☐ Keep this drug and all medications out of the reach of children. As iron can be very toxic, seek emergency medical help immediately if you suspect that a child has taken this preparation unsupervised.
- ☐ As iron can interfere with the absorption of some drugs, do not take iron at the same time as *tetracycline* or *antacids.* These drugs must be taken during intervals when iron is not in the stomach.
- ☐ If Lisa is depressed then education may be difficult.

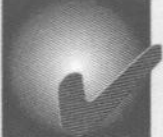

CHECK YOUR UNDERSTANDING

Answers to the questions in this chapter may be found in the Answer Key in the back of the book.

Multiple Choice

Select the most appropriate response to the following.

1. The rate of red blood cell production is controlled by
   a. iron.
   b. folic acid.
   c. erythropoietin.
   d. vitamin B_{12}.
2. Red blood cells must be continually produced by the body because
   a. the iron within the RBC wears out.
   b. with no nucleus, the RBC cannot maintain itself and wears out over time.
   c. there is continual loss of RBCs from the gastrointestinal tract of healthy adults.
   d. RBCs are processed into bile salts and must be replaced.
3. Anaemia is
   a. a decreased number of red blood cells.
   b. a lack of iron in the body.

c. a lack of vitamin B_{12} in the body.
d. an excessive number of platelets.

4. Megaloblastic anaemia is a result of insufficient folic acid or vitamin B_{12} and it affects
a. white blood cell production.
b. vegetarians.
c. all cells in the body that are rapidly turning over.
d. slow-growing cells.

5. Epoetin alfa would be the drug of choice for
a. acute blood loss during surgery.
b. replacing blood loss from traumatic injury.
c. treating anaemia during lactation.
d. the treatment of anaemia associated with renal failure.

6. A patient with anaemia who is given iron salts could expect to show a therapeutic increase in haematocrit
a. within 72 hours.
b. within 2 to 3 weeks.
c. over 6 to 10 months.
d. within 1 to 2 weeks.

7. Iron is not absorbed from the gastrointestinal tract if it is taken with
a. protein.
b. anticoagulants.
c. dairy products.
d. any other drugs.

8. A patient with pernicious anaemia would be advised to take vitamin B_{12}
a. orally with breakfast.
b. orally at bedtime.
c. subcutaneously every day.
d. intramuscularly every 5 to 10 days.

Extended Matching Questions

Select **all** that apply.

1. Clients are often given iron pills by their clinic. Instructions in giving these pills should include
a. taking the drug with milk to avoid gastrointestinal problems.
b. the potential for constipation.
c. keeping these potentially toxic pills away from children.
d. taking the drug with antacids to alleviate the gastrointestinal upset.
e. having periodic blood tests to evaluate the drug effect.
f. being aware that stools may be coloured green.

2. In a healthy person, very little iron is needed on a daily basis. Loss of iron is associated with which of the following?
a. Heavy menstrual flow
b. Bile duct obstruction
c. Internal bleeding
d. Traumatic injury and loss of blood
e. Bone marrow suppression
f. Alcoholic cirrhosis

True or False

Indicate whether the following statements are true (T) or false (F).

_____1. Blood is composed of a liquid plasma (containing water, proteins, glucose and electrolytes) and formed components including white blood cells, red blood cells and platelets.

_____2. RBCs are produced in the bone marrow in a process called erythropoiesis, which is controlled by intrinsic factor.

_____3. RBCs have a small nucleus and their lifespan is about 120 days.

_____4. An insufficient number or maturity of RBCs results in low oxygen levels in the tissues, with tiredness, fatigue and loss of reserve.

_____5. Anaemia can be caused by a lack of erythropoietin or by a lack of the components needed to produce RBCs.

_____6. Iron is needed to produce haemoglobin, which carries the oxygen.

_____7. Folic acid and vitamin B_6 are needed to produce a strong supporting structure in the RBC.

_____8. Pernicious anaemia is a lack of vitamin B_{12}, which is also used by the body to maintain the myelin sheath on nerve axons.

Bibliography

Adams, M. P., Josephson, D. L, & Holland, L. N. (2005). *Pharmacology for nurses: A pathophysiological approach*. New Jersey: Pearson Prentice Hall.
British Medical Association and Royal Pharmaceutical Society of Great Britain. (2008). *British National Formulary*. London: BMJ & RPS Publishing. *This publication is updated biannually: it is imperative that the most recent edition is consulted.*
British Medical Association and Royal Pharmaceutical Society of Great Britain. (2008). *British National Formulary for Children*. London: BMJ & RPS Publishing. *This publication is updated annually: it is imperative that the most recent edition is consulted.*
Galbraith, A., Bullock, S., Manias, E., Hunt, B., & Richards, A. (1997). *Fundamentals of pharmacology*. Harlow: Pearson Prentice Hall.
Ganong, W. (2005). *Review of medical physiology* (22nd ed.). New York: McGraw-Hill.
Howland, R. D., & Mycek, M. J. (2005). *Pharmacology* (3rd ed.). Philadelphia: Lippincott Williams & Wilkins.
Marieb, E. N., & Hoehn, K. (2004). *Human anatomy & physiology* (7th ed.). San Francisco: Pearson Benjamin Cummings.
Porth, C. M., & Matfin, G. (2008). *Pathophysiology: Concepts of altered health states* (8th ed.). Philadelphia: Lippincott Williams & Wilkins.
Simonsen, T., Aarbakke, J., Kay, I., Coleman, I., Sinnott, P., & Lysaa, R. (2006). *Illustrated pharmacology for nurses*. London: Hodder Arnold.

PART IX

Drugs Acting on the Renal System

CHAPTER 49

Introduction to the Kidneys and the Urinary Tract

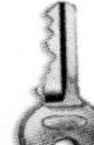

KEY TERMS

aldosterone
antidiuretic hormone (ADH)
carbonic anhydrase
countercurrent mechanism
filtration
glomerulus
nephron
prostate gland
reabsorption
renin–angiotensin system
secretion

LEARNING OBJECTIVES

Upon completion of this chapter, you will be able to:

1. Review the anatomy of the kidney and using a diagram of the nephron, explain the basic processes of the kidney and where these activities occur.
2. Explain the control of sodium, potassium, chloride and calcium in the nephron.
3. Discuss the countercurrent mechanism and the control of urine concentration and dilution and apply its effects to various clinical scenarios.
4. Describe the renin–angiotensin–aldosterone system, including controls and clinical situations where this system is active.
5. Discuss the metabolic roles of the kidney: acid–base balance, calcium regulation and red blood cell production.
6. Use the metabolic roles of the kidney to explain the clinical manifestations of renal failure.

The renal system is composed of the kidneys and the structures of the urinary tract: the ureters, the urinary bladder and the urethra. The major functions of this system in the body include:

- maintaining the volume and composition of body fluids within normal ranges, which includes clearing nitrogenous wastes from protein metabolism, maintaining acid–base balance and electrolyte levels and the excretion of various drugs and drug metabolites
- regulating blood pressure through the renin–angiotensin system
- regulating red blood cell production through the production and secretion of erythropoietin
- regulating vitamin D activation, which helps to maintain calcium levels
- regulating calcium levels

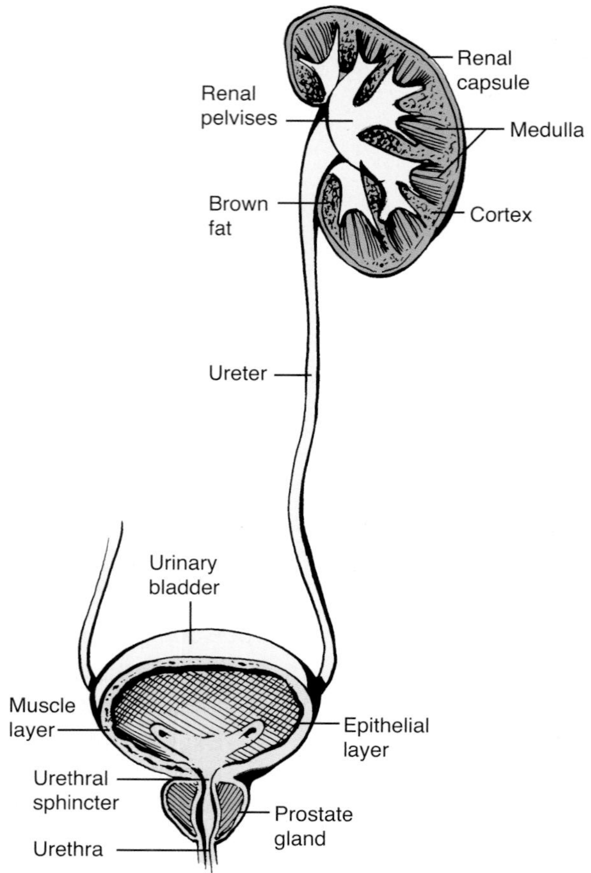

FIGURE 49.1 The kidney and organs of the urinary tract.

The Kidneys

The kidneys are two small bean-shaped organs that make up about 0.5% of the total body weight but receive about 25% of the cardiac output. Most of the fluid that is filtered out by the kidneys is returned to the body and the waste products that remain are excreted in a relatively small amount of water as urine.

The kidneys are located under the ribs for protection from injury, and have three protective layers that make up the renal capsule: a fibrous layer, a brown fat layer and the renal parietal layer. The capsule contains pain fibres, which are stimulated if the capsule is stretched secondary to an inflammatory process. The kidneys have three identifiable regions: the outer cortex, the inner medulla and renal pelvis. The renal pelvises containing calyxes drain the urine into the ureters. The ureters are muscular tubes that lead into the urinary bladder, where urine is stored until it is excreted (Figure 49.1).

The functional unit of the kidneys is called the **nephron**. There are approximately 2 million nephrons in the adult kidneys. There are two types of nephron: the cortical nephrons and the juxtamedullary nephrons, named depending on where they are found in the kidney. All nephrons filter fluid and make urine, but only the juxtamedullary nephrons can concentrate or dilute urine. It is estimated that only about 25% of the total number of nephrons are necessary to maintain healthy renal function. This means that the renal system is well protected from failure with a large backup system. However, by the time a patient has signs and symptoms of renal failure, extensive kidney damage may have already occurred.

The nephron is basically a tube (Figure 49.2). It begins with the Bowman's (glomerular) capsule, which has a fenestrated epithelium that works like a sieve to allow fluid to flow through but keeps large components (e.g. erythrocytes and large protein molecules such as albumin) from entering. The nephron then curls around in a section called the proximal convoluted tubule. From there, it narrows to form the descending and ascending loop of Henle, widens as the distal convoluted tubule, which flow into the collecting ducts, these meet at the renal pelvises. Each section of the tubule functions in a slightly different manner to maintain fluid and electrolyte balance in the body.

Renal Blood Flow

The blood flow to the nephron is unique. The renal arteries branch directly off the aorta and enter each kidney. As a renal artery enters each of the kidneys, it divides to form interlobar arteries, which become smaller arcuate (bowed) arteries, then afferent arterioles. The afferent arterioles branch to form the **glomerulus** inside Bowman's capsule. The glomerulus is like a knot of blood vessels with a capillary-like endothelium that allows easy passage of fluid and waste products. The efferent arteriole *exits* from the glomerulus and branches into the peritubular capillary system, which returns fluid and electrolytes that have been reabsorbed from the tubules to the bloodstream. These capillaries flow

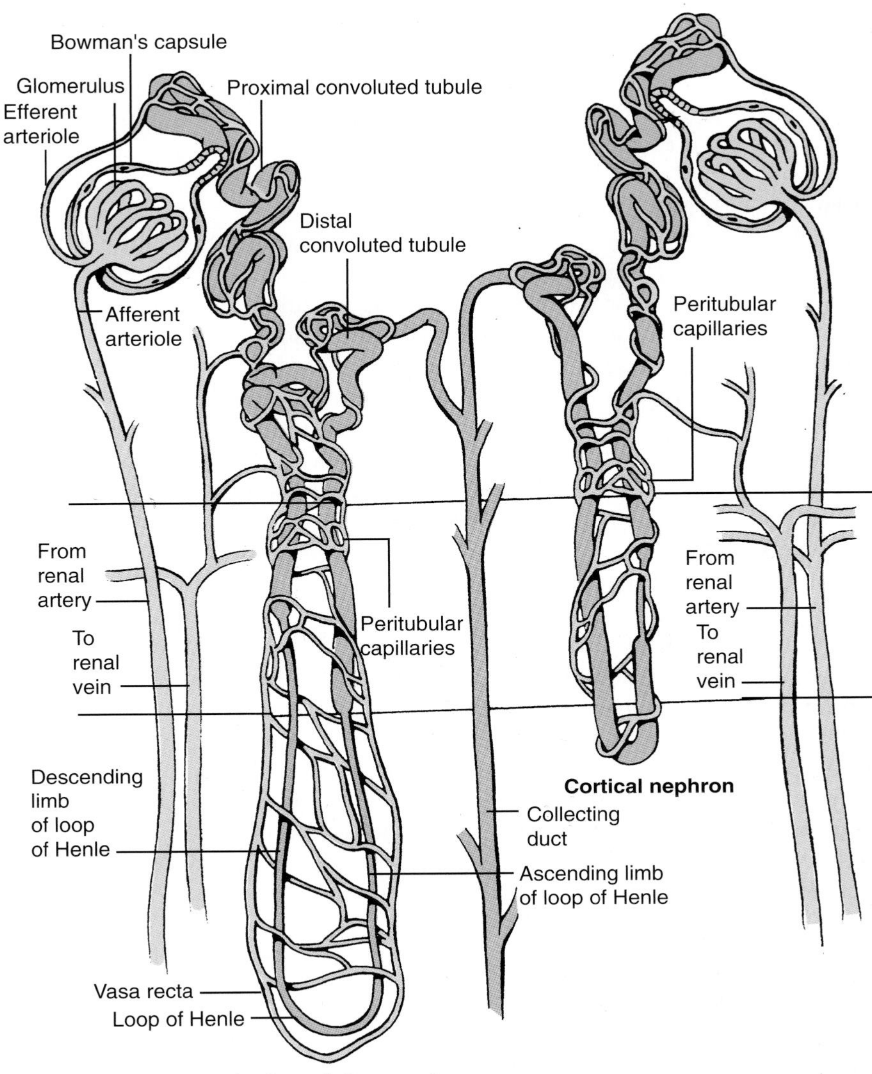

FIGURE 49.2 The nephron, the functional unit of the kidneys. Secretion and reabsorption of water, electrolytes and other solutes in the various segments of the renal tubule, the loop of Henle, and the collecting duct can be influenced by diuretics, other drugs and endogenous substances, including certain hormones. In the kidneys, the distal convoluted tubule wraps around and is actually next to the afferent arteriole to form the juxtamedullary complex.

into the *vasa recta*, which flow into intralobar veins and, in turn, drain into the inferior vena cava. The two arterioles (afferent and efferent) around the glomerulus work together to closely regulate the flow of fluid into the glomerulus, by increasing or decreasing pressure as needed, that is autoregulation.

A small group of cells, called the juxtaglomerular apparatus, connects the afferent arteriole to the distal convoluted tubule; here erythropoietin and renin are produced. These cells, in close proximity to the afferent arteriole, are especially sensitive to the volume and quality of blood flow into the glomerulus. The surrounding area to the nephrons is called the *macula densa*.

Renal Processes

The functions of the nephrons can be described using three basic processes: glomerular **filtration** (filters fluid entering the nephron), tubular **secretion** (actively removing components from the capillary system and depositing them into the tubule) and tubular **reabsorption** (removing components from the tubule to return them to the capillary system and circulation).

Glomerular Filtration

The glomerulus acts as a filter for all of the blood that flows into it. The semipermeable membrane keeps blood cells, proteins and lipids inside the vessel, whereas the hydrostatic pressure from the blood pushes water and smaller components of the plasma into the tubule. A clinical sign of renal damage is blood cells or protein in the urine. This can happen if the semipermeable membrane is scarred, swollen or damaged, allowing the larger plasma components to escape into the filtrate. The large size of these components prevents them from being reabsorbed by the tubule and they are lost in the urine.

Approximately 125 ml of fluid is filtered out each minute, or 180 l/day. About 99% of the filtered fluid is returned to the bloodstream as the filtrate progresses through the renal tubule. Approximately 1% of the filtrate, less than 2 litres of fluid, is excreted each day in the form of urine.

Tubular Reabsorption

The cells lining the renal tubule reabsorb water and various essential substances from the filtrate back into the vascular system. About 99% of the water filtered at the **glomerulus** is reabsorbed. Other filtrate components that are reabsorbed regularly include vitamins, glucose, electrolytes, sodium bicarbonate and sodium chloride. The reabsorption process uses a series of transport systems that exchange needed ions for unwanted ones (see Chapter 6 for a review of cellular transport systems). Drugs that affect renal function frequently overwhelm one of these transport systems or interfere with its normal activity, leading to an imbalance in acid–base or electrolyte levels.

Tubular Secretion

The epithelial cells that line the renal tubule can secrete substances from the blood into the tubular fluid. This is an energy-using process that allows active transport systems to remove electrolytes, some drugs and their metabolites and uric acid from the surrounding capillaries and secrete them into the filtrate. For instance, the epithelial cells can use tubular secretion to help maintain acid–base levels by secreting hydrogen ions as needed.

Maintenance of Volume and Composition of Body Fluids

The kidneys regulate the composition of body fluids by balancing the levels of the key electrolytes, secreting or absorbing these electrolytes to maintain the desired levels. The volume of body fluids is controlled by diluting or concentrating the urine.

Sodium Regulation

Sodium is one of the body's major cations (positively charged ions). It filters through the glomerulus and enters the renal tubule. In the proximal convoluted tubule it is actively reabsorbed into the peritubular capillaries. As sodium is actively moved out of the filtrate, it takes chloride ions and water with it. This occurs by passive diffusion as the body maintains the osmotic and electrical balances on both sides of the tubule.

Sodium ions are also reabsorbed via a transport system that functions under the influence of the catalyst **carbonic anhydrase** (CA see Equation 1) which allows carbon dioxide and water to combine, forming carbonic acid. The carbonic acid immediately dissociates to form sodium bicarbonate, using a sodium ion from the renal tubule and a free hydrogen ion (an acid). The hydrogen ion is then left in the filtrate, causing the urine to be slightly acidic. The bicarbonate is stored in the renal tubule as the body's alkaline reserve, for use when the body becomes too acidic and a buffer is needed.

$$\mathbf{CO_2 + H_2O \overset{CA}{\longleftrightarrow} H_2\,CO_3 \longleftrightarrow H^+ + HCO_3^-} \qquad \text{Equation 1.}$$

The distal convoluted tubule acts to further adjust the sodium levels in the filtrate under the influence of **aldosterone** (a hormone produced by the *zona glomerulosa* of the adrenal cortex) and **atrial natriuretic peptide** (**ANP**; produced by the atrial cells in the heart). Aldosterone is released into the circulation in response to high potassium levels, low sodium levels, sympathetic stimulation or angiotensin II and III. Aldosterone stimulates a sodium–potassium exchange pump in the cells of the distal tubule, which reabsorbs sodium in exchange for potassium. It also increases the number of sodium channels inserted into the distal convoluted tubule. As a result more sodium is reabsorbed into the system and potassium is lost in the filtrate.

ANP has opposing effects. It is released when the atria are stretched and blood volume is high. It causes a decrease in sodium reabsorption from the distal tubules; more sodium is lost in the urine accompanied by water therefore an increased volume of urine is produced. This aims to reduce body fluid levels.

Countercurrent Mechanism

Sodium is further regulated in the juxtamedullary nephrons in what is known as the **countercurrent mechanism** in the loop of Henle. In the descending loop of Henle, the cells are freely permeable to water and sodium. Sodium is actively reabsorbed into the surrounding peritubular tissue and water flows out of the tubule into this sodium-rich tissue to maintain osmotic balance. The filtrate at the end of the descending loop of Henle is concentrated in comparison to the rest of the filtrate.

In contrast, the ascending loop of Henle is impermeable to water, so water that remains in the tubule is trapped there. Chloride is actively transported out of the tubule using energy in a process that is referred to as the chloride pump; sodium and potassium leave with the chloride to maintain electrical neutrality. As a result, the fluid in the ascending loop of Henle becomes hypotonic in comparison to the hypertonic situation in the peritubular tissue.

Antidiuretic hormone (**ADH**; also known as vasopressin) is produced by the hypothalamus and stored in the posterior pituitary gland, is important in maintaining fluid balance. ADH is released in response to falling blood volume, sympathetic stimulation or rising sodium levels (concentration changes are sensed by osmoreceptors in the hypothalamus).

If ADH is present at the distal convoluted tubule and the collecting duct, the permeability of the membrane to water is increased due to the presence of aquaporins or water channels. Consequently, the water remaining in the tubule

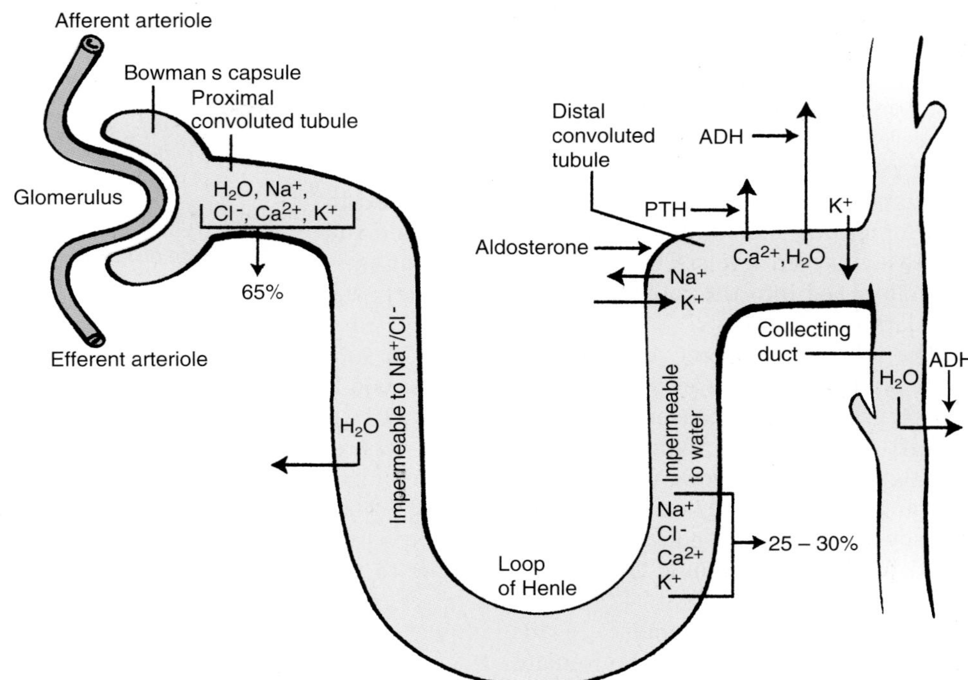

FIGURE 49.3 Nephron and points of regulation of sodium, chloride, potassium, calcium, and water. ADH, antidiuretic hormone; PTH, parathyroid hormone.

rapidly flows into the hypertonic tissue surrounding the loop of Henle, where it is either absorbed by the peritubular capillaries or re-enters the descending loop of Henle in a countercurrent style. The resulting urine is hypertonic and of small volume. If ADH is not present, the tubule remains impermeable to water. The water that has been trapped in the ascending loop of Henle passes into the collection duct, resulting in hypotonic urine of greater volume. This countercurrent mechanism allows the body to finely regulate fluid volume by regulating the control of sodium and water (Figure 49.3).

Potassium Regulation

Potassium is another cation that is vital to proper functioning of the nervous system, muscles and cell membranes. About 65% of the potassium that is filtered at the glomerulus is reabsorbed at the Bowman's capsule and the proximal convoluted tubule. Another 25% to 30% is reabsorbed in the ascending loop of Henle. The fine tuning of potassium levels occurs in the distal convoluted tubule, where aldosterone activates the sodium–potassium exchanger, leading to a loss of potassium. If potassium levels are very high, the retention of sodium in exchange for potassium also leads to retention of water and a dilution of blood volume, which further decreases the potassium concentration (Figure 49.3).

Chloride Regulation

Chloride is an important negatively charged ion that helps to maintain electrical neutrality with the movement of cations across the cell membrane. Chloride is primarily reabsorbed in the loop of Henle, where it promotes the movement of sodium out of the cell.

Regulation of Vitamin D Activation

Calcium is another important cation that is regulated by the kidneys. The absorption of calcium from the gastrointestinal (GI) tract is regulated by absorbed dietary vitamin D, which must be activated in the kidneys to calcitriol, a form that will promote calcium absorption.

Calcium Regulation

Calcium is important in muscle function, blood clotting, bone formation, contraction of cell membranes and muscle movement. Calcium is filtered at the glomerulus and mostly reabsorbed in the proximal convoluted tubule and ascending loop of Henle. Calcium levels are maintained within a very tight range by the activity of the hormones, **parathyroid hormone (PTH)** and **calcitonin**. Fine tuning of calcium reabsorption occurs in the distal convoluted tubule, where the presence of PTH stimulates reabsorption of calcium to increase serum calcium levels when they are low (see Figure 49.3 and Chapter 36).

Blood Pressure Control: Renin–Angiotensin System

The nephrons require a constant supply of blood and are equipped with a system to ensure that they are perfused.

This mechanism, called the **renin–angiotensin**– aldosterone **system** involves a response to decreased blood flow to the nephrons.

Whenever blood flow or oxygenation to the nephron is decreased (due to haemorrhage, shock, congestive heart failure, or hypotension), **renin** is released from the juxtaglomerular cells. These cells, positioned next to the glomerulus, are stimulated by decreased stretch and decreased oxygen levels. The released renin is immediately absorbed into the capillary system and enters the circulation.

The released renin activates angiotensinogen, a substrate produced in the liver, which becomes **angiotensin I**. Angiotensin I is then converted into **angiotensin II** by a converting enzyme found in the lungs and some vessels. Angiotensin II is a very powerful vasoconstrictor, combining with angiotensin II receptor sites in blood vessels to cause vasoconstriction. This powerful vasoconstriction raises blood pressure and should increase blood flow to the kidneys.

Angiotensin II is degraded in the adrenal gland to **angiotensin III** and both stimulates the release of aldosterone from the adrenal cortex. Aldosterone acts on the renal tubules to retain sodium and therefore water. This increases blood volume and further increases blood pressure, which should increase blood flow to the kidneys. The osmotic centre in the hypothalamus senses the increased sodium levels and releases ADH, leading to a further retention of water and a further increase in blood volume and pressure, which should again increase blood flow to the kidneys.

The renin–angiotensin system constantly works to maintain blood flow to the kidneys (see Figure 49.4). For example, an individual rising from a lying position experiences a drop in blood flow to the kidneys as blood pools in the legs because of gravity. This causes a massive release of renin and activation of this system to ensure that blood pressure is maintained and the kidneys are perfused. Blood loss from injury or during surgery also activates this system to increase blood flow through the kidneys.

Regulation of Red Blood Cell Production

When blood flow or oxygenation to the nephron is decreased, the hormone erythropoietin is released from the juxtaglomerular cells. This hormone stimulates the bone marrow to increase production of red blood cells, which act to bring additional oxygen to the kidneys. Erythropoietin is the only known factor that can regulate the rate of red blood cell production. When a patient develops renal failure and the production of erythropoietin drops, the production of red blood cells falls and the patient becomes anaemic.

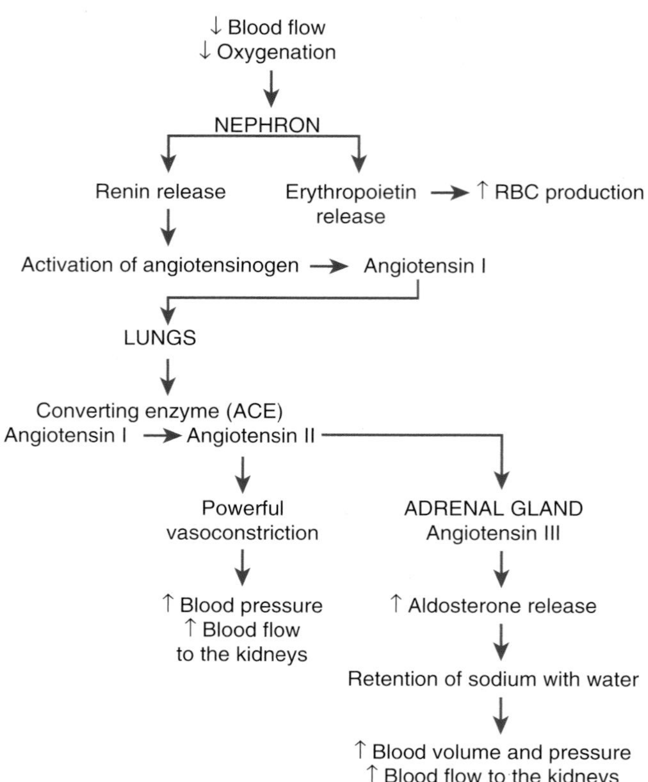

FIGURE 49.4 The renin–angiotensin system for the reflex maintenance of blood pressure control.

The Urinary Tract

As noted previously, the urinary tract is composed of the ureters, urinary bladder and urethra (see Figure 49.1). One ureter exits each kidney, draining the filtrate from the collecting ducts. The ureters have a smooth-endothelial lining and circular-muscular layers. Urine entering the ureter stimulates a peristaltic wave that pushes the urine down towards the urinary bladder. The urinary bladder is a muscular pouch that stretches and holds the urine until it is excreted from the body. Control of bladder emptying is a learned control over the urethral sphincter; once it is established, a functioning nervous system is necessary to maintain control.

Urine is usually a slightly acidic fluid; this acidity helps to maintain the normal transport systems and to destroy bacteria that may enter the bladder. In females, the urethra is very short and leads to an area populated by normal flora including *Escherichia coli*, which can cause frequent bladder infections or cystitis. In males, the urethra is much longer and passes through the **prostate gland**, a small gland that produces an acidic fluid that is important in maintaining the sperm and lubricating the tract. Enlargement and infection in the prostate gland are often problems in older males.

Points to Remember

- The kidneys are two small organs that receive about 25% of the cardiac output.
- The functional unit of the kidneys is called the nephron; it is composed of the Bowman's capsule, proximal convoluted tubule, loop of Henle, distal convoluted tubule and the collecting duct.
- The blood flow to the nephron is unique, allowing autoregulation of blood flow through the glomerulus.
- The nephrons utilize three basic processes: glomerular filtration, tubular secretion and tubular reabsorption.
- Sodium levels are regulated throughout the tubule by active and passive movement and are modulated by the presence of aldosterone in the distal tubule.
- The countercurrent mechanism in the juxtamedullary nephrons allows for the concentration or dilution of urine under the influence of ADH secreted by the hypothalamus.
- Potassium concentration is regulated throughout the tubule, with aldosterone being the strongest influence for potassium loss.
- The kidneys play a key role in the regulation of calcium by activating vitamin D to allow calcium reabsorption in the GI tract and by reabsorbing or excreting calcium from the tubule under the influence of PTH.
- The kidneys influence blood pressure control, releasing renin to activate the renin–angiotensin system, which leads to increased blood pressure and volume and a resultant increased blood flow to the kidney. The balance of this reflex system can lead to water retention or excretion and has an impact on drug therapy that promotes water or sodium loss.
- The ureters, urinary bladder and urethra make up the rest of the urinary tract. The longer male urethra passes through the prostate gland, which may enlarge or become infected, a problem often associated with advancing age.

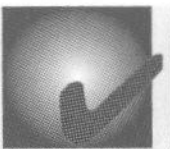

CHECK YOUR UNDERSTANDING

Answers to the questions in this chapter may be found in the answer key in the back of the book.

Multiple Choice

Select the most appropriate response to the following.

1. During severe exertion, a person may lose large amounts of hypotonic sweat. This loss would result in
   a. decreased plasma volume.
   b. decreased plasma osmolality.
   c. decreased circulating levels of ADH.
   d. Increased circulating levels of ANP

2. Urine passes through the ureter by
   a. osmosis.
   b. air pressure.
   c. filtration.
   d. gravity and peristalsis.

3. Renal reabsorption
   a. is the movement of substances from the renal tubule into the blood.
   b. is the movement of substances from the blood into the renal tubule.
   c. of water is increased in the absence of ADH.
   d. of sodium occurs only in the proximal tubule.

4. The major reason older adults should monitor their intake of fluids is that
   a. older people have decreased levels of ADH.
   b. fluids do not shift between compartments so easily.
   c. total body water decreases with age and restoration of homeostasis is slower.
   d. older people lose more fluid through the skin as it becomes thinner.

5. Blood flow to the nephron differs from blood flow to other tissues in that
   a. the venous system is not involved.
   b. there are no capillaries in the nephron.
   c. efferent and afferent arterioles allow for autoregulation of blood flow through the glomerulus.
   d. the capillary bed has a fenestrated membrane.

6. Concentration and dilution of urine is controlled by
   a. afferent arterioles.
   b. the renin–angiotensin system.
   c. aldosterone release.
   d. the countercurrent mechanism in medullary nephrons.

7. Women tend to have more problems with bladder infections than men because:
   a. women have *E. coli* in the urinary tract.
   b. females have a short urethra, making access to the bladder easier for bacteria.
   c. prostate gland secretes a substance that protects men from bladder infections.
   d. bacteria prefer the more acidic environment of the female bladder

Extended Matching Questions

Select **all** that apply.

1. Considering the metabolic functions of the kidneys, renal failure would be expected to cause which of the following?
   a. Anaemia.
   b. Loss of calcium regulation.
   c. Urea build-up on the skin.
   d. Respiratory alkalosis.
   e. Metabolic acidosis.
   f. Changes in the function of blood cells.

2. During severe diarrhoea, there is a loss of water, bicarbonate and sodium from the GI tract. Physiological compensation for this would probably include which of the following?
   a. Increased alveolar ventilation.
   b. Decreased hydrogen ion secretion by the renal tubules.
   c. Decreased urinary excretion of sodium and water.
   d. Increased renin secretion.
   e. Increased hydrogen ion secretion by the renal tubules.
   f. Increased ADH levels.

3. Maintenance of blood pressure is important in maintaining the fragile nephrons. Reflex systems that work to ensure blood flow to the kidneys include
   a. the renin–angiotensin system causing vasoconstriction.
   b. baroreceptor monitoring of the renal artery.
   c. aldosterone release secondary to angiotensin stimulation.
   d. ADH release in response to decreased blood volume with increased osmolarity.
   e. release of erythropoietin.
   f. local response of the afferent arterioles.

Fill in the Blanks

1. The kidneys are two small organs that receive approximately _________ of the cardiac output.

2. The functional unit of the kidney is called the _________, which is composed of _________, the proximal convoluted tubule, the _________, the distal convoluted tubule and the _________.

3. The nephrons function by using three basic processes: ___________________, _________ _________ and ___________________.

4. Sodium levels are regulated throughout the tubule by active and passive movement and are fine-tuned by the presence of _________ in the distal tubule.

5. The countercurrent mechanism in the medullary nephrons allows for the _________ or _________ of urine under the influence of ADH secreted by the hypothalamus.

6. Potassium concentration is regulated throughout the tubule, with _________ being the strongest influence for potassium loss.

7. The kidneys play a key role in the regulation of calcium by activating ___________.

8. The kidneys have an important role in blood pressure control, releasing ________ to activate the renin–angiotensin system.

Bibliography

British Medical Association and Royal Pharmaceutical Society of Great Britain. (2008). *British National Formulary*. London: BMJ & RPS Publishing. *This publication is updated biannually: it is imperative that the most recent edition is consulted.*

British Medical Association and Royal Pharmaceutical Society of Great Britain. (2008). *British National Formulary for Children*. London: BMJ & RPS Publishing. *This publication is updated annually: it is imperative that the most recent edition is consulted.*

Ganong, W. (2005). *Review of medical physiology* (22nd ed.). New York: McGraw-Hill.

Howland, R. D., & Mycek, M. J. (2005). *Pharmacology* (3rd ed.). Philadelphia: Lippincott Williams & Wilkins.

Marieb, E. N., & Hoehn, K. (2004). *Human anatomy & physiology* (7th ed.). San Francisco: Pearson Benjamin Cummings.

Porth, C. M., & Matfin, G. (2008). *Pathophysiology: Concepts of altered health states* (8th ed.). Philadelphia: Lippincott Williams & Wilkins.

Simonsen, T., Aarbakke, J., Kay, I., Coleman, I., Sinnott, P., & Lysaa, R. (2006). *Illustrated pharmacology for nurses.* London: Hodder Arnold.

CHAPTER 50

Diuretic Agents

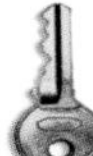

KEY TERMS

alkalosis

fluid rebound

high-ceiling diuretics

hyperaldosteronism

hypokalaemia

renin–angiotensin system

oedema

osmotic pull

LEARNING OBJECTIVES

On completion of this chapter, you will be able to:

1. Define the term diuretic.
2. Describe the therapeutic actions, indications, pharmacokinetics, associated with thiazide and thiazide-related diuretics, loop diuretics, carbonic anhydrase inhibitors, potassium-sparing diuretics and osmotic diuretics.
3. Describe the contraindications, most common adverse reactions and important drug–drug interactions associated with thiazide and thiazide-related diuretics, loop diuretics, carbonic anhydrase inhibitors, potassium-sparing diuretics and osmotic diuretics.
4. Compare and contrast the drugs hydrochlorothiazide, furosemide, acetazolamide, spironolactone and mannitol with other agents in their class.
5. Outline the nursing considerations, including important teaching points for patients receiving diuretic agents.

THIAZIDE DIURETICS

bendroflumethiazide

hydrochlorothiazide

hydroflumethiazide

THIAZIDE-RELATED DIURETICS

chlorthalidone

indapamide

metolazone

LOOP DIURETICS

bumetanide

furosemide

torsemide

CARBONIC ANHYDRASE INHIBITORS

acetazolamide

methazolamide

POTASSIUM-SPARING DIURETICS

amiloride

spironolactone

triamterene

OSMOTIC DIURETICS

mannitol

There are five classes of diuretics, each working at specific sites in the nephron, utilizing different mechanisms. Diuretic classes include the thiazide and thiazide-related diuretics, loop diuretics, carbonic anhydrase inhibitors, potassium-sparing diuretics and the osmotic diuretics. The overall nursing care of the majority of adult patients receiving any diuretic is similar; however, there are differences across the lifespan.

Diuretic Agents

Diuretic agents are usually drugs that increase the volume of urine produced by the kidneys. However, the clinical significance of diuretics is their ability to increase sodium excretion. A comparison of some of types of diuretics can be seen in Table 50.1.

Therapeutic Actions and Indications

Diuretics prevent the cells of the renal tubules from reabsorbing an excessive proportion of the sodium ions (Na^+) in the glomerular filtrate. As a result, sodium and other ions (and the water in which they are dissolved) are excreted in the urine instead of being returned to the blood.

Diuretics are indicated for the treatment of **oedema** associated with congestive heart failure acute pulmonary oedema, liver disease (including cirrhosis), renal disease and for the management of chronic hypertension. They are also used to decrease fluid pressure in the eye [intraocular pressure (IOP)], which is useful in treating glaucoma. Diuretics that decrease potassium levels may also be indicated in the treatment of conditions that cause hyperkalaemia.

Diuretics are routinely prescribed to treat hypertension. The aim of this treatment is to reduce the higher-than-normal blood pressure (diastolic >90 mmHg – The British Hypertensive Society 2004), which can damage organs and lead to serious cardiovascular disorders. Diuretics decrease blood volume, which then decreases pressure in the cardiovascular system. Now several other classes of drugs, including angiotensin-converting enzyme (ACE) inhibitors, angiotensin receptor blockers, β-blockers and calcium channel blockers, are also used for the initial treatment of hypertension. However, the use of diuretics is still the most effective way of treating initial hypertension and it is therefore the first line of treatment. Diuretics are also often used in combination with other treatments to improve the effectiveness of these other drugs.

Congestive heart failure can cause oedema as a result of several factors. The failing heart muscle does not pump sufficient blood to the kidneys, causing activation of the **renin–angiotensin system** and resulting in increases in blood volume and sodium retention. The failing heart muscle cannot respond to the usual reflex stimulation, therefore the increased volume is slowly pushed out into the capillary level as venous pressure increases because the blood is not being pumped effectively (Chapter 44). Pulmonary oedema, or left-sided coronary heart failure develops when the increased volume of fluids backs up into the lungs. The fluid pushed out into the capillaries in the lungs interferes with gas exchange. Congestive heart failure can also lead to peripheral oedema such as ankle oedema.

Patients with liver failure and cirrhosis often present with oedema (ascites). This is caused by reduced plasma protein production, and hence less oncotic pull in the vascular system. Fluid is lost at the capillary level and obstructed blood flow through the portal system, which is caused by increased pressure from congested hepatic vessels.

Renal disease produces oedema because of the loss of plasma proteins into the urine when there is damage to the glomerular basement membrane. Other types of renal diseases produce oedema because of the activation of the renin–angiotensin system as a result of decreasing blood volume (associated with the loss of fluid into the urine), which causes a drop in blood pressure; or because of failure of the renal tubules to regulate electrolytes effectively.

Glaucoma is an eye disease characterized by increased IOP in the eye, which can cause optic nerve atrophy and blindness. Diuretics are used to provide **osmotic pull** to remove some of the fluid from the eye and decrease the IOP.

Contraindications and Cautions

Diuretic use is contraindicated in the presence of allergy to any of the drugs given. Other conditions in which diuretics are contraindicated include fluid and electrolyte imbalances, which can be potentiated by the fluid and electrolyte changes caused by the diuretics, and severe renal disease, which may prevent the diuretic from working. Certain diuretics would be contraindicated if patient has hypokalaemia, hyponatraemia, severe renal and/or hepatic impairment, a patient with severe renal disease could deteriorate into a crisis stage by the blood flow changes brought about by the diuretic.

Caution should be used with the following conditions: systemic lupus erythaematosus (SLE), which frequently causes glomerular changes and renal dysfunction that could precipitate renal failure in some cases; glucose tolerance abnormalities or diabetes mellitus, which is worsened by the glucose-elevating effects of many diuretics; gout, which reflects an abnormality in normal tubule reabsorption and secretion; liver disease, which could interfere with the normal metabolism of the drugs, leading to an accumulation of the drug or toxicity; if a patient is hypotensive and/or hypovolaemic; pregnancy and lactation.These are the conditions that could be jeopardized by changes in fluid and electrolyte balance.

Adverse Effects

The most common adverse effects seen with diuretics include gastrointestinal (GI) upset, fluid and electrolyte imbalances (Box 50.1), hypotension and electrolyte disturbances. Adverse effects associated with diuretics are specific to the particular

Table 50.1 Comparison of Diuretics

Diuretic Class	Major Site of Action	Usual Indications	Major Adverse Effects
Thiazide, thiazide-like	Distal convoluted tubule	Oedema of congestive heart failure liver and renal disease Adjunct for hypertension	GI upset, CNS complications, hypovolaemia
Loop	Loop of Henle	Acute CHF Acute pulmonary oedema Hypertension Oedema of CHF, renal and liver disease	Hypokalaemia, volume depletion, hypotension, CNS effects, GI upset, hyperglycaemia
Carbonic anhydrase inhibitors	Proximal tubule	Glaucoma Diuresis in CHF Mountain sickness Epilepsy	GI upset, urinary frequency
Potassium-sparing	Distal tubule and collecting duct	Adjunct for oedema of CHF, liver and renal disease Treatment of hypokalaemia Adjunct for hypertension Hyperaldosteronism	Hyperkalaemia, CNS effects, diarrhoea
Osmotic	Glomerulus, tubule	Reduction of intracranial pressure Prevention of oliguric phase of renal failure Reduction of intraocular pressure Renal clearance of toxic substances	Hypotension, GI upset, fluid and electrolyte imbalances

class used. For details, see the section on adverse effects for each class of diuretics discussed in this chapter.

Clinically Important Drug–Drug Interactions

When diuretics are used, there is a potential for interactions with drugs that depend on a particular electrolyte balance for their therapeutic effects (e.g. antiarrhythmics such as digoxin), with drugs that depend on urine alkalinity for proper excretion (e.g. quinine) and with drugs that depend on normal reflexes to balance their effects (e.g. antihypertensives, antidiabetic agents).

Always check the most up-to-date copy of the British National Formulary (BNF) for interactions and contraindications

BOX 50.1 FOCUS ON **CLINICAL SKILLS**

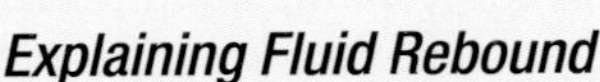

Explaining Fluid Rebound

Care must be taken when using diuretics to avoid **fluid rebound**, which is associated with fluid loss. If a patient stops taking in water and takes the diuretic, the result will be a more concentrated plasma of reduced fluid volume. The decreased volume is sensed by the nephrons, which activate the renin–angiotensin system. When the concentrated blood is sensed by the osmotic centre in the brain, antidiuretic hormone (ADH) is released to retain water and dilute the blood. The result can be a "rebound" oedema as fluid is retained.

Many patients who are taking diuretics often decrease their fluid intake so as to decrease the number of trips to the toilet. This results in rebound water retention as the plasma osmolality increases. It is important to highlight to patients taking diuretics that it is very important to continue taking in fluids to prevent this rebound retention of fluid and to re-establish fluid and electrolyte balance. It is important to be able to explain this effect. Teaching patients about balancing the desired diuretic effect with the actions of the normal reflexes is a clinical skill.

Thiazide and Related Diuretics

Bendroflumethiazide the most frequently used thiazide diuretic, is often used in combination with other drugs for the treatment of hypertension. Thiazides are also often used to relieve oedema due to coronary heart failure.

Therapeutic Actions and Indications

The thiazide diuretics aim to reduce sodium reabsorption at the beginning of the distal convoluted tubule, they exert their action by blocking the chloride pump. Chloride is actively pumped out of the tubule by cells lining the ascending limb of the loop of Henle (the nephron) and the distal tubule. Sodium passively moves with the chloride to maintain electrical neutrality. Chloride is a negative ion and sodium is a positive ion. Blocking of the chloride pump keeps the chloride and the sodium in the tubule to be excreted in the urine, thus preventing the reabsorption of both chloride and sodium in the vascular system (Figure 50.1). As these segments of the tubule are impermeable to water, there is little increase in the volume of urine produced but it will contain high levels of sodium. Thiazides are considered to be mild diuretics compared with the more potent loop diuretics.

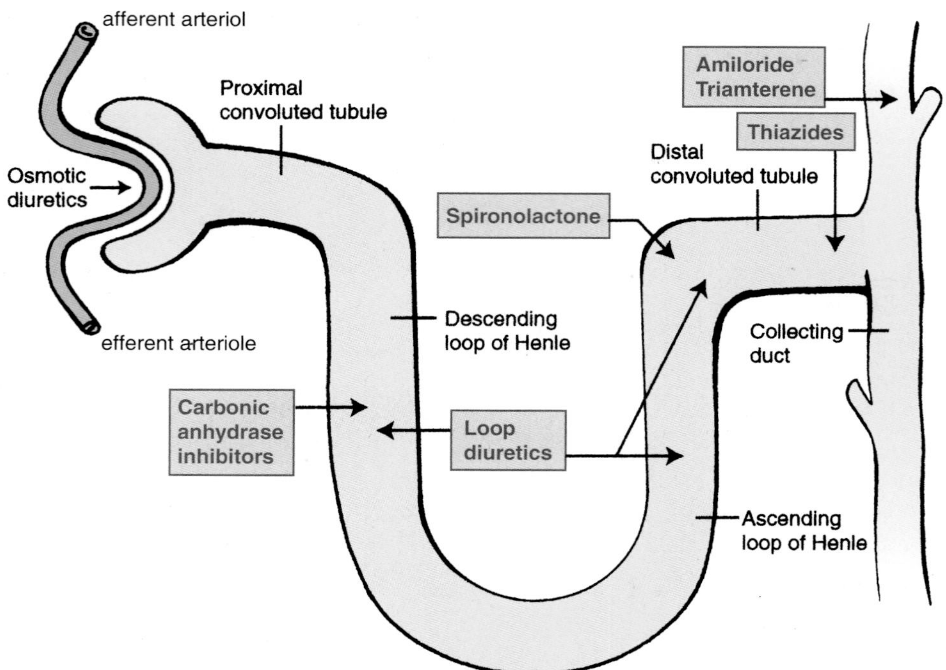

FIGURE 50.1 Sites of action of diuretics in the nephrons.

Thiazides are usually indicated for the treatment of oedema associated with coronary heart failure or with liver or renal disease. These drugs also are used on their own or in combination with other drugs for the treatment of hypertension.

Pharmacokinetics

Thiazide diuretics are well absorbed from the GI tract, with onset of action ranging from 1 to 3 hours. They are metabolized in the liver and excreted in the urine. These diuretics cross the placenta and enter breast milk. Therefore, routine use during pregnancy is not appropriate. If one of these drugs is needed during lactation, another method of feeding the baby should be used because of the potential for adverse effects on fluid and electrolyte changes in the baby.

Contraindications and Cautions

Thiazide and thiazide-related diuretics are contraindicated with fluid or electrolyte imbalances (i.e. refractory hypokalaemia, hyponatraemia, hypercalcaemia. and renal and liver disease, symptomatic hyperuricaemia and Addison's disease) Additional cautions include gout, systemic lupus SLE, diabetes, hyperparathyroidism, bipolar disorder, elderly patients, pregnancy and lactation.

Adverse Effects

Thiazides can cause **hypokalaemia** (low blood levels of potassium). Signs and symptoms of hypokalaemia include weakness, muscle cramps and arrhythmias. Another adverse effect is decreased calcium excretion, which leads to increased calcium levels. Uric acid excretion is also decreased, because the thiazides interfere with its secretory mechanism. High levels of uric acid can result in gout.

If these drugs are used over a prolonged period, blood glucose levels may increase. This may result from the change in potassium levels (which keeps glucose out of the cells).

When thiazides are used the urine will be slightly alkalinized, because they block the reabsorption of bicarbonate. This effect can cause problems for patients who are susceptible to bladder infections and for those taking quinine, which requires acidic urine for excretion. Other key side-effects include postural hypotension, mild GI effects, hypomagnesaemia and hyponatraemia.

Clinically Important Drug–Drug Interactions

Decreased absorption of these drugs may occur if they are combined with colestyramine or colestipol (anion-exchange resins used in the management of hypercholesterolaemia). If this combination is used, a 2-hour interval should be taken between these drugs.

The risk of digoxin toxicity increases due to potential changes in potassium levels; serum potassium should be monitored if this combination is used.

Decreased effectiveness of antidiabetic agents may occur related to the changes in glucose metabolism; dosage adjustment of those agents may be needed.

The risk of lithium toxicity may increase if these drugs are combined. Serum lithium levels should be monitored and appropriate dosage adjustment be made as needed.

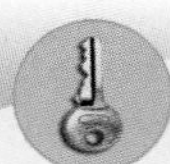

Prototype Summary: *Bendroflumethiazide*

Indications: Oedema associated with mild-or-moderate congestive heart failure alone due to the treatment of hypertension or in combination with other antihypertensives

Actions: Inhibits reabsorption of sodium and chloride in distal convoluted tubules, increasing the excretion of sodium, chloride and water by the kidneys

Pharmacokinetics:

Route	Dose	Duration
Oral for oedema	5–10 mg daily/every	48 hrs.
Oral for hypertension	2.5 mg daily	

$T_{1/2}$: 5.6–14 hours; metabolized in the liver and excreted in urine

Side-effects: postural hypotension, nausea, anorexia, vomiting, diarrhoea, hypokalaemia, hyponatraemia, hypomagnesaemia, hyperuricaemia, gout, hyperglycaemia.

Always consult the current edition of the BNF for further information on contraindications and side-effects.

Loop Diuretics

Loop diuretics are so named because they work on the loop of Henle in the nephron. Furosemide, the most commonly used loop diuretic, is less powerful than the new loop diuretics, bumetanide and torsemide, and therefore has a larger margin of safety (Critical Thinking Scenario 50-1).

Therapeutic Actions and Indications

Loop diuretics are also referred to as **high-ceiling diuretics** because they cause a greater degree of diuresis than other diuretics. These drugs block the chloride pump in the ascending loop of the nephron, where normally 30% of all filtered sodium is reabsorbed. This action decreases the reabsorption of sodium and chloride. The loop diuretics have a similar effect in the distal convoluted tubule, resulting in the production of a copious amount of sodium-rich urine. These drugs work even in the presence of acid–base disturbances, renal failure, electrolyte imbalances or nitrogen retention.

These drugs can produce a loss of fluid of up to 9 kg/day, loop diuretics are the drugs of choice when a rapid and extensive diuresis is needed. In cases of severe oedema or acute pulmonary oedema, it is important to remember that these drugs can have an effect only on the blood that reaches the nephrons. A rapid diuresis occurs, producing a more hypertonic intravascular fluid. In pulmonary oedema, this fluid then circulates back to the lungs, pulls fluid out of the interstitial spaces by its oncotic pull, and delivers this fluid to the kidneys, where the water is pulled out, completing the cycle. In the treatment of pulmonary oedema, it can sometimes take hours to move all of the fluid out of the lungs, because the fluid must be pulled out of the interstitial spaces in the lungs before it can be circulated to the kidneys for removal. Remembering how the drugs work and the way in which fluid moves in the vascular system will make it easier to understand the effects to anticipate.

Loop diuretics are commonly indicated for the treatment of acute coronary heart failure acute pulmonary oedema, oedema associated with congestive heart failure or with renal or liver disease, and hypertension.

Pharmacokinetics

The pharmacokinetics of loop diuretics is similar to thiazide diuretics (previous section).

Contraindications and Cautions

Amongst the contraindications to these drugs are, allergy to a loop diuretic, electrolyte depletion, severe renal failure, hepatic coma and pregnancy and lactation. Cautious use is recommended for patients with systemic lupus SLE, gout or diabetes mellitus. These drugs should also be used with caution in patients with hypotension, hypovolaemia and prostatic enlargement.

Adverse Effects

Adverse effects are related to the imbalance in electrolytes and fluid that these drugs cause for example hypokalaemia, alkalosis, hypocalcaemia and hypotension. Hypokalaemia occurs because potassium is lost when the transport systems in the tubule try to save some of the sodium being lost. **Alkalosis**, or a drop in serum pH, occurs as bicarbonate is lost in the urine. Calcium is also lost in the tubules along with the bicarbonate, which may result in hypocalcaemia and tetany. The fast loss of fluid can result in hypotension and dizziness if it causes a rapid imbalance in fluid levels. Long-term use of these drugs may also result in hyperglycaemia because of the diuretic effect on blood glucose levels, so susceptible patients need to be monitored for this effect. Other side-effects include hypomagnesaemia, GI disturbance and a temporary increase in plasma cholesterol and triglyceride concentration.

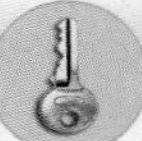

Prototype Summary: *Furosemide*

Indications: Treatment of oedema associated with coronary heart failure acute pulmonary oedema, hypertension

Actions: Inhibits the reabsorption of sodium and chloride from the loop of Henle, leading to a sodium-rich diuresis

Pharmacokinetics:

Route	Dose	
Oral	For oedema	40 mg daily/every 48 h.
	For hypertension	20–40 mg daily
IM	20 mg initially	
IV	(doses greater than 50 mg) adults max 1.5 g daily.	

Note Drug acts within 1 hour or oral administration and if given IV within 30 minutes.

$T_{1/2}$: 120 minutes; metabolized in the liver and excreted in urine

Adverse effects: electrolyte disturbances – hypokalaemia, hyponatraemia, hypocalcaemia, hypomagnesia, dizziness, vertigo, hypotension, thrombophlebitis, nausea, anorexia, vomiting, constipation, hyperglycaemia, urinary bladder spasm, leucopaenia, anaemia, thrombocytopenia, muscle cramps, and spasms, hypersensitivity and rashes.

Carbonic Anhydrase Inhibitors

Therapeutic Actions and Indications

The carbonic anhydrase inhibitors are relatively mild diuretics. The enzyme **carbonic anhydrase** is a catalyst for the formation of sodium bicarbonate, which is stored as the alkaline reserve in the renal tubule, and for the excretion of hydrogen, which results in a slightly acidic urine. Diuretics that block the effects of carbonic anhydrase slow down the movement of hydrogen ions; as a result, more sodium and bicarbonate are lost in the urine.

Acetazolamide is used to treat glaucoma, in conjunction with other drugs to treat epilepsy, and to treat mountain sickness.

Pharmacokinetics

These drugs are rapidly absorbed and widely distributed. They are excreted in urine. Some of these agents have been associated with foetal abnormalities, and they should not be used during pregnancy. As there is the potential for adverse effects on the baby; another method of feeding the infant should be used if one of these drugs is needed during lactation.

Contraindications and Cautions

Allergies to the drug or to antibacterial sulphonamides, thiazides or chronic noncongestive angle closure glaucoma are contraindications for use. Cautious use is recommended in patients who are breast-feeding or who have fluid or electrolyte imbalances, renal or hepatic disease, adrenocortical insufficiency, respiratory acidosis or chronic obstructive pulmonary disease.

Adverse Effects

Adverse effects of carbonic anhydrase inhibitors are related to the disturbances in acid–base and electrolyte balances. Metabolic acidosis is a relatively common and potentially dangerous effect that occurs when bicarbonate is lost. Hypokalaemia is also common, because potassium excretion is increased as the tubule loses potassium in an attempt to retain some of the sodium that is being excreted. Patients also complain of paresthesia (tingling) of the extremities, confusion, and drowsiness, all of which are probably related to the neural effect of the electrolyte changes.

Clinically Important Drug–Drug Interactions

There may be an increased excretion of salicylates and lithium if they are combined with these drugs. Caution should be used to monitor serum levels of patients taking lithium.

Always check the most up-to-date copy of the British National Formulary (BNF) for interactions and contraindications

Potassium-Sparing Diuretics

The potassium-sparing diuretics include amiloride and spironolactone. They are used for patients who are at a high risk of hypokalaemia associated with diuretic use, for example patients with cardiac arrhythmias receiving digitalis. These diuretics are not as powerful as the loop diuretics, but they retain potassium instead of promoting excretion.

Therapeutic Actions and Indications

Spironolactone acts as an aldosterone antagonist, blocking the actions of aldosterone in the distal convoluted tubule.

Amiloride blocks potassium secretion through the tubule. The diuretic effect of these drugs comes from the balance achieved in losing sodium to offset potassium retained.

Potassium-sparing diuretics are often used as adjuncts with thiazide or loop diuretics or in patients who are especially at risk if hypokalaemia develops, such as patients taking certain antiarrhythmics or digoxin and those who have particular neurological conditions. Spironolactone, the most frequently prescribed of these drugs, is the drug of choice for treating **hyperaldosteronism**, a condition where there is an over secretion of aldosterone, hyperaldosteronism is often seen in cirrhosis of the liver and nephritic syndrome.

Pharmacokinetics

These drugs are well absorbed and widely distributed bound to protein. They are metabolized in the liver and primarily excreted in urine. These diuretics cross the placenta and enter breast milk. Routine use during pregnancy is not appropriate and should be saved for situations in which the mother has pathological reasons for use.

Contraindications and Cautions

These drugs are contraindicated for use in patients with allergy to the drug, hyperkalaemia, renal disease or anuria. They are also contraindicated in patients taking amiloride. They are given cautiously during pregnancy and lactation, in patients with diabetes mellitus and the elderly.

Adverse Effects

The most common adverse effect of potassium-sparing diuretics is hyperkalaemia, which can cause lethargy, confusion, ataxia, muscle cramps and cardiac arrhythmias. Patients taking these drugs need to be evaluated regularly for signs of increased potassium and informed about the signs and symptoms to watch for. They should also be advised to avoid foods that are high in potassium.

Clinically Important Drug–Drug Interactions

The diuretic effect decreases if potassium-sparing diuretics are combined with salicylates. Dosage adjustment may be necessary to achieve therapeutic effects. Potassium supplements must not be given with potassium-sparing diuretics. Administration of a potassium-sparing diuretic to a patient receiving an ACE inhibitor or an angiotensin II receptor antagonist can cause severe hyperkalaemia.

Always check the most up-to-date copy of the British National Formulary (BNF) for interactions and contraindications

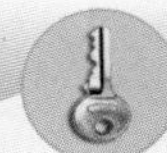

Prototype Summary: *Spironolactone*

Indications: Primary hyperaldosteronism, adjunctive therapy in the treatment of oedema associated with coronary heart failure, nephritic syndrome, hepatic cirrhosis; essential hypertension.

Actions: Competitively blocks the effects of aldosterone in the renal tubule, causing loss of sodium and water and retention of potassium. Cautions in the elderly; porphyria, hepatic and renal impairment pregnancy and breast-feeding.

Pharmacokinetics:

Route	Onset	Peak	Duration
Oral	24–48 h	48–72 h	48–72 h

$T_{1/2}$: 20 hours; metabolized in the liver and excreted in urine

Adverse effects: Dizziness, headache, drowsiness, rash, cramping, diarrhoea, hyperkalaemia, hirsutism, deepening of the voice, irregular menses, hyponatraemia, hepatotoxicity, osteomalacia and blood disorders.

Osmotic Diuretics

Osmotic diuretics pull water into the renal tubule without sodium loss. They are the diuretics of choice in cases of increased cranial pressure or acute renal failure due to shock, drug overdose or trauma. They may also be used to reduce IOP in the treatment of glaucoma. Osmotic diuretics are rarely used in heart failure as they may acutely expand blood volume.

Therapeutic Actions and Indications

Mannitol is a sugar that is not well reabsorbed by the tubules; it acts to pull large amounts of fluid into the urine by the osmotic pull of the large sugar molecule. The result is loss of large amounts of fluid in the urine. The effects of these osmotic drugs are not limited to the kidneys, because the injected substance pulls fluid into the vascular system from extra-vascular spaces, including the aqueous humour. Therefore, these drugs are often used in acute situations when it is necessary to decrease IOP before eye surgery or during acute attacks of glaucoma. Mannitol is also used to decrease intracranial pressure, to prevent the oliguric phase of renal failure and to promote the movement of toxic substances through the kidneys.

Pharmacokinetics

These drugs are freely filtered at the renal glomerulus, poorly reabsorbed by the renal tubule, not secreted by the tubule, and resistant to metabolism. Their action depends on the concentration of the osmotic activity in the solution. It is not known whether these drugs can cause foetal harm, so their use during pregnancy should be limited to situations in which the benefit to the mother outweighs the potential risk to the foetus. Effects of these drugs during lactation are not well understood; because of the potential for risk to the neonate or changes in the fluid balance of the mother, caution should be used if one of these drugs is needed during lactation.

Contraindications and Cautions

Renal disease and anuria from severe renal disease, pulmonary oedema, intracranial bleeding, dehydration and coronary heart failure are contraindications for use.

Always check the most up-to-date copy of the British National Formulary (BNF) for interactions and contraindications

Adverse Effects

The most common and potentially dangerous adverse effect related to osmotic diuretics is the sudden drop in body fluid levels. Nausea, vomiting, hypotension, light-headedness, chills and fever, confusion and headache can be accompanied by hypovolaemic shock. Patients receiving these drugs should be closely monitored for fluid and electrolyte imbalance.

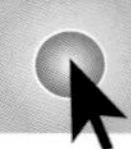

WEB LINKS

Health care providers and patients may want to consult the following Internet sources:

http://www.bpassoc.org.uk/BloodPressureandyou/Thebasics/Whatishigh The Blood Pressure Association provides guidance and information relating to hypertension and the measurement of blood pressure.

http://www.bnf.org.uk The BNF provides UK health care professionals with authoritative and practical information on the selection and clinical use of medicines.

http://cks.library.nhs.uk The NHS Clinical Knowledge Summaries provides evidence-based practical information on the common conditions observed in primary care.

http://www.nhsdirect.nhs.uk The NHS Direct service provides patients with information and advice about health, illness and health services.

http://www.nice.org.uk The NICE is an independent organization responsible for providing national guidance on promoting good health and preventing and treating ill health.

Points to Remember

- Diuretics are drugs that increase the excretion of sodium, and therefore water, from the kidneys.
- Diuretics are used in the treatment of oedema associated with coronary heart failure and pulmonary oedema, liver failure and cirrhosis, and various types of renal disease and as adjuncts in the treatment of hypertension.
- Diuretics must be used cautiously in any condition that would be exacerbated by changes in fluid and electrolyte balance.
- Adverse effects associated with diuretics include electrolyte imbalance (potassium, sodium, chloride); hypotension and hypovolaemia; hypoglycaemia and metabolic alkalosis.
- Classes of diuretics differ in their site of action and intensity of effects. Thiazide diuretics work to block the chloride pump in the distal convoluted tubule. This effect leads to a loss of sodium and potassium and a minor loss of water. Thiazides are frequently used alone or in combination with other drugs to treat hypertension. They are considered to be mild diuretics.
- Loop diuretics work in the loop of the nephron and have a powerful diuretic effect, leading to the loss of water, sodium and potassium. These drugs are the most potent diuretics and are used in acute situations as well as chronic conditions not responsive to milder diuretics.
- Carbonic anhydrase inhibitors work to block the formation of carbonic acid and bicarbonate in the renal tubule. These drugs can cause an alkaline urine and loss of the bicarbonate buffer. Carbonic anhydrase inhibitors are used in combination with other diuretics when a stronger diuresis is needed, and they are frequently used to treat glaucoma because they decrease the amount of aqueous humour produced in the eye.
- Potassium-sparing diuretics are mild diuretics that act to spare potassium in exchange for the loss of sodium and water in the urine. These diuretics are preferable if potassium loss could be detrimental to a patient's cardiac or neuromuscular condition. Patients must be careful not to become hyperkalaemic while taking these drugs.
- Osmotic diuretics use hypertonic pull to remove fluid from the intravascular spaces and to deliver large amounts of water into the renal tubule. There is a danger of sudden change of fluid volume and massive fluid loss with some of these drugs. These drugs are used to decrease intracranial pressure, to treat glaucoma and to help push toxic substances through the kidney.
- Patients receiving diuretics need to be monitored for fluid loss and retention (daily weights, blood pressure, skin evaluation, urinary output) have periodic electrolyte evaluations; particularly potassium levels and blood glucose determinations; and have evaluations of the effectiveness of their teaching programme.

CRITICAL THINKING SCENARIO 50-1

Using Furosemide in Congestive Heart Failure

The Situation

Mary is a 68-year-old woman with rheumatic mitral valve heart disease. She has refused any surgical intervention and has developed progressively worsening coronary heart failure. Recently furosemide, 40 mg/day (to be taken in the morning) was prescribed for her along with digoxin. After 10 days with the new prescription, Mary presents herself at the NHS walk-in centre and reports extensive ankle swelling and difficulty in breathing. She is referred to A&E for immediate review.

Critical Thinking

Think about the physiology of mitral valve disease and the progression of coronary heart disease in this patient. *How does furosemide work in the body?*

Discussion

An incompetent mitral valve leads to turbulent blood flow in the left atria, this in turn leads to congestion in the pulmonary system. This pulmonary congestion will eventually lead to systemic congestion (*think about the organization of the systemic and pulmonary circulations*). Over time this will lead to an enlarged and overworked left ventricle. Drug therapy for a patient with this disorder is usually aimed at decreasing the workload of the heart as much as possible to maintain cardiac output. Digoxin increases the contractility of the heart muscle, leads to an increase in cardiac output, which should improve perfusion of the kidneys.

Furosemide, a loop diuretic, acts on the loop of the nephron to block the reabsorption of sodium and hence water which leads to diuresis, this decreases the volume of blood the heart needs to pump thus reducing workload on the heart. As the blood becomes more hypertonic, it draws fluid from the tissues into circulation therefore reducing peripheral oedema where it can be acted on by the kidney, leading to further diuresis.

Mary should be encouraged to maintain fluid intake and her potassium levels should be monitored regularly (this is especially important because she is also taking digoxin, which is very sensitive to potassium levels), her oedematous limbs should be elevated periodically during the day and she should monitor her sodium intake. Coronary heart failure is a progressive, incurable disease, so patient education is a very important part of the overall management regimen.

Nursing Care Guide for Mary: Diuretic Agents

Clinically Important Drug–Drug Interactions

The risk of ototoxicity increases if loop diuretics are combined with aminoglycosides or cisplatin. Anticoagulation effects may increase if these drugs are given with anticoagulants. There may also be a decreased loss of sodium and decreased antihypertensive effects if these drugs are combined with indomethacin, ibuprofen, salicylates or other NSAIDS. The patient receiving this combination should be monitored closely and appropriate dosage adjustments should be made.

Assessment: History and Examination

Assess Mary's health history including allergies to diuretics, fluid or electrolyte disturbances, gout, glucose tolerance abnormalities, liver disease, systemic lupus erythematosus.

Focus the physical examination on the following areas:

- Skin: colour, texture, oedema
- Cardiovascular: blood pressure, pulse, cardiac and pulmonary auscultation
- GI: liver function and blood glucose levels.
- GU: urinary output

Laboratory tests: ECG, haematology, serum electrolytes, cardiac enzymes, glucose, uric acid, liver function tests, chest X-ray, arterial blood gases.

Nursing Diagnoses

- Risk for deficient fluid volume related to diuretic effect
- Impaired urinary elimination
- Imbalanced nutrition: reduced intake related to GI upset and metabolic changes
- Patient deficient in knowledge regarding drug therapy

Implementation

Obtain daily weights and monitor urine output.

Administer drug early in day.

Provide support and reassurance to deal with drug effects and lifestyle changes.

Provide patient education regarding drug name, dosage, side-effects, precautions, warnings to report, daily weighing and recording dietary changes as needed.

(continued)

Using Furosemide in Congestive Heart Failure *(continued)*

Evaluation

Evaluate drug effects: urinary output, weight changes, status of oedema, blood pressure changes and electrolyte imbalance.

Monitor for adverse effects: hypotension, hypokalaemia, hyperkalaemia, hypocalcaemia, hypercalcaemia, hyperglycaemia, increased uric acid levels.

Monitor for drug–drug interactions as indicated.

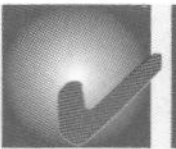

CHECK YOUR UNDERSTANDING

Answers to the questions in this chapter may be found in the answer key in the back of the book.

Multiple Choice

Select the most appropriate response to the following:

1. Most diuretics act in the body to cause
   a. loss of water.
   b. loss of sodium.
   c. retention of potassium.
   d. retention of chloride.

2. Diuretics cause a loss of blood volume in the body. The drop in volume activates compensatory mechanisms to restore the volume, including
   a. suppression of ADH release.
   b. suppression of aldosterone release.
   c. activation of the renin–angiotensin system with increased ADH and aldosterone.
   d. stimulation of the countercurrent mechanism.

3. Thiazide diuretics are considered mild diuretics because they
   a. block the sodium/potassium/chloride pump in the loop of the nephron.
   b. block the chloride pump, which causes loss of sodium and chloride but little water.
   c. do not cause a fluid rebound when they work in the kidneys.
   d. have no effect on electrolytes.

4. A loop diuretic would be the drug of choice in treating
   a. hypertension.
   b. shock.
   c. pulmonary oedema.
   d. fluid retention during pregnancy.

5. Any patient receiving a loop diuretic needs to have regular monitoring of
   a. sodium levels.
   b. bone marrow function.
   c. calcium levels.
   d. potassium levels.

6. The diuretic of choice for treating hyperaldosteronism would be
   a. spironolactone.
   b. furosemide.
   c. hydrochlorothiazide.
   d. acetazolamide.

7. A patient with severe glaucoma who is about to undergo eye surgery would benefit from a decrease in intraocular fluid. This is often best accomplished by giving the patient
   a. a loop diuretic.
   b. a thiazide diuretic.
   c. a carbonic anhydrase inhibitor.
   d. an osmotic diuretic.

8. Patients receiving diuretics should be taught to report
   a. improved vision.
   b. weight loss of 0.5 kg/day.
   c. muscle pain or cramping.
   d. increased urination.

Extending Matching Questions

Select all that apply.

1. Diuretics are currently recommended for the treatment of which of the following?
   a. Hypertension
   b. Renal disease
   c. Obesity
   d. Severe liver disease
   e. Fluid retention during pregnancy
   f. coronary heart failure

2. Routine nursing care of a client receiving a diuretic would include which of the following?
   a. Daily weights
   b. Tight fluid restrictions

c. Periodic electrolyte evaluations
d. Monitoring of urinary output
e. Regular IOP testing
f. Teaching the patient to report muscle cramping

Definitions

Define the following terms.

1. Oedema ______________________
2. Fluid rebound ______________________
3. Thiazide diuretic ______________________
4. Hypokalaemia ______________________
5. High-ceiling diuretics ______________________
6. Alkalosis ______________________
7. Hyperaldosteronism ______________________
8. Osmotic pull ______________________

Matching

Match the diuretic with the appropriate class. Some classes can be used more than once.

1. __________ acetazolamide
2. __________ furosemide
3. __________ bendroflumethiazide
4. __________ mannitol
5. __________ spironolactone
6. __________ hydrochlorothiazide
7. __________ amiloride
8. __________ bumetanide

A. Osmotic
B. Thiazide
C. Loop
D. Potassium-sparing
E. Carbonic anhydrase inhibitor

Bibliography and References

British Medical Association and Royal Pharmaceutical Society of Great Britain. (2008). *British National Formulary*. London: BMJ & RPS Publishing. *This publication is updated biannually: it is imperative that the most recent edition is consulted.*

British Medical Association and Royal Pharmaceutical Society of Great Britain. (2008). *British National Formulary for Children*. London: BMJ & RPS Publishing. *This publication is updated annually: it is imperative that the most recent edition is consulted.*

British Hypertension Society. (2004). *Latest British Hypertension Society guidelines for the management of hypertension.* Available from http://www.bhsoc.org

Ganong, W. (2005). *Review of medical physiology* (22nd ed.). New York: McGraw-Hill.

Howland, R. D,. & Mycek, M. J. (2005). *Pharmacology* (3rd ed.). Philadelphia: Lippincott Williams & Wilkins.

Marieb, E. N,. & Hoehn, K. (2004). *Human anatomy & physiology* (7th ed.). San Francisco: Pearson Benjamin Cummings.

Porth, C. M., & Matfin G. (2008). *Pathophysiology: Concepts of altered health states* (8th ed.). Philadelphia: Lippincott Williams & Wilkins.

Simonsen, T., Aarbakke, J., Kay, I., Coleman, I., Sinnott, P., & Lysaa, R. (2006). *Illustrated pharmacology for nurses.* London: Hodder Arnold.

CHAPTER 51

Drugs Affecting the Urinary Tract and the Bladder

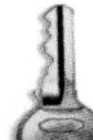

KEY TERMS

acidification

antispasmodics

benign prostatic hyperplasia (BPH)

cystitis

dysuria

nocturia

pyelonephritis

urgency

urinary frequency and incontinence

LEARNING OBJECTIVES

Upon completion of this chapter, you will be able to:

1. Describe four common problems associated with the urinary tract and the clinical manifestations of these problems.
2. Describe the therapeutic actions, indications, pharmacokinetics, contraindications, most common adverse reactions and important drug–drug interactions associated with urinary tract antispasmodics, anti-infectives, analgesics and drugs used to treat benign prostatic hyperplasia.
3. Discuss the use of drugs affecting the urinary tract and bladder across the lifespan.
4. Compare and contrast the key drugs norfloxacin, oxybutynin and doxazosin with other agents in their class.
5. Outline the nursing considerations, including important teaching points, for patients receiving drugs affecting the urinary tract and bladder.

URINARY TRACT ANTI-INFECTIVES

methenamine hippurate

nalidixic acid

nitrofurantoin

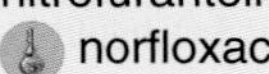 norfloxacin

URINARY TRACT ANTISPASMODICS

flavoxate

oxybutynin

solifenacin

propiverine

trospium

tolterodine

DRUGS USED TO TREAT BENIGN PROSTATIC HYPERPLASIA

alfuzosin

doxazosin

dutasteride

finasteride

tamsulosin

terazosin

One of the most common infections affecting the British population is acute urinary tract infections (UTIs). Females, with shorter urethras, are particularly vulnerable to repeated bladder and even kidney infections. Children also may have frequent problems. Patients with indwelling catheters or intermittent catheterizations are often affected by bladder infections or **cystitis**, resulting from bacteria introduced into the bladder by these devices. Blockage anywhere in the urinary tract can lead to back-flow problems and the spread of bladder infections into the kidney.

The signs and symptoms of a UTI are uncomfortable and include **urinary frequency and incontinence**; **urgency**; burning on urination (associated with cystitis); and chills, fever, lumbar (loin) pain and tenderness (associated with acute **pyelonephritis** infection of the kidney). To treat these infections, clinicians use antibiotics (see Chapter 8), as well as specific agents that reach antibacterial levels only in the kidney and bladder and are thought to sterilize the urinary tract. The use of urinary tract agents across the lifespan are discussed in Box 51.1.

Drugs are also available to block spasms of the urinary tract muscles, decrease urinary tract pain, protect the cells of the bladder from irritation and treat enlargement of the prostate gland. All of these agents are discussed in this chapter.

Urinary Tract Anti-infectives

Urinary tract anti-infectives are of two types. One type is the antibiotics, which include the following:

- Norfloxacin, a newer and more broad-spectrum drug, is effective against a wide range of gram-negative strains. This drug is rapidly absorbed and undergoes hepatic metabolism and renal excretion. Dosage must be reduced in the presence of renal impairment. This drug crosses the placenta and enters breast milk and should not be used during pregnancy or lactation unless the benefit to the mother clearly outweighs the potential risk to the foetus or neonate.
- Nalidixic acid is an older drug that is not effective against as many strains of gram-negative bacteria as the other antibiotics used for UTIs. This drug is rapidly absorbed, metabolized in the liver and excreted in urine. It has a short half-life – 1 to 2.5 hours. It is known to cross the placenta and to enter breast milk, so it should not be used during pregnancy or lactation. It is available in a suspension form and has an established dosage for children ages 3 months to 12 years.
- Nitrofurantoin is another older drug with a very short half-life (20–60 minutes). It is not effective against as many gram-negative bacteria as the newer drugs are, but it has been successfully used for suppression therapy in adults and children with chronic UTIs. It is metabolized in the liver and excreted in urine. It is not recommended during pregnancy or lactation because of the potential for adverse effects on the neonate or baby.

The other type of urinary tract anti-infective works to acidify the urine, killing bacteria that might be in the bladder. This group includes the following drug:

Methenamine hippurate undergoes metabolism in the liver and is excreted in urine. It crosses the placenta and enters breast milk and should not be used during pregnancy or lactation. Methenamine hippurate requires acid urine to

BOX 51.1 DRUG THERAPY ACROSS THE LIFESPAN

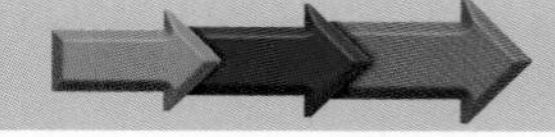

Urinary Tract Agents

CHILDREN

Children often have cystitis and need to be treated with a urinary tract agent. Some children, because of congenital problems or indwelling catheters, require other urinary tract agents.

Children need to be instructed in proper hygiene and should not be given bubble baths if UTIs occur. They should be encouraged to avoid the alkaline juices and urged to drink lots of water.

If an antispasmodic is needed, oxybutynin is indicated for children >5 years of age and flavoxate can be used in children >12 years. The child and parent/guardian should be warned the medication may cause a change in urine colour.

When administering any drug to children, always consult the most recent edition of the British National Formulary (BNF) for Children.

ADULTS

Adults need to be advised about the various measures that can reduce the risks of developing a UTI. They should be encouraged to drink plenty of fluids to maintain bladder health.

If taking an anticholinergic to block spasm, adult patients need to be advised of other precautions to take when the parasympathetic system is blocked.

Adult men being treated for benign prostatic hyperplasia (BPH) need to be aware of the possibility of decreased sexual function, as well as fatigue, lethargy and the potential for dizziness, which could interfere with working or activities of daily living.

The use of urinary tract agents during pregnancy should be approached with caution.

OLDER ADULTS

Older adults often have other medical conditions. They are also more likely to have renal or hepatic impairment, which requires caution in the use of these drugs. Older adults should be started on the lowest possible dose of the drug and it should be titrated slowly based on patient response. Special precautions to monitor cardiac function, intraocular pressure, blood pressure and bladder emptying need to be taken when using α-adrenergic blockers with these patients. Older patients may have a difficult time maintaining fluid intake and might benefit from extra encouragement to drink fluids.

be effective (BNF, 2008). It does seem to partially create acid urine via hippuric acid; however, acidification of urine could be ensured by the administration of ammonium chlorine or ascorbic acid (BNF, 2008). Methenamine hippurate has established dosage guidelines for children and comes in a suspension form.

Therapeutic Actions and Indications

Urinary tract antibacterial drugs act specifically within the urinary tract to destroy bacteria, either through a direct antibiotic effect or through **acidification** of the urine. They do not generally have an antibiotic effect systemically, being activated or effective only in the urinary tract (Figure 51.1). They are used to treat chronic UTIs, as adjunctive therapy in acute cystitis and pyelonephritis and as prophylaxis with urinary tract anatomical abnormalities and residual urine disorders.

Contraindications and Cautions

These drugs should be used with caution in the presence of renal dysfunction, which could interfere with the excretion and action of these drugs and with pregnancy and lactation because of the potential for adverse effects on the foetus or neonate.

Adverse Effects

Likely effects associated with these drugs include nausea, vomiting, diarrhoea, anorexia, bladder irritation and dysuria.

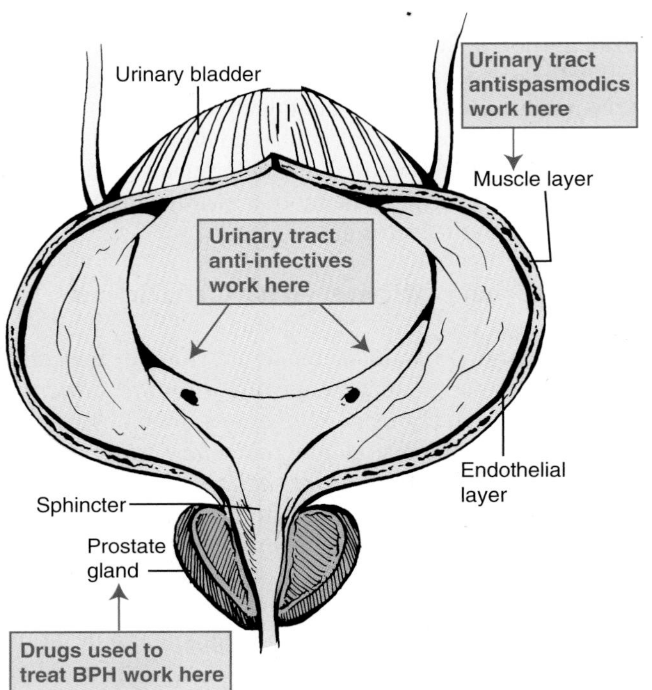

FIGURE 51.1 Sites of action of drugs acting on the urinary tract.

These effects may result from GI irritation caused by the agent, therefore it should be recommended the drug is taken with food. Other symptoms include headache, dizziness, nervousness and confusion.

Nursing Considerations for Patients Receiving Urinary Tract Anti-infectives

Assessment: History and Examination

Screen for the following conditions:

- history of allergy
- liver or renal dysfunction
- pregnancy and lactation.

Physical assessment should be done to establish baseline data for assessing the effectiveness of the drug and the occurrence of any adverse effects associated with drug therapy. Assess for the following:

- skin, to evaluate for the development of rash or hypersensitivity reactions
- orientation and reflexes, to evaluate any CNS effects of the drug
- renal and hepatic function tests, to determine baseline function of these organs.

Establish if patient is currently taking other medications or herbal therapies which may potentially interact with the urinary tract anti-infectives.

Nursing Diagnoses

The patients may have symptoms related to drug therapy:

- Acute pain related to GI, CNS or skin effects of drug
- Disturbed sensory perception (kinaesthetic, tactile, visual) related to CNS effects
- Deficient knowledge regarding drug therapy

Implementation With Rationale

- Ensure that culture and sensitivity tests are performed before therapy begins and repeated if the response is not as expected, to ensure appropriate treatment of the infection.
- Administer the drugs with food to decrease GI adverse effects if they occur.
- Advise patients to complete the full course of medication prescribed and not to stop taking it as soon as the uncomfortable signs and symptoms have resolved, to ensure elimination of the infection and prevent reoccurrence or the development of resistant strains of bacteria.

- Encourage the patient to drink lots of fluids (unless contraindicated by other conditions) to flush the bladder and urinary tract frequently and decrease the opportunity for bacteria growth.
- Educate patients with chronic UTIs about additional activities that can facilitate acidic urine to increase the effectiveness of urinary tract anti-infectives. For example, all patients should
  - avoid foods that cause an alkaline ash and produce alkaline urine (e.g. antacids).
  - drink high-acid cranberry juice.
  - empty the bladder after sexual intercourse, to help clear any invading organisms.
  - in addition, women should avoid baths if possible, especially bubble baths (because the bubbles act as transport agents to deliver bacteria through the short urethra).
  - after visiting the toilet, wipe front to back and never back to front, which introduces *Escherichia coli* and other agents to the urethra.
- Provide thorough patient education, including the drug name and prescribed dosage, measures to help avoid adverse effects, warning signs that may indicate problems and the need for periodic monitoring and evaluation, to enhance patient knowledge about drug therapy and to promote compliance.

Evaluation

- Monitor patient response to the drug (resolution of UTI and relief of signs and symptoms); repeat culture and sensitivity tests are recommended for evaluation of the effectiveness of all of these drugs.
- Monitor for adverse effects (skin evaluation, orientation and reflexes, GI effects).
- Evaluate the effectiveness of the teaching plan (patient can name drug, dosage, adverse effects to watch for, specific measures to avoid adverse effects and measures to take to increase the effectiveness of the drug).

Urinary Tract Antispasmodics

Urinary tract **antispasmodics** block the spasms of urinary tract muscles caused by various conditions. Examples of these drugs include the following:

- Flavoxate prevents smooth muscle spasm specifically in the urinary tract, but it is associated with central nervous system (CNS) effects (blurred vision, dizziness, confusion).
- Oxybutynin is a potent urinary antispasmodic, but it has numerous anticholinergic effects, decreased sweating, urinary retention, tachycardia and changes in GI activity. It is available in an oral as well as a dermal patch form for the treatment of overactive bladder.
- Tolterodine, solifenacin and propiverine are newer agents that block muscarinic receptors, preventing bladder contraction and spasm. They are indicated for the treatment of overactive bladder in patients who exhibit urinary frequency, urgency, or incontinence.
- Trospium is the newest drug approved to block urinary tract spasms. It also specifically blocks muscarinic receptors and reduces the muscle tone of the bladder. It is specifically indicated for the treatment of overactive bladder with symptoms of urge urinary incontinence, urgency and urinary frequency.

Therapeutic Actions and Indications

Inflammation in the urinary tract, such as cystitis, prostatitis, urethritis and urethrocystitis/urethrotrigonitis, causes smooth muscle spasms along the urinary tract. Irritation of the urinary tract leading to muscle spasm also occurs in patients with neurogenic bladder. These spasms lead to the uncomfortable effects of **dysuria** (pain or discomfort with urination), urgency, incontinence, **nocturia** (recurrent night time urination) and suprapubic pain. The urinary tract antispasmodics relieve these spasms by blocking parasympathetic activity and relaxing the detrusor and other urinary tract muscles (see Figure 51.1).

Pharmacokinetics

These drugs are rapidly absorbed, widely distributed, metabolized in the liver and excreted in urine. Caution should be used in the presence of hepatic or renal impairment because of the potential of alterations in metabolism or excretion of the drugs. They cross the placenta and are found in breast milk, so they should be used during pregnancy and lactation only if the benefit to the mother clearly outweighs the potential risk to the foetus or neonate.

Contraindications and Cautions

These drugs are contraindicated with pyloric or duodenal obstruction or recent surgery *because the anticholinergic effects can cause serious complications;* with obstructive urinary tract problems, *which could be further aggravated by the blocking of muscle activity;* and with glaucoma, myasthenia gravis, or acute haemorrhage, *which could all be exacerbated by the anticholinergic effects of these drugs.* Caution should be used in patients with renal or hepatic dysfunction, *which could alter the metabolism and excretion of the drugs;* and in pregnant and lactating patients *because of potential adverse effects on the foetus or neonate secondary to the anticholinergic effects of the drugs.*

Adverse Effects

Adverse effects of urinary tract antispasmodics are related to the blocking of the parasympathetic system and include nausea, vomiting, dry mouth, nervousness, tachycardia and vision changes.

Clinically Important Drug–Drug Interactions

Decreased effectiveness of phenothiazines and haloperidol has been associated with the combination of these drugs with oxybutynin. If any such combinations must be used, the patient should be monitored closely and appropriate dosage adjustments made.

Always check the most up-to-date edition of the British National Formulary (BNF) for interactions and contraindications.

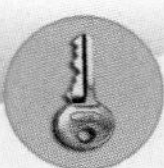

Key Drug Summary: *Oxybutynin*

Indications: Relief of symptoms of bladder instability associated with uninhibited neurogenic and reflex neurogenic bladder; treatment of signs and symptoms of overactive bladder

Actions: Acts directly to relax smooth muscle in the bladder; inhibits the effects of acetylcholine at muscarinic receptors

Pharmacokinetics:

Route	Onset	Peak	Duration
Oral	30–60 min	3–6 h	6–10 h

$T_{1/2}$: Unknown; metabolized in the liver and excreted in urine

Adverse effects: Drowsiness, dizziness, blurred vision, tachycardia, dry mouth, nausea, urinary hesitancy and decreased sweating

Nursing Considerations for Patients Receiving Urinary Tract Antispasmodics

Assessment: History and Examination

Screen for the following conditions:

- history of allergy
- pyloric or duodenal obstruction or other GI lesions or obstructions
- obstructions of the lower urinary tract
- glaucoma, which requires caution because of the blockage of the parasympathetic nervous system and the potential for increased intraocular pressure
- pregnancy or lactation, which require caution if using these drugs.

Physical assessment should be done to establish baseline status for assessing the effectiveness of the drug and the occurrence of any adverse effects associated with drug therapy. Assess the following: skin, to evaluate for the development of rash or hypersensitivity reactions; orientation and reflexes, *to evaluate any CNS effects of the drug*; ophthalmological examination including intraocular pressure, to assess for any *developing glaucoma*; and pulse, *to establish a baseline for evaluating the extent of parasympathetic blockade.*

Establish if patient is currently taking other medications or herbal therapies which may potentially interact with urinary tract antispasmodics.

Nursing Diagnoses

The patient receiving a urinary tract antispasmodic may have the following nursing diagnoses related to drug therapy:

- Acute pain related to GI, CNS
- Disturbed sensory perception (visual) related to CNS or ophthalmological effects
- Deficient knowledge regarding drug therapy

Implementation With Rationale

- Arrange for appropriate treatment of any underlying UTI, which may be causing the spasm.
- Arrange for an ophthalmological examination at the beginning of therapy and then periodically during long-term treatment to evaluate drug effects on intraocular pressure so that the drug can be stopped if intraocular pressure increases.
- Encourage the patient to continue treatment for the underlying cause of the spasm to treat the cause and prevent the return of the signs and symptoms.
- Provide patient teaching, including the drug name and prescribed dosage, measures to help avoid adverse effects, warning signs that may indicate problems and the need for periodic monitoring and evaluation to enhance patient knowledge about drug therapy and to promote compliance.

Evaluation

- Monitor patient response to the drug
- Repeat culture and sensitivity tests are recommended for evaluation of the effectiveness of all of these drugs
- Monitor for adverse effects

Drugs for Treating Benign Prostatic Hyperplasia

Two types of drugs are currently used to relieve the symptoms of **benign prostatic hyperplasia (BPH)**, which is also called benign prostatic hypertrophy or enlarged prostate. α-Adrenergic blockers doxazosin, tamsulosin, alfuzosin and terazosin *are* used to block the dilation of arterioles in the bladder and urinary tract. Tamsulosin was developed specifically for the treatment of BPH and is not associated with as many adverse adrenergic-blocking effects as the other agents. Finasteride is specifically used to treat BPH by blocking testosterone production and is associated with more androgen-blocking effects than the other drugs. Dutasteride is the newest androgen hormone inhibitor used to treat BPH.

Therapeutic Actions and Indications

BPH is a common problem in men and it increases in incidence with age. This enlargement of the gland surrounding the urethra leads to discomfort, difficulty in initiating a stream of urine, feelings of bloating and an increased incidence of cystitis. α-Adrenergic blockers are indicated for the treatment of symptomatic BPH. These drugs block postsynaptic α_1 adrenergic receptors, which results in dilation of arterioles and veins and a relaxation of sympathetic effects on the bladder and urinary tract. These drugs are also indicated for treating hypertension (see Chapter 42).

Finasteride and dutasteride inhibit the intracellular enzyme that converts testosterone to a potent androgen dihydrotestosterone (DHT), which the prostate gland depends on for its development and maintenance (see Figure 51.1). They are used for long-term therapy to shrink the prostate and relieve the symptoms of hyperplasia. Finasteride is also used to prevent male pattern baldness in patients with a strong family history.

When any of these drugs are used, it is important to make sure that the prostate enlargement is benign and not caused by cancer, infection, stricture, or hypotonic bladder. Patients receiving long-term therapy need to be reassessed periodically.

Pharmacokinetics

The α_1-selective adrenergic-blocking agents are well absorbed and undergo extensive hepatic metabolism. Therefore, they must be used with caution in patients with hepatic impairment. They are excreted in urine. Finasteride and dutasteride are rapidly absorbed from the GI tract, undergo hepatic metabolism and are excreted in faeces and urine. Women must be cautioned not to touch finasteride or dutasteride because of the risk of absorption through the skin.

Contraindications and Cautions

These drugs are contraindicated in patients who are allergic to the drugs. Caution should be used in patients with hepatic or renal dysfunction, *which could alter the metabolism and excretion of the drugs.* The adrenergic blockers should be used with caution in patients with congestive heart failure or known coronary disease.

Adverse Effects

Adverse effects of α-adrenergic blockers include headache, fatigue, dizziness, postural dizziness, lethargy, tachycardia, hypotension, GI upset and sexual dysfunction, all of which are effects seen with blockade of the α-receptors. Finasteride and dutasteride are associated with decreased libido, impotence and sexual dysfunction, all of which are related to decreased levels of DHT. Patients using either of these drugs cannot donate blood for 6 months after the last dose to protect potential blood recipients.

Clinically Important Drug–Drug Interactions

There is a possibility of decreased theophylline levels if it is combined with these drugs. The patient should be monitored and appropriate dosage adjustments made if this combination is used.

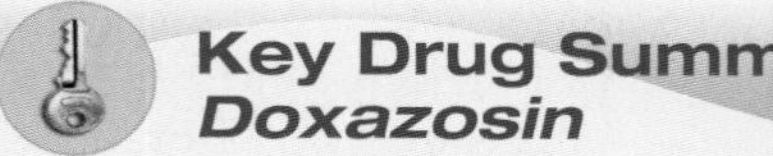

Key Drug Summary: Doxazosin

Indications: Treatment of benign prostatic hyperplasia (BPH)

Actions: Blocks postsynaptic α_1-adrenergic receptors, which results in a dilation of arterioles and veins and a relaxation of sympathetic effects on the bladder and urinary tract.

Pharmacokinetics:

Route	Onset	Peak
Oral	Varies	2–3 h

$T_{1/2}$: 22 hours; metabolized in the liver and excreted in urine, bile and faeces

Adverse effects: Headache, fatigue, dizziness, postural dizziness, lethargy, vertigo, tachycardia, palpitations, nausea, dyspepsia, diarrhoea, erectile dysfunction, rash, depression, oedema, blurred vision. This drug should be avoided in patients with a history of postural hypotension.

Nursing Considerations for Patients Receiving Drugs to Treat Benign Prostatic Hyperplasia (BPH)

Assessment: History and Examination

Screen for the following conditions:

- History of allergy
- History of congestive heart failure
- Renal or hepatic failure, *which would require caution when using these drugs.*

Physical assessment should be done *to establish baseline status for assessing the effectiveness of the drug and the occurrence of any adverse effects associated with drug therapy.* Assess the following:

- Blood pressure, pulse, cardiac/chest auscultation and perfusion, *to evaluate the cardiovascular effects of α-adrenergic blockade*
- Urinalysis and normal urinary function
- Prostate palpation and prostate-specific antigen (PSA) blood levels, *to evaluate prostate problems.*

Establish if patient is currently taking other medications or herbal therapies which may potentially interact with drugs used to treat BPH.

Nursing Diagnoses

The patient receiving a drug to treat BPH may have the following nursing diagnoses related to drug therapy:

- Sexual dysfunction related to drug effects
- Acute pain related to headache, CNS effects and GI effects of the drug
- Deficient knowledge regarding drug therapy

Implementation With Rationale

- Determine the presence of BPH and periodically evaluate through prostate examination and measurement of PSA levels *to reconfirm that no other problem is occurring.*
- Administer the drug without regard to meals, but give with meals *if GI upset is a problem.*
- Provide thorough patient teaching, including the drug name and prescribed dosage, measures to help avoid adverse effects, warning signs that may indicate problems and the need for periodic monitoring and evaluation, *to enhance patient knowledge about drug therapy and to promote compliance.*
- Offer support and encouragement *to help the patient cope with potential decreases in sexual functioning.*

Evaluation

- Monitor patient response to the drug (relief of signs and symptoms of BPH, improved urine flow, decrease in discomfort).
- Monitor for adverse effects.

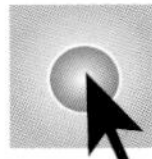

WEB LINKS

Health care providers and patients may want to consult the following Internet sources:

http://cks.library.nhs.uk The National Health Service Clinical Knowledge Summaries provides evidence-based practical information on the common conditions observed in primary care.

http://www.bnf.org.uk The BNF provides UK health care professionals with authoritative and practical information on the selection and clinical use of medicines.

http://www.cancerbackup.org.uk The UK's leading cancer information site: with over 6500 pages of up-to-date cancer information, practical advice and support for cancer patients, their families and carers.

http://www.christie.nhs.uk The Christie Hospital in Manchester is one of the leading cancer centres in Europe offering: high-quality diagnosis, treatment and care for cancer patients; world-class research and education in all aspects of cancer.

http://www.nhsdirect.nhs.uk The National Health Service Direct service provides patients with information and advice about health, illness and health services.

http://www.nice.org.uk National Institute for Health and Clinical Excellence is an independent organization responsible for providing national guidance on promoting good health and preventing and treating ill health.

Points to Remember

- Acute UTIs are second in frequency to respiratory tract infections in the British population.
- Urinary tract antibacterial agents are drugs used to kill bacteria in the urinary tract by producing acidic urine, which is undesirable to bacteria growth, or by acting to destroy bacteria in the urinary tract.
- Many activities are necessary to help decrease the bacteria in the urinary tract (e.g. hygiene measures, proper diet, forcing fluids), to facilitate the treatment of UTIs and help the urinary tract anti-infectives be more effective.
- Inflammation and irritation of the urinary tract can cause smooth muscle spasms along the urinary tract. These

spasms lead to the uncomfortable effects of dysuria, urgency, incontinence, nocturia and suprapubic pain.

- The urinary tract antispasmodics act to relieve spasms of the urinary tract muscles by blocking parasympathetic activity and relaxing the detrusor and other urinary tract muscles.
- BPH is a common enlargement of the prostate gland in older men.
- Drugs frequently used to relieve the signs and symptoms of prostate enlargement include α-adrenergic blockers, which relax the sympathetic effects on the bladder and sphincters and finasteride, which blocks the body's production of a powerful androgen. The prostate is dependent on testosterone for its maintenance and development, blocking the androgen leads to shrinkage of the gland and relief of symptoms.

CRITICAL THINKING SCENARIO 51-1

Teaching about Cystitis Treatment

The Situation

Rachel is a 6-year-old girl with a history of repeated UTIs. She is seen with complaints of dysuria, frequency, urgency and a low-grade fever. A urine sample is sent for culture and sensitivity testing. The doctor prescribes methenamine hippurate, 500 mg b.i.d. (every 12 hours) and refers Rachel and her mother to the nurse for teaching.

Critical Thinking

What is the best approach for this patient?
Think about the following points: What the drug is doing? How does it work? and How does it work best?

Discussion

Cystitis is very difficult to treat in young girls and can become a chronic problem. Patient and parent education is very important for trying to block the growth of bacteria and cure the infection.

To decrease the number of bacteria introduced into the bladder, patient education should cover the following hygiene measures: after visiting the toilet, always wipe from front to back and never from back to front, to avoid the introduction of intestinal bacteria into the urethra; avoid baths, particularly bubble baths, which facilitate the entry of bacteria into the urethra on the bubbles; and wear dry, cotton underwear to discourage bacterial growth.

Patient education should also stress the importance of avoiding alkaline foods (e.g. citrus fruits, certain vegetables) and encouraging foods that acidify the urine. Cranberry juice is often recommended as a choice of fruit juice because it helps to acidify the bladder and destroy bacteria. Fluid intake, especially water, should be encouraged as much as possible to keep the bladder flushed. Finally, the patient should be encouraged to complete the full course of medication prescribed and not to stop taking the drug when symptoms disappear.

Nursing Care Guide for Rachel: Urinary Tract Anti-Infective Methnamine Hippurate

Assessment: History and Examination

Assess Rachel's health history, particularly if she has any allergies. Assess for liver or renal dysfunction.

If Rachel were of childbearing age, you would assess pregnancy and breast-feeding status.

Focus the physical examination on the following areas:

- Skin: colour, texture
- GI: liver evaluation
- GU: urinary output
- Laboratory tests: liver function tests, urinalysis, urine culture and sensitivity testing

Nursing Diagnoses

Acute Pain related to GI, CNS, skin effects of drug

Disturbed Sensory Perception related to CNS effects

Implementation

Obtain urine sample for culture and sensitivity test.

Encourage eating acidifying foods and drinking lots of fluids.

Teach hygiene measures.

Administer medication with food if GI upset is a problem.

Provide support and reassurance to deal with drug effects

Provide patient education to Rachel and her parents/guardian regarding drug, dosage, adverse effects, precautions, warnings to report, hygiene measures and dietary changes as needed.

Evaluation

Evaluate drug effects: relief of symptoms, resolution of infection.

Monitor for adverse effects: GI upset, headache, dizziness, confusion, dysuria, urticaria.

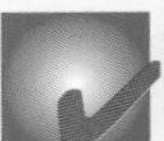

CHECK YOUR UNDERSTANDING

Answers to the questions in this chapter may be found in the answer key in the back of the book.

Multiple Choice

Select most appropriate response to the following.

1. Urinary tract. antispasmodics block the pain and discomfort associated with spasm in the smooth muscle of the urinary tract. The numerous adverse effects associated with these drugs are related to their:
   a. blockade of sympathetic β-receptors.
   b. stimulation of cholinergic receptors.
   c. stimulation of sympathetic receptors.
   d. blockade of cholinergic receptors.

2. BPH is a very common diagnosis in older men. Two types of drugs have been developed to treat the signs and symptoms of this disorder:
   a. α-adrenergic blockers and anticholinergic drugs.
   b. α-adrenergic blockers and testosterone production blockers.
   c. anticholinergic drugs and adrenergic stimulators.
   d. testosterone production blockers and adrenal androgens.

3. The drug of choice for treatment of BPH in a man with known hypotension might be
   a. doxazosin.
   b. terazosin.
   c. tamsulosin.
   d. propranolol.

4. Before administering a drug for the treatment of BPH, the nurse should ensure that the patient:
   a. has had a prostate examination and measurement of the PSA level.
   b. has not had a vasectomy.
   c. is still sexually active.
   d. is hypertensive and will tolerate the blood pressure-lowering effects.

5. A male who is very concerned about his hair loss and who is being treated for BPH might prefer treatment with
   a. doxazosin.
   b. finasteride.
   c. tamsulosin.
   d. terazosin.

Extended Matching Questions

Select **all** that apply.

1. In evaluating a client for the presence of a bladder infection, one would expect to find reports of which of the following?
   a. Frequency of urination
   b. Painful urination
   c. Oedema of the fingers and hands
   d. Urgency of urination
   e. Feelings of abdominal bloating
   f. Itching, scaly skin

2. Important educational points for clients with cystitis would include which of the following?
   a. Avoidance of bubble baths
   b. Voiding immediately after sexual intercourse
   c. After using the toilet always wiping from back to front
   d. Avoidance of foods which cause the urine to be alkaline
   e. Tight fluid restriction
   f. After using the toilet always wiping from front to back

True or False

Indicate whether the following statements are true (T) or false (F).

_____1. Acute UTIs are second in frequency to respiratory tract infections in the British population.

_____2. Urinary tract anti-infectives are used to kill bacteria in the urinary tract by producing alkaline urine or by destroying bacteria in the urinary tract.

_____3. There is nothing that can be done to help decrease the bacteria in the urinary tract.

_____4. Inflammation and irritation of the urinary tract can cause smooth muscle spasms, leading to the uncomfortable effects of dysuria, urgency, incontinence, nocturia and suprapubic pain.

_____5. The urinary tract antispasmodics relieve spasms of the urinary tract muscles by blocking sympathetic activity.

_____6. BPH is a rare condition that involves enlargement of the prostate gland in older males.

_____7. Drugs commonly used to relieve the signs and symptoms of prostate enlargement include α-adrenergic blockers, which relax the sympathetic effects on the bladder and sphincters and finasteride and dutasteride, which block the body's production of a powerful androgen.

Bibliography and References

British Medical Association and Royal Pharmaceutical Society of Great Britain. (2008). *British National Formulary*. London: BMJ & RPS Publishing. *This publication is updated biannually: it is imperative that the most recent edition is consulted.*

British Medical Association and Royal Pharmaceutical Society of Great Britain. (2008). *British National Formulary for Children*. London: BMJ & RPS Publishing. *This publication is updated annually: it is imperative that the most recent edition is consulted.*

Ganong, W. (2005). *Review of medical physiology* (22nd ed.). New York: McGraw-Hill.

Howland, R. D., & Mycek, M. J. (2005). *Pharmacology* (3rd ed.). Philadelphia: Lippincott Williams & Wilkins.

Marieb, E. N., & Hoehn, K. (2004). *Human anatomy & physiology* (7th ed.). San Francisco: Pearson Benjamin Cummings.

Porth, C. M., & Matfin G. (2008). *Pathophysiology: Concepts of altered health states* (8th ed.). Philadelphia: Lippincott Williams & Wilkins.

Simonsen, T., Aarbakke, J., Kay, I., Coleman, I., Sinnott, P., & Lysaa, R. (2006). *Illustrated pharmacology for nurses*. London: Hodder Arnold.

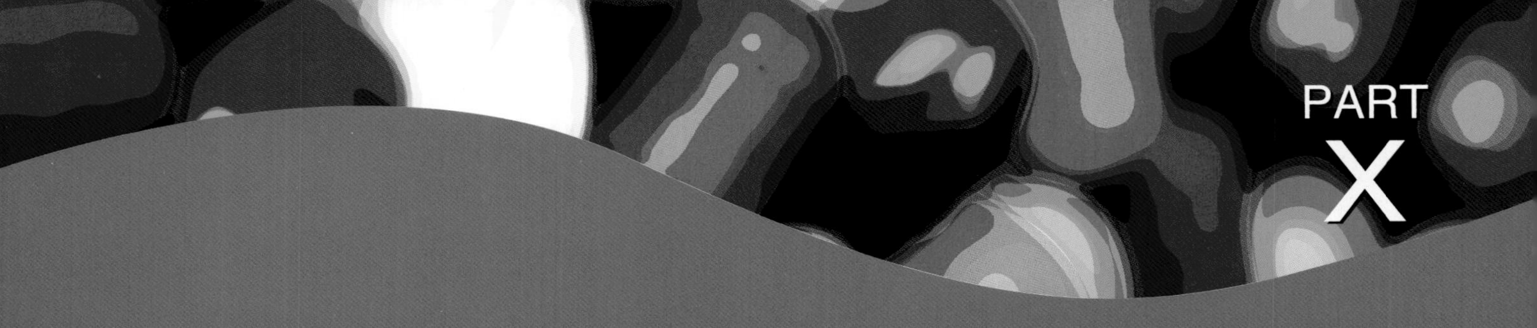

Drugs Acting on the Respiratory System

CHAPTER

52

Introduction to the Respiratory System

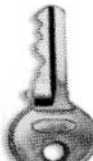

KEY TERMS

alveoli
asthma
bronchial tree
chronic obstructive pulmonary disease (COPD)
cilia
common cold
conducting zone
cough
cystic fibrosis
larynx
lower respiratory tract
pneumonia
respiration
respiratory distress syndrome (RDS)
respiratory membrane
respiratory zone
seasonal rhinitis
sinuses
sinusitis
sneeze
surfactant
trachea
upper respiratory tract
ventilation

LEARNING OBJECTIVES

Upon completion of this chapter, you will be able to:

1. Describe the parts of the respiratory system and explain the role of each part in respiration.
2. Describe the process of respiration and give clinical examples of problems that can arise with alterations in the respiratory membrane.
3. Differentiate between the common conditions that affect the upper respiratory system.
4. Identify three conditions involving the lower respiratory tract, including the clinical presentations of these conditions.
5. Discuss the process involved in obstructive respiratory diseases and correlate this to the signs and symptoms of these diseases.

The respiratory system is essential for survival. It brings oxygen into the body, allowing for the exchange of gases and expelling carbon dioxide and other waste products. The normal functioning of the respiratory system depends on an intricate balance of the nervous, cardiovascular and musculoskeletal systems. The respiratory system can be subdivided according to both position and function. When subdivided according to position, the respiratory system consists of the **upper respiratory tract** and the **lower respiratory tract.** The upper portion is composed of the nose, mouth, pharynx and larynx (Figure 52.1). The lower portion is made up of the trachea, **bronchial tree** and the **alveoli** (respiratory sacs). When the functions are considered, the respiratory system is divided into the **conducting zone** and the **respiratory zone.** The conducting zone consists of the nose, mouth, pharynx, larynx and upper bronchial tree, whereas the respiratory zone consists of respiratory bronchioles and alveolar sacs.

The Upper Respiratory Tract

Air usually moves into the body through the nose and into the nasal cavity. The nasal hairs catch and filter foreign substances that may be present in the inhaled air. The air is warmed and humidified as it passes by blood vessels close to the surface of the epithelial cells lining the nasal cavity. The epithelial lining contains goblet cells that produce mucus, which traps dust, microorganisms, pollen and any other foreign substances. The epithelial cells of this lining contain **cilia** – microscopic, hair-like projections of the plasma membrane – which are constantly moving and directing the mucus and any trapped substances down towards the throat (Figure 52.2).

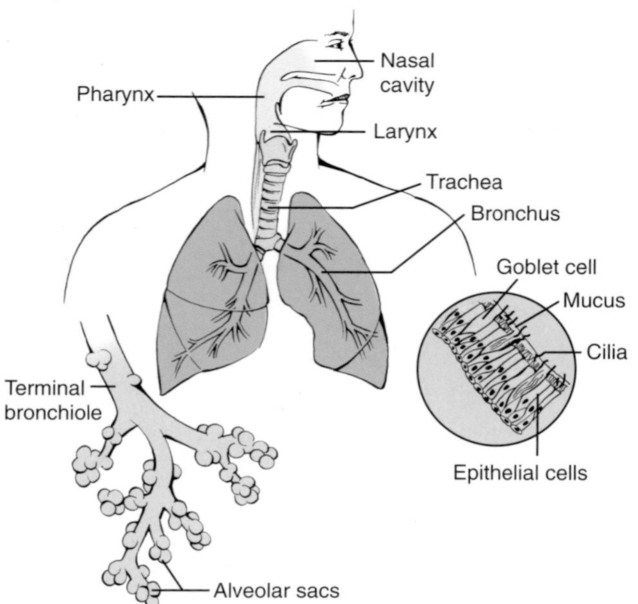

FIGURE 52.1 The respiratory tract.

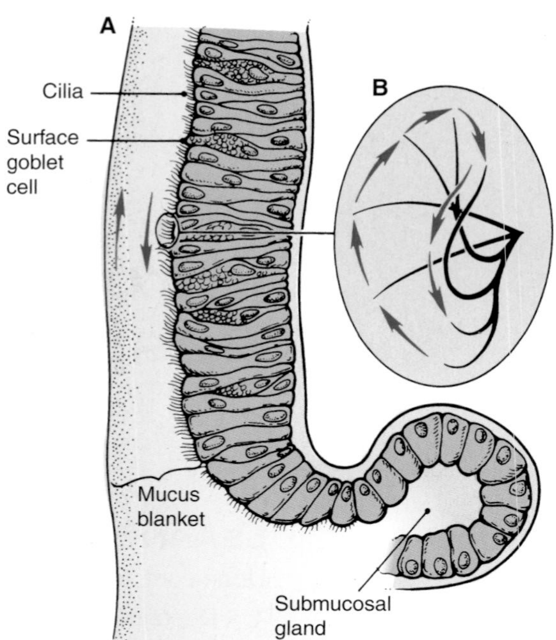

FIGURE 52.2 **(A)** The mucociliary escalator. **(B)** Conceptual scheme of ciliary movement, which allows forward motion to move the viscous gel layer and backward motion to occur entirely within the less viscous sol layer of the mucus blanket.

Air-filled passages in the skull known as **sinuses** open into the nasal cavity. Because the epithelial lining of the nasal passage is continuous with the lining of the sinuses, the mucus produced in the sinuses drains into the nasal cavity. From there, the mucus drains into the throat and is swallowed into the stomach, where gastric acid destroys foreign materials.

Air moves from the nasal cavity into the pharynx and **larynx.** The larynx contains the vocal chords and the epiglottis, which closes during swallowing to protect the lower respiratory tract from any foreign particles. From the larynx air proceeds to the **trachea,** which is lined by ciliated goblet cell-containing pseudostratified epithelium. The trachea is the main conducting airway into the lungs and the first component of the lower respiratory tract.

The Lower Respiratory Tract

The trachea divides into two main bronchi which further divide into smaller and smaller branches. All these tubes contain mucus-producing goblet cells and cilia to entrap any particles that may have escaped the upper protective mechanisms. The cilia move the mucus up the trachea and into the throat where it is swallowed.

The bronchial tubes are composed of three layers: cartilage, smooth muscle and epithelial cells. The cartilage keeps the tube open and becomes progressively less abundant as the bronchi divide and get smaller. The muscle layer keeps the bronchi open; the smooth muscle in the bronchi becomes smaller and less abundant, with only a few muscle fibres remaining in the terminal bronchi and alveoli. The epithelial cells are very similar in structure and function to the epithelial cells in the nasal passage.

The smallest bronchioles and alveoli (see Figure 52.1) are the functional units of the lungs. Within the lungs are a network of bronchi, alveoli and blood vessels. The lung tissue receives its blood supply from the bronchial artery, which branches directly off the aorta. The alveoli receive oxygen-poor blood from the right ventricle via the pulmonary artery. The delivery of this blood to the alveoli is referred to as perfusion.

Gas exchange occurs in the alveoli. In this process, oxygen is transferred into the blood and carbon dioxide is lost from the blood. The exchange of gases at the alveolar level is called **respiration**. In the alveolar sac oxygen diffuses across the **respiratory membrane** down its pressure gradient into the capillary. Oxygen is mainly transported bound to haemoglobin inside red blood cells (a small amount is transported in the plasma). In contrast, carbon dioxide, which is mostly transported as bicarbonate ions in the capillary plasma, diffuses across the membrane down its pressure gradient and enters the alveolar sac to be expired.

The respiratory membrane is made up of the capillary endothelium, the capillary basement membrane, the interstitial space, the alveolar basement membrane, the alveolar epithelium and the surfactant layer (Figure 52.3). The sac is able to stay open because the surface tension of the cells is decreased by the lipoprotein **surfactant**. Absence of surfactant leads to alveolar collapse. Surfactant is produced by the type II alveolar (septal) cells. These cells have additional metabolic functions, including the conversion of angiotensin I to angiotensin II, the degradation of serotonin and possibly the metabolism of various hormones.

The oxygen-rich blood is returned to the left atrium via the pulmonary veins; from there it is pumped throughout the body to deliver oxygen to the cells and to pick up waste products.

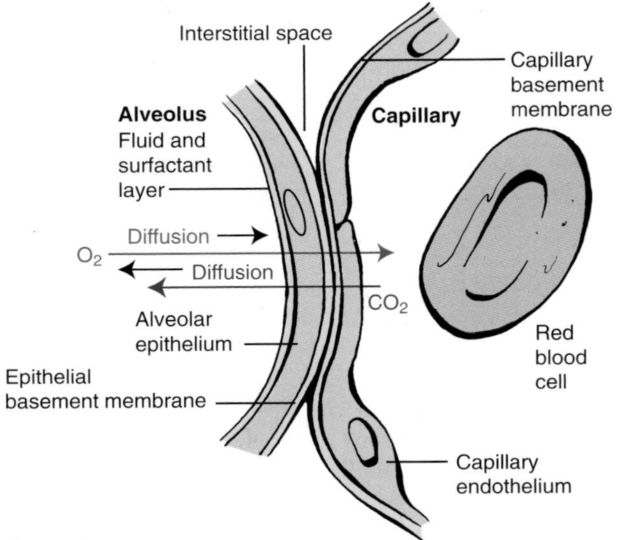

FIGURE 52.3 The respiratory membrane.

The walls of the trachea and conducting bronchi are highly sensitive to irritation. When receptors in the walls are stimulated, a central nervous system reflex is initiated and a **cough** results. The cough causes air to be pushed through the bronchial tree under tremendous pressure, forcing out any foreign irritant. This reflex, along with the similar **sneeze** reflex (which is initiated by receptors in the nasal cavity), forces foreign materials directly out of the system, opening it for more efficient flow of gas.

Throughout the airways, many macrophage scavengers freely move about the epithelium and destroy invaders. Mast cells are present in abundance and release histamine, serotonin, adenosine triphosphate (ATP) and other chemicals to ensure a rapid and intense inflammatory reaction to any cell injury. The end result of these various defence mechanisms is that the lower respiratory tract is virtually sterile – an important protection against respiratory infection that could interfere with essential gas exchange.

Ventilation

Ventilation, or the act of breathing, is controlled by the central nervous system. The inspiratory muscles – diaphragm and external intercostals – are stimulated to contract by the respiratory centres in the medulla and pons. The medulla receives input from chemoreceptors sensitive to carbon dioxide and pH levels in the cerebrospinal fluid and increases the rate and/or depth of respiration to maintain homeostasis in the body.

The vagus nerve (cranial nerve X), a predominantly parasympathetic nerve, plays a key role in stimulating diaphragm contraction and inspiration. Vagal stimulation also leads to bronchoconstriction or tightening. The sympathetic nervous system also innervates the respiratory system. Stimulation of the sympathetic system leads to increased rate and depth of respiration and dilation of the bronchi to allow greater airflow through the system.

Respiratory Pathology

This chapter will discuss the main conditions affecting the upper and lower respiratory tracts. However, it is important to recognize that the upper and lower airways do not exist as distinct areas; that is they are connected anatomically and physiologically. The continuation of the airways can explain how irritation and inflammation associated with upper respiratory tract conditions including rhinitis and sinusitis can impact upon the lower airways, in particular, bronchoconstriction and asthma. There are a number of studies that have demonstrated an association between rhinitis and asthma (reviewed by Dixon, 2009; Slavin, 2008). Treating patients for rhinitis or sinusitis could either prevent the development of asthma or improve the outcomes of those patients who already have asthma. Health care professionals should therefore examine both the upper and lower respiratory tracts.

Upper Respiratory Tract Conditions

The most common conditions that affect the upper respiratory tract involve the inflammatory response.

The Common Cold

A number of viruses cause the **common cold**. These viruses invade the tissues of the upper respiratory tract, initiating the release of histamine and prostaglandins and causing an inflammatory response. As a result of the inflammatory response, the mucous membranes become engorged with blood, the tissues swell and the goblet cells increase the production of mucus. These effects cause the person with a common cold to complain of sinus pain, nasal congestion, runny nose, sneezing, watery eyes, scratchy throat and headache. In susceptible people, this swelling can block the outlet of the eustachian tube, which drains the inner ear and equalizes pressure across the tympanic membrane. If this outlet becomes blocked, feelings of ear stuffiness and pain can occur, and the individual is more likely to develop an ear infection (otitis media).

Seasonal Rhinitis

A similar condition that afflicts many people is allergic or **seasonal rhinitis** (an inflammation of the nasal cavity), commonly called hay fever. This condition occurs when the upper airways respond to a specific antigen (e.g. pollen, mould, dust) with a vigorous inflammatory response, resulting again in nasal congestion, sneezing, stuffiness and watery eyes.

Sinusitis

Other areas of the upper respiratory tract can become irritated or infected, with a resultant inflammation of that particular area. **Sinusitis** occurs when the epithelial lining of the sinus cavities becomes inflamed. The resultant swelling often causes severe pain because the bony cavity cannot stretch, and the swollen tissue pushes against the bone and blocks the sinus passage. The danger of a sinus infection is that, if it is left untreated, microorganisms can move up the sinus passages and into brain tissue.

Pharyngitis and Laryngitis

Pharyngitis and laryngitis are infections of the pharynx and larynx, respectively. These infections are frequently caused by common bacteria or viruses. Pharyngitis and laryngitis are mostly seen with influenza, which is caused by a variety of different viruses and produces uncomfortable respiratory symptoms or other inflammations along with a fever, muscle aches and pains, and malaise.

Lower Respiratory Tract Conditions

A number of disorders affect the lower respiratory tract, including atelectasis, **pneumonia** (bacterial, viral or aspiration), bronchitis or inflammation of the bronchi (acute and chronic), bronchiectasis and the obstructive disorders – asthma, chronic obstructive pulmonary disease (COPD), cystic fibrosis and respiratory distress syndrome (RDS). Tuberculosis is a bacterial infection (see Chapter 9). All of these disorders involve, to some degree, an alteration in the ability to move gases in and out of the respiratory system.

Atelectasis

Atelectasis, the collapse of once-expanded lung tissue, can occur as a result of outside pressure against the alveoli; for example from a pulmonary tumour, a pneumothorax (air in the pleural space exerting high pressure against the alveoli) or a pleural effusion. Atelectasis most commonly occurs as a result of airway blockage, which prevents air from entering the alveoli to keep the lung expanded. This occurs when a mucus plug, oedema of the bronchioles, or a collection of pus or secretions occludes the airway and prevents the movement of air. Patients may experience atelectasis after surgery, when the effects of anaesthesia, pain and decreased coughing reflexes can lead to a decreased tidal volume and accumulation of secretions in the lower airways. Patients may present with rales (fluid accumulation in the lungs), dyspnoea, fever, cough, hypoxia and changes in chest wall movement. Treatment may involve clearing the airways, delivering oxygen and assisting ventilation.

Pneumonia

Pneumonia is inflammation of the lungs caused either by bacterial or by viral invasion of the tissue or by aspiration of foreign substances into the lower respiratory tract. The rapid inflammatory response to any foreign presence in the lower respiratory tract leads to a localized swelling, engorgement and exudation of protective sera. The respiratory membrane is affected, resulting in decreased gas exchange. Patients complain of difficulty breathing and fatigue, and they present with fever, noisy breath sounds and poor oxygenation.

Bronchitis

Acute bronchitis occurs when bacteria, viruses or foreign materials infect the inner layer of the bronchi. The person with bronchitis may have narrowed airways during the inflammatory process; this condition can be very serious in a person with obstructed or narrowed airflow. Chronic bronchitis is an inflammation of the bronchi that does not clear.

Bronchiectasis

Bronchiectasis is a chronic disease that involves the bronchi and bronchioles. It is characterized by dilation of the bronchial tree and chronic infection and inflammation of the bronchial passages. With chronic inflammation, the bronchial epithelial cells are replaced by a fibrous scar tissue. The loss of the protective mucus and ciliary movement of the epithelial cell membranes, combined with the dilation of the bronchial tree, leads to chronic infections in the now unprotected lower areas of the lung tissue. Patients with bronchiectasis often have an underlying medical condition that makes them more susceptible to infections (e.g. immune suppression, acquired immune deficiency syndrome, chronic inflammatory conditions). Patients present with the signs and symptoms of acute infection, including fever, malaise, myalgia, arthralgia and a purulent, productive cough.

Obstructive Pulmonary Diseases

As noted previously, the obstructive pulmonary diseases include asthma, cystic fibrosis, COPD and RDS.

Asthma

In the UK there are currently 5.4 million people receiving treatment for **asthma** (Asthma UK, 2008). Asthma is characterized by reversible bronchospasm, inflammation and hyper-reactive airways (Figure 52.4). The hyper-reactivity is triggered by allergens or nonallergic inhaled irritants or by factors such as exercise and emotions. The triggers cause an immediate release of histamine, which results in bronchospasm within 10 minutes. The later response (3–5 hours) is cytokine-mediated inflammation, mucus production and oedema contributing to obstruction. Appropriate treatment depends on understanding the early and late responses. The extreme case of asthma is called *status asthmaticus*; this is a life-threatening bronchospasm that does not respond to usual treatment and occludes airflow into the lungs. *Status asthmaticus* can lead to respiratory failure.

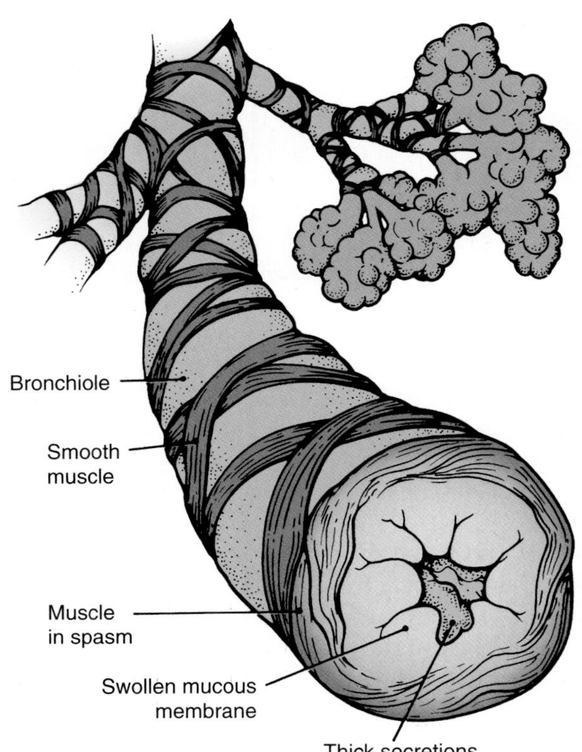

FIGURE 52.4 Asthma. The bronchiole is obstructed on expiration, particularly by muscle spasm, oedema of the mucosa and thick secretions.

Chronic Obstructive Pulmonary Disease (COPD)

Chronic obstructive pulmonary disease (COPD) is a permanent, chronic obstruction of airways, often related to cigarette smoking. COPD is the fifth most common cause of death in the UK, killing approximately 30,000 people each year. An estimated 3.7 million people have COPD; however, less than 30% of this number have had COPD diagnosed and are now receiving treatment (British Lung Foundation, 2009). It is an umbrella term used to describe a number of conditions, including emphysema and chronic bronchitis, both of which result in airflow obstruction on expiration, as well as over inflated lungs and poor gas exchange. Emphysema is characterized by loss of the elastic tissue of the lungs, destruction of alveolar walls and a resultant hyperinflation and tendency to collapse with expiration. Chronic bronchitis is a permanent inflammation of the airways with mucus secretion, oedema and poor inflammatory defences. Characteristics of both disorders are often present in patients with COPD (Figure 52.5).

Cystic Fibrosis

Cystic fibrosis is a hereditary disease that results in the accumulation of copious amounts of very thick secretions in the lungs. Eventually, the secretions obstruct the airways, leading to destruction of the lung tissue. Treatment is aimed at keeping the secretions fluid and moving and maintaining airway patency as much as possible.

Respiratory Distress Syndrome

Respiratory distress syndrome (RDS) is frequently seen in premature babies who are delivered before their lungs have fully developed and while surfactant levels are still very low. Surfactant is necessary for lowering the surface tension in the alveoli so that they can stay open to allow the flow of gases. Treatment is aimed at instilling surfactant to prevent atelectasis and to allow the lungs to expand. Adult respiratory distress syndrome (ARDS) is characterized by progressive loss of lung compliance and increasing hypoxia. This syndrome can occur as a result of a severe insult to the body,

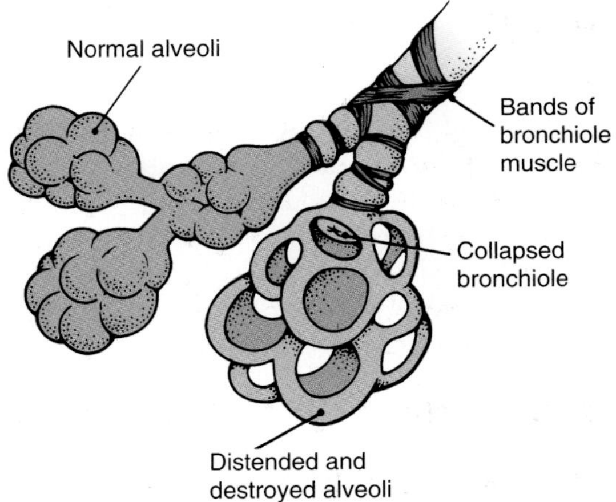

FIGURE 52.5 Distended and destroyed alveoli versus normal alveoli.

such as cardiovascular collapse, major burns, severe trauma or rapid depressurization. Treatment of ARDS involves reversal of the underlying cause of the problem combined with ventilatory support.

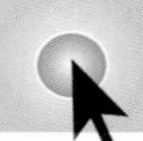

WEB LINKS

Health care providers and patients may want to consult the following Internet sources:

http://www.asthma.org.uk The charity Asthma UK works together with people with asthma, health professionals and researchers to develop and share expertise to help people increase their understanding.

http://www.innerbody.com Use this Internet source to explore the virtual respiratory tract.

http://www.lunguk.org The British Lung Foundation is a charity providing support groups and an advice helpline to people suffering from a wide range of lung diseases.

Points to Remember

- The respiratory system can be classified according to position (upper and lower respiratory tracts) and function (conducting and respiratory zones).
- The respiratory system is essential for survival; it brings oxygen into the body, allowing for the exchange of gases and the expelling of carbon dioxide and other waste products.
- The upper airways have many features to protect the fragile alveoli: hairs filter the air, goblet cells produce mucus to trap material, cilia move the trapped material towards the throat for swallowing, the blood supply close to the surface warms the air and adds humidity to improve gas movement and gas exchange and the cough and sneeze reflexes clear the airways.
- The respiratory bronchioles and alveolar sacs are where gas exchange occurs across the respiratory membrane. The alveoli produce surfactant to decrease surface tension within the sac and have other metabolic functions.
- Ventilation is controlled through the medulla and pons in the central nervous system and depends on a balance between the sympathetic and parasympathetic nervous systems and a functioning muscular system.
- Inflammation of the upper respiratory tract is seen in many uncomfortable disorders, including the common cold, seasonal rhinitis, sinusitis, pharyngitis and laryngitis.
- Inflammation of the lower respiratory tract can result in serious disorders that interfere with gas exchange, including bronchitis and pneumonia.
- Inflammation of the upper respiratory tract can impact upon the lower respiratory tract.
- Obstructive disorders interfere with the ability to deliver gases to the alveoli because of obstructions in the conducting airways and eventually in the respiratory airways. These disorders include asthma, COPD, cystic fibrosis and RDS.

CHECK YOUR UNDERSTANDING

Answers to the questions in this chapter may be found in the answer key in the back of the book.

Multiple Choice

Select the best answer to the following.

1. Sinusitis needs to be taken very seriously. The danger of a sinus infection is that
   a. it can cause a loss of sleep and exhaustion.
   b. it can lead to a painful otitis media.
   c. if left untreated, microorganisms can move up the sinus passages and into brain tissue.
   d. drainage from infected sinus membranes often leads to pneumonia.

2. Diffusion of CO_2 from the tissues into the capillary blood
   a. occurs if the concentration of CO_2 in the tissues is greater than in the blood.
   b. decreases as blood acidity increases.
   c. increases in the absence of carbonic anhydrase.
   d. is accompanied by a decrease in plasma bicarbonate.

3. The walls of the alveoli are composed of type I and type II cells. One of the functions of the type II cells is
   a. to replace mucus in the alveoli.
   b. production of serotonin.
   c. secretion of surfactant.
   d. protection of the lungs from bacterial invasion.

4. A patient who coughs has
   a. inflammation irritating the sinuses in the skull
   b. irritants affecting receptor sites in the nasal cavity
   c. pressure against the eustachian tube
   d. irritation to receptor sites in the walls of the trachea, conducting bronchi

5. For ventilation to occur, a person must have
   a. low levels of oxygen.
   b. low levels of CO_2.

c. functioning inspiratory muscles.
d. an actively functioning autonomic system.

6. The common cold is caused by
   a. bacteria that grow best in the cold.
   b. allergens in the environment.
   c. irritation of the delicate mucous membrane.
   d. a number of different viruses.

7. A patient with COPD would have
   a. a viral infection.
   b. loss of the protective respiratory mechanisms after prolonged irritation or damage.
   c. localised swelling and inflammation within the lungs.
   d. inflammation or swelling of the sinus membranes over a prolonged period.

Extended Matching Questions

Select **all** that apply.

1. Inflammation of the upper respiratory tract usually causes which of the following?
   a. A runny nose
   b. Laryngitis
   c. Sneezing
   d. Hypoxia
   e. Alveolar collapse
   f. Wheezing

2. In order for gas exchange to occur in the lungs, oxygen must pass through which of the following?
   a. 17 divisions of conducting airways
   b. The alveolar epithelium
   c. The pleural fluid
   d. The interstitial alveolar wall
   e. The capillary basement membrane
   f. The interstitial space

3. The nose performs which of the following functions in the respiratory system?
   a. Serves as a passageway for air movement
   b. Warms and humidifies the air
   c. Cleanses the air using hair fibres
   d. Stimulates surfactant release from the alveoli
   e. Initiates the cough reflex
   f. Initiates the sneeze reflex

Matching

Match the word with the appropriate definition.

1. ____________________upper respiratory tract
2. ____________________bronchial tree
3. ____________________respiratory zone
4. ____________________alveoli
5. ____________________cilia
6. ____________________sinuses
7. ____________________larynx
8. ____________________trachea
9. ____________________cough
10. ____________________respiration
11. ____________________respiratory membrane
12. ____________________surfactant

A. Air-filled passages through the skull
B. The area where gas exchange takes place
C. The vocal chords and the epiglottis
D. The conducting airways leading into the alveoli
E. Microscopic hair-like projections of the epithelial cell membrane
F. The exchange of gases at the alveolar level
G. The main conducting airway leading into the lungs
H. Lipoprotein that reduces surface tension in the alveoli
I. The surface through which gas exchange must occur
J. The respiratory sacs
K. The nose, mouth, pharynx and larynx
L. Reflex response in the respiratory membrane; results in forced air expelled through the mouth

Bibliography and References

Asthma UK. (2008). *What is asthma?* Available from http://www.asthma.org.uk

British Lung Foundation. (2009). *Chronic obstructive pulmonary disorder*. Available from http://www.lunguk.org

Dixon, A. E. (2009). Rhinosinusitis and asthma: the missing link. *Current Opinion in Pulmonary Medicine, 15,* 19–24.

Ganong, W. (2005). *Review of medical physiology* (22nd ed.). New York: McGraw-Hill.

Guyton, A., & Hall, J. (2005). *Textbook of medical physiology* (11th ed.). Philadelphia: W. B. Saunders.

Howland, R. D., & Mycek, M. J. (2005). *Pharmacology* (3rd ed.). Philadelphia: Lippincott Williams & Wilkins.

Marieb, E. N., & Hoehn, K. (2009). *Human anatomy & histology* (8th ed.). San Francisco: Pearson.

Porth, C. M., & Matfin, G. (2008). *Pathophysiology: Concepts of altered health states* (8th ed.). Philadelphia: Lippincott Williams & Wilkins.

Slavin, R. G. (2008). The upper and lower airways: the epidemiological and pathophysiological connection. *Allergy and Asthma Proceedings, 29*(6), 553–556.

CHAPTER 53

Drugs Acting on the Upper Respiratory Tract

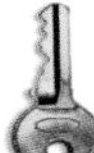

KEY TERMS

antihistamines
antitussives
decongestants
mucolytics
rebound congestion
sympathomimetic

LEARNING OBJECTIVES

Upon completion of this chapter, you will be able to:

1. Outline the underlying physiological events that occur with upper respiratory disorders.
2. Describe the therapeutic actions, indications, pharmacokinetics, contraindications, most common adverse reactions and important drug–drug interactions associated with antitussives, decongestants, topical nasal steroids, antihistamines and mucolytics.
3. Discuss the use of drugs that act on the upper respiratory tract across the lifespan.
4. Compare and contrast the key drugs pholcodine, ephedrine, beclometasone, desloratidine and carbocisteine with other agents in their class and with other classes of drugs that act on the upper respiratory tract.
5. Outline the nursing considerations, including important teaching points, for patients receiving drugs acting on the upper respiratory tract.

ANTITUSSIVES

codeine
pholcodine
dextromethorphan
morphine

DECONGESTANTS

Topical Nasal Decongestants

ephedrine
xylometazoline
ipratropium

Oral Decongestants

pseudoephedrine

Topical Nasal Steroid Decongestants

beclometasone
betamethasone
budesonide
flunisolide
fluticasone
mometasone
triamcinolone

ANTIHISTAMINES

Nonsedating Antihistamines

acrivastine
azelastine
cetirizine
desloratadine
fexofenadine
levocetirizine
loratadine
mizolastine

Sedating Antihistamines

chlorphenamine
clemastine
cyproheptadine
ketotifen
promethazine

MUCOLYTICS

carbocisteine
erdosteine
mecysteine
dornase alfa

Drugs that affect the respiratory system work to keep the airways open and gases moving efficiently. The classes discussed in this chapter include the following:

- **Antitussives**, which block the cough reflex
- **Decongestants**, which decrease the blood flow to the upper respiratory tract and decrease the overproduction of secretions
- **Antihistamines**, which block the action of histamine, a chemical released during inflammation that increases secretions and narrows airways
- **Mucolytics**, which increase or liquefy respiratory secretions to aid the clearing of the airways

Figure 53.1 displays the sites of action of these drugs. Box 53.1 discusses the use of these agents in various age groups.

The classes of drugs listed above act mainly on the upper respiratory tract and are used to treat conditions of the upper airways, for example rhinitis and sinusitis. It is important to recognize that conditions affecting the upper airways can also impact upon the lower airways as well. There is strong evidence to demonstrate that rhinitis is a risk factor for the development of asthma, a condition affecting the lower airways (Dixon *et al.,* 2006). Effective treatment of upper airways disease could therefore either prevent the development of asthma or reduce the severity of the disease.

Antitussives

Antitussives are drugs that suppress the cough reflex. Many disorders of the respiratory tract, including the common cold, sinusitis, pharyngitis and pneumonia, are accompanied by an unproductive cough. Persistent coughing can be exhausting and cause muscle strain and further respiratory tract irritation. A cough that occurs without the presence of any active disease process or persists after treatment may be a symptom of another disease process and should be investigated before any medication is given to alleviate it.

Therapeutic Actions and Indications

The traditional antitussives, including codeine, pholcodine and dextromethorphan (*Benylin* and many others), act directly on the medullary cough centre of the brain to depress the cough reflex. As they are centrally acting, they are not the drugs of choice for anyone who has a head injury or who could be impaired by central nervous system (CNS) depression. These drugs are rapidly absorbed, metabolized in the liver and excreted in the urine. They cross the placenta and enter breast milk and should not be used during pregnancy or lactation because of the potential for CNS depressive effects on the foetus or neonate.

The opioid analgesic morphine can be used to suppress cough in terminal lung cancer, however, caution should be

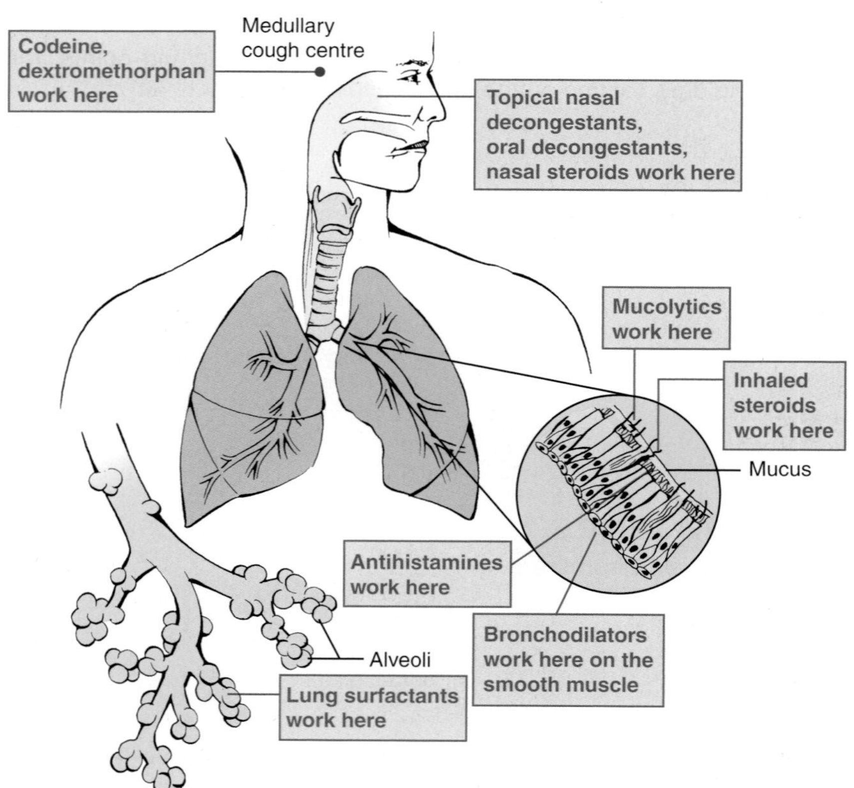

FIGURE 53.1 Sites of action of drugs acting on the upper respiratory tract.

BOX 53.1 **DRUG THERAPY ACROSS THE LIFESPAN**

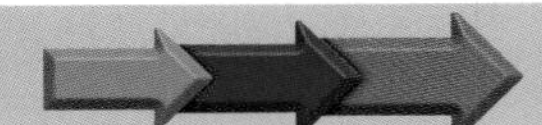

Upper Respiratory Tract Agents

CHILDREN

Antitussives containing codeine or other similar opioid analgesics are not generally recommended for use by children. Other antitussives have been used frequently with children in the past, but recent guidelines from the Commission on Human Medicines recommend that over-the-counter (OTC) cold, 'flu and cough medicines should not be used by children under the age of 6 years (Commission on Human Medicine, 2009). There is no evidence to suggest that these drugs are effective and side-effects can include allergic reactions, sleep disturbances and hallucinations. Instead, parents should be encouraged to implement nondrug measures to help the child cope with the upper respiratory problem: drink plenty of fluids, rest, use a humidifier and avoid smoke-filled areas. Paracetamol or ibuprofen can be used to reduce an elevated temperature. Antitussives are available from pharmacists for children aged 6 to 12 years. For children of this age, the risks are perceived to be lower (increased body weight and reduced number of colds), and these children are able to confirm the effectiveness of the drug.

It is important to educate parents about reading labels and following dosing guidelines to avoid potentially serious accidental overdose. Parents should always be asked specifically whether they are also giving the child an OTC or herbal remedy.

When administering any drug to children, always consult the most recent edition of the British National Formulary for Children.

ADULTS

The considerations for adults are similar to those for children. The safety of these drugs in pregnancy and breast-feeding has not been established. There is a potential for adverse effects on the foetus, especially during the first trimester, therefore drugs should only be prescribed if the expected benefit to the mother is greater than the risk to the foetus. In many cases, the amount of drug transferred into breast milk is unlikely to have a significant effect on the baby; however, it is advised that caution be used if one of these drugs is prescribed during lactation.

OLDER ADULTS

Older adults are frequently prescribed one of these drugs. Older adults are more likely to develop adverse effects associated with the use of these drugs, including sedation, confusion and dizziness. Safety measures may be needed if these effects occur and interfere with the patient's mobility and balance. These drugs should be stopped if sedation and confusion occurs.

Older adults are also more likely to have hepatic and/or renal impairment related to underlying medical conditions, which could interfere with the metabolism and excretion of these drugs. The dosage for older adults should be started at a lower level than that recommended for younger adults. The patient should be monitored closely and dosage adjustment should be based on the patient's response.

These patients also need to be alerted to the potential of polypharmacy and for toxic effects when using OTC preparations and should be advised to check with their health care provider before beginning any OTC drug regimen.

taken in administering this drug as opioids can cause respiratory failure.

Contraindications and Cautions

Antitussives are contraindicated in patients who need to cough to maintain the airways, for example postoperative patients. Careful use is recommended for patients with asthma or emphysema because cough suppression in these patients could lead to an accumulation of secretions and a loss of respiratory reserve. Caution should also be used in patients who are hypersensitive to or have a history of addiction to opioids, for example codeine. Patients who need to drive or remain alert should use codeine with extreme caution because it can cause sedation and drowsiness.

Adverse Effects

Traditional antitussives can have a drying effect on the mucous membranes and can increase the viscosity of respiratory tract secretions. Their drying effect can lead to nausea, constipation and complaints of dry mouth. Locally acting antitussives are associated with gastrointestinal (GI) upset, headache, feelings of congestion and sometimes dizziness. Centrally acting antitussives are associated with CNS adverse effects, including drowsiness and sedation.

Clinically Important Drug–Drug Interactions

The combined use of opioid antitussives with antidepressants, cimetidine, memantine (dextromethorphan) or sodium oxybate should be monitored carefully.

Always consult a current copy of the British National Formulary for further guidance.

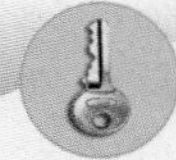

Key Drug Summary: *Pholcodine*

Indications: Control of nonproductive cough

Actions: Depresses the cough reflex in the medulla to control cough spasms

Pharmacokinetics:

Route	Onset	Peak	Duration
Oral	25–30 min	2 h	3–6 h

$T_{1/2}$: 32–43 hours; metabolized in the liver and excreted in urine

Adverse effects: Constipation, respiratory depression in sensitive patients or if given in large doses

Nursing Considerations for Patients Receiving Antitussives

Assessment: History and Examination

Screen for the following conditions, *which could be cautions or contraindications to use of the drug*: any history of allergy to any component of the drug; cough that persists longer than 1 week or is accompanied by other signs and symptoms and pregnancy or lactation. Establish if patient is currently taking other medications or herbal therapies which may potentially interact with the antitussive drug.

Physical assessment should be done *to establish baseline data for assessing the effectiveness of the drug and the occurrence of any adverse effects associated with drug therapy*. Assess the following: temperature, *to evaluate for possible underlying infection*, and respiratory rate and depth and adventitious sounds, *to assess drug effectiveness and to monitor for accumulation of secretions*.

Nursing Diagnoses

The patient receiving an antitussive may have the following nursing diagnoses related to drug therapy:

- Ineffective airway clearance related to excessive drug effects
- Disturbed sensory perception related to CNS effects (only when morphine is used for palliative care)
- Deficient knowledge regarding drug therapy

Implementation With Rationale

- Ensure that the drug is not taken any longer than recommended *to prevent serious adverse effects and increased respiratory tract problems.*
- Arrange for further medical evaluation for coughs that persist or are accompanied by high fever, rash or excessive secretions *to detect the underlying cause and to arrange for appropriate treatment.*
- Provide other measures *to help relieve cough* (e.g. humidity, cool temperatures, fluids, use of lozenges) as appropriate.
- Provide thorough patient teaching, including the drug name and prescribed dosage, measures to help avoid adverse effects, warning signs that may indicate problems and the need for periodic monitoring and evaluation, *to enhance patient knowledge about drug therapy and to promote concordance.*

Evaluation

- Monitor patient response to the drug (control of nonproductive cough).
- Monitor for adverse effects (respiratory depression, drowsiness).
- Evaluate the effectiveness of the teaching plan (patient can name drug, dosage, adverse effects to watch for, specific measures to avoid adverse effects, measures to take to increase the effectiveness of the drug).
- Monitor effectiveness of other measures to relieve cough.

Decongestants

Decongestants are usually adrenergic or **sympathomimetic** drugs, meaning that they imitate the effects of the sympathetic nervous system to cause local vasoconstriction and decreased blood flow of the irritated and dilated capillaries of the mucous membranes lining the nasal passages and sinus cavities. This vasoconstriction leads to a shrinking of swollen membranes and reduced oedema and opening of congested nasal passages, providing relief from the discomfort of a blocked nose and promoting drainage of secretions and improved airflow. An adverse effect that accompanies frequent or prolonged use of these drugs is **rebound congestion** (rhinitis medicamentosa) on withdrawal. The reflex reaction to vasoconstriction is a rebound vasodilation and temporary increase in nasal congestion. As a result, patients tend to use more drug to decrease the congestion, thus initiating a vicious cycle of congestion-drug-congestion, leading to abuse of the decongestant. Ephedrine and xylometazoline are most likely to have a rebound effect.

Topical steroids are also used as decongestants, for example mometasone. These act to directly block the effects of inflammation on the nasal mucous membranes. This inhibits the swelling, congestion and increased secretions that accompany inflammation. The end result is an opening of the nasal passage and an increase in airflow. These drugs take several weeks to be really effective and are more often used in cases of chronic rhinitis.

Topical Nasal Decongestants

Topical nasal decongestants are preferred for patients who need to avoid the systemic adrenergic effects associated with oral decongestants. Example drugs include ephedrine, xylometazoline and ipratropium. The choice of a topical nasal decongestant is individual: some patients may have no response to one and respond very well to another. Ephedrine and xylometazoline are available as OTC preparations.

Therapeutic Actions and Indications

They are available as nasal drops or sprays to relieve the discomfort of nasal congestion accompanying the common cold, sinusitis and allergic rhinitis. These drugs can also be used to relieve congestion for a short period and to allow penetration of a topical nasal corticosteroid. Topical application produces rapid effects and reduces the extent of systemic effects.

Pharmacokinetics

Although they are not generally absorbed systemically, any portion of these topical decongestants that is absorbed is metabolized in the liver and excreted in urine. There are no studies regarding the effects of these topical drugs in pregnancy or lactation. As with any drug used during pregnancy or lactation, caution should be used.

Contraindications and Cautions

Caution should be used when there is *any lesion in the mucous membranes* that could lead to systemic absorption. Caution should also be used in patients with any condition that might be exacerbated by sympathetic activity, such as glaucoma, hypertension, diabetes, thyroid disease, coronary disease or prostate problems, because these agents have adrenergic properties.

Adverse Effects

Adverse effects associated with topical decongestants include local stinging and burning, which may occur the first few times the drug is used. If the sensation does not pass, the drug should be discontinued, because it may indicate lesions or erosion of the mucous membranes. Use for longer than 3 to 5 days can lead to rebound congestion (see above). Sympathomimetic effects (e.g. increased pulse, blood pressure, urinary retention) should be monitored because some systemic absorption may occur, although these effects are less likely with topical administration than with other routes.

Clinically Important Drug–Drug Interactions

The combined use of topical nasal decongestants with any other sympathomimetic drug or sympathetic-blocking drug, *e.g.* monoamine oxidase inhibitors (MAOIs) used to treat depression; should be avoided. MAOIs inhibit monoamine oxidase resulting in an accumulation of amine neurotransmitters, including noradrenaline, dopamine and 5-HT. When MAOIs are taken together with sympathomimetics, this can lead to a hypertensive crisis. These decongestants should therefore be avoided by patients taking MAOI antidepressants.

Always consult a current copy of the British National Formulary for further guidance.

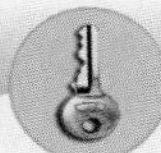

Key Drug Summary: *Ephedrine*

Indications: Symptomatic relief of nasal and nasopharyngeal mucosal congestion due to the common cold, seasonal allergic rhinitis ('hay fever') or other respiratory allergies.

Actions: Sympathomimetic effects, partly due to release of noradrenaline from nerve terminals; vasoconstriction leads to decreased oedema and inflammation of the nasal membranes

Pharmacokinetics:

Route	Onset	Duration
Topical (nasal spray)	Immediate	4–6 h

$T_{1/2}$: 0.4–0.7 hours; metabolized in the liver and excreted in urine; little is usually absorbed for systemic metabolism

Adverse effects: Local irritation, nausea, headache; tolerance with diminished effect after excessive use; cardiovascular effects also reported.

Nursing Considerations for Patients Receiving Topical Nasal Decongestants

Assessment: History and Examination

Screen for the following conditions, *which could be cautions or contraindications to use of the drug*: any history of allergy to the drug; glaucoma, hypertension, diabetes, thyroid disease, coronary disease and prostate problems, *all of which could be exacerbated by the sympathomimetic effects*; and pregnancy or lactation, *which require cautious use.*

Physical assessment should be done *to establish baseline data for assessing the effectiveness of the drug and the occurrence of any adverse effects associated with drug therapy.* Assess the following: pulse, blood pressure and cardiac auscultation *to monitor cardiovascular and sympathomimetic effects*; bladder percussion *to monitor for urinary retention related to sympathomimetic effects* and nasal mucous membrane evaluation *to monitor for lesions that could lead to systemic absorption and to evaluate decongestant effect.*

Nursing Diagnoses

The patient receiving a topical nasal decongestant may have the following nursing diagnoses related to drug therapy:

- Acute pain related to local effects of drug
- Deficient knowledge regarding drug therapy

Implementation With Rationale

- Teach the patient the proper administration of the drug *to ensure therapeutic effect* (Box 53.2).
- Caution patients not to use the drug for longer than 5 days and to seek medical care if signs and symptoms persist after that time *to facilitate detection of underlying medical conditions that may require treatment.*
- Caution patients that these drugs are found in many OTC preparations and that care should be taken not to inadvertently combine drugs with the same ingredients, *leading to overdose.*
- Introduce other measures *to help relieve the discomfort of congestion* (e.g. humidity, increased fluid intake, cool environment, avoidance of smoke-filled areas) as appropriate.
- Provide thorough patient teaching, including the drug name and prescribed dosage, measures to help avoid adverse effects, warning signs that may indicate problems, and the need for periodic monitoring and evaluation, *to enhance patient knowledge about drug therapy and to promote concordance.*
- Offer support and encouragement *to help the patient cope with the disease and the drug regimen.*

Evaluation

- Monitor patient response to the drug (relief of nasal congestion).
- Monitor for adverse effects (local burning and stinging; sympathomimetic effects such as increased pulse, blood pressure, urinary retention).
- Evaluate the effectiveness of the teaching plan (patient can name drug, dosage, adverse effects to watch for, specific measures to avoid adverse effects, measures to take to increase the effectiveness of the drug, proper administration technique).
- Monitor the effectiveness of comfort and safety measures and concordance with the regimen.

BOX 53.2 FOCUS ON CLINICAL SKILLS

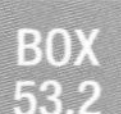

Administering Nasal Medications

Proper administration technique is very important for ensuring that drugs given nasally have the desired therapeutic effect. It is important to periodically check the nares for any lesions, which could allow systemic absorption of the drug. Most patients prefer to self-administer nasal drugs, so patient teaching is very important. Explain the technique and then observe the patient using the technique. Check the instructions given below with those supplied with the medication as some devices may require a different approach to administer the drug.

Nasal Spray

Request the patient to sit upright, tilt their head back and press a finger against one nares to close it. Hold the spray bottle upright and place the tip of the bottle about 1 cm into the open nares. Depress the canister once and inhale deeply through the nose. Repeat with the other nares.

Nasal Drops

Position the patient in the same way as for the spray. Place the tip of the bottle about 1 cm into the open nares. Firmly squeeze the bottle to deliver the drug. Caution the patient not to squeeze too forcefully, which could send the drug up into the sinuses, causing more problems. Repeat with the other nares and keep head tilted back for a few seconds after administration.

Oral Decongestants

Oral decongestants are taken to decrease nasal congestion related to the common cold, sinusitis and seasonal allergic rhinitis. The only oral decongestant currently available for use is pseudoephedrine. Pseudoephedrine is available OTC and has fewer sympathomimetic effects than some of the other sympathomimetic drugs mentioned above, for example ephedrine.

Therapeutic Actions and Indications

Oral decongestants shrink the nasal mucous membrane by stimulating α-adrenergic receptors in the nasal mucous membranes. This shrinkage results in a decrease in the size of mucous membranes, promoting drainage of the sinuses and improving airflow. As this drug is taken orally, systemic adverse effects related to the sympathomimetic effects (e.g. cardiac stimulation, feelings of anxiety) are more likely to occur.

Pharmacokinetics

Pseudoephedrine is generally well absorbed and reaches peak levels quickly in 20 to 45 minutes. It is widely distributed in the body, metabolized in the liver and primarily excreted in urine. Use during pregnancy and lactation should be reserved for situations in which the benefit to the mother outweighs any potential risk to the foetus or neonate.

Contraindications and Cautions

Pseudoephedrine has adrenergic properties; therefore, caution should be used in patients with any condition that might be exacerbated by sympathetic activity, such as glaucoma, hypertension, diabetes, hyperthyroidism, ischaemic heart disease, renal impairment and prostatic hypertrophy.

Adverse Effects

Adverse effects associated with pseudoephedrine include rebound congestion. Sympathetic effects include palpitations, anxiety, restlessness, insomnia, hallucinations (rarely) and angle-closure glaucoma (very rarely).

Clinically Important Drug–Drug Interactions

The most important interaction occurs with MAOIs used to treat depression and should therefore be avoided by patients taking MAOI antidepressants. In addition, many OTC products, including cold remedies, allergy medications and flu remedies, may contain pseudoephedrine. Taking many of these products concurrently can cause an inadvertent overdose. Patients should be advised to read the OTC labels to avoid serious adverse effects.

Always consult a current copy of the British National Formulary for further guidance.

Nursing Considerations for Patients Receiving an Oral Decongestant

Assessment: History and Examination

Screen for the following conditions which could be cautions or contraindications to use of the drug: *any history of allergy to the drug and pregnancy or lactation*, which are contraindications to drug use; *hypertension or coronary artery disease, hyperthyroidism, diabetes mellitus, susceptibility to angle-closure glaucoma or prostate enlargement*, which require cautious use, and all of which could be exacerbated by these drugs. Establish if patient is currently taking other medications or herbal therapies which may potentially interact with a decongestant drug.

Physical assessment should be done *to establish baseline data for assessing the effectiveness of the drug and the occurrence of any adverse effects associated with drug therapy.* Assess the following: skin colour and lesions *to monitor for adverse reactions*; effect *to monitor CNS effects of the drug*; blood pressure, pulse and auscultation *to monitor cardiovascular stimulations* and urinary output *to evaluate for urinary retention.*

Nursing Diagnoses

The patient receiving an oral decongestant may have the following nursing diagnoses related to drug therapy:

- Increased heart rate related to sympathomimetic actions of the drug
- Disturbed sensory perception (kinaesthetic) related to CNS effects, although hallucinations are rarely experienced
- Deficient knowledge regarding drug therapy

Implementation With Rationale

- Note that this drug is found in many OTC products, especially combination cold and allergy preparations; *care should be taken to prevent inadvertent overdose or excessive adverse effects.*
- Monitor pulse, blood pressure and cardiac response to the drug, especially in patients who are at risk of cardiac stimulation, *to detect adverse effects early and arrange to reduce dosage or discontinue the drug.*
- Encourage the patient not to use this drug for longer than 1 week and to seek medical evaluation if symptoms persist after that time *to encourage the detection of underlying medical conditions that could be causing these symptoms and to arrange for appropriate treatment.*
- Provide thorough patient teaching, including the drug name and prescribed dosage, measures to help avoid adverse effects, warning signs that may indicate problems and the need for periodic monitoring and evaluation, *to enhance patient knowledge about drug therapy and to promote concordance.*
- Offer support and encouragement *to help the patient cope with the disease and the drug regimen.*

Evaluation

- Monitor patient response to the drug (improvement in nasal congestion).
- Monitor for adverse effects (sympathomimetic reactions including increased pulse, arrhythmias, feelings of anxiety, tension).

- Evaluate the effectiveness of the teaching plan (patient can name drug, dosage, adverse effects to watch for, specific measures to avoid adverse effects, measures to take to increase the effectiveness of the drug).
- Monitor the effectiveness of comfort and safety measures and concordance with the regimen.

Topical Nasal Corticosteroid Decongestants

Topical nasal corticosteroid decongestants are currently used in the prophylaxis and treatment of seasonal allergic rhinitis. They are effective in patients who no longer obtain a response with other decongestants. Topical nasal corticosteroid decongestants include beclometasone, betamethasone, budesonide, flunisolide, fluticasone, mometasone and triamcinolone.

Therapeutic Actions and Indications

The exact mechanism of action of topical corticosteroids is not known. Their anti-inflammatory action results from their ability to produce a direct local effect that blocks many of the complex reactions responsible for the inflammatory response. As they are applied topically, there is less chance of systemic absorption and associated adverse effects. The onset of action is not immediate, and they may require up to a week to cause any changes. If no effects are seen after 3 weeks, the drug should be discontinued. In addition to treating allergic rhinitis, some nasal corticosteroids are used to shrink nasal polyps.

Pharmacokinetics

As these drugs are not generally absorbed systemically, their pharmacokinetics are not reported.

Contraindications and Cautions

As nasal corticosteroids block the inflammatory response, their use is contraindicated in the presence of acute infections. Caution should be used in any patient who has an active infection, for example pulmonary tuberculosis, because systemic absorption would interfere with the inflammatory and immune responses. Patients using nasal corticosteroids should avoid exposure to any airborne infection, such as chickenpox or measles.

Adverse Effects

The most common adverse effects associated with the use of these drugs are local irritation (burning and stinging) of the nose and throat, dryness of the mucosa, nosebleeds, ulceration (rarely) and raised intraocular pressure or glaucoma may also occur (rarely). As healing is suppressed by corticosteroids, patients who have recently experienced nasal surgery or trauma should be monitored closely until healing has occurred.

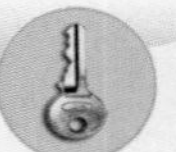

Key Drug Summary: *Beclometasone*

Indications: Prophylaxis and treatment of allergic and vasomotor rhinitis

Actions: Local anti-inflammatory action through blocking many of the complex reactions responsible for the inflammatory response

Pharmacokinetics:

Route	Onset	Peak	Duration
Topical (nasal spray)	Immediate	30 min	12 h

$T_{1/2}$: Not generally absorbed systemically

Adverse effects: Local burning, irritation, stinging, dryness of the mucosa, headache. Rare effects include anxiety, sleep disorders and behavioural changes.

Nursing Considerations for Patients Receiving Topical Corticosteroid Nasal Decongestants

Assessment: History and Examination

Screen for the following conditions, which could be cautions or contraindications to use of the drug: *any history of allergy to steroid drugs,* which would be a contraindication, and *acute untreated nasal infections,* which would require cautious use.

Physical assessment should be done *to establish baseline data for assessing the effectiveness of the drug and the occurrence of any adverse effects associated with drug therapy.* Intranasal examination should be performed *to determine the presence of any lesions that would increase the risk of systemic absorption of drug.* Assess temperature *to monitor for the possibility of acute infection.*

Nursing Diagnoses

The patient receiving topical steroid nasal decongestants may have the following nursing diagnoses related to drug therapy:

- Acute pain related to local effects of the drug
- Deficient knowledge regarding drug therapy

Implementation With Rationale

- Teach the patient how to administer these drugs properly, *which is very important to ensure effectiveness and prevent systemic effects.* A variety of preparations are available (e.g. sprays, drops). Advise the patient about the proper administration technique for whichever preparation is recommended.
- Have the patient clear nasal passages before using the drug *to improve the effectiveness of the drug.*
- Encourage the patient to continue using the drug regularly, even if results are not seen immediately, *because benefits may take 2 to 3 weeks to appear.*
- Provide thorough patient teaching, including the drug name and prescribed dosage, measures to help avoid adverse effects, warning signs that may indicate problems and the need for periodic monitoring and evaluation, *to enhance patient knowledge about drug therapy and to promote concordance.*
- Offer support and encouragement *to help the patient cope with the disease and the drug regimen.*

Evaluation

- Monitor patient response to the drug (relief of nasal congestion).
- Monitor for adverse effects (local burning and stinging).
- Evaluate the effectiveness of the teaching plan (patient can name drug, dosage, adverse effects to watch for, specific measures to avoid adverse effects, measures to take to increase the effectiveness of the drug).
- Monitor the effectiveness of comfort and safety measures and concordance with the regimen.

Antihistamines

Antihistamines are found in multiple OTC preparations that are designed to relieve respiratory symptoms and to treat allergies. These agents block the effects of histamine, bringing relief to patients suffering from itchy eyes, swelling, congestion and runny nose. Their OTC availability has led to the misuse of these drugs in treating colds and influenza.

Numerous antihistamines acting on the upper respiratory tract are available and can be divided into two classes: nonsedating and sedating antihistamines. Reduced drowsiness is reported with the nonsedating antihistamines because they have fewer anticholinergic effects in comparison to the sedating antihistamines (refer to the start of this chapter for a list of nonsedating and sedating antihistamines). When selecting an antihistamine, the individual patient's reaction to the drug is usually the governing factor. If a person needs to remain alert, one of the nonsedating antihistamines would be the drug of choice.

Therapeutic Actions and Indications

Antihistamines selectively block the effects of histamine at H_1 histamine receptors, decreasing the release of inflammatory mediators and therefore also decreasing the allergic response. They are most effective if used before the onset of symptoms. Some antihistamines also have anticholinergic (atropine-like) and antipruritic effects. Antihistamines are used for the relief of symptoms associated with seasonal allergic rhinitis (hay fever), allergic conjunctivitis, urticaria and angio-oedema. They are also used for amelioration of allergic reactions to insect bites and stings, for relief of discomfort associated with dermographism (a form of urticaria or hives where the skin is inflamed and itchy) and as adjunctive therapy in anaphylactic reactions. Other uses include alleviation of nausea and vomiting (including motion sickness) and as a premedication for surgery.

Pharmacokinetics

Oral antihistamines are well absorbed orally, with an onset of action ranging from 1 to 3 hours. They are metabolized in the liver and excreted in the urine.

Contraindications and Cautions

These drugs cross the placenta and enter breast milk and should be avoided in pregnancy and lactation unless the benefit to the mother outweighs the potential risk to the foetus or baby. They should be *used with caution in hepatic or renal impairment,* which could alter the metabolism and excretion of the drug. Special care should be taken when these drugs are used by *any patient with a history of arrhythmias or prolonged Q–T intervals* because fatal cardiac arrhythmias have been associated with the use of certain antihistamines and drugs that increase Q–T intervals, including erythromycin. As the sedating antihistamines have significant anticholinergic activity, they should be used with caution in patients with prostatic hypertrophy, urinary retention or susceptibility to angle-closure glaucoma.

Adverse Effects

The adverse effects most often seen with most of the older antihistamine drugs are drowsiness and sedation (Critical Thinking Scenario 53-1). Patients are advised to exert caution when performing skilled tasks such as driving or operating heavy machinery. The anticholinergic effects that can be anticipated include drying of the respiratory and GI mucous membranes, GI disturbances, blurred vision and urinary retention. Other adverse effects include palpitations and arrhythmias.

Clinically Important Drug–Drug Interactions

The main drug–drug interactions to consider are those with antibacterials, antifungals and antiarrhythmics. Patients should avoid consuming alcohol to minimize the risk of drowsiness and sedation.

Always consult a current copy of the British National Formulary for further guidance.

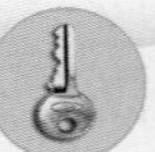

Key Drug Summary: *Desloratidine*

Indications: Symptomatic relief of seasonal rhinitis and urticaria

Actions: Competitively blocks the effects of histamine at peripheral H_1-receptor sites

Pharmacokinetics:

Route	Onset	Peak	Duration
Oral	1 h	2–4 h	24 h

$T_{1/2}$: 27 hours; metabolized in the liver and excreted in urine and faeces

Adverse effects: Fatigue, dry mouth, headache and GI disturbances

Nursing Considerations for Patients Receiving Antihistamines

Assessment: History and Examination

Screen for the following conditions, which could be cautions or contraindications to use of the drug: *any history of allergy to antihistamines; pregnancy or lactation; and prolonged Q–T interval (mizolastine),* which are contraindications to the use of the drug *and renal or hepatic impairment,* which requires cautious use of the drug. Establish if patient is currently taking other medications or herbal therapies which may potentially interact with the antihistamine drug.

Physical assessment should be done *to establish baseline data for assessing the effectiveness of the drug and the occurrence of any adverse effects associated with drug therapy.* Assess the following: orientation *to monitor for changes due to CNS effects*; and liver and renal function tests *to monitor for factors that could affect the metabolism or excretion of the drug.*

Nursing Diagnoses

The patient receiving antihistamines may have the following nursing diagnoses related to drug therapy:

- Acute pain related to GI or CNS effects of the drug
- Drowsiness or sedation related to CNS effects
- Deficient knowledge regarding drug therapy

Implementation With Rationale

- Note that a patient may have a poor response to one of these agents but a very effective response to another; the prescriber may need to try several different agents *to find the one that is most effective.*
- Patients often experience dry mouth, which may lead to nausea and anorexia; suggest lozenges *to relieve some of this discomfort.*
- Provide safety measures as appropriate, if CNS effects occur, *to prevent patient injury.* These drugs can cause drowsiness and may therefore affect the ability to drive or operation machinery.
- Increase humidity and encourage fluid intake *to decrease the problem of thickened secretions and dry nasal mucosa.*
- Have the patient empty bladder before each dose *to decrease urinary retention if this is a problem.*
- Caution the patient to avoid excessive dosage and to check OTC drugs for the presence of antihistamines, *which are found in many OTC preparations and which could cause toxicity.*
- Caution the patient to avoid alcohol while taking these drugs *because serious sedation can occur.*
- Provide thorough patient teaching, including the drug name and prescribed dosage, measures to help avoid adverse effects, warning signs that may indicate problems and the need for periodic monitoring and evaluation, *to enhance patient knowledge about drug therapy and to promote concordance.*
- Offer support and encouragement *to help the patient cope with the disease and the drug regimen.*

Evaluation

- Monitor patient response to the drug (relief of the symptoms of allergic rhinitis).
- Monitor for adverse effects (GI upset, sedation and drowsiness, urinary retention, thickened secretions, glaucoma).

- Evaluate the effectiveness of the teaching plan (patient can name drug, dosage, adverse effects to watch for, specific measures to avoid adverse effects, measures to take to increase the effectiveness of the drug).
- Monitor the effectiveness of comfort and safety measures and concordance with the regimen.

Mucolytics

Mucolytics work to break down mucus in order to aid the high-risk respiratory patient in coughing up thick, persistent secretions. The medication may be administered orally or by inhalation using a jet nebulizer. Mucolytics include carbocisteine, erdosteine, mecysteine and dornase alfa.

Therapeutic Actions and Indications

Mucolytics are usually reserved for patients who have difficulty mobilizing and coughing up secretions, such as individuals with chronic obstructive pulmonary disease (COPD), cystic fibrosis, pneumonia or tuberculosis. These drugs are also indicated for patients who develop atelectasis (the collapse of lung tissue) because of thick mucus secretions. They can be used during diagnostic bronchoscopy to clear the airway and to facilitate the removal of secretions, as well as postoperatively and in patients with tracheostomies to facilitate airway clearance and suctioning.

Carbocisteine, erdosteine and mecysteine affect the mucoproteins in respiratory secretions by splitting disulphide bonds that are responsible for holding the mucus material together. The result is a decrease in the tenacity and viscosity of the secretions. Dornase alfa is a genetically engineered version of deoxyribonuclease 1 that selectively breaks down extracellular DNA present in respiratory tract mucus. It has a long duration of action, and its fate in the body is not known. There are no data on its effects in pregnancy or lactation. All four drugs in this category are used to relieve the build-up of secretions in bronchitis, cystic fibrosis and chronic obstructive pulmonary disorder, to help keep the airways open and functioning longer.

Contraindications and Cautions

Caution should be used in patients with a history of peptic ulceration as mucolytics can disrupt the gastric mucosal barrier (carbocisteine, erdosteine and mecysteine). Caution should also be taken when prescribing these drugs to females who are either pregnant or breast-feeding.

Adverse Effects

Adverse effects most commonly associated with mucolytic drugs include nausea, vomiting, diarrhoea, abdominal pain, GI bleeding (rare), headaches, urticaria and rashes. Dornase alfa can cause pharyngitis, voice changes, chest pain, rashes, urticaria and conjunctivitis.

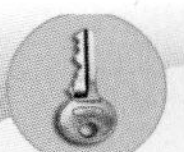

Key Drug Summary: *Carbocisteine*

Indications: Mucolytic therapy for patients with chronic bronchopulmonary disorders.

Actions: Breaks the disulphide bonds in the mucoproteins contained in the respiratory mucus secretions, decreasing the viscosity of the secretions.

Pharmacokinetics:

Route	Onset	Peak	Duration
Oral	30–60 min	2 h	Unknown

$T_{1/2}$: 2 hours; metabolized in the liver and excreted in urine

Adverse effects: GI irritation, GI bleeding (rarely) and rashes

Nursing Considerations for Patients Receiving Mucolytics

Assessment: History and Examination

Screen for the following conditions, which could be cautions or contraindications to use of the drug: *any history of allergy to the drug*, which are contraindications to the use of these drugs; *and peptic ulcer and pregnancy and breast-feeding,* which would require careful monitoring and cautious use. Establish if patient is currently taking other medications or herbal therapies which may potentially interact with the mucolytic drug.

Physical assessment should be done *to establish baseline data for assessing the effectiveness of the drug and the occurrence of any adverse effects associated with drug therapy*. Assess the following: skin colour and lesions *to monitor for adverse reactions*; and respiratory rate and depth and adventitious sounds *to monitor drug effectiveness.*

Nursing Diagnoses

The patient receiving a mucolytic may have the following nursing diagnoses related to drug therapy:

- Acute pain related to GI or skin effects of the drug
- Deficient knowledge regarding drug therapy

Implementation With Rationale

- Avoid combining with other drugs in the nebulizer *to avoid the formation of precipitates and potential loss of effectiveness of either drug.*
- Review the use of the nebulizer with patients receiving dornase alfa at home *to ensure the most effective use of the drug.* Patients should be cautioned to store the drug in the refrigerator, protected from light.
- Caution cystic fibrosis patients receiving mucolytics about the need to continue all therapies for their cystic fibrosis *because these are only a palliative therapy for improving respiratory symptoms, and other therapies are still needed.*
- Provide thorough patient teaching, including the drug name and prescribed dosage, measures to help avoid adverse effects, warning signs that may indicate problems and the need for periodic monitoring and evaluation, *to enhance patient knowledge about drug therapy and to promote concordance.*
- Offer support and encouragement *to help the patient cope with the disease and the drug regimen.*

Evaluation

- Monitor patient response to the drug (improvement of respiratory symptoms, loosening of secretions).
- Monitor for adverse effects (GI upset, skin rash).
- Evaluate the effectiveness of the teaching plan (patient can name drug, dosage, adverse effects to watch for, specific measures to avoid adverse effects, measures to take to increase the effectiveness of the drug).
- Monitor the effectiveness of comfort and safety measures and concordance with the regimen.

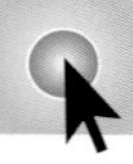

WEB LINKS

Health care providers and patients may want to consult the following Internet sources:

http://bnfc.org The BNF for Children provides UK health care professionals with authoritative and practical information on the selection and clinical use of medicines in children.

http://cks.library.nhs.uk The National Health Service Clinical Knowledge Summaries provide evidence-based practical information on the common conditions observed in primary care.

http://www.bnf.org.uk The BNF provides UK health care professionals with authoritative and practical information on the selection and clinical use of medicines.

http://www.cftrust.org.uk Information on cystic fibrosis, including research, treatments and resources.

http://www.mhra.gov.uk The Medicines and Health care products Regulatory Agency (MHRA) is the government agency responsible for ensuring that medicines and medical devises work and are safe for public use.

http://www.nhsdirect.nhs.uk The National Health Service Direct service provides patients with information and advice about health, illness and health services.

Points to Remember

- The classes of drugs that affect the upper respiratory system work to keep the airways open and gases moving efficiently.
- Antitussives are drugs that suppress the cough reflex. They can act centrally, to suppress the medullary cough centre, or locally, to increase secretion and buffer irritation or to act as local anaesthetics. These drugs should not be used longer than 1 week; patients with persistent cough after that time should seek medical evaluation.
- Decongestants are drugs that cause local vasoconstriction and therefore decrease the blood flow to the irritated and dilated capillaries of the mucous membranes lining the nasal passages and sinus cavities.
- An adverse effect that accompanies frequent or prolonged use of decongestants is rebound vasodilation, called rhinitis medicamentosa. The reflex reaction to vasoconstriction is a rebound vasodilation, which often leads to prolonged overuse of decongestants.
- Topical nasal decongestants are preferable in patients who need to avoid systemic adrenergic effects. Oral decongestants are associated with systemic adrenergic effects and require caution in patients with cardiovascular disease, hyperthyroidism or diabetes mellitus.
- Topical nasal corticosteroid decongestants block the inflammatory response from occurring. These drugs take several days to weeks to reach complete effectiveness.
- The antihistamines selectively block the effects of histamine at the H_1 receptors, decreasing the allergic response. Antihistamines are used for the relief of symptoms associated with seasonal and perennial allergic rhinitis, allergic conjunctivitis, uncomplicated urticaria or angio-oedema.

- Patients taking antihistamines may experience dryness of mucous membranes. The nurse should encourage them to drink plenty of fluids, to use a humidifier if possible and to avoid smoke-filled rooms.
- Some antihistamines should be avoided with any patient who has a prolonged Q–T interval because serious cardiac complications and even death can occur.
- Mucolytics work to break down mucus in order to aid high-risk respiratory patients in expelling thick, persistent secretions.
- Many of the drugs that act on the upper respiratory tract are found in various OTC cough and allergy preparations. Patients need to be advised to always read the labels carefully to avoid inadvertent overdose and toxicity.

CRITICAL THINKING SCENARIO 53-1

Dangers of Self-medicating for Seasonal Rhinitis

The Situation

Peter is a 46-year-old businessman who has been self-treating for seasonal rhinitis and a cold for the past 3 days. He calls the doctor's surgery for advice because he is feeling increasingly dizzy, drowsy and has been losing his balance. He is unable to drive to work or to stay awake. His wife wants to take him to Accident & Emergency (A&E) at the local hospital.

Critical Thinking

- What is the best approach for this patient?
- What crucial patient history questions should you ask before proceeding any further?
- If you do not know this patient, given his presenting story, what medical conditions would need to be ruled out before proceeding further?
- If Peter is self-medicating for the signs and symptoms of seasonal rhinitis, what could be causing his drowsiness and dizziness?
- What teaching points should be emphasized with this patient and his wife?

Discussion

There are a multitude of OTC cold and allergy remedies, most of which contain the same active drugs in varying proportions. A patient may be taking one drug to stop his runny nose, another to relieve his congestion and a third drug to treat his rhinitis. Combining OTC medications in this way puts patients at inadvertent risk of overdosing or at least allowing the medication to reach toxic levels.

In this situation, the first thing to determine is whether Peter's symptoms are caused by a neurological disorder. Careful history taking and examination will be able to rule this out. The next step is to establish which medications have been taken and the amount taken. Peter seems to have received toxic levels of antihistamines, decongestants or other upper respiratory tract agents. The nurse should encourage Peter to check the labels of any OTC medications being taken and to check with the health care provider if there are any questions. He should also be shown how to read OTC bottles or boxes for information on the contents of various preparations. In addition, he should be encouraged to use alternative methods to relieve the discomfort of seasonal rhinitis (e.g. using a humidifier, drinking lots of liquids, avoiding smoky areas) to allay the belief that many OTC drugs are needed. Finally, Peter should be advised to check with his health care provider if he has continued problems coping with seasonal allergic reactions. Other prescription medication may prove more effective.

Nursing Care Guide for Peter: Antihistamines

Assessment: History and Examination

Assess Peter's health history for allergies and bladder obstruction, renal or hepatic impairment, angle-closure glaucoma, benign prostatic hypertrophy and concurrent use of OTC allergy or cold products.

Focus the physical examination on the following areas:

- Neurological: sedation
- Skin: rash
- CV: blood pressure, pulse, peripheral perfusion
- GI: bowel sounds, abdominal examination
- Haematological: full blood count
- Respiratory: adventitious sounds
- Genitourinary: urinary output

Nursing Diagnoses

- Acute pain related to GI effects or dry mouth
- Decreased cardiac output
- Impaired sensory perception

(continued)

Dangers of Self-medicating for Seasonal Rhinitis *(continued)*

- Impaired urinary elimination
- Deficient knowledge regarding drug therapy

Implementation

- Provide comfort and safety measures, for example give drug with meals, teach about mouth care, increase humidity, institute safety measures if dizziness occurs.
- Provide support and reassurance to deal with drug effects and allergy.
- Provide patient teaching regarding drug name, dosage, adverse effects, precautions and warning signs to report.

Evaluation

- Evaluate drug effects, that is relief of nasal congestion and/or itchy eyes.
- Monitor for adverse effects: drowsiness, thickening of respiratory secretions, urinary retention and glaucoma.
- Monitor for drug–drug interactions as indicated.
- Evaluate effectiveness of support and encouragement strategies, patient teaching programme and comfort and safety measures.

Patient Teaching for Peter

- ☐ Antihistamines are commonly used to treat the signs and symptoms of various allergic reactions. Because these drugs work throughout the body, many systemic effects can occur with their use (e.g. dry mouth, drowsiness).
- ☐ Take this drug only as prescribed. Do not increase the dosage if symptoms are not relieved. Instead, consult your health care provider.
- ☐ Common effects of this drug include:
  - *Drowsiness, dizziness:* Do not drive or operate dangerous machinery if this occurs. Use caution to prevent injury.
  - *GI upset:* Taking the drug with food may help this problem.
  - *Dry mouth:* Frequent mouth care and sucking sugarless sweets may help.
  - *Thickening of the mucus, difficulty coughing, tightening of the chest:* Use a humidifier to increase the humidity of the room air (if you do not have one, place pans of water around the house); avoid smoke-filled areas; drink plenty of fluids.
  - Report any of the following to your health care provider: *difficulty breathing, difficulty in voiding, abdominal pain, visual changes, disorientation or confusion.*
- ☐ Avoid the use of alcoholic beverages while you are taking this drug. Serious drowsiness or sedation can occur if these are combined.
- ☐ Avoid the use of any OTC medication without first checking with a health care provider. Several of these medications contain drugs that can interfere with the effectiveness of this drug or they can contain very similar drugs, and you could experience toxic effects.
- ☐ Tell any doctor, nurse or other health care provider involved in your care that you are taking this drug.
- ☐ Take this drug only as prescribed. Do not give this drug to anyone else, and do not take similar preparations that have been prescribed for someone else. Keep this drug, and all medications, out of the reach of children.

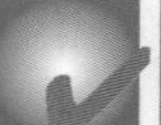

CHECK YOUR UNDERSTANDING

Answers to the questions in this chapter may be found in the answer key in the back of the book.

Multiple Choice

Select the most appropriate answer to the following.

1. A patient with sinus pressure and pain would benefit from taking
   a. an antitussive.
   b. a mucolytic.
   c. a decongestant.
   d. an antihistamine.
2. Antitussives are useful in blocking the cough reflex and preserving the energy associated with prolonged, nonproductive coughing. Antitussives are best used with
   a. postoperative patients.
   b. asthma patients.
   c. patients with a dry, irritating cough.
   d. COPD patients who tire easily.

3. Patients with seasonal allergic rhinitis experience irritation and inflammation of the nasal passages and passages of the upper airways. Treatment for these patients might include
   a. systemic corticosteroids.
   b. mucolytic agents.
   c. topical nasal steroids.
   d. an antitussive.

4. A patient taking an OTC cold medication and an OTC allergy medicine is found to be taking double doses of pseudoephedrine. As a result, the patient might exhibit
   a. ear pain.
   b. restlessness, tremors and palpitations.
   c. sinus pressure.
   d. an irritating cough.

5. Antihistamines should be used very cautiously in patients with
   a. a history of arrhythmias or prolonged Q–T intervals.
   b. COPD.
   c. asthma.
   d. angio-oedema.

6. A patient is not getting a response to the antihistamine that was prescribed. Appropriate action might include
   a. switching to a decongestant.
   b. stopping the drug and increasing fluids.
   c. trying a different antihistamine.
   d. switching to a corticosteroid.

7. Dornase alfa, because of its mechanism of action, is reserved for use in
   a. clearing secretions before diagnostic tests.
   b. facilitating removal of secretions postoperatively.
   c. relieving a dry, irritating cough.
   d. relieving the build up of secretions in cystic fibrosis.

Extended Matching Questions

Select **all** that apply.

1. Common adverse effects associated with the use of topical nasal steroids would include which of the following?
   a. Local burning and stinging
   b. Dryness of the mucosa
   c. Headache
   d. Constipation and urinary retention
   e. Fungal infections
   f. Osteonecrosis

2. An antihistamine would be the drug of choice for treating which of the following?
   a. Itchy eyes
   b. Irritating cough
   c. Nasal congestion
   d. Runny nose
   e. Idiopathic urticaria
   f. Thick, tenacious secretions

3. Additional nursing interventions for patients receiving antihistamines probably would include which of the following?
   a. Using a humidifier
   b. Advising client to suck sugarless lozenges to help relieve the dry mouth
   c. Limiting fluid intake to decrease swelling
   d. Providing safety measures to prevent falls or injury
   e. Encourage fluid intake if not on fluid restriction
   f. Leaving bowls of water around the house to increase humidity

Bibliography and References

British Medical Association and Royal Pharmaceutical Society of Great Britain. (2008). *British National Formulary*. London: BMJ & RPS Publishing. *This publication is updated biannually: it is imperative that the most recent edition is consulted.*

British Medical Association and Royal Pharmaceutical Society of Great Britain. (2008). *British National Formulary for Children*. London: BMJ & RPS Publishing. *This publication is updated annually: it is imperative that the most recent edition is consulted.*

Brunton, L., Lazo, J. S., Parker, K., Goodman, L. S., & Gilman, A. G. (2005). *Goodman and Gilman's the pharmacological basis of therapeutics* (11th ed.). London: McGraw-Hill.

Commission on Human Medicines. (2009). *Children's over-the-counter cough and cold medicines: New advice.* Available from http://www.mhra.gov.uk/.

Dixon, A. E., Kaminsky, D. A., Holbrookm J. T., Wise, R. A., Shade, D. M., & Irvin, C. G. (2006). Allergic rhinitis and sinusitis in asthma: differential effects on symptoms and pulmonary function. *Chest, 130,* 429–435.

Howland, R. D., & Mycek, M. J. (2005). *Pharmacology* (3rd ed). Philadelphia: Lippincott Williams & Wilkins.

Porth, C. M., & Matfin, G. (2008). *Pathophysiology: Concepts of altered health states* (8th ed.). Philadelphia: Lippincott Williams & Wilkins.

Rang, H. P., Dale, M. M., Ritter, J. M., & Flower, R. J. (2007). *Rang and Dale's pharmacology* (6th ed.). Philadelphia: Churchill Livingstone.

Simonsen, T., Aarbakke, J., Kay, I., Coleman, I., Sinnott, P., & Lysaa, R. (2006). *Illustrated pharmacology for nurses.* London: Hodder Arnold.

CHAPTER 54

Drugs Used to Treat Obstructive Pulmonary Disorders

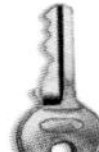

KEY TERMS

anti-inflammatory
antimuscarinics
β-adrenoceptor agonists
bronchodilators
corticosteroids
leukotriene receptor antagonists
mast cell stabilizers
sympathomimetic
xanthines

LEARNING OBJECTIVES

Upon completion of this chapter, you will be able to:

1. Describe the underlying pathophysiology involved in obstructive pulmonary disease and correlate this information with the presenting signs and symptoms.
2. Describe the therapeutic actions, indications and pharmacokinetics associated with xanthines, β-adrenoceptor agonists, antimuscarinic bronchodilators, inhaled steroids, leukotriene receptor antagonists, mast cell stabilizers and lung surfactants.
3. Describe the contraindications, most common adverse reactions and important drug–drug interactions associated with xanthines, β-adrenoceptor agonists, antimuscarinic bronchodilators, inhaled steroids, leukotriene receptor antagonists, mast cell stabilizers and lung surfactants.
4. Discuss the use of drugs used to treat obstructive pulmonary disorders across the lifespan.
5. Compare and contrast the key drugs salbutamol, beclometasone, theophylline, ipratropium, montelukast, sodium cromoglycate and beractant with other agents in their class and with other classes of drugs used to treat obstructive pulmonary disorders.
6. Outline the nursing considerations, including important teaching points, for patients receiving drugs used to treat obstructive pulmonary disorders.

β-ADRENOCEPTOR AGONISTS

bambuterol
ephedrine
fenoterol
formoterol
salbutamol
salmeterol
terbutaline

INHALED CORTICOSTEROIDS

beclometasone
budesonide
ciclesonide
fluticasone
mometasone

XANTHINES

aminophylline
theophylline

ANTIMUSCARINICS

ipratropium
tiotropium

LEUKOTRIENE RECEPTOR ANTAGONISTS

montelukast
zafirlukast

MAST CELL STABILIZERS	MONOCLONAL ANTIBODIES	LUNG SURFACTANTS
sodium cromoglicate	omalizumab	beractant
nedocromil		poractant alfa

Pulmonary obstructive diseases, including asthma and chronic obstructive pulmonary disease (COPD), cause obstruction of the major airways and are related to inflammation that results in narrowing of the interior of the airway and/or muscular constriction resulting in narrowing of the conducting tube (Figure 54.1).

The pathogenesis of *asthma* involves a genetic predisposition and a number of environmental factors including pet hair, grass pollen and house dust mites. Continued inflammatory reactions in response to allergens cause the airways to become hyper-responsive to a wide range of stimuli that nonasthmatic individuals do not respond to (e.g. cold air, exercise, cigarette smoke). The stimulus causes the bronchial smooth muscle to contract, constricting the airways leading to wheezing, a tight chest and shortness of breath.

In the majority of asthma patients, there are two phases to the asthma attack: an early and a late phase. The early phase occurs up to 20 minutes after the allergen interacts with immunoglobulin E (IgE) antibodies present on mast cells on the airway mucosa. The activated mast cells then release a number of inflammatory mediators including histamine, leukotrienes and prostaglandins which cause bronchoconstriction. In contrast to COPD, the airway constriction is reversible upon treatment with a bronchodilator.

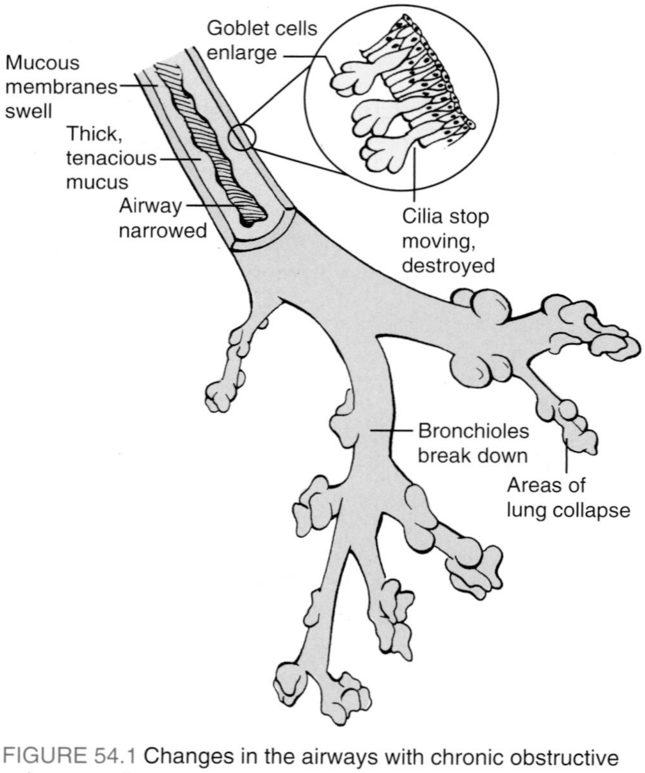

The late phase is characterized by an influx of inflammatory cells to the area, including T-lymphocytes, eosinophils and monocytes. These cells release further inflammatory mediators which damage the epithelial cells lining the airways allowing the allergen to access underlying sensory receptors. This is an important step in the development of bronchial hyper-responsiveness. Oedema of the mucosa, hypertrophy and hyperplasia of the bronchial smooth muscle and increased mucus production also occur.

For some asthmatics, avoiding exposure to the environmental stimuli known to trigger an asthma attack can improve their asthma. However, the majority of patients will require further treatment to open their conducting airways through muscular bronchodilation and/or a decrease of the effects of inflammation on the airway lining. The **β_2-adrenoceptor agonists**, leukotriene receptor antagonists and xanthines target different stages of the early phase. **Corticosteroids** are used to prevent the inflammatory processes in the late phase. The British Thoracic Society currently recommends a stepwise approach to managing asthma (see Table 54.1) where patients start treatment at the step appropriate to the severity of their asthma (British Thoracic Society and Scottish Intercollegiate Guidelines Network, 2008). Control is maintained by stepping up treatment when necessary or stepping down when control is good.

COPD is a group of diseases including emphysema and chronic bronchitis. The main cause of COPD is cigarette smoking but the disease can also result from a congenital condition known as alpha$_1$-antitrypsin deficiency (see Box 54.1). COPD is characterized by inflammatory processes mediated by macrophages, neutrophils and T-lymphocytes. There is fibrosis of the bronchial wall and an increase in the number of goblet cells, particularly in the large bronchi, resulting in increased mucus production. The release of protease enzymes from inflammatory cells leads to a loss of elastin fibres in the lung parenchyma and collapse of the airways. These pathological changes cause scarring, airway obstruction and reduced air flow where the air becomes trapped in the lower airways. There is also degeneration of the alveoli, a characteristic of emphysema, significantly reducing the surface area available for gas exchange. The permanent structural damage that occurs in COPD cannot

FIGURE 54.1 Changes in the airways with chronic obstructive pulmonary disease.

Table 54.1 Stepwise Management of Asthma in Adults. Patients should start treatment at the step most appropriate to the initial severity of their asthma. Taken from guidelines produced by the British Thoracic Society and Scottish Intercollegiate Guidelines Network (2008).

	Step 1: Mild intermittent Asthma *(Less Frequent Than Daily)*	**Step 2: Regular Preventer Therapy** *(Daily Symptoms)*	**Step 3: Initial add-on Therapy** *(Severe Symptoms)*	**Step 4: Persistent Poor Control** *(Uncontrolled Severe Symptoms With High-Dose Inhaled Corticosteroids)*	**Step 5: Continuous or Frequent use of Oral Steroids** *(Deterioration of Severe Symptoms)*
Treatment	Inhaled short-acting β_2-adrenoceptor agonist when required	Add inhaled corticosteroid (200–800 μg/day of beclometasone; but dose should be matched to severity of disease. 400 μg is an appropriate starting dose for most patients)	Add inhaled long-acting β_2-adrenoceptor agonist ***Assess asthma control:*** – If the patient responds well to the long-acting β_2-adrenoceptor agonist, continue treatment – If there is some benefit from the long-acting β_2-adrenoceptor agonist but control is still inadequate, continue β_2-adrenoceptor agonist and increase dose of inhaled corticosteroid to 800 μg/day – If the patient does not respond to the long-acting β_2-adrenoceptor agonist, stop the drug and increase dose of inhaled corticosteroid to 800 μg/day. If control is still inadequate, start trials of either a leukotriene receptor antagonist or sustained-release oral theophylline	Consider trials of: – Increasing inhaled steroid up to 2000 μg/day. – Addition of a fourth drug, for example leukotriene receptor antagonist, sustained-release oral theophylline, or oral β_2-adrenoceptor agonist	– Use daily steroid tablet in lowest dose providing adequate control – Maintain high-dose inhaled steroid at 2000 μg/day – Consider other treatments to minimize the use of steroid tablets – Refer patient for specialist care

be reversed fully even with some of the drugs described here. Patients are prone to infections, and in severe COPD, patients can develop respiratory failure and require oxygen therapy in addition to bronchodilators.

BOX 54.1 Focus on Enzyme Therapy: Alpha$_1$ (α_1)-antitrypsin Inhibitor (Human)

α_1-Antitrypsin inhibitor is produced by the liver and diffuses into the lungs from blood. In the lungs, α_1-antitrypsin inhibitor acts to inhibit neutrophil elastase, an enzyme capable of destroying the connective tissue present in alveolar walls. Neutrophil elastase levels are increased by smoking or lung infection. In the UK, one child in every 5000 is born with a hereditary, autosomal dominant deficiency of α_1-antitrypsin inhibitor and is at risk of progressive lung tissue destruction with smoking or lung infection. Not all these individuals will go on to develop any symptoms; however, those who develop breathlessness during their 30s or 40s exhibit radiographic evidence of basal emphysema. This type of emphysema is treated in the same way as other cases of emphysema; that is smoking cessation, drug therapy (bronchodilators, corticosteroids). Infusions of α_1-antitrypsin isolated from pooled human plasma (e.g. prolastin) could prove beneficial for patients with very low levels of α_1-antitrypsin. However, the enzyme therapy is not currently approved in the UK because there is insufficient data supporting the benefits of this treatment (National Institute for Health and Clinical Excellence, 2004).

Respiratory distress syndrome (RDS) in neonates causes obstruction at the alveolar level and is related to a lack of the lipoprotein surfactant, leading to an inability to maintain an open alveolus. Surfactant is essential in decreasing the surface tension in the alveolar sacs, allowing the sacs to expand and remain open. If surfactant is lacking, the alveoli collapse and gas exchange cannot occur. Pharmacological therapy for this condition involves instilling surfactant into the alveoli.

Adult respiratory distress syndrome (ARDS) is characterized by progressive loss of lung compliance and increasing hypoxia. This syndrome occurs as a result of a severe insult to the body, such as cardiovascular collapse, major burns, severe trauma and rapid depressurization. Treatment of ARDS involves reversal, where possible, of the underlying cause of the problem combined with ventilatory support.

Antiasthmatics

There are two types of antiasthmatics: **bronchodilators** and **anti-inflammatory** drugs. Bronchodilators reverse the bronchospasm and dilate the airways, providing symptomatic relief or prevention of bronchial asthma and for bronchospasm associated with COPD. Anti-inflammatory drugs inhibit the inflammatory processes underlying asthma. Some bronchodilator drugs also have anti-inflammatory actions, for example β-adrenoceptor agonists. The preferred administration route for antiasthmatics is via inhalation using inhalers or nebulizers. Inhalation has the advantage of fewer systemic adverse reactions and ensures that the drug is delivered directly to the site of action. Some antiasthmatics are administered orally (e.g. corticosteroids) or via intravenous infusion during acute severe asthma attacks. There is greater potential for systemic adverse effects via these routes. Box 54.2 discusses the use of these drugs with different age groups.

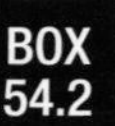

DRUG THERAPY ACROSS THE LIFESPAN

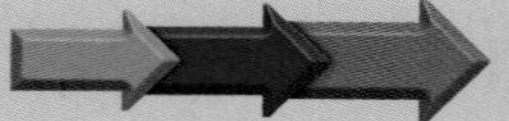

Lower Respiratory Tract Agents

CHILDREN

Premature neonates may require surfactant therapy to replace the surfactant absent from the surface of the alveoli. The parents of premature babies will require constant support and education to help them to cope with the stress of this event.

The incidence of asthma in children is rapidly increasing and antiasthmatics are frequently used. Children are usually commenced on a treatment trial to determine if their airway obstruction can be reversed by a bronchodilator (British Thoracic Society and Scottish Intercollegiate Guidelines Network, 2008). Acute episodes are best treated with a short-acting β_2-adrenoceptor agonist as required. Where possible, the drug should be administered using an inhaler to minimize adverse systemic effects. For long-term prophylaxis, the β_2-adrenoceptor agonist can be combined with an inhaled corticosteroid, a leukotriene receptor antagonist or theophylline.

Parents need to be encouraged to take measures to prevent acute attacks, including avoidance of known allergens, smoke-filled rooms and dusty areas. Parents should be cautioned about the proper way to measure liquid preparations to avoid inadvertent toxic doses or too little of the drug.

As the child grows and matures, its condition will need to be re-evaluated and dosage adjustments made to meet the needs of the growing child. Teenagers need to learn the proper administration and use of inhaled corticosteroids for prevention of exercise-induced asthma. As with other classes of medications, children may be more susceptible to the adverse effects associated with these drugs and need to be carefully monitored and evaluated.

When administering any drug to children, always consult the most recent edition of the British National Formulary for Children.

ADULTS

Adults may be able to manage their asthma quite well with the use of inhalers and avoidance of aggravating situations. Periodic review of the proper use of the various inhalers should be part of routine evaluation of these patients as should spirometry and peak expiratory flow rate (PEFR) readings to evaluate the effectiveness of the therapy.

Nicotine increases the metabolism of xanthines in the liver; xanthine dosage must be increased in patients who continue to smoke while using xanthines. In addition, extreme caution must be used if the patient decides to decrease or discontinue smoking because severe xanthine toxicity can occur.

It is important to ensure that asthma is well controlled during pregnancy to avoid maternal and foetal hypoxia during a serious asthma attack. To avoid foetal exposure to these drugs, the preferred route of administration is via inhalation. Most drugs used to treat obstructive pulmonary disorders can be taken during pregnancy and breast-feeding.

OLDER ADULTS

Older adults are frequently prescribed one or more of these drugs and are more likely to experience adverse effects, such as sedation, confusion, dizziness, urinary retention and cardiovascular effects, for example tachycardia and palpitations. Safety measures may be needed if these effects occur and interfere with the patient's mobility and balance.

Older adults are also more likely to have renal and/or hepatic impairment related to underlying medical conditions, which could interfere with the metabolism and excretion of some of these drugs. The dosage for older adults should be started at a lower level than that recommended for young adults. Patients should be monitored very closely and the dose adjusted based on patient response.

These patients also need to be alerted to the potential for toxic effects when using over-the-counter (OTC) preparations and should be advised to check with their health care provider before beginning any OTC drug regimen. Older adults with progressive COPD may be taking many combined drugs to help them maintain effective respirations. These patients should have an overall treatment plan involving complex pulmonary physiotherapy, fluids, nutrition and humidified air as well as a drug regimen to deal with the impact of this disease.

General Nursing Considerations Applicable to All Drug Classes

Assessment: History and Examination

Physical assessment should be performed *to establish baseline data for assessing the effectiveness of the drug and the occurrence of any adverse effects associated with drug therapy*, for example PEFR using a peak flow meter and forced expiratory volume in 1 second (FEV_1; the volume of air breathed out in the first second of a forced exhalation) using spirometry. The FEV_1 is normally expressed as a fraction of the forced vital capacity (FVC), the volume of air exhaled forcefully and as rapidly as possible following a maximal inhalation. A FEV_1 and/or PEFR of >80% of the predicted values for that patient indicate the asthma is well controlled (British Thoracic Society and Scottish

Intercollegiate Guidelines Network, 2008). Lung function tests should be carried out before and after treatment with the bronchodilator to assess if the bronchoconstriction is reversible.

Assess the following: respiratory rate and adventitious sounds *to establish a baseline for drug effectiveness.*

Establish if patient is currently taking other medications or herbal therapies which may potentially interact with the proposed drug treatment.

Implementation With Rationale

- Reassure the patient that the drug of choice will vary with each individual. A patient may have to try several different drugs before the most effective one is found.
- Carefully teach the patient about the proper use of the prescribed delivery system. The patient's technique should be assessed by a health care professional and review the patient's technique periodically *because improper use may result in ineffective therapy* (Box 54.3).
- Provide thorough patient teaching, including the drug name and prescribed dosage, measures to help avoid adverse effects, warning signs that may indicate problems and the need for periodic monitoring and evaluation, *to enhance patient knowledge about drug therapy and to promote concordance.* The British Thoracic Society and Scottish Intercollegiate Guidelines Network (2008) recommend a written personalized action plan for each patient.
- Offer support and encouragement *to help the patient cope with the disease and the drug regimen.*

Evaluation

- Monitor patient response to the drug: measure the FEV_1 as a fraction of the FVC and the PEFR. Both can be used to assess if the treatment has improved air flow and eased ventilation. The FEV_1 and/or PEFR should be greater than 80% of the predicted values for that patient (British Thoracic Society and Scottish Intercollegiate Guidelines Network, 2008). For COPD patients, the improvement in FEV_1 following bronchodilator therapy is likely to be small (<15%) because airway obstruction is only partly reversed in COPD.
- Evaluate the effectiveness of the teaching plan (patient can name drug, dosage, adverse effects to watch for, specific measures to avoid adverse effects, measures to take to increase the effectiveness of the drug).
- Monitor the effectiveness of other measures (e.g. allergen avoidance) to ease breathing

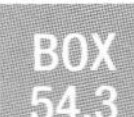

BOX 54.3 FOCUS ON **CLINICAL SKILLS**

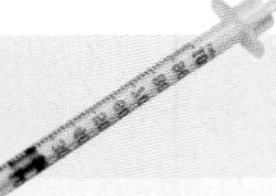

Teaching Patients to Self-administer Medication

It is important to deliver inhaled drugs into the lungs to achieve a rapid reaction and decrease the occurrence of systemic adverse effects. Patients who are self-administering inhaled drugs may be using an inhaler (with or without a spacer) or a nebulizer.

Inhalers

An inhaler is a device that allows a canister containing the drug to be inserted into a metered-dose device that will deliver a specific amount of the drug when the patient compresses the canister. The inhaler has a mouthpiece through which the drug is delivered.

Procedure for the correct use of a metered-dose inhaler (MDI):

1. Shake the inhaler and remove the cap covering the mouthpiece and check if it is clean.
2. Patient should then breathe out gently.
3. Place the mouthpiece in the mouth, ensuring that the lips form a tight seal around the mouthpiece.
4. As the patient begins to breathe in slowly and deeply, press the canister down and continue to inhale steadily and deeply.
5. The patient should hold their breath for 10 seconds or as long as is comfortable.
6. If a second dose is required, the patient must wait for approximately 30 seconds before repeating steps 2 to 5.

Spacers

Some inhalers may also have a spacer, a large plastic container with a mouthpiece at one end and a hole for the inhaler at the other. A spacer is designed to hold the dose of the drug while the patient inhales. This is advantageous if the patient has difficulty compressing the canister and inhaling at the same time or if inhaling is difficult. There are two techniques for using an inhaler with a spacer: the single breath technique and the multiple breath technique.

The single breath technique:

1. Remove the cap covering the mouthpiece and then shake the inhaler. Insert the inhaler into the appropriate end of the spacer.
2. Patient should then breathe out gently.
3. Place the mouthpiece end of the spacer in the mouth, ensuring that the lips form a tight seal around the mouthpiece.
4. The inhaler canister must be depressed once to release a single dose of the drug.
5. The patients should take one deep slow breath in and hold their breath for 10 seconds or for as long as is comfortable. The spacer can then be removed from the mouth, and the patient can breathe out.
6. If a second dose is required, the patient must wait for approximately 30 seconds before repeating steps 2 to 5.

The multiple breath technique:

1. Carry out steps 1 to 3 above.
2. The patient should start breathing in and out of the spacer slowly and gently and once a regular breathing pattern is established, the canister should be depressed once. The patient should then continue to breathe from the spacer several more times.
3. If a second dose is required, the patient must wait for approximately 30 seconds before repeating the steps above.

Nebulizers

A nebulizer uses compressed air to change a liquid drug into a fine mist for inhalation through a mask or mouthpiece. Nebulizers are more commonly used when high doses of bronchodilators require delivery in an emergency situation, for example in a clinical setting. These devices are no more effective than an inhaler and spacer for treating the majority of asthma attacks.

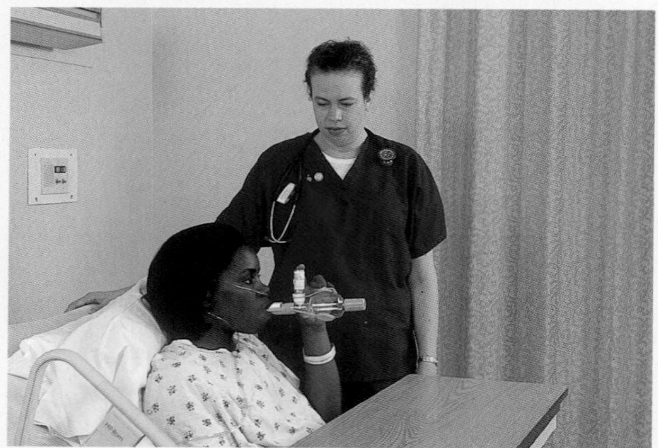

Teaching a patient to use a metered-dose inhaler. © B Proud.

β_2-Adrenoceptor Agonists

β_2-adrenoceptor agonists are **sympathomimetic** drugs that mimic the effects of the sympathetic nervous system. One of the actions of the sympathetic nervous system is dilation of the bronchi with increased rate and depth of respiration. β_2-adrenoceptor agonists act specifically on the β_2-adrenoceptors present on bronchial smooth muscle to increase the formation of the intracellular messenger cyclic AMP (cAMP). The concentration of calcium ions (Ca^{2+}) inside the smooth muscle cells is also reduced through the binding of Ca^{2+} to cytosolic proteins and by transporting Ca^{2+} across the plasma membrane. Together the increase in cAMP formation and reduction in intracellular Ca^{2+} result in smooth muscle relaxation and dilation of the airways during an asthma attack.

These drugs can be divided into two classes: short-acting drugs to provide immediate relief of symptoms and long-acting drugs which are usually used in conjunction with corticosteroid therapy as prophylactic treatment. All these drugs can be used to treat other conditions associated with reversible airways obstruction in addition to asthma.

Short-acting drugs (duration of action is 3–5 hours) include:

- *Fenoterol*, administered by inhalation, is available as a compound preparation combined with ipratropium (an **antimuscarinic** bronchodilator).
- *Salbutamol* is available in inhaled, oral, intravenous and intramuscular forms; however, the inhalation route is preferred; can be used as prophylaxis for exercise-induced asthma.
- *Terbutaline* can be used orally, parenterally or by inhalation (preferred route).

Long-acting drugs (duration of action is 8–12 hours) include:

- *Bambuterol* (prodrug of terbutaline) is delivered orally and recommended for adult use only.
- *Formoterol* is an inhaled drug used for maintenance treatment of asthma and prevention of bronchospasm in patients older than 5 years of age who have reversible obstructive airway disease and for prevention of exercise-induced bronchospasm in patients older than 6 years of age. Formoterol can be added to inhaled corticosteroid therapy in the long-term management of chronic asthma.
- *Salmeterol* is an inhaled drug successfully used to treat nocturnal asthma and prevent exercise-induced asthma and for the prophylaxis of bronchospasm in selected patients older than 4 years of age. Salmeterol is slower to act than either salbutamol or terbutaline and should not be used for the treatment of an acute asthma attack. Like formoterol, salmeterol can also be added to inhaled corticosteroid therapy.

Ephedrine and adrenaline (epinephrine) are also β-adrenoceptor agonists; however, they are used less frequently to treat obstructive airway disorders because of their wider systemic sympathomimetic effects, including arrhythmias. Adrenaline (epinephrine) is the drug of choice in adults and children for the treatment of acute bronchospasm associated with anaphylactic shock.

Therapeutic Actions and Indications

Most of the sympathomimetics used as bronchodilators are β_2-selective adrenergic agonists. That means that at therapeutic levels, their actions are specific to the β_2-receptors found in the bronchi (see Chapter 29). This specificity is lost at higher levels, and other systemic effects of sympathomimetics include increased blood pressure and heart rate, vasoconstriction and decreased renal and gastrointestinal (GI) blood flow – all actions of the sympathetic nervous system. These overall effects limit the systemic usefulness of these drugs in certain patients. However, β_2-adrenoceptor agonists can also play a useful role in the treatment of premature contractions in pregnant women where salbutamol and terbutaline are used to relax uterine smooth muscle.

Pharmacokinetics

Inhalation is the preferred route of administration for β-adrenoceptor agonists (see Box 54.3) so the inhaled drug is rapidly absorbed into the lung tissue. This route is also preferred during pregnancy to minimize exposure to the foetus. These drugs can be taken as normal during breast-feeding. Some β-adrenoceptor agonists, for example salbutamol, can also be administered by subcutaneous, intramuscular or intravenous injection and orally. Any absorbed drug is mostly excreted unchanged in the urine, and the rest is transformed in the liver to metabolites that are excreted in the urine.

Contraindications and Cautions

β-adrenoceptor agonists are contraindicated or should be used with caution, depending on the severity of the underlying condition, *in conditions that would be aggravated by the sympathetic stimulation*, for example hyperthyroidism, ischaemic heart disease, arrhythmias and hypertension. Patients requiring high doses of β-adrenoceptor agonists during pregnancy should have the drug administered via inhalation only. If given parenterally, the β-adrenoceptor agonists can cause tachycardia, arrhythmias and myocardial ischaemia and can also reduce the contractility of the myometrium. Diabetic patients should also use β-adrenoceptor agonists cautiously because there is a risk of hyperglycaemia and ketoacidosis. The blood glucose levels of diabetic patients should be monitored.

Adverse Effects

Adverse effects of these drugs, which can be attributed to sympathomimetic stimulation, include nervous tension, tremor (particularly the hands), headache, palpitations, tachycardia, cardiac arrhythmias, peripheral vasodilation (and therefore hypotension), paradoxical bronchospasm and sleep disturbances. High doses of β-adrenoceptor agonists can cause hypokalaemia.

Clinically Important Drug-Drug Interactions

Special precautions should be taken to avoid the combination of sympathomimetic bronchodilators with the antihypertensive, methyldopa. The peripheral vasodilation and consequent fall in blood pressure associated with long-term use of β-adrenoceptor agonists (particularly salbutamol) together with methyldopa will cause hypotension. The risk of hypokalaemia is increased if patients are taking a β-adrenoceptor agonist together with theophylline, corticosteroids and diuretics. Plasma potassium levels should be monitored.

Always consult a current copy of the British National Formulary for further guidance.

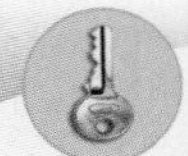

Key Drug Summary: *Salbutamol*

Indications: Asthma and other conditions associated with reversible airways obstruction; premature labour.

Actions: Predominantly binds to β-adrenoceptors in the airway smooth muscle to cause dilation of the airways

Pharmacokinetics:

Route	Onset	Peak	Duration
Oral	30 min	2 h	4–8 h
Sub-cut or IM	5–10 min	20 min	4–8 h
Inhalation	Minutes	30 min	3–6 h
IV	Minutes	Minutes	4–8 h

$T_{1/2}$: ~4 hours. If taken orally, approximately half is excreted unchanged in the urine, and the rest is metabolized by the liver and the metabolites excreted in the urine.

Adverse effects: Fine tremor (of the hands in particular), nervous tension, headache, muscle cramps, palpitations, tachycardia, arrhythmias and peripheral vasodilation.

Nursing Considerations for Patients Receiving β_2-adrenoceptor Bronchodilators

Assessment: History and Examination

Screen for the following conditions, *which are cautions to use of the drug*: allergy to any sympathomimetic; cardiovascular disease, hypertension, arrhythmias, diabetes, renal or hepatic impairment and hyperthyroidism, *which may be exacerbated by sympathomimetic effects*.

Assess the following: pulse, blood pressure and, in certain cases based on medical history, a baseline ECG *to monitor the cardiovascular effects of sympathetic stimulation* and liver function tests *to assess for changes that could interfere with drug metabolism and require dosage adjustment.*

Nursing Diagnoses

The patient receiving a sympathomimetic bronchodilator may have the following nursing diagnoses related to drug therapy:

- Increased cardiac output related to sympathomimetic effects (e.g. tachycardia, palpitations)
- Acute pain related to cardiovascular effects of the drug
- Deficient knowledge related to drug therapy

Implementation With Rationale

- Advise patients to use the minimal amount needed for the shortest period necessary *to prevent adverse effects and accumulation of drug levels.*
- Teach patients who use one of these drugs for exercise-induced asthma to use it immediately before exercising *to ensure peak therapeutic effects when they are needed.*

Evaluation

- Monitor for adverse effects (increased pulse and blood pressure).

Inhaled Corticosteroids

Inhaled corticosteroids are a very effective treatment for reversible and irreversible bronchospasm. Note that these drugs are not bronchodilators as such; instead, these drugs treat the underlying inflammation associated with asthma and COPD. By reducing inflammatory pathways, oedema and mucus secretion are also reduced. Drugs approved for this use include beclometasone, budesonide, ciclesonide, fluticasone and mometasone. A more detailed description of corticosteroids is given in Chapter 35, but it is important to note that the mechanism of action of these drugs is in regulating gene expression which will take hours rather than minutes to take effect: benefits are usually observed between 3 and 7 days. Therefore, corticosteroids are used to prevent attacks rather than in the acute management of an attack. Some patients may find a compound preparation of a corticosteroid combined with a long-acting β_2-adrenoceptor agonist effective (see Box 54.4). Patients with persistently poor control of their asthma may benefit from an oral corticosteroid, such as prednisolone (Table 54.1; Step 5).

BOX 54.4 Compound Bronchodilator Preparations

Some asthma treatments are available as a combined preparation of two drugs. There are no proven advantages to taking a compound preparation in comparison to single-ingredient preparations; however, a compound preparation may be appropriate for patients already taking the two asthma drugs separately. Patients should be stabilized on each drug separately before switching to the combination drug.

- Fenoterol (a β_2-adrenoceptor agonist) plus ipratropium (an antimuscarinic agent). Unsuitable for children.
- Formoterol (a β_2-adrenoceptor agonist) plus budesonide (a corticosteroid). Unsuitable for children.
- Salbutamol (a β_2-adrenoceptor agonist) plus ipratropium.
- Salmeterol (a β_2-adrenoceptor agonist) plus fluticasone (a corticosteroid).

Therapeutic Actions and Indications

Inhaled corticosteroids decrease the inflammatory response in the airway by reducing the number of eosinophils and other inflammatory cells attracted to the area. Production of the prostaglandins associated with vasodilation and hence oedema and swelling are also reduced. In airways that are swollen and narrowed by inflammation and swelling, both actions will increase air flow and facilitate ventilation. Corticosteroids can also increase the number of β_2-adrenoceptors to promote smooth muscle relaxation and inhibit bronchoconstriction (see Figure 54.2).

Pharmacokinetics

The majority (75–90%) of the inhaled dose adheres to the oral cavity and is swallowed. The remainder of the drug is absorbed well from the respiratory tract. Any systemically absorbed drug undergoes first-pass metabolism in the liver and is excreted in the urine. In pregnancy where the benefits to the mother outweigh the risk, corticosteroids delivered by inhalation are suitable. Only a small amount of inhaled drug is likely to be present in breast milk, and therefore the risk to the neonate during breast-feeding is likely to be negligible.

Contraindications and Cautions

Inhaled corticosteroids are not used during either an acute asthma attack or for emergency use in acute severe asthma (previously known as status asthmaticus). Corticosteroids delivered intravenously (hydrocortisone) are more appropriate for the latter. These preparations should be used with caution in any patient who has an

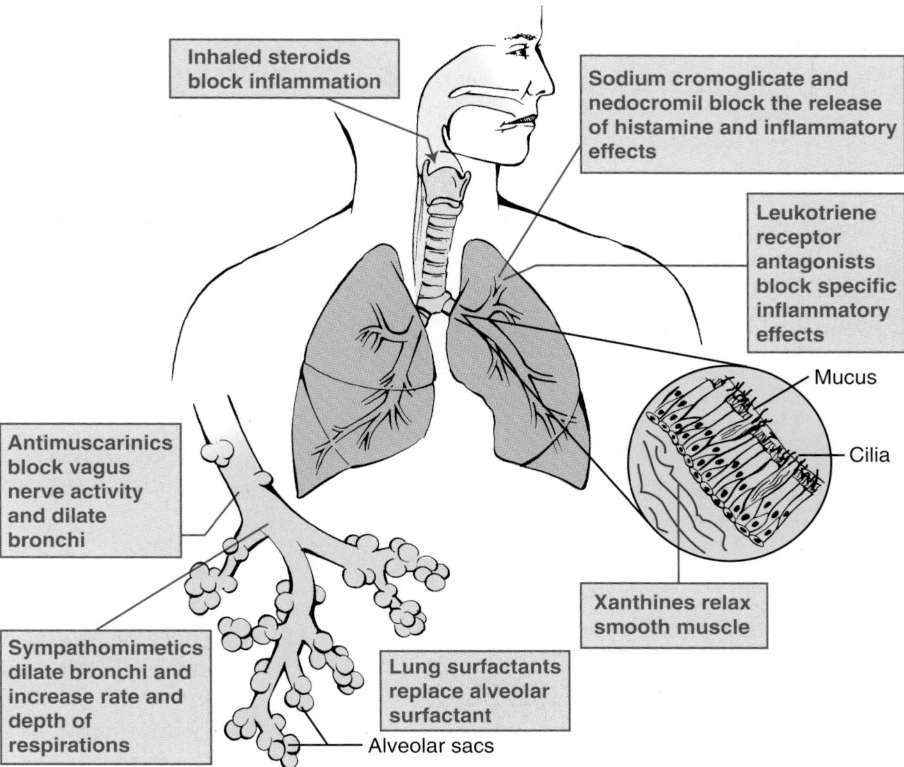

FIGURE 54.2 Sites of action of drugs used to treat obstructive pulmonary disorders.

active infection of the respiratory system because the depression of the inflammatory response could result in serious illness.

Adverse Effects

Inhalation of corticosteroids tends to decrease the numerous systemic effects associated with steroid use, and health care professionals should use the lowest dose necessary to control symptoms. High doses of inhaled corticosteroids can induce adrenal suppression, and patients should carry a 'steroid card' (see Chapter 35). Long-term administration can also lead to osteoporosis and possibly growth restriction in children. Sore throat, hoarseness and fungal infections of the oral mucosa (candidiasis) are the most common adverse effects encountered. Candidiasis can be reduced by either using a spacer or rinsing the mouth out or cleaning the teeth after delivery. If a patient does not administer the drug appropriately or develops lesions that allow absorption of the drug, the systemic side-effects associated with steroids may occur. There is a small risk of glaucoma and cataracts with inhaled corticosteroids.

Clinically Important Drug–Drug Interactions

The interactions with other drugs are less important when using inhaled corticosteroids. The key corticosteroid–drug interactions include antibacterials, antifungals and antivirals; anticoagulants, antiepileptics, barbiturates, methotrexate and vaccines.

Always consult a current copy of the British National Formulary for further guidance.

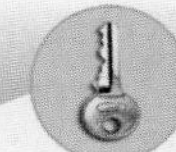

Key Drug Summary: *Beclometasone*

Indications: Prevention and treatment of asthma as an adjunct therapy for patients whose asthma is not controlled by traditional bronchodilators

Actions: Decreases the inflammatory response in the airway; this action will increase air flow and facilitate respiration in an airway narrowed by inflammation

Pharmacokinetics:

Route	Onset	Peak	Duration
Inhalation	Slow	30 min	8–12 h

$T_{1/2}$: 2.7 hours; metabolized in the liver and other tissues; excreted mainly in faeces

Adverse effects: adrenal suppression (high doses); osteoporosis; slower growth in children; sore throat, hoarseness, fungal infections of the oral mucosa and rarely anxiety, sleep disorders and behavioural changes.

Nursing Considerations for Patients Receiving Inhaled Corticosteroids

Assessment: History and Examination

Screen for the following conditions, *which could be cautions or contraindications to use of the drug*: acute asthmatic attacks and allergy to the drugs and systemic infections, *which require cautious use.*

Assess the following: temperature *to monitor for possible infections.*

Nursing Diagnoses

The patient receiving an inhaled steroid may have the following nursing diagnoses related to drug therapy:

- Risk of injury related to immunosuppression
- Deficient knowledge regarding drug therapy

Implementation With Rationale

- Do not administer the drug to treat an acute asthma attack or status asthmaticus *because these drugs are not intended for treatment of acute attack.*
- The lowest possible dose of inhaled steroid should be maintained for each patient. The patient should be re-assessed every 3 months to determine if the dose can be decreased.
- Taper systemic steroids carefully during the transfer to inhaled steroids; *deaths have occurred from adrenal insufficiency with sudden withdrawal.*
- Have the patient use decongestant drops before using the inhaled steroid *to facilitate penetration of the drug if nasal congestion is a problem.*
- Have the patient rinse the mouth after using the inhaler *because this will help to decrease oral fungal infections.*
- Monitor the patient for any sign of respiratory infection; *continued use of steroids during an acute infection can lead to serious complications related to the depression of the inflammatory and immune responses.*
- Monitor blood glucose levels in patients with diabetes *because corticosteroids can cause hyperglycaemia.*

Evaluation

- Monitor for adverse effects (sore throat, hoarseness, candidiasis).

Xanthines

The **xanthines** were once the main treatment choices for asthma and bronchospasm. Theophylline and aminophylline (a combination of theophylline and ethylenediamine) are the main drugs in this class where aminophylline is more soluble than theophylline alone. This group of drugs has a relatively narrow margin of safety (therapeutic window), and they interact with many other drugs, therefore they are no longer considered the first-choice bronchodilators. However, they can be used in addition to corticosteroids by patients for whom β_2-adrenoceptor agonists are ineffective (see Table 54.1; Step 3).

Therapeutic Actions and Indications

Xanthines are indicated for the symptomatic relief of acute severe bronchial asthma and for reversal of bronchospasm associated with stable COPD. Xanthines are not generally effective in exacerbations of COPD. The mechanism of action of xanthines is unknown, but the outcome is direct relaxation of the smooth muscle of the bronchi and vasculature (Figure 54.2). Smooth muscle relaxation increases the vital capacity that has been impaired by bronchospasm or air trapping. Theophylline also increases the contractility of the diaphragm further increasing the vital capacity. Xanthines may also have some anti-inflammatory action.

Pharmacokinetics

The xanthines are rapidly absorbed from the GI tract, reaching peak levels within 2 hours. They are widely distributed and metabolized in the liver and excreted in urine. Xanthines can cross the placenta, and the foetus is at greatest risk in the third trimester of pregnancy. They have been associated with foetal abnormalities and breathing difficulties at birth in animal studies. Although no clear studies are available in human pregnancy, use should be limited to situations in which the benefit to the mother clearly outweighs the potential risk to the foetus. Xanthines can also enter breast milk and cause neonatal irritability. The mother may choose to use another method of feeding the baby if these drugs are needed during lactation.

Contraindications and Cautions

Caution should be taken with any patient with cardiac disease, hypertension, fever, GI problems (e.g. peptic ulcer), hepatic disease, alcoholism or hyperthyroidism because the half-life of xanthines is affected by these conditions (see Adverse Effects below). Xanthines are available for oral and parenteral use; the drugs are too irritating for intramuscular injection and, when given intravenously, must be through slow infusion (greater than 20 minutes).

Adverse Effects

The adverse effects associated with xanthines are related to theophylline levels in the blood (Critical Thinking Scenario 54-1). Therapeutic plasma theophylline levels are from 10 to 20 mg/l, and plasma theophylline concentrations must be monitored after the initial dose and at least 5 days after starting treatment. With increasing levels, adverse effects are seen ranging from GI upset, nausea, irritability, insomnia and tachycardia to convulsions, arrhythmias and even death.

Clinically Important Drug–Drug Interactions

A number of beverages, including coffee, cola, chocolate and tea, contain caffeine or other xanthine derivatives, and, if taken together with theophylline, can lead to signs of toxicity. Xanthines are metabolized in the liver by cytochrome P450 enzymes. Many drugs are known to inhibit or induce these enzymes and therefore affect the half-life of xanthines. For example, heavy smoking and drinking induces liver enzymes (increases their activity) and ultimately decreases the half-life of xanthines and the plasma concentrations. Other important interactions include antibacterials, antifungals and antivirals; antidepressants, calcium channel blockers and cimetidine.

Always consult a current copy of the British National Formulary for further guidance.

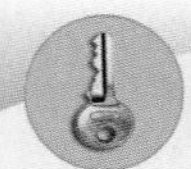

Key Drug Summary: *Theophylline*

Indications: Symptomatic relief of acute severe bronchial asthma and reversible airways obstruction associated with chronic bronchitis and emphysema

Actions: Directly relaxes bronchial smooth muscle, causing bronchodilation and increasing vital capacity; may also have an anti-inflammatory action

Pharmacokinetics:

Route	Onset	Peak	Duration
Oral	Varies	2 h	Varies

$T_{1/2}$: 3 to 15 hours (nonsmoker), 4 to 5 hours (smoker); metabolized in the liver and excreted in urine

Adverse effects: tachycardia, palpitations, nausea, GI disturbances, headache, central nervous system (CNS) stimulation, insomnia, arrhythmias and convulsions

Nursing Considerations for Patients Receiving Xanthines

Assessment: History and Examination

Screen for the following conditions, *which could be cautions to use of the drug*: any known allergy to one of the xanthines; cigarette use, *which would affect the metabolism of the drug;* peptic ulcer, epilepsy, hypertension, hyperthyroidism, coronary disease and hepatic dysfunction.

Perform the following assessments: blood pressure, pulse, cardiac auscultation and peripheral perfusion *to provide a baseline for effects on the cardiovascular system;* and liver evaluation and blood tests *to provide a baseline for hepatic function.* In addition, evaluate plasma theophylline levels *to provide a baseline reference.*

Nursing Diagnoses

The patient receiving a xanthine bronchodilator may have the following nursing diagnoses related to drug therapy:

- Acute pain related to headache and GI upset
- Disturbed sensory perception (kinaesthetic) related to CNS effects
- Deficient knowledge regarding drug therapy

Implementation With Rationale

- Administer oral drug with food or milk *to relieve GI irritation, if GI upset is a problem.*
- Provide comfort measures, including dietary control of caffeine and headache therapy as needed, *to help the patient cope with the effects of drug therapy.*
- Provide periodic follow-up, including blood tests, *to monitor plasma theophylline levels.*

Evaluation

- Monitor for adverse effects (CNS effects, cardiac arrhythmias, GI upset).
- Monitor for potential drug–drug interactions; consult with the prescriber to adjust dosages as appropriate.

Antimuscarinic Bronchodilators

Although sympathomimetic bronchodilators are the preferred asthma treatment as they are more effective, antimuscarinic bronchodilators can be useful in cases of severe asthma when used in combination with other standard therapies.

Therapeutic Actions and Indications

Antimuscarinics are used as bronchodilators because of their antagonism of muscarinic acetylcholine receptors in the parasympathetic nervous system (see Figure 54.2). Normally, vagal stimulation and release of acetylcholine result in contraction of the bronchial smooth muscle and bronchoconstriction. By blocking the muscarinic receptors and the vagal effect, relaxation of smooth muscle in the bronchi occurs, leading to bronchodilation. Both ipratropium and tiotropium are used in the maintenance treatment of patients with COPD, including bronchospasm and emphysema. Ipratropium can also be used in the treatment of an acute asthma attack and can be combined with β_2-adrenoceptor agonists in compound preparations (see Box 54.4).

Pharmacokinetics

Ipratropium has an onset of action of approximately 15 minutes when inhaled, and its peak effects occur in 30 to 60 minutes with a duration of effect of 3 to 6 hours. The drug is poorly absorbed, and therefore the effects of ipratropium are localized to the airways. Tiotropium also has a rapid onset of action with a longer duration than ipratropium with a half-life of 5 to 6 days. It is excreted unchanged in urine.

Contraindications and Cautions

Caution should be used in any condition *that would be aggravated by the antimuscarinic or atropine-like effects of the drug*, such as angle-closure glaucoma *(drainage of the vitreous humour can be blocked by smooth muscle relaxation)*, bladder outflow obstruction or benign prostatic hypertrophy *(relaxed muscle causes decreased bladder tone)* and conditions aggravated by dry mouth and throat.

Adverse Effects

Adverse effects are related to the antimuscarinic effects of the drug if it is absorbed systemically. The most common adverse effect is a dry mouth, but other rarer effects include nausea, headache, constipation, tachycardia, blurred vision and urinary retention.

Clinically Important Drug–Drug Interactions

When combining two or more antimuscarinic drugs, the side-effects associated with antimuscarinics are increased. Because both ipratropium and tiotropium are both inhaled drugs, the typical drug–drug interactions observed with antimuscarinics are not generally observed.

Always consult a current copy of the British National Formulary for further guidance.

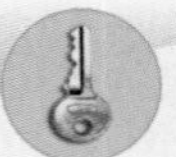

Key Drug Summary: *Ipratropium*

Indications: Maintenance treatment of bronchospasm associated with COPD, rhinitis

Actions: Antimuscarinic that blocks vagally mediated reflexes by antagonizing the action of acetylcholine

Pharmacokinetics:

Route	Onset	Peak	Duration
Inhalation	15 min	30–60 min	3–6 h

$T_{1/2}$: Unknown; metabolized by neural pathways

Adverse effects: dry mouth, nausea, headache, constipation, tachycardia, palpitations, paradoxical bronchospasm, blurred vision, angle-closure glaucoma, urinary retention and hypersensitivity reactions (e.g. rash).

Nursing Considerations for Patients Receiving an Antimuscarinic Bronchodilator

Assessment: History and Examination

Screen for the following conditions, *which could be cautions or contraindications to use of the drug*: allergy to antimuscarinics; acute bronchospasm, *which would be a contraindication;* angle-closure glaucoma *(drainage of the vitreous humour can be blocked by smooth muscle relaxation)*, bladder outflow obstruction or benign prostatic hypertrophy *(relaxed muscle causes decreased bladder tone)* and conditions aggravated by dry mouth and throat, *all of which could be exacerbated by the use of this drug;* and pregnancy and lactation, *which would require cautious use of tiotropium.*

Assess the following: orientation *to evaluate CNS effects*, pulse and blood pressure *to monitor cardiovascular effects of the drug* and urinary output and prostate palpation as appropriate *to monitor antimuscarinic effects.*

Nursing Diagnoses

The patient receiving an antimuscarinic bronchodilator may have the following nursing diagnoses related to drug therapy:

- Acute pain related to CNS, GI, GU or respiratory effects of the drug

- Imbalanced nutrition: less than body requirements, related to dry mouth and GI upset
- Deficient knowledge regarding drug therapy

Implementation With Rationale

- Recommend patient maintains adequate hydration *to make the patient more comfortable.*
- Recommend small, frequent meals and sugarless sweets *to relieve dry mouth and GI upset.*
- Encourage the patient to empty bladder before each dose of medication *to prevent urinary retention related to drug effects.*
- Provide safety measures if blurred vision occurs *to prevent patient injury.* Advise the patient not to drive or use hazardous machinery.

Evaluation

- Monitor for adverse effects (CNS effects, increased pulse, GI upset, dry mucous membranes).

Leukotriene Receptor Antagonists

A newer class of drugs, the **leukotriene receptor antagonists**, was developed to act more specifically at the site of the problem associated with asthma. Zafirlukast was the first drug of this class to be developed. Montelukast is the other drug currently available in this class.

Therapeutic Actions and Indications

Leukotriene receptor antagonists selectively and competitively block receptors for the leukotrienes C_4, D_4 and E_4 released during inflammation (see Figure 54.2). As a result, these drugs block many of the signs and symptoms of asthma, such as neutrophil and eosinophil migration, neutrophil and monocyte aggregation, leukocyte adhesion, increased capillary permeability and smooth muscle contraction. These factors contribute to inflammation, oedema, mucus secretion and bronchoconstriction seen in patients with asthma. The leukotriene receptor antagonists are indicated for the prophylaxis and chronic treatment of bronchial asthma in adults and children. Taking longer to produce an effect than the sympathomimetics, the leukotriene receptor antagonists are not indicated for the treatment of acute asthmatic attacks. However, they may be of use in preventing exercise-induced asthma and treating patients with concomitant rhinitis.

Pharmacokinetics

Taken orally, these drugs are rapidly absorbed from the GI tract. The lukasts are extensively metabolized in the liver by the cytochrome P450 enzyme system and are primarily excreted in the faeces.

Contraindications and Cautions

These drugs should be used cautiously in patients with hepatic or renal impairment *because these conditions can affect the drug's metabolism and excretion.* Both drugs can cross the placenta and enter breast milk. Montelukast should be avoided unless essential in pregnancy and lactation. The use of zafirlukast during pregnancy is only advised if the potential benefit outweighs the risk and should be avoided while breast-feeding.

Adverse Effects

Adverse effects associated with leukotriene receptor antagonists include headache, dizziness, nausea, vomiting, diarrhoea, abdominal pain, hepatic disorders, generalized pain, myalgia and very rarely Churg–Strauss syndrome, characterized by eosinophilia, vasculitis and a deterioration of pulmonary symptoms.

Clinically Important Drug–Drug Interactions

Use caution if aspirin is taken with these drugs because increased toxicity can occur. The therapeutic effect of lukasts can also be reduced by erythromycin, primidone and phenobarbital. Lukasts can also affect the plasma concentration of warfarin and theophylline, and so decreased dosage of either drug may be necessary.

Always consult a current copy of the British National Formulary for further guidance.

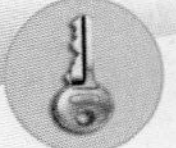

Key Drug Summary: *Montelukast*

Indications: Prevention and long-term treatment of asthma in adults and children

Actions: Specifically blocks receptors for leukotrienes, reducing airway oedema and inflammatory processes in the airway

Pharmacokinetics:

Route	Onset	Peak	Duration
Oral	Rapid	2–2.5 h	Unknown

$T_{1/2}$: 2.7–7 hours; metabolized in the liver and excreted mostly in faeces

Adverse effects: Include abdominal pain, thirst, headache, diarrhoea, dyspepsia, nausea, vomiting, hepatic disorders, palpitations, oedema, increased bleeding, Churg–Strauss syndrome, dizziness, generalized pain and fever

Nursing Considerations for Patients Receiving Leukotriene Receptor Antagonists

Assessment: History and Examination

Screen for the following conditions, *which could be cautions or contraindications to use of the drug*: allergy to the drug, pregnancy or lactation, *all of which would be contraindications to the use of the drug;* and impaired renal and liver function, *which could alter the metabolism of the drug and might require an adjustment in dose.*

Assess the following: orientation and effect *to monitor for CNS effects of the drug;* liver function tests *to assess for impairment if the patients medical notes suggest a history of hepatic dysfunction.*

Nursing Diagnoses

The patient receiving a leukotriene receptor antagonist may have the following nursing diagnoses related to drug therapy:

- Acute pain related to headache, GI upset or myalgia
- Risk of injury related to CNS effects
- Deficient knowledge regarding drug therapy

Implementation With Rationale

- Caution the patient that these drugs are not to be used during an acute asthmatic attack or bronchospasm; *instead, regular emergency measures will be needed.*
- Caution the patient to take the drug continuously and not to stop the medication during symptom-free periods *to ensure that therapeutic levels are maintained.*
- Provide appropriate safety measures if dizziness occurs *to prevent patient injury.*
- Inform patients of the signs of liver dysfunction including nausea, vomiting, malaise or jaundice. Patients should consult a health care professional.
- Urge the patient to avoid OTC preparations containing aspirin, *which might interfere with the effectiveness of these drugs.*

Evaluation

- Monitor for adverse effects [drowsiness, headache, abdominal pain, myalgia, Churg–Strauss syndrome (eosinophilia, rash, deteriorating pulmonary symptoms)]. Also monitor for signs of infection (e.g. elevated body temperature) as patients are at an increased risk of infection.

Mast Cell Stabilizers

The drugs sodium cromoglicate and nedocromil are both **mast cell stabilizers** used in the treatment of asthma and allergy. The use of this class of drugs has reduced in recent years mostly because of the improved efficacy of inhaled corticosteroids over mast cell stabilizers.

Therapeutic Actions and Indications

Although the precise mechanism of action of these drugs is not fully understood, they prevent the release of the inflammatory and bronchoconstricting substance, histamine, when the mast cells are stimulated by irritation or the presence of an antigen. By blocking the release of histamine, sodium cromoglicate prevents the allergic asthmatic response when the respiratory tract is exposed to the offending allergen. Administered by an inhaler, sodium cromoglicate may not reach its peak effect for 1 week. It is recommended for prophylaxis of asthma, exercise-induced asthma, allergic conjunctivitis and allergic rhinitis. This class of drugs should not be used in the treatment of acute asthma attacks.

Nedocromil inhibits the mediators of a variety of inflammatory cells, including eosinophils, neutrophils, macrophages and mast cells (see Figure 54.2). By blocking these effects, nedocromil decreases the release of histamine and blocks the overall inflammatory response. This drug is indicated for the prophylaxis of asthma in adult patients and children above 6 years of age.

A new approach to reducing the release of bronchoconstrictors from mast cells using monoclonal antibodies is described in Box 54.5.

Pharmacokinetics

Sodium cromoglicate is primarily active in the lungs, and most of the inhaled dose is excreted during exhalation or, if swallowed, excreted in urine and faeces. Nedocromil, when absorbed, is excreted primarily unchanged in urine. Sodium cromoglicate is not known to be harmful during pregnancy and is unlikely to be present in milk and is therefore safe for use in pregnancy and lactation. Nedocromil should be used with caution during pregnancy but is safe to use when breast-feeding.

BOX 54.5 Focus on Monoclonal Antibodies: Omalizumab

The antibody immunoglobulin E, or IgE, plays an important role in the inflammatory processes underlying asthma in some patients. Inhaled allergens, such as pet hair and dust mites, can bind to the IgE molecules on mast cells, causing the release of the bronchoconstrictors histamine and leukotriene B_4. Omalizumab is a humanized monoclonal anti-IgE antibody designed to bind to both circulating IgE and IgE molecules bound to mast cells, therefore preventing the release of chemical mediators from the mast cells.

Early studies have demonstrated that omalizumab may be beneficial to those patients (adults and children over 12 years) with poorly controlled allergic asthma where the patient has had a number of asthma attacks requiring hospital admission (Nowak, 2006). Administered subcutaneously every 2 to 4 weeks, the most common adverse effects are bruising, erythema and pain at the injection site. Rare adverse effects, including anaphylaxis, can occur in the first few days following injection.

Contraindications and Cautions

Neither sodium cromoglicate nor nedocromil is effective during an acute asthma attack, and patients need to be instructed in this precaution. Both drugs are safe for use by adults and children over the age of 6 years.

Adverse Effects

Few adverse effects have been reported with the use of sodium cromoglicate; those that do occur on occasion include coughing, throat irritation and a short-lived bronchospasm which can be avoided if a β_2-adrenoceptor agonist is administered beforehand. In addition to these adverse effects observed with sodium cromoglicate, nedocromil can also cause headache, nausea, vomiting, dyspepsia and abdominal pain.

Clinically Important Drug–Drug Interactions

There are no known drug–drug interactions with either sodium cromoglicate or nedocromil reported in the *British National Formulary*.

Always consult a current copy of the British National Formulary for further guidance.

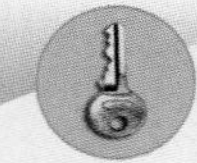

Key Drug Summary: *Sodium cromoglicate*

Indications: Prophylaxis of severe bronchial asthma, prevention of exercise-induced asthma, food allergy and allergic conjunctivitis and rhinitis

Actions: Inhibits the allergen-triggered release of histamine and other inflammatory mediators from mast cells, decreases the overall allergic response in the airways

Pharmacokinetics:

Route	Onset	Peak	Duration
Inhaled	Slow	15 min	6–8 h

$T_{1/2}$: 80 min; mainly excreted unchanged via exhalation

Adverse effects: Coughing, throat irritation and a short-lived bronchospasm

Nursing Considerations for Patients Receiving Mast Cell Stabilizers

Assessment: History and Examination

Screen for the following conditions, *which could be cautions or contraindications to use of the drug*: allergy to sodium cromoglicate or nedocromil.

Assess the following: respiratory rate and depth and adventitious sounds *to evaluate drug effectiveness*.

Nursing Diagnoses

The patient receiving a mast cell stabilizer may have the following nursing diagnoses related to drug therapy:

- Acute pain related to local effects, headache or GI effects
- Deficient knowledge regarding drug therapy

Implementation With Rationale

- Caution the patient not to discontinue use abruptly; sodium cromoglicate and nedocromil should be tapered slowly if discontinuation is necessary *to prevent rebound adverse effects.*
- Caution the patient to continue taking this drug, even during symptom-free periods, *to ensure therapeutic levels of the drug.*

Evaluation

- Monitor for adverse effects (headache, GI upset, local irritation).

Lung Surfactants

Lung surfactants are naturally occurring compounds or lipoproteins containing lipids and apoproteins that reduce the surface tension within the alveoli, allowing expansion of the alveoli for gas exchange. The two drugs currently available for use are beractant and poractant alfa. Poractant alfa is used in the treatment of adult RDS and in adults after cases of near-drowning where water has been aspirated.

Therapeutic Actions and Indications

These drugs are used to replace the surfactant that is missing in the lungs of neonates with RDS (see Figure 54.2). They are indicated for either the rescue treatment of infants who have developed RDS or in the prophylactic treatment of preterm neonates considered at risk of RDS. Neonates must have a birth weight of over 700 g. The parents of premature babies undergoing surfactant therapy will also require consistent support and education to help them to cope with the stress of this event.

Pharmacokinetics

These drugs are administered via endotracheal tubes directly into the bronchial tree and begin to act immediately. They are metabolized in the lungs by the normal surfactant metabolic pathways.

Contraindications and Cautions

Neonates must be continuously monitored to avoid hyperoxaemia resulting from a rapid improvement in arterial oxygen concentration.

Adverse Effects

The main adverse effect associated with the use of lung surfactants is pulmonary haemorrhage, especially in the more preterm neonates. This effect may be related to the immaturity of the patient, the invasive procedures used or reactions to the lipoprotein. The endotracheal tube may become blocked by mucus secretions.

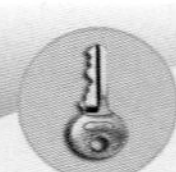

Key Drug Summary: *Poractant alfa*

Indications: Prophylactic treatment of preterm neonates at high risk for developing RDS, rescue treatment of infants who have developed RDS

Actions: Natural porcine compounds of lipoproteins that reduce the surface tension and allow expansion of the alveoli; replaces the surfactant that is missing in infants with RDS

Pharmacokinetics:

Route	Onset	Peak
Endotracheal	Immediate	Hours

$T_{1/2}$: Unknown; metabolized by surfactant pathways

Adverse effects: pulmonary haemorrhage

Nursing Considerations for Patients Receiving Lung Surfactants

Assessment: History and Examination

Screen for time of birth and exact weight *to determine appropriate dosages.* There are no contraindications to screen for as this drug is used as an emergency treatment.

Physical assessment should be done *to establish baseline data for assessing the effectiveness of the drug and the occurrence of any adverse effects associated with drug therapy.*

Assess the following: skin temperature and colour *to evaluate perfusion;* respirations, adventitious sounds, endotracheal tube placement and patency and chest movements *to evaluate the effectiveness of the drug and drug delivery;* blood pressure, pulse and arterial pressure *to monitor the status of the infant;* blood gases and oxygen saturation *to monitor drug effectiveness* and temperature and complete blood count *to monitor for sepsis.*

Nursing Diagnoses

The patient receiving a lung surfactant may have the following nursing diagnoses related to drug therapy:

- Decreased cardiac output related to cardiovascular and respiratory effects of the drug
- Risk of injury related to prematurity and risk of infection
- Ineffective airway clearance related to the possibility of mucous plugs
- Deficient knowledge regarding drug therapy (for parents)

Implementation With Rationale

- Monitor the patient continuously during administration and until stable *to provide life-support measures as needed.*

- Ensure proper placement of the endotracheal tube with bilateral chest movement and lung sounds *to provide adequate delivery of the drug.*
- Suction the infant immediately before administration, but do not suction for 2 hours after administration unless clinically necessary *to allow the drug time to work.*
- Provide support and encouragement to parents of the patient, explaining the use of the drug, *to help them cope with the diagnosis and treatment of their infant.*
- Continue other supportive measures related to the immaturity of the infant *because this is only one aspect of medical care needed for premature infants.*

Evaluation

- Monitor patient response to the drug (improved breathing, alveolar expansion).
- Monitor for adverse effects.
- Evaluate the effectiveness of the teaching plan and support parents as appropriate.
- Monitor the effectiveness of other measures to support breathing and stabilize the patient.
- Evaluate effectiveness of other supportive measures related to the immaturity of the infant.

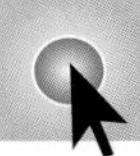

WEB LINKS

Health care providers and patients may want to consult the following Internet sources:

http://bnfc.org The BNF for Children provides UK health care professionals with authoritative and practical information on the selection and clinical use of medicines in children.

http://cks.library.nhs.uk The National Health Service Clinical Knowledge Summaries provide evidence-based practical information on the common conditions observed in primary care.

http://www.asthma.org.uk The charity Asthma UK works together with people with asthma, health professionals and researchers to develop and share expertise to help people increase their understanding.

http://www.bnf.org.uk The BNF provides UK health care professionals with authoritative and practical information on the selection and clinical use of medicines.

http://www.brit-thoracic.org.uk This site is run by The British Thoracic Society and provides current guidelines on the management of asthma.

http://www.nhsdirect.nhs.uk The National Health Service Direct service provides patients with information and advice about health, illness and health services.

http://www.nice.org.uk/guidance The National Institute for Clinical and Health Excellence provides specific guidance on the management of COPD in primary and secondary care.

http://www.sign.ac.uk The Scottish Intercollegiate Guidelines Network is involved in the preparation of clinical guidelines based on current evidence.

Points to Remember

- Pulmonary obstructive diseases include asthma, emphysema and chronic bronchitis which cause obstruction of the major airways; and RDS, which causes obstruction at the alveolar level.
- Drugs used to treat asthma and COPD include drugs to block inflammation and drugs to dilate bronchi and bronchioles.
- The xanthine derivatives have a direct effect on the smooth muscle of the respiratory tract, both in the bronchi and in the blood vessels.
- The side-effects and adverse effects of the xanthines are directly related to the theophylline concentration in the blood and are a feature of the narrow therapeutic window.
- β_2-adrenoceptor agonists mimic the effects of the sympathetic nervous system and dilate the bronchi to increase the rate and depth of respiration.
- Antimuscarinics can be used as bronchodilators because of their effect on the vagus nerve, resulting in a relaxation of smooth muscle in the bronchi, which leads to bronchodilation.
- Steroids are used to decrease the inflammatory response in the airway. Inhaling the steroid tends to decrease the numerous systemic effects that are associated with their use.
- Leukotriene receptor antagonists block or antagonize receptors for the production of leukotrienes D_4 and E_4, thus blocking many of the signs and symptoms of asthma.
- The mast cell stabilizers are antiasthmatic drugs that block mediators of inflammation and help to decrease swelling and blockage in the airways.
- Lung surfactants are instilled into the respiratory system of premature infants who do not have enough surfactant to ensure alveolar expansion.

CRITICAL THINKING SCENARIO 54-1

Toxic Reaction to Theophylline

The Situation

Rita has a medical diagnosis of chronic bronchitis and has been stabilized on theophylline for the past 3 years. She has been labelled as noncompliant with medical therapy because she continues to smoke more than 20 cigarettes per day, knowing that she has a progressive pulmonary disease. During a recent check-up, the nurse discussed the importance of smoking cessation, and Rita made a determined effort to cut down her cigarette intake. Several weeks later, Rita presented to Accident & Emergency (A&E) with complaints of dizziness, nausea, vomiting, confusion and palpitations. Her admission heart rate was 96 beats/min with occasional-to-frequent premature ventricular contractions.

Critical Thinking

- What probably happened to Rita?
- What information should the nurse have known before conducting the teaching programme?
- How could that information have been included in the patient teaching programme?
- What would the best approach be to this patient now?

Discussion

Rita probably did cut down on her smoking. However, she was not aware that cigarette smoking increases the metabolism of theophylline and that she had been stabilized on a dose that took that information into account. When she cut down on smoking, theophylline was not metabolized as quickly and began to accumulate, leading to the toxic reaction that brought Rita into A&E. This reaction illustrates the narrow therapeutic window of theophylline, that is, the difference between a dose that has a therapeutic effect and one which has a toxic effect is small.

Staff should be educated on the numerous variables that affect drug therapy and encouraged to check drug interactions frequently when making any changes in a patient's regimen. Regular follow-up and support will be important to help Rita continue her progress in cutting down smoking. Frequent checks of theophylline levels should be done while Rita is cutting back, and dosage adjustments should be made by her prescriber to maintain therapeutic levels of theophylline and avoid toxic levels.

Nursing Care Guide for Rita: Xanthines

Assessment: History and Examination

Assessment parameters include a health history focused particularly on allergies, peptic ulcer, hepatic dysfunction, coronary disease, cigarette use, pregnancy and lactation, as well as concurrent use of antibacterials, antidepressants, antiepileptics, antifungals, antivirals, barbiturates, calcium channel blockers and ulcer healing drugs. Always consult an up-to-date version of the British National Formulary for a comprehensive list of drug interactions.

Screen for the following conditions, *which could be cautions to use of the drug*: any known allergy to one of the xanthines; cigarette use, *which would affect the metabolism of the drug*; peptic ulcer, epilepsy, hypertension, hyperthyroidism, coronary disease and hepatic dysfunction.

Physical assessment should be performed *to establish baseline data for assessing the effectiveness of the drug and the occurrence of any adverse effects associated with drug therapy;* for example PEFR, spirometry readings. Perform the following assessments: blood pressure, pulse, cardiac auscultation and peripheral perfusion *to provide a baseline for effects on the cardiovascular system;* and liver evaluation and blood tests *to provide a baseline for hepatic function.* In addition, evaluate plasma theophylline levels *to provide a baseline reference.*

Focus the physical examination on the following areas:

- Neurological: orientation, effect, co-ordination
- Respiratory: respiratory rate and character, adventitious sounds
- Skin: colour
- CV: blood pressure, pulse, peripheral perfusion, baseline ECG
- GI: bowel sounds, abdominal examination
- Laboratory tests: serum theophylline levels, hepatic function test

Toxic Reaction to Theophylline *(continued)*

Nursing Diagnoses

- Acute pain related to GI effects
- Decreased cardiac output
- Impaired sensory perception (kinaesthetic)
- Deficient knowledge regarding drug therapy

Implementation

Provide supportive care with comfort and safety measures:

- Give drug with meals.
- Allow for rest periods.
- Provide a quiet environment.
- Ensure dietary control of caffeine.
- Provide headache therapy as needed.
- Provide reassurance to deal with drug effects and lifestyle changes.
- Provide patient teaching regarding drug name, dose, adverse effects, precautions, warnings to report, dietary cautions and need for follow-up.

Evaluation

- Evaluate drug effects: relief of respiratory difficulty, improvement of air movement.
- Monitor for adverse effects: GI upset, CNS effects, cardiac arrhythmias; monitor for drug–drug interactions as appropriate.
- Evaluate effectiveness of patient teaching programme and comfort and safety measures.

Patient Teaching for Rita

- ☐ The drug that has been prescribed for you, theophylline, is called a bronchodilator. Bronchodilators work by relaxing the airways, helping to make breathing easier and to decrease wheezes and shortness of breath. To be effective, this drug must be taken exactly as prescribed.
- ☐ This drug should be taken on an empty stomach with a full glass of water. If GI upset is severe, you can take the drug with food. Do not chew the modified-release capsules or tablets – they must be swallowed whole to be effective.
- ☐ Common effects of this drug include:
  - *GI upset, nausea*: Taking the drug with food may help this problem.
  - *Restlessness, difficulty in sleeping*: The body often adjusts to these effects over time. Avoiding other stimulants, such as caffeine, may help decrease some of these symptoms.
  - *Headache*: This often goes away with time. If headaches persist or become worse, notify your health care provider.
  - Report any of the following to your health care provider: *vomiting, severe abdominal pain, pounding or fast heart beat, confusion, unusual tiredness, muscle twitching, skin rash, hives.*
- ☐ Many foods can change the way that your drug works; if you decide to change your diet, consult with your health care provider.
- ☐ Adverse effects of the drug can be avoided by avoiding foods that contain caffeine or other xanthine derivatives (coffee, cola, chocolate, tea) or by using them in moderate amounts. This is especially important if you experience nervousness, restlessness or insomnia.
- ☐ Cigarette smoking affects the way your body uses this drug. If you decide to change your smoking habits, such as increasing or decreasing the number of cigarettes you smoke each day, consult with your health care provider regarding the possible need to adjust your dosage. Otherwise you could experience adverse drug effects.
- ☐ Avoid the use of any OTC medication without first checking with your health care provider. Several of these medications can interfere with the effectiveness of this drug.
- ☐ Tell any doctor, nurse or other health care provider involved in your care that you are taking this drug.
- ☐ Keep this drug, and all medications, out of the reach of children.

CHECK YOUR UNDERSTANDING

Answers to the questions in this chapter may be found in the answer key in the back of the book.

Multiple Choice

Select the most appropriate answer to the following.

1. Treatment of obstructive pulmonary disorders is aimed at
   a. opening the conducting airways through muscular bronchodilation or by decreasing the effects of inflammation on the lining of the airway.
   b. blocking the autonomic reflexes that alter respirations.
   c. blocking the effects of the immune and inflammatory systems.
   d. altering the respiratory membrane to increase flow of oxygen and carbon dioxide.

2. The xanthines
   a. block the sympathetic nervous system.
   b. stimulate the sympathetic nervous system.
   c. directly affect the smooth muscles of the respiratory tract.
   d. act in the CNS to cause bronchodilation.

3. Your patient has been maintained on theophylline for many years and has recently taken up smoking. The theophylline levels in this patient would be expected to
   a. rise, because nicotine prevents the breakdown of theophylline.
   b. stay the same, because smoking has no effect on theophylline.
   c. fall, because the nicotine stimulates liver metabolism of theophylline.
   d. rapidly reach toxic levels.

4. A person with hypertension and known heart disease has frequent bronchospasms and asthma attacks that are most responsive to sympathomimetic drugs. This patient might be best treated with
   a. an inhaled sympathomimetic to decrease systemic effects.
   b. a xanthine.
   c. no sympathomimetics because they would be contraindicated.
   d. an antimuscarinic.

5. A patient with many adverse reactions to different bronchodilator drugs is tried on an inhaled corticosteroid to prevent asthma attacks. For the first 3 days, the patient does not notice any improvement. You should
   a. switch the patient to a xanthine.
   b. encourage the patient to continue the drug for 2 to 3 weeks; if no response is noted by then, try another inhaled steroid.
   c. switch the patient to a sympathomimetic.
   d. try the patient on surfactant.

6. Leukotriene receptor antagonists act to block production of several inflammatory leukotrienes. They are most beneficial in treating
   a. seasonal allergic rhinitis.
   b. pneumonia.
   c. COPD.
   d. asthma.

7. Respiratory distress syndrome occurs in
   a. babies with frequent colds.
   b. babies with genetic allergies.
   c. premature babies and those with low birth weight.
   d. babies stressed during the pregnancy.

8. Lung surfactants used therapeutically are
   a. injected into a developed muscle.
   b. instilled via a nasogastric tube.
   c. injected into the umbilical artery.
   d. instilled into an endotracheal tube properly placed in the baby's lungs.

Extended Matching Questions

Select **all** that apply

1. Patients who are using inhalers require careful teaching about which of the following?
   a. Avoiding food 1 hour before and 2 hours after dosing
   b. Storage of the drug
   c. Administration techniques to promote therapeutic effects and avoid adverse effects
   d. Lying flat for as long as 2 hours after dosing
   e. Timing of administration
   f. The difference between rescue treatment and prophylaxis

2. A child with repeated asthma attacks may be treated with which of the following drugs?
   a. A leukotriene receptor antagonist
   b. A β-blocker
   c. An inhaled corticosteroid
   d. An inhaled β agonist
   e. A surfactant
   f. A mast cell stabilizer

True or False

Indicate whether the following statements are true (T) or false (F).

_____ 1. Pulmonary obstructive diseases include asthma, emphysema, COPD, respiratory distress syndrome and seasonal rhinitis.

_____ 2. Drugs used to treat asthma and COPD include agents that block inflammation and dilate bronchi.

_____ 3. The xanthine derivatives have a direct effect on the smooth muscle of the respiratory tract.

_____ 4. The adverse effects of the xanthines are directly related to the theophylline levels.

_____ 5. Sympathomimetics mimic the effects of the sympathetic nervous system and are used to dilate the bronchi.

_____ 6. Antimuscarinics can be used as bronchodilators because of their effect on the sympathetic nervous system receptor sites.

_____ 7. Steroids are used to decrease the inflammatory response in the airway.

_____ 8. Leukotriene receptor antagonists block or antagonize receptors for the production of leukotrienes C_4, D_4 and E_4, thus blocking many of the signs and symptoms of asthma.

Bibliography and References

British Medical Association and Royal Pharmaceutical Society of Great Britain. (2008). *British National Formulary*. London: BMJ & RPS Publishing. *This publication is updated biannually: it is imperative that the most recent edition is consulted.*

British Medical Association and Royal Pharmaceutical Society of Great Britain. (2008). *British National Formulary for Children*. London: BMJ & RPS Publishing. *This publication is updated annually: it is imperative that the most recent edition is consulted.*

British Thoracic Society and Scottish Intercollegiate Guidelines Network. (2008). British guidelines on the management of asthma. *Thorax, 63* (Suppl. 4), iv1–121.

Devereux, G. (2006). ABC of chronic obstructive pulmonary disease. Definition, epidemiology, and risk factors. *British Medical Journal, 332*(7550), 1142–1144.

Global Initiative for Chronic Obstructive Lung Disease. (2008). Global strategy for the diagnosis, management and prevention of chronic obstructive pulmonary disease. Available from http://www.gold.copd.com.

Ganong, W. (2005). *Review of medical physiology* (22nd ed.). New York: McGraw-Hill.

Howland, R. D., & Mycek, M. J. (2005). *Pharmacology* (3rd ed.). Philadelphia: Lippincott Williams & Wilkins.

Marieb, E. N., & Hoehn, K. (2009). *Human anatomy & histology* (8th ed.). San Francisco: Pearson.

National Collaborating Centre for Chronic Conditions. (2004). National clinical guideline on management of chronic obstructive pulmonary disease in adults in primary and secondary care. *Thorax, 59*(Suppl 1), 1–3, 192–194

National Institute for Health and Clinical Excellence. (2004). Chronic obstructive pulmonary disease: management of chronic obstructive pulmonary disease in adults in primary and secondary care. Available from http://www.nice.org.uk.

Nowak, D. (2006). Management of asthma with anti-immunoglobulin E: a review of clinical trials of omalizumab. *Respiratory Medicine, 100*(11), 1907–1917.

Porth, C. M., & Matfin, G. (2008). *Pathophysiology: Concepts of altered health states* (8th ed.). Philadelphia: Lippincott Williams & Wilkins.

Rang, H. P., Dale, M. M., Ritter, J. M., & Flower, R. J. (2007). *Rang and Dale's pharmacology* (6th ed.). Philadelphia: Churchill Livingstone.

Simonsen, T., Aarbakke, J., Kay, I., Coleman, I., Sinnott, P., & Lysaa, R. (2006). *Illustrated pharmacology for nurses*. London: Hodder Arnold.

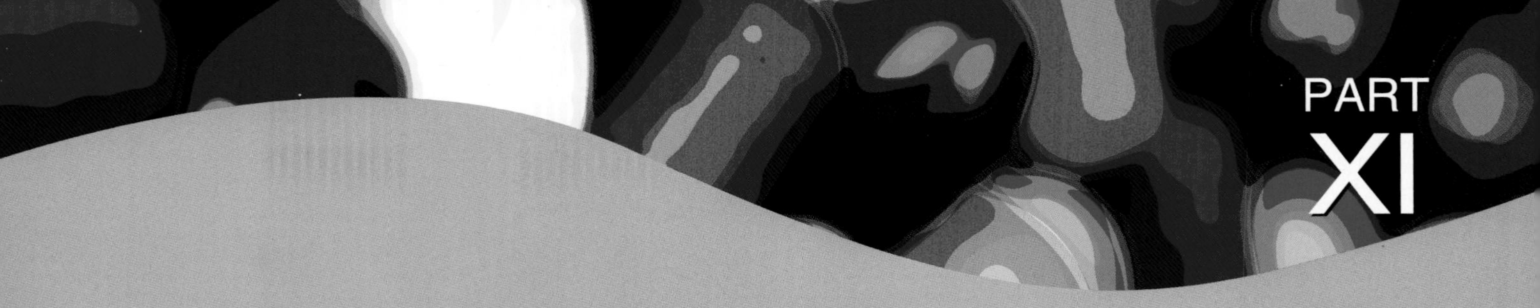

PART XI

Drugs Acting on the Gastrointestinal Tract

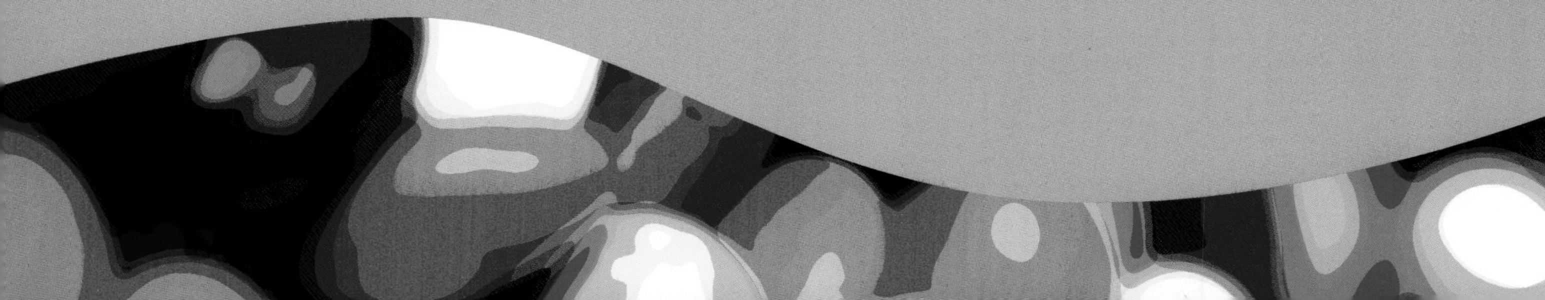

CHAPTER

55

Introduction to the Gastrointestinal Tract

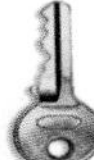

KEY TERMS

bile

chemoreceptor trigger zone (CTZ)

chyme

gallstones

gastrin

histamine H_2 receptors

hydrochloric acid

muscarinic receptors

nerve plexus

pancreatic enzymes

pepsin

peristalsis

saliva

segmentation

swallowing

vomiting

LEARNING OBJECTIVES

Upon completion of this chapter, you will be able to:

1. Label the parts of the gastrointestinal (GI) tract on a diagram and describe secretions, absorption, digestion and type of motility that occurs in each part.
2. Discuss the nervous control of the GI tract, including influences of the autonomic nervous system on GI activity.
3. List three of the local GI reflexes and describe the clinical application of each.
4. Describe the vomiting reflex and list three factors that can stimulate the reflex.
5. Outline the steps involved in swallowing and describe two factors that can influence this reflex.

The gastrointestinal (GI) tract is the only system in the body that is open at both ends to the external environment. Composed of one continuous tube beginning at the mouth, the GI tract progresses through the pharynx, oesophagus, stomach, small intestine (duodenum, jejunum and ileum), large intestine (caecum; ascending, transverse and descending colon; sigmoid colon) and ends at the rectum and anus. The pancreas, liver and gallbladder are accessory organs supporting the functions of the GI tract (Figure 55.1). The GI tract has four major activities:

- *Secretion* of enzymes, acid, bicarbonate and mucus
- *Absorption* of water and almost all of the essential nutrients needed by the body
- *Mechanical and chemical breakdown* of food into usable and absorbable components
- *Motility* and movement of food and secretions through the system (what is not used is excreted as faeces)

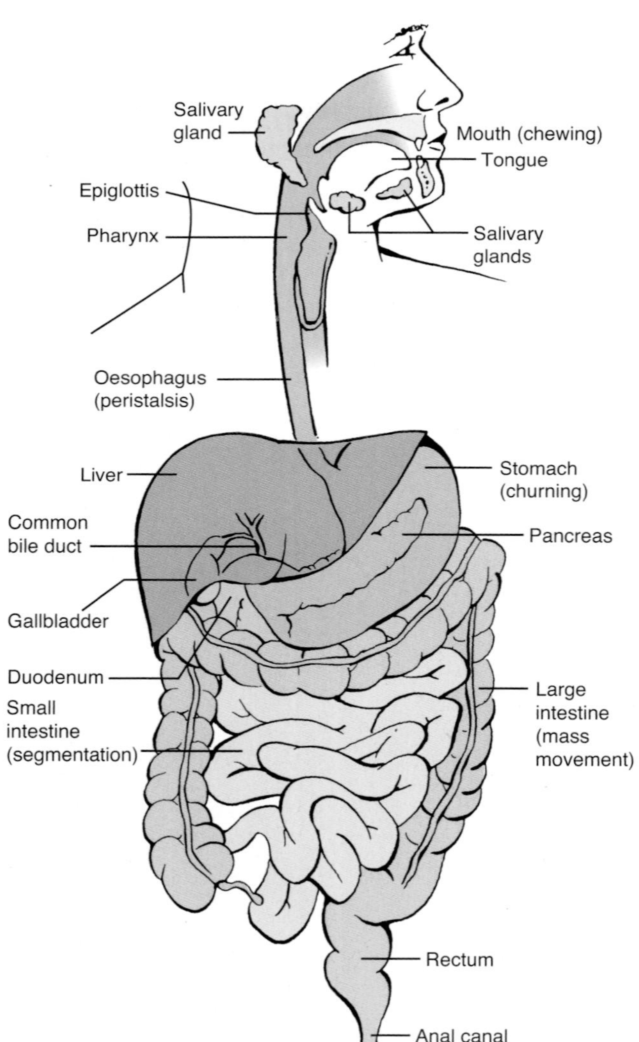

FIGURE 55.1 The gastrointestinal tract.

The GI tract is responsible for only a very small part of waste excretion. The kidneys and lungs are responsible for excreting most of the waste products of normal metabolism.

Composition of the Gastrointestinal Tract

As the GI tract is continuous with the external environment, the GI tract is exposed to many foreign agents and bacteria that are not found in the rest of the body. The peritoneum is a serous membrane with an inner *visceral* layer which wraps around the abdominal organs and an outer *parietal* layer attached to the abdominal wall. The peritoneal cavity forms the space between the two layers. The peritoneum helps keep the GI tract in place and prevents a build-up of friction with movement. The greater and lesser omenta hang from the stomach over the lower GI tract and are full of lymph nodes, lymphocytes, monocytes and other components of the mononuclear phagocyte system. This barrier provides rapid protection for the rest of the body if any of the bacteria or other foreign agents in the GI tract should be absorbed into the body.

The GI tract is composed of four layers: the mucosa, muscularis mucosa, **nerve plexus** and adventitia (Figure 55.2).

- The mucosal layer provides the inner lining of the GI tract and has a lining of epithelial cells and an underlying connective tissue component. This layer can be seen in the mouth and is fairly consistent throughout the tract. When assessing a patient, if the mouth is very dry or full of lesions, this is a reflection of the state of the entire GI tract and may indicate that the patient has difficulty digesting or absorbing nutrients.
- The muscularis mucosa layer is made up of muscles. Most of the GI tract has two muscle layers. One layer runs circularly around the tract, helping keep the tract open and squeezing the tract to aid digestion and motility. The other layer runs horizontally, which helps propel the GI contents down the tract. The stomach has a third

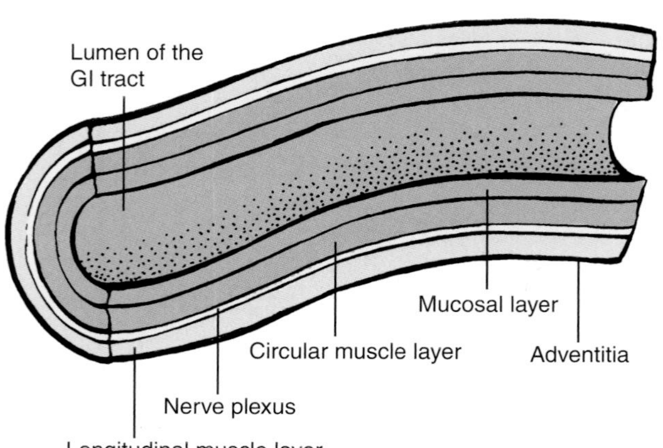

FIGURE 55.2 Layers of the gastrointestinal tract.

layer of muscle, running obliquely and gives the stomach the ability to move contents in a churning motion.

- The nerve plexus has two layers of nerves: one submucosal layer and one myenteric layer. These nerves give the GI tract local control of movement, secretions and digestion. The nerves respond to local stimuli and act on the contents of the GI tract accordingly. The GI tract is also innervated by the sympathetic and parasympathetic nervous systems. The sympathetic system is stimulated during times of stress (e.g. 'fight-or-flight' response) when digestion is not a priority. To slow the GI tract, the sympathetic system decreases muscle tone, secretions and contractions and increases sphincter tone. A reduction in GI activity saves the body energy for other activities. In contrast, the parasympathetic system ('rest and digest' response) stimulates the GI tract, increasing muscle tone, secretions and contractions and decreasing sphincter tone. Note that neither system can initiate local activity.
- The adventitia, the outer layer of the GI tract, serves as a supportive layer and helps the tract maintain its shape and stay in position.

Gastrointestinal Activities

The GI tract has four functions: secretion, digestion, absorption and motility. Each function is discussed in detail in the following sections.

Secretion

The GI tract secretes various compounds to aid the movement of the food bolus through the tract to protect the inner layer of the GI tract from injury and to facilitate the digestion and absorption of nutrients (see Figure 55.1). Secretions begin in the mouth. Saliva, secreted from the salivary glands (parotid, submandibular and sublingual), contains water and the digestive enzymes amylase (breaks down starch) and lingual lipase (breaks down fats) to begin the digestive process and to facilitate swallowing by making the bolus slippery. Mucus is also produced in the mouth to protect the epithelial lining and aid swallowing. The oesophagus produces mucus to protect the inner lining of the GI tract and to further facilitate the movement of the bolus.

The stomach produces gastric or **hydrochloric acid** (HCl) and digestive enzymes. In addition, it generates a large amount of mucus to protect the stomach lining from the acid and the enzymes. Secretion begins with what is called the cephalic phase of digestion. The sight, smell or taste of food stimulates the stomach to begin secreting before any food reaches the stomach. Once the bolus of food arrives at the stomach, the hormone **gastrin** is secreted from G cells in the stomach and duodenum. Gastrin stimulates the stomach muscles to contract, the parietal cells to release hydrochloric acid and the chief cells to release pepsinogen. Pepsinogen is the inactive form of **pepsin,** an enzyme which digests proteins. The pepsinogen molecules are activated by hydrochloric acid in the stomach.

The production of hydrochloric acid by the gastric parietal cells is a multistep process which occurs when gastrin, acetylcholine or histamine bind to **gastrin, muscarinic** and **histamine H_2 receptors**, respectively. Binding of the transmitter to their respective receptor results in a cytoplasmic signalling cascade which concludes with activation of the hydrogen–potassium adenosine triphosphatase (H^+/K^+-ATPase or 'proton pump') located in the apical membrane of the parietal cell. This proton pump exchanges intracellular H^+ for K^+ from the stomach lumen. The H^+ are generated in the cytoplasm from combining carbon dioxide (CO_2) and water (H_2O) to form carbonic acid (H_2CO_3). This process occurs under the action of the enzyme carbonic anhydrase. The carbonic acid then dissociates to form H^+ and bicarbonate ions (HCO_3^-).

The chloride ions required to form the hydrochloric acid are initially transported into the cell across the basolateral membrane in exchange for the bicarbonate ions produced by the dissociation of carbonic acid. Once in the cytoplasm, the chloride ions are transported out again across the apical membrane and into the stomach lumen via another exchange mechanism. Once in the stomach lumen, the H^+ and the chloride ions combine to form hydrochloric acid.

Peptic ulcers can develop when there is a decrease in the protective mucosal layer or an increase in acid production. Understanding the mechanism of acid production has led to the development of antihistamines, histamine H_2 receptor antagonists and proton pump inhibitors which can reduce the acid production (see Chapter 56).

When the now acidic bolus leaves the stomach and enters the duodenal section of the small intestine, *secretin* is released, which stimulates the pancreas to secrete large amounts of *sodium bicarbonate* (to neutralize the acid bolus), the pancreatic enzymes *chymotrypsin* and *trypsin* (to breakdown proteins to smaller amino acids), *lipases* (to breakdown fat) and *amylases* (to breakdown carbohydrates). These enzymes are delivered to the GI tract through the common hepatic duct, which is shared with the gallbladder.

When fat is present in the bolus, the gallbladder contracts and releases **bile** into the small intestine. Bile contains a detergent-like substance that breaks fat molecules apart for processing and absorption. Bile is produced by the liver during normal metabolism and delivered to the gallbladder for storage. In the gallbladder, the bile is concentrated by the removal of water by the walls of the gallbladder. Some people are prone to develop **gallstones** in the gallbladder when the cholesterol in the bile crystallizes. These stones can move down the duct and cause severe pain or even blockage of the bile duct. See Box 55.1 for information on methods of removing gallstones.

BOX 55.1 Treatment of Gallstones

Cholecystectomy (removal of the gall bladder) is usually the treatment of choice for patients with symptomatic gallstones. Severe pain, nausea and vomiting usually accompany an acute gallbladder attack (biliary colic), and removal is desirable. Some patients are not suitable for surgery because of other underlying medical conditions. These patients might benefit from either shock wave lithotripsy or gallstone solubilizers to dissolve certain gallstones. Only one drug, ursodeoxycholic acid, is available to dissolve gallstones and is best used when the gallstones are small (<10 mm in diameter) and nonobstructive. It may take several months of therapy for the gallstones to dissolve, and there is a high relapse rate.

Digestion

Digestion is the process of breaking down food into usable, absorbable nutrients. Digestion begins in the mouth, with the enzymes in the saliva starting the process of breaking down starch and a small amount of fat, and the mechanical digestion through chewing. The stomach continues the digestion process with muscular churning, breaking down some foodstuffs while mixing them thoroughly with the hydrochloric acid and enzymes. The acid and enzymes further break down sugars and proteins into building blocks and separate vitamins, electrolytes, minerals and other nutrients from ingested food for absorption. The beginning of the small intestine introduces bile to the food bolus, which is now called **chyme**. Bile breaks down fat molecules for processing and absorption into the bloodstream. Digestion is finished at this point, and absorption of the nutrients begins.

Absorption

Absorption is the active process of removing water, nutrients and other elements from the GI tract and delivering them to the bloodstream for use by the body. Some absorption of highly lipid-soluble substances such as alcohol occurs in the lower end of the stomach. The majority of fluid is absorbed in the small intestine. Here, the mucosal layer is specially designed to facilitate this absorption, with long villi on the epithelial layer providing a vast surface area for absorption. Between 6.5 and 7.5 l of fluid, including nutrients, drugs and anything that is taken into the GI tract, plus secretions, are absorbed each day. The large intestine reabsorbs approximately 1200 ml/day, mostly sodium and water. The portal system drains the entire lower GI tract and delivers what is absorbed into the venous system directly to the liver. The liver filters, clears and further processes most of what is absorbed before it is delivered to the body.

Motility

The GI tract depends on an inherent motility to keep things moving through the system. The nerve plexus maintains a basic electrical rhythm, much like the pacemaker rhythm in the heart. This rhythm maintains the tone of the GI tract muscles and can be affected by local or autonomic stimuli to increase or decrease the rate of firing.

The basic movement seen in the oesophagus is **peristalsis**, a constant wave of contraction that moves from the top to the bottom of the oesophagus. The act of **swallowing**, a response to a food bolus in the back of the throat, stimulates the peristaltic movement that directs the food bolus into the stomach. The stomach uses its three muscle layers to produce a churning action. This action mixes the digestive enzymes and acid with the food to increase digestion. Contraction of the lower end of the stomach pushes the chyme into the small intestine.

The small intestine uses a process of **segmentation** with an occasional peristaltic wave to clear the segment. Segmentation involves contraction of one segment of small intestine while the next segment is relaxed. The contracted segment then relaxes, and the relaxed segment contracts. This action exposes the chyme to a vast surface area to increase the absorption. The small intestine maintains a rhythm of 11 contractions per minute.

The large intestine uses a process of mass movement with an occasional peristaltic wave. When the initial segment of the large intestine is stimulated, it contracts and sends a massive peristaltic movement throughout the entire large intestine. The end result of the mass movement is usually excretion of waste products. Rectal distension after mass movement stimulates a defaecation reflex that causes relaxation of the external and internal sphincters. Control of the external sphincter is a learned behaviour. Receptors in the external sphincter adapt relatively quickly and will stretch and require more and more distension to stimulate the reflex if the reflex is ignored.

Local Gastrointestinal Reflexes

Stimulation of local nerves within the GI tract causes increased or decreased movement within the system, maintaining homeostasis. Loss of reflexes or stimulation can result in *constipation* and a lack of movement of the bolus along the GI tract, or *diarrhoea* with increased motility and excretion. In constipation, the faecal bolus remains in the large intestine for an extended period of time. During this time, more sodium and water is reabsorbed, and the stools become harder and more difficult to pass. It is important to note that individuals will have their own normal bowel movements: some will pass stools on a daily basis, whereas others will defaecate every 3 to 4 days. Patients with constipation will have noted that passing stools has become more difficult than it used to be.

Diarrhoea can be caused by stress or a viral or bacterial infection and leads to the chyme rushing through the large intestine, leaving insufficient time for nutrient and water reabsorption. This results in nutrient loss and watery stools. Prolonged diarrhoea can result in dehydration and electrolyte imbalance (loss of potassium) and can be particularly serious in infants, the frail and the elderly.

There are many local GI reflexes, and some knowledge of how they operate makes it easier to understand what happens when the reflexes are blocked or overstimulated and how therapeutic measures are often used to cause reflex activity.

- *Gastroenteric reflex:* Stimulation of the stomach by stretching, the presence of food or cephalic stimulation causes an increase in activity in the small intestine. It is thought that this prepares the small intestine for the coming chyme.
- *Gastrocolic reflex:* Stimulation of the stomach also causes increased activity in the colon, again preparing to empty any contents to provide space for the new chyme.
- *Duodenal-colic reflex:* The presence of food or stretch in the duodenum stimulates colon activity and mass movement, again to empty the colon for the new chyme.

It is important to remember the gastroenteric, gastrocolic and duodenal reflexes when helping patients to maintain GI movement. Taking advantage of stomach stimulation (e.g. having the patient drink orange juice or hot water or eat fibre-rich food) and providing the opportunity of time and privacy for a bowel movement encourages normal reflexes to keep things in control.

Central Reflexes

Two centrally mediated reflexes, swallowing and vomiting, are very important to the functioning of the GI tract. The *swallowing reflex* is stimulated whenever a food bolus stimulates pressure receptors in the back of the throat and pharynx. These receptors send impulses to the medulla, which stimulates a series of nerves that cause the following actions: the soft palate elevates and seals off the nasal cavity; respirations cease in order to protect the lungs; the larynx rises and the glottis closes to seal off the airway and the pharyngeal constrictor muscles contract and force the food bolus into the top of the oesophagus, where pairs of muscles contract in turn to move the bolus down the oesophagus into the stomach.

This reflex can be facilitated in a number of ways if swallowing (food or medication) is a problem. Cooling the tongue by sucking on an ice cube blocks external nerve impulses and allows this more basic reflex to respond. Keeping the head straight (not turned to one side) also allows the muscle pairs to work together and helps the process. Providing stimulation of the receptors in the mouth through temperature variations and textured foods helps initiate the reflex. Patients who do not produce their own saliva can be given artificial saliva to lubricate the food bolus and aid the swallowing reflex.

The *vomiting reflex* is another basic reflex that is centrally mediated and important in protecting the system from unwanted irritants. If irritating stimuli are sensed in the pharynx, oesophagus, stomach or upper regions of the small intestine, signals are sent to the **vomiting centre** in the medulla, and in turn impulses are sent to abdominal muscles and the diaphragm. Reverse peristalsis occurs which can quickly push the gastric contents of the small intestine back to the stomach. The sphincter between the oesophagus and stomach then relaxes allowing the contents to enter the oesophagus. At this stage, the patient takes one deep inspiration; the glottis closes and the palate rises, trapping the air in the lungs and sealing off entry to the lungs. The abdominal and thoracic muscles contract, and intra-abdominal pressure increases. The oesophageal sphincter relaxes completely, and the gastric contents are forced upwards through the oesophagus and mouth. With nothing in the stomach, this movement is known as retching and can be quite tiring and uncomfortable.

Vomiting can also be stimulated by:

- Tactile stimulation of the back of the throat, a reflex to get rid of something that is too big or too irritating to be swallowed
- Excessive stomach distension
- An increase in bowel movement (a possible explanation for vomiting in early pregnancy)
- Increasing intracranial pressure by direct stimulation
- Stimulation of the vestibular receptors in the inner ear (a reaction often accompanied by dizziness)
- Intense pain fibre stimulation
- Direct stimulation by various chemicals, including fumes, certain drugs and debris from cell death (a reason for vomiting after chemotherapy or radiation therapy that results in cell death).

Stimulation of a second area in the medulla, known as the **chemoreceptor trigger zone (CTZ)**, can also induce vomiting. Impulses pass from the CTZ to the vomiting centre, and the sequences of events described above are elicited. Some drugs, including morphine, can stimulate the CTZ directly.

Vomiting is a complex and protective reflex ridding the body of offending irritants, but it can also be undesirable in certain clinical situations, for example when the stimulant is not something that can be vomited or when the various components of the vomiting reflex could be detrimental to a patient's health status.

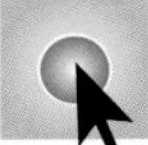

WEB LINK

To explore a virtual GI system, consult the following Internet source:
http://www.innerbody.com.

Points to Remember

- The GI tract is composed of one long tract that starts at the mouth; includes the oesophagus, the stomach, the small intestine and the large intestine and ends at the anus. The GI system is responsible for digestion and absorption of nutrients.
- Secretion of digestive enzymes, acid, bicarbonate and mucus facilitates the digestion and absorption of nutrients.
- The GI tract is controlled by a nerve plexus, which maintains a basic electrical rhythm and responds to local stimuli to increase or decrease activity. The autonomic nervous system can influence the activity of the GI tract, with the sympathetic system slowing and the parasympathetic system increasing activity. Initiation of activity depends on local reflexes.
- A series of local reflexes within the GI tract helps maintain homeostasis within the system. A change in stimulation of any of these reflexes can result in constipation (underactivity) or diarrhoea (overactivity).
- Swallowing is a centrally mediated reflex that is important in delivering food to the GI tract for processing. It is controlled by the medulla and involves a complex series of timed reflexes.
- Vomiting is controlled by the vomiting centre and CTZ in the medulla. The vomiting centre is stimulated by several different processes and initiates a complex series of responses that first prepare the system for vomiting and then cause a strong backward peristalsis to rid the stomach of its contents.

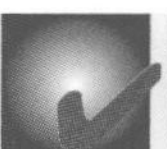

CHECK YOUR UNDERSTANDING

Answers to the questions in this chapter may be found in the Answer Key in the back of the book.

Multiple Choice

Select the best response to the following.

1. Constipation
   a. results from increased peristaltic activity in the intestinal tract.
   b. occurs only if one does not have a bowel movement at least once a day.
   c. leads to decreased salt and water absorption from the large intestine.
   d. symptoms can be artificially induced by increasing the volume of the large intestine.

2. The pancreas
   a. is only an endocrine gland.
   b. secretes enzymes in response to an increased plasma glucose concentration.
   c. neutralizes the hydrochloric acid secreted by the stomach.
   d. produces bile.

3. Gastrin
   a. stimulates acid secretion in the stomach.
   b. secretion is blocked by the products of protein digestion in the stomach.
   c. secretion is stimulated by acid in the duodenum.
   d. is responsible for the chemical or gastric phase of intestinal secretion.

4. The activities of the GI tract, movement and secretion are controlled by
   a. the sympathetic nervous system.
   b. the parasympathetic nervous system.
   c. local nerve reflexes initiated in the nerve plexus layer of the GI tract.
   d. the medulla.

5. The presence of fat in the duodenum causes
   a. acid indigestion.
   b. decreased acid production.
   c. increased gastrin release.
   d. contraction of the gallbladder.

6. The basic type of movement that occurs in the small intestine is
   a. peristalsis.
   b. mass movement.
   c. churning.
   d. segmentation.

7. Most of the nutrients absorbed from the GI tract pass immediately into the portal venous system and are processed by the liver. This is possible because almost all absorption occurs through the
   a. lower section of the stomach.
   b. top section of the large intestine.
   c. small intestine.
   d. ileum.

Extended Matching Questions

Select all that apply.

1. The vomiting centre in the brain is activated by which of the following?
   a. Stretch of the stomach
   b. Decreased GI activity
   c. Radiation
   d. Cell death
   e. Extreme pain

2. Acid production in the stomach is stimulated by which of the following?
   a. Protein in the stomach
   b. High levels of acid in the stomach
   c. Alcohol in the stomach
   d. Low levels of acid in the stomach
   e. Histamine H_2 receptor stimulation

3. Pancreatic digestive enzymes help in the breakdown of which of the following?
   a. Gastric acid
   b. Proteins
   c. Carbohydrates
   d. Bile
   e. Lipids

Matching

Match the following words with the appropriate definition.

1. ____________________bile
2. ____________________chyme
3. ____________________gallstones
4. ____________________gastrin
5. ____________________histamine H_2 receptors
6. ____________________hydrochloric acid
7. ____________________nerve plexus
8. ____________________pancreatic enzymes
9. ____________________peristalsis
10. ____________________segmentation

A. Acid released in response to gastrin
B. Sites on the parietal cells of the stomach that cause the release of hydrochloric acid into the stomach.
C. Contents of the stomach
D. Trypsin, pancreatic amylase and pancreatic lipase
E. Network of nerve fibres running through the wall of the GI tract
F. Fluid stored in the gallbladder
G. Crystallization of cholesterol in the gallbladder
H. Secreted by the stomach to stimulate the release of hydrochloric acid
I. GI movement characterized by contraction of one segment of small intestine while the next segment is relaxed
J. GI movement characterized by a progressive wave of muscle contraction

Fill in the Blanks

1. The GI system is composed of one long tract and is responsible for____________________and ____________________of nutrients.

2. Secretion of digestive enzymes,____________________, bicarbonate and____________________facilitates the digestion and absorption of nutrients.

3. The GI system is controlled by a ____________________ which maintains a basic electrical rhythm and responds to local stimuli to increase or decrease activity.

4. The autonomic system can influence the activity of the GI tract; the____________________system slows it and the____________________system increases activity.

5. Initiation of activity in the GI tract depends on ____________________.

6. Over stimulation of any of the GI reflexes can result in____________________(underactivity) or ____________________(overactivity).

7. Swallowing is a centrally mediated reflex that is important in delivering food to the GI tract for processing. It is controlled by the____________________.

8. Vomiting is controlled by the____________________ and the ____________________ in the medulla.

Bibliography

Ganong, W. (2005). *Review of medical physiology* (22nd ed.). New York: McGraw-Hill.

Guyton, A., & Hall, J. (2005). *Textbook of medical physiology* (11th ed.). Philadelphia: W. B. Saunders.

Howland, R. D., & Mycek, M. J. (2005). *Pharmacology* (3rd ed.). Philadelphia: Lippincott Williams & Wilkins.

Marieb, E. N., & Hoehn, K. (2009). *Human anatomy & histology* (8th ed.). San Francisco: Pearson.

Porth, C. M., & Matfin, G. (2008). *Pathophysiology: Concepts of altered health states* (8th ed.). Philadelphia: Lippincott Williams & Wilkins.

CHAPTER 56

Drugs Affecting Gastrointestinal Secretions

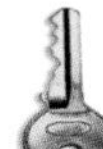

KEY TERMS

acid rebound

histamine (H_2) receptor antagonists

peptic ulcer

prostaglandin analogues

proton pump inhibitor

LEARNING OBJECTIVES

Upon completion of this chapter, you will be able to:

1. Describe the current theories on the pathophysiological process responsible for the signs and symptoms of peptic ulcer disease.
2. Describe the therapeutic actions, indications, pharmacokinetics, contraindications, most common adverse reactions and important drug–drug interactions associated with agents used to affect gastrointestinal secretions and digestive enzymes.
3. Discuss the drugs used to affect gastrointestinal secretions across the lifespan.
4. Compare and contrast the key drugs compound alginates, cimetidine, omeprazole, misoprostol and pancreatin with other drugs in their class and with other classes of drugs used to affect gastrointestinal secretions.
5. Outline the nursing considerations, including important education points, for patients receiving drugs used to affect gastrointestinal secretions.

ANTACIDS

aluminium salts

compound alginates

magnesium salts

HISTAMINE H_2 RECEPTOR ANTAGONISTS

cimetidine

famotidine

nizatidine

ranitidine

PROTON PUMP INHIBITORS

esomeprazole

lansoprazole

omeprazole

pantoprazole

rabeprazole

ANTIPEPTIC AGENT

bismuth chelate

misoprostol

sucralfate

tripotassium dicitratobismuthate

DIGESTIVE ENZYMES

pancreatin

Gastrointestinal (GI) disorders are among the most common complaints seen in clinical practice. Many products are available for the self-treatment of upset stomach and dyspepsia, commonly known as indigestion or heartburn. The underlying causes of these disorders can range from dietary excess, stress, hiatus hernia, oesophageal reflux and adverse drug effects, to the more serious peptic ulcer disease.

Drugs that affect GI secretions can decrease GI secretory activity, block the action of GI secretions, form protective coverings on the GI lining to prevent erosion from GI secretions or replace missing GI enzymes that the GI tract or ancillary glands and organs can no longer produce (Figure 56.1). These drugs are used with all age groups (Box 56.1).

Digestive Enzyme Dysfunction

Some patients require a supplement to the production of digestive enzymes. Patients with strokes, salivary gland disorders or surgery of the head and neck may not be able to produce saliva. Saliva is important in initiating the digestion of starch and, to a lesser extent lipids, and is essential in lubricating the bolus of food and initiating the swallowing reflex. Artificial saliva may be necessary for these patients to aid swallowing. Patients with common duct problems, pancreatic disease or cystic fibrosis may not be able to produce or secrete pancreatic enzymes.

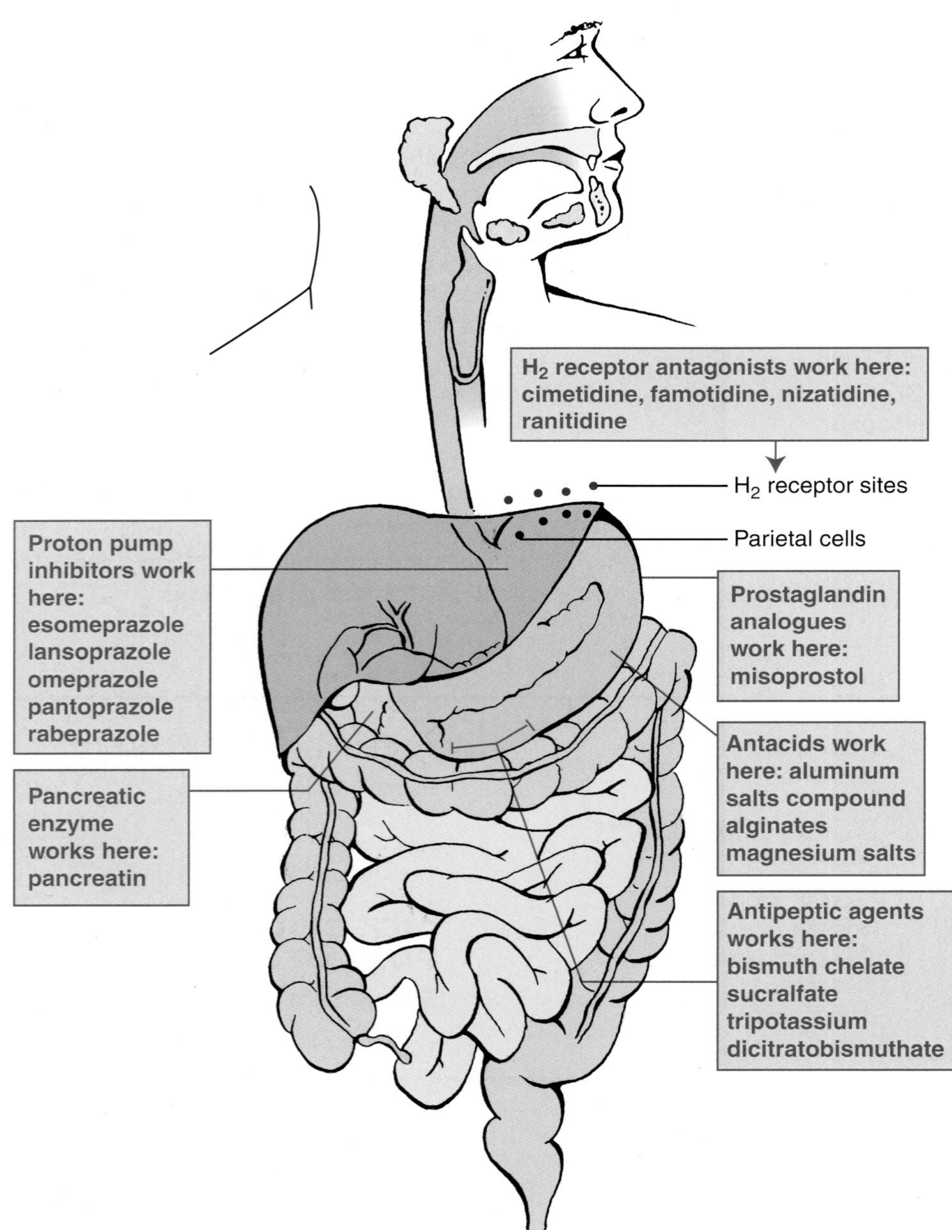

FIGURE 56.1 Sites of action of drugs affecting gastrointestinal secretions.

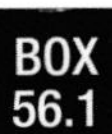

BOX 56.1 DRUG THERAPY ACROSS THE LIFESPAN

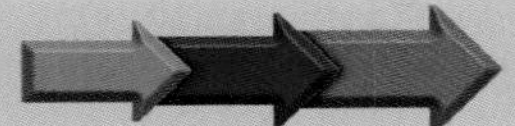

Agents That Affect Gastrointestinal Secretions

CHILDREN

Antacids may be used in children who complain of upset stomach or who are receiving therapy known to increase acid production. Children diagnosed with oesophagitis (inflammation of the oesophagus) may require an H_2-receptor antagonist (e.g. cimetidine) to reduce acid secretion. If the oesophagitis is resistant to inhibition of the H_2-receptors, a proton pump inhibitor such as omeprazole or lansoprazole may be used. Lansoprazole has established paediatric dosages. Special caution should be used with any of these agents to prevent electrolyte disturbances or any interference with nutrition, which could be especially detrimental to children.

ADULTS

Adults should be cautioned not to overuse drugs that modify GI secretions and to check with their health care provider if GI discomfort continues after repeated use of any of these drugs. Patients should be monitored for any electrolyte disturbances, for example antacids containing magnesium salts may lead to hypermagnesaemia in patients with renal dysfunction. Antacids may also interfere with the absorption or action of other drugs and should, therefore, be spaced 1 to 2 hours before or after the use of other drugs.

The safety of these drugs during pregnancy and lactation has not been established. Misoprostol is an abortifacient and should never be used during pregnancy. Women of childbearing age who use this drug should be advised to use barrier-type contraceptives. Use of these agents should be reserved for those situations in which the benefit to the mother outweighs the potential risk to the foetus. The drugs may enter breast milk and may also alter electrolyte levels or gastric secretions in the neonate. It is advised that caution should be used if one of these drugs is prescribed during lactation.

OLDER ADULTS

Older adults are frequently prescribed one or more of these drugs. There is potential for serious drug–drug interactions between drugs prescribed to modify GI secretions and drugs prescribed for other conditions. Older adults are more likely to develop adverse effects associated with the use of these drugs, including sedation, confusion, dizziness, urinary retention and cardiovascular effects. Safety measures may be needed if these effects occur and interfere with the patient's mobility and balance.

Older adults are also more likely to have renal and/or hepatic impairment related to underlying medical conditions, which could interfere with the metabolism and excretion of these drugs. Patients should be monitored very closely, and dosage adjustment should be made based on patient response.

These patients also need to be alerted to the potential for toxic effects when using over-the-counter (OTC) preparations that may contain the same ingredients as many of these agents. They should be advised to check with their health care provider before beginning any OTC drug regimen.

Proton pump inhibitors may be the best choice for treating gastro-oesophageal reflux disease in older patients because of fewer adverse effects and better therapeutic response with these drugs.

These enzymes may need to be administered to allow normal digestion and absorption of nutrients.

Peptic Ulcers

Erosions in the lining of the stomach and adjacent areas of the GI tract are called **peptic ulcers**. Ulcer patients present with a gnawing, burning pain, often occurring a few hours after meals. Many of the drugs used to affect GI secretions are designed to prevent, treat or aid in the healing of these ulcers. The actual cause of chronic peptic ulcers is not completely understood. For many years it was believed that ulcers were caused by excessive acid production, and treatment was aimed at neutralizing acid or blocking the parasympathetic nervous system to decrease normal GI activity and secretions. Further research led many to believe that, because acid production was often normal in ulcer patients, ulcers were caused by a defect in the mucous lining that coats the inner lumen of the stomach to protect it from acid and digestive enzymes. Some of the risk factors that were suggested to be linked to causing an ulcer were a family history of peptic ulcers, smoking, drugs such as nonsteroidal anti-inflammatory drugs (NSAIDs) and stress. Treatment was aimed at improving the balance between the acid produced and the mucous layer that protects the stomach lining. The focus of treatment today is on eradicating the cause of the ulcer instead. It is now known that the primary cause of chronic ulcers may result from bacterial infection by *Helicobacter pylori* bacteria. Chronic ulcers caused by *H. pylori* can be effectively treated by a combination of antibiotics and inhibition of acid production.

Acute ulcers, or 'stress ulcers', are often seen in situations that involve acute stress, such as trauma, burns or prolonged critical illness. The activity of the sympathetic nervous system during stress decreases blood flow to the GI tract, leading to weakening of the mucosal layer of the stomach and erosion by acid in the stomach. Many of the drugs available for treating various peptic ulcers act to alter acid-producing activities of the stomach. Five types of drugs are used in the treatment of ulcers:

- *Antacids*, which interact with acids at the chemical level to neutralize them
- *Histamine H_2 receptor antagonists*, which block the release of hydrochloric acid in response to gastrin
- *Proton pump inhibitors*, which suppress the secretion of hydrochloric acid into the lumen of the stomach via inhibition of the H^+/K^+-ATPase pump
- *Antipeptic agents*, which coat any injured area in the stomach to prevent further injury from acid

- *Prostaglandin analogues*, which inhibit the secretion of gastrin and increase the secretion of the mucous lining of the stomach, providing a buffer.

The National Institute for Health and Clinical Excellence provide current guidelines for the management and treatment of ulcers in adults (NICE, 2004).

Antacids

The antacids are a group of inorganic chemicals usually containing aluminium or magnesium that are alkaline in nature and used to neutralize stomach acid. Antacids are available over-the-counter (OTC), and many patients use them to self-treat a variety of GI symptoms. Antacids are not recommended as the sole treatment of peptic ulcer disease and patients should seek medical attention if symptoms persist or reoccur.

Administering an antacid frequently causes **acid rebound**. Neutralizing the stomach contents to an alkaline level stimulates gastrin production to cause an increase in acid production and return the stomach to its normal acidic state. In many cases, the acid rebound causes an increase in symptoms, resulting in an increased intake of the antacid. This leads to more acid production and a cycle develops.

The choice of an antacid depends on adverse effect and absorption factors. Available agents include the following:

- Sodium bicarbonate, the oldest drug in this group, is readily available in many preparations for indigestion. However, this drug should no longer be prescribed alone for the relief of dyspepsia and should be avoided by patients on a low sodium diet, for example patients with renal impairment.
- Calcium carbonate is actually precipitated chalk. The main drawbacks to this agent are acid rebound and constipation. It can be absorbed systemically and cause calcium imbalance. When absorbed, it is metabolized in the liver and excreted in urine and faeces. Known to cross the placenta and enter breast milk, this drug should be used with caution during pregnancy and lactation.
- Magnesium salts are very effective in buffering acid in the stomach but have been known to cause diarrhoea. These agents are not generally absorbed systemically and therefore may be a drug of choice if an antacid is needed during pregnancy or lactation.
- Aluminium salts do not cause acid rebound but are not very effective in neutralizing acid. They are bound in faeces for excretion and have been related to severe constipation. Aluminium binds dietary phosphates and can cause hypophosphataemia, which can then cause calcium imbalance throughout the system. For that reason, this drug should be used with caution during pregnancy and should be avoided during lactation because of the potential for adverse effects on the foetus and neonate.
- Aluminium–magnesium complexes minimize the GI effects of constipation and diarrhoea by combining these two salts but may cause rebound hyperacidity and alkalosis.

Antacids can greatly affect the absorption of other drugs from the GI tract. Most drugs are prepared for an acidic environment, and an alkaline environment can prevent them from being broken down for absorption or can actually neutralize them so that they cannot be absorbed. Patients taking antacids should be advised to separate them from any other medications by 1 to 2 hours.

Antacids can be combined with an alginate. Alginates increase both the viscosity and the adherence of mucus to the mucosa of the oesophagus thus protecting the mucosa from acid reflux. Many antacids in combination with alginates are available without prescription.

Therapeutic Actions and Indications

Antacids neutralize stomach acid by a direct chemical reaction (see Figure 56.1). They are recommended for the symptomatic relief of upset stomach associated with hyperacidity, as well as the hyperacidity associated with peptic ulcer, gastritis, peptic oesophagitis, gastric hyperacidity and hiatus hernia.

Contraindications and Cautions

The antacids are contraindicated in the presence of any known allergy to antacid products. Caution should be used in the following instances: any condition that can be exacerbated by electrolyte or acid–base imbalance; any electrolyte imbalance; hypophosphataemia; GI obstruction, *which could cause systemic absorption*; allergy to any component of the drug; renal dysfunction, *which could lead to electrolyte disturbance if any absorbed antacid is not neutralized properly* and pregnancy and lactation *because of the potential for adverse effects on the foetus or neonate.*

Adverse Effects

The adverse effects associated with these drugs relate to their effects on acid–base levels and electrolytes. Rebound acidity, in which the stomach produces more acid in response to the alkaline environment, is common. Alkalosis, where the pH of the blood becomes more alkaline; with resultant metabolic changes (nausea, vomiting, neuromuscular changes, headache, irritability, muscle twitching and even coma) may occur. Prolonged high doses of calcium salts may lead to hypercalcaemia and milk-alkali syndrome (seen as alkalosis, renal calcium deposits or severe electrolyte disorders). Constipation or diarrhoea may result, depending on the antacid being used. Combining an antacid with simeticone can reduce the flatulence associated with antacids resulting from the production of carbon dioxide as the antacids neutralize stomach acid. Hypophosphataemia can occur with the use of aluminium or magnesium salts. Finally, fluid retention and congestive heart failure can occur with sodium bicarbonate because of its high sodium content.

Clinically Important Drug–Drug Interactions

Antacids can affect the absorption of many other drugs and preferably should not be taken at the same time as other drugs, such as tetracyclines, phenothiazines and ketoconazole, and is why they should be taken 2 hours before or 2 hours after other medications are taken. If the pH of urine is affected by large doses of antacids, plasma levels of drugs, such as salicylates may decrease as a greater quantity of the drug is excreted in the urine.

Always consult a current copy of the British National Formulary for further guidance.

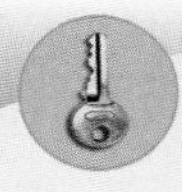

Key Drug Summary: *Compound Alginates (antacid plus alginate)*

Indications: Nonerosive gastro-oesophogeal reflux, dyspepsia and ulcer dyspepsia

Actions: The antacid neutralizes or reduces gastric acidity, resulting in an increase in gastric pH; and the alginate increases the viscosity of the stomach contents which protects the oesophageal mucosa

Pharmacokinetics:

Route	Onset	Peak	Duration
Oral	Rapid	30 min	1–3 h

$T_{1/2}$: Unknown; excreted unchanged in faeces

Adverse effects: Compounds containing magnesium or aluminium can cause diarrhoea or constipation, respectively. Those containing calcium can cause gastric acid rebound, hypercalcaemia and alkalosis; and those containing magnesium salts may lead to hypermagnesaemia in patients with renal dysfunction. Preparations containing sodium bicarbonate should be avoided in patients on low-sodium diets.

Nursing Considerations for Patients Receiving Antacids

Assessment: History and Examination

Screen for the following conditions which could be cautions or contraindications to use of the drug: any history of allergy to antacids; renal dysfunction *that might interfere with the drug's excretion*; electrolyte disturbances *that could be exacerbated by the effects of the drug*; and pregnancy or lactation, *which would require caution*. Establish if patient is currently taking other medications or herbal therapies which may potentially interact with the antacid.

Include screening for baseline data *to assess the effectiveness of the drug and the occurrence of any adverse effects associated with drug therapy*. Assess the following: active bowel sounds, *to ensure GI motility*; and serum electrolytes and renal function tests.

Nursing Diagnoses

The patient receiving antacids may have the following nursing diagnoses related to drug therapy:

- Diarrhoea related to GI effects
- Risk of constipation related to GI effects
- Imbalanced nutrition: less than body requirements, related to GI effects
- Risk for imbalanced fluid volume related to systemic effects
- Deficient knowledge regarding drug therapy

Implementation With Rationale

- Administer the drug apart from any other oral medications (1–2 hours before or 2 hours after) *to ensure adequate absorption of the other medications.*
- Have patients chew tablets thoroughly and follow with water *to ensure therapeutic levels reach the stomach.*
- Assess patients for any signs of acid–base or electrolyte imbalance *to arrange for appropriate interventions.*
- Provide thorough patient education, including drug name, prescribed dosage, measures for avoidance of adverse effects and warning signs that may indicate possible problems *to enhance patient knowledge about drug therapy and to promote concordance.*
- Offer support and encouragement *to help patients cope with the disease and the drug regimen.*

Evaluation

- Monitor patient response to the drug (relief of GI symptoms caused by hyperacidity).

- Monitor for adverse effects (GI effects, acid–base levels, signs of renal insufficiency and hypermagnesaemia).
- Evaluate effectiveness of education plan (patient can give the drug and dosage, as well as describe adverse effects to watch for, specific measures to avoid adverse effects and to increase the effectiveness of the drug).
- Monitor effectiveness of comfort measures and concordance with regimen.

Histamine H_2 Receptor Antagonists

The **histamine H_2 receptor antagonists** selectively block histamine H_2 receptors. These receptors are located on the parietal cells. Blocking these receptors prevents histamine-, gastrin- and acetylcholine-stimulated hydrochloric acid production and can also promote healing of duodenal ulcers. Four H_2 receptor antagonists are currently available, in both oral and parenteral forms. These drugs should be used with caution in pregnancy and lactation as all four are known to cross the placenta and to also enter breast milk.

- *Cimetidine* was the first drug in this class to be developed. In rare cases cimetidine has been associated with androgenic effects, including gynaecomastia and impotence. It is metabolized mainly in the liver and can slow the metabolism of many other drugs that use the same metabolizing enzyme system, for example warfarin, phenytoin and theophylline. The potential for numerous drug–drug interactions has reduced the frequency of prescribing cimetidine for treatment of ulcers.
- *Ranitidine*, which is longer acting and more potent than cimetidine, is not associated with the marked slowing of metabolism in the liver.
- *Famotidine* is similar to ranitidine in terms of its actions and adverse effects, but it is much more potent than either cimetidine or ranitidine. Metabolized by the liver, famotidine is then excreted in urine.
- *Nizatidine*, the newest drug in this class, is similar to ranitidine in its effectiveness and adverse effects.

Therapeutic Actions and Indications

H_2 receptor antagonists selectively block histamine H_2 receptors causing a reduction in gastric acid secretion. H_2 receptors are also found in the heart where histamine is known to increase both the heart rate and cardiac output. High levels of H_2 receptor antagonists can, therefore, produce bradycardia and cardiac arrhythmias.

These drugs are used in the following conditions:

- Short-term treatment of benign gastric or duodenal ulcers: a reduction in the overall acid level can promote healing and decrease discomfort (see Critical Thinking Scenario 56-1).
- Treatment of pathological hypersecretory conditions such as Zollinger–Ellison syndrome in which increased levels of gastrin are secreted leading to overproduction of hydrochloric acid.
- Prophylactic use to reduce the frequency of gastroduodenal erosions in hepatic failure and other conditions requiring intensive care: blocking the production of acid protects the stomach lining, which is at risk because of decreased mucus production associated with extreme stress.
- Treatment of erosive gastro-oesophageal reflux: decreasing the acid regurgitated into the oesophagus will promote healing and decrease pain.
- Relief of symptoms of heartburn, acid indigestion and hyperacidity as OTC preparations.

Pharmacokinetics

H_2 receptor antagonists are readily absorbed after oral administration. They cross the placenta and enter breast milk. They are metabolized in the liver and excreted in urine.

Contraindications and Cautions

Patients with hepatic or renal dysfunction could experience problems with drug metabolism and excretion. Hepatic dysfunction is a greater problem with cimetidine. Care should also be taken if prolonged or continual use of these drugs is necessary because they may be masking serious underlying conditions, in particular gastric cancer. Histamine H_2 receptor antagonists should be used with caution during pregnancy and while breastfeeding.

Adverse Effects

The adverse effects most commonly associated with H_2 receptor antagonists include plasma and other GI disturbances, dizziness, headache, rash and tiredness. More rare side-effects include confusion, depression or even hallucinations (thought to be related to possible H_2 receptor effects in the CNS); cardiac arrhythmias and bradycardia (related to H_2 cardiac receptor blocking; more commonly seen with intravenous or intramuscular administration or with prolonged use); gynaecomastia (more common with long-term use of cimetidine) and impotence; blood disorders and skin reactions.

Clinically Important Drug–Drug Interactions

Cimetidine can slow the metabolism of the following drugs, leading to increased plasma levels and possible toxic reactions: opioid analgesics, some antiarrhythmics, some antibacterials, anticoagulants, antidepressants, antidiabetics, antiepileptics, antimalarials, antipsychotics, benzodiazepines, β-adrenergic blockers, calcium channel blockers, ciclosporin, cilostazol, cytotoxics and theophylline. It is a good idea to review a patient's other medications carefully any time an H_2 antagonist is prescribed or a patient reports taking an OTC form.

Always consult a current copy of the British National Formulary for further guidance.

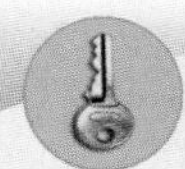

Key Drug Summary: *Cimetidine*

Indications: Benign gastric and duodenal ulcers, reflux oesophagitis, treatment of pathological hypersecretory conditions (Zollinger–Ellison syndrome), prophylaxis of stress-induced ulcers, relief of symptoms of heartburn and acid indigestion

Actions: Inhibits the actions of histamine at H_2 receptor sites of the stomach, inhibiting gastric acid secretion

Pharmacokinetics:

Route	Onset	Peak	Duration
Oral	Varies	1–1.5 h	4–5 h
IM, IV	Rapid	1–1.5 h	4–5 h

$T_{1/2}$: 2 hours; metabolized in the liver and excreted in urine

Adverse effects: Diarrhoea and other GI disturbances, altered liver function, headache, dizziness, rash and tiredness. Rare side-effects include acute pancreatitis, bradycardia, cardiac arrhythmias, confusion, depression and hallucinations particularly in the elderly or the very ill. Occasional reports of gynaecomastia, impotence and alopecia

Nursing Considerations for Patients Receiving Histamine H_2 Receptor Antagonists

Assessment: History and Examination

Screen for the following conditions, *which could be cautions or contraindications to use of the drug*: history of allergy to any H_2 receptor antagonists; impaired renal or hepatic function; pregnancy or lactation; and a detailed description of the GI problem, including length of time of the disorder and medical evaluation. Establish if patient is currently taking other medications or herbal therapies which may potentially interact with the histamine H_2 receptor antagonist.

Include screening for baseline pulse and blood pressure, electrocardiogram (if intravenous use is needed); liver and abdominal examination; and liver and renal function tests if the patient's history indicates hepatic or renal dysfunction.

Nursing Diagnoses

The patient who is receiving any H_2 receptor antagonist may have the following nursing diagnoses related to drug therapy:

- Acute pain related to CNS and GI effects
- Disturbed sensory perception (kinaesthetic, auditory) related to CNS effects
- Decreased cardiac output related to cardiac arrhythmias
- Deficient knowledge regarding drug therapy

Implementation With Rationale

- Administer oral drug with or before meals and at bedtime (exact timing varies with product) *to ensure therapeutic levels when the drug is most needed.*
- Arrange for decreased dosage in cases of hepatic or renal dysfunction *to prevent serious toxicity.*
- Monitor patient continually if giving intravenous doses *to allow early detection of potentially serious adverse effects, including cardiac arrhythmias.*
- Assess patient carefully for any potential drug–drug interactions if giving in combination with other drugs *because of the drug effects on liver enzyme systems.*
- Provide comfort measures, including analgesics *to improve patient tolerance of the drug and drug effects.*
- Arrange for regular follow-up *to evaluate drug effects and the underlying problem.* Persistent pain or dyspepsia may be symptoms of a more serious disease.
- Provide thorough patient education, including drug name, prescribed dosage, measures for avoidance of adverse effects and warning signs that may indicate possible problems to *enhance patient knowledge about drug therapy and to promote concordance.*

- Offer support and encouragement *to help patients cope with the disease and the drug regimen.*

Evaluation

- Monitor patient response to the drug (relief of GI symptoms, ulcer healing, prevention of ulcer progression).
- Monitor for adverse effects (dizziness, confusion, hallucinations, GI alterations, cardiac arrhythmias, hypotension, gynaecomastia).
- Evaluate effectiveness of education plan (patient can name drug, dosage, adverse effects to watch for and specific measures to avoid adverse effects).

Proton Pump Inhibitors

The gastric acid pump or **proton pump inhibitors** suppress gastric acid secretion by specifically inhibiting the hydrogen–potassium adenosine triphosphatase (H^+/K^+-ATPase or 'proton pump') enzyme system on the apical membrane of the gastric parietal cells. This action blocks the final step of acid production (see Chapter 55), lowering the acid levels in the stomach. Five proton pump inhibitors are currently available:

- *Omeprazole* is a fast-acting and quickly excreted drug. Available OTC for the relief of heartburn.
- *Esomeprazole* is a longer acting drug; it is not broken down as fast in the liver compared with the parent drug omeprazole.
- *Lansoprazole* is available in a delayed-release form and is approved for use in children.
- *Pantoprazole* is available in parenteral form for short-term use when the oral form cannot be tolerated.
- *Rabeprazole* is available only in a delayed-release form and is used to heal and maintain gastro-oesophogeal reflux disease, for the healing of duodenal ulcers, and for the treatment of pathological hypersecretory conditions.

Therapeutic Actions and Indications

Proton pump inhibitors act at specific secretory surface receptors to prevent the final step of acid production and thereby decrease the level of acid in the stomach. They are recommended for the short-term treatment of gastric and duodenal ulcers, dyspepsia, gastro-oesophageal reflux disease, erosive oesophagitis and benign gastric ulcer; for the long-term treatment of pathological hypersecretory conditions (Zollinger–Ellison syndrome); as maintenance therapy for healing of erosive oesophagitis and ulcers; and in combination with amoxicillin and clarithromycin for the treatment of *H. pylori* infection.

With many patients taking NSAIDs over a long term for a variety of conditions, including arthritis and cancers, the incidence of GI ulceration and bleeding could increase. Many health care providers will, therefore, prescribe a proton pump inhibitor as well to protect the patient from gastric erosion (NICE, 2004).

Pharmacokinetics

These drugs are acid labile and are rapidly absorbed from the GI tract. They undergo extensive metabolism in the liver and are excreted in urine. There are no adequate studies of these drugs during pregnancy and lactation. Caution should be used, however, because of the potential for adverse effects on the foetus or neonate. Only omeprazole and lansoprazole can be used by children.

Contraindications and Cautions

These drugs are contraindicated in the presence of known allergy to either the drug or the drug components. Caution should be used in pregnant or lactating women and in patients with liver disease. It is possible these drugs may mask the symptoms of more serious conditions, for example gastric cancer. These conditions should be ruled out before treatment is commenced.

Adverse Effects

The adverse effects associated with these drugs are related to their effects on the H^+/K^+-ATPase pump on parietal and other cells. Less frequent side-effects of this group of drugs include GI disturbances (nausea, vomiting, abdominal pain, flatulence, diarrhoea and constipation), dizziness and headache. More rare side-effects include dry mouth and taste disturbances, insomnia, drowsiness, apathy, blurred vision, muscular and joint pain, hypersensitivity reactions including rash and pruritis (itchy sensations), liver dysfunction and peripheral oedema.

Clinically Important Drug–Drug Interactions

Some of the proton pump inhibitors can affect the plasma concentration of a number of different drug groups, including anticoagulants, antiepileptics and antivirals. The plasma concentration of cilostazol is also increased by concomitant use of omeprazole.

Always consult a current copy of the British National Formulary for further guidance.

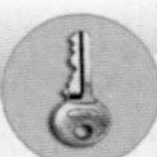

Key Drug Summary: *Omeprazole*

Indications: Short-term treatment of active duodenal ulcer or active benign gastric ulcer; treatment of heartburn or symptoms of gastro-oesophageal reflux; treatment of pathological hypersecretory syndromes; eradication of *H. pylori* infection as part of combination therapy

Actions: Specifically inhibits the H^+/K^+-ATPase enzyme system on the secretory surface of the gastric parietal cells, blocking the final step in acid production and decreasing gastric acid levels.

Pharmacokinetics:

Route	Onset	Peak	Duration
Oral	Varies	0.5–3.5 h	Varies

$T_{1/2}$: 30–60 minutes; metabolized in the liver and excreted in urine and bile

Adverse effects: Paraesthesia (tingling), headache, dizziness, vertigo, insomnia, rash, diarrhoea, abdominal pain, nausea, vomiting

Nursing Considerations for Patients Receiving Proton Pump Inhibitors

Assessment: History and Examination

Screen for any history of allergy to a proton pump inhibitor, pregnancy, or lactation, *which could be cautions or contraindications to use of the drug.* Establish if patient is currently taking other medications or herbal therapies which may potentially interact with the proton pump inhibitor.

Include screening *to establish baseline data for assessing the effectiveness of the drug and the occurrence of any adverse effects associated with drug therapy.* Assess skin colour, as well as affect and orientation. In addition, complete an abdominal examination.

Nursing Diagnoses

The patient receiving proton pump inhibitors may have the following nursing diagnoses related to drug therapy:

- Diarrhoea related to GI effects
- Risk of constipation related to GI effects
- Imbalanced nutrition: less than body requirements, related to GI effects
- Disturbed sensory perception (kinaesthetic, auditory) related to CNS effects
- Deficient knowledge regarding drug therapy

Implementation With Rationale

- Administer drug 30 minutes before meals; ensure that the patient does not open, chew or crush capsules; they should be swallowed whole *to ensure maximum absorption and therapeutic effectiveness of the drug.*
- Provide appropriate safety and comfort measures if CNS effects occur *to prevent patient injury.*
- Arrange for medical follow-up if symptoms are not resolved after 4 to 8 weeks of therapy *because serious underlying conditions could be causing the symptoms.*
- Provide thorough patient education, including drug name, prescribed dosage, measures for avoidance of adverse effects and warning signs that may indicate possible problems. Instruct patients about the need for periodic monitoring and evaluation *to enhance patient knowledge about drug therapy and to promote concordance.*
- Offer support and encouragement *to help patients cope with the disease and the drug regimen.*

Evaluation

- Monitor patient response to the drug (relief of GI symptoms caused by hyperacidity; healing of erosive GI lesions).
- Monitor for adverse effects (GI effects, CNS changes, dermatological effects, respiratory effects).
- Monitor liver function and serum gastrin levels. Over secretion of gastrin can occur with constant acid suppression.
- Evaluate effectiveness of education plan (patient can name the drug and dosage and describe adverse effects to watch for, specific measures to avoid adverse effects, and measures to take to increase the effectiveness of the drug).
- Monitor effectiveness of comfort and safety measures and concordance with regimen.

Cytoprotective Agents

These agents are responsible for protecting eroded ulcer sites in the GI tract from further damage by acid and digestive enzymes. Drugs belonging to this group include sucralfate, bismuth chelate (tripotassium dicitratobismuthate) and the **prostaglandin analogue**, misoprostol.

Therapeutic Actions and Indications

Sucralfate, a complex of aluminium hydroxide and sulphated sucrose, is recommended for the short-term treatment of duodenal ulcers. In the acid environment of the stomach, the aluminium component is released and binds to protein molecules (albumin and fibrinogen) released from the ulcer site. A protective layer is then formed at duodenal ulcer sites, protecting the sites against acid, pepsin and bile salts. This action prevents further breakdown of the area and promotes ulcer healing. Secretion of mucus and prostaglandins is stimulated, whereas pepsin activity in gastric juices is reduced, preventing further breakdown of proteins in the stomach, including the stomach wall (see Figure 56.1).

Bismuth chelate is commonly used in the healing of gastric and duodenal ulcers and can be used in combination with other drugs to eradicate *H. pylori*. It is thought to coat the base of the ulcer, and also adsorb pepsin, increase prostaglandin synthesis and secretion of bicarbonate to neutralize gastric acid.

Prostaglandin E_1 is known to inhibit gastric acid secretion and increase bicarbonate and mucus production in the stomach, thus protecting the stomach lining (see Figure 56.1). *Misoprostol*, a prostaglandin E_1 analogue, is used to prevent NSAID-induced gastric ulcers in patients who are at high risk of complications from a gastric ulcer (e.g. elderly or debilitated patients who cannot stop taking NSAIDs). In the past, this drug has also been used as an abortifacient to induce labour; however, this is no longer a licensed indication.

Pharmacokinetics

In the stomach, sucralfate forms a viscous paste and a significant proportion of the drug remains in the stomach after oral administration; only a small amount (3%–5%) is absorbed. The small amount of drug reaching the systemic circulation is metabolized in the liver and excreted in faeces and urine. The risks to the unborn child and the neonate during breast-feeding are unknown and, therefore, caution should be taken if prescribing during pregnancy or lactation unless the benefit to the mother clearly outweighs the potential adverse effects.

The pharmacokinetics of bismuth chelate is similar to that of sucralfate. If renal excretion is impaired, the plasma concentration of bismuth can increase causing encephalopathy.

Misoprostol is rapidly absorbed from the GI tract, metabolized in the liver and excreted in urine. Caution should be used in hepatic or renal impairment, which could interfere with the effective drug metabolism and excretion.

Contraindications and Cautions

Sucralfate should not be given to any person with known allergy to the drug or any of its components. It should not be given to individuals with renal failure or undergoing dialysis *because a build-up of aluminium may occur if it is used with aluminium-containing products*. Seriously ill patients receiving enteral feeds and those with delayed gastric emptying should use sucralfate with caution. Caution should also be used in patients who are pregnant or lactating.

Bismuth chelate should not be given to patients with severe renal impairment. Bismuth is known to have a teratogenic effect and should not be used in pregnancy.

Misoprostol is contraindicated during pregnancy *because it is an abortifacient and potential teratogen*. It is advised that misoprostol should only be used if the patient uses barrier contraceptives during therapy and has been advised of the risks of taking the drug while pregnant. The manufacturer also advises that the drug should not be used during lactation. Misoprostol should be used with caution by patients with conditions which could be complicated by a drop in blood pressure, for example cardiovascular or cerebrovascular disease.

Adverse Effects

Most of the adverse effects of these drugs are primarily related to their GI effects. With sucralfate, constipation is the most frequently seen adverse effect. Diarrhoea, nausea, indigestion, gastric discomfort and dry mouth may also occur. Other adverse effects that have been reported with this drug include dizziness, drowsiness, vertigo, skin rash and back pain. Bismuth chelate can cause nausea and vomiting. The patients tongue may also darken and faeces may blacken. For misoprostol, refer to Key Drug Summary.

Clinically Important Drug–Drug Interactions

If aluminium salts are combined with sucralfate, there is a risk of high aluminium levels and aluminium toxicity. Extreme care should be taken if this combination is used. Sucralfate is also known to reduce the absorption of a number of drug groups including antibacterials anticoagulants and antiepileptics. Decreased serum levels and drug effectiveness may result.

Always consult a current copy of the British National Formulary for further guidance.

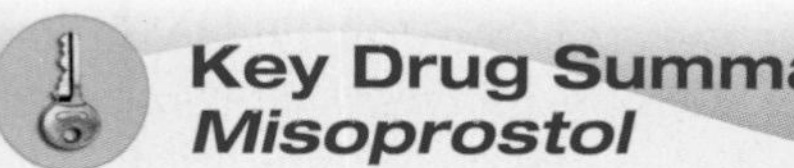

Key Drug Summary: *Misoprostol*

Indications: Promotes healing of gastric and duodenal ulcers; prophylaxis of nonsteroidal anti-inflammatory induced ulcers

Actions: Stimulates prostaglandin receptors and therefore lowers gastric acid production

Pharmacokinetics:

Route	Onset	Peak	Duration
Oral	30 min	1–1.5 h	Up to 3 h

$T_{1/2}$: 20–40 minutes; metabolized in the liver and excreted mostly in urine

Adverse effects: nausea, diarrhoea, abdominal pain, flatulence, vomiting, dyspepsia and constipation. Genitourinary effects, which are related to the actions of prostaglandins on the uterus, include miscarriages, excessive bleeding, spotting, cramping, hypermenorrhoea, dysmenorrhoea and other menstrual disorders. Women taking this drug should be notified, both in writing and verbally, of the potential adverse effects of this drug.

Nursing Considerations for Patients Receiving Cytoprotective Agents

Assessment: History and Examination

Screen for the following conditions, *which could be cautions or contraindications to use of the drug*: any history of allergy to sucralfate, bismuth or misoprostol, renal dysfunction or dialysis, and pregnancy or lactation. Establish if patient is currently taking other medications or herbal therapies which may potentially interact with the cytoprotective drug.

Include screening *to establish baseline information for assessing the effectiveness of the drug and the occurrence of any adverse effects associated with drug therapy*. Assess the following: skin colour; affect and orientation; and abdominal examination. For misoprostol, complete abdominal examination and pregnancy test.

Nursing Diagnoses

The patient receiving sucralfate/bismuth/misoprostol may have the following nursing diagnoses related to drug therapy:

- Diarrhoea related to GI effects
- Risk for constipation related to GI effects
- Imbalanced nutrition: less than body requirements, related to GI effects
- Disturbed sensory perception (kinaesthetic) related to CNS effects
- Sexual dysfunction related to genitourinary effects (misoprostol only)
- Deficient knowledge regarding drug therapy

Implementation With Rationale

For sucralfate and bismuth:

- Administer drug on an empty stomach, 1 hour before or 2 hours after meals and at bedtime, *to ensure therapeutic effectiveness of the drug.*
- Monitor patient for GI pain, *and arrange to administer antacids to relieve pain if needed.*
- Administer antacids between doses of sucralfate, not within 30 minutes of a sucralfate dose, *because sucralfate can interfere with absorption of oral agents.*
- Provide comfort and safety measures if CNS effects occur *to prevent patient injury.*

For misoprostol:

- Administer to patients at high risk of NSAID-induced ulcers during the full course of NSAID therapy *to prevent the development of gastric ulcers.* Administer four times a day, with meals and at bedtime.
- Arrange for a serum pregnancy test within 2 weeks before beginning treatment; begin therapy on the second or third day of the menstrual period *to ensure that women of childbearing age are not pregnant and to prevent abortifacient effects associated with this drug.*
- Provide patient with both written and verbal information regarding the associated risks of pregnancy *to ensure that the patient understands the risks involved*; advise the use of barrier contraceptives during therapy *to ensure prevention of pregnancy.*

In addition:

- Assess nutritional status if GI effects are severe *in order to arrange for appropriate measures to relieve discomfort and ensure nutrition.*
- Provide frequent mouth care (for sucralfate); bowel programme as needed; and small, frequent meals *if GI effects are uncomfortable.*
- Provide thorough patient education, including drug name, prescribed dosage, measures for avoidance of adverse effects and warning signs that may indicate possible problems. Instruct patients about the need for periodic monitoring and evaluation to enhance patient knowledge *about drug therapy and to promote concordance.*
- Offer support and encouragement *to help patients cope with the disease and the drug regimen.*

Evaluation

- Monitor patient response to the drug (relief of GI symptoms caused by hyperacidity; healing of erosive GI lesions, prevention of GI ulcers related to NSAIDs).

- Monitor for adverse effects (GI effects, CNS changes, dermatologic effects, genitourinary).
- Evaluate effectiveness of education plan (patient can name drug and dosage and describe adverse effects to watch for, specific measures to avoid adverse effects and measures to take to increase the effectiveness of the drug).
- Monitor effectiveness of comfort and safety measures and concordance with regimen.

Digestive Enzymes

Some patients, for example those with cystic fibrosis or pancreatic dysfunction; may require digestive enzyme supplements. In conditions where there is a lack of pancreatic lipase, pancreatin is used to aid the digestion and absorption of fats, proteins and carbohydrates.

Therapeutic Actions and Indications

The pancreatic enzymes are replacement enzymes that help the digestion and absorption of fats, proteins and carbohydrates (see Figure 56.1). They are used as replacement therapy in patients with cystic fibrosis, and following pancreatectomy, gastrectomy or chronic pancreatitis.

Contraindications and Cautions

Pancreatin is inactivated by gastric acid. It is therefore best to take the supplements either with food, or immediately before or after. This enzyme is inactivated by heat; therefore patients should ensure that the drug is not mixed with hot liquids or foods. Pancreatin should not be used where there is a known allergy to pork products as the drug is derived from pigs. In addition, they should be used with caution in lactation.

Clinically Important Drug–Drug Interactions

Pancreatin should not be taken with the antidiabetic, acarbose.

Always consult a current copy of the British National Formulary for further guidance.

Adverse Effects

The adverse effects that most often occur are related to GI irritation and include nausea, vomiting and abdominal cramps.

Nursing Considerations for Patients Receiving Digestive Enzymes

Assessment: History and Examination

Screen for the following conditions, *which could be cautions or contraindications to use of the drug*: any history of allergy to any of the drugs or to pork products; pregnancy or lactation. Establish if patient is currently taking other medications or herbal therapies which may potentially interact with the pancreatin.

Include screening *for baseline information for assessing the effectiveness of the drug and the occurrence of any adverse effects associated with drug therapy*. Assess the following: abdominal examination, mucous membranes, blood pressure, cardiac evaluation, and pancreatic enzyme levels.

Nursing Diagnoses

The patient receiving digestive enzymes may have the following nursing diagnoses related to drug therapy:

- Diarrhoea related to GI effects
- Imbalanced nutrition: less than body requirements, related to GI effects
- Deficient knowledge regarding drug therapy

Implementation With Rationale

- If necessary, use a saliva substitute *to coat the mouth and ensure therapeutic effectiveness of the drug.*
- Monitor swallowing *because it may be impaired and additional therapy may be needed.*
- Administer pancreatic enzymes with meals and snacks so that enzyme is available when it is needed. Avoid spilling powder on the skin *because it may be irritating.* Do not crush the capsule or allow the patient to chew it; it must be swallowed whole *to ensure full therapeutic effects.*
- Assess nutritional status if there are GI effects *in order to arrange for appropriate measures to relieve discomfort and ensure nutrition.*
- Ensure patient maintains an adequate level of hydration if prescribing high-strength preparations of pancreatin.
- Provide thorough patient education, including drug name, prescribed dosage, measures for avoidance of adverse effects and warning signs that may indicate possible problems. Instruct patients about the need for periodic monitoring and evaluation *to enhance patient knowledge about drug therapy and to promote concordance.*

- Offer support and encouragement *to help patients cope with the disease and the drug regimen.*

Evaluation

- Monitor patient response to the drug (e.g. relief of dry mouth and throat; digestion of fats, proteins, and carbohydrates).
- Monitor for adverse effects (e.g. electrolyte imbalance, GI effects).
- Evaluate effectiveness of education plan (patient can name the drug and dosage and describe adverse effects to watch for, specific measures to avoid adverse effects and measures to take to increase the effectiveness of the drug).
- Monitor effectiveness of comfort/safety measures and concordance with regimen.

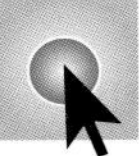

WEB LINK

Health care providers and patients may want to consult the following Internet sources:

http://bnfc.org The British National Formulary for Children provides UK health care professionals with authoritative and practical information on the selection and clinical use of medicines in children.

http://cks.library.nhs.uk The National Health Service Clinical Knowledge Summaries provides evidence-based practical information on the common conditions observed in primary care.

http://www.bnf.org.uk The British National Formulary provides UK health care professionals with authoritative and practical information on the selection and clinical use of medicines.

http://www.nhsdirect.nhs.uk The National Health Service Direct service provides patients with information and advice about health, illness and health services.

Points to Remember

- GI complaints are some of the most common symptoms seen in clinical practice.
- Peptic ulcers may result from increased acid production, decrease in the protective mucous lining of the stomach, infection with *H. pylori* bacteria, or a combination of these.
- Agents used to decrease the acid content of the stomach include H_2 receptor antagonists, which block the release of acid in response to gastrin or parasympathetic release; antacids, which chemically react with the acid to neutralise it; and proton pump inhibitors, which block the last step of acid production to prevent release.
- Acid rebound occurs when the stomach produces more gastrin and more acid in response to lowered acid levels in the stomach. Balancing the reduction of the stomach acid without increasing acid production is a clinical challenge.
- The cytoprotective drugs form a protective coating over the eroded stomach lining to protect it from acid and digestive enzymes and to aid healing.
- The prostaglandin analogue misoprostol blocks gastric acid secretion while increasing the production of bicarbonate and mucous lining in the stomach.
- Digestive enzymes such as pancreatic enzymes may be needed if normal enzyme levels are very low and proper digestion cannot take place.

CRITICAL THINKING SCENARIO 56-1

Histamine H_2 Receptor Antagonists

The Situation

William, a 48-year-old travelling salesman, had experienced increasing epigastric discomfort during a 7-month period. When he finally sought medical care, the diagnosis was a duodenal ulcer. He began taking a compound alginate (e.g. Gaviscon) for relief of his immediate discomfort, as well as cimetidine. William was referred to the nurse for patient education and given an appointment for a follow-up visit in 3 weeks.

Critical Thinking

- Think about the physiology of duodenal ulcers and the various factors that can contribute to aggravating the problem.
- What patient education points should be covered with this patient regarding diet, stress factors, and use of alcohol and tobacco?
- What adverse effects of the drugs should this patient be aware of?

(continued)

Histamine H_2 Receptor Antagonists *(continued)*

- How should this patient be monitored?
- What lifestyle changes may be necessary to ensure ulcer healing, and how can William be assisted in making these changes fit into the demands of his job?

Discussion

Further examination indicated that William is a healthy man except for the ulcer. As he is basically healthy and did not seek medical care until he became very uncomfortable (7 months of pain), he may find it difficult to comply with his drug therapy and any suggested lifestyle changes.

William requires information on duodenal ulcers; ways to decrease acid production (such as avoiding cigarettes, acid-stimulating foods, alcohol and caffeine); and ways to improve the protective mucous layer of the stomach by reducing stress. Cimetidine (and other H_2 receptor antagonists) can cause dizziness and drowsiness, which could be a major problem if William needs to drive to meet his clients. If driving is important for his job, he may want to explore other means of dealing with his ulcer pain and healing.

In addition, spacing of the cimetidine and antacid doses should be stressed. Cimetidine should be taken 1–2 hours before or 2 hours after any antacids because they can interfere with the absorption of cimetidine and the patient may not receive a therapeutic dose. William should be encouraged to avoid OTC medications and self-medication because several of these products contain ingredients that could aggravate his ulcer or interfere with the effectiveness of the drugs that have been prescribed. William should be encouraged to return for regular medical evaluation of his drug therapy and his underlying condition.

Finally, William should feel that he has some control over his situation. Allow him to suggest ways to decrease stress, ways to cut down on smoking or the use of alcohol without interfering with the demands of his job. He will learn which foods and situations irritate his condition. However, research has shown that bland or restrictive diets are not particularly effective in decreasing ulcer pain or spread, and they may actually increase patient anxiety. William should be encouraged to jot down the situations or times of day that seem to cause him the most problems. This information can help to provide a guide for adjusting lifestyle and/or dietary patterns to aid ulcer healing and prevent further development of ulcers.

Nursing Care Guide for William: Histamine H_2 Receptor Antagonists

Assessment: History and Examination

Assess William's health history for allergies to any of these drugs, renal or hepatic failure, and other drugs being taken, such as antiarrhythmics (e.g. amiodarone), oral anticoagulants, antidepressants, antiepileptics, antifungals, antipsychotics, ciclosporin, cilostazol, cytotoxics, ergot alkaloids and theophylline.

Focus the physical examination on the following areas:

- Neurological: orientation, affect
- Skin: colour, lesions
- Cardiovascular: pulse, cardiac auscultation
- GI: liver evaluation
- Laboratory tests: full blood count, liver, renal function tests if the patient's history suggests hepatic or renal dysfunction

Nursing Diagnoses

- Acute pain related to GI or CNS effects
- Disturbed sensory perception (kinaesthetic, auditory) related to CNS effects
- Decreased cardiac output related to cardiac effects
- Deficient knowledge regarding drug therapy

Implementation

- Administer with meals and at bedtime.
- Arrange for decreased dose in renal/hepatic disease.
- Provide support and reassurance to deal with drug effects and lifestyle changes.
- Provide patient education regarding drug name, dosage, adverse effects, precautions and warnings to report.

Evaluation

- Evaluate drug effects: relief of GI symptoms, ulcer healing, prevention of ulcer progression.
- Monitor for adverse effects: dizziness, confusion, gynaecomastia, arrhythmias, GI alterations.
- Monitor for drug–drug interactions as listed.
- Evaluate effectiveness of patient education programme.

Histamine H_2 Receptor Antagonists *(continued)*

Patient Education for William

- ☐ The drug that has been prescribed for you, cimetidine, is called a histamine H_2 receptor antagonist. A histamine H_2 receptor antagonist decreases the amount of acid that is produced in the stomach. It is used to treat conditions that are aggravated by excess acid.
- ☐ Some of the following adverse effects may occur with this drug:
  - *Diarrhoea*: have ready access to bathroom facilities. This usually becomes less severe over time.
  - *Dizziness, feeling faint on arising, headache*: these usually lessen as your body adjusts to the drug. Change positions slowly. If you feel drowsy, avoid driving or dangerous activities.
  - Report any of the following to your health care provider: *sore throat, unusual bleeding or bruising, confusion, muscle or joint pain, heart palpitations.*
- ☐ Avoid taking any OTC medication without first checking with your health care provider. Several of these medications can interfere with the effectiveness of this drug. If an ant acid has been ordered for you, take it exactly as prescribed.
- ☐ Tell any clinician, nurse, or other health care provider involved in your care that you are taking this drug.
- ☐ If you are taking any other medications, do not vary the drug schedules.
- ☐ It is important to have regular medical follow-up while you are taking this drug to evaluate your response to the drug and any possible underlying problems.
- ☐ Keep this drug, and all other medications, out of the reach of children.

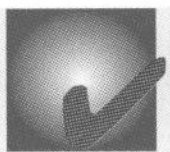

CHECK YOUR UNDERSTANDING

Answers to the questions in this chapter may be found in the answer key in the back of the book.

Multiple Choice

Select the most appropriate response to the following:

1. Histamine H_2-antagonists act to
   a. block the release of gastrin.
   b. selectively block histamine receptors, reducing swelling and inflammation.
   c. selectively block histamine receptors, leading to a reduction in gastric acid secretion and reduction in pepsin production.
   d. are effective only with long-term use.

2. H_2 receptors are found predominantly in the
   a. nasal passages, upper airways and stomach.
   b. CNS and upper airways.
   c. respiratory tract and the heart.
   d. heart, CNS and stomach.

3. A patient receiving intravenous cimetidine for an acute ulcer problem needs to be monitored for
   a. GI upset.
   b. gynaecomastia.
   c. cardiac arrhythmias.
   d. constipation.

4. Acid rebound is a condition that occurs when
   a. lowering gastric acid to an alkaline level stimulates the release of gastric acid.
   b. raising gastric acid levels causes heartburn.
   c. combining protein, calcium and smoking greatly elevates gastric acid levels.
   d. eating citrus fruit neutralises gastric acid.

5. A nurse taking care of a patient who is receiving a proton pump inhibitor should teach the patient to
   a. take the drug after every meal.
   b. chew or crush tablets to increase their absorption.
   c. swallow tablets or capsules whole.
   d. stop taking the drug after 3 weeks of therapy.

6. Misoprostol is a prostaglandin that is used to
   a. prevent uterine contractions.
   b. prevent NSAID-related gastric ulcers in patients at high risk.

c. decrease hyperacidity with meals.
d. relieve the burning associated with hiatus hernia at night.

7. A nurse caring for a patient receiving pancreatic enzymes as replacement therapy should be assessing the patient for
a. hypertension.
b. cardiac arrhythmias.
c. excessive weight gain.
d. signs of GI irritation.

Extended Matching Questions

Select **all** that apply.

1. Patients who use antacids frequently can be expected to experience which of the following adverse effects?
a. Systemic alkalosis
b. Electrolyte imbalances
c. Hyperkalaemia
d. Metabolic acidosis
e. Constipation or diarrhoea
f. Muscle weakness

Matching

Match the following drugs with the appropriate class of drugs used to affect GI secretions. Some classes may be used more than once.

1. ____________________ misoprostol
2. ____________________ lansoprazole
3. ____________________ sucralfate
4. ____________________ cimetidine
5. ____________________ aluminium salts
6. ____________________ sodium bicarbonate
7. ____________________ pancreatin
8. ____________________ omeprazole
9. ____________________ famotidine
10. ____________________ bismuth chelate

A. Histamine (H_2) antagonists
B. Antacids
C. Proton pump inhibitors
D. Cytoprotective agent
E. Prostaglandin analogue
F. Digestive enzymes

Bibliography and References

British Medical Association and Royal Pharmaceutical Society of Great Britain. (2008). *British National Formulary*. London: BMJ & RPS Publishing. *This publication is updated biannually: it is imperative that the most recent edition is consulted.*

British Medical Association and Royal Pharmaceutical Society of Great Britain. (2007). *British National Formulary for Children*. London: BMJ & RPS Publishing. *This publication is updated annually: it is imperative that the most recent edition is consulted.*

Brunton, L., Lazo, J. S., Parker, K., Goodman, L. S., & Gilman, A. G. (2005). *Goodman and Gilman's the pharmacological basis of therapeutics* (11th ed.). London: McGraw-Hill.

Ganong, W. (2005). *Review of medical physiology* (22nd ed.). New York: McGraw-Hill.

Howland, R. D., & Mycek, M. J. (2005). *Pharmacology* (3rd ed.). Philadelphia: Lippincott Williams & Wilkins.

National Institute for Health and Clinical Excellence. (2004). Dyspepsia: Management of dyspepsia in adults in primary care. Available from http://www.nice.org.uk

Porth, C. M., & Matfin, G. (2008). *Pathophysiology: Concepts of altered health states* (8th ed.). Philadelphia: Lippincott Williams & Wilkins.

Rang, H. P., Dale, M. M., Ritter, J. M., & Flower, R. J. (2007). *Rang and Dale's pharmacology.* (6th ed.). Philadelphia: Churchill Livingstone.

Simonsen, T., Aarbakke, J., Kay, I., Coleman, I., Sinnott, P., & Lysaa, R. (2006). *Illustrated pharmacology for nurses.* London: Hodder Arnold.

CHAPTER
57

Laxative and Antimotility Agents

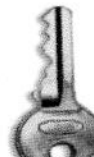

KEY TERMS

antimotility drug
bulk stimulant
cathartic dependence
constipation
diarrhoea
lubricant

LEARNING OBJECTIVES

Upon completion of this chapter, you will be able to:

1. Describe the underlying processes in diarrhoea and constipation and correlate this with the types of drugs used to treat these conditions.
2. Describe the therapeutic actions, indications and pharmacokinetics, associated with stimulant laxatives, bulk-forming laxatives, osmotic laxatives, gastrointestinal stimulants and antimotility drugs.
3. Describe the contraindications, most common adverse reactions and important drug–drug interactions associated with stimulant laxatives, bulk-forming laxatives, osmotic laxatives, gastrointestinal stimulants and antimotility drugs.
4. Discuss the use of laxatives and antimotility agents across the lifespan.
5. Compare and contrast the key drugs glycerol, lactulose, metoclopramide and loperamide with other agents in their class and with other classes of laxatives and antimotility agents.
6. Outline the nursing considerations, including important teaching points, for patients receiving laxatives and antimotility agents.

LAXATIVES

Stimulant Laxatives
bisacodyl
dantron
docusate
glycerol
sodium picosulphate

Bulk-forming Laxatives
ispaghula husk
methylcellulose
sterculia

Osmotic Laxatives
lactulose
macrogols
magnesium salts
phosphates
sodium citrate

Faecal Softeners
arachis oil

GASTROINTESTINAL STIMULANTS

metoclopramide
domperidone

ANTIMOTILITY DRUGS

codeine phosphate
co-phenotrope
loperamide
morphine

Drugs used to affect the motor activity of the gastrointestinal (GI) tract can do so in several different ways. They can be used to speed up or improve the movement of intestinal contents along the GI tract when movement becomes too slow or sluggish (as in **constipation**). This allows for proper absorption of nutrients and excretion of waste. Drugs are also used to increase the tone of the GI tract and to stimulate motility throughout the system. They can also be used to decrease movement along the GI tract when rapid movement decreases the time for absorption of nutrients, leading to a loss of water and nutrients and the discomfort of **diarrhoea** (Figure 57.1). All of these drugs are used with people of all ages (Box 57.1).

Laxatives

Laxative drugs are used in several ways to speed the passage of the intestinal contents through the GI tract. Laxatives may be either ***stimulant laxatives***, which increase the intestinal motility, ***bulk-forming stimulants*** (also called mechanical stimulants), which cause the faecal matter to increase in bulk or **lubricants**, which help the intestinal content move more smoothly, such as ***osmotic laxatives*** and *faecal softeners*.

Stimulant Laxatives

Stimulant laxatives, as the name suggests, stimulate motility of the gut. One side-effect is that they can cause abdominal cramps, and they should not be used in patients with intestinal obstruction. Such laxatives include the following agents:

- Dantron is only used to treat constipation in terminally ill patients due to its potential carcinogen risk.
- Glycerol is a hyperosmotic laxative available as glycerol suppository. Glycerol acts as a mild stimulant to gently evacuate the rectum without higher systemic effects in the GI tract.

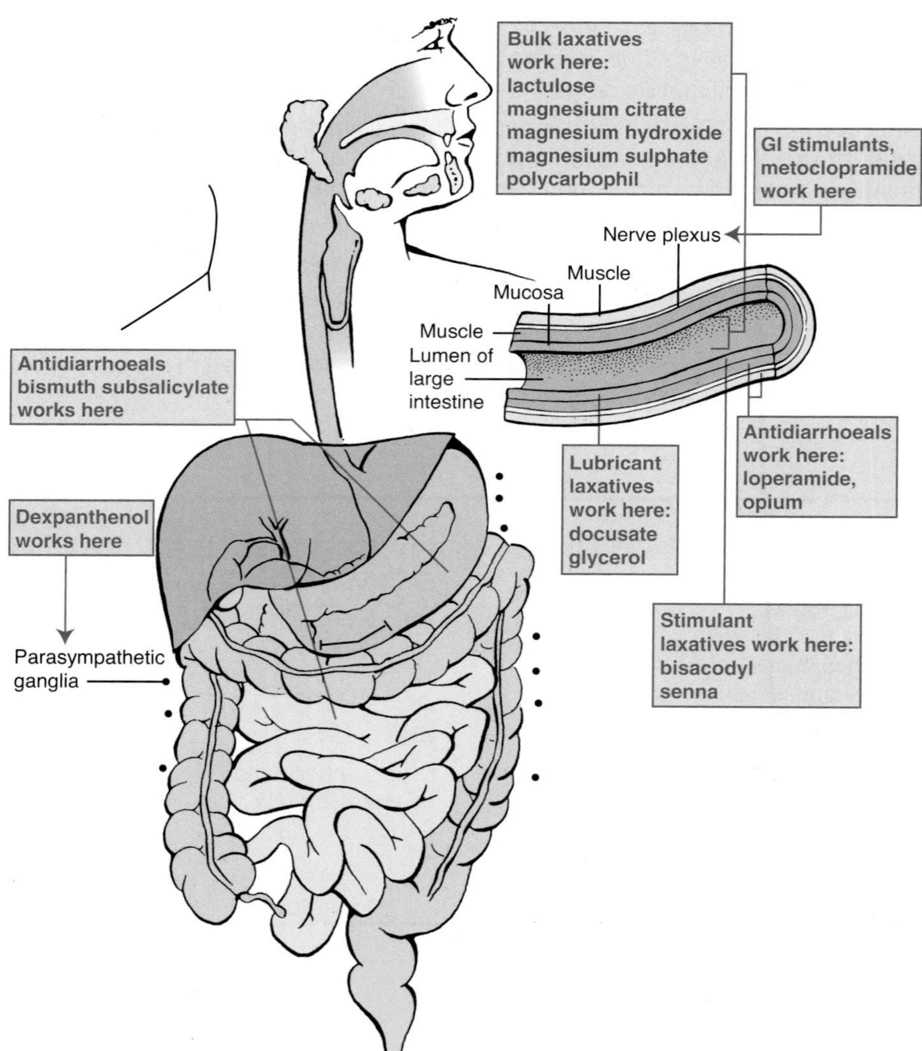

FIGURE 57.1 Sites of action of drugs affecting gastrointestinal motility.

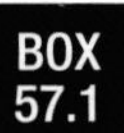

BOX 57.1 DRUG THERAPY ACROSS THE LIFESPAN

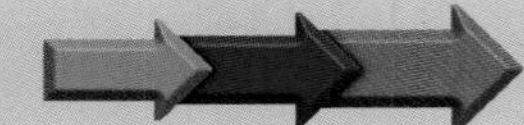

Laxatives and Antimotility Agents

CHILDREN

Laxatives should not be used in children routinely. Dietary changes including fibre, plenty of fluids and plenty of exercise should be tried first if a child has a tendency to become constipated. Stool softeners can be used in older children, but harsh stimulants should be avoided. Children with encopresis, however, are often given senna preparations to help them evacuate the massive stool.

Children receiving these agents should only use them for a short period and should be investigated for potential underlying medical or nutritional problems if they are not able to return to normal function.

Loperamide may be the antimotility of choice in children >4 years of age if such a drug is needed. Special precautions need to be taken to monitor for electrolyte and fluid disturbances and supportive measures taken as needed.

When administering any drug to children, always consult the most recent edition of the British National Formulary for Children.

ADULTS

Adults who use laxatives need to be cautioned not to become dependent. Proper diet, exercise and adequate intake of fluids should keep the GI tract functioning normally. If an antimotility agent is needed, adults should be carefully instructed about the proper dosing of the drug and monitoring of their total use to avoid excessive dosage.

The safety of these drugs during pregnancy and lactation has not been established. Use should be reserved for those situations in which the benefit to the mother outweighs the potential risk to the foetus. A mild stool softener is often used after delivery. The drugs may enter breast milk and may also affect GI activity in the neonate. It is advised that caution be used if one of these drugs is prescribed during lactation.

OLDER ADULTS

The older adult should be encouraged to drink plenty of fluids to exercise every day and to get plenty of roughage in the diet. Many older adults have established routines, such as drinking warm water or prune juice at the same time each morning, that are disrupted with illness or hospitalization. These patients should be encouraged and helped to try to maintain their usual protocol as much as possible.

Older patients may be taking other drugs that are associated with constipation, and they may need help to prevent severe problems from developing. They are more likely to have renal and/or hepatic impairment related to underlying medical conditions, which could interfere with the metabolism and excretion of these drugs. The dosage for older adults should be started at a lower level than that recommended for younger adults. The patient should be monitored very closely, and dosage adjustment should be made based on patient response.

Older adults are more likely to develop adverse effects associated with the use of these drugs, including sedation, confusion, dizziness, electrolyte disturbances, fluid imbalance and cardiovascular effects. Safety measures may be needed if these effects occur and interfere with the patient's mobility and balance.

These patients also need to be alerted to the potential for toxic effects when using over-the-counter (OTC) preparations and should be advised to check with their health care provider before beginning any OTC drug regimen.

A psyllium product is the agent of choice with older adults because there is less risk of adverse reactions. The patient needs to be cautioned to drink plenty of fluid after taking one of these agents to prevent problems that can occur if the drug starts to pull in fluid while still in the oesophagus.

- Sodium picosulphate is also used to evacuate the bowel prior to surgical, radiological or endoscopic procedures. It is administered orally.
- Docusate has a detergent action on the surface of the intestinal bolus, increasing the admixture of fat and water and making a softer stool. This drug is frequently used as prophylaxis for patients who should not strain (such as after surgery, myocardial infarction or obstetrical delivery).
- Senna is a natural leaf product. Found in many OTC preparations, it is available as tablet, granule and oral liquid form. It usually takes between 8 and 10 hours to take effect.
- Bisacodyl is often the drug of choice to empty the bowel before surgery or diagnostic tests, such as barium enema. It may be administered orally or rectally.

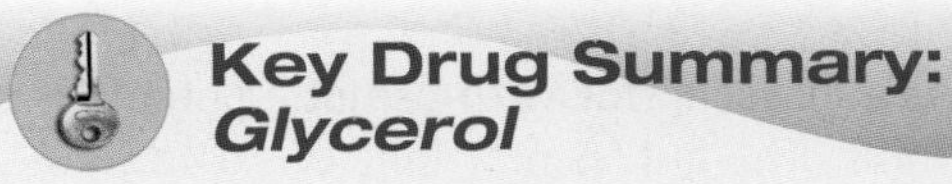

Key Drug Summary: *Glycerol*

Indications: Constipation.

Actions: Increases electrolyte and water secretion by the gut mucosa; increases peristalsis

Pharmacokinetics:

Route	Onset	Peak
Rectal	15–30 min	45 min–1 h

$T_{1/2}$: unknown

Adverse effects: mild abdominal cramps.

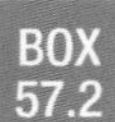

BOX 57.2 Irritable Bowel Syndrome

IBS is a very common disorder, striking three times as many women as men and reportedly accounting for half of all referrals to GI specialists. The disorder is characterized by abdominal distress, bouts of diarrhoea or constipation, bloating, nausea, flatulence, headache, fatigue, depression and anxiety. No anatomical cause has been found for this disorder. Underlying causes might be stress related. Patients with this disorder have often suffered for years, not enjoying meals or activities because of their GI pain and discomfort.

Support and symptomatic relief remain the mainstays of treating this disorder. Stress management and a consistent relationship with a health care provider may help to relieve some of the problems associated with this common, although not entirely understood disorder.

Bulk-forming Stimulants

Bulk stimulants increase the motility of the GI tract by increasing the faecal mass; this in turn will increase peristalsis in the large intestine. Available bulk stimulants include ispaghula husk, methylcellulose and sterculia. The effects of these agents often take several days to develop. These agents are often used for patients suffering from, for example, irritable bowel syndrome (IBS) (see Box 57.2), haemorrhoids, colostomy or ileostomy. Patients should be encouraged to maintain an adequate fluid intake to prevent intestinal obstruction.

Osmotic Laxatives

These laxatives increase the motility of the GI tract by increasing the amount of fluid in the intestinal contents by drawing fluid into the intestine or retaining fluid there. This will stimulate local stretch receptors and activate local activity. Available osmotic diuretics include the following agents:

- Lactulose is a disaccharide with osmotic potential as it draws fluid into the gut. It may take up to 48 hours to take effect. This agent is given orally, and it should not be used in patients who are lactose intolerant.
- Macrogols, for example. polyethylene glycol: restores water in the large intestine. This agent may be associated with abdominal distension and pain. Patients should be encouraged to take it with plenty of fluids. This agent is given orally.
- Magnesium salts: these agents provide a rapid bowel evacuation. Care must be taken to avoid these substances being abused. Adequate fluid intake should accompany the administration of these oral agents. Patients with renal impairment should avoid these agents due to the risk of magnesium accumulation.
- Phosphates are useful for rapid bowel evacuation prior to surgery, endoscopy or abdominal radiological investigations. These agents are administered as a suppository or as an enema.
- Sodium citrate may also be used as an enema for rapid bowel evacuation. It may be administered to adults and children over 3 years old.

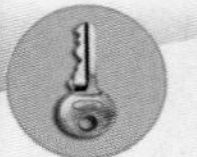

Key Drug Summary: *Lactulose*

Indications: Constipation and hepatic encephalopathy.

Actions: Draws fluid from the body into the bowel.

Pharmacokinetics:

Route	Onset
Oral	Can take 2–3 days to act

$T_{1/2}$: unknown; metabolized by bacteria in large intestine

Adverse effects: Flatulence, cramps and abdominal discomfort.

Faecal Softeners

Some drugs are used to soften the faecal matter during severe constipation. Liquid paraffin used to be the traditional lubricant of choice but this has been associated with irritation after prolonged use and is no longer recommended. Instead, agents such as arachis oil (peanut oil) within an enema have been shown to soften impacted faeces. Other laxatives such as docusate are also used for this purpose as they too have faecal-softening properties.

Therapeutic Actions and Indications

Laxatives work in three ways by:

- Direct stimulation of the GI tract,
- Production of bulk or increased fluid in the lumen of the GI tract, leading to stimulation of local nerve receptors,
- Lubrication of the intestinal bolus to promote passage through the GI tract (see Figure 57.1).

Laxatives are indicated for the short-term relief of constipation to prevent straining when it is clinically undesirable (such as after surgery, myocardial infarction or obstetrical delivery), to evacuate the bowel for diagnostic procedures, to remove ingested poisons from the lower GI tract and as an adjunct in anthelmintic therapy (agents that kill parasitic worms) when it is desirable to flush helminths from the GI tract. Measures, such as proper diet and exercise and taking advantage of the actions of the intestinal reflexes, have eliminated the need for laxatives in many situations; therefore, these agents are used less frequently than they once were in clinical practice.

Most laxatives are available in OTC preparations, and they are often abused by people who then become dependent on them for stimulation of GI movement. Such individuals may develop chronic intestinal disorders as a result. Patients suffering from constipation should initially be encouraged to alter their diet (to include more fibre such as vegetables, bran or fruit juice) and to increase their exercise regimen before taking laxatives.

Pharmacokinetics

Most of these agents are only minimally absorbed and exert their therapeutic effect directly in the GI tract. Changes in absorption, water balance and electrolytes resulting from GI changes can have adverse effects on patients with underlying medical conditions that are affected by volume and electrolyte changes. Use with caution during pregnancy and lactation because of the lack of studies regarding the effects of these drugs. Magnesium laxatives can cause diarrhoea in the neonate.

Contraindications and Cautions

Laxatives are contraindicated in acute abdominal disorders, including appendicitis, diverticulitis and ulcerative colitis, *when increased motility could lead to rupture or further exacerbation of the inflammation*. Laxatives should be used with great caution during pregnancy and lactation. In some cases, stimulation of the GI tract can precipitate labour, and many of these agents cross the placenta and are excreted in breast milk.

Adverse Effects

The adverse effects most commonly associated with laxatives are GI effects such as diarrhoea, abdominal cramping and nausea. Central nervous system (CNS) effects, including dizziness, headache and weakness, are not uncommon and may relate to loss of fluid and electrolyte imbalances that may accompany laxative use. Sweating, palpitations, flushing and even fainting have been reported after laxative use. These effects may be related to a sympathetic stress due to the loss of fluid and electrolyte imbalance.

A very common adverse effect that is seen with frequent laxative use or laxative abuse is **cathartic dependence**. This reaction occurs when patients use laxatives over a long period, and the GI tract becomes dependent on the forceful stimulation of the laxative. Without this stimulation, the GI tract does not move for a period of time (i.e. several days), which could lead to constipation and drying of the stool and ultimately to impaction.

Clinically Important Drug–Drug Interactions

As laxatives increase the motility of the GI tract and some interfere with the timing or process of absorption, it is advisable not to take laxatives with other prescribed medications. The administration of laxatives and other medications should be separated by at least 30 minutes.

Always consult a current copy of the British National Formulary for further guidance.

Nursing Considerations for Patients Receiving Laxatives

Assessment: History and Examination

Screen for the following conditions, *which could be cautions or contraindications to use of the drug*: history of allergy to laxative, faecal impaction or intestinal obstruction; acute abdominal pain, nausea or vomiting and pregnancy or lactation.

Include screening for baseline pulse rate; abdominal examination, including bowel sounds and serum electrolyte levels.

Establish if patient is currently taking other medications or herbal therapies which may potentially interact with laxatives.

Nursing Diagnoses

The patient receiving any laxative may have the following nursing diagnoses related to drug therapy:

- Acute pain related to CNS and GI effects
- Diarrhoea related to drug effects
- Deficient knowledge regarding drug therapy

Implementation With Rationale

- Administer only as a temporary measure *to prevent development of cathartic dependence*.
- Arrange for appropriate dietary measures, exercise and environmental controls *to encourage return of normal bowel function*.
- Administer with a full glass of water and caution the patient not to chew tablets *to ensure that laxative reaches the GI tract to allow for therapeutic effects*. Encourage fluid intake throughout the

day as appropriate *to maintain fluid balance and improve GI movement*.

- Do not administer in the presence of acute abdominal pain, nausea or vomiting, *which might indicate a serious underlying medical problem that could be exacerbated by laxative use*.
- Monitor bowel function *to evaluate drug effectiveness*. If diarrhoea or cramping occurs, discontinue the drug *to relieve discomfort and to prevent serious fluid and electrolyte imbalance*.
- Provide comfort and safety measures *to improve patient compliance and to ensure patient safety*, Offer support and encouragement *to help patient deal with the discomfort of the condition and drug therapy*.
- Provide thorough patient education, including name of drug, dosage prescribed, proper administration, measures to avoid adverse effects, warning signs of problems and the importance of periodic monitoring and evaluation, *to enhance patient knowledge about drug therapy and promote compliance with the drug regimen*.
- Offer support and encouragement *to help patient deal with the diagnosis and the drug regimen*.

Evaluation

- Monitor patient response to the drug (relief of GI symptoms, absence of straining, evacuation of GI tract).
- Monitor for adverse effects (dizziness, confusion, GI alterations, sweating, electrolyte imbalance, cathartic dependence).
- Evaluate effectiveness of teaching plan (patient can name the drug and dosage as well as describe adverse effects to watch for and specific measures to use to avoid adverse effects).
- Monitor effectiveness of comfort measures and compliance with the regimen

Gastrointestinal Stimulants

Some drugs are available for more generalized GI stimulation that results in an overall increase in GI activity and secretions. These drugs stimulate parasympathetic activity or make the GI tissues more sensitive to parasympathetic activity. Both domperidone and metoclopramide are dopamine antagonists that stimulate gastric emptying by blocking dopamine receptors and making the GI cells more sensitive to acetylcholine. This leads to increased GI activity and rapid movement of food through the upper GI tract.

Therapeutic Actions and Indications

By stimulating parasympathetic activity within the GI tract, these drugs increase GI secretions and motility and exert their effects throughout the tract (see Figure 57.1). These drugs are indicated when more rapid movement of GI contents is desirable. Domperidone and metoclopramide are both indicated for relief of symptoms of gastro-oesophageal reflux disease, for prevention of nausea and vomiting after emetogenic chemotherapy or after surgery and for the promotion of GI movement during small bowel intubation or to promote rapid movement of barium.

Pharmacokinetics

These drugs are rapidly absorbed, metabolized in the liver and excreted in urine. They can cross the placenta and enter breast milk. No adequate studies are available on their effects during pregnancy and lactation, but they should be used only if the benefit to the mother clearly outweighs the potential risk to the foetus or neonate.

Contraindications and Cautions

GI stimulants should not be used in patients with any GI obstruction or perforation. They should be used with caution during pregnancy or lactation.

Adverse Effects

The most common adverse effects seen with GI stimulants include nausea, vomiting, diarrhoea, intestinal spasm and cramping. Other adverse effects, such as declining blood pressure and heart rate, weakness and fatigue, may be related to parasympathetic stimulation.

Clinically Important Drug–Drug Interactions

Increased sedation can occur if either of these drugs is combined with alcohol or other CNS sedative drugs. Metoclopramide has been associated with increased absorption of aspirin from the GI tract; patients taking this combination should be monitored carefully.

Decreased immunosuppressive effects and increased toxicity of cyclosporin have occurred when these drugs were combined. This combination should be avoided.

Always consult a current copy of the British National Formulary for further guidance.

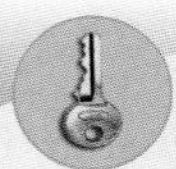

Key Drug Summary: Metoclopramide

Indications: Relief of acute and chronic diabetic gastroparesis, short-term treatment of gastro-oesophageal reflux disorder in adults who cannot tolerate standard therapy, prevention of postoperative nausea and vomiting, facilitation of small bowel intubation, stimulation of gastric emptying to speed the intestinal transit of barium. Short-term treatment for severe vomiting during pregnancy and migraine.

Actions: Stimulates movement of the upper GI tract without stimulating gastric, pancreatic or biliary secretions; appears to sensitize tissues to the effects of acetylcholine

Pharmacokinetics:

Route	Onset	Peak	Duration
Oral	30–60 min	60–90 min	1–2 h
IM	10–15 min	60–90 min	1–2 h
IV	1–5 min	60–90 min	1–2 h

$T_{1/2}$: 5–6 hours; metabolized in the liver and excreted in urine

Adverse effects: Restlessness, drowsiness, fatigue, extrapyramidal effects, Parkinsonian-like reactions, nausea, diarrhoea, hyperprolactinaemia, depression.

Nursing Considerations for Patients Receiving Gastrointestinal Stimulants

Assessment: History and Examination

Screen for the following conditions, *which could be cautions or contraindications to the use of the drug*: any history of allergy to these drugs; intestinal obstruction, bleeding or perforation and pregnancy or lactation.

Include screening *to establish baseline data for assessing the effectiveness of the drug and the occurrence of any adverse effects associated with drug therapy*. Perform an abdominal examination, checking bowel sounds *to ensure GI motility*; assess pulse and blood pressure *to monitor for adverse effect*.

Establish if patient is currently taking other medications or herbal therapies which may potentially interact with GI stimulants.

Nursing Diagnoses

The patient receiving GI stimulants may have the following nursing diagnoses related to drug therapy:

- Diarrhoea related to drug effects
- Acute pain related to GI effects
- Deficient knowledge regarding drug therapy

Implementation With Rationale

- Usual administration is at bedtime *to ensure therapeutic effectiveness*.
- Provide thorough patient education, including name of drug, dosage prescribed, proper administration, measures to avoid adverse effects, warning signs of problems and the importance of periodic monitoring and evaluation, *to enhance patient knowledge about drug therapy and promote compliance with the drug regimen*.
- Offer support and encouragement *to help the patient deal with the diagnosis and the drug regimen*.

Evaluation

- Monitor patient response to the drug (increased tone and movement of GI tract).
- Monitor for adverse effects (GI effects, parasympathetic activity).
- Evaluate effectiveness of the teaching plan (patient can name the drug and dosage, as well as describe adverse effects to watch for and specific measures to take to avoid adverse effects and increase the effectiveness of the drug).
- Monitor the effectiveness of comfort measures and compliance with the regimen.

Antimotility Drugs

Antimotility drugs that block stimulation of the GI tract are used for symptomatic relief from acute diarrhoea. Fluid and electrolyte replacement therapy may be necessary in patients suffering from dehydration. Antimotility agents are not recommended for use in children (National Institute for Health & Clinical Excellence, 2009). Available agents include the following:

- Loperamide is the drug of choice for travellers' diarrhoea. It acts on opiate receptors in the gut and has a direct effect on the muscle layers of the GI tract to slow peristalsis and allow increased time for absorption of fluid and electrolytes. Loperamide does not directly cross the blood–brain barrier so it does not affect the CNS and has localized actions in the gut.

- Codeine phosphate is used as cough suppressant as well as for analgesia. It inhibits gut motility by acting on opioid receptors. It is administered orally but is not recommended for use in children.
- Morphine is another opioid agonist, but its actions on the GI tract are more complex. It increases tone on the smooth muscles but reduces the propulsive activity. It also causes contraction of the GI tract sphincters. The overall actions are constipated.
- Co-phenotrope is a mixture of diphenoxylate and atropine sulphate and is used as an adjunct to rehydration therapy in acute diarrhoea and to control faecal consistency following bowel surgery.

Therapeutic Actions and Indications

Antimotility agents slow down the motility of the GI tract through direct action on the lining of the GI tract to inhibit local reflexes (bismuth subsalicylate), through direct action on the muscles of the GI tract to slow activity (loperamide) or through action on CNS centres that cause GI spasm and slowing (opium derivatives). These drugs are indicated for the relief of symptoms of acute and chronic diarrhoea, reduction of volume of discharge from ileostomies and prevention and treatment of traveller's diarrhoea (see Figure 57.1).

Pharmacokinetics

In general, the pharmacokinetics of antimotility agents varies depending on the agent.

- Loperamide is absorbed from the GI tract and undergoes some first-pass metabolism in the liver. Only a small amount of the intact drug reaches the systemic circulation. The metabolites are excreted in the faeces via bile.
- Codeine phosphate is absorbed from the GI tract and is metabolized in the liver. Codeine and its salts are absorbed from the GI tract. Metabolites are excreted via the urine.
- Morphine is prepared as a suspension with kaolin. The kaolin is not absorbed and acts as an adsorbent in the GI tract. Kaolin is excreted unchanged in faeces. Morphine is well absorbed from the GI tract and is metabolized by the liver. The metabolites are mostly excreted in urine.
- Co-phenotrope is well absorbed from the GI tract and undergoes extensive metabolism by the liver. The metabolites are mainly excreted in the faeces.

Contraindications and Cautions

Antimotility should be used with caution in pregnancy and lactation. Care should also be taken in individuals with any history of GI obstruction, acute abdominal conditions or diarrhoea due to poisonings.

Adverse Effects

The adverse effects associated with antimotility drugs, such as constipation, distension, abdominal discomfort, nausea, vomiting and dry mouth, are related to their effects on the GI tract. Other adverse effects that have been reported include fatigue, weakness, abdominal bloating and dizziness.

Clinically Important Drug–Drug Interactions

Loperamide is known to increase the plasma levels of desmopressin. The most significant drug interactions with codeine phosphate, morphine and co-phenotrope include antidepressants, antipsychotics, anxiolytics and hypnotics, β-blockers (morphine), sodium oxybate and cimetidine.

Always consult a current copy of the British National Formulary for further guidance.

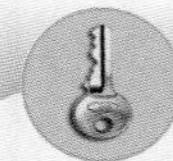

Key Drug Summary: *Loperamide*

Indications: Control and symptomatic relief of acute, nonspecific diarrhoea and chronic diarrhoea associated with irritable bowel syndrome; reduction of volume of discharge from ileostomies

Actions: Inhibits intestinal peristalsis through direct effects on the longitudinal and circular muscles of the intestinal wall, slowing motility and movement of water and electrolytes

Pharmacokinetics:

Route	Onset	Peak
Oral (capsule)	Varies	5 h

$T_{1/2}$: 10.8 hours; metabolized in the liver and excreted in urine and faeces

Adverse effects: Abdominal pain, distension or discomfort; dry mouth; nausea; constipation; dizziness; tiredness; drowsiness

Nursing Considerations for Patients Receiving Antimotility drugs

Assessment: History and Examination

Screen for the following conditions, *which could be cautions or contraindications to the use of the drug*: any history of allergy to these drugs, acute abdominal conditions, poisoning and pregnancy or lactation.

Include screening *to establish baseline data for assessing the effectiveness of the drug and the occurrence of any adverse effects associated with drug therapy*. Perform an abdominal examination, including bowel sounds, assess orientation and affect.

Establish if patient is currently taking other medications or herbal therapies which may potentially interact with antimotility drug.

Nursing Diagnoses

The patient receiving antimotility drugs may have the following nursing diagnoses related to drug therapy:

- Constipation related to GI slowing
- Acute pain related to GI effects
- Disturbed sensory perception (i.e. gustatory) related to CNS effects
- Deficient knowledge regarding drug therapy

Implementation With Rationale

- Monitor response carefully. If no response is seen within 48 hours, *the diarrhoea could be related to an underlying medical condition*. Arrange to discontinue the drug and arrange for medical evaluation *to allow for diagnosis of underlying medical conditions*.
- Provide appropriate safety and comfort measures if CNS effects occur *to prevent patient injury*.
- Administer drug after each unformed stool *to ensure therapeutic effectiveness*. Keep track of exact amount given *to ensure that dosage does not exceed recommended daily maximum dose*.
- Provide thorough patient education, including name of drug, dosage prescribed, proper administration, measures to avoid adverse effects, warning signs of problems and the importance of periodic monitoring and evaluation, *to enhance patient knowledge about drug therapy and promote compliance with the drug regimen*.
- Offer support and encouragement *to help the patient deal with the diagnosis and the drug regimen*.

Evaluation

- Monitor patient response to the drug (relief of diarrhoea).
- Monitor for adverse effects (GI effects, CNS changes, dermatologic effects).
- Evaluate effectiveness of teaching plan (patient can name the drug and dosage, as well as describe adverse effects to watch for, specific measures to use to avoid adverse effects and measures to take to increase the effectiveness of the drug).
- Monitor effectiveness of comfort and safety measures and compliance with the regimen.

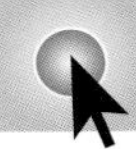

WEB LINKS

Health care providers and patients may want to consult the following Internet sources:

http://cks.library.nhs.uk The National Health Service Clinical Knowledge Summaries provides evidence-based practical information on the common conditions observed in primary care.

http://www.bnf.org.uk The BNF provides UK health care professionals with authoritative and practical information on the selection and clinical use of medicines.

http://www.nhsdirect.nhs.uk The National Health Service Direct service provides patients with information and advice about health, illness and health services.

http://www.nathanac.org This is a comprehensive site providing advice from the UK Health Protection Agency's National Travel Health Network and Centre.

http://www.nice.org.uk The National Institute for Health and Clinical Excellence (NICE) provides guidance on best practice.

Points to Remember

- Laxatives are drugs used to stimulate movement along the GI tract and to aid excretion. They may be used to prevent or treat constipation.
- Laxatives can be stimulants, which directly irritate the local nerve plexus, bulk stimulants, which increase the size of the food bolus and stimulate stretch receptors in the wall of the intestine or lubricants, which facilitate movement of the bolus through the intestines.

- Use of proper diet and exercise, as well as taking advantage of the actions of the intestinal reflexes, has eliminated the need for laxatives in many situations.
- Cathartic dependence can occur with the chronic use of laxatives, leading to a need for external stimuli for normal functioning of the GI tract.
- GI stimulants act to increase parasympathetic stimulation in the GI tract and to increase tone and general movement throughout the GI system.
- Antimotility drugs are used to soothe irritation to the intestinal wall, block GI muscle activity to decrease movement or affect CNS activity to cause GI spasm and stop movement.

CRITICAL THINKING SCENARIO 57-1

Traveller's Diarrhoea

The Situation

Penny arranged a week's holiday in the sun to celebrate her graduation from university. On the fourth day of the trip, Penny began experiencing nausea, some vomiting and a low-grade fever. Several hours later, she began experiencing intense cramping and diarrhoea; she was feeling very nauseous and complained of a headache. For the next 2 days, Penny felt so ill that she was unable to leave her hotel room. The next morning she returned home.

Critical Thinking

- What is probably happening to Penny? *Think about the GI reflexes and explain the underlying cause for her signs and symptoms.*
- What treatment should be started now?
- What could have been done to prevent this problem from occurring?
- What possible drug therapy might have been helpful for Penny?

Discussion

Penny is probably experiencing the common disorder called traveller's diarrhoea. This disorder occurs when pathogens found in the food and water of a foreign environment are ingested. As these pathogens are commonly found in the environment, they do not normally cause problems for the people who live in the area. When the pathogen, usually a strain of *Escherichia coli*, enters a host that is not accustomed to the bacteria, it releases enterotoxins and sets off an intestinal reaction in the host.

The intestinal–intestinal reaction results in a reduction of activity above the point of irritation (which causes nausea and in some cases vomiting) and an increase in activity below the point of irritation. The body is trying to flush the invader from the body. A low-grade fever may occur as a reaction to the toxins released by the bacteria. Muscle aches and pains, malaise and fatigue are often common symptoms. It is important at this stage of the disease to maintain fluid intake to prevent dehydration from occurring.

Once traveller's diarrhoea is diagnosed, loperamide can be taken. It should not be used if the patient has bloody diarrhoea or diarrhoea that worsens or persists for more than 48 hours. The best course of action, however, is prevention. Several measures can be taken to avoid ingestion of the local bacteria: drinking only bottled or mineral water, avoiding fresh fruits and vegetables that may have been washed in the local water (unless they are peeled), avoiding ice cubes in drinks because the ice cubes are made from the local water, avoiding any food that might be undercooked or rare, including shellfish and even being cautious about using water to brush teeth or gargle. People who have suffered a bout of traveller's diarrhoea are very cautious about exposure to local bacteria when they travel again, with careful avoidance of local pathogens. Penny can be reassured that in a few days the diarrhoea and associated signs and symptoms should pass and she will regain her strength and energy.

Nursing Care Guide for Penny: Loperamide

Assessment: History and Examination

Assess the patient's health history for allergies to loperamide, liver disease or pregnancy.

Focus the physical examination on the following:

- Neurological: orientation
- GI: abdominal examination, bowel sounds
- Laboratory tests: serum electrolyte levels
- CVS: pulse, BP
- Renal: urinalysis
- Skin check for hydration
- Other: temperature

Traveller's Diarrhoea *(continued)*

Nursing Diagnoses

- Acute pain related to GI, CNS effects
- Diarrhoea related to GI effects
- Deficient knowledge regarding drug therapy

Implementation

- Administer antimotility agent only as a temporary measure.
- Provide comfort and safety measures, including assistance, access to bathroom, safety precautions if necessary.
- Monitor bowel function.
- Provide support and reassurance for coping with drug effects and discomfort.
- Provide patient education regarding drug name and dosage, adverse effects and precautions, warning signs of serious adverse effects to report.

Evaluation

- Evaluate drug effects: relief of GI symptoms.
- Monitor for adverse effects: GI alterations, dizziness, skin reactions.
- Monitor for drug–drug interactions as indicated.
- Evaluate effectiveness of patient education programme and comfort and safety measures.

Patient Education for Penny

☐ The drug prescribed for you is called loperamide, an antimotility agent. It relaxes the smooth muscle in the bowel and reduces peristalsis.

☐ Take this drug exactly as indicated. If using the liquid preparation, shake the bottle well before use.

☐ Common effects of this drug include:

- Abdominal cramps and bloating, dizziness, drowsiness and skin reactions.

☐ Report any of the following conditions to your health care provider: *diarrhoea that does not stop within 2 days, fever and/or intense abdominal pain.*

☐ Stay away from any food or beverage that may be contaminated with bacteria. Use bottled water for drinking, as well as for brushing your teeth. Do not wash fruit or vegetables with water from the local supply.

☐ Tell any doctor, nurse or other health care provider involved in your care that you are taking this drug.

☐ Keep this drug and all medications out of the reach of children.

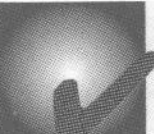

CHECK YOUR UNDERSTANDING

Answers to the questions in this chapter may be found in the answer key in the back of the book.

Multiple Choice

Select the most appropriate response to the following.

1. Laxatives are drugs used to
   a. increase the quantity of wastes excreted.
   b. speed the passage of the intestinal contents through the GI tract.
   c. increase digestion of intestinal contents.
   d. increase the water content of the intestinal contents.

2. Cathartic dependence can occur when patients:
   a. do not use laxatives and become very constipated.
   b. chronically use laxatives which leads to a reliance on the intense stimulation of laxatives to cause movement.
   c. maintain a good diet including roughage.
   d. start an exercise programme.

3. Drugs that stimulate parasympathetic activity are used to increase GI activity and secretions. This could be therapeutic in the treatment of
   a. duodenal ulcers.
   b. gastric ulcers.
   c. signs and symptoms of gastro-oesophageal reflux disease.
   d. poisoning to induce nausea and vomiting.

4. The drug of choice for treating traveller's diarrhoea would be
   a. loperamide.
   b. opium.
   c. bisacodyl.
   d. codeine.

Extended Matching Questions

Select **all** that apply.

1. A nurse is preparing a teaching plan for a client who has been prescribed a laxative. The teaching plan should include the
   a. importance of proper diet and fluid intake
   b. need to take the drug for several weeks to get the full effect
   c. importance of exercise
   d. need to take advantage of natural reflexes by providing privacy and time to allow them to work
   e. need to limit fluids
   f. importance of limiting the duration of laxative use

2. When explaining the actions of laxatives to a client, the nurse would state that they can work by
   a. acting as chemical stimulants.
   b. acting as lubricants of the intestinal bolus.
   c. acting to increase bulk of the intestinal bolus and stimulate movement.
   d. stimulating CNS centres in the medulla to cause GI movement.
   e. blocking the parasympathetic nervous system.
   f. causing central nervous system depression.

True or False

Indicate whether the following statements are true (T) or false (F).

_____1. Laxatives are used to stop movement along the GI tract.

_____2. Laxatives are used to prevent or treat constipation.

_____3. Chemical stimulants directly irritate the local nerve plexus of the GI tract.

_____4. Bulk stimulants decrease the size of the food bolus and stimulate stretch receptors in the intestinal wall.

_____5. For many patients, eating a proper diet, exercising and taking advantage of the actions of the intestinal reflexes has eliminated the need for laxatives.

_____6. Cathartic dependence can occur with the occasional use of laxatives, leading to a need for external stimuli for normal functioning of the GI tract.

_____7. GI stimulants act to increase sympathetic stimulation in the GI tract.

_____8. Antimotility drugs are used to soothe irritation to the intestinal wall, block GI muscle activity to decrease movement or affect central nervous system activity to cause GI spasm and stop movement.

Bibliography and References

British Medical Association and Royal Pharmaceutical Society of Great Britain. (2008). *British National Formulary*. London: BMJ & RPS Publishing. *This publication is updated biannually: it is imperative that the most recent edition is consulted.*

British Medical Association and Royal Pharmaceutical Society of Great Britain. (2008). *British National Formulary for Children*. London: BMJ & RPS Publishing. *This publication is updated annually: it is imperative that the most recent edition is consulted.*

Ganong, W. (2005). *Review of medical physiology* (22nd ed.). New York: McGraw-Hill.

Howland, R. D., & Mycek, M. J. (2005). *Pharmacology* (3rd ed.). Philadelphia: Lippincott Williams & Wilkins.

Marieb, E. N., & Hoehn, K. (2004). *Human anatomy & physiology* (7th ed.). San Francisco: Pearson Benjamin Cummings.

National Institute for Health & Clinical Excellence. (2009). Diarrhoea and vomiting caused by gastroenteritis: diagnosis, assessment and management in children younger than 5 years. Available from http://www.nice.org.uk/CG084.

Porth, C. M., & Matfin, G. (2008). *Pathophysiology: Concepts of altered health states* (8th ed.). Philadelphia: Lippincott Williams & Wilkins.

Simonsen, T., Aarbakke, J., Kay, I., Coleman, I., Sinnott, P., & Lysaa, R. (2006). *Illustrated pharmacology for nurses*. London: Hodder Arnold.

CHAPTER 58

Antiemetic Agents

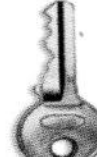

KEY TERMS

antiemetic

chemoreceptor trigger zone (CTZ)

intractable hiccups

vestibular

vomiting centre

LEARNING OBJECTIVES

Upon completion of this chapter, you will be able to:

1. Outline the vomiting reflex, including factors that stimulate it and how measures used to block it work.
2. Describe the therapeutic actions, indications, pharmacokinetics, contraindications, most common adverse effects and important drug–drug interactions associated with antiemetic agents.
3. Discuss the use of antiemetics across the lifespan.
4. Compare and contrast the key drugs metoclopramide, cyclizine, ondansetron and aprepitant with other agents in their class and with other classes of antiemetics.
5. Outline the nursing considerations, including important teaching points, for patients receiving antiemetics.

ANTIEMETIC AGENTS

Dopamine D_2 Receptor Antagonists

domperidone
haloperidol
metoclopramide
Phenothiazine derivatives
chlorpromazine
levomepromazine
perphenazine
prochlorperazine
trifluoperazine

Antimuscarinics & Antihistamines

cinnarizine
cyclizine
hyoscine
promethazine hydrochloride
promethazine teoclate

Serotonin 5-HT_3 Receptor Antagonists

dolasetron mesilate
granisetron
ondansetron
palonosetron
tropisetron

Substance P/Neurokinin 1 Receptor Antagonist

aprepitant

Cannabinoids

nabilone

One of the most common and most uncomfortable complaints encountered in clinical practice is that of nausea and vomiting. Feelings of nausea usually precede vomiting. Vomiting is a complex reflex reaction to various stimuli, including stress, pain, shock, bacterial toxins associated with food poisoning, drug overdose, motion sickness, migraine headaches and ear disorders which affect the vestibular apparatus. Distension or inflammation of the gastrointestinal (GI) tract can also cause nausea.

The vomiting reflex is controlled by two areas in the brain: the **chemoreceptor trigger zone (CTZ)** on the floor of the fourth ventricle and the **vomiting centre** in the medulla. The CTZ is bathed in cerebrospinal fluid and therefore detects drugs or toxins which have entered the cerebrospinal fluid via the blood. The vomiting centre receives sensory input from the CTZ, the GI tract, cerebral cortex and vestibular apparatus. Stimulation of the vomiting centre causes wavelike contractions of the diaphragm and abdominal muscles, relaxation of the gastro-oesophageal sphincter and subsequent expulsion of the stomach contents.

Although vomiting can be a useful way of ridding harmful substances from the upper GI tract, in many clinical conditions, vomiting is uncomfortable and even clinically hazardous to the patient's condition, leading to dehydration and abnormal electrolyte levels. In such cases, an **antiemetic** is used to decrease or prevent nausea and vomiting. Antiemetic agents can be centrally or locally acting, and they have varying degrees of effectiveness. These drugs are used with all age groups (Box 58.1).

Antiemetic Agents

Drugs used in managing nausea and vomiting are called antiemetics. Most of these drugs act centrally to block dopamine, serotonin/5-HT, opioid or acetylcholine receptors in the CTZ or suppress the vomiting centre (Figure 58.1). Centrally acting antiemetics can be classified in several groups: dopamine receptor antagonists, serotonin (5-HT_3) receptor antagonists, substance P/neurokinin 1 (NK1) receptor antagonists, anticholinergics/antihistamines and cannabinoids. The class of antiemetic prescribed will depend on the cause of the nausea: for example nausea induced by motion sickness is usefully treated with either an antihistamine or anticholinergic, whereas nausea induced by opioid analgesics or antineoplastic drugs is effectively managed with a dopamine receptor antagonist. Some of the drugs within these classes also work peripherally to reduce distension or irritation of the gut and therefore prevent signals being sent to the vomiting centre.

BOX 58.1 **DRUG THERAPY ACROSS THE LIFESPAN**

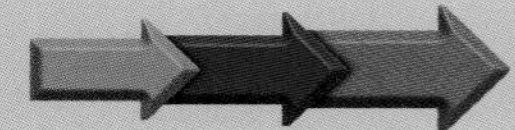

Antiemetic Agents

CHILDREN

In infants and children, vomiting is a relatively common symptom in association with either a generalized illness or an underlying GI condition. If an infant or child is vomiting persistently, it is important to seek medical help; newborns and infants in particular can become rapidly dehydrated. In all cases, it is important to ensure the correct cause of vomiting is identified as quickly as possible; antiemetics should not be prescribed before a diagnosis is completed. Premature treatment with an antiemetic can increase the time it takes to reach a diagnosis.

Children are most likely to require an antiemetic to prevent motion sickness. In this case, an antihistamine such as cyclizine or cinnarizine is recommended as both have lower sedating effects. Antiemetics should be used with caution in children who are at higher risk of adverse effects, including central nervous system (CNS) effects such as dystonia, as well as fluid and electrolyte disturbances.

When administering any drug to children, always consult the most recent edition of the British National Formulary for Children.

ADULTS

Antiemetics are often used after surgery to treat postoperative nausea and vomiting (PONV) or as an adjunct treatment in chemotherapy (see Chapter 13). PONV is a relatively common occurrence following surgery, affecting approximately 30% of all surgical patients. These patients are at increased risk of bleeding from the site of surgery, stomach contents entering the respiratory system, electrolyte imbalance and dehydration. This can lead to extended stays in hospital and considerable discomfort to the patient. Patients should be administered either one of the phenothiazines, a 5-HT_3 antagonist, an antihistamine or dexamethasone.

In any medical situation, precautions should be used to ensure that the CNS effects associated with antiemetics do not interfere with mobility or other activities.

The safety of some of these drugs during pregnancy has been established. The antihistamines cyclizine, promethazine hydrochloride and promethazine teoclate are safe for use during pregnancy and lactation. If necessary, promethazine can be used to reduce nausea and vomiting in the first trimester of pregnancy. Hyoscine hydrobromide is also safe to use during lactation. The other antiemetic drugs should only be used in those situations where the benefit to the mother outweighs the potential risk to the foetus or neonate.

OLDER ADULTS

Older adults are more likely to develop adverse effects associated with the use of these drugs including sedation, confusion, dizziness, fluid imbalance and cardiovascular effects. Safety measures may be needed if these effects occur and interfere with the patient's mobility and balance. Older adults are also more likely to have renal and/or hepatic impairment related to underlying medical conditions, which could interfere with the metabolism and excretion of these drugs. The patient should be monitored very closely, and dosage adjustment should be made based on patient response.

Dopamine D_2 receptor antagonists: chlorpromazine, domperidone, haloperidol, levomepromazine, metoclopramide, prochlorperazine, promethazine
Brain
5-HT_3 receptor antagonists work here: dolasetron granisetron ondansetron palonosetron tropisetron
Nabilone works here
CTZ & vomiting centre
Anticholinergic & antihistamines antiemetics work here: cinnarizine, cyclizine, promethazine, hyoxine
Substance P/neurokinin 1 receptor antagonist works here: aprepitant
Dopamine D_2 receptor antagonists work here: domperidone metaclopramide
5-HT_3 receptor antagonists work here: andansetron
anticholinergics work here: hyoscine

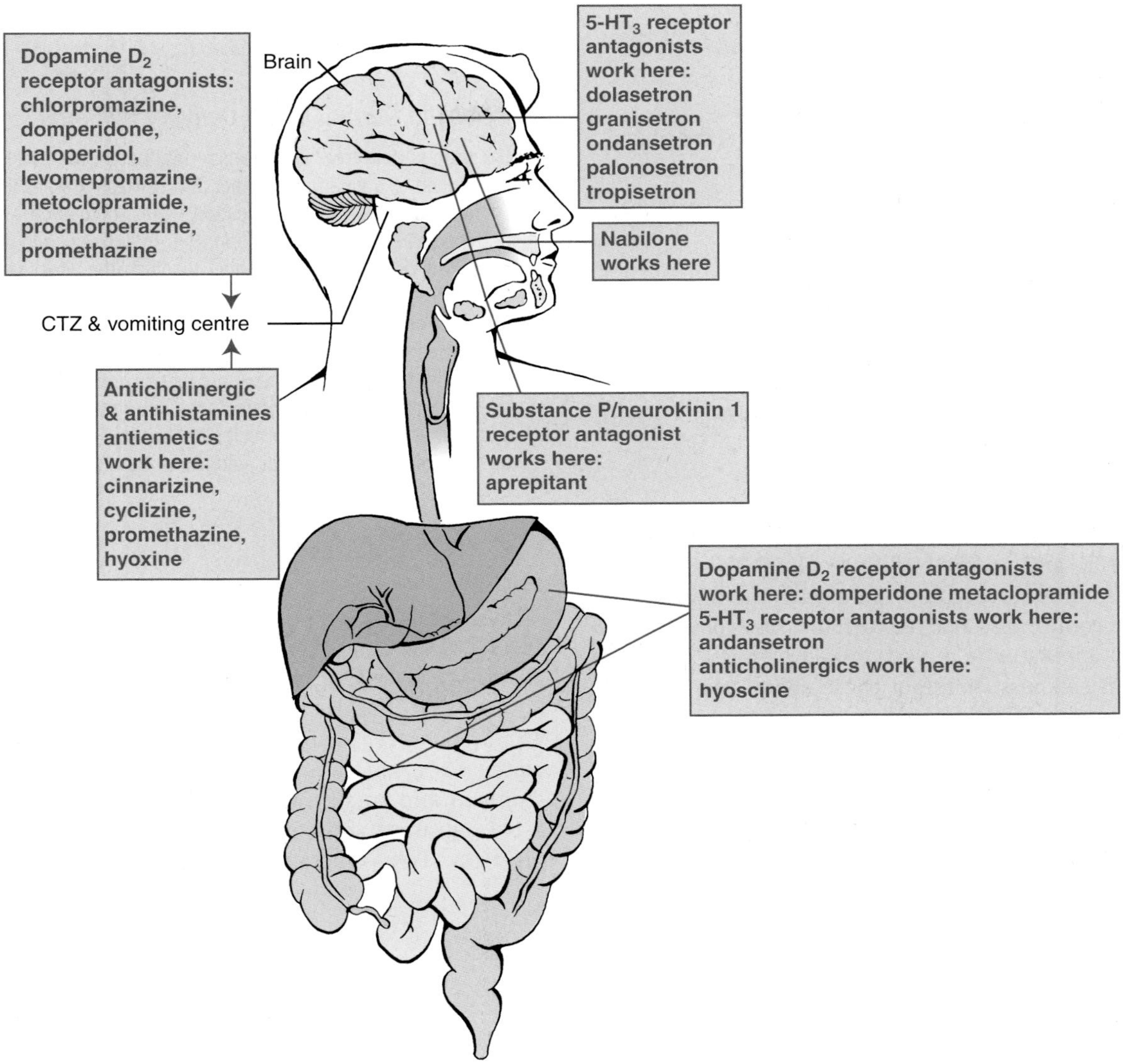

FIGURE 58.1 Sites of action of antiemetics. CTZ, chemoreceptor trigger zone.

Therapeutic Actions and Indications: Dopamine D_2 Receptor Antagonists

The CTZ is rich in dopamine D_2 receptors. Antagonists of these receptors reduce the responsiveness of nerve cells in the CTZ area to circulating chemicals that induce vomiting. Some of the drugs in this class also target receptors in the vomiting centre and GI tract. These drugs are effective in treating the nausea and vomiting associated with radiotherapy, chemotherapy and general anaesthesia. The phenothiazines prochlorperazine (see Critical Thinking Scenario 58-1), perphenazine and trifluoperazine exhibit reduced sedative effects compared to other drugs in the class. Chlorpromazine is also used to treat **intractable hiccups**, caused by persistent diaphragmatic spasm.

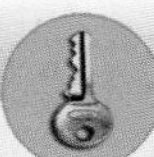

Key Drug Summary: *Metoclopramide*

Indications: Prevention of nausea and vomiting associated with GI disorders, chemotherapy, radiotherapy and migraine

Actions: Increases peristalsis and emptying of the upper GI tract

Pharmacokinetics:

Route	Onset	Peak	Duration
Oral	30–60 min	60–90 min	1–2 h
IM	10–15 min	60–90 min	1–2 h
IV	1–3 min	60–90 min	1–2 h

$T_{1/2}$: 4–6 hours; metabolized in the liver and excreted mainly in urine

Adverse effects: Extrapyramidal symptoms (especially in children and young adults), drowsiness, restlessness, diarrhoea, depression, rashes, pruritis (itching), oedema, cardiac conduction abnormalities [intravenous (IV) administration only]

Therapeutic Actions and Indications: Antimuscarinics & Antihistamines

The antihistamines used to prevent or treat nausea and vomiting include cinnarizine, cyclizine, promethazine hydrochloride and promethazine teoclate. These antagonists of histamine H_1 receptors are used in the treatment of nausea and vomiting associated with disorders of **vestibular** (inner ear) apparatus (e.g. vertigo and Ménière's disease) and motion sickness. Some of these agents are available over the counter (OTC) in a reduced dose for prevention of motion sickness.

Some of the antihistamines also have some action on muscarinic acetylcholine receptors. Hyoscine hydrobromide is an anticholinergic drug, used in the treatment of motion sickness and also as a premedication before surgery. Hyoscine hydrobromide is available in a transdermal form (Box 58.2) which must be applied 5 to 6 hours before travelling.

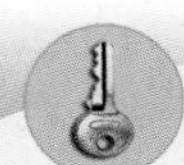

Key Drug Summary: *Cinnarizine*

Indications: Prevention of nausea and vomiting associated with vestibular disorders such as vertigo, tinnitus and Ménière's disease; motion sickness

Actions: Blocks muscarinic receptors located in the central and peripheral nervous system

Pharmacokinetics:

Route	Onset	Peak	Duration
Oral	1–2 h	2 h	8–10 h

$T_{1/2}$: 3–6 hours; metabolism probably by the liver; excreted in faeces mainly as unchanged drug and in the urine as metabolites

Adverse effects: Drowsiness, headache, urinary retention, dry mouth and GI disturbances.

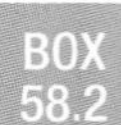

BOX 58.2 FOCUS ON **CLINICAL SKILLS**

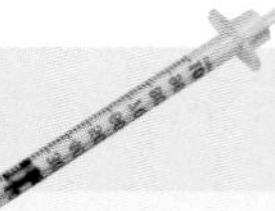

Applying Dermal Patch Delivery Systems

If a drug is delivered via a transdermal patch, the patch should be applied to a clean, dry, intact and hairless area of the body. Do not shave an area of application – that could abrade the skin and lead to increased absorption. Hair may be clipped if necessary. Peel off the backing without touching the adhesive side of the patch. Place the patch at a new site each time to avoid skin irritation or degradation. Remove the old patch and clean the area when putting on a new transdermal patch. It is important to remember that many transdermal systems contain an aluminized barrier that could cause an electrical charge with arcing, smoke and severe transdermal burns if a defibrillator is discharged over it. Remove any transdermal patches in the area if a defibrillator is to be used.

Therapeutic Actions and Indications: 5-HT_3 Receptor Antagonists

The 5-HT_3 receptor blockers block those receptors associated with nausea and vomiting in the CTZ and in the stomach and small intestine. These drugs include dolasetron, granisetron, ondansetron, palonosetron and tropisetron. They are rapidly absorbed from the GI tract,

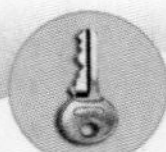

Key Drug Summary: *Ondansetron*

Indications: Control of severe nausea and vomiting associated with emetogenic cancer chemotherapy, radiotherapy; prevention and treatment of PONV

Actions: Blocks 5-HT_3 receptor sites associated with nausea and vomiting, peripherally and in the CTZ

Pharmacokinetics:

Route	Onset	Peak	Duration
Oral	30–60 min	60–90 min	1.7–2.2 h
IV	Immediate	60–90 min	Duration of infusion

$T_{1/2}$: 3.5–5 hours; metabolized in the liver and excreted in urine

Adverse effects: Headache, constipation, flushing and pain at injection site. Less common adverse effects include hiccups, hypotension, bradycardia, chest pain, arrhythmias, movement disorders, seizures. IV administration can also cause dizziness and visual disturbances

metabolized in the liver and excreted in urine and faeces. This class of drugs is especially helpful in treating the nausea and vomiting associated with antineoplastic chemotherapy and PONV. These drugs are known to cross the placenta and enter breast milk, and manufacturers advise that their use should be avoided during pregnancy and lactation or limited to situations in which the benefit to the mother outweighs the potential risk to the foetus or neonate.

Therapeutic Actions and Indications: Substance P/NK1 Receptor Antagonist

The first drug in the newest class of drugs for treating nausea and vomiting is the substance P/NK1 receptor antagonist aprepitant. This drug acts directly in the CNS to block receptors associated with nausea and vomiting with little to no effect on 5-HT, dopamine or corticosteroid receptors. It is approved for use in treating the nausea and vomiting associated with highly emetogenic antineoplastic chemotherapy, including cisplatin therapy. It is given orally, usually in combination with dexamethasone and a 5-HT_3 receptor antagonist. This drug is known to cross the placenta and to enter breast milk and should not be used during pregnancy unless the benefits to the mother clearly outweigh the risk to the foetus. Aprepitant should not be used during lactation.

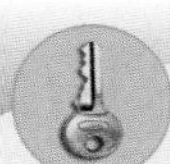

Key Drug Summary: *Aprepitant*

Indications: In combination with dexamethasone and a 5-HT_3 antagonist for prevention of acute and delayed nausea and vomiting associated with moderate and severely emetogenic chemotherapy

Actions: Selectively blocks human substance P/NK1 receptors in the CNS, blocking the nausea and vomiting caused by highly emetogenic chemotherapeutic agents

Pharmacokinetics:

Route	Onset	Peak
Oral	Rapid	4 h

$T_{1/2}$: 9–13 hours; metabolized in the liver and excreted in urine and faeces

Adverse effects: More common adverse effects include hiccups, dyspepsia, diarrhoea, constipation, anorexia, physical weakness, headache and dizziness

Therapeutic Actions and Indications: Cannabinoids

Nabilone, a synthetic cannabinoid with properties similar to the active component of marijuana, is believed to stimulate cannabinoid receptors around the vomiting centre. This drug is approved for use in managing the nausea and vomiting associated with cancer chemotherapy in cases that have not responded to other treatment. Patients receiving nabilone should be kept under close observation, preferably in a hospital setting. It is readily absorbed and metabolized in the liver, with excretion via bile in faeces (mainly) and in urine.

Contraindications and Cautions with Antiemetics

In general, antiemetic drugs should not be used in patients with coma or severe CNS depression or in those who have experienced brain damage or injury *because of the risk of further CNS depression*. Other contraindications include severe hypotension or hypertension and severe liver dysfunction, *which might interfere with the metabolism of the drug*. Caution should be used in individuals with renal dysfunction, active peptic ulcer or pregnancy and lactation.

Adverse Effects with Antiemetics

Adverse effects associated with antiemetic drugs are linked to their interference with normal CNS stimulation or response. Drowsiness, dizziness, weakness, tremor and headache are common adverse effects. As previously stated, some of the antiemetics are thought to have fewer CNS effects. Other less common adverse effects include hypotension, hypertension and cardiac arrhythmias. When the anticholinergics and antihistamines are used as antiemetics, autonomic effects such as dry mouth, blurred vision, photosensitivity (increased sensitivity to the sun and ultraviolet light) and urinary retention can occur but are rare side-effects.

Clinically Important Antiemetic–Drug Interactions

Additive CNS depression can be seen with any of the antiemetics if they are combined with other CNS depressants, including alcohol. Patients should be advised to avoid this combination and any OTC preparation unless they check with their health care provider.

Always consult a current copy of the British National Formulary for further guidance.

Nursing Considerations for Patients Receiving an Antiemetic

Assessment: History and Examination

Screen for the following conditions, *which could be cautions or contraindications to the use of the drug*: history of allergy to antiemetic; impaired renal or hepatic function; pregnancy or lactation; coma or semiconscious state, epilepsy; CNS depression; hypotension; cardiovascular disease (including prolonged QT interval and other conduction disorders) and GI obstruction. Establish if patient is currently taking other medications or herbal therapies which may potentially interact with the antiemetic drug.

Include screening for orientation and affect: baseline pulse and blood pressure, liver and abdominal examination and liver and renal function tests if the patient's history suggests potential problems.

Nursing Diagnoses

The patient receiving an antiemetic may have the following nursing diagnoses related to drug therapy:

- Acute pain related to CNS and GI effects
- Risk of injury related to CNS effects
- Decreased cardiac output related to cardiac effects
- Deficient knowledge regarding drug therapy

Implementation With Rationale

- Assess the patient carefully for symptoms precipitating the vomiting or that are occurring concurrently.
- Assess for any potential drug–drug interactions if giving antiemetics in combination with other drugs *to avert potentially serious drug–drug interactions*.
- Administer antiemetic only when the patient is alert to reduce the risk of aspiration.
- Provide comfort and safety measures, including mouth care, ready access to bathroom facilities and remedial measures to treat dehydration if it occurs, *to protect patient from injury and to increase patient comfort*.
- Provide support and encouragement, as well as other measures (quiet environment, deep breathing), *to help the patient cope with the discomfort of nausea and vomiting and drug effects*.
- Provide thorough patient teaching, including name of drug, dosage prescribed, proper administration, measures to avoid adverse effects, warning signs of problems, the importance of periodic monitoring and evaluation, and the need to avoid overdose, *to enhance patient knowledge about drug therapy and promote compliance with the drug regimen*.

Evaluation

- Monitor patient response to the drug (relief of nausea and vomiting).
- Monitor for adverse effects (dizziness, confusion, GI alterations, cardiac arrhythmias, hypotension).
- Evaluate effectiveness of teaching plan (patient can name the drug and dosage as well as describe adverse effects to watch for and specific measures to avoid these adverse effects).
- Monitor effectiveness of comfort measures and compliance with the regimen.

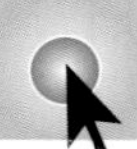

WEB LINKS

Health care providers and patients may want to consult the following Internet sources:

http://bnfc.org The BNF for Children provides UK health care professionals with authoritative and practical information on the selection and clinical use of medicines in children.

http://www.bnf.org.uk The BNF provides UK health care professionals with authoritative and practical information on the selection and clinical use of medicines.

http://cks.library.nhs.uk The National Health Service Clinical Knowledge Summaries provides evidence-based practical information on the common conditions observed in primary care.

http://www.nhsdirect.nhs.uk The National Health Service Direct service provides patients with information and advice about health, illness and health services.

Points to Remember

- Antiemetics are used to manage nausea and vomiting in situations in which these actions are not beneficial and could actually cause harm to the patient.
- Antiemetics act by depressing the hyperactive vomiting reflex, either locally or through alteration of CNS actions.
- The choice of an antiemetic depends on the cause of the nausea and vomiting and the expected actions of the drug.
- Most antiemetics cause some CNS depression with resultant dizziness, drowsiness and weakness. Care must be taken to protect the patient and advise him or her to avoid dangerous situations, for example driving, performing hazardous tasks.

CRITICAL THINKING SCENARIO 58-1

Handling Postoperative Nausea and Vomiting

The Situation

Andy is a 19-year-old boy who has undergone reconstructive knee surgery after a football injury. After the surgery, Andy complains of nausea and vomits three times in 2 hours. He becomes increasingly agitated. An intramuscular injection of prochlorperazine is ordered to relieve the nausea, to be followed by an oral order when tolerated. The prochlorperazine is somewhat helpful in relieving the nausea.

Critical Thinking

- What are the important nursing implications in this case?
- What other measures could be taken to relieve Andy's nausea?

Discussion

It is often impossible to pinpoint an exact cause of a patient's nausea and vomiting in a hospital setting. For example, the underlying cause may be related to the pain or a reaction to the pain medication being given. A combination of factors should be considered when dealing with nausea and vomiting. The administration of IM prochlorperazine may take the edge off the nausea, although Andy will have to be reminded that the drug he is being given may make him dizzy, weak or drowsy and that he should ask for assistance if he needs to move.

Once the nausea and vomiting resolves, it will be possible to try other interventions to help stop the vomiting reflex. Administration of pain medication, as prescribed, may relieve the CTZ stimulus that comes with intense pain. Other interventions include encouraging Andy to take slow, deep breaths, which stimulate the parasympathetic system (vagus nerve) and partially override the sympathetic activity stimulated by the CTZ to activate vomiting. For many patients, mouth care, ice cubes or small sips of water may also help to relieve the discomfort and ease the sensation of nausea.

Nursing Care Guide for Andy: Antiemetics

Assessment: History and Examination

Assess Andy's medical history for allergies to any antiemetic, coma, CNS depression, cardiovascular disease, severe hypotension, hepatic or renal dysfunction, epilepsy and concurrent use of anticholinergic drugs and barbiturate anaesthetics.

Focus the physical examination on the following areas:

- Neurological: orientation, affect
- Skin: colour, lesions
- CV: pulse, blood pressure, orthostatic blood pressure
- GI: abdominal and liver evaluation

Nursing Diagnoses

- Acute pain related to GI, CNS effects
- Risk for injury related to CNS, CV effects
- Deficient knowledge regarding drug therapy

Implementation

- Administer antiemetics only as a temporary measure.
- Provide comfort and safety measures including assistance with mobility, access to bathroom, mouth care and ice cubes.
- Monitor Andy's hydration status and electrolyte levels. Provide remedial measures as needed.
- Provide support and reassurance for coping with drug effects and discomfort.
- Provide patient teaching regarding drug name, dosage, adverse effects, precautions, warning to report.

Evaluation

- Evaluate drug effects, for example relief of nausea and vomiting.
- Monitor for adverse effects, including extrapyramidal symptoms and dystonia, GI alterations, hypotension, dizziness, confusion, sensitivity to sunlight and dehydration.
- Monitor for drug–drug interactions as appropriate.
- Evaluate effectiveness of patient teaching programme and comfort and safety measures.

Patient Teaching for Andy

- ☐ The drug that has been prescribed for you is called prochlorperazine. It belongs to a class of drugs called antiemetics. An antiemetic helps resolve nausea and vomiting and the discomfort they cause.

(continued)

Handling Postoperative Nausea and Vomiting *(continued)*

- ☐ Common effects of this drug include:
  - *Dizziness, weakness:* Change positions slowly. If you feel drowsy, avoid tasks requiring co-ordination.
  - *Sensitivity to the sun:* Avoid exposure to the sun and ultraviolet light.
  - *Dehydration:* Avoid excessive heat exposure and try to drink fluids as much as possible.
  - Report any of the following conditions to your health care provider: *fever, rash, yellowing of the eyes or skin, dark urine, pale stools, easy bruising, rash and vision changes*.
- ☐ Avoid OTC medications. If you feel that you need one, check with your health care provider first.
- ☐ Tell any doctor, nurse or other health care provider that you are taking this drug.
- ☐ Keep this drug and all medications out of the reach of children.

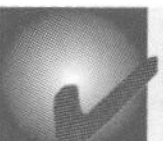

CHECK YOUR UNDERSTANDING

Answers to the questions in this chapter may be found in the answer key in the back of the book.

Multiple Choice

Select the most appropriate response to the following.

1. Prochlorperazine would be the antiemetic of choice for
   a. nausea and vomiting after anaesthesia.
   b. nausea and vomiting associated with cancer chemotherapy.
   c. motion sickness.
   d. intractable hiccups.

2. Most antiemetics work with the CNS to decrease the activity of the
   a. medulla.
   b. CTZ.
   c. respiratory centre.
   d. sympathetic nervous system.

3. The 5-HT_3 receptor blockers, including ondansetron and granisetron, are particularly effective in decreasing the nausea and vomiting associated with
   a. vestibular problems.
   b. emetogenic cancer chemotherapy.
   c. pregnancy.
   d. severe pain.

Extended Matching Questions

Select **all** that apply.

1. Nursing interventions for the patient receiving an antiemetic drug would include which of the following?
   a. Frequent mouth care and ice chips to suck.
   b. Bowel programme to deal with constipation.
   c. Protection from falls or injury.
   d. Fluids to guard against dehydration.
   e. Protection from sun exposure.
   f. Quiet environment and temperature control.

2. Palonosetron would be a drug of choice for a patient with which of the following problems?
   a. Nausea and vomiting associated with cancer chemotherapy.
   b. A prolonged QT interval.
   c. Postoperative nausea and vomiting.
   d. Difficulty swallowing.
   e. Hypokalaemia.
   f. Hypomagnesaemia.

Fill in the Blanks

1. ________________ are used to manage nausea and vomiting in situations in which they are not beneficial and could actually cause harm to the patient.

2. Antiemetics act by depressing the ________________, either locally or through alteration of CNS actions.

3. Vomiting is a complex reflex mediated through the ________________ located in the ________________.

4. The CTZ can be stimulated by ________________, ________________, ________________ or several other mechanisms.

5. Most antiemetics cause some________________, with resultant dizziness, drowsiness and weakness.

6. ________________is another common adverse effect with antiemetics. Patients should be protected from exposure to the sun and ultraviolet light.

Bibliography

British Medical Association and Royal Pharmaceutical Society of Great Britain. (2008). *British National Formulary*. London: BMJ & RPS Publishing. *This publication is updated biannually: it is imperative that the most recent edition is consulted.*

British Medical Association and Royal Pharmaceutical Society of Great Britain. (2007). *British National Formulary for Children*. London: BMJ & RPS Publishing. *This publication is updated annually: it is imperative that the most recent edition is consulted.*

Ganong, W. (2005). *Review of medical physiology* (22nd ed.). New York: McGraw-Hill.

Brunton, L., Lazo, J. S., Parker, K., Goodman, L. S., & Gilman, A. G. (2005). *Goodman and Gilman's the pharmacological basis of therapeutics* (11th ed.). London: McGraw-Hill.

Howland, R. D., & Mycek, M. J. (2005). *Pharmacology* (3rd ed.). Philadelphia: Lippincott Williams & Wilkins.

Marieb, E. N., & Hoehn, K. (2009). *Human anatomy & physiology* (8th ed.). San Francisco: Pearson Benjamin Cummings.

Porth, C. M., & Matfin, G. (2008). *Pathophysiology: Concepts of altered health states* (8th ed.). Philadelphia: Lippincott Williams & Wilkins.

Simonsen, T., Aarbakke, J., Kay, I., Coleman, I., Sinnott, P., & Lysaa, R. (2006). *Illustrated pharmacology for nurses*. London: Hodder Arnold.

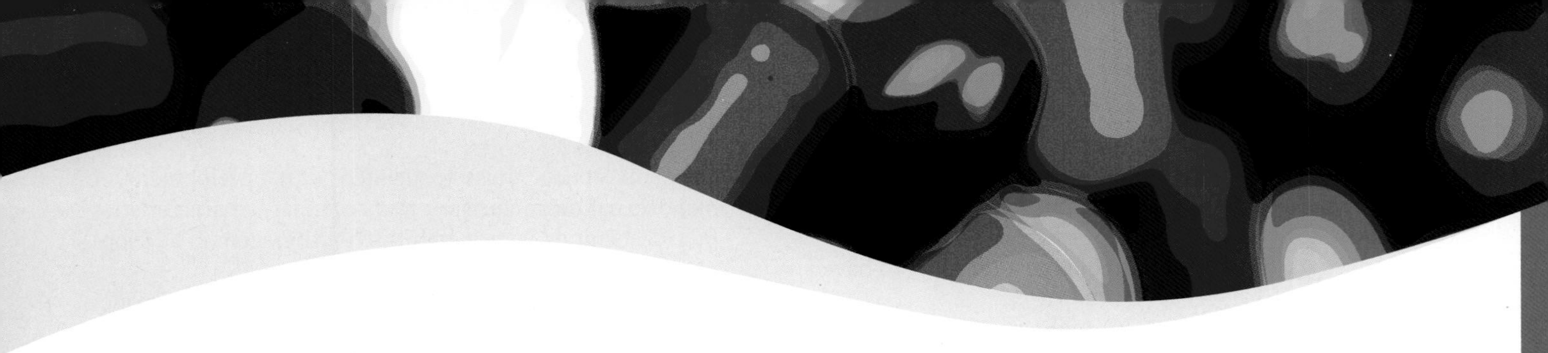

Glossary

A

A fibres large-diameter nerve fibres that carry peripheral impulses associated with touch and temperature to the spinal cord

absence seizure type of generalized seizure that is characterized by sudden, temporary loss of consciousness, sometimes with staring or blinking for 3 to 5 seconds; formerly known as a petit mal seizure

absolute refractory period the time when it is impossible to stimulate an area of cell membrane following an action potential

absorption what happens to a drug from the time it enters the body until it enters the blood; intravenous administration causes the drug to directly enter the blood, bypassing the many complications of absorption from other routes

ACE inhibitor drug that blocks the enzyme responsible for converting angiotensin I to angiotensin II in the lungs; preventing the vasoconstriction and aldosterone release related to angiotensin II

acetylcholine receptor site area on the plasma membrane where acetylcholine (ACh) binds to a specific receptor site to cause stimulation of the cell in response to nerve activity

acetylcholinesterase enzyme responsible for the immediate breakdown of ACh when released from the nerve ending; prevents overstimulation of cholinergic receptor sites

acid rebound reflex response of the stomach to lower than normal acid levels; when acid levels are lowered through the use of antacids, gastrin production and secretion are increased to return the stomach to its normal acidity

acidification the process of increasing the acid level; used to treat bladder infections, making the bladder an undesirable place for bacteria

acidosis state of having too many hydrogen ions or excess acid in the extracellular fluid; can occur during severe asthma attacks and in chronic obstructive pulmonary disorder

acquired immunodeficiency syndrome (AIDS) collection of opportunistic infections and cancers that occurs when the immune system is severely depressed by a decrease in the number of functioning helper T cells; caused by infection with human immunodeficiency virus (HIV)

acromegaly thickening of bony surfaces in response to excess growth hormone after the epiphyseal plates have closed

actin thin filament that makes up a sarcomere or muscle unit

action potential sudden change in electrical charge of a nerve cell membrane caused by the influx of Na^+ ions into the cell; the electrical signal by which neurons send information

active immunity the formation of antibodies secondary to exposure to a specific antigen; leads to the formation of plasma cells, antibodies, and memory cells to immediately produce antibodies if exposed to that antigen in the future; imparts lifelong immunity

active transport the movement of substances across a cell membrane against the concentration gradient; this process requires the use of energy in the form of adenosine triphosphate (ATP)

A-delta and C fibres small-diameter nerve fibres that carry peripheral impulses associated with pain to the spinal cord

adrenal cortex outer layer of the adrenal gland; produces glucocorticoids and mineralocorticoids in response to adrenocorticotropic hormone stimulation

adrenal medulla inner layer (middle) of the adrenal gland; a sympathetic ganglion, it releases noradrenaline and adrenaline into circulation in response to sympathetic stimulation

adrenergic agonist a drug that stimulates the adrenergic receptors of the sympathetic nervous system (SNS), either directly (by binding to receptor sites) or indirectly (by increasing noradrenaline levels)

adrenergic blocking agents drugs which bind to adrenergic receptors (α and/or β) and prevent adrenaline or noradrenaline binding

adrenergic receptor sites on effectors that respond to noradrenaline/adrenaline

adverse drug reaction a potentially harmful reaction to a medicine; there may be a requirement to reduce the dose of the drug administered or complete withdrawal

adverse effects drug effects that are not the desired therapeutic effects; may be unpleasant or even dangerous

aerobic bacteria that depend on oxygen for survival
afferent neurons or groups of neurons that bring information to the central nervous system; sensory nerve
agonist a drug or ligand that binds to a receptor to have an effect
AIDS-related complex (ARC) collection of less serious opportunistic infections with HIV infection; the decrease in the number of helper T cells is less severe than in fully developed AIDS
aldosterone hormone produced by the adrenal cortex that causes the distal tubule to retain sodium, and therefore water, while losing potassium into the urine
alkalosis state of not having enough acid to maintain normal homeostatic processes
alopecia hair loss; a common adverse effect of many antineoplastic drugs, which are more effective against rapidly multiplying cells such as those of hair follicles
alpha(α)-agonist drug that specifically stimulates the α-receptors within the sympathetic nervous system, causing body responses seen when the α-receptors are stimulated
alpha (α)-receptor adrenergic receptors that are found on specific tissues, including vascular smooth muscle, bronchi, gastrointestinal tract, male and female reproductive tracts, bladder and eye
alpha$_1$(α_1)-selective adrenergic blocking agents drugs that block the postsynaptic α_1-receptor sites, causing a decrease in vascular tone and a vasodilation that leads to a fall in blood pressure; these drugs do not block the presynaptic α_2-receptor sites, and therefore the reflex tachycardia that accompanies a fall in blood pressure does not occur
alternative medicine including herbs and other natural products that fall outside conventional medicine and are used to treat patients; these products are not controlled or tested by the regulatory authorities
alveoli the respiratory sac, the smallest unit of the lungs where gas exchange occurs
Alzheimer's disease degenerative disease of the cerebral cortex with loss of ACh-producing cells and cholinergic receptors; characterized by progressive dementia
amoebiasis amoebic dysentery, which is caused by intestinal invasion of the trophozoite stage of the protozoan *Entamoeba histolytica*
amnesia loss of memory
anabolic steroids androgens developed with more anabolic or protein-building effects than androgenic effects
anaerobic bacteria that survive without oxygen, which are often seen when blood flow is cut off to an area of the body
analgesia loss of pain sensation
analgesic compounds with pain-blocking properties, capable of producing analgesia
anaphylaxis an acute allergic reaction where mast cells release inflammatory substances, including histamine and bradykinin; characterized by vasodilation and bronchoconstriction
anaplasia loss of organization and structure; property of cancer cells
androgenic effects those associated with development of male sexual characteristics and secondary characteristics (e.g. deepening of voice, hair distribution, genital development, acne)
androgens male sex hormones, primarily testosterone; produced in the testes and adrenal cortex
anaemia a decrease in the number of red blood cells (RBCs), or haemoglobin concentration of whole blood leading to a reduced oxygen carrying capacity of the blood
angina pectoris pain caused by the imbalance between oxygen being supplied to cardiac muscle and demand for oxygen by cardiac muscle
angiogenesis the generation of new blood vessels; cancer cells release an enzyme that will cause angiogenesis or the growth of new blood vessels to feed the cancer cells
angiotensin II receptors specific receptors found in blood vessels and in the adrenal cortex that bind angiotensin II to cause vasoconstriction and release of aldosterone
Anopheles mosquito type of mosquito that is essential to the life cycle of *Plasmodium*; injects the protozoa into humans for further maturation
anterior pituitary lobe of the pituitary gland that produces stimulating hormones, as well as growth hormone, prolactin and melanocyte-stimulating hormone
antiarrhythmics drugs that affect the action potential of cardiac cells and are used to treat arrhythmias and return normal rate and rhythm
antibacterial a chemical that is able to inhibit the growth of specific bacteria or cause the death of susceptible bacteria
antibiotic chemicals produced by micro-organisms to inhibit the growth of specific bacteria or cause the death of susceptible bacteria
antibodies immunoglobulins; produced by B cell plasma cells in response to a specific protein; bind to that protein to cause its destruction directly or through activation of the inflammatory response
anticoagulants drugs that block or inhibit any step of the coagulation process, preventing or slowing clot formation
antidiuretic hormone (ADH) hormone produced by the hypothalamus and stored in the posterior pituitary gland; important in maintaining fluid balance; causes the distal tubules and collecting ducts of the kidney to become permeable to water, leading to an antidiuretic effect and fluid retention
antiemetic drug that blocks the hyperactive response of the chemoreceptor trigger zone (CTZ) to various stimuli, the response that produces nausea and vomiting
antigen foreign protein
antihistamine drug that blocks the release or action of histamine, a chemical released during inflammation that increases secretions and narrows airways
anti-inflammatory blocking the effects of the inflammatory response
antimotility drug a drug that blocks the stimulation of the gastrointestinal tract, leading to decreased activity and increased time for reabsorption of needed nutrients and water

antimuscarinic drug that opposes the effects of ACh at muscarinic ACh receptor sites; also known as anticholinergics

antineoplastic drug used to combat cancer or the growth of neoplasms

antipeptic drug that coats any damaged area in the stomach to prevent further injury from acid or pepsin

antipsychotic drug used to treat disorders involving thought processes; dopamine receptor blocker that helps affected people organize their thoughts and respond appropriately to stimuli

antipyretic blocking fever, often by direct effects on the thermoregulatory centre in the hypothalamus or by blockade of prostaglandin mediators

antiseizure agent drug used to treat the abnormal and excessive energy bursts in the brain that are characteristic of epilepsy

antispasmodics drugs which block muscle spasm associated with irritation or neurological stimulation

antitoxins immune sera that contains antibodies to specific toxins produced by invaders; may prevent the toxin from adhering to body tissues and causing disease

antitussives drugs that block the cough reflex

apoptosis the process of programmed cell death; occurs in cells infected with a virus or irreparable cells

atrial natriuretic peptide (ANP) released from the atria when blood volume is high. It causes an increase in sodium excretion from the distal tubules

anxiety unpleasant feeling of tension, fear, or nervousness in response to an environmental stimulus, whether real or imaginary

anxiolytic drug used to depress the central nervous system (CNS); prevents the signs and symptoms of anxiety

arachidonic acid released from damaged cells to stimulate the inflammatory response through activation of various chemical substances

arrhythmia a disruption in cardiac rate or rhythm

arteries vessels that take blood away from the heart; muscular, resistance vessels

assessment information gathering regarding the current status of a particular patient, including evaluation of past history and physical examination; provides a baseline of information and clues to effectiveness of therapy

asthma disorder characterized by recurrent episodes of bronchospasm (i.e. bronchial muscle spasm leading to narrowed or obstructed airways); a reversible disease of the airways

atheroma plaque in the endothelial lining of arteries; contains lipids, blood cells, inflammatory agents, platelets; leads to narrowing of the lumen of the artery, stiffening of the artery and loss of distensibility and responsiveness

atherosclerosis narrowing of the arteries caused by build-up of atheromas, swelling and accumulation of platelets; leads to a loss of elasticity and responsiveness to normal stimuli

atrium upper chambers of the heart; right atrium receives deoxygenated blood from the systemic circulation (via both vena cava and the left atrium receives oxygenated blood from the pulmonary circulation via the pulmonary veins

attention-deficit hyperactivity disorder (ADHD) behavioural syndrome characterized by an inability to concentrate for longer than a few minutes and excessive activity

auricle appendage on the atria of the heart, holds blood to be pumped into the ventricles with atrial contraction

autoimmune disease a disorder that occurs when the body responds to specific self-antigens to produce antibodies or cell-mediated responses against its own cells

automaticity property of muscle cells, where cardiac cells generate an action potential without an external stimulus

autonomic nervous system portion of the central and peripheral nervous systems that, together with the endocrine system, functions to maintain internal homeostasis

autonomy loss of the normal controls and reactions that inhibit growth and spreading; property of cancer cells

axon long projection from a neuron that carries information from one nerve to another nerve or effector

azoles a group of drugs used to treat fungal infections

B

B cells lymphocytes programmed to recognize specific proteins; when activated, these cells cause the production of antibodies which recognize the protein

bactericidal substance that causes the death of bacteria, usually by interfering with cell membrane stability or with proteins or enzymes necessary to maintain the cellular integrity of the bacteria

bacteriostatic substance that prevents the replication of bacteria, usually by interfering with proteins or enzyme systems necessary for reproduction of the bacteria

balanced anaesthesia use of several different types of drugs to achieve the quickest, most effective anaesthesia with the fewest adverse effects

barbiturate former mainstay drug used for the treatment of anxiety and for sedation and sleep induction; associated with potentially severe adverse effects and many drug–drug interactions, which makes it less desirable than some of the newer agents

baroreceptor pressure receptor; located in the arch of the aorta and in the carotid artery; responds to changes in pressure and influences the medulla to stimulate the sympathetic system to increase or decrease blood pressure

basal nuclei lower area of the brain associated with co-ordination of unconscious muscle movements that involve movement and position

benign prostatic hyperplasia (BPH) enlargement of the prostate gland, associated with age and inflammation; also called benign prostatic hypertrophy

benzodiazepine drug that acts in the limbic system and the reticular activating system to make gamma-aminobutyric acid (GABA), an inhibitory neurotransmitter; more effective, causing interference with neuron firing; depresses CNS to block the signs and symptoms of anxiety and may cause sedation and hypnosis (extreme sedation with further CNS depression and sleep) in higher doses

beta-(β) adrenergic agonist specifically stimulating to the β-receptors within the sympathetic nervous system, causing body responses seen when the β-receptors are stimulated

beta-(β) adrenergic blocking drugs at therapeutic levels, selectively block the β-receptors of the sympathetic nervous system

beta-(β) receptors adrenergic receptors that are found in the heart, lungs and vascular smooth muscle

$beta_1$-(β_1) selective adrenergic blocking drugs, at therapeutic levels, specifically block the β_1-receptors in the sympathetic nervous system, while not blocking the β_2-receptors and resultant effects on the respiratory system

bile fluid stored in the gallbladder that contains cholesterol and bile salts; essential for the emulsification and absorption of fats

bile acids cholesterol-containing acids found in the bile that act like detergents to break up fats in the small intestine

bipolar affective disorder formerly known as manic depression; patients may alternate between periods of elevated mood or mania and depression

biological weapons so-called germ warfare; the use of bacteria, viruses and parasites on a large scale to incapacitate or destroy a population

biopharmaceutical proteins or nucleic acids produced by genetic engineering methods for therapeutic purposes

bisphosphonates drugs used to block bone resorption and lower serum calcium levels in several conditions

blood dyscrasia bone marrow depression caused by drug effects on the rapidly multiplying cells of the bone marrow; lower-than-normal levels of blood components can be seen; any abnormal or pathological condition of the blood

body surface area the surface area of the body is calculated using the patient's body weight and height; some drugs are administered according to body surface area

bone marrow suppression inhibition of the blood-forming components of the bone marrow; a common adverse effect of many antineoplastic drugs, which are more effective against rapidly multiplying cells, such as those in bone marrow; also seen in anaemia, thrombocytopenia, and leucopenia

bradycardia slower than normal heart rate (usually <60 beats per minute)

bradykinesia difficulty in performing intentional movements and extreme slowness and sluggishness; characteristic of Parkinson's disease

brain stem an area of the brain connecting the cerebral hemispheres with the spinal cord

British National Formulary (BNF) used by health care professionals, including doctors, nurses and pharmacists, to provide up-to-date information on the range of medicines available for prescribing; information enables selection of the most appropriate medicines

bronchial tree the conducting airways of the respiratory system leading into the alveoli; they branch smaller and smaller, appearing much like a tree

bronchodilation relaxation of the muscles in the bronchi and bronchioles, resulting in a widening airways; an effect of sympathetic stimulation

bronchodilator medication used to facilitate respiration by dilating the airways; helpful in symptomatic relief or prevention of bronchial asthma and bronchospasm associated with chronic obstructive pulmonary disease

bulk stimulant drug that increases in bulk, frequently by osmotic pull of fluid into the faeces; the increased bulk stretches the gastrointestinal wall, causing stimulation and increased gastrointestinal movement

C

calcitonin hormone produced by the parafollicular (C) cells of the thyroid; counteracts the effects of parathyroid hormone to maintain calcium levels in the blood

Candida fungus that is normally found on mucous membranes; can cause yeast infections or thrush (Candida albicans) of the gastrointestinal tract and vagina in immunosuppressed patients

capacitance (venous) system refers to the venous system, as it is derived from the fact that veins have the capacity to hold large quantities of fluid as they distend with fluid volume

capillary small vessel made up of loosely connected endothelial cells that connect arterioles to venuoles

carbonic anhydrase an enzyme that speeds up the chemical reaction combining water and carbon dioxide, which react to form carbonic acid; this immediately dissociates to form bicarbonate and H^+

carcinoma tumour that originates in epithelial cells

cardiac cycle a period of cardiac muscle relaxation (diastole) followed by a period of contraction (systole) in the heart

cardiac output the amount of blood the heart can pump out per unit time (millilitres per minute); influenced by the coordination of cardiac muscle contraction, heart rate and blood return to the heart

cardiomegaly enlargement of the heart, seen with chronic hypertension, valvular disease and congestive heart failure

cardiomyopathy a disease of the heart muscle that leads to an enlarged heart and eventually to complete heart muscle failure and death

cardiovascular (vasomotor) centre area of the medulla oblongata in the brain at which stimulation will activate the SNS to increase blood pressure, heart rate and so on

carrier molecules transmembrane proteins that are used to transport lipid insoluble substances across the plasma membrane

catecholamine-*O*-methyl transferase (COMT) an enzyme responsible for the metabolism of catecholamines, that is noradrenaline

cathartic dependence overuse of laxatives that can lead to the need for strong stimuli to initiate movement in the intestines; local reflexes become resistant to normal stimuli after prolonged use of harsher stimulants, leading to further laxative use

cell cycle life cycle of a cell, which includes the phases G_0, G_1, S, G_2 and M; during the M phase, the cell divides into two identical daughter cells

cerebellum lower portion of the brain associated with coordination of muscle movements, including voluntary motion, as well as extrapyramidal control of unconscious muscle movements

cerebral hemispheres the two cerebral hemispheres form the cerebrum, the largest area of the brain

cestode tapeworm with a head and segmented body parts that is capable of growing to several yards in the human intestine

C (unmyelinated) fibres respond to stimulation by generating nerve impulses that produce pain sensations

chemical name a name that reflects the chemical structure of a drug

chemical stimulant agent that stimulates the normal gastrointestinal reflexes by chemically irritating the lining of the gastrointestinal wall, leading to increased activity in the gastrointestinal tract

chemoreceptor trigger zone (CTZ) an area in the brain sensitive to circulating chemicals; when stimulated triggers the vomiting centre to generate feelings of nausea and vomiting

chemotaxis property of drawing neutrophils to an area

chemotherapeutic agents synthetic chemicals used to interfere with the functioning of foreign cell populations; this term is frequently used to refer to the drug therapy of neoplasms, but it also refers to drug therapy affecting any foreign cell

Cheyne–Stokes respiration abnormal pattern of breathing characterized by apnoeic periods followed by periods of tachypnoea; may reflect delayed blood flow through the brain

cholesterol necessary component of human cells that is produced and processed in the liver, a lipid that is essential for the formation of steroid hormones and cell membranes; it is produced in cells and taken in by dietary sources

cholinergic responding to ACh; refers to receptor sites stimulated by ACh, as well as neurons that release ACh

cholinergic neuron a neuron that manufactures and releases ACh

cholinergic receptor sites on effectors that respond to ACh

chronic obstructive pulmonary disease (COPD) chronic condition that occurs over time; often the result of chronic bronchitis, emphysema or repeated and severe asthma attacks; leads to destruction of the respiratory defence mechanisms and physical structure

chrysotherapy treatment with gold salts; gold is taken up by macrophages, which then inhibit phagocytosis; it is reserved for use in patients who are unresponsive to conventional therapy and can be very toxic

chylomicron carrier for lipids in the bloodstream, consisting of proteins, lipids and cholesterol

chyme contents of the stomach containing ingested food and secreted enzymes, water and mucus

cilia microscopic, hair-like projections of the epithelial cell membrane lining the upper respiratory tract, which are constantly moving and directing the mucus and any trapped substance toward the pharynx

cinchonism syndrome of quinine toxicity characterized by nausea, vomiting, tinnitus and vertigo

clotting factors substances formed in the liver, that react in a cascading sequence to cause the formation of thrombin from prothrombin; thrombin then breaks down fibrin threads from fibrinogen to form a clot

coagulation the process of blood changing from a fluid state to a solid state to plug injuries to the vascular system

common cold viral infection of the upper respiratory tract that initiates the release of histamine and prostaglandins and causes an inflammatory response

common pathway the shared pathway for the 'intrinsic' and 'extrinsic' coagulation pathways involving the conversion of prothrombin to thrombin

competitive antagonist a drug molecule that binds to a receptor preventing another the ligand or another drug from binding to the receptor, reducing the probability of receptor activation

complement system series of cascading proteins that combine with the antigen–antibody complex to destroy the protein or stimulate an inflammatory reaction

compliance applies when a patient follows medical advice given by a health care professional

concordance an approach to involve patients in the treatment process and therefore improve compliance to treatment

conducting zone an area of the respiratory tract consisting of the nose, mouth, pharynx, larynx and upper bronchial tree; conducts air to and from the respiratory zone where gas exchange occurs

conductivity property of heart cells to rapidly conduct an action potential of electrical impulse

congestive heart failure (CHF) a condition in which the heart muscle fails to adequately pump blood around the cardiovascular system, leading to a backup or congestion of blood in the systemic circulation

constipation slower than normal evacuation of the large intestine, which can result in increased water absorption from the faeces and can lead to impaction

conversion finding the equivalent values between two systems of measure

convulsion (tonic–clonic) muscular reaction to excessive electrical energy arising from nerve cells in the brain

coronary artery disease (CAD) characterized by progressive narrowing of coronary arteries, leading to a decreased delivery of oxygen to cardiac muscle cells; leading killer of adults in the Western world

corpus luteum remains of follicle that releases mature ovum at ovulation; becomes an endocrine gland producing oestrogen and progesterone

corpus striatum part of the brain that connects with the substantia nigra to maintain a balance of suppression and stimulation

corticosteroids steroid hormones produced by the adrenal cortex; include androgens, glucocorticoids and mineralocorticoids

cough reflex response to irritation in the respiratory membrane, results in expelling of forced air through the mouth

countercurrent mechanism process used by medullary nephrons to concentrate or dilute the urine in response to body stimuli to maintain fluid and electrolyte balance

culture sample of the bacteria (e.g. from sputum, cell scrapings, urine) to be grown in a laboratory to determine the species of bacteria that is causing an infection

cycloplegia inability of the lens in the eye to accommodate to near vision, causing blurring and inability to see near objects

cystic fibrosis a hereditary disease that results in the accumulation of copious amounts of very thick secretions in the lungs, which will eventually lead to obstruction of the airways and destruction of the lung tissue

cystitis inflammation of the bladder, caused by infection or irritation

cytokines important chemical mediators involved in the immune response

cytomegalovirus (CMV) DNA virus that accounts for many respiratory, ophthalmic and liver infections

cytoplasm interior of a cell; contains organelles for producing proteins, energy, and so on

D

decongestants drugs that decrease the blood flow to the upper respiratory tract and decrease the overproduction of secretions

dendrite short projection on a neuron that transmits information

dendritic cells form part of the immune system; these cells phagocytose antigenic material and following migration to lymph nodes present the antigen to lymphocytes

depolarization opening of the sodium channels in a nerve membrane to allow the influx of positive sodium ions (Na^+), reversing the membrane charge from negative to positive

depolarizing neuromuscular junction (NMJ) blocker stimulation of a muscle cell, causing it to contract, with no allowance for repolarization and restimulation of the muscle; characterized by contraction and then paralysis

depression affective disorder in which a person experiences sadness that is much more severe and long-lasting than is warranted by the event that seems to have precipitated it; the condition may not even be traceable to a specific event or stressor

dermatological reactions skin reactions commonly seen as adverse effects of drugs; can range from simple rash to potentially fatal exfoliative dermatitis

diabetes insipidus lack of antidiuretic hormone (ADH), which results in the production of copious amounts of dilute glucose-free urine

diabetes mellitus a metabolic disorder characterized by high blood glucose levels and altered metabolism of proteins and fats; associated with thickening of the basement membrane, leading to numerous complications

diapedesis the movement of white blood cells (WBCs) from blood vessels into the tissues

diarrhoea more frequent than normal bowel movements, often characterized as fluid-like and watery because as food passes through the intestines there is not enough time for absorption of fluid

diastole resting phase heart during the cardiac cycle; blood is returned to the heart during this phase

diencephalon an area of the brain containing the thalamus, hypothalamus and epithalamus

diffusion movement of solutes from an area of high concentration to an area of low concentration across a semipermeable membrane

distribution movement of a drug to body tissues; the places where a drug may be distributed depend on the drug's solubility, perfusion of the area, cardiac output and binding of the drug to plasma proteins

diurnal rhythm response of the hypothalamus and then the pituitary and adrenals to wakefulness and sleeping; normally, the hypothalamus begins secretion of melatonin–corticotropin-releasing factor (CRF) in the evening, peaking at about midnight; adrenocortical peak response is between 6 and 9 a.m.; levels fall during the day until evening, when the low level is picked up by the hypothalamus and CRF secretion begins again

dopa-decarboxylase inhibitors drugs that target the enzyme dopa-decarboxylase which is responsible for the conversion of dopa to dopamine; used in the treatment of Parkinson's disease to prevent the metabolism of levodopa in the periphery

dopaminergic drug that increases the effects of dopamine at receptor sites

drug allergy formation of antibodies to a drug or drug protein; causes an immune response when the person is next exposed to that drug

drugs chemicals that are introduced into the body to bring about some sort of change

dwarfism small stature, resulting from lack of growth hormone in children

dyspnoea discomfort with respirations, often with a feeling of anxiety and inability to breathe, seen with left-sided CHF

dysrhythmia a disruption in cardiac rate or rhythm, also called an arrhythmia

dysuria painful urination

E

ectopic focus where there is a shift in the pacemaker of the heart from the sinoatrial node to some other site

effective concentration the amount of a drug required to cause a therapeutic effect

effector cell stimulated by a nerve; may be a muscle, a gland, or another nerve

efferent neurons or groups of neurons that carry information from the central nervous system to an effector; motor neurons

electrocardiogram (ECG) an electrical recording reflecting the conduction of an electrical impulse through the heart muscle; does not reflect mechanical activity

endocrine relating to a system of glands (endocrine glands) that release hormones (chemical messengers) into the blood to maintain homeostasis

endocytosis engulfing substances and moving them into a cell by extending the cell membrane around the substance; pinocytosis and phagocytosis are two kinds of endocytosis

endorphins naturally occurring peptides that bind to opioid receptors

enkephalins naturally occurring peptides that bind to opioid receptors

epilepsy collection of various syndromes, all of which are characterized by seizures

ergosterol steroid-type protein found in the cell membrane of fungi; similar in configuration to adrenal hormones and testosterone

ergot derivative drug that causes a vascular constriction in the brain and the periphery; relieves or prevents migraine headaches but is associated with many adverse effects

erythrocytes or red blood cells (RBCs) contain haemoglobin and are responsible for carrying oxygen to the tissues and removing carbon dioxide; have no nucleus and live approximately 120 days

erythropoiesis process of red blood cell production and life cycle; formed by megaloblastic cells in the bone marrow, using iron, folic acid, carbohydrates, vitamin B_{12} and amino acids; they circulate in the vascular system for about 120 days, then are lysed and recycled

erythropoietin glycoprotein produced by the kidneys, released in response to decreased blood flow or oxygen tension in the kidney; controls the rate of red blood cell production in the bone marrow

essential hypertension sustained blood pressure above normal limits with no discernible underlying cause

evaluation part of the nursing process; determining the effects of the interventions that were instituted for the patient and leading to further assessment and implementation

excretion removal of a drug from the body; primarily occurs in the kidneys but can occur through the skin, lungs, bile, sweat or faeces

exocrine a system of glands that secrete substances via a duct

exocytosis removal of substances from a cell by pushing them through the cell membrane

extrapyramidal tract cells from the cortex and subcortical areas, including the basal nuclei and the cerebellum, which co-ordinate unconsciously controlled muscle activity; allows the body to make automatic adjustments in posture or position and balance

extrinsic pathway of coagulation occurs following damage of blood vessel factors; the mechanism that produces fibrin following tissue injury, beginning with formation of an activated complex between tissue factor and factor VII and leading to activation of factor X

facilitated diffusion a process whereby large molecules are moved across the plasma membrane into the cytoplasm using a carrier molecule

fertility drugs used to stimulate ovulation and pregnancy in women with functioning ovaries who are having difficulty conceiving

fibrillation rapid, irregular stimulation of the cardiac muscle resulting in lack of pumping activity

filtration passage of fluid and small components of the blood through the glomerulus into the nephron's proximal convoluted tubule

first-pass effect a phenomenon in which drugs given orally are carried directly to the liver after absorption, where they may be largely inactivated by liver enzymes before they can enter the general circulation; oral drugs frequently are given in higher doses than drugs given by other routes because of this early breakdown

flatworms platyhelminths, including the cestodes or tapeworms; a worm that can live in the human intestine or can invade other human tissues (flukes)

fluid rebound reflex reaction of the body to the loss of fluid or sodium; the hypothalamus causes the release of ADH, which retains water, and stress related to fluid loss combines with decreased blood flow to the kidneys to activate the renin–angiotensin system, leading to further water and sodium retention

flukes belong to the family of platyhelminth or flatworms

focal seizure involves one area of the brain and does not spread throughout the entire brain; also known as a partial seizure

follicle (ovarian) storage site of each ovum in the ovary; allows the ovum to grow and develop, produces oestrogen and progesterone

follicles structural unit of the thyroid gland; cells arranged in a circle

forebrain upper level of the brain; consists of the two cerebral hemispheres, where thinking and coordination of sensory and motor activity occur

fungus a cellular organism with a hard cell wall that contains chitin and many polysaccharides, as well as a cell membrane that contains ergosterols

G

G-proteins a large family of proteins involved in intracellular signalling pathways

gallstones a crystalline solid found in the gallbladder or common bile duct; can cause jaundice if the bile duct is obstructed

gamma-aminobutyric acid (GABA) the main inhibitory neurotransmitter in the central nervous system

ganglia a closely packed group of nerve cell bodies found within the central nervous system

gastrin secreted by the stomach in response to many stimuli; stimulates the release of hydrochloric acid from parietal cells and pepsin from chief cells; causes histamine release at histamine-2 receptors to effect the release of acid

gate control theory a theory stating that the transmission of a nerve impulse can be modulated at various points along its path by descending fibres from the brain that close the 'gate' and block transmission of pain information and by A fibres that are able to block transmission in the dorsal horn by closing the gate for transmission for the A-delta and C fibres

general anaesthetic drug that induces a loss of consciousness, amnesia, analgesia and loss of reflexes to allow performance of painful surgical procedures

generalized seizure that begins in one area of the brain and rapidly spreads throughout both hemispheres

generic drugs sold by their chemical name; not trade (or brand) name products

generic name the original designation that a drug is given when the drug company that developed it applies for the approval process

genetic engineering process of altering DNA, usually of bacteria, to produce a chemical to be used as a drug

giardiasis protozoal intestinal infection that causes severe diarrhoea and epigastric distress; may lead to serious malnutrition

gigantism response to excess levels of growth hormone before the epiphyseal plates close

glomerulus the knot of capillaries of blood vessel between the afferent and efferent arterioles in the nephron; the fenestrated membrane of the glomerulus allows filtration of fluid from the blood into the nephron tubule

glucocorticoids steroid hormones released from the adrenal cortex; they increase blood glucose levels, fat deposits and protein breakdown for energy

glycogen storage form of glucose; can be broken down for rapid glucose level increases during times of stress

glycogenolysis breakdown of stored glucose to increase the blood glucose levels

glycosuria presence of glucose in the urine

glycosylated haemoglobin a blood glucose marker that provides a 3-month average of blood glucose levels

Gram-negative bacteria that accept a negative stain and are frequently associated with infections of the genitourinary or gastrointestinal tract

Gram-positive bacteria that take a positive stain and are frequently associated with infections of the respiratory tract and soft tissues

grand mal seizure *see tonic–clonic seizure*

granulocytes a type of white blood cell (leukocytes) characterized by the presence of granules in the cytoplasm, for example basophil, eosinophil and monophils

H

haemodynamics the study of the forces moving blood throughout the cardiovascular system

haemoptysis blood-tinged sputum, seen in left-sided CHF when blood accumulates in the pulmonary circuit and fluid leaks out into the lung tissue

haemorrhagic disorders characterized by a lack of clot-forming substances, leading to states of excessive bleeding

haemostasis stopping bleeding; vasoconstriction, platelet aggregation, and thrombin and fibrin synthesis all prevent bleeding and blood loss

haemostatic drugs that stop blood loss, usually by blocking the plasminogen mechanism and preventing clot dissolution

half-life the time it takes for the amount of drug in the body to decrease to one-half of the peak level it previously achieved

heart block a block of the conduction of an impulse through the cardiac conduction system; can occur at the atrioventricular node, interrupting conduction from the atria into the ventricles, or in the bundle branches within the ventricles, preventing the normal conduction of the impulse

helminth worm that can cause disease by invading the human body

helper T cell human lymphocyte that helps initiate immune reactions in response to tissue invasion

herpes virus DNA virus that accounts for many diseases, including shingles, cold sores, genital herpes and encephalitis

high-ceiling diuretics powerful diuretics that work in the loop of Henle to inhibit the reabsorption of sodium and chloride, leading to a sodium-rich diuresis

high-density lipoprotein (HDL) loosely packed chylomicron containing fats but with a high protein/fat ratio; able to absorb fats and fat remnants in the periphery; thought to have a protective effect, decreasing the development of coronary artery disease

hirsutism hair distribution associated with male secondary sex characteristics (e.g. increased hair on trunk, arms, legs, face)

histamine a chemical mediator that causes acid secretion in the stomach, vasodilation and smooth muscle contraction; also released from mast cells during inflammatory response

histamine (H_2) receptor antagonist drug that blocks the H_2 receptor sites; used to decrease acid production in the stomach (H_2 sites are stimulated to cause the release of acid in response to gastrin or parasympathetic stimulation)

histamine (H_2) receptors sites near the parietal cells of the stomach which, when stimulated, cause the release of hydrochloric acid into the lumen of the stomach; also found near cardiac cells

histocompatibility antigens proteins found on the surface of the cell membrane, which are determined by genetic code; provide cellular identity as self-cell

HMG-CoA reductase enzyme that regulates the last step in cellular cholesterol synthesis

hormones chemical messengers working within the endocrine system to communicate within the body

human immunodeficiency virus (HIV) retrovirus that attacks helper T cells, leading to a decrease in immune function and AIDS or ARC

human leukocyte antigen genes found on chromosome 6 that code for proteins in the cell that transport antigens from within the cell to the cell surface; product of the major histocompatibility complex
hydrochloric acid released by the parietal cells of the stomach in response to gastrin release or parasympathetic stimulation; makes the stomach contents more acidic to aid digestion and breakdown of food products and to kill ingested bacteria
hyperaldosteronism excessive output of aldosterone from the adrenal gland, leading to increased sodium and water retention and loss of potassium
hypercalcaemia an excess of calcium in the plasma
hyperglycaemia elevated blood glucose levels (>110 mg/dl) leading to multiple signs and symptoms and abnormal metabolic pathways
hyperlipidaemia increased levels of lipids in the serum, associated with increased risk of coronary artery development
hyperparathyroidism excessive parathyroid hormone
hypersensitivity excessive responsiveness to either the primary or the secondary effects of a drug; may be caused by a pathological or individual condition
hypertension constant, excessive high blood pressure (SBP >140 mmHg, DBP >90 mmHg)
hyperthyroidism excessive levels of thyroid hormones
hypertonia state of excessive muscle response and activity
hypnosis extreme sedation resulting in CNS depression and sleep
hypnotic drug used to depress the CNS; causes sleep
hypocalcaemia low levels of calcium in the plasma
hypoglycaemia lower than normal blood sugar (<40 mg/dl); often results from imbalance between insulin or oral agents and patient's eating, activity and stress
hypogonadism underdevelopment of the gonads (testes in the male)
hypokalaemia low potassium in the blood, which often occurs after diuretic use; characterized by weakness, muscle cramps, trembling, nausea, vomiting, diarrhoea and cardiac arrhythmias
hypoparathyroidism rare condition of absence of parathyroid hormone; may be seen after thyroidectomy
hypopituitarism lack of adequate function of the pituitary; reflected in many endocrine disorders
hypotension sustained blood pressure that is lower than that required to adequately perfuse all of the body's tissues
hypothalamus 'master gland' of the neuroendocrine system; regulates both nervous and endocrine responses to internal and external stimuli
hypothalamic-pituitary axis (HPA) interconnection of the hypothalamus and pituitary to regulate the levels of certain endocrine hormones through a complex series of negative feedback systems
hypothyroidism lack of sufficient thyroid hormone to maintain metabolism

I

immune stimulant drug used to energize the immune system when it is exhausted from fighting prolonged invasion or needs help fighting a specific pathogen or cancer cell
immune suppressant drug used to block or suppress the actions of the T cells and antibody production; used to prevent transplant rejection and to treat autoimmune diseases
immune system body system that helps the body defend itself against invasion of foreign proteins; fights infection; involves lymphocytes (B and T) lymph nodes and lymphoid tissue
immunoglobulin preformed antibodies found in sera from animals or humans who have had a specific disease and developed antibodies to it
immunization the process of stimulating active immunity by exposing the body to weakened or less toxic proteins associated with specific disease-causing organisms; the goal is to stimulate immunity without causing the full course of a disease
incontinence the involuntary leakage of urine from the bladder
induction time from the beginning of anaesthesia until achievement of surgical anaesthesia
influenza A RNA virus that invades tissues of the respiratory tract, causing the signs and symptoms of the common cold or influenza
inhalation breathing of air or a compound into the lungs through the nose and mouth
inhibin oestrogen-like substance produced by seminiferous tubules during sperm production; acts as a negative feedback stimulus to decrease release of follicle-stimulating hormone (FSH)
inhibiting hormones released from one body structure to inhibit the release of hormones from another body structure
insulin hormone produced by the β cells in the pancreas; stimulates insulin receptor sites to move glucose into the cells thus lowering plasma glucose levels: promotes storage of fat and glucose in the body
interferons tissue hormone that is released in response to viral invasion; blocks viral replication
interleukins chemicals released by white blood cells to communicate with other white blood cells and to support the inflammatory and immune reactions
interneuron neuron in the central nervous system that communicates with other neurons, not with muscles or glands
interstitial or Leydig cells part of the testes that produce testosterone in response to stimulation by luteinizing hormone (LH)
interstitial cystitis chronic inflammation of the interstitial connective tissue of the bladder; may extend into deeper tissue
intervention action undertaken to meet a patient's needs, such as administration of drugs, comfort measures or patient teaching

intractable hiccups repetitive stimulation of the diaphragm that leads to hiccups, a diaphragmatic spasm that persists over time

intrinsic factor produced by the parietal cells in the stomach required for absorption of vitamin B_{12}

intrinsic pathway cascade of clotting factors leading to the formation of a clot within a damaged vessel

iodine important dietary element used by the thyroid gland to produce thyroid hormone

iron deficiency anaemia low red blood cell count with low iron available because of high demand, poor diet, or poor absorption; treated with iron replacement

K

ketoacidosis an accumulation of ketone bodies in the blood; can occur in uncontrolled diabetes mellitus

ketosis breakdown of fats for energy, resulting in an increase in ketone bodies to be excreted from the body

kinin system activated by Factor XII as part of the inflammatory response; includes bradykinin

L

labour inducers can be used to bring on labour if the pregnancy over runs or if the pregnancy is terminated

larynx the vocal chords and the epiglottis, which close during swallowing to protect the lower respiratory tract from any foreign particles

leishmaniasis skin, mucous membrane, or visceral infection caused by a protozoan passed to humans by the bites of sand flies

leukocytes or white blood cells; can be neutrophils, basophils, eosinophils, lymphocytes or monocytes

leukotriene receptor antagonists drugs that selectively and competitively block or antagonize receptors for the production of leukotrienes D_4 and E_4

levothyroxine a synthetic salt of thyroxine (T_4), a thyroid hormone, the most frequently used replacement hormone for treating thyroid disease

ligand can be either a neurotransmitter, peptide or hormone

ligand-gated ion channels are pores in the plasma membrane permeable to ions such as sodium, potassium and chloride; the opening of the channel is regulated by binding of a specific ligand

limbic system area in the midbrain that is rich in adrenaline, noradrenaline and serotonin and seems to control emotions

liothyronine (T3) the most potent thyroid hormone, with a short half-life of 12 hours

lipoprotein structure composed of proteins and lipids; bipolar arrangement of the lipids monitors substances passing in and out of the cell

loading dose a higher dose of drug than that usually used for treatment; used when specific drugs take a prolonged period of time to reach critical concentrations in the plasma

local gastrointestinal reflex response to various stimuli that allows the gastrointestinal tract local control of its secretions and movements based on the contents or activity of the whole gastrointestinal system

local anaesthetic powerful nerve blocker that prevents depolarization of nerve membranes, blocking the transmission of pain stimuli and, in some cases, motor activity

loss of sensation the inability to feel touch, pressure or pain

low-density lipoprotein (LDL) tightly packed fats that are thought to contribute to the development of CAD when remnants left over from the LDL are processed in the arterial lining

lower respiratory tract the trachea, bronchial tree and the alveoli (respiratory sacs) that make up the lungs

lubricant drug that increases the viscosity of the faeces, making it difficult to absorb water from the bolus and easing movement of the bolus through the intestines

lymphocytes white blood cells with large, varied nuclei; can be T cells or B cells

lysosomes encapsulated digestive enzymes found within a cell; they digest old or damaged areas of the cell and are responsible for destroying the cell when the membrane ruptures and the cell dies

M

macrophages mature leukocytes that are capable of the phagocytosis of an antigen (foreign protein); also called monocytes or mononuclear phagocytes

major histocompatibility complex (MHC) a set of molecules found on the cell surface that are responsible for lymphocyte recognition and 'antigen presentation.' The MHC molecules regulate the immune response through recognition of 'self' and 'non-self' and, consequently, play a role in transplantation rejection

major tranquilizer former name of antipsychotic drugs; no longer used because it implies that its primary effect is sedation, which is no longer thought to be the desired therapeutic action

malaria protozoal infection with *Plasmodium*, characterized by cyclic fever and chills as the parasite is released from ruptured red blood cells; causes serious liver, central nervous system, heart and lung damage

malignant hyperthermia reaction to some neuromuscular junction drugs in susceptible individuals; characterized by extreme muscle rigidity, severe hyperpyrexia, acidosis and in some cases death

mania state of hyperexcitability; one phase of bipolar affective disorder, which alternate between periods of severe depression and mania

mast cell stabilizer drug that works at the cellular level to inhibit the release of histamine (released from mast cells in response to inflammation or irritation)

Medicines and Healthcare products Regulatory Agency (MHRA) the regulatory authority controlling the procedures and protocols in clinical trials

megaloblastic anaemia caused by lack of vitamin B_{12} and/or folic acid, in which red blood cells are larger in size, fewer in number have a weak stroma and a short lifespan; treated by replacement of folic acid and vitamin B_{12}

menopause depletion of the female ova; results in lack of oestrogen and progesterone

menstrual cycle cycling of female sex hormones in interaction with the hypothalamus and anterior pituitary feedback systems

metabolism rate at which the cells burn energy; the process by which drugs are converted into less chemically active substances that can be more easily excreted from the body

metastasis ability to enter the circulatory or lymphatic system and travel to other areas of the body that are conducive to growth and survival; property of cancer cells

metric system the most widely used system of measure, based on the decimal system; all units in the system are determined as multiples of ten

midbrain the middle area of the brain; it consists of the hypothalamus and thalamus and includes the limbic system

migraine headache a headache characterized by severe, unilateral, pulsating head pain associated with systemic effects, including gastrointestinal upset and sensitization to light and sound; related to a hyperperfusion of the brain from arterial dilation

mineralocorticoids steroid hormones released by the adrenal cortex; they cause sodium and water retention and potassium excretion

miosis constriction of the pupil; relieves intraocular pressure in some types of glaucoma

mitochondria membrane-bound organelles; that produce ATP for energy within the cell

mitral or bicuspid valve, is situated between the left atrium and the left ventricle in the heart and is composed of two leaflets or cusps

monoamine oxidase (MAO) enzyme that breaks down catecholamines to make them inactive; there are two forms of the enzyme: monoamine oxidase-A (MAO-A) and monoamine oxidase-B (MAO-B)

monoamine oxidase inhibitor (MAOI) drug that prevents the enzyme monoamine oxidase from breaking down noradrenaline (NAdr), leading to increased NAdr levels in the synaptic cleft; relieves depression and also causes sympathomimetic effects

monoclonal antibodies specific antibodies produced by a single clone of B cells to bind to very specific antigen

mononuclear phagocytes collection of macrophages derived from monocytes found in the alveoli of the lungs, kupffer cells of the liver and microglia

mononuclear phagocyte system (MPS) a family of cells comprising of cells that originate in the bone marrow blood monocytes and tissue macrophage

motor neuron carries impulses away from the brain and spinal cord to the target site; efferent neuron

mu-(μ)receptors primarily pain-blocking receptors that respond to naturally occurring enkephalins and endorphins and opioid drugs

mucolytics drugs that increase or liquify respiratory secretions to aid the clearing of the airways

muscarinic receptors cholinergic receptors that also respond to stimulation by muscarine

mutagen has an adverse effect on genetic material

myasthenia gravis autoimmune disease characterized by antibodies to cholinergic receptor sites, leading to destruction of the receptor sites and decreased response at the neuromuscular junction; it is progressive and debilitating, leading to paralysis

mycosis disease caused by a fungus

mydriasis relaxation of the muscles around the pupil, leading to pupil dilation

myelin sheath a phospholipid and protein sheath wrapped around the outside of some neurons; acts as an insulator that speeds up nerve impulse conduction

myelocytes leukocyte-producing cells in the bone marrow that can develop into neutrophils, basophils, eosinophils, monocytes or macrophages

myeloid cells are all derived from the bone marrow; these cells include megakaryocytes, erythrocyte precursors, mononuclear phagocytes and all the polymorphonuclear granulocytes

myocardial infarction end result of vessel blockage in the heart; leads to ischaemia and then necrosis of the area cut off from the blood supply; the area can heal, with the dead cells replaced by scar tissue

myocardium the muscle of the heart

myometrial relaxants used to relax the uterus to prolong pregnancy

myosin thick filament with projections that makes up a sarcomere or muscle unit

myxoedema severe lack of thyroid hormone in adults

N

narcolepsy mental disorder characterized by daytime sleepiness and periods of sudden loss of wakefulness

National Institute for Health and Clinical Excellence (NICE) provides guidance to health care professionals and also members of the public through the sharing of best practise

natural killer cells are cytotoxic lymphocytes that constitute a major component of the innate immune system; targeting tumour cells and protecting against a wide variety of infectious microbes

negative feedback a control system in which increasing levels of a hormone lead to decreased levels of releasing and stimulating hormones, leading to decreased hormone levels, which stimulates the release of releasing and stimulating hormones; allows tight control of the endocrine system

nematode a roundworm such as whipworm, threadworm, *Ascaris* or hookworm

neoplasm new or cancerous growth; occurs when abnormal cells have the opportunity to multiply and grow

nephron functional unit of the kidney, composed of Bowman's capsule, the proximal and distal convoluted tubules, the loop of Henle and the collecting duct

nerve a bundle of neurons running parallel to one another
nerve gas irreversible acetylcholinesterase inhibitor used in warfare to cause paralysis and death by prolonged muscle contraction and parasympathetic crisis
nerve plexus network of nerve fibres running through the wall of the gastrointestinal tract that allows local reflexes and control
neuroendocrine system the combination of the nervous and endocrine systems, which work closely together to maintain regulatory control and homeostasis in the body
neuroleptic a drug with many associated neurological adverse effects that is used to treat disorders that involve thought processes (e.g. schizophrenia)
neuron structural unit of the nervous system
neurotransmitter chemical produced by a nerve and released when the nerve is stimulated; binds to a specific receptor site to cause a reaction
nicotinic receptors cholinergic receptors that also respond to stimulation by nicotine
nitrates drugs used to cause direct relaxation of smooth muscle, leading to vasodilation and decreased venous return to the heart with decreased resistance to blood flow; this rapidly decreases oxygen demand in the heart and can restore the balance between blood delivered and blood needed in the heart muscle of patients with angina
nocturia getting up to urinate at night, reflecting increased renal perfusion with fluid shifts in the supine position when a person has gravity-dependent oedema related to coronary heart failure; other medical conditions, including urinary tract infection and enlargement of the prostate gland, increase the need to get up and urinate
nomogram can be used to determine body surface area using the patients height and weight
noncompetitive antagonists bind to a region on the target protein distinct from the agonist-binding site; changes the conformation of the target protein preventing effective binding of the agonist
nondepolarizing neuromuscular junction (NMJ) blocker no stimulation or depolarization of the muscle cell; prevents depolarization and stimulation by blocking the effects of acetylcholine
non-nucleoside reverse transcriptase inhibitors inhibit the enzyme reverse transcriptase, preventing the transcription of viral RNA into DNA
nonsteroidal anti-inflammatory drugs (NSAIDs) drugs that block prostaglandin synthesis and act as anti-inflammatory, antipyretic and analgesic agents
normal flora microorganisms normally found in the human body; some have beneficial functions
nucleoside reverse transcriptase inhibitors are nucleoside analogues which are incorporated into the viral DNA, preventing extension of the DNA chain and leading to viral death
nuclear receptors are protein molecules located in the cytoplasm; when bound to hormones, the hormone–receptor complex moves into the nucleus to regulate gene expression and cellular activity
nucleus the part of a cell that contains the DNA and genetic material; regulates cellular protein production and cellular properties
nursing the skill of caring and administering to the sick combined with the scientific application of chemistry, anatomy, physiology, biology, nutrition, psychology and pharmacology to the particular clinical situation
nursing diagnosis statement of an actual or potential problem, based on the assessment of a particular clinical situation, which directs needed nursing interventions
nursing process the problem-solving process used to provide efficient nursing care; it involves gathering information, formulating a nursing diagnosis statement, carrying out interventions and evaluating the process

O

oedema movement of fluid into the interstitial spaces; occurs when the balance between osmotic pull (from plasma proteins) and hydrostatic push (from blood pressure) is disturbed
oestrogen hormone produced by the ovary, placenta and adrenal gland; stimulates development of female characteristics and prepares the body for pregnancy
off-label uses of a drug that are not part of the stated therapeutic indications for which the drug was approved
oncogenesis the process by which cells become cancerous and begin to develop into tumours
oncotic pressure the pulling pressure of the plasma proteins, responsible for returning fluid to the vascular system at the capillary level
opioid agonists drugs that bind to opioid receptor sites to stimulate the effects of the receptors
opioid agonists–antagonists drugs that bind to some opioid receptor sites to stimulate their activity and at other opioid receptor sites to block activity
opioid antagonists drugs that block the opioid receptor sites; used to counteract the effects of narcotics or to treat an overdose of narcotics
opioid receptors receptor sites on nerves that endorphins and enkephalins bind to; the receptors are receptive to opioids
opioids drugs originally derived from opium that are used to treat many types of pain; bind to specific opioid receptors throughout the body
organelles distinct structures found within the cell cytoplasm
orphan drugs that have been discovered but are not available for use by those who could benefit from them, usually because they are not financially profitable
orthopnoea difficulty breathing when lying down, often referred to by the number of pillows required to allow a person to breath comfortably
osmosis movement of water from an area of low solute concentration to an area of high solute concentration in an attempt to equalize the concentrations
osmotic pull drawing force of large molecules on water, pulling it into a tubule or capillary; essential for maintaining normal

fluid balance within the body; used to draw out excess fluid into the vascular system or the renal tubule

OTC drugs see *over-the-counter (OTC) drugs*

ova eggs; the female gamete; contain half of the information needed in a human nucleus

ovaries female sexual glands that store ova and produce oestrogen and progesterone

over-the-counter (OTC) drugs that are available without a prescription for self-treatment of a variety of complaints

ovulation the release of an ovum from the follicles in the ovary usually on day 14 of the menstrual cycle

oxytocics drugs that act like the hypothalamic hormone oxytocin; they stimulate uterine contraction and contraction of the lacteal glands in the breast, promoting milk ejection

P

Paget's disease a genetically linked disorder of overactive osteoclasts that are eventually replaced by enlarged and softened bony structures

pancreatic enzymes digestive enzymes secreted by the exocrine pancreas which are needed for the correct digestion of lipids, proteins, carbohydrates and nucleic acids

paralysis lack of muscle function

parasympathetic division of the autonomic nervous system; 'rest and digest' response mediator that contains central nervous system cells from the cranium or sacral area of the spinal cord, long preganglionic axons, ganglia near or within the effector tissue, and short postganglionic axons which release acetylcholine

parasympatholytic preventing parasympathetic effects

parasympathomimetic mimicking the effects of the parasympathetic nervous system bradycardia, hypotension, pupil constriction, increased gastrointestinal secretions and activity, increased bladder tone, relaxation of sphincters, bronchoconstriction

parathyroid hormone a hormone produced by the parathyroid glands; responsible for maintaining calcium levels in conjunction with calcitonin

Parkinson's disease debilitating disease, characterized by progressive loss of co-ordination and function, which results from the degeneration of dopamine-producing cells in the substantia nigra

partial seizures also called focal seizures; seizures involving one area of the brain that do not spread throughout the entire organ

passive diffusion movement of substances across a semipermeable membrane with the concentration gradient; this process does not require energy

passive immunity the injection of preformed antibodies into a host at high risk for exposure to a specific disease; immunity is limited by the amount of circulating antibody

penile erectile dysfunction condition in which the corpus cavernosum does not fill with blood to allow for penile erection; can be related to ageing or to neurological or vascular conditions

pepsin an enzyme responsible for the digestion of proteins

peptic ulcer erosion of the lining of stomach or duodenum; results from imbalance between acid produced and the mucous protection of the gastrointestinal lining, or possibly from infection by *Helicobacter pylori* bacteria

peripheral resistance force that resists the flow of blood through the vessels, mostly determined by the arterioles, which contract to increase resistance; important in determining overall blood pressure

peristalsis type of gastrointestinal movement that moves a food bolus forward; characterized by a progressive wave of muscle contraction

pernicious anaemia megaloblastic anaemia characterized by lack of vitamin B_{12} secondary to low production of intrinsic factor by gastric cells; vitamin B_{12} must be replaced by intramuscular injection or nasal spray because it cannot be absorbed through the gastrointestinal tract

petit mal seizure see *absence seizure*

phaeochromocytoma a tumour of the chromaffin cells of the adrenal medulla that periodically releases large amounts of noradrenaline and adrenaline into the system with resultant severe hypertension and tachycardia

phagocytes neutrophils that are able to engulf and digest foreign material

phagocytosis the process of engulfing and digesting foreign material

pharmacodynamics the science that deals with the interactions between the chemical components of living systems and the foreign chemicals, including drugs, that enter living organisms; the way a drug affects a body

pharmacogenomics the study of genetically determined variations in the response to drugs

pharmacokinetics the way the body deals with a drug, including absorption, distribution, metabolism and excretion

pharmacology the study of the biological effects of chemicals

pharmacotherapeutics clinical pharmacology, the branch of pharmacology that deals with drugs; chemicals that are used in medicine for the treatment, prevention and diagnosis of disease in humans

phase I study a pilot study of a potential drug done with a small number of selected, healthy human volunteers

phase II study a clinical study of a drug by selected physicians using actual patients who have the disorder the drug is designed to treat; patients must provide informed consent

phase III study use of a drug on a wide scale in the clinical setting with patients who have the disease the drug is thought to treat

phase IV study continual evaluation of a drug after it has been released for marketing

phenothiazine anxiolytic drug that blocks the responsiveness of the chemoreceptor trigger zone to stimuli, leading to a decrease in nausea and vomiting

phospholipids lipid molecules that also contain phosphate groups; reside in the plasma membrane photosensitivity hypersensitive reaction to the sun or ultraviolet light, seen as an adverse reaction to various drugs; can lead to severe skin rash and lesions as well as damage to the eye

pituitary gland found in the sella turcica of the brain; produces hormones, endorphins and enkephalins and stores two hypothalamic hormones

placebo a substance or treatment the patient believes will have a therapeutic effect

placebo effect documented effect of the mind on drug therapy; if a person perceives that a drug will be effective, the drug is much more likely to actually be effective

plasma the liquid part of the blood; consists mostly of water and plasma proteins, glucose and electrolytes

plasma cell white blood cells producing large quantities of antibodies

plasma esterase enzyme found in plasma that immediately breaks down ester-type local anaesthetics

plasma membrane lipoprotein structure that separates the interior of a cell from the external environment; regulates what can enter and leave a cell

plasminogen natural clot-dissolving system; converted to plasmin (also called fibrinolysin) by many substances to dissolve clots that have formed and to maintain the patency of damaged vessels

Plasmodium a protozoan that causes malaria in humans; its life cycle includes the *Anopheles* mosquito, which injects protozoa into humans

platelets cell fragments found in blood; involved in haemostasis

platelet aggregation property of platelets to adhere to a damaged surface and then attract other platelets, which clump together or aggregate at the area, plugging up an injury to the vascular system

platyhelminth flatworm or fluke such as the tapeworm

Pneumocystis pneumonia (PCP) opportunistic infection by the fungus *Pneumocystis jiroveci* that occurs when the immune system is depressed; a frequent cause of pneumonia in patients with AIDS and in those who are receiving immunosuppressive therapy

pneumonia inflammation of the lungs that can be caused by bacterial or viral invasion of the tissue or by aspiration of foreign substances

poisoning overdose of a drug that causes damage to multiple body systems and the potential for fatal reactions

polydipsia increased thirst; seen in diabetes when loss of fluid and increased tonicity of the blood lead the hypothalamic thirst centre to make the patient feel thirsty

polymorphic having multiple alleles of a gene expressing different phenotypes

polyphagia increased hunger; sign of diabetes when cells cannot use glucose for energy and feel that they are starving, causing hunger

positive feedback a control system in which increasing levels of a hormone/process leads to an increased levels of another hormone or process

positive inotropic causing an increased force of contraction

posterior pituitary lobe of the pituitary that receives antidiuretic hormone and oxytocin via neurons from the hypothalamus and stores them to be released when stimulated by the hypothalamus

postmenopausal osteoporosis dropping levels of oestrogen allow calcium to be pulled out of the bone, resulting in a weakened and honeycombed bone structure

preclinical test initial trial of a chemical thought to have therapeutic potential; uses laboratory animals, not human subjects

premature atrial contraction (PAC) caused by an ectopic focus in the atria that stimulates an atrial response

premature ventricular contraction (PVC) caused by an ectopic focus in the ventricles that stimulates the cells and causes an early contraction

premedication drugs given before surgery to sedation and reducing anxiety

Prinzmetal's angina drop in blood flow through the coronary arteries caused by a vasospasm in the artery, not by atherosclerosis

proarrhythmic tending to cause arrhythmias; many of the drugs used to treat arrhythmias have been found to generate arrhythmias

prodrug a drug that is administered in an inactive or less active form; once absorbed the drug is metabolized to produce the active form of the drug

progesterone hormone produced by the ovary, placenta and adrenal gland; promotes maintenance of pregnancy

progestin female sex hormone; important in maintaining a pregnancy and supporting many secondary sex characteristics

progestogens group of hormones of which progesterone is an example; used in the oral contraceptive pill

prophylaxis treatment to prevent an infection before it occurs, as in the use of antiprotozoals to prevent malaria

prostaglandin a number of tissue hormones that have local effects on various systems and organs of the body, including vasoconstriction, vasodilation, increased or decreased gastrointestinal activity, and increased or decreased pancreatic enzyme release

prostaglandin analogues these are drug molecules which mimic the actions of naturally produced prostaglandins

prostate gland located around the male urethra; responsible for producing a slightly acidic fluid that maintains sperm and forms the bulk of seminal fluid

protease inhibitors drugs that block the activity of the enzyme protease in HIV; protease is essential for the maturation of infectious virus, and its absence leads to the formation of an immature and noninfective HIV particle

protein kinase an enzyme that modifies other proteins by adding phosphate groups; involved in many intracellular signalling pathways

proton pump inhibitor drug that blocks the H^+/K^+-ATPase enzyme system on the secretory surface of the gastric parietal cells, thus interfering with the final step of acid production and lowering acid levels in the stomach

protozoa single-celled organisms that pass through several stages in its life cycle, including at least one phase as a human parasite; found in areas of poor sanitation and hygiene and crowded living conditions

puberty point at which the hypothalamus starts releasing gonadotropin-releasing factor to stimulate the release of follicle-stimulating hormone and luteinizing hormone and begin sexual development

pulmonary oedema severe left-sided coronary heart failure with backup of blood into the lungs, leading to loss of fluid into the lung tissue

pulse pressure the systolic blood pressure minus the diastolic blood pressure; reflects the filling pressure of the coronary arteries

pyelonephritis inflammation of the pelvis of the kidney, frequently caused by backward flow problems or by bacteria ascending the ureter

pyramidal tract fibres within the central nervous system that control precise, intentional movement

pyrogen substance that resets the thermoregulatory centre in the hypothalamus to elevate the body temperature, thus speeding metabolism; some pyrogens are released by active neutrophils as part of the inflammatory response

R

ratio and proportion an equation in which the ratio containing two known equivalent amounts is on one side of the equation and the ratio containing the amount desired to convert and its unknown equivalent is on the other side

reabsorption the movement of substances from the renal tubule back into the vascular system

rebound congestion occurs when the nasal passages become congested as the effect of a decongestant drug wears off; patients tend to use more drug to decrease the congestion and a vicious circle of congestion, drug, and congestion develops, leading to abuse of the decongestant; also called rhinitis medicamentosa

receptor a protein that binds specifically to other molecules; for example neurotransmitters, hormones. May be either integrated within the plasma membrane or located within the cytoplasm

receptor sites on plasma membranes where specific chemicals bind to cause an effect; a drug may be effective because it binds to a specific receptor site on particular cells in the body

recombinant DNA technology use of bacteria to produce chemicals normally produced by human cells

reflex arc simple reflexes involving sensory receptors in the periphery and spinal motor nerves, responsible for maintaining muscle tone and keeping an upright position against the pull of gravity

releasing hormones chemicals released by the hypothalamus into the anterior pituitary to stimulate the release of anterior pituitary hormones

renin enzyme released from granular cells in the kidney; causes the conversion of angiotensinogen to angiotensin I

renin–angiotensin system compensatory process that leads to increased blood pressure and blood volume to ensure perfusion of the kidneys; important in the day-to-day regulation of blood pressure

repolarization return of a membrane to a resting state, with more sodium ions outside the membrane and a relatively negative charge inside the membrane

resistance ability of bacteria over time to adapt to an antibacterial and produce cells that are no longer affected by a particular drug

resistance system the arteries; the muscles of the arteries provide resistance to the flow of blood, leading to control of blood pressure

respiration the transport of oxygen from the atmosphere to the tissues and the transport of carbon dioxide from the tissues to the atmosphere

respiratory distress syndrome (RDS) disorder found in premature neonates whose lungs have not had time to mature and who are lacking sufficient surfactant to maintain open airways to allow for respiration

respiratory membrane area through which gas exchange must be made; made up of the surfactant layer, alveolar endothelium, alveolar basement membrane, capillary basement membrane and capillary endothelium

respiratory zone an area of the respiratory tract consisting of the respiratory bronchioles and alveolar sacs; gas exchange takes place here

reticulocyte red blood cell that has lost its nucleus and entered the circulation but is not yet fully matured

reverse transcriptase inhibitors drugs that block the transfer of both RNA- and DNA-dependent DNA polymerase activities; prevents the transfer of information that allows the virus to replicate and survive

rhinitis medicamentosa reflex reaction to vasoconstriction caused by decongestants; a rebound vasodilation that often leads to prolonged overuse of decongestants; also called rebound congestion

ribosomes membranous structures that are the sites of protein production within a cell

risk factors that have been identified to increase the risk of the development of a disease; for coronary artery disease, risk factors include genetic predisposition, gender, age, high-fat diet, sedentary lifestyle, gout, hypertension, diabetes and oestrogen deficiency

roundworm worm such as *Ascaris* that causes a common helmintic infection in humans; can cause intestinal obstruction as the adult worms clog the intestinal lumen or severe pneumonia when the larvae migrate to the lungs and form a pulmonary infiltrate

S

salicylates salicylic acid compounds, used as anti-inflammatory, antipyretic and analgesic agents; they block the prostaglandin system

saliva fluid produced by the salivary glands in the oral cavity in response to tactile stimuli and cerebral stimulation; contains enzymes to begin digestion as well as water, lysosymes, immunoglobulin E and mucus to lubricate the food bolus for ease of swallowing

sarcoma tumour that originates in the mesenchyme and is made up of embryonic connective tissue cells

sarcomere functional unit of a muscle cell, composed of actin and myosin molecules arranged in layers to give the unit a striped or striated appearance

schistosomiasis infection with a blood fluke that is carried by a snail; it poses a common problem in tropical countries, where the snail is the intermediary in the life cycle of the worm; larvae burrow into the skin in fresh water and migrate throughout the human body, causing a rash and then symptoms of diarrhoea and liver and brain inflammation

schizophrenia the most common type of psychosis; characteristics include hallucinations, paranoia, delusions, speech abnormalities and affective problems

Schwann cell insulating cell found around nerve axons in the peripheral nervous system; speeds the transmission of information

seasonal rhinitis inflammation of the nasal cavity, commonly called hay fever; caused by reaction to a specific antigen

secretion the active movement of substances from the blood into the renal tubule; also refers to the movement of cellular products from within the cell to the exterior, for example enzymes and fluid from salivary glands

sedation loss of awareness of and reaction to environmental stimuli

sedative drug that depresses the CNS; produces a loss of awareness of and reaction to the environment

segmentation gastrointestinal movement characterized by contraction of one segment of small intestine while the next segment is relaxed; the contracted segment then relaxes, and the relaxed segment contracts; exposes the chyme to a vast surface area to increase absorption

seizure sudden discharge of excessive electrical energy from nerve cells in the brain

selective serotonin reuptake inhibitor (SSRI) drug that specifically blocks the reuptake of serotonin and increases its concentration in the synaptic cleft; relieves depression and is not associated with anticholinergic or sympathomimetic adverse effects

selective toxicity property of a chemotherapeutic agent that affects only systems found in foreign cells, without affecting healthy human cells (e.g. specific antibiotics can affect certain proteins or enzyme systems used by bacteria but not by human cells)

self-care tendency for patients to self-diagnose and determine their own treatment needs

seminiferous tubules part of the testes that produce sperm in response to stimulation by follicle stimulating hormone

sensitivity testing evaluation of bacteria obtained in a culture to determine to which antibiotics the organisms are sensitive to and which agent would be appropriate for treatment of a particular infection

sensory neuron carries sensory information to the brain and spinal cord

sertoli cells found in the seminiferous tubules produce oestrogens and inhibin

shock severe hypotension that can lead to accumulation of waste products (e.g. lactic acid) and cell death

sinoatrial (SA) node the normal pacemaker of the heart; composed of primitive cells that constantly generate an action potential

sinuses air-filled passages through the skull that open into the nasal passage

sinus rhythm (normal) a normal ECG pattern and heart rate

sinusitis inflammation of the epithelial lining of the sinus cavities

sliding filament theory explains muscle contraction as a reaction of actin and myosin molecules when they are freed to react by the inactivation of troponin after calcium is allowed to enter the cell during depolarization

sneeze reflex response to irritation in the nasal passages; results in expelling of forced air through the nose

soma cell body of a neuron; contains the nucleus, cytoplasm and various granules

spasticity sustained muscle contractions

spectrum range of bacteria against which an antibacterial is effective (e.g. broad-spectrum antibacterials are effective against a wide range of bacteria)

sperm male gamete; contains half of the information needed for a human cell nucleus

spinothalamic tract nerve pathway from the spine to the thalamus along which pain impulses are carried to the brain

stable angina chest pain associated with activity or stress comes under the umbrella term of acute coronary syndrome

Starling's law of the heart addresses the contractile properties of the heart: the more the muscle is stretched, the stronger it will contract, until it is stretched to a point at which it will not contract at all

status epilepticus state in which seizures rapidly recur; most severe form of generalized seizure

stomatitis inflammation of the mucous membranes related to drug effects; can lead to alterations in nutrition and dental problems

stroke volume the amount of blood pumped out of the ventricle with each beat; important in determining blood pressure

substantia nigra a part of the brain rich in dopamine and dopamine receptors; site of degenerating neurons in Parkinson's disease

sulphonylureas oral antidiabetic agents used to stimulate the pancreas to release more insulin

superinfections infections caused by the destruction of bacteria of the normal flora by certain drugs, which allows other bacteria to enter the body and cause infection; may occur during the course of antibacterial therapy

supraventricular arrhythmias irregular or abnormal heartbeat that occurs above the ventricles

surfactant lipoprotein that reduces surface tension in the alveoli, allows airways to remain open for gas exchange

swallowing complex reflex response to a bolus in the back of the throat; allows passage of the bolus into the oesophagus and movement of ingested contents into the gastrointestinal tract

sympathetic division of the autonomic nervous system; 'fight or flight' response mediator; composed of central nervous system cells from the thoracic or lumbar areas, short preganglionic axons, ganglia near the spinal cord and long postganglionic axons

sympatholytic a drug that inhibits or blocks the effects of the sympathetic nervous system

sympathomimetic drugs that mimic the effects of the sympathetic nervous system

synapse junction between a nerve and an effector; consists of the presynaptic nerve ending, a space called the synaptic cleft, and the postsynaptic cell

syncytium intertwining network of muscle fibres that make up the atria and the ventricles of the heart; allows for a co-ordinated pumping contraction

synergy drugs that work together to increase drug effectiveness

systole contracting phase of the heart, during which blood is pumped out of the heart

T

T cells lymphocytes that originate in the thymus gland to recognize self-cells; may be effector T cells, helper T cells, or suppressor T cells

tachycardia faster than normal heart rate (usually >100 beats per minute)

tachypnoea rapid and shallow respirations, seen with left-sided coronary heart failure

tapeworm a form of flatworm that can live in the intestines following the ingestion of infected meat products

teratogen having adverse effects on the foetus

testes male sexual gland that produces sperm and testosterone

testosterone male sex hormone; produced by the interstitial or Leydig cells of the testes and in the adrenal cortex

therapeutic index a ratio of the minimum effective dose and the maximum tolerated dose; gives an indication of the relative safety of the drug; where the index is large there is a greater margin of safety between the minimum effective dose and the toxic dose and vice versa for a small therapeutic index

thiazide type of diuretic acting in the renal tubule to block the chloride pump, which prevents reabsorption of sodium and chloride, leading to a loss of sodium and water in the urine

thioamides drugs used to prevent the formation of thyroid hormone in the thyroid cells, lowering thyroid hormone levels

threadworm (or pinworms) is a common nematode infection amongst school-age children

thrombin factor X cleavage prothrombin (factor II) to thrombin (factor IIa). Thrombin catalyses the conversion of fibrinogen (factor I), a soluble plasma protein to insoluble fibrin

thromboembolic disorders characterized by the formation of clots or thrombi on damaged blood vessels with potential breaking of the clot to form emboli that can travel to smaller vessels, where they become lodged and occlude the vessel

thrombolytic drugs lyse, or break down, a clot that has formed; these drugs activate the plasminogen mechanism to dissolve fibrin threads

thyroxine (T_4) a thyroid hormone that is converted to triiodothyronine (T_3) in the tissues; it has a half-life of 1 week

tinea fungus called ringworm that causes infections such as athlete's foot

tocolytics drugs used to relax the gravid uterus to prolong pregnancy

tolerance the decreased effect over time of a drug used on a continual basis

tonic–clonic seizure type of generalized seizure that is characterized by serious clonic–tonic muscular reactions and loss of consciousness, with exhaustion and little memory of the event on awakening; formerly known as a grand mal seizure

trachea the main conducting airway leading into the lungs

trade name the name given to an approved drug by the pharmaceutical company that developed it; also called brand name

trichinosis disease that results from ingestion of encysted roundworm larvae in undercooked pork; larvae migrate throughout the body to invade muscles, nerves and other tissues; can cause pneumonia, heart failure and encephalitis

trichomoniasis infestation with a protozoan that causes vaginitis in women but no signs or symptoms in men

tricyclic antidepressant (TCA) drug that blocks the reuptake of noradrenaline and serotonin; relieves depression and has anticholinergic and sedative effects

triptan $5HT_1$ agonists selective serotonin receptor agonists that cause a vascular constriction of cranial vessels; used to treat acute migraine attacks

trophozoite a developing stage of a parasite, which uses the host for essential nutrients needed for growth

troponin a complex of regulatory proteins that prevent the interaction between actin and myosin, leading to muscle relaxation; it is inactivated by calcium during muscle stimulation to allow actin and myosin to interact, causing muscle contraction

trypanosomiasis African sleeping sickness, which is caused by a protozoan that inflames the central nervous system and is spread to humans by the bite of the tsetse fly; also

Chagas' disease, which causes a serious cardiomyopathy after the bite of the house fly.

tyramine an amine found in food that causes vasoconstriction and raises blood pressure; ingesting foods high in tyramine while taking an monoamine oxidase inhibitor poses the risk of a severe hypertensive crisis

type 1 insulin-dependent diabetes mellitus (IDDM) an autoimmune disease that results in the destruction of β cells in the pancreatic islets of Langerhans; the resultant lack of insulin produces high levels of blood glucose; usually develops before the age of 15

type 2 noninsulin-dependent diabetes mellitus (NIDDM) the insulin receptors are unresponsive to circulating insulin; there is a genetic predisposition to diabetes mellitus for some patients; overweight patients with a sedentary lifestyle are also predisposed to this form of diabetes

U

unconsciousness loss of awareness of one's surroundings

unstable angina acute chest pain caused by lack of oxygen supply to the myocardium; occurs without cause

upper respiratory tract composed of the nose, mouth, pharynx and larynx

urgency the feeling that one needs to urinate immediately; associated with infection and inflammation in the urinary tract

urinary frequency the need to urinate often; usually seen in response to irritation of the bladder, age and inflammation

uterus a female reproductive organ (the womb); site of growth and development of the embryo and foetus

V

vaccine immunization containing weakened or altered protein antigens to stimulate a specific antibody formation against a specific disease; refers to a product used to stimulate active immunity

vagus nerve the tenth cranial nerve

veins vessels that return blood to the heart; distensible tubes

vena cava all of the deoxygenated blood from the body flows into the right atrium from the inferior and superior vena cava

ventilation the movement of air through the airways; the act of breathing

ventricle lower chambers of the heart, which contract to pump blood out of the heart either to the lungs (right ventricle) or around the body in the systemic circulation (left ventricle)

vesicular transport the use of vesicles to transport molecules across the plasma membrane

vestibular referring to the apparatus of the inner ear that controls balance and sense of motion; stimulus to this area can cause motion sickness

virion a complete virus particle with its DNA or RNA core and protein coat; also known as a viral particle

virus particle of DNA or RNA surrounded by a protein coat that survives by invading a cell to alter its functioning

volatile drugs liquid drugs that are unstable at room temperature and release vapours; used as inhaled general anaesthetics, usually in the form of a halogenated hydrocarbon

vomiting complex reflex mediated through the medulla after stimulation of the chemoreceptor trigger zone; protective reflex to remove possibly toxic substances from the stomach

W

whipworm worm that attaches itself to the intestinal mucosa and sucks blood; may cause severe anaemia and disintegration of the intestinal mucosa

X

xanthines naturally occurring substances, including caffeine, that have a direct effect on smooth muscle of the bronchi and in the blood vessels

Y

yeast a eukaryotic microorganism belonging to the fungi kingdom; some species can cause opportunistic infections, for example *C. albicans* and oral thrush

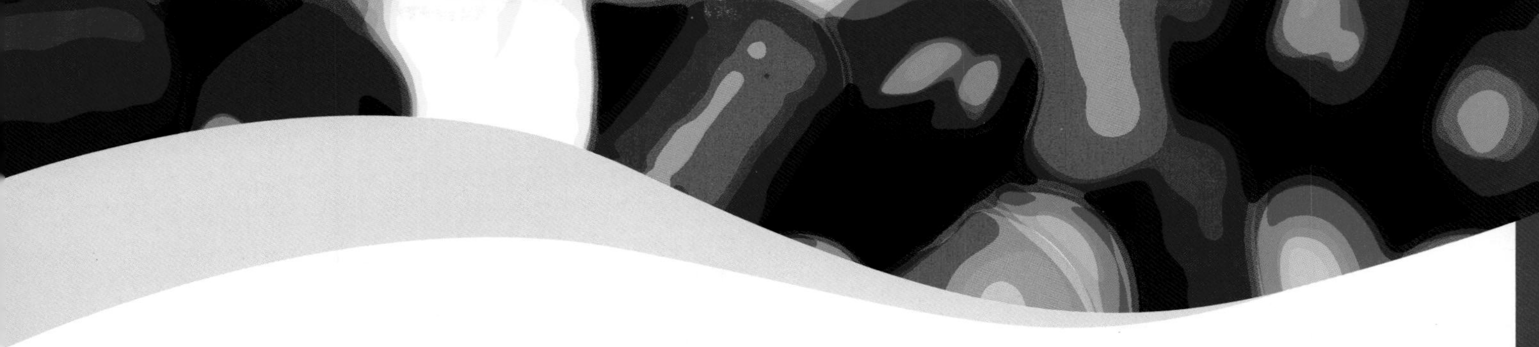

Answer Key

Chapter 1

Multiple Choice
1. b 2. d 3. c 4. d 5. b 6. c

Extended Matching Questions
1. c, d, e, f, g
2. a, c, d, f

Matching
1. G 2. F 3. A 4. H 5. E 6. I 7. C 8. J 9. B 10. D

Chapter 2

Multiple Choice
1. c 2. b 3. d 4. b 5. c 6. a 7. b

Extended Matching Questions
1. c, e
2. a, d, e, f
3. b, e, f

Fill in the Blanks
1. pharmacodynamics
2. pharmacokinetics
3. chemotherapeutic drugs
4. effective concentration
5. absorption, metabolism, distribution, excretion
6. first-pass effect
7. enzyme induction
8. half-life

Chapter 3

Multiple Choice
1. c 2. d 3. b 4. d 5. b 6. c

Extended Matching Questions
1. a, b, f
2. a, b, c, d, e, f
3. a, d, e, f
4. b, c, d, e

Matching
1. e 2. c 3. a 4. f 5. b 6. d

Fill in the Blanks
1. gentamicin
2. hypoglycaemia
3. chloroquine
4. ototoxicity
5. blood dyscrasia
6. dizziness, drowsiness, confusion

Chapter 4

Multiple Choice
1. c 2. a 3. a 4. d 5. c 6. a

Extended Matching Questions
1. a, b, c
2. b, c, d
3. a, b, d, e

Complete the List
1. Correct drug and patient
2. Correct storage of the drug
3. Correct and most effective route
4. Correct dosage
5. Correct preparation
6. Correct timing
7. Correct recording of administration

Fill in the Blanks
1. assessment
2. evaluation
3. nursing diagnoses
4. over-the-counter drugs or herbal therapies
5. dose
6. avoid driving a car or operating dangerous machinery

Chapter 5

Multiple Choice
1. a 2. b 3. c 4. c 5. b 6. d

Complete the Problems
1. a. 0.1 g b. 1.5 kg c. 1000 ml d. 0.5 l
2. 0.65 ml
3. 0.67 ml
4. 1.6 ml
5. 50 ml

Chapter 6

Multiple Choice
1. d 2. a 3. c 4. b 5. c 6. b

Extended Matching Questions
1. b, c, e, f
2. b, d, e
3. a, d, f

Matching
1. E 2. D 3. B 4. C 5. A

Chapter 7

Multiple Choice
1. c 2. c 3. a 4. c 5. b 6. c 7. d

Extended Matching Questions
1. a, b, c
2. a, c, d

Definitions
1. culture: sample of bacteria (from sputum, cell scraping, urine, etc.) to grow in a laboratory to determine the species of bacteria that is causing an illness
2. prophylaxis: treatment to prevent an infection before it occurs, as in the use of antiprotozoals to prevent malaria
3. resistance: ability of bacteria over time to adapt to an antibacterial and produce cells that are no longer affected by the drug
4. selective toxicity: antibacterial property that allows them to disturb certain proteins or enzyme systems used by bacteria but not by human cells, sparing the human cells from the destructive effects of the antibacterial
5. sensitivity testing: evaluation of bacteria obtained in a culture to determine to which antibacterial the organisms are sensitive and which agent would be appropriate for treatment of a particular infection
6. spectrum: range of bacteria against which an antibacterial is effective (e.g. broad-spectrum antibacterials are effective against a wide range of bacteria)

Chapter 8

Multiple Choice
1. d 2. c 3. b 4. a 5. d 6. d 7. b 8. c 9. c 10. b

Extended Matching Questions
1. b, d, f
2. a, b, c, f

True or False
1. T 2. F 3. F 4. T 5. F 6. T 7. F 8. T

Matching
1. G 2. K 3. I 4. A 5. B 6. J 7. C 8. D 9. E 10. C 11. A 12. H

Chapter 9

Multiple Choice
1. c 2. d 3. c 4. b 5. a 6. b

Extended Matching Questions
1. a, d, e, f
2. a, e, f

Fill in the Blanks
1. zanamivir
2. ribavirin
3. foscarnet
4. famciclovir/inosine pranobex/valaciclovir
5. aciclovir
6. zidovudine
7. penciclovir

Chapter 10

Multiple Choice
1. b 2. d 3. c 4. c 5. b 6. c

Extended Matching Questions
1. a, d, f
2. a, c, f

Fill in the Blanks
1. hard, ergosterol
2. mycosis
3. hepatic, renal
4. Candida
5. tinea
6. systemically
7. wounds
8. burning, irritation, pain

Chapter 11

Multiple Choice
1. d 2. b 3. d 4. b 5. c 6. d 7. d 8. a 9. c

Extended Matching Questions
1. b, c, d, f

Matching
1. A 2. B 3. A 4. B and C 5. A 6. D 7. B 8. D

Chapter 12

Multiple Choice
1. b 2. a 3. c 4. d 5. a 6. b 7. a

Extended Matching Questions
1. a, c, f

Definitions
1. cestode: tapeworm with a head and segmented body parts that is capable of growing to several metres in the human intestine
2. trematode: commonly known as flukes; nearly all trematodes infect molluscs as the definitive host
3. nematode: roundworm such as the commonly encountered whipworm, threadworm, Ascaris or hookworm
4. threadworm: nematode that causes a common helminthic infection in humans; lives in the colon and causes anal and possible vaginal irritation and itching
5. roundworm: worm such as *Ascaris* that causes a common helminthic infection in humans; can cause intestinal obstruction because the adult worms clog the intestinal lumen or severe pneumonia when the larvae migrate to the lungs and form a pulmonary infiltrate
6. schistosomiasis: infection with blood fluke that is carried by a snail, poses a common problem in tropical countries, where the snail is the intermediary in the life cycle of the worm; larvae burrow into the skin in fresh water and migrate throughout the human body, causing a rash and then symptoms of diarrhoea and liver and brain inflammation
7. trichinosis: disease that results from ingestion of encysted roundworm larvae in undercooked pork; larvae migrate throughout the body to invade muscle and nervous tissue; can cause pneumonia, heart failure and encephalitis.
8. whipworm: worm that attaches itself to the intestinal mucosa and sucks blood from the host; may cause severe anaemia and rectal prolapse

Chapter 13

Multiple Choice
1. c 2. d 3. a 4. c 5. b 6. b 7. b 8. c

Matching
1. D 2. G 3. C 4. E 5. F 6. A 7. H 8. B

Chapter 14

Multiple Choice
1. d 2. b 3. b 4. b 5. d 6. b 7. d 8. a

Extended Matching Questions
1. a, b, c
2. a, b, d

True or False
1. T 2. F 3. T 4. F 5. F 6. F 7. F 8. T 9. F 10. T

Definitions
1. interleukin: chemical released by WBCs to communicate with other WBCs and to support the inflammatory and immune reactions
2. pyrogen: substance that resets the thermoregulatory centre in the hypothalamus to elevate body temperature, thus speeding metabolism; some pyrogens are released by active neutrophils as part of the inflammatory response
3. antibody: an immunoglobulin; produced by B cell plasma cells in response to specific protein; reacts with that protein to cause its destruction directly or through activation of the inflammatory response
4. chemotaxis: property of drawing neutrophils to an area
5. neutrophil: white blood cell that is the first responder to an inflammatory reaction, undergoes phagocytosis to remove invading pathogens, injured cells
6. antigen: foreign protein

Chapter 15

Multiple Choice
1. d 2. c 3. d 4. b 5. d 6. a 7. c

Extended Matching Questions
1. a, b, c, f

Matching
1. D 2. G 3. E 4. C 5. B 6. F 7. A

Chapter 16

Multiple Choice
1. d 2. c 3. d 4. a 5. d 6. c

Extended Matching Questions
1. a, b, d
2. a, c, d

Definitions
1. autoimmune: having antibodies to self-cells or self-proteins; leads to chronic inflammatory disease and cell destruction
2. interferon: protein released by cells in response to viral invasion, prevents viral replication in other cells
3. interleukin: 'between white cells'; substance released by active white cells to communicate with other white cells and support the inflammatory and immune reaction
4. monoclonal antibodies: specific antibodies produced by a single clone of B cells to react with a specific antigen
5. immune suppressant: drugs used to block or suppress the actions of the T cells and antibody production; used to prevent transplant rejection and treat autoimmune disease

Fill in the Blanks
1. monoclonal antibodies
2. basiliximab, daclizumab, muromonab CD3
3. Crohn's
4. respiratory syncytial virus
5. trastuzumab
6. rituximab
7. omalizumab
8. alemtuzumab

Chapter 17

Multiple Choice
1. b 2. a 3. d 4. b 5. d 6. b 7. a

Extended Matching Questions
1. a, b, c, f
2. c, e, f
3. b, c

True or False
1. F 2. T 3. T 4. T 5. T 6. T 7. F

Chapter 18

Multiple Choice
1. b 2. c 3. a 4. b 5. c 6. a

Extended Matching Questions
1. a, b, c

Matching
1. G 2. C 3. B 4. J 5. I 6. H 7. A 8. F 9. E 10. D

Definitions
1. neuron: structural unit of the nervous system
2. neurotransmitter: chemical produced by a nerve and released when a nerve is stimulated; binds to a specific receptor site to cause an action
3. limbic system: area of the brain above the hypothalamus, rich in noradrenaline neurons; thought to be the site of emotions in the human brain
4. Schwann cell: insulating cell found on neuronal axons in the peripheral nervous system; allows 'leaping' electrical conduction to speed the transmission of information
5. myelination: property of a neuronal axon that has Schwann cells or oligodendrocytes
6. soma: cell body of a neuron; contains the nucleus, cytoplasm and various granules
7. synapse: junction between a nerve and an effector; consists of the presynaptic nerve ending, a space called the synaptic cleft, and the postsynaptic cell
8. repolarization: return of a membrane to a resting state, with more sodium ions outside the membrane and a relatively negative charge inside the membrane

Chapter 19

Multiple Choice
1. d 2. a 3. a 4. c 5. c 6. d 7. a

Extended Matching Questions
1. a, b, c, e
2. a, b, c, f

Fill in the Blanks
1. anxiety
2. motivator
3. sedatives
4. hypnotics
5. tension, fear
6. sedation
7. depress
8. benzodiazepines

Chapter 20

Multiple Choice
1. c 2. c 3. d 4. b 5. d 6. b 7. d 8. c

Extended Matching Questions
1. a, c, d
2. a, c, d

Fill in the Blanks
1. noradrenaline, dopamine, serotonin
2. breakdown, synaptic cleft
3. reuptake
4. noradrenaline, serotonin
5. tyramine
6. antimuscarinic

Chapter 21

Multiple Choice
1. c 2. a 3. b 4. c 5. d 6. b 7. a

Extended Matching Questions
1. a, b, c, d
2. a, b, d

Matching
1. E 2. C 3. B 4. F 5. A 6. D

Chapter 22

Multiple Choice
1. c 2. d 3. b 4. a 5. a 6. c 7. b

Extended Matching Questions
1. b, e
2. b, c, d

Fill in the Blanks
1. epilepsy
2. seizure
3. convulsion
4. antiseizure agents
5. grand mal seizure
6. absence seizure
7. myoclonic seizures
8. febrile seizures
9. status epilepticus
10. focal

Chapter 23

Multiple Choice
1. c 2. c 3. c 4. a 5. c 6. b

Extended Matching Questions
1. a, b, c
2. a, b, c, f

Chapter 24

Multiple Choice
1. a 2. c 3. b 4. c 5. b 6. a

Extended Matching Questions
1. a, b, c

Chapter 25

Multiple Choice
1. c 2. d 3. d 4. c 5. d 6. c 7. c

Extended Matching Questions
1. a, b, d, f
2. a, c, d, e, f

Matching
1. C 2. E 3. H 4. F 5. A 6. B 7. G 8. D

True or False
1. F 2. T 3. F 4. F 5. T 6. F 7. T 8. F 9. T 10. F

Chapter 26

Multiple Choice
1. b 2. c 3. c 4. c 5. b 6. d 7. b 8. c

Extended Matching Questions
1. b, c, d, e
2. a, c, f

Definitions
1. A fibres: large-diameter nerve fibres that carry peripheral impulses associated with touch and temperature to the spinal cord
2. A-delta and C fibres: small-diameter nerve fibres that carry peripheral impulses associated with pain to the spinal cord
3. gate-control theory: theory that the transmission of nerve impulses can be modulated at several points along its path by the closing and opening of 'gates'
4. migraine headache: headache characterized by severe, unilateral, pulsating head pain and associated with systemic effects, including GI upset, light and sound sensitization
5. opioids: drugs originally derived from opium that react with specific opioid receptors in the body
6. opioid agonist: drugs that act at opioid receptors to simulate the effects of the receptors
7. opioid agonist-antagonists: drugs that act at some opioid receptors to stimulate activity and at other opioid receptors to block activity
8. opioid antagonists: drugs that block opioid receptors, used to counteract the effects of narcotics and to treat narcotic overdose
9. opioid receptors: receptor sites on nerves that react with enkephalins and endorphins and that are receptive to narcotic drugs
10. triptan: selective serotonin receptor blocker that causes a vascular constriction of cranial vessels, used to treat acute migraine attacks

Chapter 27

Multiple Choice
1. b 2. c 3. b 4. a

Extended Matching Questions
1. a, b, d, f
2. a, b, d, e
3. a, b, c, f

Fill in the Blanks

1. pain relief, analgesia, amnesia, unconsciousness
2. loss of sensation, death
3. induction of anaesthesia
4. balanced anaesthesia
5. depolarization of the nerve membrane
6. central nervous system depression
7. sensation, mobility, the ability to communicate
8. skin breakdown, self-injury, biting oneself

Chapter 28

Multiple Choice

1. c 2. b 3. d 4. c 5. d 6. b 7. d 8. a

Extended Matching Questions

1. a, b, f
2. a, e, f

Matching

1. J 2. B 3. E 4. A 5. H 6. F 7. G 8. I 9. D 10. K
11. C

Chapter 29

Multiple Choice

1. c 2. b 3. c 4. d 5. c 6. a

Extended Matching Questions

1. c, e, f

Definitions

1. adrenergic agonist: a drug that stimulates the adrenergic receptors of the sympathetic nervous system, either directly, by reacting with the receptor site, or indirectly by increasing noradrenaline levels
2. α-agonist: specifically stimulating the α-receptors within the sympathetic nervous system, causing body responses seen when the α-receptors are stimulated
3. β-agonist: specifically stimulating the beta receptors within the sympathetic nervous system, causing body responses seen when the β-receptors are stimulated
4. glycogenolysis: breakdown of stored glucose to increase the blood glucose levels
5. sympathomimetic: a drug that mimics the effects of the sympathetic nervous system

Chapter 30

Multiple Choice

1. d 2. c 3. a 4. b 5. a 6. c 7. d 8. c

Extended Matching Questions

1. a, b, d, f
2. a, b, d, f

True or False

1. F 2. T 3. F 4. T 5. T 6. F 7. T 8. T

Chapter 31

Multiple Choice

1. b 2. c 3. a 4. c 5. b 6. b 7. b 8. c

Extended Matching Questions

1. a, b, d
2. a, b, d

Matching

1. D 2. B, C 3. B 4. A, C 5. E 6. E

Fill in the Blanks

1. acetylcholine
2. parasympathomimetic
3. direct-acting
4. indirect-acting
5. Alzheimer's disease
6. myasthenia gravis
7. nausea, vomiting, diarrhoea, increased salivation
8. bradycardia, hypotension, heart block

Chapter 32

Multiple Choice

1. a 2. c 3. d

Extended Matching Questions

1. a, b, c
2. a, e, f

Fill in the Blanks

1. acetylcholine
2. parasympatholytic
3. increase, decrease
4. sweating
5. cyclopegia
6. mydriatic
7. dry mouth, difficulty swallowing

Chapter 33

Multiple Choice

1. d 2. b 3. a 4. c 5. d 6. d 7. c

Extended Matching Questions

1. a, b, e, f
2. a, b, d
3. c, e, f

Matching

1. D 2. H 3. F 4. A 5. G 6. C 7. E 8. B

Chapter 34

Multiple Choice

1. a 2. c 3. d 4. b 5. c 6. c 7. d 8. b

Extended Matching Questions

1. d, e, f
2. c, e

Chapter 35

Multiple Choice

1. b 2. c 3. d 4. a 5. a 6. d 7. a 8. c

Extended Matching Questions

1. a, b, c, f
2. a, b, d, f

True or False

1. F 2. F 3. F 4. T 5. T 6. F 7. F 8. T 9. T 10. T

Chapter 36

Multiple Choice

1. b 2. c 3. c 4. b 5. c

Extended Matching Questions
1. a, c, d
2. b, c, d

Matching
1. E 2. A 3. F 4. B 5. J 6. C 7. H 8. D 9. G 10. I

Chapter 37

Multiple Choice
1. c 2. c 3. a 4. b 5. b 6. d

Extended Matching Questions
1. a, b, c, e, f
2. a, b, d, f

Fill in the Blanks
1. insulin, glucagons, somatostatin
2. glycogen, lipids, proteins
3. glycosuria
4. polyphagia
5. polydipsia
6. ketosis
7. sulphonylureas
8. metformin

Chapter 38

Multiple Choice
1. a 2. b 3. b 4. c 5. b 6. c

Extended Matching Questions
1. a, b, c, f
2. a, c, d, e

True or False
1. F 2. T 3. T 4. F 5. T 6. F 7. F 8. T

Chapter 39

Multiple Choice
1. b 2. c 3. a 4. b 5. b 6. c

Extended Matching Questions
1. b, c, e, f
2. a, b, c, e, f
3. a, b, d, e

Fill in the Blanks
1. oxytocics
2. tocolytics
3. osteoporosis, hot flushes, coronary artery disease
4. thrombi, emboli
5. raloxifene
6. injection
7. fertility drugs
8. labour inducers/abortifacients

Chapter 40

Multiple Choice
1. a 2. d 3. c 4. b 5. c 6. a

Extended Matching Questions
1. a, b, d
2. b, d, e, f

True or False
1. T 2. F 3. T 4. T 5. F 6. F 7. T 8. T 9. F 10. F

Fill in the Blanks
1. androgenic
2. anabolic
3. testosterone
4. erectile penile dysfunction
5. prostaglandin, injected
6. ildenafils

Chapter 41

Multiple Choice
1. c 2. c 3. d 4. c 5. a 6. b 7. a 8. c 9. c

Extended Matching Questions
1. a, b, c, e, f
2. a, b, c, f

Definitions
1. troponin: chemical in muscle that prevents actin and myosin from reacting, leading to muscle relaxation; inactivated by calcium during muscle stimulation to allow actin and myosin to react, causing muscle contraction
2. actin: thin filament that makes up a sarcomere or muscle unit
3. myosin: thick filament that makes up a sarcomere or muscle unit
4. arrhythmia: a disruption in cardiac rate or rhythm
5. Starling's Law of the Heart: addresses the contractile properties of the heart; the more the muscle is stretched, the stronger it will react until stretched to a point at which it will not react at all
6. fibrillation: rapid, irregular stimulation of the cardiac muscle resulting in lack of pumping activity
7. capillary: small vessel made up of loosely connected endothelial cells that connect arteries to veins
8. resistance system: the arteries; the muscles of the arteries provide resistance to the flow of blood, leading to control of blood pressure

Matching
1. H 2. C 3. F 4. E 5. D 6. L 7. J 8. A 9. K 10. G
11. I 12. B

Chapter 42

Multiple Choice
1. b 2. b 3. d 4. d 5. c 6. b 7. c

Extended Matching Questions
1. a, b, c, e
2. a, b, d, e

Matching
1. B 2. A 3. E 4. B 5. D 6. D 7. A 8. B 9. C

True or False
1. F 2. T 3. F 4. F 5. T 6. F 7. T 8. T 9. F 10. T

Chapter 43

Multiple Choice
1. b 2. c 3. a 4. c 5. d 6. b 7. c 8. b

Extended Matching Questions
1. a, b, c
2. a, c, d, e

Chapter 44

Multiple Choice
1. d 2. c 3. d 4. a 5. d

Extended Matching Questions
1. a, c, d, f
2. a, b, c, e, f

Fill in the Blanks
1. tachycardia, bradycardia
2. cardiac output
3. action potential
4. automaticity
5. β-receptor
6. digoxin
7. lidocaine

Chapter 45

Multiple Choice
1. a 2. b 3. d 4. b 5. d

Extended Matching Questions
1. a, b, d, e, f
2. a, b, c, f
3. a, b, d, e
4. c, e, f

Matching
1. C 2. F 3. E 4. G 5. A 6. D 7. H

True or False
1. F 2. T 3. F 4. T 5. F 6. F 7. T 8. T

Chapter 46

Multiple Choice
1. b 2. b 3. c 4. d 5. b 6. c 7. d

Extended Matching Questions
1. a, b, f
2. a, b, e, f

Chapter 47

Multiple Choice
1. c 2. b 3. c 4. d 5. b 6. c

Extended Matching Questions
1. a, b, c
2. b, c, d
3. a, b, c, f
4. a, b, c, e, f

True or False
1. T 2. F 3. T 4. F 5. T 6. F 7. T 8. F 9. F 10. T

Chapter 48

Multiple Choice
1. c 2. b 3. a 4. c 5. d 6. c 7. c 8. d

Extended Matching Questions
1. b, c, e, f
2. a, c, d

True or False
1. T 2. F 3. F 4. T 5. T 6. T 7. F 8. T

Chapter 49

Multiple Choice
1. a 2. d 3. a 4. c 5. c 6. d 7. b

Extended Matching Questions
1. a, b, c, e, f
2. a, c, d, e, f
3. a. c, f

Fill in the Blanks
1. 25%
2. nephron, Bowman's capsule, loop of Henle, collecting duct
3. glomerular filtration, tubular secretion, tubular reabsorption
4. aldosterone
5. concentration, dilution
6. aldosterone
7. Vitamin D
8. renin

Chapter 50

Multiple Choice
1. b 2. c 3. b 4. c 5. d 6. a 7. d 8. c

Extended Matching Questions
1. a, b, d, f
2. a, c, d, f

Definitions
1. oedema: movement of fluid into the interstitial spaces; occurs when the balance between osmotic pull and hydrostatic push is upset
2. fluid rebound: reflex reaction of the body to the loss of fluid or sodium; hypothalamus causes the release of ADH, which leads to the retention of water and stress related to the fluid loss combines with decreased blood flow to the kidneys to activate the renin–angiotensin–aldosterone system, leading to further sodium and water retention
3. thiazide: type of diuretic acting in the renal tubule to block the chloride pump, which prevents reabsorption of sodium and chloride, leading to a loss of sodium and water in the urine
4. hypokalaemia: low potassium in the blood; often occurs with diuretic use; characterized by weakness, muscle cramps, trembling, nausea, vomiting, diarrhoea and cardiac arrhythmias
5. high-ceiling diuretics: powerful diuretics that work in the loop of Henle to inhibit the reabsorption of sodium and chloride, leading to a sodium-rich diuresis
6. alkalosis: state of not having enough acid to maintain normal homeostatic processes; seen with loop diuretics, which cause the loss of bicarbonate in the urine
7. hyperaldosteronism: excessive output of aldosterone from the adrenal gland, leading to an increased sodium and water retention and loss of potassium
8. osmotic pull: drawing force of large molecules on water; pulling it into the tubule or capillary; essential for maintaining normal fluid balance within the body; used to draw excessive fluid into the vascular system or the renal tubule

Matching
1. E 2. C 3. B 4. A 5. D 6. B 7. D 8. C

Chapter 51

Multiple Choice
1. d 2. b 3. d 4. b 5. a 6. a

Extended Matching Questions
1. a, b, d, e
2. a, b, d, f

True or False
1. T 2. F 3. F 4. T 5. F 6. T 7. F

Chapter 52

Multiple Choice
1. c 2. a 3. c 4. d 5. c 6. d 7. b

Extended Matching Questions
1. a, b, c
2. a, b, d, e
3. a, b, c, f

Matching
1. K 2. D 3. B 4. J 5. E 6. A 7. C 8. G 9. L 10. F
11. I 12. H

Chapter 53

Multiple Choice
1. c 2. c 3. c 4. b 5. a 6. c 7. d

Extended Matching Questions
1. a, b, c, e
2. a, c, d, e
3. a, b, d, e, f

Chapter 54

Multiple Choice
1. a 2. c 3. c 4. a 5. b 6. d 7. c 8. d

Extended Matching Questions
1. b, c, e, f
2. a, c, d

True or False
1. F 2. T 3. T 4. T 5. T 6. F 7. T 8. T

Chapter 55

Multiple Choice
1. d 2. c 3. a 4. c 5. d 6. d 7. c

Extended Matching Questions
1. a, b, d, e
2. a, c, d, e
3. b, c, e

Matching
1. F 2. C 3. G 4. H 5. B 6. A 7. E 8. D 9. J 10. I

Fill in the Blanks
1. digestion, absorption
2. acid, mucus
3. nerve plexus
4. sympathetic, parasympathetic
5. local reflexes
6. constipation, diarrhoea
7. medulla
8. vomiting centre, chemoreceptor trigger zone (CTZ)

Chapter 56

Multiple Choice
1. c 2. d 3. c 4. a 5. c 6. b 7. d

Extended Matching Questions
1. a, b, c, e, f

Matching
1. E 2. C 3. D 4. A 5. B 6. B 7. F 8. C 9. A 10. D

Chapter 57

Multiple Choice
1. b 2. b 3. c 4. a

Extended Matching Questions
1. a, c, d, f
2. a, b, c

True or False
1. F 2. T 3. T 4. F 5. T 6. F 7. F 8. T

Chapter 58

Multiple Choice
1. a 2. b 3. b

Extended Matching Questions
1. a, c, d, e, f
2. a, c

Fill in the Blanks
1. antiemetics
2. vomiting reflex
3. CTZ, medulla
4. pain, chemicals, debris from cell death
5. CNS depression
6. photosensitivity

Index

Note: Page numbers followed by f indicate figures; those followed by t indicate tables; and those followed by b indicate boxed text.

A

Q

R

S